Veterinary Emergency and Critical Care Medicine

Veterinary Emergency and Critical Care Medicine

Robert J. Murtaugh, D.V.M., M.S.
Associate Professor
Department of Medicine
Tufts University
School of Veterinary Medicine
North Grafton, Massachusetts
Diplomate, American College of Veterinary Internal Medicine
Diplomate, American College of Veterinary Emergency and Critical Care

Paul M. Kaplan, D.V.M.
Mobile Referral Consultant
Cardiac and Abdominal Imaging Service of New England
Westford, Massachusetts
Diplomate, American College of Veterinary Internal Medicine (Cardiology)

*With **263** illustrations*

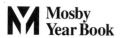
Mosby
Year Book

St. Louis Baltimore Boston Chicago London Philadelphia Sydney Toronto

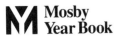

Mosby
Year Book
Dedicated to Publishing Excellence

Editor Robert W. Reinhardt
Assistant Editor Melba Steube
Project Manager Gayle May Morris
Editing York Production Services
Designer David Zielinski

Printed in the United States of America

Mosby-Year Book, Inc.
11830 Westline Industrial Drive
St. Louis, Missouri, 63146

Library of Congress Cataloging in Publication Data

Murtaugh, Robert J.
    Veterinary emergency and critical care medicine / Robert J.
Murtaugh, Paul M. Kaplan.
        p.   cm.
    Includes bibliographical references and index.
    ISBN 0-8016-6399-7
    1. Veterinary emergencies.   2. Veterinary critical care.
I. Kaplan, Paul M.   II. Title.
SF778.M87 1992
636.089'602'5—dc20   91-37
                                                                      C

92 93 94 95 96 CL/MV 9 8 7 6 5 4 3 2 1

Contributors

Alan Bachrach, Jr., V.M.D., Dip. ACVO
Clinical Associate Professor,
Tufts University,
School of Veterinary Medicine,
North Grafton, Massachusetts

E. Murl Bailey, Jr., D.V.M., M.S., Ph.D.
Professor,
Department of Veterinary Physiology/
  Pharmacology,
Texas A&M University,
College of Veterinary Medicine,
College Station, Texas

John Berg, D.V.M., M.S., Dip. ACVS
Assistant Professor,
Department of Surgery,
Tufts University,
School of Veterinary Medicine,
North Grafton, Massachusetts

Randy J. Boudrieau, D.V.M., Dip. ACVS
Assistant Professor,
Department of Surgery,
Tufts University,
School of Veterinary Medicine,
North Grafton, Massachusetts

Marjory Brooks, D.V.M., Dip. ACVIM
Research Associate,
Comparative Hematology Laboratory,
Wadsworth Center for Labs and Research,
Albany, New York

Dennis J. Chew, D.V.M., Dip. ACVIM
Professor,
Department of Veterinary Clinical Sciences,
Ohio State University,
College of Veterinary Medicine,
Columbus, Ohio

Michael H. Court, B.V.Sc., Dip. ACVA
Assistant Professor,
Department of Surgery,
Director of Clinical Anesthesia,
Tufts University,
School of Veterinary Medicine,
North Grafton, Massachusetts

**C. Guillermo Couto, D.V.M., Dip. ACVIM
  (Oncology)**
Associate Professor,
Department of Veterinary Clinical Sciences,
Ohio State University,
College of Veterinary Medicine,
Columbus, Ohio

M. Susan Crisp, D.V.M., Dip. ACVIM
Assistant Professor and Director,
Intensive Care Unit,
Department of Veterinary Clinical Sciences,
Ohio State University,
College of Veterinary Medicine,
Columbus, Ohio

**Dennis T. Crowe, Jr., D.V.M., Dip. ACVS,
  Dip. ACVECC**
Director of Surgery,
The Animal Emergency Center and The
  Veterinary Institute of Trauma, Emergency,
  and Critical Care,
Milwaukee, Wisconsin;
Formerly, Associate Professor of Surgery and
  Chief, Emergency and Critical Care Services,
The University of Georgia,
College of Veterinary Medicine,
Athens, Georgia

**Deborah J. Davenport, D.V.M., M.S., Dip.
  ACVIM**
Mark Morris Associates,
Topeka, Kansas

Stephen P. DiBartola, D.V.M., Dip. ACVIM
Associate Professor,
Department of Veterinary Clinical Sciences,
Ohio State University,
College of Veterinary Medicine,
Columbus, Ohio

Tam Garland, D.V.M.
Research Assistant,
Department of Veterinary Physiology/
  Pharmacology,
Texas A&M University,
College of Veterinary Medicine,
College Station, Texas

Geoffrey Gibbons, B.V.Sc., FRCVS, MACVSc
Goddard Veterinary Group, New Wanstead,
Wanstead, England;
Formerly, Staff Veterinarian,
Foster Hospital for Small Animals,
Tufts University,
School of Veterinary Medicine,
North Grafton, Massachusetts

Alan S. Hammer, D.V.M.
Assistant Professor,
Department of Veterinary Clinical Sciences,
Ohio State University,
College of Veterinary Medicine,
Columbus, Ohio

Elizabeth M. Hardie, D.V.M., Ph.D.
Associate Professor, Surgery,
Department of Companion Animals and Special
  Species Medicine,
North Carolina State University,
College of Veterinary Medicine,
Raleigh, North Carolina

**Paul M. Kaplan, D.V.M., Dip. ACVIM
  (Cardiology)**
Mobile Referral Consultant,
Cardiac and Abdominal Imaging Service of New
  England,
Westford, Massachusetts

Gretchen E. Kaufman, D.V.M.
Staff Veterinarian,
Exotic Animal Medicine,
Tufts University,
School of Veterinary Medicine,
North Grafton, Massachusetts

**Lawrence J. Kleine, D.V.M., M.S., Dip.
  ACVR**
Associate Professor and Head of Radiology,
Tufts University,
School of Veterinary Medicine,
North Grafton, Massachusetts;
Research Associate,
Harvard Medical School and Brigham and
  Women's Hospital,
Boston, Massachusetts

Mary Anna Labato, D.V.M.
Clinical Assistant Professor,
Department of Medicine;
Staff Clinician,
Foster Hospital for Small Animals,
Tufts University,
School of Veterinary Medicine,
North Grafton, Massachusetts

M. J. LaRue, D.V.M.
Derry Animal Hospital,
Derry, New Hampshire

David E. Lee-Parritz, D.V.M.
New England Regional Primate Research Center,
Southborough, Massachusetts

**Aunna C. Lippert, D.V.M., M.S., Dip.
  ACVA**
Allied Veterinarians Referral Services,
Dearborn Heights, Michigan

Robert A. Martin, D.V.M., Dip. ACVS
Associate Professor and Section Chief of Small
  Animal Surgery and Anesthesiology,
Virginia Tech and University of Maryland,
Virginia-Maryland Regional College of
  Veterinary Medicine,
Blacksburg, Virginia

Rebecca May, B.A.
Museum Coordinator for the Kansas Department
  of Wildlife and Parks,
Pratt, Kansas

**Matthew W. Miller, D.V.M., Dip. ACVIM
  (Cardiology)**
Assistant Professor,
Department of Small Animal Medicine and
  Surgery,
Texas A&M University,
College of Veterinary Medicine;
Staff Cardiologist,
Texas Veterinary Medical Center,
College Station, Texas

**Bradley L. Moses, D.V.M., Dip. ACVIM
  (Cardiology)**
Clinical Assistant Professor,
Department of Medicine,
Tufts University,
School of Veterinary Medicine,
North Grafton, Massachusetts;
Roberts Animal Hospital,
Hanover, Massachusetts

Robert J. Murtaugh, D.V.M., Dip. ACVECC
Associate Professor,
Department of Medicine,
Tufts University,
School of Veterinary Medicine,
North Grafton, Massachusetts

Michael M. Pavletic, D.V.M., Dip. ACVS
Associate Professor,
Department of Surgery,
Head, Section of Small Animal Surgery,
Tufts University,
School of Veterinary Medicine,
North Grafton, Massachusetts

Dominique G. Penninck, D.V.M., Dip. ACVR
Assistant Professor,
Department of Surgery,
Tufts University,
School of Veterinary Medicine,
North Grafton, Massachusetts

Mark A. Pokras, D.V.M., B.S.
Assistant Professor,
Wildlife Clinic,
Tufts University,
School of Veterinary Medicine,
North Grafton, Massachusetts

**Marc R. Raffe, D.V.M., M.S., Dip. ACVA,
Dip. ACVECC**
Associate Professor of Anesthesia/Critical Care,
University of Minnesota,
College of Veterinary Medicine,
St. Paul, Minnesota

Keith P. Richter, D.V.M., Dip. ACVIM
Staff Internist,
Veterinary Specialty Hospital of San Diego,
Rancho Santa Fe, California

**James N. Ross, Jr., D.V.M., M.Sc., Ph.D.,
Dip. ACVIM, Dip. ACVECC**
Professor and Chairman,
Department of Medicine,
Tufts University,
School of Veterinary Medicine,
North Grafton, Massachusetts

Linda A. Ross, D.V.M., M.S., Dip. ACVIM
Associate Professor,
Department of Medicine;
Chief of Staff,
Foster Hospital for Small Animals,
Tufts University,
School of Veterinary Medicine,
North Grafton, Massachusetts

**John E. Rush, D.V.M., M.S., Dip. ACVIM
(Cardiology)**
Assistant Professor of Cardiology/Critical Care,
Tufts University,
School of Veterinary Medicine,
North Grafton, Massachusetts

**Michael Schaer, D.V.M., Dip. ACVIM, Dip.
ACVECC**
Professor and Associate Chairman,
Department of Small Animal Clinical Sciences,
University of Florida, College of Veterinary
Medicine,
Gainesville, Florida

Eric R. Schertel, D.V.M., Ph.D.
Assistant Professor,
Department of Veterinary Clinical Sciences,
Ohio State University,
College of Veterinary Medicine,
Columbus, Ohio

**Kenneth Lee Schunk, D.V.M., Dip. ACVIM
(Neurology)**
Hillsborough County Veterinary Hospital,
Amherst, New Hampshire

David C. Seeler, D.V.M., M.Sc., Dip. ACVA
Associate Professor,
University of Prince Edward Island,
Atlantic Veterinary College,
Charlottetown, Prince Edward Island, Canada

Frances O. Smith, D.V.M., Ph.D., Dip. ACT
Crossroads Animal Hospital,
Burnsville, Minnesota

Joseph Taboada, D.V.M., Dip. ACVIM
Department of Veterinary Clinical Sciences,
Louisiana State University,
School of Veterinary Medicine,
Baton Rouge, Louisiana

Robin E. Wall, D.V.M.
Resident,
Emergency Medicine/Critical Care,
Tufts University,
School of Veterinary Medicine,
North Grafton, Massachusetts

**Wendy A. Ware, D.V.M., M.S., Dip.
ACVIM (Cardiology)**
Associate Professor,
Department of Veterinary Clinical Sciences,
Iowa State University,
College of Veterinary Medicine,
Ames, Iowa

Stephen D. White, D.V.M., Dip. ACVD
Associate Professor,
Veterinary Teaching Hospital,
Colorado State University,
College of Veterinary Medicine and Biomedical
Sciences,
Fort Collins, Colorado

This text is dedicated to our loves, Deb and Brenda, for their understanding and patience during its preparation, and to the compassionate and conscientious critical care and emergency veterinary technicians past and present at Tufts University School of Veterinary Medicine for their unceasing efforts: Sharon, Celeste, Sheila, Donna B., Dee, Ellen, Therese, Robin, Deb C., Chris, Jean, Deb D., Donna E., Evelyn, Kris, Spider, and Soo.

Preface

This text represents the culmination of many great efforts by the contributors to bring the reader state-of-the art information and reference material on veterinary emergency and critical care medicine topics. We have accomplished our goal of providing complete discussions of: (1) current management for specific emergencies such as trauma and sepsis, surgical conditions (gastric-dilatation volvulus, intervertebral disc herniation), and many species (avian, wildlife) or organ system–oriented emergencies; (2) crucial, pertinent critical care topics such as transfusion medicine, nutritional support, and cardiopulmonary resuscitation; and (3) important aspects of emergency and critical care practice such as patient monitoring, clinical decision making, client relations, and ethics. We hope that you will find this text as enlightening to read and use as we found it to compile for the benefit of our colleagues in this exciting arena of our veterinary profession.

Robert J. Murtaugh
Paul M. Kaplan

Contents

SECTION ONE

The Emergency/Critical Care Environment

1 Establishing the Critical Care Facility

Paul M. Kaplan

Intensive care/emergency facilities and the practice of critical care medicine are no longer confined to larger institutions but are becoming available in veterinary private practice throughout the United States. Increased public awareness of the necessity and availability of critical care/emergency services obliges veterinarians to provide these services or access to them. The rapidly expanding field of critical care medicine is placing new demands on veterinarians and veterinary technicians. Most of our patients do not have scheduled appointments but arrive at our emergency clinics with critical life-threatening conditions. Consequently, the critical care/emergency facility is often a fast-paced, stressful environment for the staff as well as the patient and pet owner. The critical care facility should be designed to handle acute emergency situations efficiently and to provide continuous care for the critically ill. Sophistication and technology in critical care medicine is increasing and so are the costs of this medical care. The growth and survival of critical care facilities depends on improved efficiency and economic considerations for all aspects of operation (medical records, personnel, equipment, laboratory testing, and facility design, to name a few). Some critical care facilities are established to provide critical care at a central location to a large number of veterinary hospitals. This helps alleviate time on-call for some practitioners while providing intensive care for their patients.

A variety of diseases prompt admission to the critical care/emergency facility. Animals admitted to the critical care facility can generally be grouped into three categories: animals requiring extensive nursing care, animals that are physiologically stable but that require intense monitoring or observation, and animals that are physiologically unstable and require constant veterinary critical care. Hospitalization in a general hospital setting (ward area) is not conducive to the staff and time commitment required for intensive patient treatment.

Extensive nursing care ranges from calculating intake and output fluid measurements every few hours in a dog with acute renal failure, to administering ophthalmic ointments every hour to a dog with a deep corneal ulcer. These animals are stable but require a large amount of nursing/clinician time and effort.

Physiologically stable animals may be admitted to the intensive care unit (ICU) for monitoring or observation if complications from their disease are possible (e.g., seizure disorders, intermittent cardiac arrhythmias). The recognition and treatment of these complications are more likely in the ICU than in a general hospital setting, decreasing the morbidity and mortality rates for these animals.

The single most time-consuming disease process for the emergency veterinary clinician is trauma. Often, traumatized animals are in shock and require extensive treatment to correct their abnormal hemodynamic state. These patients present with multiple problems and often require interventions such as thoracocentesis and/or tube thoracostomy for resolution of pneumothorax. It is this group of animals that demands constant care by the attending emergency clinician until the animal achieves a "stable" status. Frequent physical examinations and serial monitoring of various parameters is important, as some of these patients will become progressively unstable (e.g., from continual abdominal bleeding) requiring changes in medical management or immediate surgical intervention.

Although changing technology has provided critical care clinicians with many new diagnostic tools, the value of clinical intuition and clinical assessment cannot be underestimated. The critical care patient should have multiple physical examinations and frequent updating of its clinical status.

THE PHYSICAL PLANT

A critical care/emergency facility ideally should be located central to the veterinary hospitals or area that it services, with easy access from major roadways. The hospital should be clearly identified and the entrance to the reception area easily noticed. An inclined ramp into the reception area is often necessary for large nonambulatory dogs who must be brought into the hospital on a gurney. Some space in the reception area should be devoted to client education—not only describing the triage procedure (treatment in order of severity of injury) but also describing some common first-aid procedures for simple emergencies. This serves to minimize owner anxiety while waiting to be seen, as well as providing for and improving client education. Examination rooms should be situated between the reception area and the treatment/ICU area.

One area within the ICU should be set up to enable rapid treatment of acute life-threatening situations such as cardiac arrest. Direct access from the reception area to the ICU in these situations is critical. The necessary emergency equipment (laryngoscope, endotracheal tubes, etc.) should be readily accessible in this area at all times. A complete checklist of drugs and equipment for this emergency area should be reviewed daily, and the area should be restocked after each use.

The function of the critical care/emergency facility should revolve around the ICU. The ICU should be a highly visible, easily accessible ward that is central to all other ancillary areas (Fig. 1-1). The critical care facility is dependent on ancillary services. Complete laboratory capabilities and radiographic support services should be available within this facility (Chapter 3). The surgical suite should be located close to the ICU, minimizing transport time of postsurgical patients to ICU. If space within the facility is available, a special procedures area can be set up for advanced diagnostic and therapeutic interventions (endoscopy, ultrasonography). An isolation ward should be close to but distinctly separate from the ICU and other hospital areas. A closed-circuit television linkage or viewing window connected to the ICU is useful to observe patients in isolation.

The floor plan of the ICU should allow for constant visualization of all patients from a central work area. In preexisting buildings, the use of wide-angle mirrors in the ICU may be useful to

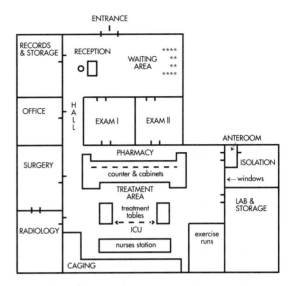

Fig. 1-1 Floor plan for an emergency clinic incorporating easy access to service areas, with easy visualization of hospitalized animals from treatment area and nurses' station. (From Murtaugh RJ. Emergency medicine. In Ettinger SJ, ed. Textbook of veterinary internal medicine, ed 3, vol 1, Philadelphia, WB Saunders, 1989; 1:212.)

achieve this goal. Multiple sources (wall-mounted, portable) of oxygen and suction are necessary for easy access when treating more than one animal. In addition, ample lighting and several electrical outlets should be available. Ceiling track mounts may be used to suspend intravenous fluids administration sets. The intensive care unit should have an emergency generator in the event of power failure.

DRUGS

Essential drugs that should be available in a critical care facility are listed alphabetically in Table 1-1. Storage of these drugs in an organized fashion is essential to facilitate easy access for use by the staff. Narcotic drugs and other classified drugs should be kept in a double-locked storage cabinet or safe. An accompanying log should specify patient name and identification number, date and time of usage, amount of drug used, amount of drug remaining in bottle, and signature of the clinician requiring these drugs. As the number of drugs in our armamentarium increases, so do the possibilities for drug interactions. A listing of common drug interactions should be available in the critical care unit. In addition, poison control telephone numbers should be posted in an accessible place.

Table 1-1 Alphabetical list of drugs recommended for use in veterinary emergency facilities*

Fluids	Dipyrone
Blood (A-negative)	Dobutamine
Dextrans	Doxapram
5% dextrose	Enteral nutrition for-
2.5% dextrose and	mulas
0.45% saline	Emeraid II (birds)
50% dextrose in	Ensure plus
water	Epinephrine
Lactated Ringer's	Ethanol
Mannitol	Euthanasia solution
Potassium chloride	Fenbendazole
0.9% saline	Florinef
Sodium bicarbonate	Flunixin meglumine
Sterile water for	Furosemide
injection	Heparin
Acetylcysteine	Hydralazine
Acepromazine	Hydralazine injection
Activated charcoal	Inhalation anesthetic
Aminophylline	Isoproterenol
Amrinone	Ketamine
Antibiotics (assorted	Lactulose
types, dosage	Lidocaine
forms)	Magnesium sulfate
Antihistamine(s)	Metoclopramide
Apomorphine	Morphine
Aquamephyton	Nalorphine
Ascorbic acid	Naloxone
Assorted eye and ear	Neostigmine
medications	Neuromuscular
Atropine	blocking agent
Bismuth subsalicylate	Nitroglycerin ointment
(Pepto-Bismol)	Oxymorphone
Butorphanol	Oxytocin
(analgesic)	Phenobarbital
Calcium gluconate	Phenylephrine
Calcium chloride	Pralidoxime (organo-
CaNa$_2$ EDTA	phosphate antidote)
Captopril	Prednisolone succinate
Carbonic anhydrase	Procainamide
inhibitor	Propranolol
Chlorpromazine	Quinidine
Desoxycorticosterone	Sulfadimethoxine
Dexamethasone	Sodium nitroprusside
Digoxin (injectable	Thiobarbiturate
and oral)	Valium
Dimercaprol (other	Verapamil
antidotes based on	Vinegar (neutralization
type practice	of alkali)
caseload)	Vitamins A, B, D, and
	E, injectable
	Xylazine (emetic in
	cats)

*From Murtaugh RJ. Emergency medicine. In Ettinger SJ, ed. Textbook of veterinary internal medicine, ed 3, vol 1, Philadelphia, WB Saunders, 1989, 214.

PERSONNEL

Staffing for critical care facilities is often composed of a relatively small number of people. The success of a critical care facility is largely dependent on the personnel staffing the facility, their interrelationships, and their willingness to work toward the common goal of coordinated veterinary care. Each member of the team has a set of individual tasks to perform to ensure proper daily patient care and continual smooth operation of the facility. Selection of personnel for a critical care facility should be largely based on an individual's experience, ability to work under stress, and ability to maintain good communicative skills with other members of the team in this stressful environment. The minimum number of team members necessary for optimal operation of a critical care facility at any given time should include a receptionist, two nurses, a surgeon available on-call, and a primary care veterinary clinician.

The role of the receptionist is multifactorial. He/she must be adept at recognizing and prioritizing emergencies (triage) and skillful in client communication. Pet owners with critically ill animals are extremely anxious. It is the receptionist's role to calm the owners and keep them updated on their pet's status. The receptionist serves as liaison between the veterinarian and owner when the veterinarian is unavailable to talk with the owner. The receptionist should be skilled in the recognition of life-threatening emergencies and be trained in the principles of cardiopulmonary resuscitation (CPR) as he/she is the first staff member to make contact with the patient and owner. The receptionist must communicate on the telephone with referring veterinarians and clients and be able to clearly and concisely obtain and relay patient information and clinical data. The receptionist (or other hospital administrator) should be responsible for discussing financial arrangements, leaving the veterinarian free to care for the patient. Financial "surprises" are a continual problem in critical care medicine, as critical patients usually require extensive monitoring, diagnostics, and therapeutics, leading to higher costs than those incurred for routine veterinary services. The initial estimate should be continually reviewed and revised, and the client should be updated about any changes necessary.

Important members of the critical care team are the ICU nurses. Their responsibilities include direct patient care, such as monitoring of vital signs, attending to the patients' physiologic and psychologic needs, administering medication, and keeping clear and concise records.[1] The ICU nurse is usually the first person to recognize sudden changes in the patient's condition and is acutely aware of the actual status of the patient. Emergency clinicians must be willing and eager to consider recommendations and observations made by these highly trained nurses. Additional responsibilities delegated to the ICU nurses include maintenance of the equipment and training of new critical care personnel. The ICU nursing position can be highly stressful and demanding. It is up to the clinical director to ensure adequate compensation for these important members of the team. Continuing education should be available and mandatory for ICU nurses in order to encourage further development and satisfaction from their nursing position. Low personnel turnover is paramount to a smoothly operating critical care facility. Two ICU nurses or technicians are essential to aid the attending veterinarian in the treatment of emergency patients and in the performance of ancillary diagnostic testing (radiology, laboratory testing, etc.) while ensuring that a technician/nurse is available to attend to the needs of the other inpatients. All personnel should be skilled in aseptic techniques, as higher infection rates in the critically ill are directly related to poor hygienic practices.[2,3]

Responsibilities of the critical care veterinary clinician include treatment of patients, coordination of the critical care facility, and counseling the client. A critical care clinician should be efficient and competent in the diagnosis and treatment of trauma patients, which constitute the majority of critical care cases seen on an emergency basis. The attending clinician is considered the "quarterback" of the critical care team. It is up to him/her to make critical decisions governing patient care and changes in patient treatment. In addition, the clinician must delegate duties and responsibilities to co-workers as necessary. Good communicative skills are extremely important in a critical care facility, where tension and stress are high.

The need for an emergency surgeon at a critical care facility is often sporadic; however, a surgeon should be available on-call at all times to handle diseases requiring immediate surgical intervention (i.e., acute abdomen).

Critical care "burn-out" is a very real phenomenon among all members of the team. It is often the result of working on your days off, working double shifts, or working extended periods without a day off. It may also occur as a result of constant high tension and stress in the working environment. "Burn-out" can be avoided by having additional trained personnel available to fill in when necessary (vacations, sick days, personal days) and by having regularly scheduled meetings for continuing education, to discuss grievances, and to solicit suggestions from the staff members.

REFERENCES
1. Livingston MS. The nurse and critical patient care. J Am Anim Hosp Assoc 1972;8:420-424.
2. Thorp JM, Richards WC, Telfer ABM. A survey of infection in an intensive care unit. Anaesthesia 1979;34:643-650.
3. Burrows CF. Inadequate skin preparation as a cause of intravenous catheter-related infection in the dog. J Am Vet Med Assoc 1982;180:747-749.

SUGGESTED READING
Haskins SC. Overview of emergency and intensive care in contemporary issues in small animal practice. In Sherding RG, ed. Medical emergencies. New York, Churchill Livingston, 1985;1-35.

2 Medical Records

Robert J. Murtaugh

The medical record represents a critically important link to the patient. Medical records contain the historical perspective on each patient and a chronology of the approach to the medical care administered to that patient. The importance of good medical records cannot be overemphasized with respect to the practice of critical care and emergency medicine. The medical record is an important key to the continuity of care required for critical care patients. The systematic approach required for producing and maintaining quality medical records helps ensure quality veterinary medical care. Attention to the details of medical record keeping provides for a thoughtful, complete, systematic, and progressive approach to the delivery of patient care. Good medical record keeping will not guarantee the practice of good medicine, but disorganized and incomplete medical records can result in compromised patient care.[1]

The format and style used for medical records can be varied for several reasons, including the needs of the veterinarian(s), the size of a particular practice, and the type of caseload involved. A good medical record should be simple, complete, and easy to understand. An individual unfamiliar with a particular case should be able to go to the medical record and retrieve the necessary information required to provide the continuity of care for a particular patient. The practice of good medical record keeping requires veterinarians to adhere to certain specific standards with respect to the generation and maintenance of medical records.

STANDARD MEDICAL RECORD FORMAT

There are several important functions of the medical record. It provides documentation of the clinical course of the patient—what was done, the results, and the treatments performed. The medical record (including results of tests and examinations) enables the clinician to plan and document future care of the patient. An organized approach to the medical record solidifies the clinician's stepwise approach to the care of a patient. The medical record permits review of the case by another clinician unfamiliar with the patient. This function preserves the continuity of care within a hospital or at another hospital should the patient be transferred to the care of another veterinarian. The medical record is a legal document and is significant in the defense of a clinician's actions. A poorly maintained medical record can be a significant hindrance to defending oneself should that circumstance arise.[2] Medical record data that are easily retrievable provide a means for education and retrospective research endeavors. Although this function is used primarily in academic environments, critical medical record reviews can provide insight into improving the medical care provided in any veterinary practice. Since medical records serve many purposes, veterinary clinicians must ensure that specific aspects of medical record keeping are incorporated into their practice.

Medical record identification

A separate medical record should be initiated and maintained on each animal examined or hospitalized. Medical records must be clearly and legibly identified. Handwritten or typewritten identification (case numbers and names) can be misprinted or misinterpreted, leading to errors or incompleteness in a medical record. Plastic cards embossed with the patient case number, name, and demographic data are recommended for imprinting medical record data sheets (Fig. 2-1). The increased efficiency and accuracy of this system warrants consideration for its implementation in any practice. Regardless of the identification sys-

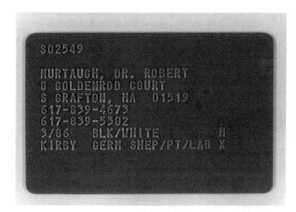

Fig. 2-1 Demographic information is imprinted on a plastic card that resides in the medical record folder or the medical record tinback during hospitalization of the patient.

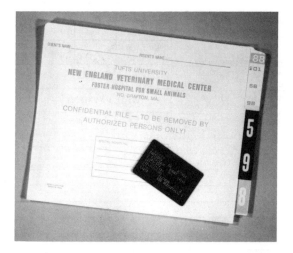

Fig. 2-2 Example of cardboard folder with embossed case numbers and hospital identification that can serve the functions of medical record organization and protection.

Table 2-1 Guidelines for collation of medical records

Left-hand side (top to bottom)
(Chemotherapy chart—only if needed)
Master problem list
Outpatient prescription list
Referring veterinarian information

Right-hand side (top to bottom)*
Discharge orders
History
Physical examination
Client communication sheet
ICU daily records (ICU ward treatment/monitoring flow sheet) ⎫
Medication records (general ward treatment flow sheet) ⎬ in chronologic order
Progress notes ⎭
Electrocardiographic tracings
Laboratory reports
   Hematology
   Chemistry
   Urinalysis
   Cytology
   Miscellaneous laboratory work (serology, microbiology, etc.)
Pathology (biopsy or necropsy)
Radiology reports
Nuclear medicine report
Ultrasound report
Surgery report
Anesthesia report
Consultation reports
Transfer sheet
Estimate
Euthanasia request
Consent to treat

---

*Each visit is compiled individually, separated from other visits by dividers, and filed chronologically with reference to previous visits (last visit on top).

tem employed, all patient information and demographic data should be carefully proofread with the client at the time of each visit.

Content and structure of the medical record

The content and structure of a medical record will depend to a certain extent on the needs, size, and type of caseload of each practice. Cardboard folders with embossed case numbers provide a protective cover that allows organization of the medical record for collation and filing (Fig. 2-2). Medical record forms may be maintained in the medical record folder by an H-style clip placed through prepunched holes in the forms. When an animal

is hospitalized, pertinent medical records and the patient's identification card may be kept in a medical record holder (tinback) that accompanies the animal. A standard approach to collation of the medical record forms is recommended (Table 2-1). The complexity of medical record data requires, in most cases, that separate medical record forms be used for recording various types of information in order to ensure clarity, consistency, and organization in the medical record. The efficiency of a single (multiple copy) form that serves the function of recording history, physical examination, owner consent, progress notes, financial data, and referral summary/discharge in-

ANIMAL EMERGENCY FACILITY

			APPROX. COST	FINAL COST

LAST NAME	FIRST NAME	MIDDLE NAME	DATE-LAST VACCINATION	EMER. EXAM FEE / INJECTIONS/ MEDICATION/ TREATMENT

STREET ADDRESS — DISTEMPER / PARVO

CITY   STATE   ZIP — RABIES / FELINE SERIES

ADMISSION DATE   TIME   A.M. P.M.   WORK PHONE   HOME PHONE — LAB. / X-RAY

PATIENT NAME   SPECIES   BREED   M SEX F / ALTERED   AGE   COLOR — FLUIDS/ IV. CATH.

REFERRING OR FAMILY VETERINARIAN   PAYMENT PREFERENCE   CASH ○ CHECK ○ B/A ○ M/C ○ — SEDATION/ ANESTHESIA / SURGERY

AUTHORIZATION FOR MEDICAL AND/OR SURGICAL TREATMENT

I HEREBY AUTHORIZE THE DOCTOR ON DUTY (AND ASSISTANTS THE DOCTOR MAY DESIGNATE) TO ADMINISTER TREATMENT AS IS CONSIDERED THERAPEUTICALLY AND/OR DIAGNOSTICALLY NECESSARY ON THE BASIS OF FINDINGS DURING THE COURSE OF SAID EVALUATION. I ALSO CONSENT TO THE ADMINISTRATION OF SUCH ANESTHETICS AS ARE NECESSARY AND SURGICAL PROCEDURES OF AN EMERGENCY NATURE.

— SURG. ROOM/ MATERIALS / INTENSIVE CARE

I HEREBY CERTIFY THAT I HAVE READ AND FULLY UNDERSTAND THE ABOVE AUTHORIZATION FOR MEDICAL AND/OR SURGICAL TREATMENT THE REASONS WHY THE SURGERY IS CONSIDERED NECESSARY, ITS ADVANTAGES AND POSSIBLE COMPLICATIONS IF ANY, AS WELL AS POSSIBLE ALTERNATIVE MODES OF TREATMENT, WHICH ARE EXPLAINED TO ME BY THE DOCTOR, I ASSUME FINANCIAL RESPONSIBILITY FOR ALL CHARGES INCURRED TO PATIENT, CONSENT TO RELEASE OF MEDICAL INFORMATION AND AUTHORIZE DIRECT PAYMENT TO THE ABOVE NAMED HOSPITAL OR CLINIC.

— HOSPITALIZATION

I UNDERSTAND THAT EMERGENCY PATIENTS MUST BE REMOVED FROM THE CLINIC DAILY BY 8:00 A.M. THOSE RECEIVED ON SATURDAY OR SUNDAY MAY, IF NECESSARY, BE HELD UNTIL MONDAY AT 8:00 A.M. IF I FAIL TO REMOVE SAID ANIMAL BY THAT TIME I WILL BE RESPONSIBLE FOR ADDITIONAL CHARGES FOR TRANSPORTATION TO THE HUMANE SOCIETY, POUND, OR S.P.C.A.

X _____
SIGNATURE OF OWNER OR RESPONSIBLE AGENT

— TOTAL CHARGES

X _____
WITNESS   ALL PRICES OF TAXABLE ITEMS INCLUDE REIMBURSEMENT FOR SALE TAX COMPUTED TO THE NEAREST MILL.

— MC   V / CK   CA — DEPOSIT

	☐ Normal ☐ Abnormal	INTEGU-MENTARY	☐ Normal ☐ Abnormal	MUSCULO-SKELETAL	☐ Normal ☐ Abnormal	BALANCE
CARDIO-VASCULAR	☐ Normal ☐ Abnormal	RESPIRA-TORY	☐ Normal ☐ Abnormal	DIGESTIVE	☐ Normal ☐ Abnormal	**TOTAL PAYMENT**
URO-GENITAL	☐ Normal ☐ Abnormal	EARS EYES	☐ Normal ☐ Abnormal	NERVOUS SYSTEM	☐ Normal ☐ Abnormal	DISCHARGE STATUS: / Unimproved

TEMP.   HR.   PULSE   RESP.   MM — No Change / Expired

① HISTORY   ② PHYSICAL FINDING ·   ③ DIAGNOSIS   ④ TREATMENT — Improved / Euthanasia

_____

℞ ITEM & SIZE

_____

RETURN TO REFERRING VETERINARIAN ON:
RELEASE TO: OWNER/AGENT

_____DATE _____TIME_____   A.M. P.M.   **NUMBER** **Nº 003018**   VETERINARIAN

TECHNICIAN

WHITE: HOSPITAL COPY   CANARY: REF. D.V.M.   PINK: OWNER COPY   GOLDENROD: ADMINISTRATIVE

Fig. 2-3 Emergency record that can simplify and ensure medical record keeping in this type of practice situation. (From Duppong BL, Ettinger SJ: The medical record. In Ettinger SJ, ed. Textbook of veterinary internal medicine, ed 2, Philadelphia, WB Saunders, 1983.)

structions may be adequate for medical record keeping in the context of an overnight emergency clinic (Fig. 2-3). The scope of this discussion on medical records does not allow for in-depth review of all possible forms used in a complete medical record.[3,4] Figs. 2-4 through 2-7 provide examples of forms that are of particular importance to the veterinarian involved in emergency and critical care medicine.

Medical records should be separated from billing records in most situations. The medical record appears more professional to the client when this practice is followed, that is, a record of the patient's medical care versus a billing worksheet. There is a significant chance that charges may be lost in the medical record (by omission or commission) when billing data is stored in the medical record. Separation of billing records from the medical record provides an additional means of enhancing medical record retrieval when case record numbers are unavailable from a client and cross-reference indexes fail.

DATE:		LOCATION:	DIET:		WATER:			
TREATMENT PLAN	TREAT #							
	8 AM							
	9							
	10							
	11							
	12							
	1 PM							
	2							
	3							
	4							
	5							
	6							
	7							
	8							
	9							
	10							
	11							
	12							
	1 AM							
	2							
	3							
	4							
	5							
	6							
	7							

TIME	URINATION	STOOL	VOMIT	OTHER

Medication Record

Fig. 2-4 Flow sheet used to record treatments and to follow trends in various parameters that are monitored. Clinician's orders are numbered and described in the left-hand column. The corresponding numbers are listed at the top of the columns across the page, and desired times for each order to be carried out are highlighted down each corresponding column. When an order has been carried out, the box corresponding to that time for each order is checked off and initialed, and results are written in or alongside that box (i.e., CVP reading, results of PCV/TS, urine output reading). Additional observations on the patient are recorded at the bottom of the page.

ANIMAL EMERGENCY
    FACILITY

Time and date admitted: _____

Admitting Clinician: _____ Date Transferred:_____

Attending Clinician: _____

Patient Location: Ward _____ Cage _____ Stall _____

Initial Estimate $ _____ Revised Estimate $ _____

Please Inform Client ☐ and RDVM ☐ of Transfer/Estimate Revision

History and physical exam summary:_____
_____
_____
_____
_____
_____
_____
_____

Patient location and condition/initial and current therapy: _____
_____
_____
_____

Diagnostic completed and pending/Additional requests submitted: _____
_____
_____
_____

Preliminary diagnostic results: _____
_____
_____
_____

Prognosis given owner/client and referring veterinarian communication status: _____
_____
_____
_____

Call owner/billing before proceeding ☐   Owner's telephone _____
                                          from _____ to _____

Fig. 2-5 Summary sheet that can be used to supplement other medical record entries when a case is transferred from one clinician to another within the same hospital. This form provides improved continuity of patient care in these circumstances.

ANIMAL EMERGENCY
FACILITY

WARD: CAGE: CLINICIAN:

Date	D = Direct T = Telephone	Summary of communication (include comments made on patient progress, test interpretation, prognosis and treatment cost.) **Each entry must be signed by the student or clinician.**

CLIENT AND REFERRING VETERINARIAN COMMUNICATION SHEET

Fig. 2-6 Client communication sheets are recommended as part of a complete medical record. Records of communication with clients help ensure continuity/consistency in the communication to clients during hospitalization of their animals. These records can serve an important function in legal defense of your position when billing disputes or other issues related to the care of a patient occur.

ANIMAL EMERGENCY
FACILITY

Date Admitted _____ Date Discharged _____ ☐ Medication to go

Diagnosis _____

Home Instructions _____
_____
_____
_____
_____
_____

Medication Dispensed _____	Amount _____	Size _____	Instructions _____
_____	_____	_____	_____
_____	_____	_____	_____
_____	_____	_____	_____
_____	_____	_____	_____

Additional Instruction Sheets ☐ _____

Follow-up Visits ☐   at TNEVMC ☐   at Ref. Vet. ☐   Date _____ Time _____

For _____

Owner to call Clinician _____ Date _____ Time _____

PROFESSIONAL REPORT (to Referring Veterinarian only)

Diagnostic Procedures and Findings _____
_____
_____
_____
_____
_____
_____

Surgical Procedure _____

Medical Treatment _____

Prognosis and Follow-up Care _____
_____
_____
_____

Thank you for the referral.

_____

ATTENDING CLINICIAN

DISCHARGE ORDERS   MEDICAL RECORDS

Fig. 2-7 Example of multiple-part form that can be used to provide client discharge instructions, pharmacy requisition, referring veterinarian communication, and a summary for the medical record.

Review of the medical record system

A method for purging and coding (diagnoses, procedures, anatomic locations) medical records must be developed for any medical record system. These methods can be developed to varying degrees depending on the consideration of legal issues related to medical record keeping, space constraints of a practice, and the desires of the involved veterinarians to be able to retrieve case material for review (education/research). As with any aspect of a veterinary medical practice, the medical record format employed should be under continual review to ensure that content, clarity, and completeness are maintained. The medical records must be able to perform the functions desired/required, but should not be allowed to become more complex unnecessarily—redundancy should be avoided and simplicity preserved whenever possible.

PROBLEM-ORIENTED MEDICAL RECORD KEEPING

The format of problem-oriented medical record keeping encourages an organized, consistent, and logical approach to the treatment of a veterinary patient. This medical record structure lends itself to quick and easy retrieval of information and ready assessment of the animal's current health status and the plans needed to address unresolved medical problems.[4] The problem-oriented medical record has four components—data base, problem list, initial plans, and progress notes.[2]

Data base

A standard data base may vary depending on the needs of the practice or patient (age, chief complaint, etc.). The data base represents the initial information accumulated on a patient and generally includes history, physical examination, complete blood count, urinalysis, serum biochemical profile, and possibly, chest/abdominal radiographs. The problems identified from the initial data base are numbered and listed on a problem list in as refined a form as possible (Fig. 2-8). Initial problems are often broadly defined, for example, a physical examination finding (lymphadenopathy) or an abnormal laboratory result (increased serum hepatic enzyme activities).

The problem list

The problem list is vital to the organization and application of the problem-oriented approach to

ANIMAL EMERGENCY
FACILITY

PROBLEM			DATE ENTERED	DATE RESOLVED
1. Pruritus	4/25/89	see problem 9	4/23/89	4/25/89
2. Hematuria	4/26/89	see problem 10	4/23/89	4/26/89
3. Stranguria	4/26/89	" "	4/23/89	4/26/89
4. Pyuria	4/26/89	" "	4/23/89	4/26/89
5. Azotemia	4/26/89	" "	4/23/89	4/26/89
6. Leukocytosis	4/26/89	" "	4/23/89	4/26/89
7. Increased SAP Enzyme Activity	4/27/89	see problem 11	4/23/89	4/26/89
8. Progressive retinal atrophy	4/23/89	inactive	4/23/89	
9. Generalized demodicosis and secondary pyoderma			4/25/89	6/20/89
10. Pyelonephritis – E.coli			4/26/89	5/19/89
11. Pituitary dependent Cushing's	6/3/89	see problem 12	4/27/89	6/3/89
12. Pituitary dependent Cushing's controlled with Lysodren			6/3/89	
13.				
14.				
15.				

Fig. 2-8 The problem list should reflect a summation of the course of events related to the identification and resolution of the patient's disease(s); that is, it should be a table of contents for the medical record.

medical problems and medical records. Initial problem lists should be updated and refined throughout the course of medical/surgical treatment of a patient. Initial broad-based problems will be more narrowly defined as additional subjective and objective data are obtained and patient reassessment occurs. Problems can be resolved, redefined and updated, combined with other problems, inactivated, or left unresolved (Fig. 2-8).[4]

Initial plans

Initial plans (diagnostic and therapeutic) are formulated and clearly identified in the record for each problem. Initial diagnostic plans normally include a listing of differential diagnosis and the corresponding tests required to rule in or out each differential diagnosis for a particular problem. Initial therapeutic plans are formulated and clearly identified in the record for each specific problem. These plans address which treatments are indicated based on the problems initially derived from the patient data base. These plans should include specification as to how response to therapy and side effects of therapy will be assessed.

Progress notes

Following formulation of the data base, initial problem list, and initial diagnostic/therapeutic plans, daily progress notes are entered in the medical record for each active problem. Progress notes are written in a standard format with four main components (*s*ubjective data, *o*bjective data, *a*ssessment of the problem, and *p*lans [SOAP]). Subjective data include historical information on the patient as well as ongoing subjective observations related to the animal's attitude and constitution following hospitalization. Objective data include physical examination findings and results of laboratory and diagnostic imaging tests. Assessment represents the synthesis of past and present subjective/objective data into a refined problem (definitive diagnosis, if possible). Diagnostic, therapeutic, and client education plans for each problem are updated as the course of patient treatment progresses and problems are revised to a more refined (definitive) form. The progress notes should reflect any resolution of a problem and the explanation of that resolution.

REFERENCES

1. Wilson JF. The diagnostic reasons for medical recordkeeping. Compend Contin Ed Pract Vet 1984;6:405-413.
2. Wilson JF. The business reasons for medical recordkeeping. Compend Contin Ed Pract Vet 1984;6:526-534.
3. Duppong BL, Ettinger SJ. The medical record. In Ettinger SJ, ed. Textbook of veterinary internal medicine, ed 2 Philadelphia: WB Saunders, 1983:3-29.
4. Saidla JE. Problem-oriented veterinary medical record. In Ettinger SJ, ed. Veterinary internal medicine, ed 2 Philadelphia: WB Saunders, 1983:29-37.

3 Equipment, Laboratory, and Diagnostic Capabilities

Paul M. Kaplan

An emergency facility must be able to provide essential emergency diagnostic procedures as well as offer therapeutic interventions (surgical or medical) during all hours of operation. The emergency facility should be well stocked with essential drugs (Chapter 1) and have capabilities for in-house laboratory testing essential in the critical care patient. The guidelines established by the Veterinary Emergency Critical Care Society classify emergency facilities as Categories I to IV. These categorizations depend on the staffing (doctors and technicians), equipment (see the boxes that follow), and ancillary capabilities of the facility.[1] This discussion will focus on the necessary and optional laboratory and ancillary diagnostic capabilities required for a Category I (complete) critical care unit.

LABORATORY DIAGNOSTIC CAPABILITIES

Basic laboratory tests to be performed on all critical care/emergency patients following admission should include packed cell volume, total solids, blood glucose determination, blood urea nitrogen determination, and urine specific gravity. Blood urea nitrogen and blood glucose may be determined using reagent strip testing (e.g., Azostix for blood urea nitrogen, Chemstrip bG for blood glucose determination). The results of these five tests in conjunction with the physical examination of the critical care patient often provide valuable information regarding the physiologic status of the patient. Results of these simple tests may identify a cause of the patient's critical state (e.g., hyperglycemic coma) or may suggest a diagnostic approach in search of the cause (e.g., decreased packed cell volume and total solids suggestive of acute blood loss).

Hematology

A complete blood count (including blood smear evaluation) should be performed within 1 to 2 hours of admission. A pretreatment blood sample should be submitted for serum biochemical analysis. Many in-house serum biochemical analyzers (e.g., Kodak Ektachem DT-60, Dupont Analyzer system) are available and are cost effective. These analyzers provide various serum biochemical determinations (e.g., creatinine, blood urea nitrogen, calcium, electrolytes, liver enzyme tests, etc.) depending on the equipment purchased. These analyzers accommodate add-on features for additional serum biochemical determinations, if needed. The results obtained are quantitatively more accurate than the reagent strip determinations employed as initial screening tests (e.g., Azostix, Chemstrip bG).

Cytology

Cytologic evaluation of any fluid and tissue samples obtained from an animal is paramount to appropriate critical care patient treatment (e.g., differentiating a transudate from an exudate). A slide preparation of an aliquot of fluid, tissue aspirate, or touch imprint of any biopsy obtained should be stained (e.g., Harleco's Diff-Quik) and evaluated microscopically. A Gram stain should be applied to slide preparations of any exudate obtained. A Gram stain of the material will aid in identifying septic inflammation (presence of organisms) and identify staining characteristics of organisms (gram-positive or gram-negative) that can guide empirical antibiotic therapy.

Microbiology

Aerobic (blood agar plates, MacConkey's media) and anaerobic cultures should be performed for

EQUIPMENT RECOMMENDED FOR A VETERINARY EMERGENCY CLINIC

AMBU bag
Anesthesia machines (isoflurane vaporizer)
Autoclave
Bandage scissors
Blender
Blood banking equipment
    Blood receptacle containers (glass vacuum bottle,
        plastic bags, plastic syringes)
    Centrifuge for component separation
    Anticoagulant
    Refrigerator for blood storage
Blood donor animals
Blood gas analyzer
    1 and 3 ml syringes
    25-gauge needles
    Heparin
Buckets (stainless steel)
Cages (dogs, cats, birds, reptiles)
Circulating warm-water blanket
Clinical laboratory equipment
Compression cuff for rapid intravenous fluid adminis-
    tration
Crash cart
Central venous pressure equipment
    Manometer
    Tubing
    Three-way stopcocks
    Jugular catheter
Direct-current defibrillator (external and internal pad-
    dles)
Direct arterial pressure monitoring equipment
    Arterial catheters
    Pressure transducer
    Electronic monitoring device
Disposable three-bottle suction units for chest drains
Electric hair clippers
Electrocardiography machine
Electronic thermometer (70°-100° F)
Endoscopy equipment
    Rigid and flexible endoscope
    Flexible bronchoscope
    Retrieval and biopsy instruments
    Suction apparatus
    Light source
Endotracheal tubes (various sizes)
Enema can and tubing
Esophageal stethoscope
Face masks (for oxygen and anesthetic administration)
Fluid-warming chamber
Heat lamp
Hemostats
Incubator for neonates

Indirect blood pressure monitoring equipment
    Doppler blood flow detector
    Sphygmomanometer, various sizes of blood pres-
        sure cuffs
Instrument packs (see box on p. 18)
Instrument stand
Intravenous fluid administration sets
Intravenous fluid infusion pump
Intravenous stands/poles
Laryngoscopes
Mechanical ventilator
Mouth speculums
Oscilloscope monitor with printout capacity
Ophthalmoscope/otoscope
Oxygen cage
Penlight
Portable lighting
Radiographic equipment
    300-mA x-ray machine with fluoroscopy
    Automatic film processor
    Film cassettes and film
    Cerebrospinal fluid needles
    Iodinated and noniodinated contrast media (myelo-
        graphy, cystography, intravascular pressure,
        etc.)
    Barium
    Catheters (pacing, flow-directed pulmonary artery,
        etc.)
    Sandbags for positioning
Refrigerator
Retrieval forceps (Forrester sponge forceps, etc.)
Shiotz tonometer
Stethoscope
Stomach pump (large animal)
Stomach tubes
Stretcher/mobile gurney
Suction unit
Surgery table
Surgical packs (see box on p. 18)
Transvenous and/or transthoracic pacing catheters
Ultrasonic nebulizer
Ultrasound equipment
    Two-dimensional real-time sector scanner with Dop-
        pler capability
    Video recorder
    Video printer
    Acoustic coupling gel
Vacuum sweeper
Vaginal speculum
Wastebaskets
Water bed
Weighing scales (kilogram/gram scale for birds)
Woods lamp

GENERAL SUPPLIES RECOMMENDED FOR A VETERINARY EMERGENCY FACILITY

Adhesive tape
Alcohol
Baby food
Bandage material (see box on p. 18)
Bandage scissors
Biohazardous-waste container
Blood collection and administration sets
Catheter caps
Clinical laboratory supplies (see box below)
Cotton-tipped applicators
Diagnostic peritoneal lavage catheters
Disposable gloves
Extension tubing
Fluorescein stain
Graduated burettes for small-volume infusions
Heimlich one-way valves
Hydrogen peroxide
Intravenous catheters (various gauges)
    Over-the-needle cannulas
    Inside-the needle cannulas
    Wing-tipped catheters
Intravenous fluids
    Lactated Ringer's
    Acetated Ringer's
    Ringer's
    0.9% sodium chloride
    0.45% sodium chloride
    Hypertonic (7%) sodium chloride
    2.5%, 5%, 50% dextrose solutions
    2.5% dextrose in half-strength lactated Ringer's

    5% dextrose in lactated Ringer's
    2.5% dextrose in 0.45% sodium chloride
    5% dextrose in 0.9% sodium chloride
Irrigation solution
Latex gloves (sterile)
Lubricating jelly (sterile)
Nasogastric feeding tubes
Nasal oxygen catheters
Paper coveralls for isolation
Penrose drains
Peritoneal dialysis catheters
Plastic cadaver bags
Plastic garbage bags
Prescription diets
Scalpel blades
Schirmer tear test strips
Surgical gowns, masks, caps, shoe covers
Surgical scrub and disinfectant solutions
Suture material
Syringes, hypodermic needles
Thermometers
Thoracostomy tubes (Argyle, various sizes)
Three-way stopcocks
Tongue depressor blades
Tracheal suction catheters
Tracheostomy tubes
Urinary catheters (red rubber, Foley, tom-cat, etc.)
Urine collection bags (sterile for closed collection
    system)
Urine specimen containers

CLINICAL LABORATORY EQUIPMENT AND SUPPLIES RECOMMENDED FOR A VETERINARY EMERGENCY FACILITY

Activated clotting time tubes
Blood gas analyzer
Blood collection tubes
Blood culture tubes
Bunsen burner
Centrifuges (blood tubes, hematocrit)
Coulter counter/hemocytometer
Culture transport media (aerobic and anaerobic)
Culture loop
Culture plates (blood agar, MacConkey's agar)
Culture broth (thioglycolate)
Cotton-tipped applicators
Fecal containers and solution

Gram-staining solution
Incubator for culture plates
Microhematocrit tubes
Microscope
Microscope slides and coverslips
Pipettes
Quick staining solutions (Diff-Quik, New Methylene
    Blue)
Reagent strips (blood glucose, blood urea nitrogen)
Refractometer
Spectrophotometer, flame photometer
Serum biochemical analyzer and reagents
Urinalysis reagent strips (dipsticks)

EMERGENCY SURGICAL PACKS

Ophthalmic pack

1 Adson tissue forceps
1 Adson dressing forceps
4 Halsted mosquito forceps
1 Mayo scissors
1 iris scissors
1 needle holder
1 Metzenbaum scissors
1 scalpel handle
1 eyelid retractor
1 strabismus hook
4 towels
4 towel clamps
1 eye drape
Sterile cotton-tipped applicators
Gauze sponges (4-by-4-in.)

Thoracostomy pack

4 towels (drape)
4 towel clamps
1 scalpel handle
1 rib retractor (Finochetto rib spreader)
1 rat tooth tissue forceps
1 Mayo scissors
1 Metzenbaum scissors
1 Satinsky clamp
1 needle holder
4 Halsted mosquito forceps
Gauze sponges (4-by-4-in.)

Tracheostomy pack

4 towels (drape)
4 towel clamps
1 scalpel handle
2 mosquito forceps
1 Metzenbaum scissors
1 rat tooth tissue forceps
2 Allis tissue forceps
1 small Weitlander retractor
1 large Weitlander retractor
Gauze sponges (4-by-4-in.)

Laceration pack

4 towels
4 towel clamps
1 scalpel handle
1 Brown Adson forceps
3 curved mosquito forceps
2 Crile forceps (straight or curved)
1 Mayo scissors
1 Metzenbaum scissors
1 needle holder
Gauze sponges (4-by-4-in.)

BANDAGE MATERIALS

Sterile

Packages of 4-by-4-in. gauze sponges
Paper drapes
Kling (2 in., 4 in.)
Nonadherent pads (several sizes)
Adaptic nonadherent dressing

Nonsterile

Porous tape (1 in., 2 in.)
Waterproof tape (1 in., 2 in.)
Tongue depressors
Elasticon (elastic tape, 2 in., 3 in., 4 in.)
Vetrap (conforming bandage, 2 in., 4 in.)
Gauze sponges (4-by-4-in.)
Cast padding (2 in., 3 in., 4 in., 6 in.)
Kling (conforming gauze bandage, 2 in., 3 in., 4 in.)
1-lb. cotton roll
Stockinette (2 in., 3 in., 4 in.)
Fiberglass or plaster casting tape (2 in., 3 in., 4 in.)
Cast cutter
Cast spreader
Mason Meta splints (several sizes)
1/8 in., 1/4 in. malleable aluminum rods

more definitive evaluation of fluid or tissue samples demonstrating septic inflammation. At a minimum, appropriate samples should be placed in appropriate culture transport media and submitted to a diagnostic microbiology laboratory. An in-house microbiology laboratory decreases the turn-around time for obtaining results. Culture results are usually available within 24 to 48 hours. Microorganism identification and antibiotic sensitivity kits may be employed if space, time, and trained support staff are available.

Hemostasis

Bleeding diatheses are common in critical patients as primary (e.g., vitamin K antagonists) or secondary (e.g., disseminated intravascular coagulation) disturbances (Chapters 23 and 27). In patients suspected of having a bleeding diathesis, a bleeding time, platelet count and blood smear examination, activated clotting time, and evaluation for fibrin degradation products should be performed immediately. Blood samples should be submitted for laboratory determination of prothrombin time and partial thromboplastin time.

The bleeding time is a measure of in vivo platelet function. A small wound is inflicted, using a standardized stylet on the mucous membrane surface of the inner lip, and the time to cessation of hemorrhage is measured. The cuticle bleeding time is a variation of the skin bleeding time. The test involves cutting a toenail and measuring the time to cessation of bleeding.[2,3] The major drawbacks of both these procedures are nonreproducibility of results and nonstandardization of technique. Prolonged bleeding time occurs with quantitative (thrombocytopenia) and qualitative (platelet function) platelet dysfunction as well as with abnormalities in blood vessel walls. Platelet numbers should be estimated on a blood smear examination and if thrombocytopenia is suspected, a quantitative platelet evaluation should be performed.

Activated clotting time measures blood coagulation in vitro using a diatomaceous earth surface activated tube (Activated Clotting Tube, Becton Dickinson Vacutainer Systems, Rutherford, NJ).[4] The activated clotting time test is a rapid, easy test yielding immediate results regarding intrinsic clotting system disorders. Prolonged activated clotting time (normal mean values: dogs, 75 to 81 seconds; cats, 70 to 75 seconds) may occur with inhibition or deficiency of intrinsic or common pathway factors (disseminated intravascular coagulation, congenital factor VIII deficiency, vitamin K antagonist poisoning).[4,5] Severe thrombocytopenia may result in mild prolongation of the activated clotting time. Whole-blood clotting time, another simple screening test of the intrinsic clotting system, lacks sensitivity and is influenced by numerous variables, making this test less reliable than the activated clotting time.[5]

Determination of elevated levels of fibrin degradation products in an animal, due to ongoing or excessive fibrinolysis, is useful to the diagnosis of disseminated intravascular coagulation. Commercially available blood collection tubes and laboratory diagnostic kits are available for this determination (Thrombowellcotest, Wellcome Research Laboratories, Beckenham, England). A blood smear evaluation may suggest disseminated intravascular coagulation by demonstrating the presence of numerous fragmented red blood cells and thrombocytopenia.

These rapid, easy screening procedures should be performed to document any disorder of hemostasis. In some instances these screening tests may define the cause of the bleeding diathesis. For further evaluation of bleeding disorders an aliquot of blood should be collected in sodium citrate tubes. The plasma should be separated, stored in a freezer, and submitted for laboratory evaluation of prothrombin time and partial thromboplastin time to confirm a suspected coagulopathy. Von Willebrand's factor activity and individual coagulation factor activities should be determined if the etiology of the animal's bleeding diathesis remains undefined after completion of the screening assays.

ANCILLARY SERVICES
Radiography

A veterinary emergency/critical care facility must have complete diagnostic radiography services. These capabilities should include the expertise and equipment necessary to perform contrast radiography (cystography, myelography, gastrointestinal studies). An automatic processor for film developing is often cost effective because it increases available technician time, decreases turnaround time for film review by the clinician, and improves efficiency in patient treatment. In patients requiring cardiac pacing or invasive hemodynamic diagnostics and monitoring (e.g., measurement of pulmonary capillary wedge pressure) fluoroscopy is useful to aid in proper positioning of these catheters. However, fluoroscopic units are expensive and may not be cost effective for all veterinary facilities.

Ultrasound

Two-dimensional (real-time) ultrasonography has become an imperative service that should be available for the treatment of the critical care/emergency veterinary patient. The use of ultrasound techniques can improve diagnosis and hasten appropriate therapeutic intervention (medical or surgical) of many disease processes (see the box that follows), often leading to an increased patient survival rate.[6] The most versatile ultrasound machine for cardiac and abdominal imaging of small animals is a real-time sector scanner with M-mode capacity. Portable real-time ultrasound equipment allows imaging in the critical care unit with minimal disturbance to the patient.

Ultrasound imaging with Doppler capability (spectral and color flow doppler) allows noninvasive assessments of various blood flow parameters (pressure gradients, cardiac output, etc.) (Chapter 35). Alterations in blood flow (e.g., shock, congestive heart failure, thromboembolic disease) occur in critical care/emergency patients. Applications for Doppler ultrasound techniques include the serial monitoring of patient blood flow parameters as a means of monitoring efficacy of therapy.

Endoscopy/bronchoscopy

Foreign-body obstruction (tracheal, esophageal) is a common emergency requiring immediate intervention to prevent short-term (death due to airway obstruction) and long-term (esophageal pressure necrosis and mediastinitis) sequelae. Rigid endoscopes, flexible fiberoptic scopes, and bronchoscopes are essential equipment for the emergency facility. When purchasing flexible fiberoptic endoscopes, scope versatility is imperative. Ideally,

---

DIFFERENTIAL DIAGNOSIS OF ACUTE DISORDERS CLARIFIED BY ULTRASOUND

Cardiac

Cardiomegaly
Pericardial effusion
Chamber enlargement/hypertrophy
Peritoneopericardial diaphragmatic hernia
New or changing murmurs
Bacterial endocarditis (valvular)
Papillary muscle dysfunction
Ruptured chordae tendineae
Arrhythmias
Primary myocardial disease
Neoplasia
No apparent structural disease
Syncope/weakness
Left ventricular outflow tract obstruction
Left ventricular inflow tract obstruction

Abdominal

Prostatomegaly
Abscess
Cyst
Hypertrophy
Neoplasia
Hemoperitoneum
Presence or absence of a mass
Hepatomegaly
Focal/multifocal disease (abscess, tumor)
Diffuse disease (lipidosis, inflammatory)
Obstructive biliary disease
Renomegaly
Mass lesion
Hydronephrosis
Genital
Assess fetal viability in utero
Pyometra

---

the scope should have distal tip deflection capabilities in four directions. In addition, air insufflation, suction, and water flushing capabilities are essential features. A small-diameter fiberscope provides the greatest versatility for use in canine and feline patients (e.g., GIF-XP10 OES Small Caliber Gastrointestinal Fiberscope, Olympus Corporation, Lake Success, NY). Numerous types of specialized forceps are available for use in retrieval of foreign bodies.

Cardiopulmonary monitoring

Electrocardiographic monitoring is essential to the treatment of critical care patients manifesting or predisposed to cardiac abnormalities during diagnostic evaluations and during surgery and intensive care treatment. An oscilloscope monitor with printout capability, an electrocardiograph or telemetric monitoring may be used for monitoring the animal's heart rate and rhythm. Monitoring equipment for direct or indirect blood pressure measurements should be available (e.g., Ultrasonic Doppler Flow Detector, Parks Electronics Laboratories, Aloha, OR; Arteriosonde Sphygmomanometer, Hoffmann LaRoche, Cranbury, NJ) (Chapter 40).

A "crash cart" should be close to the patient in the event that electrocardiographic instability and hemodynamic compromise (hypotension, malignant arrhythmias) occur, necessitating immediate intubation, defibrillation, or pharmacologic intervention in the patient (Chapters 17 and 32).

Respiratory function

A blood gas analyzer (or rapid access to one) should be available at a critical care/emergency facility (e.g., IL1302, Instrumentation Laboratories, Lexington, MA). Transcutaneous sensors for measurement of tissue partial pressures of oxygen and carbon dioxide, devices for the measurement of end-tidal carbon dioxide concentrations in intubated patients, and pulse oximetry are becoming useful adjuncts for serial monitoring of an animal's cardiopulmonary status (Chapters 4 and 36).

REFERENCES

1. Kurtz S, et al. Veterinary emergency and critical care society directory. The Society. Miami FL, 1989;26.
2. Giles AR, Tinlin S, Greenwood R. A canine model of hemophilic factor (factor VIII:C deficiency) bleeding. Blood 1982;60:1135-1138.
3. Pynappels MIM, Briet E, Van der Zwet GT, et al: Evaluation of the cuticle bleeding time in canine hemophilia A. Thromb Haemost 1986;55:70-73.
4. Byars TD, Ling GV, Ferris NA, Keeton KS. Activated coagulation time (ACT) of whole blood in normal dogs. Am J Vet Res 1976;37:1359.
5. Johnstone IB: Clinical and laboratory diagnosis of bleeding disorders. Vet Clin North Am (Small Anim Pract) 1988;18:21.
6. Kaplan PM, Murtaugh RJ, Ross JN. Ultrasound in emergency veterinary medicine. Semin Vet Med Surg (Small Anim) 1988;3:245-254.

4 Monitoring

Paul M. Kaplan

Over the past 10 years, dramatic changes have occurred in the treatment of critically ill veterinary patients. Monitoring of arterial blood pressure, central venous pressure, pulmonary capillary wedge pressure, and cardiac output can be routinely performed in the veterinary critical care unit. Interpretation of the data generated often aids in appropriate treatment of critically ill patients and reflects the efficacy of emergency therapy. Despite this improved instrumentation and technology, the most important method of monitoring remains the physical examination. Noninvasive assessments and serial monitoring of temperature, pulse, respiration, urinary output, and cardiac rhythm gives clinicians valuable information about the status and progression of critical patients and their disease. Reevaluation of the critical care patient should be performed as often as the disease process dictates. Basic monitoring should be performed on the critically ill patient at least twice daily but, in many instances, more frequent or continuous monitoring may be necessary.

Invasive hemodynamic monitoring entails a small risk to the animal. Catheterization is not an innocuous procedure, and the risks to the patient must be weighed against the potential benefits. Morbidity and, less commonly, mortality may occur due to instrumentation of some critically ill patients. Routine invasive hemodynamic monitoring is not indicated in all critical care patients but is helpful in (1) assessing myocardial function and aiding in determination of causes for dyspnea and hypoxia (pulmonary versus cardiac disease); (2) guiding treatment with various cardiotonic drugs (positive inotropes, vasodilators, antiarrhythmic medications); (3) treating critically ill patients with associated cardiovascular disease; (4) monitoring changes in patient hemodynamic status during therapy; and (5) providing prognostic information about critical care patients.

This chapter will address noninvasive and invasive means of monitoring the critical care patient.

NONINVASIVE MONITORING
Temperature

An animal's normal body temperature is a function of the balance between heat loss from skin and lungs, and heat production in skeletal muscle and liver (Chapter 16).[1,2] Temperature alterations in the critically ill animal may occur following exposure to adverse environmental conditions (hypothermia or hyperthermia) and can occur secondary to disease processes (hyperthermia with status epilepticus) or medical/surgical interventions (hypothermia during general anesthesia).[3,4] As a result of prolonged severe alterations in an animal's body temperature, multiple-organ system dysfunction may occur (acute renal failure, acid-base disturbances, cardiac arrhythmias, disseminated intravascular coagulation)(Chapter 16).[5,6,7]

Frequent monitoring of body temperature in the critically ill patient is imperative. A change in an animal's body temperature may reflect a change in physiologic or metabolic status (e.g., hyperthermia with sepsis). Temperature monitoring is most commonly performed with a standard rectal thermometer. In the event of severe hypothermia or hyperthermia, rectal monitoring with a continuously recording thermometer is recommended until normothermia has returned. Standard rectal thermometers have a capability of measuring body temperatures down to 94° F (34.4° C); a thermometer capable of reading temperatures in the subnormal range (from 74° F) may be necessary to obtain an accurate rectal temperature in the hypothermic animal.

A noninvasive device employing infrared tympanic thermometry has become available for monitoring body temperature. This optical device (Exergen Veterinary Infrared Tympanic Temperature

Scanner, Newton, MA) uses state-of-the-art technology and evaluates heat radiation (in 5 seconds) from the tympanic membrane. Correlation of tympanic temperature readings with rectal temperature readings have been documented to within 0.1° C. This device is particularly useful in assessing the critical care patient because of its ease of use, accuracy, temperature operating range (0 to 43° C), and rapidity of results.

Toe-web temperature (skin temperature) provides an index for assessing an animal's cardiac output and peripheral circulation.[8] This technique may be particularly useful in the critical care veterinary patient as a means of monitoring the animal's hemodynamic response to therapy.

Accidental hypothermia has been described in people as a decrease in core body temperature without primary pathology of the hypothalamic temperature regulatory center.[9] Accidental hypothermia has been described in veterinary patients with hypothyroidism,[4] during anesthesia,[3] and following exposure to a cold environment. In the critically ill, immobile patient in the critical care unit, heat is dissipated to the environment, resulting in varying degrees of hypothermia if not closely monitored. The ability to increase cellular metabolic rate or generate heat via shivering (a normal compensatory mechanism) may be impaired in critical care patients.

Prolonged, severe hypothermia can result in profound cardiovascular effects (bradycardia, decreased cardiac output, decreased myocardial contractility, development of arrhythmias and other cardiac conduction system abnormalities,[7,10-12] neurologic dysfunction (decreased mentation, decreased peripheral nerve conduction, dilated pupils),[9] renal dysfunction ("cold diuresis," azotemia),[13] hypovolemia, metabolic acidosis, respiratory depression, and death.

Passive rewarming (e.g., covering the animal with a blanket) is easy, safe, and acceptable for rewarming mildly hypothermic patients. Metal cages, often a source of "cold environmental exposure" in the critical care unit, should be lined with insulating materials to decrease dissipation of heat from the patient.

Circulating warm-water heating pads (active external rewarming) can be used to rewarm mild to moderately hypothermic animals and to maintain normal body temperature in surgical patients.[14] Caution must be exercised when using heat lamps for rewarming because of the potential for the development of superficial burns. The use of electric heating pads is discouraged for this reason as well.

The hypothermic patient receiving external heat supplementation should be repositioned frequently to prevent superficial burns. Slow external rewarming is critical to prevent a further drop in body temperature caused by rapid external rewarming. Rapid external rewarming can cause peripheral vasodilation and transference of cool blood to the central circulation, increasing predisposition to the development of ventricular fibrillation.[15,16]

Animals presenting for severe or prolonged exposure hypothermia (temperature <90° F [32° C]) are more appropriately treated by active core rewarming (internal rewarming). This may be accomplished using warm peritoneal dialysis or warm colonic-intragastric lavage (Chapter 16).[17] Warm intravenous fluid administration will serve to raise body temperature gradually in the hypothermic patient. Active core rewarming reduces the potential for the development of the "rewarming shock" mentioned above.

Heat stroke (hyperthermia) often occurs in animals confined in a hot, humid environment with poor ventilation. Prolonged hyperthermia can lead to cerebral edema, acute renal failure, and disseminated intravascular coagulation.[18] The pathophysiology and sequelae of heat stroke are reviewed in Chapter 16.

Hyperthermic animals may be cooled by various methods, including ice baths, cold water baths, cold water enemas, and cool air flow (fans). Continuous monitoring of rectal temperature is imperative during the cooling process. Many animals tend to become hypothermic with overzealous cooling, and it is recommended to discontinue cooling procedures when the rectal temperature reaches 103° F.

Pulses and myocardial performance

Pulses. The femoral arterial pulse is the most easily palpable arterial pulse in the dog and cat. Palpation of the femoral arterial pulse provides valuable diagnostic and prognostic information regarding cardiovascular status. Light digital pressure is applied over the femoral artery using the fingertips. The arterial pulse is characterized with respect to its rate, rhythm, and quality (intensity and duration). Excessive digital pressure applied to the artery often reduces the quality/accuracy of the information obtained.

Arterial blood flow is pulsatile, and it is the difference between the systolic and diastolic pressures that is represented as the pulse pressure (the major determinant of pulse strength). The normal arterial pulse rises rapidly, reaches a peak, and subsequently declines. Pulse pressure is affected by stroke volume, ejection velocity, and arterial compliance. Alteration in one or any combination of these factors may result in changes in the character of an animal's arterial pulse.

When examining an animal's arterial pulse, the clinician should note the cardiac rhythm simultaneously; cardiac arrhythmias (ventricular premature contractions, atrial fibrillation) may cause beat-to-beat variation in the pulse amplitude (pulse deficits). In the presence of premature heartbeats, ventricular filling is incomplete. The resulting arterial pulse generated may be imperceptible or of different character than the patient's arterial pulse generated by sinoatrial node activation of a cardiac contraction. In critically ill patients, cardiac dysrhythmias are common and may be the result of primary cardiac dysfunction or cardiac dysfunction secondary to other disease processes (gastric dilatation volvulus, electrolyte imbalances).[19-22] The detection of pulse deficits associated with significant hemodynamic compromise warrants therapy for the patient involved as well as further investigation of the characteristics and cause of the cardiac arrhythmia (Chapter 17).

Hypokinetic (weak) pulses are the result of decreased left ventricular stroke volume (states of low cardiac output) associated with primary myocardial disease (dilated cardiomyopathy), decreased intravascular volume (hypovolemia), pericardial disease, and/or severe tachyarrhythmias. Left ventricular outflow obstruction (aortic stenosis) may result in a weak pulse, which rises slowly and is prolonged in duration. Shock conditions are associated with weak, "thready" pulses attributable to decreased stroke volume and intense peripheral arteriolar vasoconstriction.

Hyperkinetic (exaggerated) pulses are bounding pulses noted in any condition in which pulse pressure is increased. Hyperkinetic arterial pulses may be observed in animals with diseases associated with an increased stroke volume (aortic insufficiency or patent ductus arteriosus). In animals with these conditions there is often an increased systolic systemic arterial blood pressure (SABP) and a decrease in diastolic systemic arterial blood pressure, due to a "diastolic runoff," leading to an increased pulse pressure. Occasionally, mitral insufficiency and ventricular septal defects may produce bounding arterial pulses in animals secondary to left ventricular volume overload and increased stroke volume. Hyperkinetic circulatory states (high output states) such as fever, anemia, and thyrotoxicosis may result in bounding arterial pulses in animals.

Alternating weak and strong pulses associated with sinus rhythm in an animal is known as pulsus alternans. Pulsus alternans is related to a beat-to-beat variability in left ventricular systolic pressure.[23] This pulse abnormality can occur in the presence of severe myocardial failure (dilated cardiomyopathy) but is rarely perceptible on palpation of the peripheral arterial pulse.

A palpable decrease in pulse intensity during inspiration, as compared with the character of an animal's pulse during expiration, is known as pulsus paradoxus. In the normal animal there is a decline in systolic SABP with inspiration resulting from reduced left ventricular stroke volume due to the effects of transmission of the negative intrathoracic pressure to the aorta. This decrease in systolic SABP is not readily detectable on palpation of the femoral arterial pulse in the healthy animal. In the presence of cardiac tamponade, alteration of right and left ventricular filling (increased diastolic filling pressure) causes an exaggeration of the decrease in systolic SABP during inspiration that may become detectable on palpation of the femoral arteries.

Finally, femoral pulse characteristics should be compared bilaterally, as unilateral femoral arterial embolization can occur with various cardiac disorders and, occasionally, with primary vascular or hemostatic disorders.

Myocardial performance. Noninvasive assessments of ventricular performance can be made by auscultation of heart sound intensity, palpation of the precordium (chest wall in the area of the heart), palpation of the strength and quality of arterial pulses (see section on arterial pulses above), indirect blood pressure measurements (see section on blood pressure measurement below), and echocardiography. The generally accepted theory of heart sound production is that heart sounds are the result of vibrations of cardiac structures and blood within the heart produced by acceleration or deceleration of blood during different phases of the cardiac cycle. The heart sounds are generated by vibration of the valve leaflets, valve annulus, ventricular walls, and blood.[24] Chest-wall thickness, patient obesity, and pleural or pericardial space-occupying lesions (fluid, air, tissue) that increase the distance between the heart and stethoscope on the chest wall will affect (attenuate) the intensity of cardiac sounds. Tachyarrhythmias auscultated with poor ventricular filling, hypovolemia, and systolic dysfunction (primary myocardial disease) are also associated with decreases in heart sound intensity. The strength of the detected cardiac impulse on palpation of the chest wall can provide a crude assessment of ventricular performance. This estimation is a crude index due to variations in species/breed conformations and other individual patient variables (e.g., obesity or presence of pleural effusion). Ventricular performance can be assessed using M-mode echocardiography, most commonly by assessing fractional shortening of the left ventricle and measurement of circumferential shortening of the left ventricle, left ventricular ejection fraction, and/or systolic time intervals.[25-28] Doppler echocardiography provides a quantitative assessment of left ventricular function by noting peak velocity and peak acceleration of blood flow in the ascending aorta. Estimates of cardiac output may be determined using Doppler technology. Doppler echocardiography can also provide important information concerning cardiovascular function by detecting and quantitating alterations in patterns of normal blood flow.[29,30]

Respiration

Dyspnea is a common clinical sign in animals admitted into the critical care unit. It is defined as shortness of breath accompanied by difficult, labored, or uncomfortable breathing. After establishing an airway and adequate ventilation in the animal, further examination of the animal's respiratory system should be performed to determine the cause of the respiratory distress. The character of the animal's respiration should be noted. Inspiratory dyspnea, cyanosis, and inspiratory stridor often signal the presence of upper airway obstruction (laryngeal paralysis, foreign-body obstruction). Extrathoracic airway obstruction (collapsed trachea) produces primarily inspiratory distress, while intrathoracic airway obstruction typically produces expiratory distress in patients. Diseases that inhibit expansion of the lungs (pleural effusion, pneumothorax, diaphragmatic hernia) usually lead to inspiratory distress or a combination of inspiratory and expiratory distress. Identifying the characteristics/pattern of an animal's respiration can be a valuable aid in determining the cause and appropriate treatment for respiratory distress in an animal (Chapter 25).

In patients exhibiting upper airway obstruction, palpation of the laryngeal or upper tracheal region and digital/visual oral examination may reveal the presence of mass lesions or foreign bodies. Visual examination of the vocal folds, necessary for the diagnosis of laryngeal paralysis, usually requires sedation of the animal. In some instances upper airway obstruction may be the result of infectious disease (cats), and other confirmatory clinical signs may be noted on oral examination (lingual ulcers).

In a patient that has sustained chest trauma, thoracic-wall palpation is important, as it may reveal rib fractures, flail segments, or subcutaneous emphysema.

Auscultation. Parenchymal changes in the lung usually produce alteration of the normal breath sounds. An appreciation of normal breath sounds is necessary in order to understand and classify abnormal sounds. The normal breath sounds include bronchial, vesicular, and bronchovesicular sounds. Bronchial sounds are "tubular-type" or "harsh blowing" sounds auscultated over the larger airways and carina during inspiration and expiration. The frequency of these sounds may vary, but they are usually of higher intensity than vesicular sounds. Vesicular sounds are quiet, "rustling leaves," normal sounds of low intensity and low pitch, that are auscultatable over the thoracic regions peripheral to the carina and large airways. These sounds are auscultated during inspiration and may also be heard during early expiration. Vesicular sounds are louder and of longer duration during inspiration than expiration. Bronchovesicular sounds are normal breath sounds with intermediate characteristics.

The character of abnormal (adventitial) sounds auscultated (crackles, wheezes, friction rubs), the timing of these sounds (inspiratory, expiratory, both), and the distribution of these adventitial sounds can be very helpful in localizing, defining, and monitoring the progression or resolution of respiratory and cardiac disease processes.[31]

Crackles are intermittent, discrete sounds that have been described as having bubbling or popping qualities. These sounds are thought to be generated by a sudden opening of previously closed airways or by bubbles of secretion bursting within airways. The presence of crackles suggests interstitial or airway disease, and these sounds occur with pulmonary edema, pulmonary fibrosis, interstitial pneumonia, chronic obstructive pulmonary disease, bronchopneumonia, and feline asthma.

When air passes through a narrowed airway it will cause vibration of the airway wall. This vibration may produce a continuous whistling, musical sound (wheeze) that can be auscultated during expiration. Wheezes occur with laryngeal paralysis, bronchospasm, and mucosal edema or foreign bodies, tumors, or accumulation of secretion in airways during expiration.

Pleural friction rubs (loud, coarse, creaking sounds) are produced by contact of inflamed visceral with inflamed parietal pleura.

Reduced or muffled lung sounds may occur with the presence of fluid, air, or mass lesions in the pleural space (pneumothorax, pleural effusion, neoplasia, diaphragmatic hernia with abdominal contents in the thorax). In addition, severe pulmonary consolidation may also produce localized muffling of normal lung sounds.

Arterial blood gas analysis. Arterial blood gases have an important role in evaluation of the respiratory function of critical care patients and represent a sensitive index concerning the nature and severity of respiratory disturbances. Arterial blood gases measured at the onset of treatment aid the clinician in distinguishing between hypoxemia due to hypoventilation, right-to-left shunting, ventilation-perfusion mismatching, and diffusion impairment. Severe respiratory failure is indicated when the partial pressure of arterial oxygen (Pao_2) is less than 60 mm Hg or partial pressure of arterial carbon dioxide ($Paco_2$) is greater than 50 mm Hg. The changes in measured blood gases associated with oxygen supplementation to the patient is helpful in defining the cause of hypoxemia (shunt vs. ventilation-perfusion mismatch). Serial monitoring of the arterial blood gases is performed as a means of monitoring progression and resolution of respiratory-metabolic acid-base disorders (Chapters 36 and 38).

In the awake dog or cat, the femoral artery is the vessel of choice for arterial blood gas sampling because of its easy accessibility and size. The dorsal metatarsal, radial, brachial, and lingual arteries may be used for blood gas sampling, especially in anesthetized or comatose animals. The hair on the skin overlying the artery should be clipped, and the skin should be cleansed and sterilized. The artery is palpated using the index and second fingers. Using a heparinized 3-ml syringe with a 25-gauge needle attached, the artery is punctured perpendicular to its course between the phlebotomist's fingers. The syringe should fill easily with blood, as minimal negative pressure is required on the plunger of the syringe because of the animal's pulse pressure. Heparin should be used as the anticoagulant; it causes minimal alterations in blood gas results as compared with other anticoagulants.[32] The syringe barrel is coated with heparin, and it is squeezed out of the syringe so only the hub of the needle is filled with heparin to prevent coagulation of the sample. Following sample collection, any air bubbles present in the syringe should be evacuated to prevent erroneous blood gas results. The syringe should be immediately sealed (e.g., with a rubber stopper over the needle) to prevent exposure of the sample to air.[33] The blood should be analyzed as soon as possible, as storage of the arterial blood may change the measured values. The pH of blood in vitro decreases at a rate of 0.01 pH unit per 20 minutes at room temperature, while no measurable changes occur for 3 hours if the blood is stored at 4° C in an ice bath.[33]

Serial blood gas sampling has been the standard method of monitoring patients with respiratory dysfunction but requires repeated arterial puncture, is expensive, and provides only intermittent information regarding the animal's respiratory status. Pulse oximeters, devices that measure arterial oxygen saturation (hemoglobin-bound and solubilized oxygen) noninvasively, are used routinely in human medicine for perioperative and operative monitoring of arterial oxygen saturation.[34,35] Oxygen saturation measurements reflect the oxygen content of blood more completely than does blood gas measurement of Pao_2 (solubilized oxygen content).

All pulse oximeters work on the principle of absorption spectroscopy. Discrete wavelengths of light are used to measure the optical density of hemoglobin. Pulse oximetry relies on the difference in absorption spectra of reduced and oxygenated hemoglobin. According to the Beer-Lambert law, the oxygen saturation of hemoglobin is a logarithmic function of the intensity of light transmitted through the hemoglobin sample as long as a constant light source intensity and hemoglobin concentration are maintained. Pulse oximetry provides continuous information regarding oxygen saturation.

Pulse oximeters consist of a probe, a microprocessor, and display components. Pulse oximetry probes currently available are designed for fingertip or earlobe application in people. These probes are of two types: (1) fiberoptic reflectance probes, transmitting filtered light to and from the body of the instrument and (2) probes consisting of two light-emitting diodes and a photodetector. In anesthetized or moribund animals, application of the probe across the surface of the tongue provides reliable measurement of arterial oxygen saturation. Reliable results were obtained in the awake dog when the probe was applied to the toe-web, vulvar membranes, or to the shaved pinna of the ear.[36] In addition to oxygen saturation, most pulse oximetry units provide a display of the pulse rate or pulse wave form. With continued development in veterinary medicine, pulse oximetry should prove useful for serial noninvasive assessments of blood oxygenation in animals in the critical care unit.

Urine output

In the presence of mild to moderate decreases in SABP, glomerular filtration rate (GFR) is maintained by a variety of mechanisms including changes in afferent and efferent renal glomerular arteriolar resistance.[37] The rate of urine production in an animal is proportional to the GFR in that animal. When SABP falls below 60 mm Hg, GFR concomitantly declines, leading to a decreased urinary output. Urine production in the normal dog and cat is 1.0 to 2.0 ml/kg per hour. Reduced urinary output in the critical care patient often occurs in association with decreases in renal perfusion (e.g., hypovolemic shock), disruption of the integrity of the urinary tract, or development of intrinsic renal dysfunction (Chapter 21).

Monitoring of an animal's urinary output can be achieved using intermittent or continuous urine collection (Fig. 4-1). Consideration must be given to the need for these measurements and to the careful use of aseptic techniques in order to minimize iatrogenic urinary tract infection. Preputial or vulvar hair should be clipped and the skin and mucous membrane (prepuce, penis, vulva, vaginal vault) should be cleansed with chlorhexidine solution. Sterile urinary catheterization is easily performed with the male dog in lateral recumbency (sheath retracted), and with the female dog standing or in sternal recumbency. The clinician or technician should handle the catheter using sterile gloves, and an appropriately sized, soft urinary catheter (Foley catheter, red rubber feeding tube/catheter) should be lubricated and advanced slowly into the urethra to the urinary bladder. If the urinary catheter is to be indwelling, it is sutured to the vulva or prepuce and attached to a closed urinary collection system (Chapter 21). The urine reservoir container and collection tubing should be maintained off the floor and below the level of the urethral catheter to minimize the risk of ascending urinary tract infection developing. Catheter entry sites and the surrounding tissues should be cleansed with dilute antibacterial/antifungal solution frequently to minimize bacte-

rial contamination and infection of the patient's urinary tract.

Once a constancy for urine output is established for a particular patient, the urinary collection system should be withdrawn. Intermittent catheterization or replacement of the closed indwelling system can be considered should subsequent changes in urine output be suspected and measurement required. If an indwelling catheter is essential, serial urinalysis should be performed to monitor for the development of infection.

The animal's SABP should be measured concomitantly with urine output. Normalization of an animal's SABP and evidence of progressive azotemia without normal to increased urine production in the hydrated, oliguric animal suggests primary renal dysfunction (e.g., renal shutdown) or disruption of the urinary tract and the need for increasingly aggressive medical or surgical management (Chapter 21). Normalization of SABP with improving urinary output following fluid therapy in a previously oliguric patient is a favorable sign, suggesting that decreased renal perfusion was the cause of oliguria.

Recording the animal's urine output on flow sheets allows easy retrieval of this data and documents trends in urine production over time. When urinary output has stabilized, monitoring intervals are decreased. Initially, an animal's urine output should be monitored every hour until the clinician is assured that a steady urine output is achieved for the animal. Subsequently, urine output determinations every 6 to 8 hours are usually adequate in animals requiring continued monitoring. The indwelling urinary catheter should be removed when urine output has become constant (predictable).

Electrocardiographic monitoring

The electrocardiogram is the most important assessment in cardiac arrhythmia characterization and monitoring. Electrocardiographic (ECG) abnormalities in critical care patients result from numerous causes, including hypercapnia, hypoxia, electrolyte disturbances, traumatic myocarditis, uremia, and primary cardiac disease.[19-22] The importance of ECG abnormalities must be assessed in relation to the patient's clinical status. Understanding the physiologic importance of cardiac arrhythmias requires knowledge and understanding of the potential for progression of the arrhythmia, the hemodynamic consequences of the arrhythmia as well as its cause, and potential multisystemic effects. Specific management of cardiovascular abnormalities is discussed in Chapter 17.

A base-line electrocardiogram (multiple leads) is often warranted on critical care patients, and

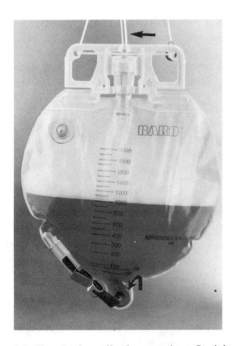

Fig. 4-1 Closed urine collection container. Straight arrow indicates tube to animal's urinary catheter; curved arrow indicates exit port for draining collection container.

continuous lead II ECG monitoring is frequently necessary. Obtaining intermittent lead II electrocardiograms for patient monitoring purposes can be cumbersome and traumatic for the animal, and may not accurately reflect the patient's predominant rhythm. Continuous ECG monitoring is recommended in animals with documented or suspected ECG abnormalities or in animals prone to the development of dysrhythmias (e.g., gastric dilatation volvulus). Continuous ECG monitoring is most easily performed by applying adherent ECG electrode patches to shaved, cleansed areas on both sides of the patient's thorax. Exact placement of electrode patches is not crucial for monitoring purposes. Clip-on ECG leads are attached to the electrode patches in a manner that provides a "clean" tracing for monitoring of the animal's cardiac rhythm. A light bandage wrap can be applied over the patches and ECG leads.

A continuous electrocardiogram is performed mainly for the purpose of monitoring disturbances in cardiac rhythm and alterations in the ST segment in critical care patients. Measurement of other ECG parameters (P-wave amplitude and duration, P-R interval, etc.) should be conducted on hard-copy electrocardiograms obtained in the standard fashion (right lateral recumbency with normal limb lead placement). Many continuous ECG monitoring units have built-in alarms that may be adjusted to signal arrhythmias or signal when preset heart rate limits (high and low) are exceeded.

Common technical problems encountered using "hard-wired" continuous ECG monitoring techniques are loosening of electrode patches, entanglement of the animal in lead wires or severance (biting) of the lead wires by the patient. An Elizabethan collar on the animal is frequently necessary to prevent the latter complication.

A more expensive, but less cumbersome, method of continuous ECG monitoring involves the use of telemetry. Telemetric ECG units allow the lead wires and patches to be retained (within a light body wrap or jacket) on the patient. The electrocardiogram obtained is transmitted to a monitor via radio frequency. This technique also allows the monitoring of numerous patients from one site (station) within the critical care unit.

A normal electrocardiogram for an animal does not imply normal mechanical activity of the heart. Severe myocardial failure (systolic or diastolic dysfunction) may be present despite a normal electrocardiogram. Proper use of ECG data involves integrating these results with a complete physical examination of the animal (including arterial pulse evaluation, auscultation, jugular pulse evaluation) and results of other ancillary evalua-

tions performed (complete blood count, serum biochemical profile, radiographs, ultrasonographs). Evaluation of the electrocardiogram and specific cardiac arrhythmias are reviewed in Chapter 17.

PACKED CELL VOLUME, TOTAL SOLIDS, BLOOD SMEAR EXAMINATION, BLOOD UREA NITROGEN DETERMINATION, URINE SPECIFIC GRAVITY, AND BLOOD GLUCOSE DETERMINATION

All patients admitted to the critical care facility should have a packed cell volume, total solids, blood urea nitrogen determination, blood glucose determination, blood smear examination, and urine specific gravity test performed. These tests can be rapidly performed (within 5 minutes) and yield valuable preliminary information about the patient's physiologic status while laboratory results (complete blood count, individual serum chemistries, and complete serum biochemical profile) are pending. Numerous in-house serum chemical analyzer machines have become available to the veterinarian, allowing more rapid determination of serum biochemical abnormalities.

Packed cell volume, total solids, and blood smear examination

When interpreting the results of a decrease in packed cell volume, it is important to interpret the results in relation to the clinical status of the patient. Patients with acute blood loss are more hemodynamically compromised than animals with chronic blood loss. This phenomenon is due in part to an absence of compensatory mechanisms with acute blood loss that occur with chronic blood loss, such as a shift in the oxygen-hemoglobin dissociation curve favoring oxygen delivery to the tissues.

An animal's packed cell volume should always be evaluated in light of results of total solids measurements (Table 4-1). Packed cell volume and total solids may be normal immediately following peracute hemorrhage, but within hours, they will be decreased concomitantly. In chronic anemia, unassociated with blood loss, packed cell volume will be decreased while total solids may be normal. A concomitant decrease in packed cell volume and total solids should prompt the clinician to search for a source of ongoing blood loss. An anemic, dehydrated patient's packed cell volume and total solids may decrease further on rehydration of the patient (hemodilution), and these changes may not necessarily reflect ongoing blood loss. Serial monitoring of an anemic animal's packed cell volume and total solids should be per-

Table 4-1 Interpretation of packed cell volume (PCV) and total solids (TS)

	Decreased PCV	Normal PCV	Increased PCV
Decreased TS	Recent blood loss (≥12 hours previous) Overhydration Peracute blood loss following volume replacement	Gastrointestinal protein loss Renal protein loss Severe liver disease	Protein loss with splenic contraction
Normal TS	Red blood cell destruction Inadequate red blood cell production Chronic blood loss	Normal Peracute blood loss	Splenic contraction Polycythemia (1 or 2 degrees) Hypoproteinemia with dehydration
Increased TS	Severe liver disease with chronic anemia Lymphoproliferative diseases Anemia of chronic disease	Anemia with dehydration Severe liver disease Hyperglobulinemias	Dehydration

formed to monitor progression or resolution of the anemia.

An increase in packed cell volume and total solids is commonly the result of dehydration in an animal (Table 4-1). Serial monitoring of packed cell volume and total solids during fluid therapy is one means of monitoring changes in patient hydration status. Serial body weight determinations represent the best means of monitoring hydration status. Hypoproteinemia in the presence of an increased or normal packed cell volume suggests the presence of plasma or protein loss, such as may occur with severe burns or with protein-losing disorders in animals.

In addition to the measurement of packed cell volume and total solids, the color and clarity of the plasma in the spun microhematocrit tube should be assessed. White, turbid plasma is indicative of lipemia, and this lipemic condition will compromise the accuracy of determinations of total solids. Possible causes for this finding include postprandial lipemia, diabetes mellitus, acute pancreatitis, liver disease, hypothyroidism, and hyperadrenocorticism. If the plasma layer appears yellow, then hyperbilirubinemia is likely. This finding may be noted in animals with liver, biliary, or hemolytic disease. A red appearance of the plasma layer is indicative of hemolysis and may be detected with various diseases (disseminated intravascular coagulation, intravascular hemolysis), or this finding may be the result of poor sample collection techniques.

The height of the buffy coat layer should be visually evaluated. An increase in the buffy coat layer suggests an increased total blood leukocyte count, while a decrease or absence of this layer suggests possible leukopenia.

A blood smear should be examined to estimate the various white blood cell, reticulocyte, and platelet numbers, and to evaluate the morphology of the white and red blood cells.

Blood urea nitrogen and urine specific gravity

Pretreatment measurements of blood urea nitrogen and creatinine concentration and measurement of an animal's urine specific gravity provide the critical care clinician with an accurate assessment of renal/prerenal dysfunction. A simple, rapid approximation of blood urea nitrogen can be obtained by employing reagent strips (e.g., Azostix) using one drop of patient blood. Serial monitoring of blood urea nitrogen and creatinine concentrations can be used to document efficacy of therapy and provides prognostic information regarding progression or resolution of renal/prerenal dysfunction.

Blood glucose

Rapid determination of blood glucose concentrations is essential to the treatment of critical care patients. Alterations in glucose homeostasis occur frequently (diabetes mellitus, hypoglycemia due to sepsis) and often result in significant clinical signs affecting multiple organ systems (Chapter 18). Reagent strips using enzymatic (glucose oxidase) methods specific for glucose determination (e.g., Chemstrip bG, Dextrostix) are available and provide rapid, semiquantitative assessment of blood glucose concentrations. These blood glucose determinations are inexpensive, require a drop of blood to assay, and are a rational approach to serial monitoring of blood glucose concentrations in critical care patients.

NEUROLOGIC MONITORING

Serial monitoring of animals with neurologic dysfunction in the critical care unit is crucial. Deterioration of patient neurologic status often results in irreversible sequelae (e.g., loss of pain sensation to the limbs of animals with spinal cord disease), and early detection of deteriorating neurologic dysfunction may allow successful medical or therapeutic intervention. A complete neurologic examination should be performed twice daily on patients with neurologic dysfunction unless the dysfunction present dictates more frequent evaluations (e.g., disk disease). The animal's pupillary size, symmetry, and response to light, and eye movement, level of consciousness, and limb movements and sensation should be serially monitored.

Evaluation of an animal's pupillary size, symmetry, and response to light aid in localization of neurologic injury and in assessment of improvement or deterioration in an animal's neurologic status.[38,39] Pupil symmetry and normal reactivity to light suggest that the third cranial nerves and upper brainstem are intact. Abnormal pupil size, the result of sympathetic-parasympathetic imbalance, may occur with lesions of varying severity at various levels of the central nervous system (Chapter 20). Miotic pupils generally suggest a better prognosis for the animal than does the presence of mydriatic pupils. Bilaterally dilated pupils that are nonresponsive to light in a comatose animal suggest severe midbrain disease, which carries a poor prognosis. Miosis that progresses to mydriasis on serial examination of the patient indicates a progressive lesion of the midbrain or bilateral tentorial herniation and a poor prognosis. Cerebral and metabolic disorders do not generally cause changes in pupillary size or responsiveness.

The "doll's head (eye) maneuver" (moving the animal's head side to side and observing the physiologic nystagmus generated) aids in evaluation of reflex (involuntary) eye movements and their nervous system pathways. This oculocephalic reflex, if present, reflects integrity of the vestibular apparatus and parts of the brainstem and is a good prognostic indicator. Abnormalities detected during evaluation of the doll's eye maneuver aid in localization of brainstem and vestibular lesions in animals.[40] Pathologic (spontaneous) nystagmus suggests vestibular dysfunction arising from inner ear, brainstem, or cerebellar involvement (Chapter 20).

A decreasing level of consciousness on serial examination of an animal suggests a progressive neurologic lesion (e.g., cerebral herniation with resultant midbrain compression, progressive midbrain hemorrhage, epidural-subdural hemorrhage or cerebral edema causing increased intracranial pressure).[39] If this animal is receiving aggressive treatment (Chapter 20) and is continuing to deteriorate neurologically, an emergency computed tomographic scan (if available) may aid in localizing the lesion, and craniotomy to relieve increased intracranial pressure may be attempted.[41]

Patients with spinal cord compression may demonstrate varying degrees of paresis. The need for surgical decompression of the spinal cord in animals with moderate to severe paresis is controversial (Chapter 11). Any animal exhibiting paresis should be closely monitored for changes in motor function and deep pain sensation of the limbs. A loss of voluntary motor function associated with decreasing pain perception should prompt an aggressive surgical approach (myelography, decompressive procedures) to relieve spinal cord compression (Chapter 11). A paretic patient with minimal voluntary motor function should be monitored hourly for preservation of neurologic function while medical therapy is attempted (Chapters 11 and 20).

INVASIVE MONITORING
Establishing central venous access

Central venous cannulation is indicated for a variety of reasons, including the following: to monitor central venous pressures, for rapid fluid administration during treatment of shock or cardiopulmonary arrest, and for administration of hypertonic alimentation solutions (Chapter 37).

Insertion of central venous catheters should be performed in an aseptic fashion. Attention to sterile technique should be no less meticulous than that associated with surgical procedures. Severely ill animals with protracted hospitalization are at increased risk for nosocomial infection (Chapter 6). Central venous catheters used for maintenance fluid administration should be removed and changed every 48 to 72 hours. If evidence of local or systemic infection is present (fever, leukocytosis with a left shift, swelling over the catheter site), the tip of the catheter should be cultured on removal. Blood cultures should be performed in this setting.

Establishment of central venous access is most commonly performed with the awake patient in lateral recumbency, using a local anesthetic block over the right jugular vein. The hair is clipped from the angle of the mandible to the thoracic inlet bilaterally, and the skin over the right jugular vein is cleansed with an antibacterial-antifungal solution (chlorhexidine).

The central venous pressure monitoring catheter used for insertion into the jugular vein should be premeasured externally on the animal to identify the approximate level of insertion required for the catheter to reach the right atrium. A small stab incision is made in the skin with a scalpel, and the catheter system introduced into the vein (clinician should be using sterile gloves). The catheter should advance with ease. Once the central venous catheter is properly positioned in the jugular vein, it should be secured to the neck and the catheter flushed with heparinized saline.

If central venous pressure (CVP) monitoring is the objective, a through-the-needle catheter system may be used (e.g., Venocath, Abbott Laboratories, North Chicago, IL). Alternatively, an over-the-needle catheter (e.g., Angio Cath, Deseret Company, Sandy, UT) may be adequate if of sufficient length. If mixed venous oximetry, pulmonary artery pressure, pulmonary capillary wedge pressure, or cardiac output determinations are the objectives, catheter insertion through a vascular sheath may be necessary (Fig. 4-2)(see section below on these determinations).

Several commercial kits are available that contain all the instruments (drapes, scalpel, bacteriocidal skin preparation, etc.) necessary for establishing vascular access. In some instances (vascular collapse, hematoma formation) a surgical approach may be necessary in order to obtain access to the jugular vein.

Central venous pressure

The CVP, measured from the intrathoracic cranial vena cava, is a reflection of intravascular volume, cardiac function, and venous compliance. Normal CVP in dogs and cats is generally between 0 and 5 cm H_2O. While single measurements of CVP may not reflect an animal's hemodynamic status, trends in CVP measurements provide the clinician with valuable information that aids in the treatment of critical care patients.

Two common causes of increased CVP are congestive heart failure and pericardial disease. This elevation in CVP is the result of decreased forward flow of blood (congestive heart failure) or is the result of increased diastolic filling pressures (increased intrapericardial pressure) in the case of pericardial effusion.

Central venous pressure will be affected by alterations in intrathoracic pressure. Inspiration may cause a decrease in CVP, while loss of normal

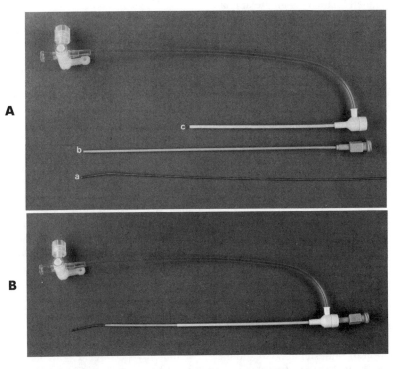

Fig. 4-2 A, Cordis vascular access system. Individual components of the system include a guide wire, a vessel dilator, and a vascular sheath with side arm port for flushing with heparinized saline. **B,** Assembled system as it would appear in the jugular vein prior to removal of the guide wire and vessel dilator (see text).

negative pleural pressure causes an increased CVP (pneumothorax, thoracotomy, positive-pressure ventilation).

It is important to remember that administration of certain drugs may alter venous compliance (cause venoconstriction), leading to increases in CVP. Hypervolemia causes an increased CVP, and this elevation can occur following intensive fluid therapy of critical care patients. For this reason, CVP measurements are particularly useful in monitoring administration of fluid therapy to animals with congestive heart failure or other critical conditions. The combination of CVP and pulmonary capillary wedge pressure measurements (see next section) provides the clinician with more complete information concerning an animal's intravascular fluid volume.

The most common cause of decreased CVP is hypovolemia. Rapid administration of fluid replacement therapy is often necessary in critical care patients, and the adequacy of volume replacement can be monitored using CVP in combination with measurements of SABP or urine output. If the CVP rises 4 to 6 cm H_2O above the initial measurement, the fluid administration rate should be decreased. Conversely, a decreasing CVP suggests that the rate of fluid administration should be increased. A CVP value of zero may be present in hypovolemia.

The development of pulmonary edema and the assessment of left heart filling pressures is more accurately determined by monitoring pulmonary capillary wedge pressure. This procedure requires passing a vascular catheter into the periphery of the pulmonary circulation and obtaining a "wedge pressure" (see next section).

For the measurement of CVP, a three-way stopcock is attached to the jugular catheter, to the administration set of the animal's intravenous fluids (isotonic saline), and to a vertically positioned manometer. The zero level of the manometer should be aligned approximately horizontal to the position of the catheter tip (the junction of the cranial vena cava and right atrium) in the patient (Fig. 4-3). The manometer is filled with crystalloid solution and the stopcock is turned off to the intravenous fluid port, allowing equilibration of the patient's cranial vena caval pressure with the saline-filled manometer. Results of measurements should be recorded on a flow sheet, enabling easy assessment of trends and changes in CVP.

Consistency in technique is important when measuring CVP. The CVP measurements should be obtained with the animal and manometer in the same position for each measurement (usually lateral recumbency). Measurements should be obtained by the same technician or staff member if possible. Verification of proper placement of the catheter for CVP measurement may be performed using radiography-fluoroscopy or by observing the meniscal fluctuation, associated with the heartbeat, within the manometer. Small fluctuations of the fluid level (2 to 5 mm) are associated with correct placement of the tip of the catheter,

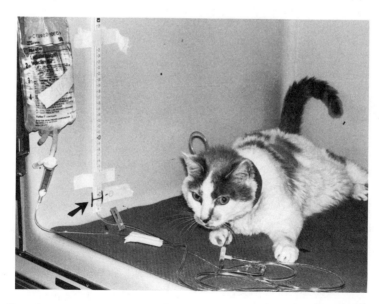

Fig. 4-3 Central venous pressure monitoring in a critically ill cat. Note that the zero level of the manometer *(arrow)* is at approximately the same level as the right atrium, where the tip of the monitoring catheter is situated.

while large fluctuations suggest the catheter has been positioned in the right ventricle. Large fluctuations may be noted when the catheter is properly positioned and severe tricuspid insufficiency is present in the animal.

Pulmonary artery pressure, pulmonary capillary wedge pressure, and cardiac output determination

Insertion of a vascular catheter is necessary to determine invasively an animal's pulmonary artery pressure, pulmonary capillary wedge pressure, or cardiac output. Surgical exposure of the jugular vein facilitates introduction of a vascular catheter (Fig. 4-4); however, percutaneous insertion of a flow-directed catheter or catheter sheath system may be accomplished using an introducer needle (e.g., Seldinger, Potts-Cournand) to aid introduction of a guide wire into the jugular vein (Fig. 4-5). Once the guide wire is positioned, a stab

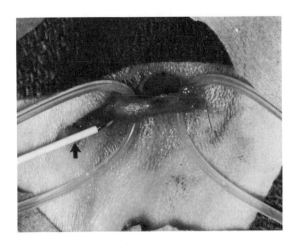

Fig. 4-4 Surgical exposure of the jugular vein prior to introduction of the vascular catheter *(arrow)*. The jugular vein is isolated and atraumatically manipulated using silastic tubing as stents.

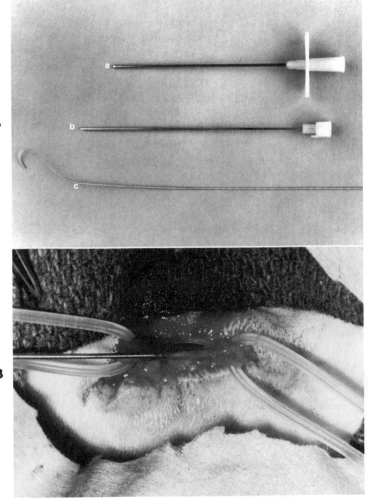

Fig. 4-5 A, Introducer needle with stylet and guide wire. Once venipuncture is performed the stylet is removed and the guide wire advanced through the needle. **B,** The guide wire is in place within the jugular vein. The introducer needle has been removed. Gentle traction on the silastic tubing prevents backbleeding from the puncture in the jugular vein. A vessel dilator would now be advanced over the guide wire to facilitate insertion of the catheter sheath.

wound is made along the wire's ventral surface where the wire enters the skin, using the point of a No. 11 scalpel blade. This incision facilitates passage of the venous dilator and catheter sheath over the guide wire and through the skin and subcutaneous tissue. (Occasionally, the edge of the catheter sheath becomes roughened and cannot be advanced through the subcutaneous tissue. In this instance, the venous dilator is removed from the catheter sheath and advanced over the wire dilating the subcutaneous tissue to create a larger subcutaneous tunnel for passage of the sheath. It may also be necessary to trim the roughened edge of the sheath to facilitate its passage.) When the catheter sheath with the dilator is fully advanced over the guide wire, and the hub of the sheath is against the patient's skin, the dilator and guide wire are removed from the catheter sheath. The catheter sheath is flushed with heparinized saline through the back bleed valve (diaphragm) or through the side arm port (Fig. 4-6). A pulmonary artery catheter may now be advanced through the catheter sheath. Pulmonary artery catheters should be flushed with heparinized saline prior to introduction through the catheter sheath. Fluoroscopic guidance aids in the proper positioning of the pulmonary artery catheter, but its use is not mandatory. Balloon-tipped flow-directed catheters (e.g., Swan-Ganz flow-directed catheter, Edwards Labs, Santa Ana, CA) may be passed while visualizing the characteristic pressure wave forms generated from the different ar-

eas of the cardiovascular system as the catheter is advanced.[42] Inflation of the balloon, with the catheter tip in the right atrium, is usually necessary to facilitate blind passage of this catheter into the pulmonary artery (Fig. 4-7).

Most monitoring systems used with indwelling pulmonary artery catheters have a fluid-filled catheter, tubing and stopcock system through which the pressures are transmitted; an electromagnetic device (transducer) that translates pres-

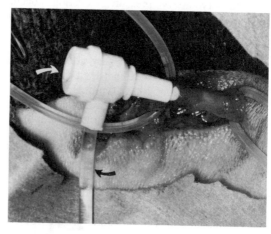

Fig. 4-6 Catheter sheath in place within the jugular vein. Vascular catheters are introduced into the top of the catheter sheath *(white arrow)* through the diaphragm. Flushing of the vascular sheath is performed through the side arm port *(black arrow).*

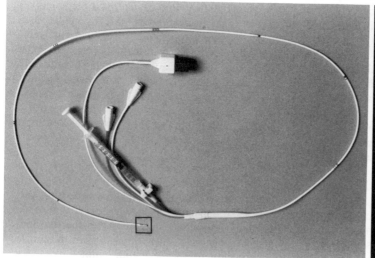
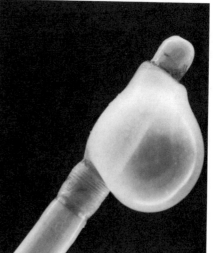

A

B

Fig. 4-7 A and **B,** 5 French multilumen balloon-tipped Swan-Ganz flow-directed catheter. Injection of air through the syringe attached to the balloon port results in inflation of the balloon tip, **B,** allowing easy passage of the catheter tip into the pulmonary artery.

sure pulses into an electrical signal; and an instrument that translates this electrical signal back into pressure readings that are displayed (pressure monitor).

Microtransducers and fiber optics reflectance oximetry systems that are attached to the tips of catheters have been developed. These instruments provide more accurate determination of pressures and pressure wave forms and allow continuous measurement of mixed venous oxygen saturation; however, these devices are expensive.

Pulmonary artery pressure elevations occur most commonly with pulmonary parenchymal and vascular disease (e.g., pulmonary embolism, pulmonary hypertension, chronic obstructive pulmonary disease). Normal pulmonary artery pressure is 20 to 40 mm Hg/5 to 10 mm Hg (systolic/diastolic), with a mean of 10 to 20 mm Hg. In the absence of pulmonary vascular disease, pulmonary artery diastolic pressure and pulmonary capillary wedge pressure are approximately equal, and pulmonary artery diastolic pressure may be followed as a reflection of mean left atrial pressure. In instances where significant differences (>5 mm Hg) between pulmonary arterial diastolic pressure and pulmonary capillary wedge pressure occur, a primary pulmonary vascular disorder should be suspected.[42]

Pulmonary capillary wedge pressure (a reflection of left atrial pressure) is obtained by advancing the catheter into a small branch of the pulmonary artery. The catheter tip balloon should be gradually inflated while monitoring the pressure tracings until a change from pulmonary artery pressure to pulmonary capillary wedge pressure configuration is noted in the wave form. On inflation of the balloon tip, blood flow between that pulmonary artery and the left atrium is halted and pressure measurements from the tip of the catheter are reflecting left atrial pressure. Measurement of mean left atrial pressure aids in defining the origin of pulmonary congestion and edema. Serial monitoring of pulmonary capillary wedge pressure in patients with cardiac disease aids in determining efficacy of therapy and the need for changes in medical treatment of the patient. Normal pulmonary capillary wedge pressure is 3 to 8 mm Hg in the dog.

The contractile state of the myocardium may be adversely affected by hypoxia, hypercapnia, metabolic acidosis, electrolyte disturbances, and other physiologic disturbances often present in critical care patients. Contractility is one of the determinants of ventricular performance and, ultimately, cardiac output (CO) in an animal. Alterations in preload, afterload, distensibility, heart rate (HR), and synergy of ventricular contraction

(SV) influence cardiac output as follows:

CO = SV (determined by preload, afterload, contractility) × HR (determined by rhythmicity and conduction, neural and humoral regulation)

Common invasive methods for determination of cardiac output include the Fick method and the indicator dilution method.

The Fick technique employs measurements of arteriovenous differences in blood oxygen content and total body oxygen consumption in order to calculate cardiac output. Although the Fick technique is a more accurate technique, it is cumbersome to perform.

The indicator dilution method of cardiac output determination requires injection of a known concentration of indicator, usually indocyanine green dye or iced saline (thermodilution technique), and subsequent downstream measurement of the change in indicator "concentration." The thermodilution method is easy to perform in a clinical setting and requires two pieces of equipment, a thermistor-tipped multiple-lumen pulmonary artery catheter to detect and record changes in the temperature of pulmonary artery blood and a computer that calculates cardiac output based on data points from the measured time-temperature curve of the pulmonary blood. A bolus of iced saline (1 to 5 ml) is injected intravenously into the proximal port of the vascular catheter, which should be located in the right atrium. The iced saline mixes with the animal's blood, lowering the temperature of the blood. The thermistor tip of the catheter located in the pulmonary artery records the temperature change, and the computer calculates cardiac output by integrating the area under the time-temperature curve. Alternatively, hand computation of the area under the curve can be utilized.[43,44] Cardiac output is most commonly determined in patients having primary cardiac disease; however, extracardiac disease (acidosis, hypovolemia) can have profound effects on cardiac output. Immediate response to medical treatment is easily gauged using serial cardiac output determinations.

Complications associated with pulmonary artery catheterization include catheter knotting, pulmonary artery thrombosis, endomyocarditis, cardiac valve damage, pulmonary artery rupture associated with balloon inflation, and the development of cardiac arrhythmias. To minimize complications associated with pulmonary artery catheterization, a few basic guidelines should be followed: (1) catheters should not be left in the wedge position for more than 15 to 20 seconds;

(2) inflation of the balloon should be done slowly and stopped when a wedge pressure tracing is obtained; (3) careful attention should be paid to the predetermined inflation volume so as not to overinflate or rupture the balloon; (4) the animal's electrocardiogram should be monitored during these invasive procedures; and (5) thoracic radiographs or fluoroscopic techniques should be used to detect catheter position after placement or when apparent problems arise.

Systemic arterial blood pressure

Systemic arterial blood pressure derangements in critical care patients are common occurrences, especially in trauma patients. When mean SABP decreases below 60 mm Hg, impairment to renal, coronary, and cerebral artery perfusion occurs. This impaired blood flow can lead to multiple-organ system failure if not corrected. Emergency clinicians must identify, treat, and monitor alterations of SABP in animal patients in order to prevent multiple-organ system failure.

Systemic arterial blood pressure may be measured directly by invasive means (arterial cannulation or arterial puncture) or indirectly by oscillometric or Doppler ultrasound techniques. Systemic arterial blood pressure measurements include measurement of systolic, diastolic, and mean arterial blood pressure. According to Spangler et al.,[45] normal SABP values in conscious dogs were: systolic 152.4 ± 27.8 mm Hg; diastolic 83.3 ± 15.3 mm Hg; and mean, 108.3 ± 19.6 mm Hg (Chapter 40). Systolic systemic arterial blood pressure is related to left ventricular stroke volume, velocity of ventricular ejection, and arterial wall compliance. Diastolic systemic arterial blood pressure is influenced by peak systolic arterial blood pressure, peripheral vascular resistance, and cardiac cycle length. An increase in stroke volume (aortic insufficiency, patent ductus arteriosus, anemia, hyperthyroidism) or a decrease in arterial compliance (vasoconstriction) results in increased systolic systemic arterial blood pressure. Systolic arterial hypertension has been documented with advanced spontaneous or experimentally induced renal failure in dogs.[45-47] Decreased SABP is most often due to hypovolemia, decreased cardiac output, or severe vasodilatation.

Pulse pressure (difference between systolic and diastolic pressures) determines the strength of the pulse palpated. The significance of alterations of pulse intensity and character have been discussed previously (see section on noninvasive monitoring).

Direct measurement. The placement of an intraarterial catheter for direct arterial blood pressure measurement allows the clinician to monitor the SABP of an animal accurately and continuously.

The two arteries most commonly used for cannulation in dogs and cats are the dorsal metatarsal artery and the femoral artery. The dorsal metatarsal artery (superficial location, ease of stabilization of the catheter to the limb) is suggested for use for long-term intraarterial monitoring associated with minimal complications. Cannulation of these arteries may be accomplished percutaneously or by surgical exposure of the artery. Local infiltration of 2% lidocaine is recommended to minimize pain and reduce reflex vasospasm, allowing vessel cannulation. If absolutely necessary, sedatives and analgesics with the least cardiovascular effects (least effects on SABP) should be employed (morphine, oxymorphone). Many critical care patients have central nervous system depression and require minimal immobilization or sedation techniques during placement of these arterial catheters.

Aseptic preparation of the artery site for cannulation is similar to that used for long-term venous cannulation. Percutaneous catheterization is easily accomplished using an over-the-needle catheter system, a through-the-needle catheter system (although bleeding around the catheter may occur), or an introducer needle and guide wire as previously discussed for pulmonary artery catheterization. End hole catheters should be avoided because falsely elevated blood pressure readings will occur due to the impact of oncoming arterial flood flow.[48]

Following insertion, the intraarterial cannula is secured to the skin, flushed with heparinized saline, and attached to fluid-filled coupling tubing and a measuring device (commercial transducer, fluid column, aneroid manometer). Transducers should be "zeroed" and calibrated prior to the onset of SABP measurements. The calibrated transducer should be placed at the level of the catheter tip with the vessel cannulated during measurement of SABP. The pressure wave form is then recorded by the measuring device and is available for interpretation.

The presence of air bubbles within the tubing greatly increases resonance (a property within a fluid-filled measuring system that produces inherent artifactual changes in the values measured). Increased resonance results in alteration of the amplitude of the systolic upstroke and dicrotic notch of measured SABP. Continuous flushing systems are useful to prevent air bubble entrapment and thrombosis in the pressure monitoring equipment.

The length and gauge of the coupling tubing from the arterial catheter to the transducer greatly influences resonance. Ideally, short, stiff, large-bore tubing should be used to minimize this effect.[48] Multiple connections have a negative influence on the accuracy of the measured SABP. The quality and reliability of the signal improve, the closer the transducer is to the catheter (signal source). Other factors that cause artifacts in the measured SABP include signal amplifications and impedance mismatch.

Many of the negative effects on blood pressure measurements are minimized using microtransducer-tipped catheters; however, these catheters can be extremely expensive.

If the monitoring system is free of air bubbles, the length of coupling tubing and number of connections is minimized, the transducer is placed at the level of the cannula, and the transducer is correctly zeroed and calibrated, then an accurate, precise SABP measurement is obtained. In situations in which the accuracy of systolic and diastolic blood pressure measurements obtained are questionable, the clinician should rely on the measured mean SABP when making decisions on therapy for the patient, as mean SABP is generally least affected by changes in resonance.

Complications of arterial cannulation are few but include catheter-related infection, vessel thrombosis, bleeding from the venipuncture site, and excessive bleeding from the arterial line or catheter should disconnection or laceration of the tubing occur.

Indirect blood pressure measurement. Indirect blood pressure measurement is technically easier to perform and is associated with minimal complications. Indirect blood pressure measurement is least accurate at low SABP and when small arteries are used for obtaining the measurements. Individual SABP measurements obtained by indirect methods tend to be less accurate than those obtained by direct measurement.[49] The trends in SABP obtained from repeated measurements by indirect methods can provide valuable information for the treatment of critical patients.

Systemic arterial blood pressure can be measured indirectly by oscillometric methods. This method involves application of a manometer incorporated in an occlusion cuff to assess oscillations of the underlying artery within the cuff (most commonly the dorsal metatarsal artery). As the cuff pressure is increased above systolic arterial blood pressure, blood flow is occluded. As the cuff pressure is slowly decreased and falls below systolic arterial blood pressure, blood begins to flow intermittently and is detected as needle oscillations on the manometer roughly corresponding to systolic arterial pressure. Recorded needle oscillations on the manometer reach a maximum

amplitude at a pressure corresponding to the mean SABP. The oscillations decrease in amplitude below the mean systolic arterial pressure. Diastolic pressure is read at the point where needle oscillations no longer decrease in magnitude. Pressure-monitoring devices that automatically inflate and deflate the occlusion cuff, and determine the mean, systolic, and diastolic blood pressure via a built-in microprocessor are available (Dinamap, Critikon, Tampa, FL).

Errors in measurement of SABP with oscillometric methods occur with the use of inappropriately sized cuffs (Chapter 40). The cuff width should approximate 40% of the circumference of the limb. Narrow cuff widths yield erroneously high values for blood pressure, while inappropriately wide cuffs yield erroneously low values.[48] Measurements of systolic arterial pressure over peripheral arteries yield slightly increased values compared with measurements of central (aortic) systolic pressure. These differences are attributable to the changes in vascular compliance and pressure wave reflections in distal arteries. Indirect systemic arterial blood pressure measurements using the proximal forelimb or hind limb are difficult to perform, and results may be inaccurate because of the inability to achieve a stable cuff position.

Doppler instrumentation, using piezoelectric crystals, for detecting blood flow or vessel-wall movement over peripheral arteries has proven to be an accurate means of measuring SABP over a wide range.[50] This technique involves the use of an occlusive cuff and placement of a piezoelectric crystal over an artery; the crystal transmits a signal (sound waves) at a certain frequency, receives the reflected signal at a different frequency, and the Doppler unit transforms this signal to audible sound and/or measurements of blood flow (Chapter 40). No vessel-wall motion or blood flow occurs in the occluded artery when cuff pressures exceed systolic arterial blood pressure. As cuff pressure is slowly decreased and pulsatile arterial blood flow begins, an audible Doppler signal is detected corresponding to systolic arterial blood pressure. Diastolic arterial blood pressure is heralded by an abrupt muffling or cessation of sound as the vibrations of the arterial wall cease.

Indirect blood pressure measurement may prove more practical for physiologically stable patients requiring only intermittent assessments of SABP. Direct arterial pressure monitoring should be considered in the hemodynamically unstable patient (shock), the unstable congestive heart failure patient receiving vasoactive drugs, or the critical care and/or cardiac patient undergoing anesthesia and surgery.

REFERENCES

1. Ganong WF. Neural centers regulating visceral function. In Ganong WF, ed. Review of medical physiology. Los Altos, CA: Lange Medical Publications, 1981;178-197.
2. Adams T. Carnivores. In Whittow GL, ed. Comparative physiology of thermoregulation, vol 2, New York, Academic Press, 1971;152-189.
3. Waterman A. Accidental hypothermia during anaesthesia in dogs and cats. Vet Rec 1975;96:308-313.
4. Noxon JO. Accidental hypothermia associated with hypothyroidism. Can Pract 1983;10:17-22.
5. Krum SH, Osborne CA. Heatstroke in the dog: a polysystemic disorder. J Am Vet Med Assoc 1977;170:531-535.
6. Smith M. Hypothermia. Compend Contin Ed Pract Vet 1985;7:321-326.
7. Zenoble RD, Hill BL. Hypothermia and associated cardiac arrhythmias in two dogs. J Am Vet Med Assoc 1979;175:840-842.
8. Kolata RJ. The significance of changes in toe web temperature in dogs in circulatory shock. Proceedings of the 28th Gaines Veterinary Symposium. 1978;21-26.
9. Reuler JB. Hypothermia: pathophysiology, clinical setting, and management. Ann Intern Med 1978;89:519-527.
10. Burch GE, Hyman A. Influence of a hot and humid environment upon cardiac output and work in normal man and in patients with congestive heart failure at rest. Am Heart J 1957;53:665.
11. Trevino A, Razi B, Beller BM. The characteristic electrocardiogram of accidental hypothermia. Arch Intern Med 1971;127:470-473.
12. Wynne NA, Fuller JA, Szekely P. Electrocardiographic changes in hypothermia. Br Heart J 1960;22:842-846.
13. Moyer JH, Morris G, Debakey ME. Hypothermia: I. Effect on renal hemodynamics and on excretion of H_2O and electrolytes in dog and man. Ann Surg 1957;145:26-40.
14. Evans AT, Sawyer DL, Krahwinkel DJ. Effect of a warm-water blanket on development of hypothermia during small animal surgery. J Am Vet Med Assoc 1973;163:147-148.
15. Zenoble RD. Accidental hypothermia. In Kirk RW, ed. Current veterinary therapy VIII. Philadelphia: WB Saunders, 1983;186.
16. Wong KC. Physiology and pharmacology of hypothermia (medical progress). West J Med 1983;138:227-232.
17. Reuler JB, Parker RA. Peritoneal dialysis in the management of hypothermia. JAMA 1978;240:2289-2290.
18. Schall WD. Heat stroke. In Kirk RW, ed. Current veterinary therapy VIII. Philadelphia: WB Saunders, 1983;183.
19. Schaer M. Hyperkalemia in cats with urethral obstruction: Electrocardiographic abnormalities and treatment. Vet Clin North Am 1977;7:407.
20. Muir WW. Gastric-dilatation-volvulus in the dog, with emphasis on cardiac arrhythmias. J Am Vet Med Assoc 1982;180:739.
21. Feldman EC, Ettinger ST. Electrocardiographic changes associated with electrolyte disturbances. Vet Clin North Am 1977;7:487.
22. Bond B, Tilley LP. Cardiomyopathy in the dog and cat. In Kirk RW, ed. Current veterinary therapy VII. Philadelphia: WB Saunders, 1980;307.
23. Abrams J. The arterial pulse. In Abrams J et al, eds. Essentials of cardiac physical diagnosis. Philadelphia: Lea & Febiger 1987;25-40.
24. Abrams J. Essentials of cardiac physical diagnosis. Philadelphia: Lea & Febiger, 1987;3-12.
25. Gibson DG, Brown DJ. Assessment of left ventricular systolic function in man from simultaneous echocardiographic and pressure measurements. Br Heart J 1976;38:8-17.
26. Lewis RP. The use of systolic time intervals for evaluation of left ventricular function. In: Fowler NO, ed. Non-invasive diagnostic methods in cardiology. Philadelphia: FA Davis, 1983;335-353.
27. Feigenbaum H. Echocardiography, ed 4, Philadelphia: Lea & Febiger, 1986.
28. Pipers FS, Andrysco RM, Hamlin RL. A totally noninvasive method for obtaining systolic time intervals in the dog. Am J Vet Res 1978;39:1822-1826.
29. Gardin JM, Iseri LT, Elkayam U, et al. Evaluation of dilated cardiomyopathy by pulsed doppler echocardiography. Am Heart J 1983;106:1057.
30. Kolittis M, Kenkins BS, Webb-Pebloe MM. Assessment of left ventricular function by indices derived from aortic flow velocity. Br Heart J 1976;38:18.
31. Roudebush P. Lung sounds. J Am Vet Med Assoc 1982;181:122-126.
32. Haskins SC. Blood gases and acid-base balance: clinical interpretation and therapeutic implications. In Kirk RW, ed. Current veterinary therapy VIII. Philadelphia: WB Saunders, 1983;215.
33. Madiero G, Sciacla R, Hause L. Air bubbles and temperature effect on blood gas analysis. J Clin Pathol 1980;33:864.
34. Taylor MB, Whitman JG. The current status of pulse oximetry. Anaesthesia 1986;41:943.
35. Ramanathan R. Pulse oximetry for continuous oxygen monitoring in sick newborn infants. J Pediatr 1986;109:1052-1056.
36. Robertson S. Personal communication. Michigan State University, February 1990.
37. Valtin H. Renal function: mechanisms preserving fluid and solute balance in health. Boston: Little, Brown, 1973.
38. Fenner WR. Head trauma and nervous system injury. In Kirk RW, ed. Current veterinary therapy VIII. Philadelphia: WB Saunders, 1983; 739-744.
39. DeLahunta A. Veterinary neuroanatomy and clinical neurology. Philadelphia: WB Saunders, 1983.
40. Chrisman CL. Problems in small animal neurology. Philadelphia: Lea & Febiger, 1982.
41. Fenner WR. Medical emergencies of the central nervous system. In Sherding RG, ed. Medical emergencies, contemporary issues in small animal practice. New York: Churchill Livingstone, 1985; 285-314.
42. Ganz P, Swan HJC, Ganz W. Balloon-tipped flow directed catheters. In Grossman W, ed. Cardiac catheterization and angiography. Philadelphia: Lea & Febiger, 1986;88-97.
43. Bradley EC, Barr JW. Fore-n-aft triangle formula for rapid estimation of area. Am Heart J 1969;78:643-648.
44. Prys-Roberts C. Measurement of cardiac output and regional blood flow. In Prys-Roberts C, ed. The circulation in anaesthesia. Oxford: Blackwell Scientific, 1980;531-560.
45. Spangler WL, Gribble DH, Weiser MG. Canine hypertension: a review. J Am Vet Med Assoc 1977;170:995.
46. Weiser MG, Spangler WL, Gribble DH. Blood pressure measurement in the dog. J Am Vet Med Assoc 1977;171:364.
47. Muirhead EE, Grollman A, Vanatta J. Hypertensive cardiovascular diseases (malignant hypertension): changes in canine tissue induced by various manipulations of the kidney with special reference to vascular and myocardial lesions. Arch Pathol 1950;51:137.
48. Kittleson MD, Olivier NB. Measurement of systemic arterial blood pressure. Vet Clin North Am 1983;13:321-336.
49. Haskins SC. Monitoring the critically ill patient. Vet Clin North Am 1989;19:1059-1077.
50. Freundlich JT, Detweiler DK, Hance KE. Indirect blood pressure determination by the ultrasonic doppler technique in dogs. Curr Ther Res 1972;14:73-80.

5 Clinical Decision Making and Delivery of Patient Care

Robert J. Murtaugh

Technologic advances in our ability to sustain vital organ function in critically ill patients, coupled with society's expectations that modern medicine can cure or reverse the most devastating illnesses, have led to the development of the "technologic imperative" (do everything possible, no matter how hopeless the situation). This principle has particular application to the practice of critical care and emergency medicine, in which the inability to predict recovery accurately for specific patients reinforces this approach. Certainly, our first priority should be to attempt to save life whenever possible; however, we must not lose sight of the reality that we are limited in resources, in knowledge, and by the severity of disease in our abilities to provide a cure for all patients. As providers of critical care services we must be able to realize when the goal of cure is not attainable (severe, acute injury; terminal disease with multiple-organ system failure) and shift our goals to alleviating patient suffering and providing emotional support to our clients—directing their decisions on limiting treatment and interventions and on euthanasia for their animals. Veterinarians practicing critical care medicine must have the technical training, experience, and awareness of the existing body of knowledge (medical, ethical, legal) in critical care medicine in order to realize this role effectively and avoid practicing "defensive medicine" (technologic imperative) at that stage of patient-care needs.

Clinicians involved in critical care medicine must realize that the resources at their disposal (personnel, equipment) are limited and exercise care in application of those resources to patients in order to maximize benefit (triage), minimize complications (iatrogenesis), and limit unnecessary expense. A critical assessment of the data pertaining to patient benefit by treatments, monitoring, and interventions is often lacking, and continual review of practice standards and examination of bedside care (amount of testing and monitoring required) must be undertaken by all involved in the delivery of critical care services. The appropriate application of resources, treatment, and interventions when cure is possible or the patient outcome is in question as well as the tempering of our approach to alleviate patient suffering when disease is irreversible or terminal represent worthwhile goals that emanate from the best traditions of medicine.[1]

THE ART AND SCIENCE OF CLINICAL DECISION MAKING IN CRITICAL CARE
Patient classification—who needs the intensive care unit (ICU)?

Animals admitted to an ICU (or emergency clinic) are dissimilar in terms of the goals of the ICU admission, the dimensions of care used, and the resources required. They can be separated by goals into three groups: animals with risk of complications admitted for intensive observation/monitoring (postoperative patient with preexisting compensated organ-system dysfunction—heart, kidney), animals that are stable physiologically but require extensive nursing care (ventilatory support), and animals requiring constant medical attention (multiple trauma patients with cardiorespiratory dysfunction).[1]

Animals are considered appropriate candidates for ICU admission for monitoring and observation alone even if they are physiologically stable. These patients must have a recognized risk of complications and should be admitted when the likelihood of recognition and successful treatment is higher in the ICU setting.[1] For example, monitoring and observation with early institution of effective treatment for simple, premonitory dysrhythmias have been well documented to reduce mortality.[1] If equivalent detection and treatment of a developed complication can be reasonably expected in both routine care areas and the ICU, no advantage can be postulated for admission of the patient to ICU.

The complexity and frequency of nursing tasks (position changes, complex wound and dressing care, intake and output measurements, laboratory testing, etc.) are legitimate motivating forces behind an ICU admission. The measures designed to improve efficiency and capability in the delivery of these services (centralization of personnel, equipment, supplies) are generally included in the overall design of an ICU. Patients needing complex nursing make up the majority of the population of patients in an ICU—a group of patients that by most indices of severity are neither very sick nor very well. These patients in the extensive care group may be physiologically stable but require careful monitoring and observation. These patients remain in the ICU for extended periods and are subjected to many complications related to the primary admitting diagnosis and subsequent failure of vital organ systems (related to interrelationships of sepsis, immune function, and nutritional state), all of which create demands on nursing resources that are best addressed in an ICU environment.[1]

Patients that are physiologically unstable do not represent a problem with respect to the appropriateness of ICU admission. Attending personnel must remain at the animal's side reacting to changes and implementing, validating, and refining further therapy. These patients conform to the popular image of intensive care, as the elements of high technology, rapid but efficient activity, crisis, and the possibility for dramatic response exist.[1] These patients remain in this category for only a short time; thereafter, the acute abnormalities are resolved successfully and the patient enters the extensive care patient group, or if initial therapy is unsuccessful the patient dies.

Prediction of outcome

Prediction of outcome fits into the broader area of clinical judgment; it is clearly one of medicine's arts. There are four elements—the patient, the disease, the veterinarian(s), and the nurse technician(s)—representing the interacting forces that result in outcome for any particular case. Clinical judgment has been shown to predict outcome accurately approximately 85% of the time.[1] This degree of uncertainty related to clinical judgment has led to the development of several quantitative

indices for evaluation of critical care human patients. The fascination with technology and the potential for generation of tremendous amounts of data in critically ill patients has relegated clinical judgment to a lesser role in many human ICU units. These quantitative indices (e.g., acute physiology score and the chronic health evaluation—APACHE; Therapeutic Intervention Scoring System—TISS) were developed to provide a more precise and accurate tool to evaluate the degree of illness and likelihood of recovery in critical care patients.[1] It was hoped that these data, when subjected to proper statistical analysis, would provide accurate predictions and replace the uncertainty of clinical judgment. Most of these systems are geared to data collection in the first 24 hours following ICU admission. Parameters reflecting the immune system, nutritional state, and organ system functions or unique determinants of outcome (catastrophic new illness, iatrogenic events) cannot be accurately measured or predicted.[1] Most predictive indices are weighted for acute physiologic changes (cardiorespiratory and oxygen transport function), and the long-term ICU patients developing sepsis or multiple-organ system failure often have these indicators normal on admission and close to normal even moments before death. The end result of these manipulations, when compared with the use of ongoing clinical judgment, is that they too only predict outcome with 85% accuracy; the 15% failure rate should not necessarily be construed as representing a shortcoming of clinical judgment or a particular index, but may be inherent in the evolution of disease.[1] Standard ICU monitoring does not tell how any particular vital organ or subunit is functioning; these functions (dysfunctions) may be the limiting factor in a patient's survival. Research in veterinary critical care aimed at developing accurate outcome predictors as a function of the initial presenting condition, diagnoses, and ongoing prognostic variables (e.g., nutritional measurements, metabolic and immune parameters) should be encouraged. Accomplishing this goal will maximize efficient use of ICU resources (focus resources/testing on patients that can be saved) and allow early recognition of terminal cases (focus patient care on alleviation of suffering and stress rather than on the continued futile pursuit of the "therapeutic imperative").

Clinical assessment in the ICU[1]

The proper delivery of patient care in critical care medicine requires that clinicians integrate all available data into the formulation of the treatment plan for each patient. Clinicians must be careful not to rely wholly on numerical reflections of a patient's state. Data derived from technologic monitoring can easily supplant careful hands-on clinical assessment in the hectic ICU environment. A balanced approach most benefits patients. It is inappropriate to exclude the value of a well-performed clinical evaluation and concentrate solely on the flow chart and vice versa. Use of one approach without the other represents an uncritical reliance on either system and does not represent the ideal technique for patient care and assessment. A complete evaluation of any patient must include careful attention to historical data and repeated, careful physical examination of the patient in conjunction with assessment of objective data from measurements of appropriate parameters. The intent is to integrate the objective with the subjective—the so-called feel of the experienced ICU clinician. It is the subjective assessment that, when appropriately applied, provides the cornerstone on which all diagnostic and therapeutic decisions should be based.

The sophistication and limitations of various monitoring systems must be understood in order for the data derived from them to be properly applied and not misinterpreted. Quantitative data obtained on patients in the ICU setting has its reproducibility and absolute accuracy reduced by many factors, including subtle changes in the electronics of monitoring systems over time, the variability in nursing staff skills, and the hectic pace within the ICU. These factors contribute to a lack of specificity in obtaining any measurement and the likelihood of random oscillations of the values for parameters measured. Interpretation of "quantitative data" on patients in the ICU should concentrate on following the trends of measured parameters over time. That is, is the patient staying about the same, or do we see an overall change that suggests a major deviation in patient condition that is occurring or has occurred? Trends in monitored parameters must always be viewed, in order to identify spurious reasons for abnormal quantitative data, in conjunction with a clinical assessment of the patient to ensure that the clinical status of the patient matches the changes in measured parameters. A noncritical interpretation of data and failure to understand the deficiencies inherent in ICU monitoring can lead to inappropriate diagnosis and care (iatrogenesis). The importance of clinical assessment is further emphasized by the fact that introduction of sophisticated, technologically derived monitoring methods has seemingly done little to decrease mortality for a variety of diseases.[1] Patient outcome or changes in patient status continue to be predicted as accurately by repeated clinical evaluation of the patient as by scoring systems based on physiologic data points that are accurately charted. The importance here is to realize that it is not monitoring alone that is beneficial or protective, but rather the integration of the data with the knowledge of the observer, who subsequently must alter treatment if outcome is to be affected.

Critical care treatment can be divided into periods of resuscitation and observation. The treatment of the critically ill patient must proceed rapidly and in an orderly fashion; in many cases this must occur before complete objective assessments or reassessments (blood test results, monitored parameters) of the patient are available. It is into this area that the clinically oriented critical care clinician fits best. Certainly it is not optimal to make a clinical decision that may later prove erroneous, but it is more important to learn how to manage resuscitation without waiting for all the data. This approach is followed by experienced critical care clinicians. Clinical intuition may be the optimism of ignorance, but clinical intuition provides the framework for diagnostic and therapeutic interventions.[1] How, then, can this intuition be learned? The skill is developed by continuous patient contact. Involvement in all aspects of the care of patients leads to insights into the tolerance and reserves of patients with various diseases. Protocols can help direct the treatment of patients with difficult diseases, but frequently, appropriate decisions are based on the experience acquired from previous treatment of patients with similar problems.

The focus of this discussion has been on the relationship of the clinical assessment of patients in the critical care environment and the commonly used adjuncts to diagnosis and care. Too frequently, laboratory data and monitored parameters (electrocardiogram, blood pressure, central venous pressure) overwhelm the importance of the clinical information derived by patient examination and observation. The collection and recording of basic physiologic variables (temperature, pulse, respiration) by technicians and clinicians, although important, serves the additional and perhaps more important function of bringing critical care providers and their patients together at regular intervals.[1] Communication between clinicians and technicians as well as repeated patient examinations, accomplished with a high level of suspicion and integrated with all ancillary data, are important for proper clinical assessment and treatment of critical care patients.

The what and when of clinical decision making

Lists of differential diagnoses and sets of diagnostic or treatment algorithms cannot fully capture the essence of clinical decision making in critical care medicine. Decision making in this environment is a process that evolves through the accumulation of additional information and is often influenced by the passage of time. Clinical decision making in critical care medicine is an ongoing process that can be viewed from separate vantage points during the course of patient treatment.[1] Reevaluation and reappraisals are required, and decision making reflects a continuously changing perception in the clinician's mind of the critical care patient. The uncertainties brought about by adding, deleting, weighing, and assessing the variables associated with this ever-changing and poorly delineated process in essence represents a major source of challenge and frustration for the critical care clinician.

There are a vast number of potentially useful diagnostic tests from which to choose. In critical care medicine, many tests may be used repetitively. The use of this diagnostic armementarium is often attributed to a heightened awareness on the part of critical care clinicians to the "proven superiority" of these tests to traditional history taking and physical examination.[1] In many cases, the proper timing, sequence, and repetition of diagnostic testing has not been critically assessed. Many tests are selected during initial patient evaluation in order to "improve efficiency" in diagnosis and treatment. This approach removes the possibility of omission, but thought (rather than automatic behavior) is the key to maximizing effective utilization of resources and patient management while minimizing unnecessary testing, expense, and delays in diagnosis and treatment.

Possible forms of therapy must constantly be evaluated in terms of projected risks and benefits inherent in the treatment itself and as influenced by the patient's current health status and disease state. Therapy implies a chance for cure, which means there should be evidence linking improved outcome to the application of the treatment. Clinicians involved in critical care medicine must guard against applying interventions associated with significant risk or unproven efficacy (see iatrogenesis) and minute-to-minute treatment interventions aimed at maintaining physiologic variables within a tight "normal" range—a practice that has minimal to no effect on outcome, but that results in increased costs and poor use of nursing and laboratory personnel.[1] It is important to identify our expectations for treatment. Short-term objectives (reversal of hypovolemic shock) may be attained through proper application of clinical decision making; however, long-term objectives (survival) may not be obtained because of the development of intervening complications (sepsis).

The failure to achieve long-term objectives should not be construed as evidence of improper short-term decision making; however, the evolution of objectives (anticipation) must be part of the temporal framework for clinical decision making from the outset in all patients.[1] An evaluation of long-term outcome must form part of the process of initiation of therapy.

The changing nature of the decision-making process in critical care medicine reflects the effects of diseases during their evolution, changes created by the introduction of therapy, and the subsequent development of complications.[1] During the course of patient care it becomes necessary to acquire new information and reassess both the choice of diagnosis and the effects of therapy. The continually updated decision will be influenced by the passage of time and the selection of objectives (cure versus alleviation of suffering) appropriate to the evolved state of illness and the patient's response to therapy. Clinical decision making in critical care medicine is concerned with appropriateness of therapy given the existing circumstances for *this* patient at *this* point in the illness. Clinicians must consider decision making at all stages of treatment in the context of effecting a balance between the probable effects of disease and the wishes of the client (Chapter 7). The first goal of critical care medicine providers is the preservation of life; clients must be given options, recommendations, and counsel, as they must ultimately influence the clinical decision-making process. When the possibility of death increases, decisions should depart from the illness-based algorithm approach, which concentrates on diagnosis and treatment, and focus on caring for the patient (alleviation of suffering, rather than ordering new drugs, tests, and procedures) and client (communication, clarification, and explanation).

IATROGENESIS[1]

Iatrogenic illness can be defined as any illness that results from a diagnostic procedure, from any form of therapy, or from harmful occurrences (e.g., injury from a fall) during hospitalization that are not a direct consequence of a patient's disease. The term "iatrogenic" does not imply negligence in the delivery of care, as certain complications can be expected despite appropriate precautions associated with the application of appropriate diagnostic tests or treatments. The patients requiring the greatest intensity of care (multiple drugs, prolonged hospital stay, invasive procedures) are those most likely to suffer iatrogenic complications. In 1983, Eugene Robin described four types of harm that can occur to patients. These concepts of iatrogenesis included technical errors in the laboratory leading to erroneous results and treatment, the poor application of science or technology ("iatrodemics") leading to interpretive errors (misdiagnosis) and incorrect decisions (mismanagement), physical injuries that result from invasive procedures selected or performed inappropriately, and informational overload (the plethora of data that impedes correct identification and selection of priorities for the patient).[1]

Clinicians in critical care medicine must exercise care in clinical decision making in order to minimize the potential for iatrogenesis. Once a diagnostic "label" has been attached to a specific patient, the thought process and investigation expended to uncover unknown factors usually ceases.[1] Important aspects of the patient's illness may elude identification and continue to exert their effects unabated, undiagnosed, and untreated. Continued reevaluation of patients is required in clinical decision making in order to prevent, among other things, perpetuation of erroneous "labels"; many specific diagnoses have similar presentations, and individual cases rarely present in a "classical fashion." Similarly, the number of diagnostic tests and "therapeutic" interventions carried out on individual patients should be critically evaluated for benefit versus risk. Manipulations that do not affect outcome (successful treatment) can only have potentially deleterious results. Critical care clinicians must learn to distinguish the necessary elements of patient care from those which are unnecessary and contain the potential only for harm. The data collected on patients in the ICU must be organized to determine its usefulness and relevance. A necessary and sufficient data base for different categories of patients must be defined. A proper evaluation of potential outcome in patients must allow discrimination between curable patients and those dying and beyond therapy. One of the important issues faced in veterinary critical care medicine is the distinction between therapeutic efforts that may return a patient to a good quality of life and ineffective efforts that only increase the risk for patient suffering and prolong a patient's dying. Improving efficiency in use of resources and a better focus for patient care are attainable objectives. Diminishing unnecessary activity will decrease complications and have a salutary effect. Having additional time for patients and their owners will fulfill the important goal of caring and decrease our sense of failure when confronted with the death of our patients. Clinicians in critical care must concentrate their efforts on thinking, assessing, and decision making rather than on frenetically ordering, reacting, and intervening.[1] An ultimate effect in purifying, clarifying, distilling, and delineating proper ICU patient care will be the elimination of misinterpretations, misdirections, and misadventures—iatrogenesis.[1]

THE DELIVERY OF PATIENT CARE
The team

An ICU is a high-tension environment, where uncertainty about patient survival ("Are we doing the right things?") is coupled with the random appearance of unpredictable crises. The stressors in an ICU cannot be eliminated. Knowing how we handle stress and how it handles us can benefit all members of the ICU team. Different people handle stress in different ways—joking, shouting, or becoming quiet and withdrawn. The emphasis of teamwork should be on doing what is right for the patient. Clinicians and technicians must have the same goal; however, dealing with the different personalities requires a delicate balance of tact and diplomacy. Factors influencing the ability of the team to perform satisfactorily include a clear understanding of the team's objectives, role delineation, technician-clinician collaboration, and communication skills.[1]

The goal of an ICU is the safe delivery of coordinated medical care. All team members are important, contributing their skills and expertise to complete this objective. The critical care clinician is the quarterback; the other team members look to that person for the plan of therapy (decision making) and support for their cause (delivery of patient care). Each member of the team is responsible for individual tasks but will continually monitor the entire patient care process to ensure that daily goals are being achieved. Inquiries about therapy are generally not intended to question an individual's judgment, but to ensure that the plan of care is consistent with the goals of patient care.

The team, which relies on individual commitment to a common goal, establishes behaviors and expectations such as honesty, sound judgment, satisfactory job performance, an attitude of caring, a strong desire to do what is right for the patient, an attention to detail, and an acknowledgment of the importance of the team approach.[1] Team spirit develops in this type of practice and enhances the morale of clinicians and technicians involved in caring for a specific group of patients. The team spirit becomes difficult to maintain if dissension develops. Team membership has to be earned. Participation in unit activities demonstrates acknowledgment of the team and its importance in the overall functioning of the unit, even when particular procedures seem wrong. Deviation from established protocols is often considered unwillingness to be part of the team, not evidence of a superior way to do a task. This approach can be disruptive to morale, can heighten organizational stress, and can ultimately obstruct the delivery of patient care. Initially, it is easiest to accept the team's "correct" way and after acceptance to the team have one's ideas evaluated on their merit.[1] Correcting "errors" and introducing new (better?) ways, before "joining" the team, leads to defensiveness and hostility instead of trust and acceptance.[1]

Controlling chaos—organization and prioritization[1,2]

Organization is one of the keys to success. The best-planned or best-organized schedule may be difficult to accomplish because of multiple ongoing emergencies. Planning the workday in an ICU is important; establishing priorities becomes imperative. The daily schedule includes rounds to provide a basis and plan for therapy, communication of this plan in the form of orders, completion of general tasks (obtaining samples and results, treatments, nursing care) and special procedures, accepting new admissions, and responding to crises. As all of these events occur each day, chaos can easily result unless each day evolves in a planned fashion and certain protocols are adhered to. Patient orders should be written (not just verbalized), a treatment schedule should be used, and observations and measurements should be recorded as they occur or as they are completed. Prioritization of daily tasks must be established for each member of the team with respect to each patient in the unit. The goals of patient care (resource utilization) must be defined for each patient and between patients. The frequent unpredictable events of the day will add confusion to the best-organized schedule. Disruptions (crises) in the prioritized routine create the potential for mistakes of omission and commission. Clinicians and technicians must remain in control, working quickly and efficiently—completion of each prioritized task should be accomplished before proceeding to the next, whenever possible, in order to minimize errors and maximize delivery of the appropriate level of patient care.

Communication and documentation

The smooth functioning of any system is dependent on effective communication. This is the keystone in critical care patient treatment; its importance needs only to be underscored by the reality that mistakes resulting from miscommunication may be life threatening and lethal. The various members of the ICU team must be in contact throughout the day on the various aspects of each

patient's condition. The critical care clinician has the central role in coordinating all communication, as that individual has the overall responsibility in the clinical decision making for and the welfare of the patient. Open communication between all members of the critical care team generates the most effective patient treatment, as all relevant data passes among the key individuals before decision making occurs. The clinician must serve as the repository of information—collecting and collating data from various sources and serving as a conduit for its distribution to the client and to the various individuals involved in each patient's care.[1] In view of the complexity of care in many cases, well-constructed documentation in the medical record is an excellent means of facilitating communication and maintaining the continuity of care required.

Adequate record keeping is crucial for transmitting information from one caregiver to another. All observations, treatments, results, and interventions (and their complications) must be thoroughly documented for each patient. In order to write good progress notes (containing information, assessment, and plan), the material must be gathered and processed in the mind of the writer. Good documentation is a stimulus to good thought processes and is evidence of same. Progress notes should be written at least every 24 hours, and good progress notes may take 15 to 20 minutes to complete.[1] Progress notes should contain impressions and judgments along with observations and data; that is, the medical record should reflect the clinical decision-making process for the patient.

Rounds, conducted at the time of work shift changes, serve to maintain continuity of patient care and supplement medical record communications. Reports on patients should be communicated beginning with the animal's signalment and reason for presentation (problem list) followed by a synopsis of what has been done to the patient and the results of tests and interventions. The report is completed with an up-to-the-minute assessment of the patient, plans for the day, and expected course of disease (prognosis). Clinicians and technicians giving reports should be prepared to explain and defend their actions and be willing to change treatment plans if better ideas are expressed by colleagues.

Allocation of resources[1,3-5]

Intensive care is a limited resource, with the principal limitation being the extent to which nurse technicians can be "stretched" before patient care begins to suffer. Critical care clinicians should examine their role in the utilization of nursing resources by carefully considering the necessity for admission of each patient and the extent of nursing care, treatments, tests, and interventions requested for each patient admitted to the ICU. Patients should be categorized into the groups mentioned previously (monitoring/observation, extensive nursing, and constant care) and orders written to meet the physiologic needs of the patient. Clinicians must disavow the belief that a lengthy order sheet is a good reflection of thoroughness and learn the role that inappropriate order writing plays in confusing activity with productivity.[1] Proper classification of patients and the design of efficient care protocols for these patients in various groups achieve the goals of ICU care—maximization of benefit to the patient and minimization of the risks for iatrogenesis, unnecessary expense to the client, and inappropriate utilization of ICU resources.

Patient stress

Patients in the ICU require attention to their psychologic well-being in addition to the continued attempts to correct their physiologic disturbances. Clinicians and technicians must make attempts to befriend the animals by alleviating the discomforts of pain, fear, unfamiliar surroundings, interrupted sleep patterns, and other psychologic disturbances. The care factor in critical care medicine must remain paramount in the endeavors and clinical decision making of critical care providers.

REFERENCES

1. Civetta JM, Taylor RW, Kirby RR. Critical Care. Philadelphia: JB Lippincott, 1988.
2. Bliven MT. Animal health technicians in the emergency hospital. In Wingfield WE, ed. Veterinary clinics of North America—small animal practice, Philadelphia: WB Saunders, 1981;11:9-22.
3. Civetta JM, Hudson-Civetta JA. Maintaining quality of care while reducing charges in the ICU—Ten ways. Ann Surg 1985;202:524-530.
4. Engelhardt HT, Rie MA. Intensive care units, scarce resources, and conflicting principles of justice. JAMA 1986;255:1159-1164.
5. Strauss MJ, LoGerfo JP, Yeltatzie JA, Temkin N, Hudson LD. Rationing of intensive care unit services—An everyday occurrence. JAMA 1986;255:1143-1146.

6 Nosocomial Disease

Robert J. Murtaugh

Nosocomial infections are defined as infections that were not present or were not incubating in patients at the time of admission to the hospital.[1] These hospital-acquired infections are most commonly caused by single or multiple bacteria (staphylococcus or enterobacteriaceae most commonly) that manifest resistance to several antibiotics and are difficult to treat. Host and environmental factors, along with virulence of the organism, are involved in the development of nosocomial infections in hospitalized animals. The common sites of nosocomial infections include the respiratory and urinary tracts, surgical wounds, and indwelling catheter/tube sites.[2,3] Septicemia and subsequent multiple-organ failure resulting in death of the patient is the primary sequela of concern in patients in whom nosocomial infections develop.[2] The mortality rate in human patients with nosocomial infections approaches 44%.[4] The incidence, prevalence, and mortality rates for nosocomial infections in veterinary patients have not been established. However, reports of nosocomial infections in veterinary teaching hospitals have begun to appear in the literature (Fig. 6-1).[3,5] The development of nosocomial infections and a strategy for control of such infections will be outlined in this chapter.

DEVELOPMENT OF NOSOCOMIAL DISEASE

Nosocomial infections in human hospitals are estimated to affect 5% to 10% of all patients hospitalized.[3] The prevalence of infections is highest in patients hospitalized in intensive care wards (18%) as compared with patients hospitalized in general medical or surgical wards (6%).[3] There are several factors that account for the increased prevalence of infections in the critical care patient. These factors include the following: (1) severe illness/debilitation, (2) increased use of inva-

sive monitoring and support devices, (3) frequent handling by multiple personnel, (4) prolonged hospital stays, and (5) greater use of antibiotic therapy in many of these patients as compared with other hospitalized individuals.[6]

Debilitation and disease

Diseases that compromise an animal's immune system predispose to the development of nosocomial disease (uremia, diabetes mellitus, hyperadrenocorticism, neoplastic disease, burns, and traumatic injury). Many of the treatments used to control the primary diseases in critical care patients (corticosteroids, chemotherapy) contribute to further immunosuppression. An additional fac-

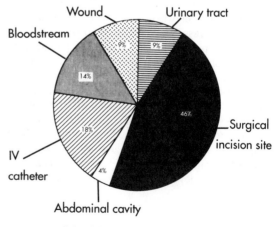

*N = 22 cases at TUSVM 1988

Fig. 6-1 Relative frequency of nosocomial infections by site of infection. (From Murtaugh RJ, Mason GD. In Kirby R, ed. Critical care medicine, Veterinary clinics of North America—small animal practice, Philadelphia: WB Saunders, 1989;19:1269.)

tor that contributes to the potential for nosocomial disease in many of these patients is their negative nutritional state. This factor results in further immunocompromise by several mechanisms, including the following: (1) decreasing liver synthesis of acute-phase proteins; (2) limiting protein substrate for production of complement, fibronectin, cytokines, antibodies, and other immunoregulatory substances; and (3) altering the production and synthetic capabilities of many immunocompetent cells.

Tubes and devices

Critical care patients are subjected to monitoring, support, and treatment measures that require placement of catheters, tubes, and drains into the animal. These devices provide potential avenues for bacterial colonization and eventual infection of the animal with nosocomial pathogens. Aseptic technique in placement and management of catheters, tubes, and drains, accompanied by their prudent usage and limitation of dwell times minimizes the risks for nosocomial disease. Equipment that is used on multiple patients (nebulizers, clipper blades, oxygen and suction lines, respirator tubes, etc.) represent additional potential sources for spread of nosocomial pathogens between patients when proper preventive measures are not employed.

Personnel

The spread of nosocomial pathogens, with resultant colonization and infection of patients, occurs most commonly through the handling of multiple patients by clinicians and personnel inattentive to proper hygiene practices.[7-9] The admonition "wash hands between each patient contact" is easy to express, universally acknowledged, yet difficult to practice.[7] The number of patient contacts per shift and occurrence of sudden emergencies in a critical care setting make it extremely difficult to adhere to the precept of handwashing between each patient and between different procedures on the same patient.[7] The difficulty does not diminish the importance of doing so. This point can be best emphasized by realizing the magnitude and importance of the problems associated with the development of nosocomial sepsis in a patient.[7]

Antibiotics

Use of antibiotics exerts profound influences on the nature of host microflora, and though this may not directly augment host susceptibility to infection, it appears to influence directly the nature of the organisms that colonize and subsequently infect hospital patients.[3,10] Almost all antibiotics in therapeutic doses precipitate various changes in the microflora of the skin, upper respiratory tract, gastrointestinal tract, and the urogenital tract. Resistant organisms, whether present or acquired, are selected to multiply and replace the susceptible organisms that are inhibited by antibiotic therapy. In some patients serious or fatal infections develop.[3,10]

Antibiotics are presently one of the most frequently prescribed groups of drugs in both human and veterinary medicine.[3] The common practice of prescribing antibiotics to "see if the patient gets better," does not constitute rational drug therapy. In two surveys, reviewers from human infectious disease departments judged the use of antibiotics to be inappropriate in 52% of patients in one hospital,[10] and in 62% of patients in a second hospital.[11] Many physicians and veterinarians assume that a fever, for instance, represents a treatable bacterial infection and, hence, may dispense antibiotics without any further diagnostic tests. Many gastrointestinal upsets are similarly treated with antimicrobials, when in fact, the majority are not due to specific bacterial agents. In these cases, drug therapy can do more harm than good by inhibiting normal gut flora and facilitating the growth of resistant organisms.[3]

Evidence exists to support the consideration that antibiotic usage is associated with the emergence of antimicrobial resistance in the environmental microflora of hospitals.[3,10,12] Antimicrobial resistance is more commonly found among bacteria causing nosocomial infections than among those causing community-acquired infections. In nosocomial infection outbreaks, patients infected with resistant strains are more likely to have received previous antimicrobial therapy than are patients colonized or infected with susceptible strains for the same species. Changes in antimicrobial use are reflected by similar changes in the prevalence of resistance to that particular antibiotic. The areas of human hospitals with the highest prevalence of resistant bacteria are usually those with the most extensive antibiotic usage (e.g., burn units, critical care units, and oncology units). An increasing probability of patient colonization or infection with resistant organisms occurs with increasing duration of exposure to antibiotics in the hospital. The increased risk appears to apply whether or not the particular patient has received antibiotic therapy. In general, a dose-response relationship seems to hold true, in that increasing dosage of antimicrobials increases the patient's risk of superinfection or colonization with resistant organisms. Finally, as mentioned previously, antibiotic therapy produces marked effects on the host's endogenous flora, especially that of the skin and gastrointestinal tract, and exerts selective pressure in favor of resistant organisms.

NOSOCOMIAL INFECTIONS
Respiratory

The clinical diagnosis of nosocomial pneumonia includes fever, leukocytosis, purulent tracheobronchial secretions, new or progressive infiltrates on chest radiographs, and isolation of pathogenic bacteria in tracheobronchial secretions. Pneumonia is considered the most common cause of fatality associated with hospital-acquired infection in humans (mortality rates of 33% to 70% for patients with gram-negative pneumonias), causing mortality in 12% to 15% of all human patients in an intensive care unit.[2]

Organisms responsible for nosocomial pneumonia originate from the oropharynx and gastrointestinal tract.[2] An alteration in bacterial colonization of the oropharynx and gastrointestinal tract is possibly the most important factor contributing to the increased incidence of the bacterial species responsible for pneumonia in critically ill human patients.[2] Studies have shown that as many as 90% of critical care human patients in whom pneumonia developed had an earlier oropharyngeal colonization with the same organism.[13] The ability of various bacteria to adhere to epithelial cells is important in the pathogenesis of colonization of the oropharynx with gram-negative bacteria.[2] Gram-positive organisms normally colonize the oropharynx and may protect against adherence and colonization by gram-negative bacteria.[2] Fibronectin depletion may have a role in this phenomenon, as gram-negative bacilli adhere well to epithelial cells deficient in this glycoprotein.[14] Preventive alkalinization of the stomach may also contribute to colonization of the upper digestive tract, providing a source of organisms for subsequent aspiration.[2] Nosocomial pneumonia is not as prevalent in veterinary as it is in human critical care patients. This results from less use of ventilator therapy for respiratory disease in veterinary patients. Nonetheless, the problem is not uncommon in postoperative and other patients in veterinary intensive care units. Awareness of its significance and the need for careful attention to preventive measures must be maintained by all providers of critical care services.

Postoperative wound infections

Postoperative wound infection rates depend on several factors. Wound infection rates are similar in human and veterinary medicine with the lowest infection rates seen following clean, elective surgeries (1% to 2%) and infection rates as high as 20% to 40% expected with contaminated or dirty surgical procedures (often performed in emergency or trauma situations).[15,16] Risk factors in human patients with traumatic injuries include multiple-organ injury, shock on presentation, multiple-transfusion requirement, increasing age, therapeutic delay, and degree of bacterial contamination.[15] Proper use of prophylactic and therapeutic antibiotic therapy is required to minimize the potential for postoperative wound infections. The choice of antibiotic, route of administration, and duration of administration are all important considerations.[3,15]

A number of factors not related to antibiotics can influence postoperative infection rates following clean surgical procedures in which bacterial contamination was absent or minimal. The duration of preoperative hospitalization is directly related to the rate of infection; in human patients the rate doubles for each week of hospitalization prior to surgery.[17] In addition, many intensive care patients are colonized by nosocomial pathogens within 2 weeks of admission.[18] Preoperative shaving of the surgical site on the day before surgery increases infection rates because of enhanced growth and multiplication of skin organisms in damaged epithelium.[19] The duration of surgery plays a significant part in determining the potential for postoperative infections as a result of waning effects of prophylactic antibiotics and increased opportunity for bacterial colonization of the wound. Infection rates generally double with each added hour of surgery time.[15] Significant increases in postoperative wound infections can be expected when an elective procedure is performed in the presence of an active remote infection. It is prudent to resolve urinary, pulmonary, or skin infections prior to elective surgical procedures.[15]

Catheter-related septicemia

Intravenous and intraarterial catheters, although necessary, are invasions of the normal skin barrier. The major risk from intravascular infusion devices is local infection or bacterial dissemination in the bloodstream. Organisms can be isolated from up to 58% of indwelling plastic intravenous catheters; however, the rate of septicemia from local colonizations is only about 10%.[15]

Phlebitis is strongly associated with subsequent infection. A local thrombus, developing from chemical or physical irritation, may become infected and is the usual source of catheter-related septicemia. Catheter-related infection rates increase when multiple attempts are required to place a catheter successfully in a site and with dwell times exceeding 48 to 72 hours. There is also a striking relationship between the hospital day on which a catheter is placed and the risk of infection. Significant differences in infection rates exist when comparing patients with catheters placed on Day 0 to 6 versus Day 7 to 13 versus Day 14 and later.[2] The use of multiple-lumen catheters appears to be associated with a catheter-related infection rate comparable to that of single-lumen catheters.[2]

Skin bacteria surrounding the catheter site are the most common pathogens. For this reason, catheters should be inserted with strict aseptic technique, and the surrounding area should be kept clean with dressings and antiseptic solutions. Remote infections occasionally result in contamination of the catheter tip. Infusions through surgical cutdowns in the lower extremities have higher infection rates.[2,15]

The type of infusion fluid may also influence the development of contamination and subsequent infection. Fluids that require the addition of other substances (e.g., vitamins, electrolytes) increase the risk of external contamination. Hypertonic solutions, such as those used in hyperalimentation, often result in chemical phlebitis, which predisposes to infection.

Any febrile spike in a patient with an indwelling intravenous catheter should suggest the possibility of catheter-related sepsis. After other causes of fever have been investigated and ruled out, blood cultures should be obtained and all catheters removed and cultured.[15]

Catheter cultures should be taken from an intracutaneous portion of the catheter using a semi-quantitative culture technique.[20] Blood cultures should not be taken through catheters suspected of being the source of catheter-related infections, and the tips of removed catheters should not be cultured, as these results can be misleading.[3]

The majority of catheter-associated septicemias are self-limiting following catheter removal. Febrile episodes usually cease following catheter removal, and systemic antibiotics are rarely necessary for successful treatment. If the infected catheter is left in place, however, metastatic infections may result from continued septicemia. No evidence has shown that "prophylactic" systemic antibiotic administration reduces, or in any way alters, the incidence of catheter-associated infection.

NOSOCOMIAL DISEASE PREVENTION PROTOCOL[21]

A restricted program of antibiotic use should be practiced. Prophylactic antibiotic therapy for surgical patients is administered perioperatively only. Administration of amikacin and second- or third-generation cephalosporins is prohibited un-less multiple antibiotic resistant organisms are identified by culture as resistant to other alternative treatments. Injectable antibiotic doses are drawn up daily and stored in a single drawer of the intensive care unit (ICU) refrigerator or in bags in the individual patients' drug boxes. No antibiotic solutions are discarded down sinks or drains.

Several procedures are followed in an attempt to prevent animal-to-animal spread of infection. Disposable gloves are worn by all personnel, and gloves are changed between animals.[8] All personnel are instructed to wash their hands before handling medications, fluids, and intravenous lines and between patients before putting on a new pair of disposable gloves. At-risk patients are treated first and those with known or suspected colonization or infection with multiple antibiotic resistant organisms are treated last. Cohort nursing (same nurse treats same cases each time) may also help limit spread of nosocomial pathogens.[8] Injection ports are swabbed with disinfectant before intravenous administration of medications. Intravenous catheters used to administer maintenance fluids are ideally not used as access for medication administration. Total parenteral nutrition catheters are not, under any circumstance, used for medication administration. Clipper blades, electrocardiographic clips, and blood pressure cuffs are all cleaned and disinfected between uses. Surgical drains are bandaged, and dressings are changed frequently to prevent "strike through." Soiled bedding and bandages should be placed in appropriate receptacles and not left on floors or counters. Disposable thermometers and lubrication containers are not shared between patients. Diagnostic and therapeutic interventions on patients (aside from intravenous catheter placement) are performed outside the ICU whenever possible. Intravenous catheters, urinary catheters, and chest drains are placed using aseptic technique.

Short, over-the-needle catheters are not used for maintenance fluid administration. Intravenous catheters are covered with a bandage, and catheters are removed and replaced every 48 to 72 hours. Bandages are not disturbed unless they become soiled. Animals with indwelling intravenous catheters that experience fever spikes generally have the catheter removed, provided no other identifiable cause for the fever can be detected. The catheter segment and blood are cultured. Empirical antibiotics are started if the animal appears septic or when the fever fails to resolve within 12 to 24 hours of catheter removal. Disconnection of intravenous catheters from administration sets is minimized (not allowed with total parenteral nutrition catheters), and when it is done aseptic technique is used (ends are plugged or covered with sterile materials). Intravenous fluid administration lines are changed every 24 to 48 hours (at the time when a new fluid setup is started). Routine addition of glucose and other medications to isotonic intravenous fluid preparations is not allowed; resultant hypertonicity can predispose a patient to thrombophlebitis and catheter-related infections. Intravenous catheters used for fluid administration are not used for blood sampling.

The use of indwelling urinary catheters is discouraged; when used, closed collection systems are mandatory. Routine urinalyses are performed every 36 hours, and urine cultures are submitted when pyuria is detected on urinalysis and/or when the catheter is removed. Similar protocols are followed for indwelling chest and abdominal (dialysis) catheters. Flushing into chest drains or urinary catheters is discouraged. Indwelling urinary catheter or chest drain placement is minimized to ≤5 days whenever possible, as infection rates escalate when this limit is exceeded. Similarly, the length of patient stays in the ICU has direct correlation to the potential for development of nosocomial disease (≥5 days).

Immobile patients are repositioned regularly, and convalescing patients are encouraged to ambulate early to minimize retention of respiratory secretions, which predispose to pneumonia.[9]

A standardized environmental surveillance and cleaning and disinfection protocol are adhered to in the ICU. All table tops and cages are cleaned and disinfected between patients. Chlorhexidine and bleach are two disinfectants recommended. Runs and cages are allowed to stand dry for several hours before they are used again. Drying kills enteric (multiple antibiotic resistant organism) bacteria. All multiple-use equipment (nebulizer, oxygen and suction lines, respirator tubes, vacuum cleaner, etc.) are disassembled, cleaned, and disinfected/sterilized between uses. All storage containers (for swabs, gauze, etc.) are cleaned and sterilized weekly; no food storage or consumption is allowed in the ICU. Environmental cultures are performed bimonthly as a check on cleaning/disinfection protocols and for identification of new isolates and assessment of the overall environmental "load" of multiple antibiotic resistant organisms.

Treatment of nosocomial infections[3]

Because of the resistant nature of many nosocomial pathogens, treatment can be difficult. The most important consequence of nosocomial infection, especially that caused by gram-negative organisms, is septicemia. In human patients, gram-negative septicemia is associated with a high prevalence of shock and death. The eventual outcome of septicemia was found to be directly related to the degree of underlying disease. It is therefore necessary to be aggressive with respect to medical therapy in these instances.

Blood cultures are strongly recommended as part of the diagnostic approach, as they frequently provide accurate information about the source of the infection, as well as identification of the pathogen. If the offending organism has been isolated in culture, the choice of an appropriate antibiotic therapy is based on sensitivity tests. Otherwise, empirical treatment of serious nosocomial infections should include antimicrobials effective against gram-negative organisms (e.g., aminoglycosides). Gram stains of purulent drainage or infected body fluids are often a helpful guide to drug selection pending results of blood and site cultures. The patient should be completely assessed for potential sources of infection, especially with regard to invasive procedures. If the site of infection can be determined, potential pathogens identified from that source will help in drug selection as well. Whenever possible, abscesses or empyemas are best treated by drainage and lavage.

A combination of amikacin and cephalothin (with metronidazole when anaerobes suspected) is the current choice in our hospital, based on cumulative sensitivities of nosocomial infections. Only 9% of multiple antibiotic resistant organisms that caused nosocomial infections at Tufts University School of Veterinary Medicine were found to be resistant to amikacin, despite the fact that 38% were resistant to gentamicin (Murtaugh and Mason, unpublished data). These figures are similar to those obtained by Roudebush and Fales,[22] who studied gentamicin-resistant isolates from 26 small animal patients. It has been suggested that amikacin is effective for treating resistant gram-negative bacilli because of its relative resistance to plasmid-mediated enzymes.[10]

Septicemia in hospital patients requires intensive supportive care as well as antimicrobial therapy. Patients with signs of impending shock should be treated accordingly. Fluid therapy not only maintains blood pressure and cardiac output, but also protects tissue perfusion and thus optimizes drug distribution. If the patient does not respond adequately to the prescribed course of treatment, the clinician should reassess the original diagnosis, reculture to exclude the possibility of a resistant or new pathogen, and search for other complicating factors.

SUMMARY

Nosocomial infection control programs of various types have been implemented in human hospitals since the staphylococcal pandemic of the 1950s. The prevalence of hospital infections is expected to increase in veterinary medicine with the advent of sophisticated invasive monitoring techniques, lengthier patient hospital stays, and the widespread use of antimicrobial agents. In order to monitor and control nosocomial infection outbreaks, the hospital staff must regard strategic measures as a priority.

REFERENCES

1. Gardner P, Causey WA. Hospital-acquired infections. In Petersdorf RG, Adams RD, Beaunwald E, et al, ed. Harrison's principles of internal medicine, ed 10, New York: McGraw-Hill, 1983;855.
2. Norwood SH. The prevalence and importance of nosocomial infections. In Civitta JM, Taylor RW, Kirby RR, eds. Critical care. Philadelphia: JB Lippincott, 1988;757-767.
3. Murtaugh RJ, Mason GD. Antibiotic Pressure and Nosocomial Disease. In Kirby R, ed. Critical care medicine, veterinary clinics of North America—small animal practice. Philadelphia: WB Saunders, 1989;19:1259-1274.
4. Bryan CS, Reynolds KL, Brenner ER. Analysis of 1,186 Episodes of gram-negative bacteria in non-university hospitals: The effects of antimicrobial therapy. Rev Infect Dis 1983; Suppl:629.
5. Lippert AC, Fulton RB, Parr AM. Nosocomial infection surveillance in a small animal intensive care unit. J Am Anim Hosp Assoc 1988;24:627-636.
6. Jones RL. Control of nosocomial infections. In Kirk RW, ed. Current veterinary therapy IX. Philadelphia: WB Saunders, 1986;19-24.
7. Hudson-Civetta JA, Civetta JM. Clean and aseptic technique at the bedside. In Civetta JM, Taylor RW, Kirby RR, eds. Critical care. Philadelphia: JB Lippincott, 1988;183-195.
8. Klein BS, Perloff WH, Maki DG. Reduction of Nosocomial infection during pediatric intensive care by protective isolation. N Engl J Med 1989;320:1714-1721.
9. Haskins SC. Overview of emergency and intensive care. In Sherding RG, ed. Medical emergencies, contemporary issues in small animal practice. New York: Churchill Livingstone, 1985;1-35.
10. Eickhoff TC. Antibiotics and nosocomial infections. In Bennett JV, Brachman PS, eds. Hospital infections. Boston: Little, Brown 1979;171-192.
11. Stevens GP, Jacobson JA, Burke JP. Changing patterns of hospital infections and antibiotic use. Arch Intern Med 1981;141:589-592.
12. McGowan JE: Antimicrobial resistance in hospital organisms and its relation to antibiotic use. Rev Infect Dis 1983;5:1033-1044.
13. Johanson WG, Pierce AK, Sanford JP, et al. Nosocomial respiratory infections with gram-negative bacilli. Ann Intern Med 1972;77:701.
14. Woods DE, Bass JA, Johanson WG, et al. Role of adherence in the pathogenesis of *Pseudomonas aeruginosa* lung infection in cystic fibrosis patients. Infect Immun 1980;30:694.
15. Nichols RL, Rush DS. Bacterial infectious disease considerations in the surgical patient. In Civetta JM, Taylor RW, Kirby RR, eds. Critical care. Philadelphia: JB Lippincott, 1988;817-828.
16. Daly WR. Wound infections. In Slatter DH, ed. Textbook of small animal surgery. Philadelphia: WB Saunders, 1985;37-51.
17. Cruse PJE, Foord R. A five-year prospective study of 23,649 surgical wounds. Arch Surg 1973;107:206.
18. Northey D. Microbial surveillance in a surgical intensive care unit. Surg Gynecol Obstet 1974;139:321.
19. Seropian R, Reynolds BM. Wound infections after preoperative depilatory versus razor preparation. Am J Surg 1971;121:251.
20. Maki DG, Weis CE, Sarafin HW. A semiquantitative culture method of identifying intravenous catheter-related infections. N Engl J Med 1977;296:1305.
21. Murtaugh RJ. Hospital borne infection: Its role in critical care. Proceedings of the Eastern States Veterinary Conference, Orlando FL, 1989;41-42.
22. Roudebush P, Fales WH. Antibacterial susceptibility of gentamicin resistant organisms recovered from small companion animals. J Am Anim Hosp Assoc 1982;18:649-652.

7 Client Relations and Ethics

Robert J. Murtaugh

The client is the most important person in our business.
He is not dependent on us—we depend on him.
He is not an interruption in our work—he is the very purpose of it.
He does us a favor when he calls—we are not doing him a favor when we serve him.
He is not just a cold statistic, but a real flesh and blood human, just like you and me.
He is a vital part of our business—not an outsider.
He is not a name, a fact, or a number on a ledger.
He is not a person to argue or match wits with.
He is a person who brings to us his needs and wants. Our job is to fulfill them.
He is the very lifeblood of our community.
He is the one who buys our services—pays our salaries.
He deserves the most courteous and attentive treatment we can give him.

TAPREL LOOMIS

The March 1986 Newsletter for the Idaho Veterinary Medical Association reprinted the results of an informal, nationwide survey conducted by a national health care publication to assess the reasons that clients do not return to a clinic. Improper medical treatment for the patient was not listed among the eight most common reasons for client dissatisfaction. Eighty percent of the respondents registered complaints about "officious, overbearing" staff members. Seventy percent of the clients surveyed objected to the manner in which fees were explained. More than 50% of these clients mentioned dehumanizing factors (office staff failing to treat client as an individual) and having to wait for the doctor as reasons for dissatisfaction.

The results of this survey emphasize the importance of establishing good rapport and communication with clients. Success in veterinary medicine is commonly linked to how medicine is practiced, not necessarily to its quality.

Critical care and emergency medicine is ripe with the potential for conflict and frustration in the area of client communication and client relations. Clinicians involved in the delivery of this veterinary care must have a clear understanding of the issues and be accomplished in the art of establishing and maintaining good client relations. Significant impairments to the successful treatment of critical care patients can result from failure to achieve these goals.

TALKING TO CLIENTS— COMMUNICATION BEHAVIOR

Veterinary clinicians are intently focused on keeping up with the ever-expanding body of scientific knowledge and technical skills required to deliver the best in patient care. In this pursuit of clinical excellence clinicians can easily lose sight of the importance of developing and maintaining our human relation aptitudes (compassion, gentleness, empathy) and communication capabilities.[1] These factors are the key elements to establishing a good doctor-client relationship. A good communicator will strengthen, while a poor communicator will weaken, the doctor-client bond.[2] What is stated and how it is communicated will either fortify or cripple the relationship. The clinician has to strive to make the client understand the patient's condition while understanding, appreciating, and respecting the client's interests and needs. Uneasiness experienced by clinicians is attributable to a variety of factors, including incomplete understanding of the animal's condition, unpleasant subject matter (terminal disease), or a difficult client. This uneasiness is natural to feel, but when communicating with clients it must be overcome by the realization that the client and patient need us and must be served.[3]

One of the best ways to reinforce the doctor-client bond is to ask questions that elicit the expression of the client's feelings.[2] Some of the most important feelings are the fears and anxieties concerning what the doctor has in mind. Questions posed to clients concerning their fears about the treatment plan, costs, and their role in decision-making processes have a cohesive and firming influence on the doctor-client bond.[2] Some of these client anxieties may be subconscious. Clinicians must make conscious efforts to address these issues and get the client to express these concerns.

Terms such as castration, amputation, enucleation, and anesthesia may have quite different meanings to the doctor from what they do to the client. The client's prior experiences with health care professionals, superstitions, and indoctrinations by parents and relatives color their perceptions of a clinician's attempted communication.[2] An object of good communication is to ensure that client and doctor mutually understand (share) the meanings of the words that are spoken. Distinguishing between private and shared meanings is an art, and the best way to determine whether the client understands the clinician's intent is for the doctor to ask the client for their interpretation of the transmission (feedback).[2] This approach to communication facilitates client consent, minimizes subsequent misunderstanding, and allows the clinician to formulate the best possible treatment plan for the patient *and* client.

There are several useful techniques and strategies that can be employed by clinicians to aid in effective communications with clients. Client participation should be stimulated by making comments and questions open-ended.[3] Voluntary or solicited client contributions often answer specific diagnostic questions that clinicians may not think to ask. The more important the clinical issues, the more important it is for the clinician to concentrate on making the necessary statements and avoid rambling, which may exacerbate client anxiety.[3] The client's main interest is in the patient. A clinician should concentrate on projecting the idea that he/she cares about the patient and should avoid monologues (only tangentially associated with the patient) on his/her achievements, skills, and equipment.[3] Most clients are concerned with an assessment of prognosis for the animal and the economics of proposed options for treatment. Attempts should be made by the clinician to get to these points, using logic and empathy, as quickly as possible.[3] Veterinarians should exercise care and good judgment in "filtering" what is said to clients.[3] Clinicians must provide information and recommendations to clients, but do so without appearing condescending or insensitive.

Clinicians can attenuate their own anxiety by making every effort to put their clients at ease. The use of deliberate relaxation (taking a few deep breaths before starting the conversation) improves a clinician's ability to communicate in difficult situations.[2] Redirecting attention outward and making the attempt to offer the client needed support makes a doctor's imagined shortcomings and feelings of inadequacy fade away when confronted with difficult clinical or client situations.[2] It is important to speak slowly, look directly into the client's eyes, and say only what one sincerely believes.[2] Veterinarians must dare to be personal and offer clients heartfelt warmth and closeness during clinician-client interactions.

Clinicians who fancy themselves great communicators are usually speaking of their transmission capability (ability to talk at the client).[2] Feedback is a response relevant to the preceding transmission[2]—communication is a two-way street. Engaging in an aspect of communication behavior in a doctor-client interaction (transmission) does not necessarily constitute communication with the client.[2]

Listening, compassion, concern

The inability to be good listeners appears to be a universal human failing, and it is easy to understand why a bulk of client complaints boil down to a perception by clients that "clinicians don't listen."[4] There are several factors that may impede good listening behavior. There is a clear dysjunction between the speeds at which we speak (120 to 150 words per minute) and think (500 to 750 words per minute).[4] The average person has the capacity (attention span) to listen effectively for only about 7 minutes out of each half hour of hearing.[4] These factors, coupled with the potential for other distractions during the course of an examination room dialogue between clients and clinicians, make it difficult for clients and clinicians to be effective listeners.

Clients prefer clinicians who demonstrate a sincere interest in their wishes, needs, and hopes. For clinicians to demonstrate this required compassion and concern they must be effective and productive listeners. When clinicians listen attentively, it is apparent that the clinician values the client's story and the client; the bond between doctor and client thus becomes firmer.[3,4]

There are several key elements to developing effective and productive listening skills. The clinician's verbal input to any conversation with a client should amount to 50% or less.[4] Clinicians should frame their questions and responses in shorter sentences than the ones the client has just finished. Clinicians must be aware of a client's reluctance to ask questions or seek clarifications. Clinicians should solicit questions from the client concerning the diagnosis and plans proposed in order to ensure that the client understands the patient's condition. After summarizing his/her assessment and treatment plan the clinician should ask the client to review the alternatives verbally and select the plan to be implemented.[4] The client speaks last and enjoys becoming the most important person in the visit. Clinicians must be active listeners, redirecting the client to the discussion of relevant material and maintaining eye contact as a signal that the clinician is interested in the client, the animal, and in what the client is saying. Clients will resent being interrupted unless it is accomplished tactfully. Clinicians should realize that an important reason why clients will depart from addressing the central issues of the visit and discussion is indecision. Clinicians should wait for a break in a client's narrative or interrupt in a courteous fashion by initiating verbal input with "excuse me" or "pardon me for interrupting." This stops the flow of conversation in a friendly way and provides an opening for redirecting the discussion and ascertaining why a client may appear indecisive. Several techniques can be used to facilitate the switch (e.g., clarifying—"It seems to me that you want to . . .").[4]

The art of listening is a valuable tool in any human relations setting, and veterinarians owe it to their clients and to themselves to become proficient in this important skill.

The difficult client

Ideally, veterinarians should expect the same communication behavior and listening skills from their clients as clinicians would of themselves. All clinicians know from experience that this idealized image of the client will not necessarily manifest itself in reality. The success of a client visit is the clinician's responsibility; it is a veterinarian's obligation to ensure that doctor-client interactions are successful and productive. Veterinarians must understand the psychologic basis for client resistance, anger, and other factors that contribute to the makeup of "difficult" clients. Clinicians must develop the communication skills necessary to deal with these individuals in order to discharge their responsibilities effectively.

Veterinarians can be disconcerted by indifferent clients or those possessed with superstitions, preconceived notions, or hearsay.[5] Clinicians must guard against turning to ridicule as a defense for this frustration ("How could that person be so stupid?"). A lack of education or experience regarding medical conditions and terms should not be confused with stupidity.[5] Veterinarians must realize that an emotional reaction would be counterproductive, and in these circumstances doctors must spend the time necessary to educate the client concerning their animal's condition. This explanation should include assessments of the expected time frame for response to proposed treatments and the potential for frustrations and complications during the course of treatment. The time devoted to productive discussions of this nature at the beginning of client/doctor interactions will go a long way toward promoting a strong doctor-client bond, minimizing client resistance to proposed treatment plans, and eliminating client misconceptions leading to client dissatisfaction during the course of patient care. This approach aids in ensuring that the client will remain with the clinician when treatment "A" does not work for their animal rather than branding the clinician as "incompetent" and changing veterinarians— possibly jeopardizing the care of their animal.[6,7] Dealing with fallacious client contentions while maintaining cordial relations with the client can be difficult; although clinicians may be certain of where the truth lies they must still convince the client of it in a sensitive, sincere, nondenigrating manner.[8]

Understanding client resistance. Client consent can be elusive.[6] Veterinarians often feel that a particular patient has an urgent need for diagnostic or therapeutic intervention. The sincerest expression of this urgency can be misunderstood by the client, for a variety of reasons, as unwanted pressure.[6]

Veterinarians cannot promise absolute recovery of a patient, exact healing time, or infallible diagnostic genius.[6] These inputs (approximations) often yield similar or ambiguous client outputs (client resistance) that can become a source of frustration or anger to veterinarians attempting to help the client and animal. Reluctance of clients to proceed may be based in common causes for resistance to consent—insufficient funds, genuine fear of anesthesia, etc.[6] In situations involving multiple family members, family disunity concerning the "best" approach for care of the patient often manifests. Clinicians should address their advice, admonitions, and guidance to the dominant family member. This individual is the most self-assured (least tense) and can usually be identified as the person manifesting the fewest displacement behaviors (throat clearing, hair smoothing, clothing adjustment).[6] Clinicians must deliver a clear charge to this individual, making him/her responsible for the cooperation of the rest of the group. Clinicians must counsel in these situations to the best of their abilities and direct the clients' attention to the plight of the patient, not permitting a struggle for dominance among family members.

Clinicians usually have little difficulty comprehending and dealing with the obvious expressions of reluctance. Frustration is encountered by clinicians when they are confronted with irrational client views for opposition to consent, despite overwhelming evidence against the validity of these views.[6]

The "mysterious" resistances (repression, denial, projection, rationalization) exhibited by clients can be termed defense mechanisms. The responses are automatic, involuntary, unconscious ways in which the client is reacting to a threatening situation in order to preserve self-image. Clients manifesting these behaviors are attempting to avoid conflict and to avoid facing reality but attempting to remain convinced that they are acting in the best interest of their animals.[6]

Repression is an unconscious "putting-out-of-the-mind" process.[6] The requirement for a client's decision on a proposed plan for patient care, or the specifics of a proposed option (surgery) given to the client by the clinician for care of the animal, so disturbs the client that he/she unconsciously forgets about it and does not act on the matter as he/she should. Arguing the point with the client or attempting to psychoanalyze for the client's benefit are unproductive approaches and must be avoided.[6] Clinicians should accept the excuse and retrace the necessary steps with the client in order to bring the indefinite matter to an immediate and distinct conclusion. This form of client resistance is unlikely to be encountered by critical care clinicians in an examination room setting (during the provision of emergency care), but could certainly be encountered during the extended care of critical care patients.

Denial, the first reaction to loss, is simply the refusal to accept things as they are.[6] Clients will often exhibit this behavior when confronted with the reality of serious or terminal disease in their pet. Frontal attack ("believe this now") on the client exhibiting denial behavior that is blocking decision making with respect to the patient can only result in defeat.[6] Clients must be allowed time to accommodate unpleasant information. Clinicians should maintain a logical approach to supporting the patient and express understanding and compassion for the client during this time, rather than arguing with the client's delusion. Failure by a clinician to follow a tactful approach in this circumstance can lead to a client's demand for release of the animal, at great risk to the animal, and "hospital-hopping" as the client searches for veterinary care from an individual tuned into their defensive needs.[6]

Projection is the mind's way of casting out undesirable thoughts and displacing them onto others (e.g., "I can't leave my animal here because the staff aren't the type of people he's used to").[6] These objections should be acknowledged and understood as a client's defense for fears concerning the pet. Allowing the client to observe the continued treatment of the patient enables him/her to observe how smoothly procedures progress (despite the patient's alleged bias). This approach often reassures the client and eliminates resistance to a veterinarian's recommendations.[6]

The list of potential defenses is long and finds frequent expression in veterinary medicine as a means of client resistance to consent. Successful responses to these client defenses by clinicians are peaceful ones.[6] The purpose of the defense mechanisms exhibited by clients is the avoidance of pain and discomfort. If pressured, the defensive client will become angry and the development of the necessary client-doctor bond will be impossible.

Combating client anger.[9] The basic idea is to learn how to prevent snapping into a fight-or-flight reaction. A clinician's approach to the angry client should be similar to that used when the clinician is confronted with a hostile animal. The animal receives tranquilization and so should the client—a verbal tranquilizer. Clinicians intuitively know the proper approach to the "angry" animal, but often react in an opposite fashion to the hostile client—with argument (the wrong treatment). Client anger often stems from an incorrect assessment or an incorrect approach to a client's needs (compassion, understanding) and/or poor communication between the client and the doctor and staff. The best treatment for the client is to understand the situation and to address it appropriately. A verbal tranquilizer must nourish and elevate the client, must justify his/her behavior, and must show that the clinician understands and sympathizes with the client's point of view.[9] A veterinarian must assist deescalation of this situation by imparting a tone and verbal substance to which the client can relate.[9] Statements made by clinicians to clients in these situations must be genuine and sincere: acknowledging the client's right to be angry, expressing an appreciation for how they feel, seeking clarification from the client as to the cause of the anger, and seeking the client's input on how the problems can be resolved. The goal should be reasonable negotiation between the client and doctor, resulting in the development of a mutually beneficial and satisfactory understanding ("common ground"). Clinicians are not obligated to grant every whim set forth by an abrasive or demanding client, but angry clients often present clinicians with an opportunity to take action to preserve the client-doctor relationship—the question to be answered by the clinician is "at what cost?"

Narcissism. Narcissistic clients are individuals with an inflated sense of self-importance and an insatiable need to be the center of attention.[10] Individuals with these tendencies are not uncommon in the veterinary practice setting. The client who insists the patient is "special," when in fact it is not, most likely has narcissistic tendencies.[10] These are the same individuals who may drop-in unexpectedly and demand immediate attention, may demonstrate insensitivity to the needs and feelings of others (including family members and the patient), and may fly into a rage when the doctor cannot come to the phone immediately. Narcissistic clients require a considerable effort on the part of clinicians and staff just to maintain a cordial relationship. Recognition of the narcissistic tendencies of a client allows clinicians to adopt approaches that utilize the individuals' tendencies for the benefit of the patient, rather than allowing these tendencies to lead to detrimental patient care. A productive approach with these clients is to emphasize their importance to the decision-making process and successful treatment of the patient.[10] Praise in advance for future involvement (at-home care) is also helpful in focusing the narcissistic client on the tasks at hand. Criticism should be avoided, as the narcissistic client can be crushed by the faintest hint of criticism.[10] The clinician's approach to a narcissistic client who may have failed to perceive his/her animal's needs or to deliver the prescribed treatment should be similar to the following: "We both know that no one can change the past. We need to concentrate on the present, and I'm certain you will do your part exceptionally well due to your desire and intelligence."[10] These clients need continual reassurance of their value, as their self-esteem is usually low. If the clinician fails to deliver repeated verbal support, the narcissistic client will feel rejected. This leads to anger, resistance, and lack of cooperation in the treatment of the patient. The clinician's challenge is clear: work for the patient through the client's personality smokescreen.[10]

Empathy and sympathy

Psychologists differentiate between empathy (ability to feel with a person) and sympathy (ability to feel for another person). Empathy is the ability to put yourself in the other person's place and appreciate that person's situation without becoming so emotionally involved that your judgment is affected.[11] In as much as empathy is a rational or intellectual (cognitive) skill, then it is a learnable trait. Studies on human patients reveal that satisfaction with the physician is a greater function of the use of a caring approach by the doctor than it is a function of success in treatment. Patients were more satisfied when they were allowed to tell their stories in their own words, and when they perceived that the doctors were listening and understanding.[11]

Veterinarians should develop empathy for their clients *and* patients. Individuals have difficulty learning empathy when they depersonalize their subjects (patients).[11] Pet ownership by veterinarians tends to personalize the doctor-patient relationship, facilitating empathy for patients.

To cultivate empathy for the client, clinicians must consciously make the effort to listen, pay attention, and respond with signals that let the client know the clinician is "tuning in."[11] In following this practice, empathy eventually becomes a part of a clinician's general approach to clients, and this process serves to reverse depersonalization, promote understanding, and increase the satisfaction level for clinicians involved in doctor-client-patient relationships.

The veterinarian as counselor[12]

Veterinarians are often confronted with clients demonstrating strong emotional reactions. These situations tend to make clinicians feel awkward and uncomfortable. Veterinarians must overcome their own uneasiness and develop a sense of responsibility to react appropriately (empathy) to help the client in these circumstances. Many clients require counseling during the course of doctor-client interactions, and clinicians cannot avoid the role of counselor. Certainly some clients may require more expertise than a clinician can offer (e.g., those with pathologic grief), but appropriate responses to a client's emotional distress can have a profound influence on a client's emotional well-being and serve to support most clients through difficult, emotional periods.

Antemortem counseling. Veterinarians confronted with a patient with a terminal disease must communicate this information and must also be prepared to offer emotional support to the client in this circumstance. Helping clients decide whether to discontinue the patient's treatment, who signs the euthanasia consent form, who should be present at the time of the euthanasia, what to do with the pet's remains, how to memorialize the pet, and other related matters demands more than medical counseling.[12] Clinicians cannot ignore the psychologic elements in all these issues and must provide the necessary mental health counseling to the client as well.

The issues of death and dying

Recognition of the grief process. Clinicians must familiarize themselves with the signs and stages of grief; they are not always obvious, but their recognition is vital. Symptoms of grief in clients can be physical (crying, fatigue, insomnia), intellectual (confusion, inability to concentrate, denial), emotional (sadness, anger, depression, guilt, hopelessness), social (withdrawal, alienation), and spiritual (changes in religious beliefs, visions).[13] Clients can experience anticipatory grief when terminal illness or a critical condition has been diagnosed in their animal, and clinicians must be aware of this possibility in order to act and react appropriately. The first stage in the grief or mourning process is denial, and this reaction can often occur prior to the death of the pet. Anger follows denial, and the anger can be directed at innocent parties (veterinarians, family members). Clients may be angry with themselves for not recognizing the pet's illness sooner or for being careless and allowing the pet to be injured. Bargaining and depression follow, and it is during this period that clients will feel the greatest sense of loss. Finally, clients experiencing a healthy mourning process will come to terms with their feelings and accept their pet's death. Grieving is a personal process and different people will progress through the process at different rates and in different fashions. Some individuals may skip steps, reverse the order of stages, and some individuals may never reach the desired endpoint—acceptance.[12]

Role of the veterinarian in the grief process. When interacting with clients who are experiencing manifestations of grief, clinicians should do the following: (1) reassure clients that the emotions they are experiencing and expressing are normal responses; (2) comfort clients and relieve client guilt when possible ("It's no sin to mourn him for as long as it takes, but you have absolutely no reason to feel guilty as no one could have foreseen this."[12]); (3) encourage clients to discuss their feelings with family members, friends, and the clinician; (4) acknowledge the importance of the client's loss ("It's always difficult to lose a longtime friend. I understand how you must feel."[4]); and (5) dare to be compassionate (show emotions, closeness) while maintaining professionalism. Clinicians must take steps to ensure the start of normal mourning and limit the escalation of guilt that could lead to pathologic mourning.[8] Clients will feel rejected and angry when clinicians appear not to have time to get involved with clients in these situations. Likewise, too rapid a referral to a professional counselor may be viewed by the client as rejection or an indication that their behavior is viewed as unhealthy.[12]

The decisions and process associated with the procedure of euthanasia of a client's animal have several implications for the clinician. A client may ask the veterinarian to make the euthanasia decision: "Doctor, what would you do if it were your pet?" The client must not be made to feel pressured into a decision when the veterinarian's response is to recommend euthanasia. Clients should understand the euthanasia procedure, and explanations should be made using easily understood terminology. Clinicians should avoid the use of euphemisms that may seem insincere and insensitive;[12] "painless death" should be used descriptively instead of "put to sleep" or "gone to doggie heaven," and "handling of remains" should be substituted for "disposal of the body" (connotes an equivalence between the pet and garbage). Some clients will desire to remain with the pet during the animal's euthanasia procedure. These clients should be instructed that the animal can sense their emotions and that the client can assist by providing calm emotional support to the pet. Potential physiologic responses (urinations, agonal gasps, muscle tremors) by the animal should be explained to these clients prior to performing the euthanasia of the pet. Following the euthanasia, owners may receive reinforcement of their confidence in having made the right choice for their animal by being allowed a few quiet minutes alone with the pet for personal reflection and remembrance. Sensitivity to what the client needs and wants is more important than expediency and efficiency during the euthanasia procedure. Clinicians must assess these client needs and wants, not simply assume what they will be. These highly charged emotional moments will live forever in a client's consciousness, and a veterinarian can determine how he/she will be immortalized in this memory. Condolence cards, follow-up telephone calls, and donations to animal research foundations in memory of the pet are good methods to reinforce a clinician's empathy with clients following death or euthanasia of the client's animal.

The "traumatized" client[14]—special considerations for the emergency clinic

In addition to experiencing the emotional reactions discussed previously, clients of emergency clinics are experiencing stressors that are not necessarily present for clients in nonemergency care settings. These clients may experience a wide range of emotional trauma, which sets the stage for potentially unpleasant examination room client-doctor interactions. Emergency clinic clients may be experiencing emotional distress for a variety of reasons, including uncertainty about the condition of their pet, the fact that their regular veterinarian is unavailable, concerns about the additional costs of emergency care, unfamiliarity with utilizing emergency clinics, disruption in their social and/or business schedule, and guilt over feeling responsible for an animal's injuries.[14] In addition to recognition of a client's underlying feelings (listening, observing the verbal and nonverbal clues, and gentle questioning) and empathetic response to the client's emotional needs, emergency clinic clinicians should actually undertake several preventive measures in order to reduce client "trauma."[14] These client relations steps include helpful, pleasant phone contact (avoid "telephone diagnosis," provide clear directions and statements of financial policies); easy access; a clean, attractive facility; an internal decor that facilitates client comfort; efficient triage (rapid initial evaluation, explanation of delays, posted sign explaining that animals are treated in order of seriousness of condition, not arrival); providing the client with estimates (and timely reestimates) of anticipated costs; maintaining good client communication during an animal's hospitalization (set times for telephone contact, clearly written discharge instructions, being present to discuss matters with the client at time of patient discharge, preparing client for appearance of wounds and bandages); cleaning animals prior to their discharge; and maintaining the necessary follow-up communication with the client's regular veterinarian.[14]

ETHICS
Animal, client, and veterinarian interest[15]

The relative importance of the interests of the involved parties in a doctor-client-patient relationship present the potential for ethical dilemmas for clinicians involved in critical care medicine. These legitimate interests of animal, client, and veterinarian must be weighed carefully, as options for initiation of care, continued care, and euthanasia are considered for each circumstance. The interests of the animal patient include freedom from or alleviation of pain, minimization of stress and suffering (intensity and duration), the attempted correction of the disease or injury involved when a reasonable prognosis for return to function and good quality of life exists, and humane euthanasia when indicated.

There are limits to the interests of the animals involved. Client interests (e.g., accessible and competent veterinary services, expense, family pressures, psychologic well-being, ability to handle extended home treatment) and clinician's interests (e.g., monetary gain and ability and willingness to provide financial arrangements, client satisfaction, animal welfare) must be considered in conjunction with the interests of the animal patient. Critical care clinicians must wage this ethical battle when confronted with various situations, including animals presented as strays or belonging to indigent clients, consideration for refusal of service to a known "bad debt" or "difficult" client, confidentiality and loyalty to clients in cases of owner neglect or abuse of the animal patient, euthanasia of animals with terminal or treatable maladies, and decisions on limitation of care and do-not-resuscitate orders in presumed terminal patients. When considering refusal of service due to client indigence or obnoxiousness, the doctor has the moral obligation to consider the urgency of the animal's condition.[15] Alleviation of the animal's suffering may take moral precedence, requiring the veterinarian to lay aside, at least until the animal is stabilized, his/her interest in not serving a particular client (Chapter 8).[15]

Obligations to the client

Individuals who become clients of veterinarians are entitled to have certain interests respected, as the client has employed the veterinarian for his/her services. Clinicians who accept clients have agreed to serve the clients to the best of their abilities and have a moral and ethical obligation to honor the client's interests. This tenet holds importance regardless of whether the client is receiving gratuitous service or is paying full fees for the services of the veterinarian. This principle of ethics may require that a veterinarian act differently than he/she would when considering only the interests of the animal or his/herself.

Clients are entitled to expect clinicians to be honest and trustworthy; demonstrate loyalty and protect client confidences; charge reasonable fees; demonstrate an attitude of courtesy, caring, and respect; and recognize the client's right to be consulted and to provide informed consent on diagnosis and treatment plans for their animal.[15] Clients must receive information that allows them to determine how their animal is doing and whether continued economic and emotional investments are appropriate for them.[15] Clinicians are obligated to provide competent and caring services for the animal entrusted to their care. Examples of dishonest or untrustworthy behaviors on the part of veterinarians include charging for services not performed, recommending unnecessary procedures, failure to provide clean bedding and a supply of water, and performing an autopsy on an animal without the client's consent.[15] Clients are entitled to courteous treatment (time to make difficult decisions, the undivided attention of the clinician in the examination room, having phone calls returned). The animal belongs to the client, and clinicians are obligated to respect the client's right to decide on what services are to be provided for an animal by the veterinarian. Clinicians are obligated to provide clients with the necessary information, in a manner that the client will understand, on which they can make decisions concerning treatment for their animal (informed consent).

Facilitating client decision making

Clinicians must attempt to permit clients to make their own informed, rational, and voluntary decisions on what is to be done with their animal.[15] Clients are not always rational or able to comprehend explanations when confronted with the emotional trauma of bringing their ill or injured pet to an emergency clinic. Clinicians must be careful not to direct a client's choices or force "hasty" decisions; this can be difficult in situations in which indecision may result in delayed care for or prolonged suffering by the animal patient. Identification and involvement of a relative or close friend of the client in the decision-making process may help expedite client decision making. These individuals are often more aware of the client's interests than the clinician is.[15] When the ani-

mal's condition allows time for postponing a decision, the clinician should consider continued supportive care for the patient and involvement of an empathetic third party as counselor for the client.

Protecting the patient[15]

The welfare of the animal patient is usually of paramount concern to the client and to the veterinarian. In the eyes of clinicians, some clients may not exhibit behavior that reflects appropriate concern for the animal or general societal values. Clinicians in this situation are faced with the dilemma of advocating on behalf of the animal's interests and the risk of alienating the client, possibly to the further detriment of the animal. Neglect of the animal patient associated with ignorance or laziness on the part of the client can be addressed through client education and encouragement by the clinician. Confrontation of the client in situations of abuse of the animal may be pointless, as these clients may be incapable of caring. Veterinarians are not obligated by law, in many states, to report instances of abuse or neglect of animals by their owners. If authorities are informed, there may be no assurance that the animal will be cared for properly. Euthanasia of the animal may be the end result, which is not necessarily an option in the best interest of the animal. Clinicians may suggest that the client give up the animal for adoption or insist on a particular course of action if the client wants to retain the clinician's services. The potential range of ethical approaches available to clinicians in these situations are varied, and each circumstance must be assessed carefully and individually.

The previous veterinarian

The "Principles of Veterinary Ethics" (AVMA Directory, 1989) devote a considerable amount of attention to guidelines related to handling clients of colleagues—referred or not referred. The code discusses a veterinarian's obligation to "safeguard the public and the profession against veterinarians deficient in moral character or professional competence," but at the same time "veterinarians should not belittle or injure the professional standing of another member of the profession or unnecessarily condemn the character of that person's professional acts." The code of ethics states "to criticize or disparage another veterinarian's service to a client is unethical." These sections are inconsistent, and it remains unclear how a veterinarian can safeguard the public and profession without ever injuring any doctor's professional standing. The principle that one may never criticize a colleague to or in front of a client fails to do justice under certain circumstances.[15] Clients might wonder whether such an approach or attitude reflects the loyalty they assume to be part of the veterinarian-client-patient relationship they are paying for and expect.

When clinicians, as often happens in critical care medicine, are confronted with clients that are angry at the previous veterinarian or by situations that suggest incompetence or negligence by the previous veterinarian, clinicians must weigh the interests of the previous veterinarian, the client, and the animal patient in deciding on the appropriate approach. Clinicians should avoid quick criticism of the previous veterinarian; listen to the client and deal with the patient/client based on the circumstances at hand.[15,16] It is often difficult to know precisely what was presented to the previous veterinarian when he/she saw the patient. The client might be confused or dishonest about the circumstances. Conferring with the previous veterinarian is required to get the facts straight, to avoid unjustified criticism of the previous veterinarian, and to help the patient.[15]

When confronted with clients who are angry at the previous veterinarian, taking time to listen to the client will help attenuate the client's anger (allow the client to calm down).[16] This practice makes clinicians uncomfortable (we have all been previous veterinarians), but usually allows the clinician the opportunity to redirect the client's energy and focus to the problems at hand.[16] Directing the client's attention to the animal's present condition and needs will allow the veterinarian to sidestep the issue of the previous veterinarian's treatment.[16] The clinician is obligated (client-patient interests) to contact the previous veterinarian to ascertain the complete view of the previous circumstances. The clinician has an obligation to ascertain for the client whether the previous veterinarian did indeed act incorrectly and determine whether the client has justification for legal or disciplinary action against the previous veterinarian. The veterinarian must decide whether to discuss "wrongdoings" with the colleague, inform the client of his/her findings of competence (most likely) or "incompetence" on the part of the previous veterinarian, and when indicated, whether to report the previous veterinarian to the appropriate regulatory agencies. The issues are rarely black and white. For this reason, many veterinarians may elect to remain silent and forgo pursuit of these issues, choosing simply to deal with the client and patient in medical terms. However, it can be argued that clinicians owe it to their colleagues to defend them when indicated and owe it to their clients and their profession to report the misdeeds of colleagues when appropriate.[15,16]

Indigent clients and stray animals

Veterinary medicine is not heavily involved in providing gratuitous service to needy individuals, but a strong moral argument can be made that veterinarians and society have an obligation to provide or consider subsidized veterinary services.[15] The interests of veterinarians and society in cultivating the importance of the human-animal bond and attending to the welfare of animals are involved in this issue.

An important consideration is that a veterinarian entering into a client-doctor relationship involving gratuitous service has an obligation to provide service to the best of his/her abilities. Unless the client explicitly consents to less extensive services than would normally be provided to the animal involved, the clinician is required by law to provide for these clients' and animals' interests as he/she would for clients paying the full fees.[15]

Clinicians in emergency practice are often faced with the situation in which a stray animal, or one whose owner is not yet known or present, is brought in and requires emergency treatment.[15] The veterinarian has interests in being paid for services rendered and in helping injured animals. The likelihood of even partial recovery of the costs of services provided in these circumstances is often remote. Owners may be found, claim their animals, and not feel obligated to reimburse the clinician for his/her treatment of the animal. The courts and laws in some jurisdictions may permit recovery of fees by the veterinarian in these circumstances,[15] but not always, and probably not without a legal confrontation with the owner. These are considerations that go through the minds of clinicians confronted with stray or "ownerless" animals presented for treatment. The ethical considerations of the animal's interests also enter into a clinician's deliberation on how to handle these occurrences. There are legal and moral obligations for veterinarians in these situations, and care must be exercised in arriving at appropriate resolution for each circumstance (Chapter 8). Ideally, clinicians, hospital, and veterinary associations should consider a proactive approach to these dilemmas, establishing a fund (donations) to offset the costs of these services and removing economic considerations from the equation.

Initiation of treatment, discontinuation of treatment (passive euthanasia), and do-not-resuscitate (DNR) orders

The ethical considerations associated with decisions regarding initiation of treatment, discontinuation of treatment, and DNR orders in critical care medicine are similar in veterinary and human medicine and have sparked considerable debate among clinicians, lawyers, philosophers, and the general public.[17-23] The striking developments and technologic advances in intensive care medicine have increased clinicians' abilities to preserve and extend the lives of their patients. Unfortunately, the quality of the additional life so skillfully sought can range from marginally tolerable to positively miserable.[24] What many people dread (for their pets and themselves), more than death itself, is protraction of the process of dying by artificial means.[25,26] There are situations in which the benefits of intensive care medicine are far outweighed by the harm inflicted in attempting to realize them.[25] There are moments when death should not be resisted by any and all means, moments in which the clinician should focus on the realization that death of the patient is inevitable. The clinician's attention must be placed on alleviation of the patient's suffering and preparation of the client for the eventual outcome.

Many clinicians have difficulty in admitting or accepting their inability to cure all of their patients. These individuals view this occurrence as a failure, not realizing that the patient's disease or injuries are the basis for the patient's demise. Clinicians have traditionally been instructed and programmed to do everything possible for their patients. This code of ethics has been and is interpreted to mean "do everything possible to sustain life." Many individuals have advocated that this tenet to do everything for the patient includes an obligation to facilitate "death with dignity" when death is inevitable. Veterinarians have to realize that situations arise in which a patient's disease or injuries exceed the clinician's ability to correct the patient's problems. The issues of proper utilization of limited resources present additional ethical dilemmas in this arena of clinical decision making (Chapter 5).

Veterinarians have a responsibility to their patients and clients to consider appropriate decisions on initiation of treatment, withdrawal or limitation of treatment, or resuscitation of patients with severe or terminal disease. These considerations must include reflection on the severity of the patient's disease (salvageability), realistic expectations for quality of life of patients with treatment, the risks of doing more harm than good with interventions, client economic concerns, and the potential for clinician fallibility. The unknown factors associated with a patient—certainty of diagnosis and prognosis and fear of incorrect assessment—often lead to uneasiness on the part of the doctors contemplating DNR or limitation-of-treatment orders.

Clients and patients look to the veterinarian for direction and input on decision making involving the sensitive issues of initiation or discontinuation of therapy in apparently terminal patients. There are no easy answers to these ethical issues, and careful, complete communication with clients and foresight on the part of the clinician are required. Veterinarians must anticipate and address with clients beforehand, whenever possible, circumstances that may arise requiring life and death decisions in the intensive care unit.

Euthanasia

There are a myriad of ethical issues associated with a veterinarian's role in the euthanasia process for a client's animal. Jerrold Tannenbaum explores many of these issues, and their permutations, in his book *Veterinary Ethics*.[15] This discussion will focus on some of the ethical considerations surrounding euthanasia of critically ill or injured animals.

Clinicians in critical care medicine face daily interactions with clients considering the option of euthanasia for their animals. These are not easy interactions, and many doctors are uncomfortable handling this very important aspect of the doctor-client-patient relationship. Veterinarians must be prepared to handle these situations with empathy, patience, and understanding. These client interactions are unavoidable in the setting of critical care medicine. Veterinarians who maintain that they cannot become involved in the psychosocial dynamics of their clients' emotions are fooling themselves; they are already involved and might as well be involved skillfully and compassionately.[15]

Veterinarians must consider the interests of the client and animal when the decision of euthanasia for the animal is contemplated. Clinicians must facilitate the client's understanding of the animal's condition. A discussion should not be initiated with the mention of euthanasia; clients must be prepared for the discussion of that option for their pet through a clinician's description of the animal's diagnosis and prognosis. The decision to perform euthanasia of the animal must be made by the owner. The clinician must provide the client with a comfortable environment in which to discuss options, be prepared to answer client questions, assist in the initiation of the grief process, and must allow the client the time required to accommodate the decision of euthanasia for the animal. The clinician can advocate on behalf of the animal, pointing out that the animal is suffering when the situation is hopeless and allaying the fears of the client concerning outcome and treatment when a decision against euthanasia may be in the best interest of the animal. As veterinarians, we value the lives of our animal patients and do not have to grant without question the wishes of clients opting for euthanasia of their animal when the potential exists to restore the animal to health or a good quality of life. The options of treatment alternatives, payment arrangements, adoption of the animal, and other possibilities should be explored in these cases. The client must realize that they are making the decision to euthanize their animal, that the decision is final, that the animal has interests and value, that all options have been explored, and that the decision is in the best interests of the animal and themselves.

When the decision to euthanize the animal has been made, the clinician must conduct the procedure with empathy and professionalism. The process should not be hurried, and the clinician should avoid distractions during this procedure and should devote his/her attention to the client. Clients should be given the opportunity to be with the animal during the euthanasia procedure. The client should be instructed on what to expect (agonal gasps, muscle twitches, open eyes) during the euthanasia of their pet, if they choose to observe. Veterinarians must assure clients that these reflex responses occur following death and the animal is not feeling discomfort. Clinicians should allow the client to be with the animal for a few minutes of quiet reflection following euthanasia. The animal's remains should be handled with dignity, and veterinarians should be willing to assist clients in making necessary arrangements. Clinicians should demonstrate genuine concern and compassion; varying degrees of counseling and follow-up communication by the doctor will be required with each client. Veterinarians should dare to be personal in these circumstances by reassuring clients that their decision was the right one and that it represented a true reflection of their lifelong devotion, respect, and compassion for their pet.

REFERENCES

1. Antelyes J. On being compassionate. J Am Vet Med Assoc 1987;190:1534-1536.
2. Antelyes J. Communication behavior vs. communication. J Am Vet Med Assoc 1988;193:178-180.
3. Antelyes J. Talking to clients. J Am Vet Med Assoc 1988;193:1502-1504.
4. Antelyes J. Listening: heart and soul of doctor/client relationships. J Am Vet Med Assoc 1989;194:205-207.
5. Antelyes J. Idealized Image. J Am Vet Med Assoc 1987;191:400-412.
6. Antelyes J. Understanding Client Resistance. J Am Vet Med Assoc 1988;192:1690-1692.
7. Snyder G. Keep 'em Coming back for More. DVM 1986; June:11-12.
8. Antelyes J. Self delusion/self defeat. J Am Vet Med Assoc 1988;192:490-492.
9. Antelyes J. Using an old skill-anew. J Am Vet Med Assoc 1987;190:1270-1272.
10. Antelyes J. Narcissistic clients. J Am Vet Med Assoc 1989;194:1032-1034.
11. Antelyes J. Empathy—Innate Gift or Learnable Skill? J Am Vet Med Assoc 1988;192:1373-1375.
12. Antelyes J. The veterinarian as counselor. J Am Vet Med Assoc 1989;195:732-734.
13. Lagoni L, Hetts S. Pet loss counseling in veterinary medicine. Trends 1989;5:33-36.
14. Milligan JA. Care of the traumatized client. J Vet Emerg Crit Care Soc 1986;3:18-21.
15. Tannenbaum J. Veterinary ethics. Baltimore: Williams & Wilkins, 1989.
16. Antelyes J. The previous veterinarian. J Am Vet Med Assoc 1989;195:194-195.
17. Paris JJ, Reardon FE. Dilemmas in intensive care medicine: An ethical and legal analysis. J Int Care Med 1986;1:75-90.
18. Richards EP. Critical care decision-making. J Int Care Med 1986;1:297.
19. Tomlinson T, Brody H. Ethics and communication in do-not-resuscitate orders. N Engl J Med 1988;318:43-46.
20. Zimmerman JE, Knaus WA, Sharpe SM, Anderson AS, Draper EA, Wagner DP. The use and implications of do not resuscitate orders in intensive care units. JAMA 1986;255:351-356.
21. Seravalli EP. The dying patient, the physician, and the fear of death. N Engl J Med 1988;319:1728-1730.
22. Ruark JE, Raffin TA. Initiating and withdrawing life support—Principles and practice in adult medicine. N Engl J Med 1988;318:25-30.
23. Schneiderman LJ, Spragg RG. Ethical decisions in discontinuing mechanical ventilation. 1988;318:984-988.
24. Pepe PE. Whom to resuscitate. In Civetta JM, Taylor RW, Kirby RR, eds. Critical care. Philadelphia: JB Lippincott, 1988:93-102.
25. Young EWD. Life and death in the ICU: Ethical considerations. In Civetta JM, Taylor RW, Kirby RR, eds. Critical care. Philadelphia: JB Lippincott, 1988:39-49.
26. Snider GL. "The do-not-resuscitate order": ethical and legal imperative or medical decision? Am Rev Respir Dis 1991; 143:665-674.

8 Legal Considerations in Critical Care and Emergency Medicine

Robert J. Murtaugh

There are several aspects associated with the practice of critical care and emergency medicine that carry with them important legal ramifications that need to be considered by the veterinarian. There are many legal considerations, such as advertising, sanitation and waste disposal, employee issues, fee collection, Good Samaritan laws, libel and slander issues, animal cruelty, and others that have been previously discussed in the veterinary literature. The specific areas that will be addressed in this chapter include negligence (including lack of informed consent), premises and public liability issues, drug liabilities, medical records, communication issues, euthanasia and animal carcass disposal issues, stray and unclaimed animal issues, and emergency telephone and treatment concerns.

NEGLIGENCE

The simplified definition of negligence states that this form of malpractice occurs when a veterinarian deviates from the accepted standards for diagnosis, treatment, or monitoring of a patient under his/her care. For a client to recover damages, negligence must be established, and it must be demonstrated that this deviation from acceptable practice resulted in injury or damage to the patient and/or client. If it can be demonstrated, contributory negligence on the part of a client may decrease the liability of the veterinarian, for example, if the client does not come in for scheduled follow-up visit.

An individual who represents him/herself as a specialist will be held to a higher standard of practice than the generalist when professional negligence is alleged. The generalist is expected to recognize problems that may be beyond his/her capabilities and offer referral to a specialist when circumstances (a specialist in the area) provide this option.

Traditionally, accepted standards of veterinary practice had been based on the concept of the "locality rule." The "locality rule" holds that a veterinarian's professional competence will be judged against his/her peers in the same or similar locality. In the present circumstances of advanced communication networks, national continuing education programs, and the burgeoning amount of scientific information available, practitioners, especially specialists, should expect to be held to the standards of a national locality rule. Veterinarians are obligated to be aware of, and to incorporate into their practice, advances and changes in the practice standards of their profession.

Failure to arrive at a correct diagnosis does not necessarily constitute negligence. If a veterinary clinician has followed prudently the accepted standards in approach to diagnosis (obtains a good history, performs a complete physical examination, and obtains the proper ancillary diagnostic evaluations, and exercises acceptable skill and judgment in interpreting the findings), a misdiagnosis or missed diagnoses may not constitute negligence. Veterinarians are not held to a standard of perfection in determining what ails an animal. The yardstick is the standard generally followed by veterinarians, and expert testimony is required, unless the negligence is obvious or flagrant and "speaks for itself" (res ipsa loquitur), to determine what this standard is. Veterinarians are obligated to keep their knowledge current and to avoid taking "short cuts" with their patients. Many veterinarians find themselves taking shortcuts in order to save the client a few dollars. Unless the client is informed of the options and consents to this approach, the potential for allegations of negligence exist should misdiagnosis occur.

In addition to the potential liability associated with undertaking improper or unnecessary treatment, veterinarians can be sued for negligence related to improper care or monitoring of the patient during treatment. This potential for liability is illustrated well by considering the surgical patient. Once the patient enters surgery, it should not be left without professional observation until it is safe to do so. The veterinarian is liable for the negligence of others that assist in the surgery. The veterinarian should have at hand and use all equipment and materials that might be needed to prevent or care for complications that arise during surgery. Care should be exercised to ensure that all materials (sponges and surgical instruments) are accounted for; that is, they are not left in the patient. The surgeon should be familiar with any of the animal's allergies or conditions unrelated to the reason for surgery that may condition the response to situations arising in surgery. Veterinarians must ensure that patients receive the necessary monitoring required; for example, seizure patients should not be left unattended overnight. Allegations of negligence may arise when animals escape, injure themselves in cages, are injured during restraint, or are injured by other animals during hospitalization, or when animals contract a contagious disease during hospitalization. Veterinarians must take every precaution to prevent these occurrences in order to minimize the potential for liability should they occur.

There are statutes of limitations that apply to the period of time within which lawsuits must be commenced. Statutes related to allegations of malpractice vary from state to state, but in general they require action by the plaintiff within 1 to 3 years of the injury. Statutes of limitations may commence to run at a date later than the surgery or treatment giving rise to the injury, if the plaintiff is not remiss in discovering the cause (alleged negligence) of an injury at an earlier date (rule of discovery). The individual (client) is expected to show reasonable diligence in attempting to uncover negligence that may have caused any injury to an animal once that injury has been noted by the client. The statute of limitations related to contractual liability is generally of longer duration—5 to 10 years. An argument could be made that services performed on a pet are similar to those performed on other pieces of "property," and delayed malpractice actions against veterinarians could be attempted in this fashion. It should be noted that, as a result of the increasing awareness of the sentimental and emotional value of animals, malpractice awards in veterinary medicine are moving in a direction that sets the actual value of an animal at greater than the "property value."

CONTRACTUAL LIABILITY ISSUES

The veterinarian-client relationship is based on either a verbal or written contractual agreement. Either party is entitled to seek compensation if the other party fails to perform or performs in a manner contrary to their agreement. A veterinarian in general practice is not obligated to treat an animal, even in an emergency situation (regardless of how inhumane this refusal may appear), presented to his/her hospital unless that duty has been imposed by law or regulation. A veterinarian in an emergency practice might be held to an implied contractual duty to render emergency treatment when confronted with a similar circumstance because of the nature of his/her practice. The veterinarian or his/her agent must agree to treat and/or propose a course of treatment that is agreed to by the client or his/her agent before a contract is established. A simple phone conversation resulting in agreement to examine an animal constitutes a contract.

A veterinarian-client contract can be terminated in many ways. The conclusion of treatment terminates the contract whether or not the results are successful, and the veterinarian is entitled to his/her fee. An unsuccessful treatment may spawn a malpractice action or counterclaim for the veterinarian's fees by the client. The burden is on the client to prove a deficiency in treatment by the veterinarian. The contract can be terminated at the will of the client. The veterinarian can terminate a contractual arrangement with a client provided he/she provides the client reasonable time to find another veterinarian and provided service is not discontinued at a critical phase of treatment. If an animal is at a stage of treatment at which discontinuance would be damaging, the veterinarian is obligated to continue treatment until that stage is past (regardless of the prospects for payment). The implications of a veterinarian-client contract are that the veterinarian will continue service until the animal is cured or dies, until the veterinarian has done what was promised, or until the client terminates the contract.

EMERGENCY TREATMENT
Telephone contact

Advice offered to the owner of an animal not currently under your treatment may not create a contract. If the person seeking the free advice subsequently feels they have been damaged by the advice, they have no recourse. If a client calls a veterinarian in the middle of the night and tells his veterinarian that there is an emergency; there are different considerations. If the veterinarian advises the person that it is not necessary to see the animal until some later time and the animal dies or its condition worsens in the interim, the burden would be on the veterinarian to defend his/her decision as proper.

Finances

In emergency situations, the exact fee for services rendered might not be discussed before treatment is instituted. In many situations, the veterinarian may not know at the outset exactly how much service or medication may be required to accomplish the task at hand. A veterinarian is obligated to obtain consent for treatment costs whenever possible, but in the absence of a specific agreement, the veterinarian is entitled to a reasonable fee under these circumstances. If the owner ratifies the veterinarian's action in treating the animal, a contractual relationship exists. Whether a veterinarian can or should attempt to recover his/her fee from an owner who refuses to pay under these circumstances is a mixed question of law and practice policy. It is not right for an individual to receive benefit from another at the other's expense without compensating that person, regardless of the fact that no agreement was made. Should the veterinarian, on weighing the pros and cons of the decision, decide to pursue collection of a fee in those cases, in rendering a decision the court will take into consideration the nature of the emergency, the humane aspects of the veterinarian's actions, the value of the animal, and the owner's ability to pay.

Veterinarians should get approval for treatment of an animal from the parents when an animal is brought to the clinic for treatment by a minor. Parents of a minor are not likely to be held accountable for the cost of treatment of a pet animal unless they give direct consent to the treatment. When an animal is presented for emergency treatment by a "good Samaritan" and the owner is subsequently identified, the owner may insist that he/she is not bound to pay a fee for unauthorized treatment. The courts, unless statutes specifically state otherwise, may not protect the veterinarian in the event the animal was euthanized for humane reasons before an owner was identified or should the owner feel entitled to damages because of unauthorized treatment.

INFORMED CONSENT

The doctrine of informed consent imposes two duties: to disclose so the client can understand, and to obtain specific consent for contemplated expenses, procedures, and treatments. When deviations from the original plans, especially those involving sedation and anesthesia, are contemplated or additional costly procedures are indicated, every attempt should be made to obtain additional informed consent. There may arise circumstances in which critical, immediate intervention is necessary; however, if the situation is not critical and the risks and/or costs are high, clients should be consulted. The argument that complete disclosure may be too upsetting to a client is not viewed as an adequate defense. Clients have a right to know the possible risks and complications to be expected, regardless of how that may make them feel. The use of consent forms requiring client signatures is recommended, and these forms should be explicit and specific (especially with respect to innovative or experimental treatments).

Innovative (nonstandard) approaches to patient treatment should be closely related to careful attention to informed consent guidelines. The condition of the patient should help determine how innovative an approach to the care of that patient should be. If the condition appears hopeless and all known procedures have failed or are likely to fail, a veterinarian should be encouraged to try new approaches that are rational, provided the client is consulted and agrees to the approach. Courts have protected veterinarians in these circumstances previously.

Cases presented by third parties (boarding kennels) and minors represent special circumstances in which veterinary emergency clinicians may be required, due to the critical nature of the animal's condition, to act prior to receiving informed consent from adult owners. Should these owners fail to agree to pay for services using the argument that they were not consulted and did not give consent, they may not be bound legally. However, depending on the circumstances, a court may allow collection of a fee on the principle that it is not right for one to receive benefit from another without compensating that person for the services, regardless of the fact no agreement was made.

DRUGS

A veterinarian prescribing treatment (drugs) has a duty to know the product, to know his/her patient, to inform and explain, and to properly label and prescribe. Drug products should be purchased from reliable sources and handled and stored properly to avoid deterioration, contamination, and loss (especially narcotics and other controlled substances). A veterinarian must be familiar with the indications, contraindications, side effects, and proper dosages for drugs dispensed. Clients must be informed of potential risks of prescribed treatments for their animals. Failure to test an animal for a potential allergy or failure to recognize and take corrective action for adverse reactions could be grounds for malpractice actions. Follow the patient's progress and plan to see the animal at an appropriate interval following initiation of the treatment. Drugs should be dispensed in containers with child-proof safety caps. Drug labels should clearly state the date, veterinarian's name and address, drug information (name, strength, quantity dispensed, directions for use), instructions on proper storage, and pertinent warning labels. Contributory negligence on the part of clients can be used to help defend against claims related to drug liability, for example, failure to disclose essential facts about the animal or failure to medicate as instructed.

Veterinary emergency clinicians are occasionally faced with situations (telephone calls) in which clients cannot reach their regular veterinarian and they "need a refill." Failure to examine a patient before prescribing treatment can lead to potential for liability should the patient experience an undesirable result.

Veterinarians often prescribe drugs for unapproved (other than labeled) uses. Clients should be consulted and provide informed consent, and the veterinarian should be prepared to justify the use of the drug on firm scientific rationale.

A responsible approach to the discovery of drug intoxication in a pet (marijuana, cocaine) is to share the diagnosis with the client and allow them an opportunity to respond. If the client appears to be the source of the illegal drugs, the client should be informed that future "violations" will be reported to appropriate drug authorities. There is no client-veterinarian privilege of confidentiality that the client could use as a defense in this situation.

MEDICAL RECORDS

Medical records and radiographs remain the physical property of the veterinarian. Clients are entitled to the information and to copies of the medical record and radiographs on request. Veterinarians should take care to ensure a standard, complete, retrievable, organized approach to maintaining medical records. Medical records can be an important defense against litigation, especially when records of informed consent provided by clients and records of euthanasia and disposal decisions are properly documented.

If an animal is taken out of the hospital against the advice of the veterinarian, a signed release from the client should be obtained and should be kept as part of the medical record.

As a general rule, communications between a veterinarian and a client and the medical records maintained by a veterinarian are not privileged unless there is a state statute specifically granting the privilege. Animals are property, and courts are not likely to protect the veterinarian-animal

owner relationship any more than the automobile owner-mechanic relationship. The purposes of the laws concerning professional communications are to encourage full disclosure by the client to the professional so the professional can perform his/her function and to protect the individual from disclosure of information that would be injurious. Ethical considerations should compel veterinarians to disclose medical records information only to the client unless the client consents to disclosure to other individuals or unless the veterinarian has been ordered to hand over records by the court.

EUTHANASIA AND DISPOSAL

Communication with the client becomes especially important when euthanasia of an animal is considered. Before euthanizing an animal, the consent of the rightful owner or authorized agent should be given, preferably in writing on a consent form. Failure to euthanize an animal following acceptance of the request constitutes breaking of a contract, and the veterinarian is liable. A veterinarian does not have any greater right than a lay person to euthanize for humane reasons a client's animal without consent or an injured stray animal, unless state law provides otherwise. There, undoubtedly, are situations in which killing as an act of mercy is justified, but the veterinarian is vulnerable in a legal sense unless owner consent has been obtained. Veterinarians in emergency and critical care practices are likely to find themselves in these circumstances (owner out of town, incorrect phone numbers) and should proceed cautiously in making decisions on euthanasia and other forms of treatment without informed consent of the owner. In such circumstances, the veterinarian must use good judgment about what to do and hope the client agrees. If the client disagrees and decides to attempt to collect damages, the veterinarian's defense would be that other veterinarians would have acted similarly.

Disposal of an animal's remains following its death or euthanasia must be handled properly to avoid liability claims. The client retains control of the animal's body (property), and the veterinarian must honor an owner's wishes. The veterinarian has no right to dispose of an animal's remains without consent of the owner. Showing a client the body of their pet when the veterinarian has reason to believe the client will be shocked by the experience may pose a liability risk. Nevertheless, the veterinarian is obligated to provide the body of the animal to the client, in absence of a health regulation preventing delivery (such as zoonosis), on request. The body of a dead animal should not be "held hostage" for fee collection;

refusal to yield the body to a client might be regarded as a punitive act rather than a sound collection procedure. Retention and use of an animal's body for medical purposes or autopsy without client consent could give rise to a cause for action.

COMMUNICATION—LEGAL OVERTURES

Many actions brought against veterinarians by clients are not directly related to how the animal was treated, but often are related to how they (the clients) were treated. Communication is the key to establishing good will and a successful practice. Communication is also the best way to avoid malpractice suits and complaints to the state veterinary boards. If a veterinarian is too busy to talk to a client, does not explain the risks involved in a particular procedure, does not discuss the chances for successful treatment in the context of the animal's present condition, does not take time to update the client on the patient's condition during hospitalization, and/or does not provide adequate information or instruction on aftercare required at the time of discharge of the patient from the hospital—the stage is set for potential malpractice actions (regardless of how appropriate the treatment of the animal). It is the veterinarian's responsibility to explain matters in terms the client will understand. Informed consent must be obtained, and stating the choices and the facts is not enough—they must be stated in a manner that the client understands.

A veterinarian's patience is often tried by demanding clients. These clients may even demonstrate anger toward the veterinarian. Public displays of temper by a veterinarian toward a client or in the presence of a client could result in a suit for emotional distress ("tort of outrage"). The plaintiff must prove that the action or words were "outrageous" and that emotional distress was extreme and real—not just a cause of hurt feelings. However, any veterinarian who values good client relations would do well to refrain from these outbursts regardless of the potential for liability.

ABANDONED AND STRAY ANIMALS

Occasionally, veterinary emergency clinicians may be confronted with an animal that is abandoned by its owner. Most states provide a mechanism for resolution of these circumstances. The approach required involves sending a notice to the owner, by registered mail and/or newspaper advertisement, that the animal is ready to be discharged from the hospital. The time frame required between notification and the date the veterinarian can dispose of the animal varies from state to state. Notices sent to owners of abandoned animals should specifically state deadlines for reestablishing contact, a description of the animal, the client's ongoing financial obligation, and the planned disposition of the animal. Admission forms containing a statement about disposition should the animal be abandoned helps strengthen the veterinarian's contractual rights of disposition in these situations. The methods available for disposition of abandoned animals by veterinarians varies from state to state (adoption, euthanasia, giving to a pound).

A similar approach (newspaper advertisement) is recommended for trying to contact owners of stray animals. Veterinarians are obligated to make reasonable attempts to contact possible owners of stray animals prior to making choices on disposition.

ASSISTANCE FROM CLIENT

There are legal implications to consider when a client assists the veterinarian or observes treatment or surgery being performed on an animal. Veterinary practice acts do not state that veterinarians should not use the client's assistance. There are many situations in which the use of client assistance may be reasonable and appropriate; however, veterinarians should keep in mind that any negligence or lack of foresight on the veterinarians part that might lead to a client's injury can also lead to a damage suit. When a client requests assistance in restraint, get a technician. A veterinarian's defense, in cases of owner injury from bites or scratches while helping restrain their pets, can be strengthened by asking a client before proceeding whether the animal has a fractious nature (if the answer is yes, get a technician; if no, and the animal bites, you showed foresight), warning the client of possible dangers associated with helping in restraint, and showing the owner the proper method of restraint to use. The age, experience, and size of the owner; the temperament of the animal; the particular type of treatment to be administered; and the past experiences with the animal are among the factors a veterinarian should consider when permitting an owner to participate in restraint and treatment. The veterinarian is not automatically liable just because an owner is injured under these circumstances, especially if it can be demonstrated that it is common practice among veterinarians to have clients participate in restraint during the particular treatment in question and if the client has restrained his/her animals under similar circumstances in the past.

Permitting clients or other individuals to watch surgery or participate (e.g., cesarean section) in surgery contains some legal hazards. Should the client faint and injure themselves by falling or be "shocked" by the graphic nature of the experience, the veterinarian may face a threat of legal action. Veterinarians should provide clients with the proper warnings and exercise foresight in attempting to minimize these risks and not ignore their potential significance as grounds for lawsuits.

PREMISES LIABILITY—ORDINARY NEGLIGENCE

Litigation can result from injuries received by visitors to hospital premises. The persons who enter a veterinarian's office are owed the duty of reasonable care for their safety. Reasonable care implies that the veterinarian will demonstrate foresight equal to that of other reasonably prudent people in control of property in discovering and correcting conditions on the premises that might produce injury to visitors. A veterinarian is not an insurer of the safety of visitors, but ordinary care is required, for example, in providing safe sidewalks, steps, floors, chairs, and appropriate warnings to restrain pets in the lobby. The usual rules of negligence apply—there must be demonstration of a dangerous condition that was known or should have been known, the condition must be shown to be directly involved as the cause of the claimant's injury, and the claimant must not have demonstrated contributory negligence. In premises liability suits, the length of time a hazardous condition has been permitted to exist is an important factor. This is especially true with respect to the hazard posed by less than prompt removal of ice and snow. The trend of the law has been toward greater consumer protection, and the safe course is to foresee and correct situations that may lead to negligent actions and to maintain adequate public liability insurance coverage.

INSURANCE AND GUIDELINES

Malpractice insurance represents professional liability protection—veterinarians must extend their range of insurance coverage by purchasing public liability insurance and professional extension insurance to protect against claims of ordinary negligence and loss of animals through fire, vandalism, and flood.

Concerning claims of malpractice, veterinarians are obligated to inform their insurance carriers of claims or potential claims on a timely basis; insurance companies are not obligated to settle a claim without an investigation, and insurance companies should not settle a claim without the consent of the veterinarian—that is, they are obligated to defend him/her. There are a variety of considerations to take into account when deciding to defend or settle a claim.

Veterinarians are advised to follow these guidelines in order to minimize their potential for professional liability claims: do not guarantee results, advise the client of risks before proceeding, maintain complete records, label all dispensed products, avoid having the owner assist in restraint, avoid mentioning alternative treatments after unsuccessful treatment, avoid apologetic statements (express concern for the client and animal, but do not admit fault), and be cautious about pressing an unhappy client for payment.

When confronted with an actual or potential claim, veterinarians should notify the insurance carrier promptly, cooperate with the insurance representative (do not initiate contact with the client directly), and do not discuss possible malpractice, either your own or another doctor's, with clients or attorneys.

SUPPLEMENTAL READINGS

1. Katz K. AVMA professional liability insurance trust guidelines. J Am Vet Med Assoc 1987;191:294-295.
2. Hannah HW. Legal briefs from the Journal of the American Veterinary Medical Association. Schaumburg, IL: American Veterinary Medical Association, 1986.
3. Sanberg L. Misconceptions about malpractice insurance. J Am Vet Med Assoc 1988;192:322-323.
4. Shouse D. Hang on! Is luck your best bet against lawsuits? Vet Econ 1988; April:41-45.

9 Transition of the Patient from Critical Care

Paul M. Kaplan

Admission into the intensive care unit (ICU) is no longer restricted to patients with immediately life-threatening crises. The ICU houses patients requiring various levels of intensive care. Critical care is expensive, time-consuming, and in demand. It is often obvious which patients are in need of critical care admission. Patients demonstrating an uncertain physiologic status or progression of their condition to a more unstable status, as a result of a primary disease process or complications, should be admitted to the ICU until improvement is noted. However, the final decision to transfer a patient from the ICU to the general wards is often a difficult one, despite the apparent resolution of the acute physiologic abnormalities that led to admission to the ICU. Some patients deemed stable and subsequently transferred from the ICU will die despite expectations for their survival. How then do we decide which patients may be safely transferred to the general wards? There are no clear-cut guidelines. Clinicians must rely on rational clinical decision making based on improvement in patient attitude, physiologic parameters, and laboratory parameters, along with a measure of clinical intuition. Improved instrumentation and technology enhances but does not replace clinical judgment.

INTERMEDIATE CARE WARD

The concept of an intermediate care ward providing extensive nursing care and noninvasive monitoring of a physiologically stable patient is an interesting, feasible concept. Many of our physiologically stable ICU patients have disorders requiring careful monitoring or frequent administration of medication (e.g., patient with deep corneal ulcer).

Admission to the intermediate care ward should be considered when the patient is physiologically stable, shows progressive clinical improvement, and is deemed unlikely to have complications develop during recovery, but still requires intensive nursing care. This intermediate ward allows for increased monitoring and observation of the patient over that found in general wards. This triage process serves to "free up" space, equipment, and personnel resources in the ICU for unstable patients while providing a continuum of care for these recovering patients.

The intermediate care ward should be staffed with a conscientious, competent nurse-technician who has had experience with routine nursing duties and is adept at recognizing early warning signals suggesting changes in patient status. This individual will have intimate contact with these patients and should readily recognize and report any changes in patient status to the clinician on duty. His/her responsibility should be limited to this ward to ensure that patient care is not compromised.

SUGGESTED GUIDELINES FOR DISCHARGE OR TRANSFER FROM THE INTENSIVE CARE UNIT
Cardiovascular abnormalities

The inability of an animal's heart to maintain normal circulation (heart failure) often prompts admission to the ICU. Following careful patient monitoring and the administration of various cardiac medications, clinicians must decide when the patient is stable and may be safely transferred from the critical care unit. To make this assessment, knowledge of the underlying cause and pathophysiology for the animal's cardiovascular instability, the nature of the disease process, and the responsiveness of the dysfunction to medical or surgical management must be realized.

Cardiovascular instability can result from myocardial dysfunction (systolic and diastolic), valvular abnormalities causing pressure (e.g., aortic stenosis) or volume overloads (mitral regurgitation) to the heart, dysrhythmias, high cardiac output states (hyperthyroidism, arteriovenous fistulas), and myocardial restrictive diseases (e.g., pericardial tamponade). Specific management of various cardiovascular abnormalities including congestive heart failure is discussed in Chapter 17.

The most important principle of management is to establish a proper diagnosis and initiate treatment based on the underlying pathologic and pathophysiologic mechanism responsible for the clinical signs present in the patient. Following initial treatment of the cardiovascular patient, what parameters are useful in gauging when the patient is "stable" for transfer from the critical care unit?

Serial monitoring of heart rate and rhythm, peripheral-pulse quality, indexes of peripheral perfusion, thoracic radiographs, arterial blood pressure, blood gases, serum electrolytes, and invasively monitored parameters requiring instrumentation (central venous pressure, pulmonary artery pressure, pulmonary capillary wedge pressure, cardiac output, mixed venous oxygen tension) aid in this clinical decision-making process. Flow charts are helpful in evaluating trends in these parameters.

Heart rate. Dysfunction of the cardiovascular system often leads to changes in heart rate. Heart rate in critical care patients is most commonly elevated in an attempt to improve cardiac output, restore peripheral perfusion, and/or increase systemic arterial blood pressure. Cardiac output is often depressed in animals with primary myocardial disease, valvular disease, pericardial disease, and hypovolemia (e.g., hemorrhagic shock). As arterial blood pressure decreases with compromised cardiovascular function, numerous compensatory mechanisms occur.[1,2] Carotid sinus discharge decreases, causing a decrease in vagus nerve impulses and an increase in sympathetic impulses to the heart. This adrenergic stimulation increases heart rate and increases cardiac contractility, causing an increase in systemic arterial blood pressure. Appropriate medical or surgical (e.g., pericardiectomy) intervention, leading to improved cardiac output and decreased adrenergic drive to the heart, is obvious as heart rate declines. Serial improvement or normalization of systemic arterial blood pressure and normalization of an animal's heart rate for a 24- to 48-hour period is a favorable prognostic sign.

Rhythm. Cardiac dysrhythmias resulting from cardiac and extracardiac disease are a common cause of morbidity and mortality in critical care patients. Clinicians must correctly identify the dysrhythmia, determine the hemodynamic and electrophysiologic significance of the dysrhythmia, search for an underlying cause (e.g., electrolyte imbalances, hypoxemia), and institute appropriate therapy (Chapter 17). Intermittent lead II electrocardiographic tracings are less accurate representations of the predominant cardiac rhythm in an animal, and continuous electrocardiographic monitoring should be maintained.

The ultimate therapeutic goal of reestablishing sinus rhythm may not be possible in all instances (atrial fibrillation, third-degree atrioventricular block), and achievement of a stable hemodynamic status with a "controlled" ventricular rate is the goal in these situations. For example, a large-breed dog with severe left atrial enlargement and atrial fibrillation (heart rate exceeding 250 beats per minute) will have dramatically improved ventricular diastolic filling and cardiac output following pharmacologic intervention and slowing of the heart rate to 120 to 160 beats per minute, but will likely remain in atrial fibrillation.

Coronary blood flow occurs mainly in diastole, and oxygenation of the myocardium may be compromised in animals with severe tachycardic states due to decreased time in diastole. If the tachycardia persists, myocardial irritability may be increased and the potential for perpetuation or worsening of the dysrhythmia exists.[3,4]

The initial manifestation and evidence for progression of cardiac arrhythmias are important considerations when a clinician is contemplating institution of antiarrhythmic therapy in an animal. Controversy exists concerning when antiarrhythmic therapy should be administered. Occasional atrial or ventricular premature beats in an animal with apparently normal cardiovascular status are generally not treated. Supraventricular tachycardia may occur without significant effect on cardiac output (e.g., fever, pain, excitement, hypokalemia, hypoxia) In these instances the strength of the peripheral pulse and capillary refill time are normal. Resolution of any underlying physiologic cause of the tachycardia results in normalization of heart rate. Rarely does the supraventricular tachycardia in these settings result in hemodynamic compromise. Multiform ventricular premature beats, ventricular premature beats occurring during the vulnerable period of ventricular repolarization (T wave of the previous complex), and frequent ventricular premature beats are usually treated with administration of antiarrhythmic agents (Chapter 17).

Arrhythmias are generally treated if underlying structural disease of the heart is present (e.g., primary myocardial disease), if heart failure is a possible cause of the rhythm disturbance, or if progression of the arrhythmia is possible (e.g., ventricular tachycardia to ventricular fibrillation).[5-7]

Documenting a trend toward improvement and/ or normalcy in cardiac rhythm over a 24- to 48-hour period is helpful in assessing the patient for transfer from the critical care unit. Improvement may involve a decrease in the frequency of ectopic pacemaker activity, restoration of a stable hemodynamic status with ectopic pacemaker activity present, and/or abolishment of "malignant" arrhythmias (e.g., sustained ventricular tachycardia). Thoracic radiography should be repeated if pulmonary venous congestion or pulmonary edema was previously present.

Pressures. Following treatment (e.g., pericardiectomy for constrictive pericardial disease, inotropic therapy in primary myocardial disease), a decrease in central venous pressure may be apparent with improved cardiac performance regardless of the etiology of the cardiac dysfunction. However, central venous pressure is less useful in accurately reflecting the hemodynamic status of the left side of the heart than that of the right side of the heart.

Pulmonary artery diastolic pressure (in the absence of pulmonary disease) and pulmonary capillary wedge pressure are accurate reflections of left atrial filling pressures. Dogs with congestive heart failure and pulmonary edema will typically have pulmonary capillary wedge pressure in excess of 23 mm Hg.[8] However, dogs with chronic elevations of left atrial pressure (chronic mitral valvular disease) may tolerate much higher pulmonary capillary wedge pressure without the development of pulmonary edema.[8] This tolerance is due in part to a compensatory increased pulmonary lymphatic flow above the normal resting level. Monitoring pulmonary capillary wedge pressure aids the clinician in evaluating the efficacy of the administration of various medications in decreasing left atrial filling pressures in an animal with left-sided congestive heart failure. A decrease in pulmonary capillary wedge pressure will be noted following successful treatment of an animal with congestive heart failure. A decreasing pulmonary capillary wedge pressure should be evaluated in light of the respiratory distress remaining in the animal, improvement in partial pressure of arterial oxygen (arterial blood gas), and radiographic evidence for resolution of pulmonary edema. The risks and complications associated with long-term pulmonary artery catheterizations places the use of pulmonary artery catheters as diagnostic and acute therapeutic monitoring tools.

Mixed venous oxygen tension ($P\overline{v}O_2$) correlates with cardiac output in congestive heart failure.[9,10] Mixed venous oxygen tension reflects oxygen delivery to tissues. Normal $P\overline{v}O_2$ in animals is 40 to 50 mm Hg.[11] Reduced cardiac output, leading to decreased oxygen delivery to the tissues, results in decreases in $P\overline{v}O_2$, due in part to increased extraction of oxygen by tissues. Reduced oxygen delivery to tissues can also be associated with anemia and hypoxia, resulting in similarly low $P\overline{v}O_2$. Increasing $P\overline{v}O_2$ following administration of various cardiovascular therapies implies improvement in oxygen delivery, usually as a result of improved cardiac output.[10] High or increasing levels of $P\overline{v}O_2$ values may also result from decreased tissue utilization of oxygen (septic shock, hypothermia, cyanide intoxication, arteriovenous shunting).[11]

In summary, questions to consider when assessing the clinical improvement and hemodynamic stability of the patient with cardiac dysfunction include the following:

1. Is the heart rate within an acceptable range to provide maximal cardiac performance?
2. Have cardiac arrhythmias been eliminated or decreased in frequency, resulting in decreased hemodynamic compromise?
3. Is the animal's peripheral pulse quality improved?
4. Is the animal's mucous membrane color and capillary refill time within normal limits?
5. Is there radiographic and auscultatory evidence that pulmonary edema has resolved?
6. Is the animal's central venous pressure within normal limits or stable?
7. Has the animal's pulmonary capillary wedge pressure decreased following therapeutic interventions?
8. Is the animal's systemic arterial blood pressure improved?
9. Is the animal's partial pressure of arterial oxygen within normal limits?
10. Has the animal's cardiac output increased?
11. Has the animal's $P\overline{v}O_2$ returned to the normal range following therapy?
12. Has urine output returned to normal?

Nervous system

Animals with diseases of the nervous system that prompt admission to the ICU include those with altered levels of consciousness, peripheral nerve disease affecting respiration, repetitive or sustained seizure activity (status epilepticus), or acute spinal cord dysfunction resulting in paresis or paralysis. Patients with severe neurologic dysfunction and/or neurologic dysfunction resulting from trauma, can have dramatic progression of their clinical signs in a short period.

Serial neurologic evaluations, with documentation of changes noted on flow sheets, are essential to assess improvement or deterioration of the animal's neurologic status. Neurologic monitoring in the ICU focuses on serial monitoring of the animal's limb movement, strength, pain sensation, level of consciousness, pupillary light responses, oculocephalic reflexes and on the routine monitoring of other body system parameters. Specific treatment of patients with central nervous system and spinal cord dysfunction is reviewed in Chapters 11 and 20.

Neurologic injury can result in life-threatening consequences (e.g., cerebral or brainstem herniation) or permanently disabling (e.g., paralysis) conditions. Animals with status epilepticus or severe cluster seizures may develop multisystemic complications (metabolic or respiratory acidosis, hypoxia, hyperthermia, dehydration, neurogenic pulmonary edema, cardiac dysrhythmias, hypoglycemia) or neurologic complications (blindness, cerebral edema).[12-15] Many patients with severe neurologic disease will remain in the ICU throughout their hospitalization.

Animals with neurologic dysfunction likely to be transferred from the ICU are those who have exhibited dramatic and/or sustained improvement in neurologic function and animals in which complications are unlikely (e.g., postoperative animal with disk disease). Close monitoring remains essential in these patients.

Respiratory system

Respiratory failure occurs when gas exchange is significantly impaired (partial pressure of arterial oxygen [PaO_2] <60 mm Hg, partial pressure of arterial carbon dioxide [$PaCO_2$] > 50 mm Hg) and the animal cannot maintain adequate oxygen and carbon dioxide homeostasis. The cause of respiratory failure is pursued by investigation of the respiratory system components (central nervous system inputs, chest wall and respiratory muscles, pleural space, lung), the mechanisms causing impaired gas exchange (hypoventilation, ventilation-perfusion mismatch, right-to-left shunting of blood, impaired diffusion), and the specific disease process causing the respiratory failure. Treatment and monitoring of specific respiratory system dysfunctions is reviewed in Chapters 4, 25, and 36.

The decision to transfer the patient with respiratory dysfunction from the ICU is usually not difficult and is based on serial assessment of numerous parameters, including auscultatory improvement in lung sounds, normalization of respiratory rate and pattern, radiographic improvement of any pulmonary disease, and/or improvement in other monitored parameters (e.g., tidal volume, blood gases, oxygen saturation via oximetry).

Auscultation is noninvasive, inexpensive, and provides one of the best serial assessments of an animal's pulmonary status (Chapter 4). Auscultation should be performed frequently (at least three times daily) in animals with respiratory system dysfunction.

Clinical improvement of respiratory dysfunction usually precedes appreciable evidence of radiographic improvement in patients with pulmonary dysfunction. An exception to this rule is pulmonary edema, which often resolves radiographically within 24 hours following administration of appropriate medical treatment. Initial and subsequent radiographic evaluation of the animal with severe respiratory dysfunction can be stressful and should not be performed when development of further respiratory distress is likely. Clinical assessments and the measurement of parameters that do not involve as much compromise to the patient should be used to monitor the status of these critical patients (e.g., auscultation, percussion, respiratory rate).

Arterial blood gas analysis is one of the most important laboratory tests for evaluation and monitoring of animals with respiratory and metabolic dysfunction (see Chapters 21, 25, 36, and 38). When evaluating PaO_2, the clinician must remember the significance of the sigmoid shape of the oxyhemoglobin dissociation curve (Chapter 36).

With increasing PaO_2 there is a progressive increase in the percent of hemoglobin saturated. Normal oxygen saturation of hemoglobin in arterial blood is 97% (at a PaO_2 of 100 mm Hg). Arterial oxygen content (hemoglobin saturation) often remains normal despite fluctuations in the alveolar pressure of oxygen or the development of ventilation-perfusion mismatches, intrapulmonary shunting of blood, and problems with gas diffusion across alveolar membranes. For example, despite a marked decline in alveolar pressure of oxygen (60 mm Hg), the percentage of hemoglobin saturation remains close to normal (approximately 89%), and oxygen delivery to tissues is minimally affected.

A rising PaO_2 and normalizing $PaCO_2$ suggest improved gas exchange in animals with respiratory dysfunction. Several noninvasive measures of oxygen saturation (e.g., oximetry) provide additional information regarding the adequacy of pulmonary gas exchange (Chapters 4 and 36). End tidal carbon dioxide concentration, a noninvasive reflection of mixed venous blood and tissue pressure of carbon dioxide, can also be used to aid in assessing respiratory function in intubated patients (Chapter 36).

Prior to transferring the patient with respiratory

dysfunction to the general wards the clinician must assess the animal's ventilation and gas exchange by answering the following questions:

1. Has the animal's respiratory rate decreased and is breathing regular?
2. Are the animal's mucous membrane color and perfusion normal?
3. Have any abnormal auscultatory findings resolved or decreased in severity and intensity?
4. Have any radiographic abnormalities in the thorax improved or resolved?
5. Is Pao_2 >60 mm Hg and increasing following therapeutic intervention?
6. Is $Paco_2$ within normal limits?
7. Is arterial oxygen saturation greater than 90% (normal, 95% to 98%)?

Urogenital system

Disturbances of the urogenital system resulting in admission to the ICU are usually of an acute life-threatening nature (e.g., acute renal failure, disruption of integrity of urinary tract, prostatic abscess, dystocia). Following successful emergency medical or surgical therapy, many of these patients tend to stabilize and improve rapidly from their disease without further complication. Hospitalization in the ICU is often transient (with the exception of acute renal failure) for these patients as resolution of the animal's disease or a change in its character to a chronic disease status can usually allow for continued treatment of the animal in the intermediate care ward.

Assessment of patients treated for renal dysfunction involves measurement of urine flow, serial measurement of blood urea nitrogen and serum creatinine concentrations, evaluation of systemic arterial blood pressure, and serial assessments of results of acid-base and serum electrolyte measurements.

In cases of acute renal failure, the patient's condition may be refractory to conventional medical management and may require peritoneal dialysis (Chapter 39). Peritoneal dialysis is labor intensive and is best performed in the ICU.

Morbidity and mortality is high in patients with acute renal failure. Complications of the cardiovascular (pulmonary edema, arrhythmias, hypertension), gastrointestinal (nausea, vomiting, anorexia, gastric bleeding), hematologic (anemia), and neurologic (seizures) systems are common. In addition to monitoring parameters of renal function, assessment of these systems should be routinely performed.

Questions to be answered prior to transfer of the patient with urogenital disease include the following:

1. Has the patient's primary problem prompting admission to the ICU resolved (e.g., dystocia, prostatic abscess, urethral obstruction) following appropriate intervention?
2. Is the animal's urine flow normal?
3. Is the animal's systemic arterial blood pressure normal?
4. Are the animal's blood urea nitrogen, serum creatinine, serum electrolytes, and acid-base status normalized or maximally improved?
5. Do other body system functions appear within normal limits?

Patients with chronic renal dysfunction who still require intensive fluid therapy and monitoring may be appropriately treated in an intermediate care ward.

Ophthalmic emergencies

The prime consideration when evaluating and treating animals with ophthalmic emergencies (e.g., ocular trauma, glaucoma, corneal ulceration, uveitis) is preservation of vision (Chapter 19). Frequent (often, every hour) administration of ophthalmic medications and careful monitoring is usually necessary in the patient with an acute ocular emergency. This function is best performed in the ICU so that the patient's visual status, ocular integrity, and response to treatment can be continuously evaluated and sequelae such as blindness avoided.

Patients with surgical ophthalmic emergencies (e.g., proptosis of the globe, corneal lacerations) often require intensive medical treatment preoperatively and postoperatively for 12 to 24 hours. Subsequently, these patients may have treatments and monitoring performed in an intermediate care ward or, in some cases, these animals can be more closely observed at home by their owners.

Patients with deep corneal ulcers should remain in the ICU throughout their hospitalization as complications such as corneal perforation may occur. Early surgical intervention often results in preservation of vision if a deep ulcer worsens or a descemetocele occurs despite medical therapy (Chapter 19).

SUMMARY

Transition of patients from critical care is generally based on clinical improvement and improvement in hemodynamic, physiologic, and hematologic parameters. The extent or level of care required for the animal is a key factor in considering transfer of an animal from the ICU. A clinician's knowledge of possible complications associated with the animal's condition and the response of the disease process to treatment will aid in clinical decision making concerning the transition of patient care from the ICU.

REFERENCES

1. Braunwald E. Pathophysiology of heart failure. In Braunwald E, ed. Heart disease: a textbook of cardiovascular medicine. Philadelphia: WB Saunders, 1984;446-447.
2. Hirsch AT, Dzau VJ, Creager MA. Baroreceptor function in congestive heart failure: effect on neurohumoral activation and regional vascular resistance. Circulation 1987; 75(IV):36-48.
3. Wegria R, Frank CW, Wang HH, et al. The effect of atrial and ventricular tachycardia on cardiac output, coronary blood flow and arterial blood pressure. Circ Res 1958;6:624.
4. Scherlag BJ, Lazzara R. Ischemic arrhythmias: basic mechanisms. In Mandell WJ, ed. Cardiac arrhythmias. Philadelphia: JB Lippincott, 1980;366.
5. Vlay SC, Reid PR. Ventricular ectopy: etiology, evaluation and therapy. Am J Med 1982;73:899.
6. Sisson DD. The clinical management of cardiac arrhythmias in the dog and cat. In Fox PR, ed. Canine and feline cardiology. New York: Churchill Livingstone, 1988;289-308.
7. Zipes DP. Specific arrhythmias: Diagnosis and treatment. In Braunwald E, ed. Heart disease: a textbook of cardiovascular medicine. Philadelphia: WB Saunders, 1984;683-743.
8. Guyton AC, ed. Textbook of medical physiology, ed 7, Philadelphia: WB Saunders, 1985.
9. De La Rocha AG, Edmonds JF, Williams WG, et al. Importance of mixed venous oxygen saturation in the case of critically ill patients. Can J Surg 1978;21:227.
10. Kittleson MD, Johnson LE, Oliver B. Acute hemodynamic effects of hydralazine in dogs with chronic mitral regurgitation. J Am Vet Med Assoc 1985;187:258-261.
11. Haskins SC. Monitoring the critically ill patient. Vet Clin North Am 1989;19:1054-1077.
12. Meldrum BS, Horton RW. Physiology of status epilepticus in primates. Arch Neurol 1973;28:1-9.
13. Meldrum BS, Brierley JB. Prolonged epileptic seizures in primates: ischaemic cell change and its relationship to vital physiologic events. Arch Neurol 1973;28:10-17.
14. Holiday TA. Seizure disorders. Vet Clin North Am 1980;10:3-29.
15. Brooks BR, Adams RD. Cerebrospinal fluid acid-base and lactate changes after seizures in unanesthetized man. Neurology 1975;25:935.

The Emergency and Critical Care Patient

10 Triage and Trauma Management

Dennis T. Crowe, Jr.

*Meticulous attention to detail in the operative
care of the trauma patient through innumerable
small maneuvers may avert disaster or shorten
convalescence; if neglected they may cost a
patient's life.*

ERNEST SACHS, 1945

The focus of this chapter concerns the initial assessment, triage, and treatment of animals presented for emergency care that have suffered very serious traumatic injury. These patients demand a simultaneous rapid accurate assessment and treatment aimed at stabilization and, hopefully, prevention of catastrophic consequences. Such conditions as airway obstruction, tension or open pneumothorax, major external and internal hemorrhage, deep coma following blunt head injury, and very severe intrapulmonic hemorrhage with secondary pulmonary edema following blunt chest trauma are some of the most devastating results of trauma. These all can result in traumatic cardiopulmonary failure and arrest within a short period. A brief discussion of the required resuscitation management of these conditions will be presented after a general discussion on initial care and preparedness for severe trauma.

The treatment of the seriously traumatized patient with multisystemic involvement can be thought of as the ultimate "acid test" of emergency care, testing practice readiness, assessment and triage, effective teamwork, and resuscitation skills. In patients who present with severe injuries, the speed and quality of emergency care invariably determines whether or not major complications or death will result.[1] Immediate definitive surgical intervention will often be required at the receiving hospital to achieve patient stabilization in many cases.

Following immediate successful resuscitation the patient is examined thoroughly, and monitoring is continued in order to detect and assess completely all injuries and secondary complications resulting from these injuries. Definitive emergency surgical treatment or referral for such care is often necessary following serious injury.

Postsurgical and postresuscitation treatment is another "acid test" that demands careful monitoring and supportive care. Supportive care must include aggressive nutritional therapy and physiotherapy to allow as quick and uncomplicated a recovery as possible. Experience in seriously injured human patients has proven that the earlier nutritional support and physiotherapy can be started after the injury, the greater the chance for recovery.[2] Complications of sepsis and pneumonia are much more common in patients who do not receive this support. If at all possible, it is recommended in our animal patients that protein and caloric intake (either enterally [preferred], parenterally, or a combination) should be started within 12 hours following injury. Physiotherapy, begun at the same time, should be aimed at increasing blood flow, deep breathing, and maintaining muscle tone.

Although severe injuries inherently are associated with high mortality (reportedly 75% to 95% in human trauma studies), in a well-equipped facility, coordinated trained trauma teams have been able to lower this statistic to less than 10%.[1]

It has been my experience that the same can be achieved in veterinary centers, provided owners accept the costs and the professional team is trained, experienced, and operates in an organized and adequately equipped facility.

THE "GOLDEN PERIOD" OF TRAUMA MANAGEMENT

Success in the treatment of the seriously injured patient requires immediate assessment and resuscitation, during the "golden period." The term "golden period" denotes the time following the onset of the emergency condition in which effective treatment ensures a good chance of patient survival. During this period, resuscitation to the point of stabilization must be completed.

In most seriously injured patients, because of attending respiratory and cardiovascular dysfunction, the golden period following the traumatic event is the first hour following the trauma.[2] Initiation of surgical treatment during this golden hour frequently is necessary to accomplish stabilization.

KEYS TO EMERGENCY TRAUMA MANAGEMENT

To ensure rapid and high-quality emergency care of the seriously injured patient, allowing successful stabilization during the golden period and ultimate recovery, 10 key management steps are involved. These steps are listed in the order of which they are performed:

1. Preemergent "readiness" preparation and maintenance,
2. Prehospital evaluation and first aid at the scene,
3. Transport and maintained first aid,
4. Arrival, initial evaluation (primary survey), and triage,
5. Triage of multiple patients that are injured,
6. Resuscitation (to stabilize) based on priority,

7. Complete history and physical examination (secondary survey),
8. Laboratory, radiographic, and other tests as indicated,
9. Continued monitoring and resuscitation as needed,
10. Definitive care or referral as required.

These 10 steps (see the box below) will be addressed separately in this chapter, but in actual clinical practice they tend to form one continuum of care.

TRAUMA READINESS, PREPARATION, AND MAINTENANCE
General considerations

To treat a traumatized patient urgently in need of emergency care, quickly enough to prevent catastrophic consequences, requires the hospital to be maintained in a state of readiness. For efficiency, one centralized area for initial assessment and management should be used. Often the best central "ready" area is near the operating room. All seriously injured or ill animals are initially examined and treated in this area. This location should be the area where inpatient emergencies are also treated, except for those that occur in the operating room. The operating room must be equally well equipped.

The anesthesia induction area is frequently chosen to be the "readiness" area because of easy accessibility to key supplies and pieces of equipment, for example, oxygen, intravenous fluids, catheters, etc.

All resuscitation equipment and necessary drugs should be organized in this area. These materials should be packaged or stocked to facilitate ease of location and use (Fig. 10-1). The use of a daily checklist of the ready area's equipment and drugs will ensure that the area is always prepared (Fig. 10-2). Following any use of the area for patient resuscitation the checklist is reviewed. Any materials needing restocking are then charged to the client involved and the restocking is completed. It is suggested that drugs, instruments, and equipment that may have to be shared between the ready area and the operating room should be kept on a mobile "crash cart" (Fig. 10-3).

A wall chart indicating drug dosages, standard fluid administration volumes and rates, and direct-current watt-second defibrillation levels (based on estimated body weights) is recommended (Fig. 10-4).

The ready area requires good lighting, similar to that required in the operating room. Dual lights that can be directed at divergent angles are espe-

---

KEY TRAUMA MANAGEMENT STEPS

1. Hospital readiness
2. First aid at scene
3. Transport and continued aid
4. Arrival and primary survey
5. Triage and necessary first aid
6. Resuscitation to stabilize
7. Secondary survey
8. Laboratory, imaging, and electrodiagnostic tests
9. Continued monitoring and stabilization
10. Definitive care or referral

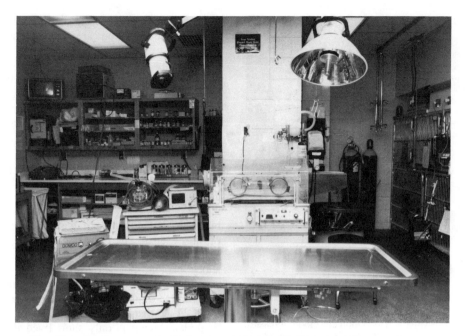

Fig. 10-1. Ready area at the University of Georgia Small Animal Teaching Hospital.

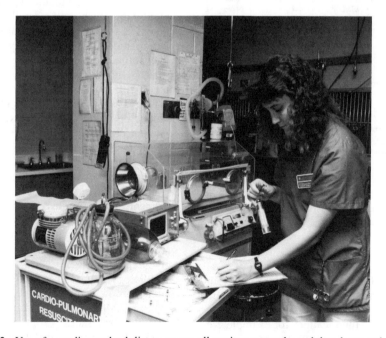

Fig. 10-2. Use of a readiness check list to ensure all equipment works and that drugs and supplies necessary for resuscitation are present. Technicians review the list daily and after every resuscitation event.

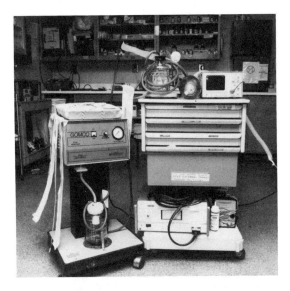

Fig. 10-3 Crash cart with necessary equipment. Note suction, oxygen, electrocardiograph, defibrillator, resuscitation bag-valve, and Doppler blood pressure monitor properly positioned, plugged in, and ready to use.

CARDIOPULMONARY RESUSCITATION: A.C.L.S. TX

Dose in ml/lb body weight by IV route   Double Dose if tracheal

Emergency Drugs/Dose		5lb	10lb	15lb	20lb	25lb	30lb	35lb	40lb	50lb	60lb	70lb	80lb	100lb
EPINEPHRINE 1:1000 1mg/ml	0.1 mg/lb 0.2 mg/kg	0.5	1	1.5	2	2.5	3	3.5	4	5	6	7	8	10ml's
ATROPINE 0.5 mg/ml	.025 mg/lb .05 mg/kg	0.25	0.5	0.75	1	1.25	1.5	1.75	2	2.5	3	3.5		5ml's
LIDOCAINE 20 mg/ml	1.0 mg/lb 2.0 mg/kg	0.25	0.5	0.75	1	1.25	1.5	1.75	2	2.5	3	3.5	4	5ml's
NA BICARB 1 meq/ml	0.5 meq/lb 1.0 meq/kg	2.5	5	7.5	10	12.5	15	17.5	20	25	30	35	40	50ml's
DEXAMETHASONE SP 4 mg/ml	2 mg/lb 4 mg/kg	2.5	5	7.5	10	12.5	15	17.5	20	25	30	35	40	50ml's
CALCIUM GLUCONATE 100 mg/ml	3 mg/lb 10 mg/kg	0.25	0.5	0.75	1	1.25	1.5	1.75	2	2.5	3	3.5	4	5ml's
COUNTER-SHOCK EXT	1-10 w's/lb	25	50	75	100	125	150	175	200	250	300	350	400	500ws
COUNTER-SHOCK INT	1-1 w's/lb	2.5	5	7.5	10	12.5	15	17.5	20	25	30	35	40	50ws

Fig. 10-4 Wall chart in ready area, used as a quick reference to indicate the amount of emergency drug or direct current required for resuscitation based on the patient's estimated body weight.

cially important for the care of the seriously injured patient. These patients frequently require emergency surgical procedures that demand the availability of good illumination, for example, venous cutdown and resuscitative tracheostomy. A focusing high-intensity cool-beam light (very useful for close and exacting or deep cavity work) and a wider-beam reflecting-dish light for general full-body illumination are recommended (Fig. 10-5).

Key items mandatory for the care of animals with catastrophic injuries include suction, oxygen, laryngoscope, major surgery pack including a curved Mayo scissors and a Balfour retractor, assorted catheters, suture, sterile towels and drapes, and emergency drugs such as epinephrine, atropine, and lidocaine (see Chapters 1 and 3). Drugs and biologics such as a first-generation cephalosporin, dextran 70 or hetastarch, plasma, and whole blood are also indispensable.

The availability of fresh homologous whole blood, in particular, is paramount in the treatment of most catastrophic injuries because severe blood loss is a common problem in these cases. In the shock patient, not suffering from severe blood loss, the need for plasma or some other colloid for volume replacement is often vital. Studies have shown that vascular compartment expansion or replenishment is only short lived if a crystalloid infusion such as lactated Ringer's solution is used.[3] In less than an hour, over 80% of the lactated Ringer's is no longer in the circulation and instead is found in the interstitium.

In the multiple-trauma patient, particularly in those with lung or head injury, the overexpansion of the interstitial space may be especially damaging. This occurs commonly with the rapid administration of "one blood volume" of crystalloid in contrast to vascular volume replenishment with a colloid with which only a small percentage of the material is in the interstitium after 12 hours. Increased amounts of interstitial water over normal values, clinically evident as edema, have been associated with higher morbidity and mortality in humans suffering from multiple trauma.[4]

There is no substitute for the rapid replacement of blood and blood components, such as plasma, in the successful resuscitation of the catastrophically injured patient.

Facility readiness

Maintaining facility readiness in regard to the treatment of the seriously injured patient applies to the operating room, intensive care, x-ray, and laboratory areas as well. In some cases the patient may go directly to the operating room for resuscitative treatment. Ideally, effective use of diagnostic radiology requires capabilities for rapid radiograph exposure and development, thus the need of at least a 200- to 300-mA x-ray unit and an automatic film processor.

In-house determinations of hematocrit, total serum solids, platelet numbers, white blood cell counts, and differential cell counts is a require-

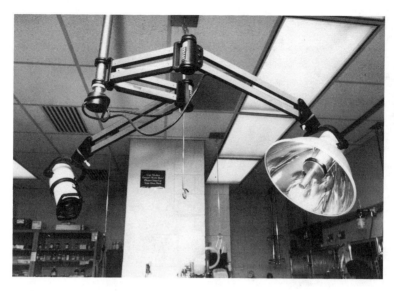

Fig. 10-5. Lighting system useful in ready area: dual-beam, combination cool-halogen focusing light and a wider-beam reflecting-disk light.

ment. Capabilities for determination of blood glucose, activated coagulation time, blood urea nitrogen, serum electrolytes, blood pH and blood gases, and cytologic evaluation of urine, body cavity fluids, or lavage samples are lifesaving in many cases. Hospitals that cannot perform these tests should make alternative arrangements, for example, setting up a protocol to have the tests performed immediately at a local human hospital or reference laboratory.

Because major surgical interventions are often required as part of the resuscitation of patients with catastrophic injury, it is important to have an operating room with the equipment and supplies necessary to perform such surgical procedures as exploratory laparotomy with autotransfusion, liver lobe resection, splenectomy and partial splenectomy, intestinal resection and anastomosis, nephrectomy, cystorrhaphy, diaphragmatic herniorrhaphy, abdominal wall herniorrhaphy, exploratory thoracotomy, lung lobectomy, chest-tube thoracostomy, wound exploration, repair or ligation of major vessel bleeding, tracheal repair and tracheostomy, and decompressive craniotomy.

Personnel and mental readiness

Readiness requires that hospital personnel be mentally and physically prepared. In-hospital training and drill sessions are recommended. Assessment and resuscitation team skills should be practiced (Fig. 10-6). When catastrophic traumatic emergencies occur everyone on the staff must know their assignment and be able to perform it well. Drill sessions facilitate the practice

of psychomotor skills and working as a team, providing for effective and efficient treatment of critical patients.

A stuffed toy dog can be used to simulate a "hit by car patient" who presents in shock and unconscious. Review sessions are held at the conclusion of the drills to evaluate team performance in a positive and constructive manner. These sessions can also be used to introduce and test the feasibility of new treatment protocols.

Trauma protocols for general assessment and management and treatment for specific catastrophic injuries are recommended. These protocols should be printed and reviewed at staff meetings. They may also be posted in key areas in the hospital or in the ready area, where they can be referred to easily. They act as guidelines and mental reminders for the staff and clinician in charge, increasing team efficiency, and helping to prevent assessment and management mistakes (see the following box).

Each trauma protocol may be organized in a numerical or alphabetical list of steps to follow (see the following box) or in an algorithm (see the following box). Protocols should be reviewed and revised as required periodically to ensure they remain current, easily understood, and effective in the setting in which they are used.

Ideally, at least three experienced professional and technical personnel should be present and involved in the treatment of animals presented following serious injury (polytrauma). Some of the required technical support can often be provided by receptionists, maintenance workers, or book-

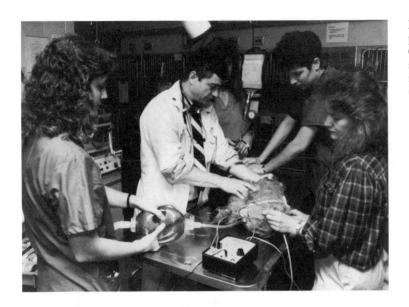

Fig. 10-6 Resuscitation being practiced at the University of Georgia in a drill session with staff using a canine cardiopulmonary resuscitation mannequin (Nasco, Fort Atkinson, WI).

CATASTROPHIC RESPIRATORY DISTRESS FOLLOWING TRAUMA: INITIAL MANAGEMENT BASED ON LEVEL OF CONSCIOUSNESS

If Animal Is Conscious or Hyperexcited

Provide high-flow oxygen by clear plastic bag hood: suggested oxygen rate, >5 L per minute for small dog, cat, or bird, >10 L per minute for medium to large dog, 15 L per minute for large dog.

Evaluate results, if there is a positive response, continue oxygen administration, place nasal catheter, and reperform careful physical examination.

If there is a poor response, perform resuscitative tracheostomy (lidocaine 1%, optional), insert cuffed endotracheal tube and secure, and begin intermittent positive-pressure ventilation with 100% oxygen at 20 to 25 breaths per minute; add positive end-expiratory pressure (5 cm H_2O), if needed.

FRACTURED CHEST-WALL MODULE

Are fractured ribs present?
↓
Yes
Is there a flail segment?

Yes — No

Does cyanosis persist despite high-flow nasal or tracheal oxygen administration?

No
Monitor blood gases; consider analgesic and oxygen administration

Yes
Perform tracheostomy, begin intermittent positive-pressure ventilation (100% oxygen, 20 breaths per minute, consider positive end-expiratory pressure, and provide analgesia through local anesthetic (bupivicaine) blocks of intercostal nerves
↓

No
Monitor blood gases; consider analgesic and oxygen administration

Reassess pulmonary and cardiovascular parameters

---

keepers. These individuals can be trained to assist with restraint and to perform basic life-support tasks (see box on p. 83). If an adequate number of professional or paraprofessional members of the team are not present, alternatives might include the following:

1. The enlistment of bystanders or the owner, although this involves an increased risk of liability and more effort on the doctor's part concerning communication and direction for these individuals.[5]
2. Calling other professionals off duty or from another practice. This can work in all but

BASIC LIFE-SUPPORT SKILLS

Provide positive pressure ventilation by squeezing the self-inflating resuscitation or rebreathing bag.

Apply direct pressure to slow or stop bleeding.

Administer emergency drugs as directed into an indwelling intravenous catheter.

Perform simple laboratory procedures, for example, plasma total solids, hematocrit, blood glucose.

Chronicle the events that occurred and treatments given on a flow chart as directed verbally by doctor.

the most catastrophic conditions, especially if an "on-call roster" and agreement is worked out ahead of time and the response time is usually under 15 to 20 minutes.

Trauma patients that require definitive body-cavity surgery as part of the resuscitation should be treated by a team that includes at least three personnel in the operating room: surgeon, assistant surgeon, and anesthetist-circulating nurse. Ventilator assistance and careful anesthesia monitoring is always required in these patients and having assistance in surgery greatly facilitates intraoperative effectiveness and speed. Provided that mechanical ventilatory assistance is available, one person may be able to function as anesthetist and circulating nurse, but this approach is still not ideal.

Equipment required for treatment of serious injuries

Effective treatment of serious injuries demands the availability of key equipment that is usually not required for the management of many other conditions. There is also often no substitute, and the lack of this equipment directly jeopardizes the patient's chances for recovery. Key equipment required is listed in the Veterinary Emergency and Critical Care Society's publication *Recommended Definitions and Guidelines for Veterinary Emergency Service Standards in the United States*[6] (Chapters 1 and 3).

An example of a key piece of equipment that is required is a suction unit for the evacuation of vomitus, blood clots, thick exudate, or saliva from the pharynx, larynx, and trachea to gain a patent airway. This instrumentation includes the suction trap bottle, suction tubing, several types of aspirator tips (Yankauer aspiratory tip for pharyngeal aspiration, dental tip for rima glottis and tracheal suctioning, and tracheal whistle-tip catheters for tracheobronchial tree aspiration), and suction capable of generating up to 300 mm Hg of vacuum that can be obtained within 4 seconds of clamping the tube[7] (Fig. 10-3). The dental suction tip is used for the aspiration of large pieces of vomitus and clot, while the whistle-tip catheters are used for the aspiration of frothy secretions, vomit, exudate, and blood.[8] An endotracheal tube with suction applied to the connecting end can also be used to evacuate particulate debris from the pharynx and upper airway[9] (Fig. 10-7).

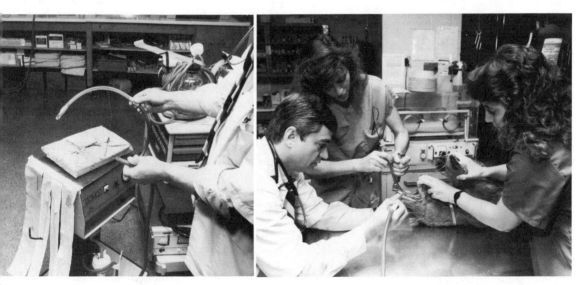

Fig. 10-7. **A,** Suction tubing attached to an endotracheal tube (endotracheal tube without Murphy eye on the end is preferred) used to aspirate and clear the pharynx of thick secretions and particulate matter (vomitus). **B,** Yankauer suction tip attached to suction unit and being used to clear material from the pharynx and facilitate intubation.

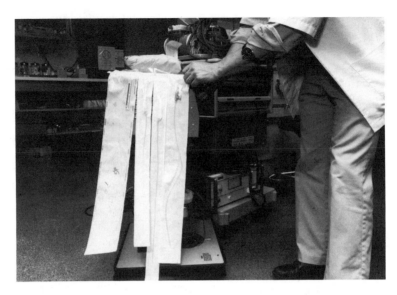

Fig. 10-8. Various-sized tracheal suction catheters fixed to the suction unit in such a way as to make rapid selection, procurement, and attachment to suction tubing possible. *Note:* these catheters can be used to deliver emergency drugs transtracheally to the bronchial bifurcation and can also be used as intravenous central lines placed by emergency venous cutdown.

Interposition of a suction trap at the base of the dental suction tip or endotracheal tube "suction tip" device will prevent clogging of the latex connecting tubing with large amounts of debris or blood clots. A trap has been described that fits directly onto the endotracheal tube. This allows effective suctioning during the act of intubation and can save valuable seconds.[9]

It is recommended for the "state of readiness" that either a Yaukauer tip, medium-sized dental suction tip, or endotracheal tube with an inflatable cuff be attached to the suction unit via a 6-in. section of ⅝-in.-diameter tubing and that the other suction attachments (tracheal suction catheter) be close at hand so exchange can be done quickly (Fig. 10-8).

Further general discussions concerning equipment, instruments, and drugs needed in the management of serious injuries are summarized in Chapters 1 and 3.

PREHOSPITAL EVALUATION AND FIRST AID CARE
General considerations

Care of the seriously traumatized pet often begins at the scene of the injury or at the owner's home following the injury. The prehospital care given may determine the outcome of the case. Appropriate immediate care can prevent further injury at the scene or during transport to the hospital. Occasionally, the type of first aid care required can

be briefly described to the caller on the telephone. An example of such may be the description to the caller of how to apply pressure around an animal's leg by squeezing with the hand proximal to a large profusely bleeding laceration deep in the foot.

At other times, proper directions on first aid cannot be described clearly enough to be used by owners that do not have a health care background. In these cases, the telephone directions are modified to keep the owner and animal safe and facilitate transport. For example, if an injury results in an obvious "bent and wobbly" distal rear leg (indicating the high probability of a severe fracture), proper application of a newspaper splint to stabilize the region and prevent further soft-tissue trauma during transport is indicated. However, if the caller has not had previous first aid training, and if it is not possible to place an effective splint (due to the animal's temperament or level of pain), then restricting the animal's movement by placement of the animal in a box may effectively limit further soft-tissue injury.

If the animal receives improper first aid or no first aid at all, the injury may become significantly worse, necessitating more extensive surgical treatment and prolonged hospitalization and increasing the risk of infection, implant failure, and even a need for amputation.

First aid recommendations given over the telephone and subsequently performed have been lifesaving. Personnel answering the hospital telephone must become knowledgeable or must direct emergency calls to someone who can provide the proper first aid recommendations. The following is an example of the difference between improper and proper first aid recommendations given over the telephone:

Two people call separate hospitals and state that their dogs, who were spayed 3 days previously, have small lumps near the incision line with a pink watery fluid seeping from the area. The receptionist, who took the call at hospital A, tells the pet owner to bring her pet in for the doctor to check it. No first aid instructions were given. The receptionist at hospital B instructs the owner to place a clean towel or bandage around the abdomen of the dog first and then to transport the dog very carefully to the hospital. The first dog, on arrival at hospital A, jumps out of the car and eviscerates its entire abdominal contents in the parking lot. The second dog arrives at hospital B with evidence of dehiscence of the deep suture line and a small amount of the subcutaneous-skin suture line disrupted, but no viscera are visible. The first dog ultimately develops peritonitis and dies, while the second makes a full recovery following reclosure of the suture line.

Key first aid care steps and procedures following trauma

The key steps outlined in detail below, except under very unusual circumstances, should always be done in this order. These steps not only apply to laypersons rendering first aid care at the scene but also to professional animal health care providers present at the scene and also when the injured animal is presented at the veterinary hospital.

Survey the scene. Initially, the first aid providers at the scene should ensure that the area and the circumstances are safe for the provider to render care. If the animal is laying in the road, before approaching first make sure that no vehicles are coming. The animal is moved off the road a safe distance before being assessed. This can be accomplished by grasping an accessible rear leg and pulling the animal while keeping the animal's head directed low and away. This approach disturbs brain blood flow the least, protects against aspiration, and keeps the spine relatively straight. Muzzling of the dog or covering the head of the animal helps gain a safe environment for the first aid provider.[10]

Call for help. First aid care to a seriously injured animal can be performed much more efficiently when two or more people are working together. If only one person is initially available to provide the care required, that person should call for help. The owner or a bystander may be asked to lend aid if professional help is not available at the scene.

An organized "on-call system" with trained technicians, lay personnel, or volunteers has been very effective in selected practices without 24-hour staffing. When severely injured animals arrive at the hospital after-hours, lay personnel and volunteers on call may include high school students, college preveterinary students, Boy Scouts, retired individuals, and off-duty police or firefighters living close to the hospital.

Initial assessment. Prehospital examination and assessment of the animal (prehospital primary survey) by the owner or other lay providers should follow the same format as recommended on initial admission to the hospital (see section on Arrival, Initial Evaluation, and Triage below).[10] The primary survey is used to determine if any immediately life-threatening conditions are apparent. This survey should be completed within 30 seconds and does not require any special equipment or in-depth knowledge. The assessment involves looking, listening, and feeling for obvious abnormalities in consciousness, breathing, circulation, and overall appearance of the traumatized animal.

Owners can be taught how to evaluate respiratory rate and effort, pulse quality and rate, heart rate, mucous membrane color, capillary refill time, and level of consciousness and to assess the appearance of the animal. The entire primary survey is completed unless airway obstruction is present and breathing or pulse is absent. If these abnormalities are detected, the survey is stopped and appropriate resuscitation is initiated.

Prehospital resuscitation. Key basic first aid procedures are required in the treatment of the traumatized pet if life-threatening conditions are present. These conditions demand immediate recognition and treatment at the scene or in the hospital on admission if successful resuscitation is to be achieved. These basic life-support techniques can be taught to the majority of laypersons and have been used successfully both at the scene and at the hospital. These procedures include the following in sequential order:

1. Airway—If airway sounds are heard and the animal is stuporous or unconscious, ensure a clear airway. This is done by carefully extending the head and neck on the same plane, pulling the tongue forward and wiping mucus, blood clots, or vomitus from the back of the mouth to clear the airway in unconscious patients. The head and neck of the unconscious animal should not be moved outside the neutral plane until cervical fractures and dislocations can be ruled out by radiographic examination.
2. Breathing—If apnea is observed, provide

positive-pressure breathing using mouth to nose and mouth (cats and small dogs) or mouth to nose (medium and large dogs) ventilatory support. In patients that have a permanent tracheostomy stoma, mouth to stoma ventilation can also be done very effectively after wiping the stoma clear of mucus. In dolichocephalic animals it is important to close the mouth with the animal's incisor teeth grasping the tongue so that the tongue occludes the rostral portion of the mouth. The dorsal and ventral labia of the animal's cheeks are grasped together to prevent air leakage. The rescuer then places his mouth over the nose of the animal, with the animal's neck extended, and gently forces breaths into the lungs of the animal. The chest of the animal should be seen to expand with successful ventilation. Ventilations are continued at 12 to 20 times per minute if spontaneous breathing, with adequate depth, does not become evident.

3. Cardiac function—Cardiac function is assessed by palpating in the groin area for a peripheral femoral artery pulse. Detection of pulses is particularly a problem in very small patients and in hypothermic individuals, in whom peripheral blood flow is dramatically decreased via physiologic vasoconstriction. A mean systemic arterial blood pressure (SABP) of at least 60 to 70 mm Hg must be present. However, with direct arterial monitoring to verify the actual pressures, a weak but present femoral pulse can be detected in thin patients with SABP as low as 40 mm Hg. If no pulses are palpable, but the patient is still conscious, a SABP of at least 50 to 60 mm Hg must be present.

If no pulses are detectable and the patient is unconscious, severe hypotension or cardiopulmonary arrest is present. As the worst should always be assumed in this situation, cardiopulmonary cerebral resuscitation (CPCR) should be instituted immediately (unless the owner decides against it at the scene or declines to start resuscitative measures at the hospital).[11]

At the scene of the injury, owners and laypersons should begin basic cardiac life-support (BCLS) procedures if no pulses are detected and the animal is unconscious. BCLS includes the ABCs: (A) Continue to ensure a patent airway through head and neck extension. (B) Continue to provide adequate breathing, giving 12 to 20 breaths per minute, via mouth to mouth and nose or

mouth to nose ventilation. These techniques are able to be successfully performed in all but the most severe airway obstructed English Bulldogs and other brachiocephalic breeds. (C) If no pulse is palpable after two breaths are given, closed-chest compressions are performed.

Closed-chest compressions are most effective in providing blood flow to the brain and heart in the smallest dogs and cats, particularly when the entire chest can be compressed in a circular fashion from 100 to 120 times per minute.[12] One ventilation is provided after every fifth compression in smaller animals. In larger animals (over 15 to 20 kg), it is recommended to provide two breaths after every 15 compressions. In these larger patients it is difficult to provide the compressive force necessary to generate adequate blood flow to the brain and heart in order to prevent irreversible global ischemia. Blood flow is best generated, using closed-chest compressions, when the compressions are performed over the widest and most "compressible" portion of the midthorax. Compressing the abdomen between chest compressions, in dogs, has also been found to increase the effectiveness of closed chest CPCR techniques. This "abdominal counterpulsation" enhances venous return and diastolic systemic arterial blood pressure, improving coronary perfusion (Crowe DT: unpublished data).* Following traumatic injury and resultant hypovolemia, it is particularly difficult to provide adequate blood flow to the brain and heart using any closed-chest compression techniques. Therefore, it is absolutely mandatory that the animal be transported in as short a time as possible to the hospital.

At the hospital, open-chest direct cardiac massage can be done if survival is believed possible. Immediate thoracotomy and direct cardiac massage is indicated on all traumatic cardiac arrest patients if prehospital resuscitation is not successful in reestablishing spontaneous, effective cardiac function. Experimental and clinical research investigations have confirmed that open chest CPCR is over three times more effective in generating brain and heart blood flow as compared with closed-chest techniques[13,14] (see also Chap-

---

*Crowe DT. Interposed abdominal counter pulsation enhances brain and heart blood flow in dogs receiving both closed and open chest CPCR. Athens, GA: University of Georgia, February 1991.

ter 32 and the section on Traumatic Cardiac Arrest below).

4. Control bleeding by compression—Direct compression or compression above and below a bleeding wound should be employed to control or limit the hemorrhage. Digital pressure of only a few pounds per square inch can effectively stop even the most profuse hemorrhage in most cases. In cases of hemorrhage from extremities, firmly holding the injured limb and wrapping a hand around the limb above the bleeding area will effectively control hemorrhage. Serious bleeding of the head and rostral cervical region can be slowed by placing inward pressure caudal to the angle of the jaw or on the carotid artery region.

Compression (tight wrapping or hand pressure) of the abdomen can be used to slow intraabdominal bleeding assumed to be occurring in animals in shock following blunt trauma or penetrating injury to the abdomen or caudal rib cage. The compression technique should include the pelvis and pelvic limbs in animals exhibiting signs of shock. This approach prevents sequestration of venous blood caudal to the abdomen and helps maintain normotension by decreasing the size of the arterioles and venules under the compressive wrap.[15] Clinical experience and research has proven how important this compression is in helping slow severe hemorrhage in the abdominal and pelvic regions. This effort is exemplified in one study in dogs, which proved that even caudal abdominal aortic hemorrhage could be completely controlled by the application of external mid-abdominal counterpressure.[16] This counterpressure, if used, should not be removed once applied until the animal has received appropriate blood volume replacement and preparations for emergent surgical intervention are completed.

Prehospital secondary survey. If airway, breathing, and circulation appear stable, then a rapid secondary survey is performed. This survey involves examination of entire animal from the tip of the nose to the tip of the tail. Although lay care providers are not expected to identify all injuries, they can recognize many obvious abnormalities and accumulate base-line information that may be helpful. Obviously, if major life-threatening problems exist, for example, shock or any other airway, breathing, or circulation abnormalities, a secondary survey should not be completed, as deterioration of the animal could occur during this reevaluation. Rapid transport and continued basic

life support is indicated in these "load-and-go" situations.

If the animal is unconscious but airway, breathing, and circulation are believed stable, a serious head injury should be suspected and monitoring should be continued, with rapid transport on a flat object.

Ancillary prehospital first aid care. Continued protection and observation of the patient should be performed and additional first aid measures should be taken as required. Important first aid care at this juncture includes the following:

5. Cover wounds—Covering open wounds with wet or moist home-made dressings or bandages prevents further contamination or drying and provides protection against further wound disruption. (A teaspoon of salt can be added to a quart of water to make saline that can be used to wet the dressing.) Wounds of the chest wall should be occluded with a dressing and pressure as soon as possible. Communication of these wounds with the pleural cavity (open pneumothorax) may be present and, if not treated quickly, this combination of injuries can lead to severe hypoxemia and death.

6. Apply cool compresses to burns—Application of a cool, wet dressing to a burn wound decreases the amount of continued thermal injury. Dressings are replaced as necessary (as they warm up) for 30 minutes.

7. Immobilize fractures—Application of a newspaper splint can help immobilize a fracture, suspected fracture, or severe sprain. Immobilization techniques should include the joint above and the joint below the suspected area of injury. This approach is particularly applicable to the large to medium-sized dog's radius and ulna, tibia, and metacarpus/metatarsus. Muzzling of the injured animal is advised prior to splint application to prevent injury to the rescuers.

Another choice for acceptable immobilization of an injured limb is the application of a mountaineering splint, which involves binding the involved limb to the opposite limb for support. In small patients simply placing the entire animal in a small box to enforce very close confinement may also be an acceptable means of "immobilizing" the injured, potentially fractured limb.

8. Prevent further heat loss—Covering the animal with a blanket prevents further heat loss and hypothermia following the injury. Covering also may help calm the animal and allow the animal to be handled. Heat loss can also be minimized by placing the animal

(except its head) in a plastic bag or by covering with plastic kitchen wrap.

9. Reexamine for further injuries—Especially following a severe traumatic event, physical examination findings can change rapidly. Continual reevaluation of the animal as transport is taking place is recommended.

Providers at the scene of the injury and those administering to the animal as it arrives in the hospital should assume that the animal is seriously hurt until proven otherwise, no matter how "well" the animal may appear.

Transport and maintained first aid care

Transport is best performed with the conscious animal in a confined area to prevent further injury. This may include a cardboard box, crate, metal cage, or pen. Transport may include the use of a flat object (stretcher), especially if the animal is unconscious or if a spinal cord injury is suspected. The animal is strapped in lateral recumbency on the object by use of tape or cord. Ideally, at least two people should be involved in the transport so that the driver will not be distracted by the animal.

Transport into and out of the vehicle should be done carefully. Animals jumping into or out of a car may start hemorrhaging following the dislodgement of internal blood clots. Rapid changes in body position in animals that are in shock or hypotensive can cause systemic arterial blood pressure to fall and bradycardia to occur secondary to gravitational effects and vagal stimulation. Transport should occur smoothly, rapidly and as safely as possible following injury, even in animals that appear stable.

ARRIVAL, INITIAL EVALUATION (PRIMARY SURVEY), AND TRIAGE
Arrival

When the emergency patient arrives, usually the first person to see the animal is the receptionist. This individual should be given basic training in the recognition of patients that require immediate care and how to summon the health care team. In small practices in which the receptionist acts as the veterinary assistant, instruction on how to perform an evaluation for life-threatening conditions and begin resuscitation is required.

Initial evaluation involves triage or "sorting into categories of seriousness" and is initially based on the animal's level of consciousness (LOC) and history. Animals that are unconscious or near unconsciousness, showing signs of extreme restlessness, tremors, or seizure activity are immediately ushered to the ready area. The hospital staff is summoned immediately and resuscita-

tion begun. Animals with a history of recent trauma are assumed to have a major life-threatening problem and are ushered to the ready area.

Front office staff should continue to provide emotional support to the owner and obtain the necessary administrative and medical information. A systems review-history sheet may be filled out by the owner to obtain a thorough medical history. The use of such a sheet helps calm the owner by demanding important information from them that may contribute to the care of their injured pet. Periodic updates on the pet's condition and what is being done is very beneficial to owners and is highly recommended, particularly when prolonged resuscitation is required. This practice communicates to the owner caring and concern and can be provided by veterinary assistants or the veterinarian.

Initial evaluation (primary survey)

First aid measures already applied should be continued as the animal is examined. The initial examination concentrates on the airway, breathing effort and rate, cardiovascular status, and the patient's LOC. The primary survey should be completed within 1 minute and should be performed uniformly each time to avoid missing serious injuries.

Life-threatening problems are treated immediately, according to their level of priority, before continuing the examination. For example, if an airway obstruction is suspected from noting severe inspiratory effort (involution of the thoracic inlet accompanying every inspiratory movement and no breath sounds heard on auscultation), resuscitative treatment to remove the obstruction is started immediately, and the animal's cardiovascular status is not immediately assessed.

A suggested standard protocol for a method of performing a primary survey is as follows:

1. Visually assess the animal from a distance, noting LOC, unusual body or limb posture, breathing effort and pattern and any audible airway sounds, the presence of blood or other materials on or around the patient, and any other gross abnormalities.

2. Approach the animal from the rostral direction, noting the patient's level of awareness and reactions to movement. Ask the owner questions concerning the animal's temperament if the animal is conscious and take appropriate safety precautions in "questionable" animals (muzzling, head covering, physical restraint).

3. Assess for hemorrhage from the nares and oral cavity and evaluate airway and breathing status by closely observing color of the

oral mucous membranes; listening for laryngeal/tracheal breath sounds (first without, then with the aid of a stethoscope); palpating the neck for jugular distention, tracheal position, tracheal/peritracheal integrity, subcutaneous emphysema, and other evidence of blunt or penetrating trauma.

4. Continue to assess the animal's breathing status by observing, palpating, and listening to the thorax. Lung and heart sounds should be auscultated bilaterally. Injuries to the skin over the thorax and cranial abdomen, subcutaneous emphysema, and loss of chest wall (muscle, rib and sternum) integrity are assessed for bilaterally by visualization and palpation.

5. Cardiovascular assessment is completed by palpating pulses during auscultation of the heart. Pulse strength, rate, rhythm, and vessel tone are easily determined in all but the very smallest animals. Assessment of heart tones, mucous membrane color, and capillary refill time are completed.

6. The primary survey ends with very rapid observation and palpation assessment of the spinal column, limbs, and abdominal, flank, and pelvic regions.

Triage of multiple patients that are injured

Location. With the arrival of more than one injured animal at the same time the veterinary assistant, technician, or veterinarian may need to complete the primary survey and triage in a secondary location, since the ready area is occupied. Initial triage by receptionist and technicians often occurs, by necessity, in the waiting area following arrival of animal patients. Secondary triage locations are ideally very close to the ready area, for example, on an examination table next to the ready area.

Procedure. Triage of multiple critically ill or injured animals involves the selection of conditions that require immediate treatment and then performing these treatments with efficient use of total manpower. Many owners can perform efficient first aid maneuvers until the veterinary team can provide the care necessary.

The amount of involvement the veterinarian has in establishing effective first aid depends on the owner, the patient, and the training of the help available. In cases in which all the skilled staff are involved with the resuscitation of an animal with a more serious condition, first aid instructions (e.g., application of pressure to a bleeding wound) may simply have to be relayed by the receptionist. Fortunately, this situation occurs infrequently in most practices, but it is in this situation

that proper triage has been lifesaving and has prevented utter chaos.

Triage classification system. When dealing with more than one injured patient a classification system based on the urgency of needed treatment is recommended; one such classification system is as follows:

Class I. Class I patients (most urgent, catastrophic) are those that must receive treatment immediately, within seconds. There are fortunately few Class I patients presented. Pets suffering from traumatic respiratory failure, cardiorespiratory arrest, or airway obstruction belong in this category. All unconscious animals should be considered Class I.

Class II. Class II patients (very severe, critical) are those in which action must be taken within minutes to an hour. All patients that suffer multiple injuries, shock, or bleeding but have "adequate" airway and ventilatory function belong in this category. Clinical research in human medicine has emphasized the importance of resuscitation within the first hour following severe trauma as a major determinant of survival.[2,17] In my experience, this so-called golden hour appears to have application in veterinary medicine as well.

Class III. Class III patients (serious, urgent) are those in which action must be taken within a few hours. Animals with severe open fractures, severe open wounds or burns, penetrating wounds to the abdomen without active bleeding, or blunt or penetrating trauma but without signs of shock or altered state of consciousness belong in this triage category.

Class IV. Class IV patients (less serious but still pressing) are those that require action within 24 hours. Most trauma patients are not in this category, but some may not be seen until the owner notices persistent health problems, for example, inability to walk on a limb, anorexia, vomiting.

The classification of each patient can change, especially during the first few hours after admission. If there is any question concerning the triage class of a patient, it is standard operating procedure to assign the more serious class. All professional and paraprofessional staff in the hospital should use the same classification system.

Classifying each patient helps with internal communications, allowing every staff member instantly to recognize the seriousness of each patient's condition, and provides administrative benefit as well. The number of animals seen, the range of charges, hospitalization days, morbidity and mortality, and number of hours of care required per case in each category can be tabulated. The triage classification presented for the traumatized patient can be applied to emergency patients with other conditions.

RESUSCITATION (TO STABILIZE)
General considerations

Goal. The goal of resuscitation is to normalize and stabilize the patient's vital physiologic functions as rapidly as possible in order to avert catastrophic consequences. This goal may be as simple as extending the head, neck, and tongue on an animal with an obstructed upper airway or as involved as having to perform major emergency surgical intervention to control continuing abdominal bleeding. *Resuscitation does not stop until the stated goal is reached, the patient dies, or the owner elects euthanasia for the animal.*

Euthanasia advised versus attempted resuscitation. Regarding this important point, there are times when owners, in the best interests of all concerned, should be advised that euthanasia is the humane course to take. However, this advice is often made too hastily or is based on the veterinarian's biases, for example, he/she thinks the owner cannot afford the costs involved.

An animal's appearance (often covered with blood, dirt, urine, and vomit) and the mental unpreparedness most people (including professionals) have for seeing and dealing with severe external injuries can cause an animal's condition to appear worse than it is. Therefore, caution should be taken to ensure that euthanasia recommendations are based on a careful and unbiased assessment and not on an initial impression. If the prognosis and costs that may be involved are unclear, this information should be communicated to the owner with an unbiased tone and inflection. Owners can be influenced significantly by the nonverbal attitude expressed by the veterinarian. Pessimism is natural, but it must be balanced with optimism when appropriate to allow a chance for pet survival.

General rules. General rules for trauma resuscitation have been developed to help prevent the rescuer from making serious mental mistakes and losing valuable time in the treatment of injured patients. These clinical protocols have been tested in both private and university emergency services.

1. Assume the injury is serious until proven otherwise.
2. Major injuries have pansystemic consequences that demand support of the ABCs plus the specific resuscitation techniques required for the primary problem (e.g., severe hemorrhagic shock therapy also requires intubation and positive-pressure ventilation).
3. Resuscitation is always followed by reassessment, and the two are always dependent on each other.
4. Monitored trends in parameters (heart and pulse rate, respiratory rate and depth, urine output, rectal and toe web temperature, mental alertness, and hematocrit and plasma total solids) are more-sensitive indicators of the success of treatment than are the actual numbers obtained for these parameters at each single measurement.
5. If the patient is not responding, assume something was missed on assessment or that the condition being treated is continuing (e.g., fracture of the pelvis with continuing blood loss).
6. The presence of shock may not indicate actual blood loss; however, blood loss should always be suspected as the primary cause of shock in all trauma patients.
7. The time required to recognize and treat the emergency condition(s) caused by trauma is one of the most important determinants that influences the likelihood of success (life) or failure (death). Therefore, *all recognized life-threatening injuries should be resolved as rapidly as possible.*
8. The number of rescuers, their training in trauma management, and the availability/organization of resuscitative drugs and equipment are key determinants of the success or failure in resuscitative treatment.
9. In trauma management, standard treatment is aggressive treatment. "Overtreatment" is often required to ensure adequate ventilation and circulation in major trauma. For example, it is better to tap the chest in the dyspneic dog than it is to wait and see if the dyspnea worsens.
10. Follow protocols that have been developed for trauma management. Do not wander. These protocols prevent unnecessary delays in detection and/or management and were developed with the intent for use by all veterinarians (experienced and inexperienced alike). Following established protocols in "the heat of the battle" prevents errors of omission and commission, both of which may kill!

The following case example is presented to illustrate the use of the general rules of trauma care.

A 4-month-old male bulldog, hit by a car 30 minutes before, was carried in by the owner. The dog demonstrates all the classic signs of shock, and no other abnormalities were obvious on the rest of the primary survey. As vital signs and observations were recorded, resuscitation was begun.

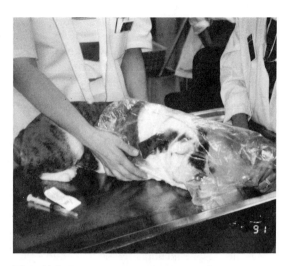

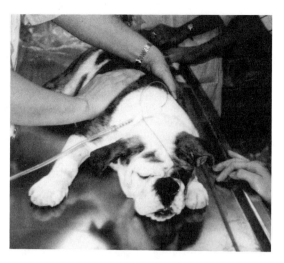

Fig. 10-9 Four-month-old English bulldog receiving high-flow oxygen (10 L/minute) using a clear plastic bag placed over his head. The "oxygen hood" was tolerated well, and his breathing rate decreased from 60 to 40 breaths per minute.

Fig. 10-10 Animal in Fig. 10-9 after placement of nasal oxygen catheter. The animal continued to receive oxygen at 4 L/minute, and a primary (repeat) survey and a secondary survey were completed.

Resuscitation was undertaken by a team of three paraprofessionals and one veterinarian. The general traumatic shock protocol was consulted. Initially, high-flow (10 L/minute) oxygen was administered into a clear plastic bag placed over the dog's head (Fig. 10-9). A nasal oxygen catheter was inserted and high-concentration oxygen supplementation was maintained at 4 L/minute (Fig. 10-10). Mild counterpressure wrapping was applied to the pelvic limbs and lower torso. A large-bore (16-gauge) cephalic-vein catheter was inserted and 5 ml of blood was withdrawn for immediate laboratory determinations.

Warmed lactated Ringer's solution was administered as rapidly as possible under 300 mm Hg pressure (estimating a rate of 8 ml/kg per minute) until the clinical signs of shock were dissipating and systemic arterial blood pressure (monitored by Doppler) was slightly above normal. As fluids were being administered to the animal, the primary survey was repeated. An increasing respiratory rate was noticed, so reexamination of the animal's respiratory tract was performed. Clinical signs of pneumothorax were present, and the right and left sides of the chest were tapped. Resuscitation and monitoring continued, and a secondary survey was performed.

This case illustrates teamwork; doing multiple resuscitation procedures simultaneously, doing the procedures in order of importance, and being aggressive with diagnosis (gathering/recording of base-line data). Aggressive resuscitation is required and is based on understanding the pathophysiologic changes occurring. Unfortunately, the commonly heard and read recommendation "to treat shock, give 1 blood volume of fluids over 1 hour" is not based on sound physiologic princi-

ples. Rather, the recommendation must be to restore intravascular blood volume as rapidly as possible and to administer as much fluid as is required to normalize or overcorrect the deficit.[17]

Resuscitation priorities (the ABCs)

Just as the primary survey and first aid management is performed with systems-oriented priorities, so is resuscitation. Airway disruption and blockage are the highest priority. Respiratory system difficulties not directly associated with airway function are the next life-threatening entities that need to be managed. Life-threatening cardiovascular system emergencies are the third priority. Resuscitation, following the ABCs, can involve first aid measures for injuries involving other systems, with the goal of stabilizing these other organ systems so that further injury and deterioration do not occur.

SPECIFIC TRAUMATIC CONDITIONS REQUIRING IMMEDIATE CARE
Upper airway blockage or disruption

Prevalence. Fortunately, airway injuries resulting in severe air exchange compromise are not common. These injuries go undiagnosed if the primary and secondary surveys do not start with assessment of the airway. Complete airway obstruction can mimic other causes of severe dyspnea. Partial obstruction may not be evident until over 75% of the airway is compromised.[18] However, once clinical signs are evident the condition easily becomes life threatening, appearing "all of a sudden" to the unsuspecting clinician.

Following complete airway obstruction, unconsciousness (in dogs previously breathing room air) begins in approximately 2 minutes, when Pao_2 reaches 30 torr (arterial oxygen saturation of 50%) or less. Increased respiratory efforts continue for another minute, with apnea beginning at 2 to 6 minutes. Pulselessness occurs at 5 to 10 minutes. Hypoxia and acidosis (from accumulation of carbon dioxide and hydrogen ions) in blood and tissues combine as a cause of circulatory failure.[19]

Pathophysiology. Following injury to the tongue, mouth, nose, and pharynx, bleeding can be significant. Clots can obstruct the airway at the larynx, trachea, or mainstem bronchi. The source of the blood resulting in these obstructing clots can be the lung–bronchi and the larynx–trachea. With the former, fine bubbles and foam are formed, potentiating airway obstruction.

Vomited food material and thick ropy saliva can cause airway obstruction. Diffuse obstruction of small airways can occur as a result of aspiration of gastric contents. Gastric emptying virtually stops following significant trauma, and if the animal is semicomatose to comatose, aspiration of passively regurgitated material is a real threat. A liquid aspirate of greater than 5 ml/20 kg of body weight with a pH less than 2.5 (common pH of stomach contents) can produce fatal obstructive bronchospasm and acute chemical pneumonitis.[20]

Anatomic disruption of the airway, from blunt or penetrating trauma, can lead to at least a partial airway obstruction that can be life threatening. The obstruction in this case works in concert with the loss of air flow through the respiratory passages secondary to the disruptive injury to cause respiratory compromise in the animal. Direct blunt trauma to the larynx can induce laryngeal spasm, which may cause partial or complete airway obstruction.

Partial to complete disruption of the trachea can lead to obstruction. Animals have been presented with complete separation of either the cervical or thoracic trachea with signs of partial obstruction. With manipulation of the animal for diagnostic purposes (e.g., radiographs) or the induction of general anesthesia and attempted intubation for repair of the recognized injury, the partial obstruction frequently can become complete.

Clinical signs. Difficulty with breathing on inspiration is the hallmark noted with severe partial airway obstructions. Airway sounds are exaggerated; the character and location of the greatest intensity of the sound helps identify the site of obstruction. Prelaryngeal airway obstruction results in sounds that are usually gurgled or sonorous;

with laryngeal and cranial tracheal obstructions, sounds are sibilant and raspy. Raspy breath sounds heard loudest at the thoracic inlet usually indicate partial obstruction at the caudal cervical or cranial thoracic trachea. Thoracic tracheal and bronchial locations usually have an exhalation component to the dyspnea.

As airway obstruction worsens, accessory muscles of respiration (face and neck) are activated. Cyanosis is a late and unreliable sign of airway obstruction (requires at least 5g/100 ml of circulating reduced hemoglobin) that is difficult to recognize in fluorescent lighting.[21] When cyanosis is present, the animal's airway demands rapid attention.

With complete obstructions, no breath sounds are heard despite attempts by the animal to ventilate. The animal is often unconscious, cyanotic (or ashen), and apneic with weak pulses. In these patients the clinical diagnosis of severe airway obstruction or disruption is not usually apparent until airway intubation and ventilation is attempted.

Resuscitation of the conscious animal with airway obstruction or disruption. If the animal is able to exchange enough air and remain conscious, the first step in treatment is to keep the animal calm. Oxygen supplementation is also of paramount importance in conscious animals with partial obstruction.

Supplemental oxygen therapy. The method of oxygen supplementation that is the best for the animal requires knowledge of the methods of oxygen supplementation available. These are described below.

Oxygen cage— A word of caution is in order if the animal is going to be placed in an oxygen cage. It is difficult to observe animals closely in an oxygen cage, and there is a danger that progressive respiratory failure can go undetected (Fig. 10-11). Other economical methods of supplementation (e.g., nasal and transtracheal catheters) that do not confine or isolate the patient are preferred.

It is not possible to monitor effectively an animal placed in an oxygen cage because the patient is isolated. When the oxygen cage door is opened, the increased oxygen in the patient's atmosphere (e.g., 40% oxygen) quickly falls, significantly stressing the animal. Nasal and transtracheal catheters allow for continued oxygen supplementation during performance of diagnostic tests (e.g., cervical and chest radiography).[22]

Oxygen bag (hood)— An alternative means of oxygen supplementation that I have found useful is a clear plastic bag placed over the patient's head and containing volume for several breath ex-

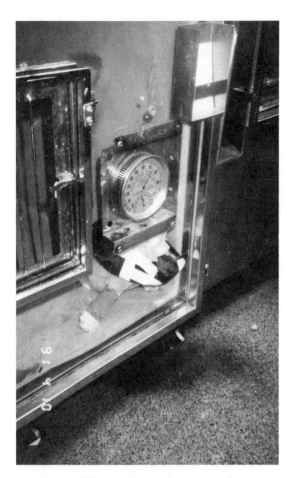

Fig. 10-11 Mixed-breed dog with increased respiratory effort, placed inside an oxygen cage receiving 10 L/ minute of oxygen. *Note:* the animal could not be observed well, and continued physical examination was not possible. Use of an oxygen hood and nasal catheter placement allowed continuation of his physical examination. Examination findings suggested pneumothorax, and this was verified by thoracocentesis.

changes. Oxygen is provided via a hose placed inside the bag near the animal's nose and administered at a minimum of 5 to 8 L per minute. The bag remains open along the animal's neck to allow gas to escape (see Fig. 10-9). This method can provide at least a 75% oxygen concentration once denitrogenation has occurred. Many animals tolerate this bag/hood method for oxygen delivery in contrast to violently objecting to the use of a face mask. This method is often used initially while nasal or transtracheal cannulation is being readied. Animals that present in a frantic state can be completely covered with a clear plastic sheet or even with a simple blanket and high-flow oxygen administered under it (15 L per minute). This approach has been very effective in helping re-store oxygenation and provides an immediate high concentration of oxygen to the animal without risking injury to providers.

Nasal catheter—This method of supplementation is tolerated very well by most animals and can be implemented easily. It involves the placement of a 5 to 8 French feeding tube (red rubber or polyvinylchloride) or commercially available oxygen catheter (6 French polyvinylchloride) into the nose of the animal following installation of a few drops of proparacaine or lidocaine. Small doses of butorphanol (0.01 to 0.05 mg/kg IV) may be required to facilitate placement in some cats. The catheter is inserted to the level of the first or second premolar in the ventral nasal meatus and secured by suturing or gluing it to the skin. The proximal end of the catheter is secured with tape around the neck and then attached to tubing leading to the humidified oxygen supply (see Fig. 10-10).

To achieve a 40% oxygen concentration in the trachea, a humidified oxygen flow rate of approximately 100 ml/kg per minute is recommended. In a research study involving nasal oxygen administration to dogs, oxygen concentrations as high as 95% were achieved with proportionally higher flow rates.

I have used the technique in over 500 dogs and cats, ranging from 300 g to 120 kg in body weight and have found patient tolerance excellent in most cases. Those that do not tolerate the catheter may require mild sedation and/or an Elizabethan collar.

Transtracheal catheter—A long intravenous catheter is placed into the trachea, following instillation of a local anesthetic, using the method recommended for diagnostic tracheal aspiration. The tracheal catheter is secured to the skin and cervical fascia with a suture and a dressing applied. Humidified oxygen is administered through the catheter at a flow rate generally sufficient to provide initially a 40% inspired oxygen concentration. Oxygen humidification prevents desiccation of the tracheal mucosa. Transtracheal catheter oxygen administration is preferred whenever epistaxis or a history of head injury is present. This technique can also be used to help alleviate breathing difficulty in animals with a laryngeal or upper tracheal obstruction or partial obstruction.

Transtracheal oxygen administration can be a helpful adjunct in the expulsion of airway foreign bodies. Oxygen, added to the trachea via this catheter, increases the amount of gas in the pulmonary airways, which would be put under compression when the chest and abdomen are squeezed. Also, the oxygen supplementation provides time for the removal of the foreign body.

Abdominal and thoracic compressions. When progressive airway obstruction signs occur and are believed to be due to foreign materials in the larynx or trachea, abdominal and thoracic compression (simultaneously performed), or back blows with the head and neck in a downward position are often useful in relieving the obstruction. Under anesthesia, airway pressures averaged 33 mm Hg generated with back blows, 15 mm Hg with abdominal thrusts, and 19 mm Hg with sternal or chest thrusts.[23] The amount of airway pressure generated by the hugging maneuver is dependent on the amount of air present in the lungs when the hug is performed.[23] Heimlich reported in a study in conscious humans that airway pressures could reach as high as 30 mm Hg.[23] Although the combination of abdominal and chest "hugs" has not been reported, this simultaneous combination may be more effective in generating pressures than the methods tested thus far.

If abdominal and thoracic "hugs" are ineffective in expelling the foreign object, oxygen can be insufflated into the trachea through a needle or catheter inserted into the trachea and the hugging reattempted.

The force of gravity may also be used to help in the removal of the foreign materials by keeping the patient's head down while the hugs are administered. The maneuvers are repeated until either the obstruction clears, clinical signs abate, or loss of consciousness occurs allowing a resuscitative tracheostomy to be performed.

Intrathoracic tracheal or mainstem bronchial injuries. Severe injuries to the intrathoracic trachea or mainstem bronchi may present with a mixture of clinical signs (e.g., muffled lung sounds unilaterally, progressive dyspnea with the accumulation of air in the pleural space, cervical region, thoracic inlet, and subcutaneous tissues of the chest wall or mediastinum). In most cases of intrathoracic or bronchial injury a resultant bronchopleural "fistula" occurs and a rapidly developing, severe unilateral pneumothorax with or without dissecting cervical subcutaneous emphysema and lung collapse (on the side of the bronchial injury) is the most common presentation.

Tension pneumothorax is a common complication that is generally treated successfully by chest-tube placement and continuous low vacuum suction (see following sections or Chapter 25). Bronchial tears generally seal spontaneously with conservative treatment (chest-tube placement and underwater suction seal and drainage) of 3 to 5 days. If the leak in the major intrathoracic airway does not slow down or stop, then an exploratory thoracotomy and direct repair of the leaking area is recommended.

Resuscitation of the unconscious patient with airway obstruction or disruption. Key steps in treatment are (1) continued attempts at chest and abdominal compressions to expel any foreign objects, (2) attempts to introduce some air or oxygen into the airway (continued first aid maneuvers until equipment and help arrive), (3) clearing of the pharynx and larynx with suctioning, (4) tracheal intubation, (5) tracheostomy, and, rarely (6) emergent cervical and parasternotomy approaches to secure the disrupted airway or open the obstructed airway. If endoscopy equipment is immediately available, application of this technique can be of benefit in selected cases.

Suction. If the airway obstruction has led to unconsciousness, then intubation, preferably with the aid of a laryngoscope, should be performed. If clots, vomit, thick saliva, or foam is causing airway obstruction or difficulty with laryngeal visualization, immediate suctioning is required. A dental suction tip with a large end hole or an endotracheal tube used as a suction tip are the best instruments for the removal of this material in the larynx or perilaryngeal area (see Fig. 10-7). A Yankauer (tonsil) suction tip is also effective for removal of less viscous pharyngeal secretions.

Intubation. Manipulation of perilaryngeal structures during intubation must be gentle, because vagal induced cardiac arrest is possible in hypoxemic and hypercarbic animals. During intubation, if possible, the patient's head should remain horizontal (not elevated) to prevent aspiration into the airway and decreased blood flow to the brain.

The best way to accomplish intubation is to place the patient in dorsal recumbency with the head at the end of the table. Animals in this position can also be intubated without assistance and with the least amount of laryngeal manipulation. Intubation without assistance may require the use of sandbags, V-shaped tray, or a surgery table with adjustable sides to maintain the patient in dorsal recumbency (Fig. 10-12). Large dogs can be left in right lateral recumbency and intubation accomplished easily with the use of the laryngoscope (Fig. 10-13).

With the animal in dorsal recumbency, the laryngoscope and the tongue are held in the left hand. The blade of the scope is inserted ventral or dorsal to the epiglottis, depending on the type of laryngoscope used. The scope is used in a leverage fashion to elevate (move ventrally) the hyoid apparatus. This maneuver brings the rima glottis rostral and opens it to facilitate the insertion of an endotracheal tube, held in the right hand (see Fig. 10-12).

Laryngoscopic intubation can be accomplished with the animal in right lateral recumbency. The

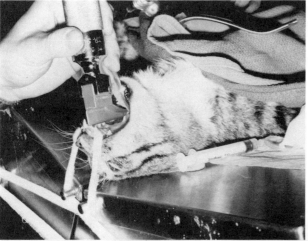

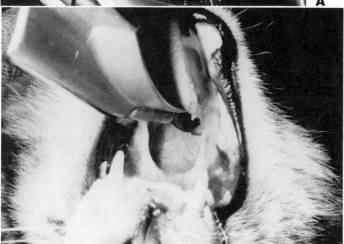

Fig. 10-12 A, Cat being intubated with the use of a laryngoscope with the patient in dorsal recumbency. Note the laryngoscope is held in the left hand, endotracheal tube in the right hand. **B,** The intubator has a clear view of the rima glottis with the use of the laryngoscope in this method, allowing intubation without undue laryngeal manipulation.

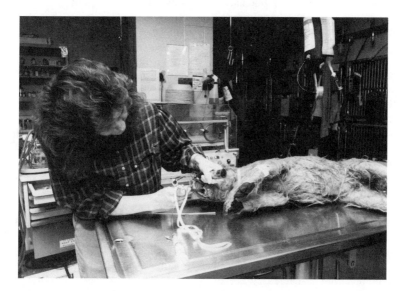

Fig. 10-13. Tracheal intubation being practiced by a veterinary technician with the patient (mannequin) in right lateral recumbency. Note that this method allows intubation to be done without assistance and keeps the patient's head nearly horizontal to maintain blood flow to the brain.

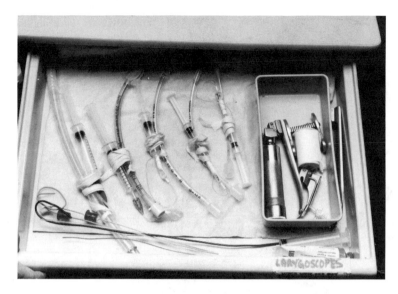

Fig. 10-14. Top drawer of crash cart containing endotracheal tubes with umbilical tape and air-filled syringe attached for rapid tube fixation and cuff inflation.

scope is held in the left hand and the endotracheal tube in the right. This approach is particularly beneficial in very large dogs when no assistance is available. If help is available, intubation is facilitated by having an assistant hold the animal's mouth open (see Fig. 10-13).

With assistance, intubation can be accomplished with the patient in ventral recumbency. However, intubating in this position decreases blood flow to the brain because the head has to be elevated. If the animal is already hypotensive, this manipulation can precipitate cardiopulmonary arrest. Elevation of the animal's head also increases the risk of aspiration of pharyngeal foreign materials.

To allow for more rapid tracheal intubation, it is recommended that each size of endotracheal tube placed in the crash cart for use on an emergent basis be fitted with an air-filled syringe for cuff inflation and umbilical tape or gauze for securing the tube following intubation of the patient. This endotracheal tube readiness will save valuable seconds when seconds really count (Fig. 10-14).

Once intubated the animal should be ventilated and auscultation used to verify that lung sounds are present bilaterally. Endotracheal tube suctioning with a dental suction tip may be required to remove pieces of food, vomitus, or blood clots in the trachea while fluid sounds or decreased breath sounds in bronchial regions indicate the need to suction using a tracheal suction cannula.

*Emergent (slash) cervical and parasternal trache-*ostomy *and tracheal intubation*. If the trachea cannot be intubated and made patent with conventional methods and the animal is dying from airway compromise (injury and obstruction), then an emergent (slash) tracheostomy is performed.

Large tracheal tears causing loss of airway continuity constitute most of the indications requiring resuscitative surgical intervention. Laryngeal injury and perilaryngeal swelling or spasm following trauma constitute other indications. Foreign-body tracheal obstruction can be an indication for emergent tracheostomy, but this circumstance is usually not associated with trauma. The consequences of losing a patent airway are grave, and airway intubation is mandatory and should be performed immediately by whatever means is required; there is no time for aseptic preparation of the animal.

Exposure to the trachea is done rapidly using a scalpel and Mayo scissors. With the animal in dorsal recumbency and the neck hyperextended, a midline or near midline skin incision is made in the midcervical region. The sternohyoideus muscles are separated on or near the midline and the trachea exposed.

Cervical tracheostomy—For a cervical tracheostomy the light peritracheal fascia is separated and an incision is made between tracheal rings or longitudinally to include two or three tracheal rings. The tip of the instrument used to enter the trachea is kept in the tracheal lumen to identify the site, and a second instrument (curved hemostat preferred) is used to separate the rings and allow ventilation. With this second instrument as a guide the trachea is intubated with a cuffed endotracheal tube or tracheostomy tube. If an endotracheal tube is used, it must be shortened and modified so it can be secured. The tracheostomy or modified endotracheal tube are secured with umbilical tape extending around the back of the patient's neck and tied in a bow.

"Awake tracheostomy"—Cervical tracheostomy is indicated in conscious patients suffering from severe dyspnea due to pulmonary contusion, edema, and intrapulmonic hemorrhage despite high-concentration oxygen supplementation. A lidocaine infiltration is placed into the surrounding soft tissues, the head and neck are extended by an assistant, and the tracheostomy is performed. Two traction sutures are inserted around the most proximal and most distal tracheal rings near the ostomy site. These sutures are left in place when the tube is inserted. These sutures are used to help guide the tube into the tracheal lumen during initial placement and during replacement following cleaning or dislodgment.

Emergent cervical tracheal exposure for disruptive wounds in the trachea—The approach is the same as for emergent tracheostomy. After exposure, major injuries to the trachea, disruptive enough to cause significant dyspnea, are generally large enough to accommodate placement of an endotracheal tube into the distal segment. Surrounding soft tissues may require retraction or debridement to allow visualization and placement of the tube. Occasionally, the opening in the trachea must be enlarged to accommodate the tube. If the injury causes substantial devitalized or crushed tissue, a completely new opening into the trachea distal to the injury may be required for the placement of an endotracheal or tracheostomy tube.

Once the trachea is intubated, ventilation is initiated and suctioning is accomplished as required. The patient is transferred to the operating room, and inhalational anesthesia is administered. The trachea is intubated by an orally placed endotracheal tube positioned through the distal segment. Passing the endotracheal tube into the distal tracheal segment often requires manipulation of this segment.

The trachea is repaired following copious irrigation and debridement of the nonvital tissues. Simple interrupted, 4-0 to 2-0, appositional monofilament nonabsorbable sutures (polypropylene or nylon) swaged on a taper or taper-cutting needle are used for repair. Sutures can enter the lumen without complication, and this procedure ensures a secure closure. When resection is required, the two tracheal rings of adjoining segments are apposed using multiple simple interrupted sutures. Half rings are created by splitting these tracheal rings circumferentially with a scalpel blade. When joined together the cut edges of hyaline cartilage from each half tracheal ring heal by primary intention with minimal scarring and stenosis.[24]

Emergency (slash) parasternotomy for thoracic tracheal exposure—Rarely, tracheal disruption occurs within the thoracic cavity from penetrating trauma, traction injuries, or blunt trauma. In these patients the lungs cannot be ventilated via a normally placed endotracheal tube. If after trying to advance the tube into the caudal thoracic trachea, beyond the injured area, difficult inspiratory ventilation remains, then an emergent caudal cervical and parasternal approach to the trachea is required. A scalpel blade is used to make the skin incision on the ventral midline or near midline. A Mayo scissors is used to separate the chondrosternal joints and soft tissues beginning at the manubrium and extending caudally at least four to five sternebrae.

While working as quickly as possible to gain tracheal exposure, great care is required to avoid injury to the bracheocephalic veins and other great vessels. Keeping the tips of the Mayo scissors as ventral as possible will help prevent injury to these vessels. Severance of the internal thoracic vein and artery on one side will be necessary and will require later ligation.

Case illustrating airway resuscitation. A 3-year-old Boston Terrier was presented with severe inspiratory dyspnea. Trauma was suspected but had not been observed. The dyspnea became progressive, resulting in cyanosis and unconsciousness. Following orotracheal intubation, lung sounds could not be heard with attempts at ventilation and a "feeling of obstruction" was detected during delivery of positive-pressure breaths. Suctioning was not productive. Respiratory arrest and deep cyanosis ensued. An emergent caudal cervical tracheal approach was made, revealing an intact trachea, and an emergent parasternotomy was accomplished.

The trachea was traced by palpation through the mediastinum to a major separation cranial to the carina. Following the discovery of a completely severed airway, placement of the end of an endotracheal tube into the distal tracheal stump and positive-pressure ventilation aborted sure cardiac arrest. The tracheal separation was repaired following careful placement of an intratracheal endotracheal tube, debridement of the ends of the trachea, and appositional suturing using a simple interrupted suture pattern of 3-0 polypropylene.

The dog was successfully resuscitated, and it

recovered with no evidence of neurologic, infectious, or residual ventilatory problems.

Prognosis. With major airway obstruction or disruption, the prognosis is often linked to the length of time before the problem was identified, the shorter the better. The greater the extent of injury and the greater the difficulty in surgically repairing the injuries, the more guarded the prognosis. Fibrosis and stricture of the lumen are sequela that can occur with circumferential injury when primary healing is not realized.

The prevalence of postoperative infection is low despite the use of resuscitative tracheostomy and parasternotomy surgical approaches through unclipped hair. This result is attributable to copious irrigation and cleaning of the exposed tissues following these surgical approaches.

Tension pneumothorax

Pathophysiology. Tension pneumothorax most commonly occurs secondary to injury to the lung parenchyma from blunt or penetrating trauma. With either form of injury a one-way valve effect is in operation, air leaks from injured bronchi or alveoli and enters the pleural space during inspiration, remaining trapped during expiration. Most instances begin as unilateral pneumothorax. Some rapidly progress to bilateral conditions due to the thin nature of the mediastinum. Eventually, pleural pressure increases and interferes with venous return to the heart. When venous return is affected, blood begins to pool in large-capacitance veins and shock ensues.

Approximately 30 ml/kg of body weight of air must be trapped within the pleural space before mild clinical signs are evident in laboratory beagles.[25] The amount of air required in the pleural space before clinical signs are observed is quite variable in traumatized animals. Animals with severe pulmonary contusions do not tolerate much pleural air accumulation before experiencing cardiopulmonary compromise. Small dogs and cats appear less tolerant to the effect of developing pneumothorax than large working breeds of dogs.[25]

Death due to cardiovascular collapse and compromised ventilation can occur within minutes after the onset of clinical signs in severe cases.

Clinical signs. Animals suffering from a tension pneumothorax appear anxious with an exaggerated respiratory effort. The main feature observed is the "all-out effort" to breathe. The animal's head and neck are extended, pectoral limbs are abducted, the chest is fully expanded, and an abdominal component to breathing is evident. Palpation of subcutaneous air in the cervical or thoracic region in dyspneic animals suggests pneumothorax. Occasionally, jugular and/or femoral venous distention (uncommon in shock caused by hemorrhage) and distention of the soft tissues at the thoracic inlet is observed with tension pneumothorax. Accessory muscles of the face and neck are activated with each attempted inspiration; for example, the commissures of the mouth are retracted with each inspiration. Cyanosis and paleness become progressively more evident and as systemic arterial blood pressure decreases, the animal becomes unconscious and respiratory arrest occurs. The chest appears expanded, mucous membranes become ashen, and the heart rate slows preterminally.

These clinical signs in an animal should prompt a tentative diagnosis of tension pneumothorax. Auscultation will confirm diminished lung sounds unilaterally or bilaterally. Chest percussion can be a very helpful diagnostic test in differentiating severe pneumothorax from fluid accumulations within the pleural space—the former providing a hollow, tympanic, resonant sound and the latter providing a dull nonresonant sound.

Diagnosis. Following recognition of the clinical signs that suggest pneumothorax, bilateral thoracocentesis is performed. The procedure should be done with minimal restraint, keeping the animal in a comfortable position. Supplemental oxygen (10 L per minute) is delivered via bag (hood) or blow-by high-flow technique (oxygen directed through a 3/8-in. tube held close and pointed toward the patient's head).

During attempted thoracocentesis, a drop of sterile fluid (saline, 1% to 2% lidocaine solution) is placed in the hub of a 20-gauge hypodermic needle following needle insertion into the skin. As the needle is advanced and enters the pleural space, the fluid moves inward, indicating a simple (normotensive) pneumothorax or normal pleura, or moves outward, indicating a tension pneumothorax. It is important not to accept "the feel" of popping through the pleura as confirmation that the pleural space was entered. A tension pneumothorax could be present, but attempted thoracocentesis could yield false negative results if steps are not taken to ensure that the pleural space was truly entered and sampled.

Following needle insertion into the pleural space, a syringe, attached by way of an extension-set and three-way stopcock, should be used in an attempt to aspirate air and fluid. The aspiration of air or blood should continue if the animal's condition begins to improve. If the animal does not appear to improve and continues to demonstrate clinical signs of shock associated with the presence of hemothorax or unrelenting aspiration of air, a large-bore (size of mainstem bronchus) chest tube (see Chapter 25) should be inserted (conscious animal) or an emergent, resuscitative thoracotomy undertaken (unconscious animal).

Radiographs are not indicated in the dyspneic patient until pneumothorax can be ruled out via thoracocentesis performed bilaterally. Supplemental oxygen via a bag (hood), mask, tracheal catheter, or nasal catheter is mandatory before undertaking thoracic radiographic evaluation.

Resuscitation of semiconscious and extremely dyspneic animals with pneumothorax. Immediate open-needle thoracocentesis, without the benefit of clipping the chest wall, is initially indicated. A plastic over-the-needle catheter (with an extra side hole added) is safer and may be more effective than a simple hypodermic needle. The needle/catheter (18-gauge minimum) used should allow rapid decompression of the pleural space. Following initial placement, a hand should be used to stabilize and prevent dislodgment or movement of the needle/catheter within the pleural space. As decompression is initiated, an extension set attached to a three-way stopcock and large syringe is connected to the needle or catheter for aspiration of air from the pleural space. In patients with severe traumatic bronchopulmonary fistulas, air will continue to accumulate, indicating the need for the placement of a large-bore chest tube (see Chapter 25). The chest-tube diameter should approximate the size of the mainstem bronchus. This ensures that aspiration will be effective for the treatment of continued leakage of air from any major traumatic airway openings.

Keeping the lung expanded and the pleural surfaces in contact helps control the leakage of air from most major pulmonary injuries. Continuous suction drainage is maintained for 2 to 4 days following the last evidence of air leakage (air bubbles arising from the underwater seal) to ensure that a firm seal between parietal and visceral pleura has formed and that recurrence of air leakage is unlikely. Underwater seal and suction drainage helps to control major air leaks from bronchial injuries, but is generally not effective in leading to a permanent seal. Persistent air leakage that does not gradually decrease over 48 to 72 hours is an indicator of such an injury. These animals often require a thoracotomy and lung lobectomy or surgical repair of bronchial injuries.

Resuscitation of unconscious animals with pneumothorax. Animals that are unconscious are intubated and receive positive-pressure ventilation. A decrease in pulmonary compliance will be noted during the ventilation of animals with severe pneumothorax. These animals will deteriorate rapidly owing to the increasing accumulation of air within the pleural space during intermittent positive-pressure breathing. In these cases, a resuscitative minithoracotomy through the unclipped chest wall is indicated. This procedure allows air within the pleural space to escape, resulting in immediate relief of the restrictive pressure within the pleural cavity.

Once the pleural pressure has normalized, improvement in cardiac function due to improved venous return and cardiac filling during diastole follows. After cardiovascular stabilization, the animal with unrelenting pneumothorax can be taken to the operating room, where exploration of the thoracic cavity should be completed in an aseptic, methodical, and thorough manner. The mediastinum should be fenestrated and the opposite side of the thoracic cavity examined as best as possible. Bronchial and pulmonary parenchymal injury should be repaired. This procedure usually requires fine monofilament suture placement and closure or the use of stapling instruments. Following thorough irrigation and the placement of a large-bore chest tube to monitor postoperative air accumulations, the thoracostomy is closed and broad-spectrum antibiotics are administered intravenously during the perioperative period. The postthoracotomy infection rate in these animals appears similar to that reported in human patients experiencing an emergent, resuscitative thoracotomy.[26,27]

Catastrophic hemorrhage

Introduction and pathophysiology. Catastrophic hemorrhage is immediately life-threatening because of (1) massive internal or external blood loss leading to vascular collapse or (2) internal blood loss into an anatomic area where space occupation by the blood causes secondary cardiovascular or neurologic malfunction, for example, pericardial tamponade or increased intracranial pressure. In trauma patients, the catastrophic hemorrhage involving massive blood loss is commonly recognized; however, the latter occurrence can be a real threat, often going unrecognized until observed at necropsy.

Immediate goals are to recognize the hemorrhage, apply temporary measures to slow the hemorrhage, provide rapid restorative therapy early in order to prevent acute death from vascular collapse and irreversible vital organ malfunction related to shock, and apply definitive measures to stop the hemorrhage.

Cardiovascular collapse from exsanguinating hemorrhage results in insufficient blood flow to the brain and profound vasodilation from persistent hypoxemia, with resultant energy failure, and metabolic acidosis.[28] Animals are often presented with extreme hypotension, bradycardia, and coma.

If 20% to 25% of the animal's blood volume is lost or sequestered over 5 to 10 minutes in a way that renders it unavailable to the circulating blood volume, catastrophic clinical signs of impending death ensue. In contrast, the same amount of hemorrhage occurring over an hour leads to only mild clinical signs (mild tachypnea and increase in capillary refill time). In the slower bleeding situation, compensatory transcapillary fluid flux and "internal autotransfusion" has an opportunity to occur.[29]

The compensatory response to rapid hemorrhage depends on the animal's ability to "mobilize" pooled red blood cells and plasma from the venous circulation and spleen. Rapid hemorrhage in a short time does not allow for adequate mobilization of interstitial fluid and pooled red blood cells into the circulation. Compensatory responses mediated by the central nervous system are also blunted due to hypoxia of the respiratory and cardiovascular centers. "Autotransfusion" capabilities vary with species, age, and factors related to the general health of the individual. For example, cats are not able to store as much blood in the spleen as dogs (5 ml/kg in cats versus 10 to 20 ml/kg in dogs). In the dog, the spleen should be thought of as an internal reservoir of a unit of packed red blood cells (packed cell volume of 70%) that can be "transfused" as the animal requires; the same cannot be stated for cats. Aged and immature animals have a smaller marginating blood pool as compared with other age groups of animals of the same species. Animals that are hypoproteinemic or malnourished are less able to tolerate hemorrhagic episodes due to an already contracted interstitial and vascular fluid volume and red blood cell mass.

Clinical signs. Physical evidence of trauma and shock with delayed capillary refill time, increased (or decreased) heart and respiratory rate, apprehension, fright, and progressive decreases in body temperature and level of consciousness is observed as bleeding continues. Pulses are not weakened and blood pressure does not decrease until late in the course of the hemorrhage and shock. Additional clinical signs depend on the location or source of the hemorrhage.

Diagnosis. Time is a key factor in the management of exsanguinating hemorrhage. The diagnosis and treatment must be aggressively pursued. Diagnosis is generally not difficult with external bleeding, whereas internal bleeding may not be readily apparent.

Generally, by the time these animals are seen, clinical signs of shock are very apparent. Animals observed immediately following injury may appear clinically stable, while profuse internal hem-

orrhage is ongoing. Clinical signs of shock take a few minutes to manifest. For example, in an experimental study in dogs, hemorrhage was induced by severing the renal artery and vein. Five minutes elapsed before signs of shock were evident.[15] Clinicians must have a high index of suspicion in animals with unknown or immediate trauma histories. This suspicion is particularly important in the first few minutes after patient admission in order to prevent delayed recognition and treatment of occult profuse hemorrhage.

If hemorrhage is inapparent in animals presented following a history of recent trauma, it should be assumed that these animals have serious ongoing internal hemorrhage until proven otherwise. These patients should be hospitalized for a minimum of a few hours for careful observation.

Exsanguinating (catastrophic) external hemorrhage. This type of hemorrhage is not difficult to assess. Specific historical data that accurately estimate the amount of blood lost prior to admission is often difficult to obtain; blood-soaked clothing, sheets, and bandages that accompany the animal provide clues. The physical examination findings of a severe external wound and shock are usually the best indications of the amount of hemorrhage that has occurred.

Exsanguinating (catastrophic) internal hemorrhage. This type of hemorrhage is hidden from sight and may occur within the thorax, peritoneum, retroperitoneum, the osseofascial compartments of the cervical area, humerus, pelvis, or femur. In traumatized patients manifesting shock without evidence of severe external hemorrhage, these areas must be investigated for evidence of blood accumulation.

Severe bleeding into the thorax and abdomen are the most common sites for occult exsanguinating hemorrhage. Although bleeding into the retroperitoneum and osseofascial compartments is not uncommon following trauma, exsanguinating hemorrhage into these areas is rare, but must be considered in all patients with severe shock.

The specific location or locations for ongoing hemorrhage are usually limited to sites of swelling, distention, bruising, or external skin lesions (puncture and bite wounds). Two patterns of bruises are specific for indicating locations of internal hemorrhage: a circular bruise centered around the umbilicus, indicating peritoneal hemorrhage, and bruising in the inguinal canal, indicating retroperitoneal hemorrhage. Clipping of the animal's hair facilitates recognition of the bruise patterns.

THORACIC HEMORRHAGE. This diagnosis is made in the seriously traumatized patient by rapid needle thoracocentesis. The needle tip must be placed correctly within the pleural space to achieve the proper diagnosis. Thoracic hemorrhage cannot be ruled out on the basis of a negative tap, as the needle may be blocked by lung or mediastinal tissues. The volume of blood within the thoracic cavity cannot be estimated based on the results of positive needle thoracocentesis.

The chances of collecting a sample are improved with the use of a multifenestrated chest tube. Additionally, this device is required to drain the pleural space effectively, a key method in the treatment of hemothorax. A large-bore chest tube (the size of the mainstem bronchus or one that will just fit between two ribs) should be inserted as quickly as possible if the animal appears to be in shock. Rapid administration of an autotransfusion using the blood removed from the thorax should be considered (see Chapter 34). If the animal is unconscious and in severe shock, with danger of immediate death, then a resuscitative thoracotomy should be performed with minimal consideration for aseptic technique.[30] Definitive diagnosis and treatment of the source of the hemorrhage is performed by a rapid exploration of the chest cavity following evacuation of the blood (see section on Resuscitative Thoracotomy below).

ABDOMINAL (PERITONEAL) HEMORRHAGE. A reliable physical examination finding associated with intraabdominal hemorrhage is a red circular discoloration centered at the patient's umbilicus.[31] It is believed this bruising is caused by an accumulation of red blood cells that move underneath the skin through a small defect in the umbilical scar.

Abdominal distention due to hemorrhage following blunt or penetrating abdominal trauma may occur, but cannot be relied on as a definitive clinical sign. To observe distention from abdominal blood accumulation in dogs requires the presence of at least 40 ml/kg of body weight of blood.[32] This amount approaches one half of an animal's blood volume. Distinct abdominal distention from acute blood loss is usually not observed unless intravenous volume replacement therapy has occurred or is ongoing.

Abdominal hemorrhage can be assumed to be the cause of abdominal distention in animals that have evidence of penetrating abdominal injury (gunshot wounds) provided percussion of the abdomen yields dullness. Resonant sounds on percussion would indicate distention caused by air, either within the stomach and intestine, or free in the peritoneal cavity (tension pneumoperitoneum—a rare consequence to disruption of the gastrointestinal tract or as the result of a "sucking" peritoneal cavity wound).

Abdominal distention can occur with enlarged abdominal organs, aerophagia with gastric distention, and with tension pneumothorax. Tension pneumothorax causes the caudal displacement of the diaphragm and visceral organs along with congestion of abdominal organs secondary to the impairment of venous return. In these cases, the erroneous diagnosis of peritoneal hemorrhage occurs when abdominocentesis of the "distended" abdomen yields blood.

To avoid errors in diagnosis and to maximize the potential for correct diagnosis a plastic multiholed catheter, with or without concomitant lavage, should be used in place of needle paracentesis in animals with suspected hemoperitoneum (Chapter 13). Numerous studies have proven that a negative needle tap tells you nothing. False positive results can also occur, particularly when congestion of abdominal veins and spleen are present.[33]

Following diagnostic peritoneal catheter placement, blood is usually easily aspirated from the abdominal cavity when severe acute peritoneal hemorrhage is present. This finding does not indicate whether the hemorrhage is continuing. In animals that are hemodynamically unstable or that remain unstable following volume replacement therapy, continued hemorrhage should be assumed. Further diagnostic tests are not indicated, and resuscitative treatment aimed at arresting the peritoneal hemorrhage should commence immediately.

In animals that cannot be operated on immediately, the hemorrhage may be slowed by rapid peritoneal infusion of physiologic saline solution through the peritoneal catheter.[32]

Diagnostic abdominal lavage catheters can be left in place for subsequent sample collection and hematocrit determinations at 10-minute intervals. In animals that are responding to volume replacement and in which the hematocrit of the lavage fluid remains within 5% of original samples, conservative, nonoperative management may be continued as hemorrhage is "controlled."

RETROPERITONEAL HEMORRHAGE. This diagnosis can be suspected in traumatized animals when a lateral-view abdominal radiograph demonstrates a depressed "psoas line" or colon. Bruising in the inguinal region suggests retroperitoneal hemorrhage as blood follows the fascia of the iliopsoas muscle to the lesser trochanter of the femur and the fascia of the femoral and inguinal canals. Catastrophic retroperitoneal hemorrhage should be suspected when a penetrating wound is present in the flank region, hemorrhage is observed from the wound, and shock is present.

Definitive diagnosis of the presence, extent,

and source for retroperitoneal hemorrhage is made during exploratory abdominal surgical intervention. Typically, the entire retroperitoneal space is filled with blood. Localized and limited hemorrhagic effusion can also be observed, especially with renal and ureteral injury.

OSSEOFASCIAL COMPARTMENT HEMORRHAGE. Severe hemorrhage into fascial compartments of the neck, flank, and inguinal region, or osseofascial compartments of the extremities can occur following blunt or penetrating trauma. This hemorrhage should be suspected if acute swelling in any of these areas is observed shortly after injury. Clipping of the swollen area should be undertaken to facilitate examination. The surface of the skin should be examined for bruises, penetrating wounds, and lacerations. If there is doubt that the swelling is due to hemorrhage, a sterile needle aspiration can be performed. The presence of a small amount of blood on aspiration confirms the diagnosis of compartmental hemorrhage.

It is important to estimate the amount of swelling present and to determine if the swelling is increasing in size, indicating continued hemorrhage into the area. An estimation of the amount of bleeding that has occurred can be made by comparing the size of the swollen area with the size of the examiner's fist. Each fist contains a volume of between 300 and 500 ml. Frequent repeated observations are then made to compare the swelling size.

Alternatively, a more accurate determination of progressive extremity swelling can be accomplished by using a tape measure to measure serially the circumference of the limb. The limb must be measured each time in the same location and with the same amount of tension to render the measurement accurate.

General management of catastrophic hemorrhage. There are four key methods of treatment for catastrophic hemorrhage and the shock syndrome that accompanies it, as listed below:

1. Application of counterpressure to the abdomen and pelvic limbs. This counterpressure slows or stops hemorrhage caudal to the diaphragm, facilitates autotransfusion of blood, and increases systemic arterial blood pressure via increasing systemic vascular resistance and venous return to the heart.
2. Rapid blood volume restitution with administration of blood, plasma, colloid plasma expanders, hypertonic saline, and/or balanced crystalloid solutions. The resuscitation should continue until systemic arterial blood pressure is stabilized slightly above normal values.
3. Rapid surgical exploration of the thorax, abdomen, or limb(s) and internal control of the hemorrhage by occlusion of the arterial blood supply leading to the site of the hemorrhage. This procedure often requires the use of vascular "loops" or temporary wide vascular tourniquets.
4. Identification, with ligation or repair, of the bleeding vessels.

All of these methods must be performed quickly because of impending vascular collapse in the vast majority of animals with severe hemorrhage. Very rapid volume restitution and the control of the hemorrhage are keys to survival. These procedures do take time to implement, and the selective use of counterpressure becomes a very important initial consideration. Counterpressure can be implemented quickly while the diagnostic approaches and more definitive treatment for catastrophic hemorrhage are initiated.

If the catastrophic hemorrhage is occurring in the thoracic cavity, counterpressure will not be effective and may cause more bleeding to occur. In these cases, a resuscitative thoracotomy should be performed and the bleeding structures temporarily occluded.

Resuscitative thoracotomy and cross clamping of the descending aorta may prove lifesaving in patients that are presented with clinical signs of severe catastrophic intraabdominal hemorrhage and impending death (e.g., unconsciousness, shallow breathing, very fast or very slow heart rate, and severe hypotension).

External counterpressure. If examination of the chest and thoracocentesis are negative (no severe chest trauma or hemorrhage), external counterpressure applied to the pelvic limbs and caudal abdomen can be very effective in temporarily raising systemic arterial and central venous blood pressures. Blood flow is preferentially redirected to the central circulation and brain. The use of counterpressure can be effective in slowing or stopping hemorrhage from or into structures under its influence, even major vessels such as the abdominal aorta and caudal vena cava.[1,15,32,34-38] Counterpressure garments have application for temporary stabilization of pelvic and femoral fractures, particularly in animals with coagulation disorders or persistent signs of shock suggesting continued hemorrhage.

Principles. Counterpressure exerts external forces on vessels, causing a decrease in diameter (radius). Blood flow through the vessels decreases significantly:

$$Q = P \times R^4/L,$$

where Q = flow, P = pressure, R = radius of the vessel, and L = length.[37] Blood flow is diverted away from the vessels under the influence of the counterpressure and systemic vascular resistance significantly increases.[37] Arterial blood pressure and flow to the areas of the body not under the influence of the counterpressure rises proportionally. Central venous pressure rises temporarily, and peripheral veins are easier to find and catheterize.[15] This effect is important in securing a large-bore venous catheter for rapid blood volume replenishment.

The return of venous blood to the heart is enhanced by the use of the counterpressure as blood pooled in the capacitance veins and venules moves into the central circulation. This form of "autotransfusion" is supposedly not as important as the influence of the increased peripheral vascular resistance.[16,36] Preliminary investigations in dogs subjected to severe hemorrhage suggests that this venous "autotransfusion" becomes more important in patients with loss of vasomotor tone, which occurs in deep shock.[15] Vascular replenishment may also be occurring by the enhanced movement of interstitial fluid into the vascular system as a result of counterpressure on increasing perivascular tissue pressure.[37]

Techniques. Counterpressure is best applied using a specially designed, commercially available, small animal "antishock" pneumatic garment (Vector, Inc., Milwaukee, WI).[39] Alternatively, wrapping elastic roller bandage on the pelvic limbs (starting at the toes), pelvis, and caudal abdomen can be used.[40] Cotton (½ to 1 pound) affixed to the ventral abdomen before applying the wide elastic bandage rolls can provide additional pressure to the splanchnic viscera, slowing hemorrhage.[39] With the former technique, the patient is wrapped in a garment that contains one to several rubber bladders. The garment is applied to include all of the pelvic limbs, the pelvis, and abdomen (to just caudal to the rib cage). After application, the bladders are inflated, starting with the most caudal or distal one, until that garment segment is visibly distended. Sequential bladders are inflated until the patient's systemic arterial blood pressure normalizes or all bladders are inflated.

Abdominal counterpressure reduces pulmonary compliance and tidal volume in spontaneously ventilating animals. Careful monitoring is required to ensure or assist ventilation as abdominal segments of the garment are inflated or as elastic bandage is applied, particularly in animals with suspected diaphragmatic hernias or pneumothorax.[41]

The pressure required to slow intraabdominal hemorrhage is 2 lb/in^2.[15,16] Correct application of counterpressure allows placement of a finger between the bandage and the skin.

Application. Counterpressure use has demonstrated efficacy in minimizing ongoing hemorrhage in several research experiments involving pigs or dogs in which bleeding from the caudal abdominal vena cava, aorta, or renal artery and vein was induced.[15,38] In many cases, bleeding produced experimentally has been completely controlled with the use of the counterpressure.[15,34]

The clinical use of the counterpressure for internal hemorrhage control has provided temporary stabilization of animals during the time required to prepare for emergent surgical intervention.[40] If surgical treatments of the animal are not an option for the owner due to cost or other factors, counterpressure may remain applied for several hours in hopes of allowing formation of a stable fibrin clot over the bleeding vessel.

In a series of 30 cases of severe hemorrhagic shock treated with counterpressure and studied by me, 20 responded with increased levels of awareness, and some animals became conscious after being completely unconscious on admission.[39] Systemic arterial blood pressure increased in all animals in which heart rate was not profoundly decreased or absent. In several animals, pulses were nonpalpable on admission but were evident following application of the garment and its inflation. Similar results have been reported following the use of the garment in human patients suffering from catastrophic hypovolemic shock. The results have been so profound in the resuscitation of trauma patients that one author on the subject stated "the development of this [external counterpressure] has as much importance to the circulatory support of the trauma patient as mouth-to-mouth breathing has to the cardiopulmonary arrest patient."[42]

The counterpressure device, once applied to the abdomen, should remain inflated until the animal's vascular volume has been restored. If unstable vital signs persist following volume replacement, continued hemorrhage requiring surgical intervention is suggested. In these patients, the counterpressure is continued until surgical approaches are initiated. Removal of counterpressure in these cases should be rapid. The abdomen is quickly entered following rapid aseptic surgical preparation undertaken while digital counterpressure remains applied over the area of suspected internal hemorrhage.

In animals in which the vital signs stabilize with the use of the counterpressure and the infusion of crystalloid or colloid solutions, the counterpressure device can be slowly removed while blood pressure and heart rate continue to be monitored. With pneumatic devices, small amounts of air are released every few minutes, provided the patient's systemic arterial blood pressure does not fall more than 5 mm Hg. If a compressive circumferential dressing was used for application of counterpressure, removal involves gradually cutting or loosening of the wrap, starting at the cranial border. If systemic arterial blood pressure decreases more than 5 mm Hg, removal of the counterpressure should be stopped and additional volume replacement instituted until pressure returns to previous levels.

Removing counterpressure devices rapidly can result in catastrophic hypotension secondary to the occurrence of a significant decrease in systemic vascular resistance.[36]

Rapid volume resuscitation. Resuscitative volume replacement should be rapid, restoring systemic arterial blood pressure and central venous pressure to slightly above normal within 15 minutes.[3,17,42] Additional indications of effective resuscitation fluid therapy include the return of mucous membrane color and normal capillary refill time, consciousness, and responsiveness.

Vascular access and administration. Peripheral *intravenous catheters*—In most animals vascular access is obtained by placement of at least one (preferably two) large-bore cephalic venous catheter(s) (14-gauge in medium to large dogs, 18- to 20-gauge in cats and very small dogs). Cephalic venous catheters are preferred so infused fluids and blood are introduced cranial to the diaphragm.

Central intravenous catheters—In animals with extreme hypotension secondary to blood loss, central venous access with a large-bore catheter or feeding tube is preferable. A large-bore feeding tube (12 French in very large dogs to 6 French in cats and small dogs) can be placed into the maxillary vein via a cutdown procedure.[39,43] The jugular vein is also readily available and easily cannulated in most animals.

Placing a catheter in the maxillary or jugular vein and advancing the tip into the cranial vena cava allows for intermittent central venous pressure monitoring. The catheters used allow rapid approximation of central venous pressure by simply lowering the fluid bag and noting the level at which fluids stop dripping into the drip chamber of the administration set.

Intraosseous administration—Resuscitative volume replacement can be administered through one or two large-bore intraosseous needles placed within the medullary canal of the humerus, femur, or tibia. These cannulas (bone marrow biopsy needles or spinal needles) are placed in the greater tubercle, trochanteric fossa, and tibial plateau, respectively.[44] Additionally, small volumes can be administered through the iliac crest without complication.

Drugs and biologic products that can be administered intravenously can be effectively administered intraosseously. In one report, drug availability was more rapid via the intraosseus route versus the intravenous (cephalic vein) route.[45] Administration rates of intraosseus routes are generally limited to slightly less than that which can be obtained with a similar sized catheter placed intravenously. In very small animals with shock, because of ease of cannula placement, intraosseus access is often preferred over intravenous access, as it is usually very difficult to establish an intravenous catheter in these animals.[46]

Volume replacement—crystalloids, colloids, and blood. Generally a polyionic balanced electrolyte solution such as lactated Ringer's solution is the initial fluid infused (90 ml/kg in dogs, 55 ml/kg in cats). In animals with severe blood loss, rapid restoration of intravascular blood volume is ideally obtained with whole-blood transfusions, autotransfusion of pooled thoracic or abdominal blood, or plasma-synthetic colloid and packed red cell administration (see Chapter 34).

The use of rapid (to effect) blood, plasma, or plasma expander administration is recommended when dealing with the severely injured and bleeding patient. This approach is preferred over the use of crystalloids. Problems with "overtransfusion" or allergic reactions in patients treated with this aggressive approach appear minimal, and it is proposed for human patients suffering from severe acute blood loss.[17]

Platelet dysfunction and the development of a coagulopathy when using dextran or hetastarch as substitutes for plasma has not been a problem in my experience as long as the total volume administered rapidly does not exceed 50% of the patient's normal plasma volume.

Hypertonic saline (7.5%) and dextran 70 (6%) solution (HSDS) has been found to be very effective in the treatment of hypovolemic shock induced through blood loss.[47] When the HSDS is infused the hypertonicity pulls interstitial fluid into the circulation very rapidly and effectively. Infusion of this solution may act through osmoreceptor and neurologically mediated influences on the cardiovascular system to stimulate a direct increase in cardiac output.[48]

The advantages of HSDS therapy is that only 5 mL/kg is required. This volume is equivalent to the infusion of one blood volume of lactated Ringer's (90 mL/kg body weight). The small amount of HSDS required allows rapid infusion as compared with the infusion of an equivalent volume of lactated Ringer's to provide the same hemodynamic response. The infusion of HSDS can also be effective if given intraosseously.

The addition of dextran or hetastarch to the hypertonic saline is important. If not used, the interstitial fluid "captured" leaves the vascular compartment as soon as the plasma osmolality normalizes (30 to 45 minutes).[48] The hemodynamic benefits of hypertonic saline infusion alone last no more than an hour. Lactated Ringer's solution similarly leaves the circulation and enters the interstitial spaces (75% within the first hour after infusion).[17] With the colloid added, especially when continued colloid is administered, sustained vascular volume expansion (2 to 5 days) has been observed in experimental studies in swine.[48]

It is important to remember that lactated Ringer's is not truly a plasma volume expander but rather is an interstitial volume expander. Overexpansion of the interstitial space has been recognized as a major problem in the resuscitation of trauma patients with crystalloids alone when estimated acute blood losses exceed 30% of blood volume.[17] This occurrence is tolerated by many traumatized patients, but also has been shown to increase morbidity and mortality in patients with head and pulmonary injuries. Therefore, particularly in these cases, blood or colloid replacement appears indicated for volume restorative therapy.[17]

Resuscitative thoracotomy. The indications for resuscitative thoracotomy other than suspected catastrophic thoracic or abdominal hemorrhage include the following: (1) a rapidly progressive tension pneumothorax in an unconscious patient; (2) cardiac arrest in a patient that has just been traumatized; and (3) cardiac arrest in which external massage and drug support had been performed and the heart is resistant to therapy.

Following tracheal intubation and institution of positive-pressure ventilation, a quick examination is performed (primary survey). If examination reveals thoracic or abdominal hemorrhage and the animal appears to be salvageable, that is, does not appear to have severe brain or spinal cord injury, then the resuscitative thoracotomy is indicated.

A scalpel is used to make an incision at approximately the fifth intercostal space on the left thoracic wall (unless otherwise indicated, e.g., because of a gunshot wound on the right). A curved Mayo scissors is used to puncture into the pleural space at the costochondral junction in order to allow air to enter the pleural space and partially collapse the left lung. With the scissor blades partially opened a pushing motion is used

to separate all layers of the thoracic musculature. The opening in the thorax is widened using fingers to stretch the tissues and the Mayo scissors for further "push" dissection. A Balfour retractor is then inserted, and the ribs are spread.

If a considerable amount of hemorrhage is present in the pleural space, the animal's body can be turned quickly to drain the pooled blood out, the blood can be aspirated for use in autotransfusion (see Chapter 34), or the blood is absorbed using laparotomy pads, sponges, towels, or cloth diapers.

If the source of hemorrhage is not obvious, absorbent material is used to pack the chest. These absorbent pressure packs are removed one by one as each quadrant is examined. As the source of bleeding is found, direct pressure is applied followed by clamping and suturing as required to control the hemorrhage definitively (see section on Thoracic Hemorrhage Management below).

Aortic occlusion (cross clamping). Aortic cross clamping directs blood flow centrally, increasing blood flow to the brain and heart significantly while decreasing hemorrhage distal to the clamped vessel. With severe hypotension, exsanguinating hemorrhage into the chest or abdomen, and cardiac arrest, the descending aorta can be cross clamped during resuscitation using a vascular clamp, Forrester sponge forceps, or rubber-covered or gauze-wrapped Allis (fascial) forceps.[34,35] If no forceps are available, a loop of umbilical tape or a feeding tube can be brought around the aorta and tightened using a hemostat in order to occlude the aorta atraumatically.

Descending thoracic aorta occlusion significantly decreases the effective size of the vascular space, increases systemic vascular resistance, and can be used to control abdominal arterial hemorrhage temporarily.[35] The aorta may remain occluded for 10 minutes without causing serious renal, spinal, or intestinal complications.[35,36] The maneuver significantly increases blood flow to the lungs, brain, and heart. When the occlusion is no longer required but has been in place over 5 minutes, gradual removal and concomitant intravenous fluid infusion is required owing to vasodilation occurring in the tissues distal to the occlusion. If aortic occlusion is required for longer than 5 to 10 minutes, it is recommended to loosen the clamp or vascular occlusive tube or tape and to allow perfusion to occur for a minute followed by reocclusion.[30] This approach minimizes the potential for renal function compromise or paraplegia, the two main complications associated with aortic occlusion.

Anesthesia. If the animal becomes arousable before necessary repairs and closure are completed, analgesia can be provided by the use of small incremental doses of intravenous narcotic-benzodiazepine combinations (oxymorphone [0.025 to 0.05 mg/kg] and diazepam [0.05 to 0.1 mg/kg]), and movement is controlled with the use of small intravenous doses of neuromuscular blocking agents (atricurium [0.25 mg/kg] or pancuronium [0.04 mg/kg]). The use of 2% lidocaine or 0.5% bupivacaine for intercostal nerve blocks and on the surface of the parietal pleura in the area of the thoracotomy provides additional anesthesia and analgesia during the intrathoracic repair, closure, and recovery period.

Following arrest of the hemorrhage, complete exploration, definitive repairs, and extensive irrigation with saline or lactated Ringer's solution (several hundred milliliters in cats and several liters in large-breed dogs), a tube thoracostomy is placed and the chest is routinely closed. Surprisingly, the infection rate with emergency thoracotomies has been low in my experience. With the use of careful cleaning, copious irrigation, and perioperative antibiotic administration (cephalothin, 40 mg/kg intravenously every 6 hours for 24 hours), wound infections developed in 2 out of 20 surviving patients. Pyothorax developed in no animals. This experience correlates with similar results reported with emergency thoracotomy in humans.[26,30]

Specific definitive hemorrhage management. In animals with catastrophic hemorrhage, the bleeding area must be approached rapidly. Occlusion of both venous and arterial structures is required, often applied blindly by simple pressure at first, followed by definitive repair or ligation.

Thoracic hemorrhage management. Following emergency thoracotomy, unless the hemorrhaging area is obvious, the pericardium is opened and the heart inspected. Myocardial punctures or lacerations are initially plugged with a finger and rapidly sutured using a simple continuous pattern. I have observed a few patients presented with myocardial punctures and although no animal survived for a long period, two were resuscitated successfully. Lack of sufficient blood available for transfusion was believed responsible for the eventual deaths in each, even though autotransfusion was used.

Left auricular access for the infusion of blood, colloids, and crystalloids can be achieved by grasping its tip with a forceps, placing a simple loop around it, cutting a small opening into the tip, and advancing a feeding tube inside. The loop is pulled tight and tied to prevent blood loss from the auricle. The suture is carried around the tube and tied to prevent the tube from backing out. Blood from within the chest can be drawn up into syringes or into a trap bottle using gentle suction and administered back through a filter and into the circulation through the atrial tube.

Injuries of the aorta and major vascular branches have been observed, but are rare. Temporary occlusion with vascular forceps or a loop of umbilical tape, feeding tube, or intravenous administration tubing is accomplished and followed by suture repair (aorta) or ligation (other vessels). Temporary occlusion of the aorta proximal (inferior) to the left subclavian artery is limited to only a few minutes (maximum) while distally aortic occlusion can be maintained for 5 to 10 minutes in most cases.[51,52] Individual variations and the differing physiologic states of animals do not allow definition of a "safe time limit" for aortic occlusion. Therefore, occlusion time should be limited to as short as possible because the need for emergency occlusion of the aorta prevents application of sophisticated electrophysiologic monitoring of evoked potentials that can be used to indicate when the time limit is being approached.[51]

The aorta tears very easily in the dog, and fine, swaged-on monofilament suture with taper needle should be used for repair attempts. Pledgets of fascia harvested from nearby muscles have been useful in stenting suture and in prevention of sutures pulling through the tissues.

Both common carotid arteries and the left subclavian artery can be ligated without complications due to the collateral circulation established through the ventral spinal artery.[50] Because of these extensive anastomoses even the brachiocephalic trunk can be ligated without complication, unless both the vertebral and carotid arteries are ligated individually, preventing arterial looping through the circulus arteriosus cerebri (circle of Willis). This arterial looping provides adequate protection against cerebral infarction and brain hypoxemia in the vast majority of animals undergoing major artery ligation.[50]

Low-pressure sources of hemorrhage can be effectively controlled initially by applying direct pressure followed by ligation or suture repair. Injury to the vena cava, brachiocephalic veins, or pulmonary arteries should be sutured. Chylothorax and craniocervical edema are complications associated with ligation of the brachiocephlic veins or proximal portion of the cranial vena cava.

With all vascular repairs, a continuous pattern using 6-0 to 3-0 polypropylene on a fine taper or or taper-cutting needle is recommended. For ligation, hand ties with 3-0 to 0 silk strands are recommended. The use of a fiberoptic head mounted surgical light and a 3 to 5× power loop is recommended to improve visualization. The use of surgical stapling devices for lung resection is an option that allows for rapid lobectomy and secure vascular and bronchial closure.[52]

Abdominal hemorrhage management. Catastrophic abdominal hemorrhage requires emergency celiotomy and is often best done following a resuscitative thoracotomy and aortic cross clamping. As soon as the abdomen is entered and the blood and fluid present is removed, systemic arterial blood pressure drops precipitously.[35] This effect can be minimized if, as soon as the abdomen is entered, a hand is inserted to compress the proximal abdominal aorta.[39] Severe arterial hemorrhage distal to the site of compression will be temporarily controlled as well.

The hand must be placed cranial to the origin of the celiac artery. This area can be located by palpating the left kidney and adrenal gland and by moving the hand to the midline just cranial to these organs. The crus of the diaphragm can also be palpated and used to locate the proximal abdominal aorta. In severe hypotensive states the aortic pulse is often not palpable. Following digital occlusion, blood flow to the heart, brain, and other structures cranial to the site of compression significantly improves. This effect can be documented by use of a Doppler blood flow detector.

Aortic occlusion does not stop severe venous bleeding; towels or laparotomy pads are inserted and packed into the abdomen. The packing will help temporarily control major venous bleeding.[39]

The incision in the abdomen is enlarged to extend from the xiphoid to near the pubis. The packs are parted to observe the aorta at the site of compression. A window in the paraaortic fascia is made with a curved forceps and a loop of umbilical tape, tape marker attached to a lap pad, or a $3\frac{1}{2}$ to 8 French feeding tube is grasped, pulled around the aorta, and held tightened with hemostats.[53,54] Packs are removed as suction and inspection is performed, quadrant by quadrant, looking for the sources of hemorrhage. Following observation and correction for severe venous bleeding the aortic occlusion is freed intermittently as each quadrant is inspected.

As each bleeding source is found, temporary hemorrhage control using a vascular occlusion method similar to that used on the aorta is applied (e.g., a feeding tube encircled around the splenic pedicle and tightened when a severely bleeding spleen is found). It has been my experience that if this method of dealing with severe intraabdominal hemorrhage is not undertaken these animals often die before all the bleeding sources are found and controlled.[39] After all major bleeding sites are temporarily controlled, definitive repair or ligation is performed.[39,55]

Liver hemorrhage. If the hemorrhage does not stop with packing, an intravenous dose of sodium penicillin (120,000 units/kg) or cephalothin (40 mg/kg) is administered and the hepatic artery isolated and temporarily occluded to remove the high-pressure source of bleeding. The antibiotic administration is necessary to prevent acute clostridia-induced hepatic necrosis.[56] If bleeding continues, the portal vein and the hepatic artery are temporarily occluded.[39] The cranial mesenteric artery should be simultaneously occluded to prevent acute portal hypertension.[57] If bleeding from the liver is still occurring, the source is a hepatic vein. This hemorrhage can be temporarily controlled by placing a tube approximately the size of the rent inside the damaged vein. A purse-string suture of 3-0 to 4-0 monofilament material (on a cardiovascular needle) is placed around the edge of the hole and as the tube is withdrawn the purse-string suture is tightened and tied. During this procedure, the tube can be used to infuse fluid and blood for volume resuscitation, including blood collected from the abdomen.[58]

Crushed liver lobes are removed by either a modified finger fracture technique, ligation at the base of the liver lobe, or stapling.[55,59]

Splenic hemorrhage. Following temporary hemorrhage control with a vascular clamp or loop on the splenic pedicle either a partial or total splenectomy is completed. Ligation with free ties of 0 to 3-0 silk is quick and efficient, and studies have shown that only six to eight double ligatures are required in splenic removal.[60] Partial splenic removal is preferred over complete removal, when possible, in order to maintain splenic function (filtration, immunoglobulin production, iron and platelet storage, etc.).[61]

Renal hemorrhage. Following temporary hemorrhage control with pressure, vascular loops, or vascular clamps, vascular repair or ligation is performed. Repair should only be attempted if renal ischemia is limited to an hour in cases of complete occlusive or separation injuries.[62] Renal arterial and venous injury repair require basic microvascular surgical knowledge, skill, instrumentation, and sutures appropriate for the size of the vessels involved.

The most common renal injury associated with severe hemoabdomen in my experience has been partial or total avulsion that cannot be repaired. If enough pedicle is present, simple double ligation of the pedicle is recommended. In cases in which the pedicle is very short or the injury extends into the junction of the renal vein-vena cava or renal artery-aorta, suture or ligation and vascular repair of the tears into the cava or aorta are required. This procedure requires the use of 4-0 to 6-0 suture, using swagged-on cardiovascular needles to place closely spaced cruciate or continuous sutures.

Retroperitoneal hemorrhage management. Intraoperative management of retroperitoneal hemorrhage is generally limited to conservative examination without further operative exploration when the source of the hemorrhage is not obvious (nonlocalized hemorrhage) and the retroperitoneal space is not expanding. These hematomas are commonly due to severance of multiple small veins and arteries that stop bleeding spontaneously. The few centimeters of water of pressure that occurs within the retroperitoneal space from this hemorrhage is sufficient to control bleeding. Exploration of the hematoma in these cases is not recommended, as this could cause recurrence of the hemorrhage. Postoperatively, treatment in these cases involves tranquilization, enforcing strict cage rest, and using pelvic limb and pelvic external counterpressure as needed. Any counterpressure applied is maintained for 24 hours, then gradually released. If pressure in the pneumatic device can be measured, it should be limited to 20 to 40 mm Hg when maintained for 24 hours.[63]

In situations of unstable hematomas (continuing expansion of the retroperitoneal space), the retroperitoneum must be explored to identify the source of the hemorrhage. The aorta should be cross clamped proximal to the hematoma prior to this surgical exploration. This procedure ensures control of brisk arterial hemorrhage, which could prevent the visual inspection required to identify the source of the bleeding. During occlusion the hematoma is carefully and gently evacuated and the source of bleeding found and ligated.

If profound arterial hemorrhage is occurring, the aorta can be ligated distal to the kidneys. However, renal compromise and rear limb ischemia is a potential complication, especially with blunt trauma and contusive injury to collateral vessels.[62]

If a hematoma is observed in the inguinal region, is not expanding, and the patient remains stable, emergency surgical exploration is often not indicated. Blunt or penetrating trauma in this region (caused, for example, by dog fights) frequently causes urogenital injury (Chapters 21 and 26) and muscle or tendon injury that leads to herniation of small intestine and/or urinary bladder. In these cases, surgical intervention should not be inordinately delayed as serious vascular compromise to the herniated and injured tissues is often present. Death of the animal due to endotoxemia may be the result when surgical treatment is delayed.

Osseofascial hemorrhage management. There are three effective methods of controlling severe hemorrhage into osseofascial compartments: (1) externally applied counterpressure (finger and hand pressure, pneumatic devices or circumferential bandaging); (2) surgical exploration with identification and ligation of the bleeding vessels; and (3) ligation of the arteries supplying blood to the area of hemorrhage. With catastrophic hemorrhage all three methods may need to be employed.

The first method is initially applied in all cases, as the other methods require an operating room setting (assistance, good lighting, suction, etc.). These approaches take time to organize. In the emergency situation, counterpressure can be applied quickly to slow the rate of bleeding and allow preparation for surgical intervention.

If a fascial compartment is observed to be enlarging quickly following a traumatic injury, indirect digital pressure should be applied to the arterial vessels supplying blood to the compartment. For example, in a dog hit by a car and showing signs of rapid hemorrhage into the right thigh (severe progressive swelling and bruising in the thigh and clinical signs of shock), pressure is applied to the right inguinal and femoral canal region, indirectly placing pressure on the deep femoral and femoral arteries. If the swelling includes these areas, then digital pressure can be applied to the external iliac artery with the tips of the fingers pushed into the lateral aspect of the caudal abdomen cranial to the inguinal canal.

Circular pressure dressings, composed of stretchable bandage material, or pneumatic antishock garments are useful for the continued control of serious hemorrhage in the extremities. This counterpressure is indicated if an expanding fascial compartment can be wrapped effectively and safely. Application of circumferential pressure bandages starts at the most distal part of the extremity involved and progresses proximally, covering the expanding region.

If the clinical signs of shock and continued hemorrhage (extremity expansion) persist following resuscitation and application of counterpressure, emergency surgical treatment with direct ligation of the involved arteries is indicated. Alternatively, surgical approach to the vessel(s) could involve placement of temporary occlusive vascular loops and exploration of the region of hemorrhage.

In most cases, primary vascular repair should not be attempted, and ligation of the major arteries and veins involved in the hemorrhage is recommended. Major vessels that are bleeding or devitalized can be ligated, as collateral blood flow will be sufficient to maintain viability. The only exceptions to this recommendation are situations in which the main collateral vessels, important in the vascular loop network supplying the tissues, are injured or compromised or when the injured vessel is believed to be repairable through suturing. Examples of pairs of vessels that can be ligated if necessary include common carotid arteries, and jugular veins; brachial arteries, brachial veins, and cephalic veins; and femoral arteries, external iliac arteries, common iliac veins, and femoral veins.

External hemorrhage management. Definitive management of severe external hemorrhage usually involves surgical intervention to expose and ligate the bleeding vessel or vessels. Direct pressure or digital occlusion of the source at a pressure point in some cases provides not only temporary but permanent arrest of the hemorrhage. Although makeshift tourniquets are not recommended in the first aid management of severe extremity hemorrhage unless the limb is expected to be lost, continued temporary hemorrhage control in the surgical treatment of salvageable extremities can be obtained using a pneumatic tourniquet.[53] The period of tourniquet-associated ischemia should be as short as possible, but up to 3 hours of ischemia results in minimal clinical abnormalities.[54]

Severe (catastrophic) traumatic shock

Definition. Severe (catastrophic) traumatic shock involves the repercussions from cellular and tissue malfunction secondary to profound peripheral and central cardiovascular collapse following severe trauma. Hypoxemia and poor glucose delivery along with the inability to remove metabolic wastes (e.g., lactic acid and carbon dioxide) lead to cellular inability to generate sufficient energy to maintain vital cellular functions. This process leads to organ system compromise and progressive organ system failure. Ultimately, enough cellular death occurs that the patient dies.[64]

Pathophysiology. Most patients suffering from severe traumatic shock have multiple pathophysiologic mechanisms involved, including the following: (1) blood loss; (2) plasma and fluid sequestration into bruised soft tissues and generalized edema secondary to leaky capillaries; (3) "pain overload" with visceral and somatic pain, causing an intense sympathetic response; (4) endotoxin and bacterial absorption (translocation) secondary to compromised gastrointestinal mucosa; (5) metabolic energy and protein substrate shortages (oxygen, glucose, and amino acids), leading to cellular malfunction and death; (6) blood flow maldistribution with tissues receiving too rapid or

too sluggish a blood flow to maintain good cellular function; and (7) diaphragmatic and cardiogenic muscular weakness, which can ultimately contribute to pulmonary and cardiovascular failure.[64]

Clinical signs. Animals presented in severe traumatic shock are very hypotensive, unconscious, or near unconsciousness with ashen, gray, white, or cyanotic mucous membranes, and weak, rapid or slow pulses. Bradycardia is generally associated with a severe leakage of blood into the abdomen, pulmonary aspiration or asphyxiation, head injury with increased intracerebral pressure, or direct cardiac injury.

Pulmonary edema may be evident in trauma patients due to direct pulmonary trauma or accompanying severe, longstanding shock associated with increased vascular permeability. Clinical signs include dyspnea, rattles, crackles, and wheezes on auscultation and frothy fluid from the patient's airways following intubation.[65]

Management. When an animal is presented with severe traumatic shock, management must be aggressively and simultaneously directed to the correction of all abnormalities if success is to be consistently attained.[17,28,29,42] The protocol is as follows:

A—Provide a patent airway. (See section on Upper Airway Blockage or Disruption above).

B—Ventilate with positive pressure using 100% oxygen. Continue ventilations at 15 to 25 per minute and consider high-frequency ventilation (100 to 150 breaths per minute with a very small tidal volume, e.g., 1 to 2 ml per kg body weight) if difficulty in obtaining adequate tidal volumes is observed (e.g., diaphragmatic hernia with gravid uterus displaced into the thoracic cavity).[42,65]

If severe respiratory compromise secondary to pulmonary contusion or traumatic-shock-induced pulmonary edema is observed, perform a tracheostomy, initiate and maintain intermittent positive-pressure ventilation with 100% oxygen, and employ 5 cm H_2O positive end-expiratory pressure (see Chapter 36). Try to wean the animal from 100% oxygen within the first 12 hours to prevent oxygen toxicity and use serial arterial blood gases to determine ventilatory therapy decisions.

C—Apply pelvic limb, pelvis, and caudal abdominal counterpressure and other cardiovascular support. (See section on Catastrophic Hemorrhage above).

Establish cardiovascular access (see section on Catastrophic Hemorrhage).

Administer a rapid infusion of hypertonic saline-dextran (5 mL/kg) and continue with whole blood (or plasma, hetastarch, or dextran as a substitute). There is no real substitute for blood in catastrophic traumatic shock when hemorrhage is involved. Circulating blood volume should be restored quickly to keep the dangerous hypoxemic episode time to a minimum.[17] Data from Shoemaker[17] suggest that due to the hyperdynamic, early compensatory mechanisms of shock, "return to circulating blood volume" should be interpreted to indicate higher than normal hemodynamic values to maximize oxygen delivery. Titration should be to control venous and systemic arterial blood pressures slightly above normal and maintained accordingly as counterpressure applied is slowly removed.[17]

Infusion volumes of blood or colloid required to bring pressures up and obtain good clinical responses are unpredictable. However, most animals require a minimum of 20 to 45 ml/kg, and those not requiring this amount are generally animals in which minimal circulating blood volume loss has occurred. A combination of fright and pain can mimic a significant internal blood loss: "weak and thready" pulse, pale mucous membranes, decreased sensorium, and delayed capillary refill time.

If blood or colloids are in short supply, administer lactated Ringer's solution (LRS) as needed (90 to 150 ml/kg). Caution is advised with lactated Ringer's solution as the sole resuscitation fluid in head, thoracic, and spinal cord injuries or in virtually all forms of cardiovascular shock except that induced by severe thermal burns. Lactated Ringer's solution, like all crystalloids, equally and rapidly distributes into all extravascular spaces following intravenous or intraosseous infusions.[3] In one study, immediately after infusion of 1 L of lactated Ringer's solution into hypovolemic human patients undergoing surgery, only 175 mL was retained in the vascular space.[3] As increasing volumes of crystalloid are administered, increasing volumes appear to remain in the vascular space for longer periods.[66] This effect may be due to the increasing interstitial hydrostatic pressure secondary to the interstitial edema induced. This edema can become a significant clinical problem, particularly in animals already suffering tissue edema following traumatic injury. The administration of large amounts of crystalloids for the treatment of hemorrhagic shock, although once commonly taught is now believed to be acceptable only if colloidal solutions and blood are not available.

Five percent dextrose in water (D_5W) does not contain electrolytes and is therefore distributed throughout the total body water space, including the intracellular space.[67] Infusion of D_5W results in comparatively small plasma volume changes and should not be used for a resuscitation fluid.

Hyponatremia, cellular swelling, and severe peripheral, splanchnic, and pulmonary edema may be a consequence of infusion with D_5W, particularly in the trauma patient.[17,64-66]

D—Provide drugs slowly (over 3 to 5 minutes) as required by intravenous or intraosseous bolus or infusion.

1. Arterial pressors—(Dopamine 10 µg/kg per minute or norepinephrine 1 to 10 µg/kg per minute).[17,68]
2. Bacteriocidal antibiotics—These are important treatments to administer to animals in severe shock as the blood supply to the gut will be compromised and bacterial translocation will occur.[69] The protocol I recommend involves administration of cephalothin (40 mg/kg first dose, followed by doses of 20 mg/kg beginning 3 hours later and four times a day for 1 day). If the respiratory or gastrointestinal tract is injured, a second-generation cephalosporin (e.g., cefoxatime or cefoxitin for increased gram-negative and anaerobic bacterial coverage) is recommended. Alternatively, the administration of gentamicin (3 mg/kg initially, followed by 1.1 mg/kg intravenously three times a day) and metronidazole (15 mg/kg initially, followed by 5 mg/kg three times a day) can be added to the cephalothin administration.[68-72] Dosage intervals or dosages may require adjustment for animals with renal compromise or conformational (thin) differences.[71,72] Ideally, dosing of antibiotics would be based on assessment of serum drug concentrations.[72] Antibiotics are discontinued following 24 hours of therapy if no other indications for use are present and shock has been successfully treated.
3. Corticosteroids—Corticosteroid use early has improved survival in experimental animal models and spontaneous cases of shock in humans.[73] Corticosteroid administration restores vascular and lysosomal membrane integrity to all organs via a number of mechanisms, including blockage of phospholipase action on membranes and by enhancing energy utilization through liberating adenosine triphosphate from the mitochondria.[68,70,73-76]

Many of the deleterious effects of shock are related to early and progressive membrane dysfunction, and the more rapidly corticosteroids are administered the greater will be the "membrane protection" provided. Data suggests corticosteroid administration prevents or lessens capillary leakage of red cells and plasma into the interstitium of lungs, intestine, liver, kidneys, and central nervous system. Improved membrane stability of leukocytes, platelets and endothelium is also responsible for decreasing aggregation, sequestration, and microthrombosis within the vascular system. Corticosteroids also act on vascular smooth muscle, causing relaxation of arterioles, precapillary sphincters, postcapillary sphincters, and venules. This action helps redistribute blood flow, which improves visceral and coronary circulation, increases cardiac output, and minimizes lactic acid production.[76]

Pharmacologic dosages (e.g., 4 to 6 mg/kg dexamethasone or 30 mg/kg methylprednisolone or prednisolone sodium succinate) are administered over a 10-minute period and only after the reconstitution of blood volume is well under way. This approach is used because the corticosteroid preparations will cause vasodilation, and very rapid injections have caused profound hypotension and death.[76]

Drugs that may be considered nonconventional but important in traumatic shock therapy in my opinion include[68,76]:

1. Anticoagulants—Anticoagulants such as heparin, as many animals in traumatic shock are in stages of disseminated intravascular coagulopathy and will benefit from the use of an antithrombin III enhancer such as heparin.[66]
2. Vasodilators—Vasodilators help decrease persistently high vascular resistance, which may occur in shock. These drugs are not used unless there is evidence of persistent peripheral vasoconstriction despite adequate volume replacement.
3. Energy substrates—Energy substrates should be supplied for use by fatigued muscle, epithelial, endothelial, and immune cells. Provided enough molecular oxygen is available, the energy substrates support immediate needs. Glucose can be added to the administered fluids to make a 5% solution.[77] Hinshaw observed in dogs that the administration of 175 mg dextrose per kilogram of body weight per hour was sufficient to prevent hypoglycemia during shock. To enhance glucose delivery into shocked cells, insulin and potassium can be added to the glucose solution (glucose-potassium-insulin [GKI]: 3 g glucose, 1 unit regular insulin, and 0.5 mEq potassium chloride per kilogram administered over 4 hours).[78] Survival rates are increased using both glucose or GKI in the treatment of experimentally induced shock in dogs.[76,77] Survival is enhanced in dogs with hemorrhagic shock given 5% fructose-1,6-diphosphate (FDP) in an electrolyte solution.[78] As acidosis progresses with shock, the glycolytic pathway "down-regulates" due to

hydrogen ion suppression of phosphofructokinase function. The FDP bypasses the portion of the glycolytic pathway most affected by acidosis. By providing FDP, energy production via the glycolytic pathway can continue despite acidosis.[79] The FDP solution can be made by dissolving 20 g of the trisodium salt of crystalline FDP (Sigma grade 98% to 100% pure) in sterile saline or LRS and passing the solution through a 0.2 micron filter. The solution must be kept out of light and refrigerated until use. It must be used within 6 months after preparation.

4. Nutritional support—Nutritional support with administration of crystalline amino acids or small peptides and essential fatty acids should be started following the injury and immediate resuscitation (usually within 12 hours). An electrolyte solution containing 3% glycerol and 3% amino acids with added potassium chloride (ProcalAmine, McGaw Laboratories) can be administered intravenously by a slow peripheral venous infusion (65 ml/kg/day). A commercial soybean or safflower oil fat emulsion can be administered with the ProcalAmine for additional nonprotein calories. To this partial parenteral nutrition protocol, enteral nutritional support (nasogastric, gastric, or jejunostomy tube) should be instituted, preferably also within the first 12 hours after injury.

   If access to the intestine is feasible, as would be the situation during an exploratory celiotomy for persistent hemorrhage, a jejunostomy tube can easily be placed and feeding started after anesthesia recovery.[80] Enteral feeding nourishes and protects the intestinal tract mucosa and greatly reduces bacterial translocation and stress ulcer formation.[81,82]

5. Analgesics—Analgesics should be administered as required for pain relief. Butorphanol (0.04 to 0.4 mg/kg intravenously) is a narcotic agonist-antagonist that can be used effectively in both cats and dogs. If necessary, for patient tolerance of the endotracheal tube and continuance of positive-pressure ventilation, low-dosage intravenous narcotic and benzodiazepine combinations (oxymorphone, 0.02 to 0.1 mg/kg, or buprenorphine, 0.005 mg/kg and diazepam 0.05 to 0.1 mg/kg) can be used.[83]
6. Neuromuscular blocking agents—These may be required to help maintain airway and pulmonary control. Atricurium (0.44 mg/kg initially and 0.1 mg/kg for repeated

doses) and pancuronium (0.05 to 0.12 mg/kg initially and one fourth this dosage for repeated doses) have been used effectively as nondepolarizing muscle blockers. Atricurium has the advantage of not requiring liver or kidney metabolism for reversal as the drug degrades within plasma associated with pH changes. Succinylcholine can be used, as a depolarizing muscle blocker, in an intravenous infusion to effect following an initial intravenous bolus administration of 0.06 to 0.07 mg/kg.

7. Superoxide radical scavengers—These may be used to help prevent reperfusion injury (chemical reactions leading to membrane damage and cellular necrosis). Drugs that have been used experimentally with success in decreasing the amount of reperfusion injury following shock include superoxide dismutase, 25 to 50 mg/kg subcutaneously, dimethylsulfoxide, 250 to 500 mg/kg intravenously, tromethamine, 0.5 to 1.0 mg/kg intravenously, and mannitol 250 to 500 mg/kg.[84] These drugs must be administered by slow intravenous drip to prevent hypotension. Greater clinical experience is required to determine the impact these drugs will have for the treatment of shock injury.

8. Superoxide radical blockade drugs—These are drugs that prevent the formation of the free oxygen radicals known to be responsible for cellular membrane dysfunction and destruction. By preventing production of these superoxide radicals, less postischemic reperfusion injury has been documented in dogs.[84] Deferoxamine, a selective chelator of ferric iron (responsible for the induction of lipid peroxidation and the production of oxygen and hydroxyl free radicals) readily crosses ischemic cell boundaries and the blood-brain barrier. Deferoxamine is administered as a slow intravenous infusion over 5 to 10 minutes, to prevent drug-induced hypotension, or the drug can be administered intramuscularly.[84] Allopurinol, a xanthine oxidase inhibitor, is another drug that has been used successfully to prevent superoxide radical production in shock models.[85] However, this drug is currently not available commercially for parenteral administration.

Severe intrapulmonic hemorrhage and traumatic pulmonary edema

Definition. This condition consists of hemorrhage and edema occurring in the lungs following severe blunt trauma and resulting in severe respiratory compromise and progressive respiratory failure.[86]

Pathophysiology. Generally this condition follows blunt trauma to the chest wall that is severe enough to injure many capillary-alveolar units. The injury occurs by three mechanisms: the sudden increase in intraalveolar pressure when the thorax is squeezed, direct concussive forces imparted to the lung tissue, and shearing forces generated by sudden movement of the lung within the chest cavity. With disruption of lung parenchyma, the capillary arterioles and venules in the immediate area become nonfunctional. Hemorrhage into the surrounding airways mixes with air and results in a myriad of small bubbles that act to obstruct small airways. As little as 4 ml/kg of blood infused into the trachea of a dog over 30 to 60 minutes reduces the partial pressure of arterial oxygen (Pao_2) below 60 torr with minimal changes in the partial pressure of arterial carbon dioxide ($Paco_2$) or airway resistance.[87] Following trauma, interstitial and alveolar edema occurs in the lung not directly injured and slowly progresses for several hours. Patients with intrabronchial bleeding tend to die from "drowning" rather than hypovolemic shock; however, the combination of shock and intrabronchial bleeding is highly lethal and can rapidly reduce oxygen transport below 25% of normal.[87]

The entire process of intraalveolar hemorrhage, small-airway blockage, and secondary edema leads to significant atelectasis and ventilation-perfusion mismatching of >2. Resultant hypoxemia causes arteriolar vasoconstriction and pulmonary hypertension. Noninjured portions of the lung become overcirculated, and the increases in hydrostatic pressure in these portions may contribute to the development of interstitial edema.[86] Atelectasis may occur secondary to decreases in surfactant. Loss of surfactant can lead to alveolar macrophage lysis and the liberation of many active eicosanoids and enzymes.[88] Decreases in surfactant occur following lung trauma from a variety of mechanisms, such as alveolar hypoxemia, microvascular thrombi from local and distant traumatized tissues, microvascular leakage, and alveolar edema.

As oxygen saturation drops below 80% it becomes increasingly difficult, if not impossible, for the animal to meet global tissue oxygen demands. Hypoxemia stimulates increased respiratory effort, and this effort increases oxygen demand, principally due to thoracic musculature activity. Severe, acute hypoxemia can lead to fulminant pulmonary edema, through centroneurogenic mediation of pulmonary hypertension. Ultimately, acute respiratory failure occurs in which hypoxemia does not respond to simple oxygen supplementation. Eventually, fatigue of the patient's respiratory musculature develops and the animal dies.

Clinical signs. Animals usually present in an anxious, almost frenzied state or in a coma. Characteristically, conscious animals extend their head and neck and appear to be using all their energy and effort just to breathe.[88] Cyanosis is usually evident, and the animal is struggling to exchange air with each breath. Radiographs of the lung fields may not reflect the severity of the injury until several hours elapse.

Earlier in the course of the development of contusion and intrapulmonic hemorrhage, animals that eventually demonstrate catastrophic signs may present with only mild respiratory dysfunction. The value of an arterial blood gas analysis for early detection cannot be overemphasized.[86] Progressive decreases in arterial oxygen tension or saturation are indicators that a profound and eventually catastrophic respiratory failure may be developing.

Management. The following protocol for the management of catastrophic respiratory failure secondary to intrapulmonic hemorrhage and edema following blunt trauma has been successful in my experience.

Supplemental oxygen is provided at high flow rates (5 to 15 L per minute) through a tube placed inside a plastic bag placed over the animal's head. If the animal becomes unconscious, intubate immediately and begin intermittent positive-pressure ventilation (IPPV). If the animal's condition is deteriorating, an emergency tracheostomy is performed and IPPV is started immediately.

If intrabronchial bleeding is severe, as evidenced by blood flowing from the endotracheal tube, it is extremely important to try to determine the lung with most of the bleeding and place the animal in lateral recumbency with this lung dependent. This procedure prevents blood from flowing through airways into the "nonhemorrhaging" lung. If a bronchoscope is available, oxygen is administered through the biopsy channel while evaluating for the source of the hemorrhage. An endotracheal tube is threaded over the scope and is visually placed into the nonhemorrhaging bronchus and the balloon is inflated. This endobronchial intubation will prevent blood from entering this less affected lung and allow ventilation to continue. If the animal cannot be stabilized by fluid resuscitation and IPPV, resuscitative thoracotomy on the side involved and removal of the severely contused and bleeding lung is indicated.[87] If the animal stabilizes, preparation continues for the possibility of surgical intervention at a later stage.

If the animal is responding well to the oxygen supplementation and IPPV (conscious, breathing spontaneously), continuous positive airway pressure (CPAP) should be considered. Continuous positive airway pressure can be performed by providing oxygen through bilateral nasopharyngeal catheters, transtracheal catheter, laryngotracheal cannula, or tracheostomy tube at such an assisted rate that during spontaneous inhalation and exhalation CPAP is maintained. Tracheostomy, performed under local block, gentle restraint, and mild sedation, provides the best method to accomplish CPAP.

Tracheobronchial suctioning is performed using a small catheter (5 to 8 French) while oxygen is insufflated into the lungs (200 ml/kg per minute, minimum). Hyperventilation is performed prior to and immediately after suctioning. While suctioning is performed, heart rhythm should be monitored for bradycardia and suctioning stopped if bradycardia occurs.

Arterial blood gases, end tidal carbon dioxide, transcutaneous oxygen tension, and oxygen saturation (pulse oximetry) can be used to determine the adequacy of the ventilations.

During this period of positive-pressure ventilation the animal should be watched carefully for signs of pneumothorax and a chest tube inserted and attached to an underwater seal and suction drainage, if necessary.[87]

Drugs can be administered to help blunt secondary bronchospasm, edema, and acute inflammatory processes. Terbutaline (a strong β_2 agonist and weak β_1 agonist) may be used to provide bronchodilation (2 to 4 mg/kg every 4 to 6 hours intravenously or 0.02 mL/kg of 1% solution diluted with 2 to 3 ml of saline, microaerosolized, every 2 to 6 hours). Isoetharine, albuterol, and metaproterenol are similar to terbutaline and can be substituted. Care should be taken in dosing to prevent complications caused by sympathetic overdrive (e.g., tachycardia).

For bronchospasm, the methylxanthines (theophylline or aminophylline) can be administered. These drugs antagonize adenosine receptors, causing bronchial smooth-muscle relaxation. These drugs improve diaphragmatic contractility and mucociliary transport and lower pulmonary artery pressure. In combination with the β-adrenergic agents these drugs provide an additive effect. Dosages for intravenous administration are 6 to 11 mg/kg three times a day (dogs) and 4 mg/kg twice a day (cats). When these drugs are administered by continuous intravenous infusion, dosage ranges from 0.3 to 1.0 mg/kg per hour. Side effects from overdosing may be severe (cardiac arrhythmias, vomiting, seizures, and sudden death) and may occur without clinical warning. Whenever these drugs are administered, serum concentrations should be determined after the first 12 to 24 hours of delivery, if possible. Although no clinical studies in dogs and cats have been reported, in children a dosage adjustment of 1 mg/kg generally changes serum levels 2 μg/mL. Since 85% of these methylxanthines are metabolized by the liver (cytochrome P-450), titration of drug dosing is especially important in cats and immature and geriatric animals.

One report suggested that 30 mg/kg of methylprednisolone will reduce the size of experimental contusions in central nervous system trauma, presumably by lysosome preservation, decreased capillary permeability through the prevention of superoxide radical formation, and antiinflammatory effects.[89] Whether this treatment would be effective in the management of pulmonary contusion remains to be determined. After the initial dose of 30 mg/kg, two doses of 15 mg/kg are administered 2 and 6 hours later. Immediately following the bolus at 6 hours, a continuous infusion of 2.5 mg/kg per hour is begun. The infusion is given for 48 hours without interruption and then is stopped abruptly without dose tapering.

Antibiotic administration remains controversial, but the amount of systemic disruption and shock suggests that their use is indicated (see section on Traumatic Shock above).

Chest physiotherapy is initiated following initial patient stabilization with postural drainage, coupage, and stimulation of deep breathing (toe pinching, getting the animal to stand, or turning the animal frequently).

Continued tracheal suctioning, intercostal nerve blocks for analgesia, nutritional support, and other therapy is performed as required. Some animals have recovered following 4 to 5 days of ventilatory support, but most that require IPPV for that duration have serious complications.

Most animals with catastrophic intrapulmonic hemorrhage and edema when presented have a slim chance for survival, but aggressive action will be necessary. Positive-pressure ventilation through a tracheostomy tube has been responsible for successful resuscitation in many animals that would otherwise have died. Most animals will require ventilatory support for at least 6 to 12 hours. Some animals respond dramatically after institution of IPPV, and it is only necessary for 2 to 3 hours.[90]

Deep coma following severe head injury

Definition. Head injury resulting in a comatose condition in which the animal does not respond or become aroused regardless of external stimulus provided.

Pathophysiology. Direct trauma to the head can lead to closed or open brain injury. In closed injury, the soft tissues surrounding the cranium may be lacerated, but the cranial vault is intact. Open injuries, by definition, communicate with the environment. Leakage of cerebrospinal fluid into the nose, ears, mouth, or outside indicates an open injury. Blunt trauma of such severity to cause a deep coma is likely to be associated with diffuse hemorrhage. Bleeding can be associated with injuries of meningeal arteries leading to epidural hematomas, dural venous sinuses leading to subdural hematomas, and subarachnoid arteries and veins leading to subarachnoid hematomas. The latter is the most rapidly fatal of these three types of hematomas.

Closed or open brain injury can be associated with fractures of the bones of the cranial vault. The weakest part of the cranial vault is the basal (or basilar) skull. This region of the skull is perforated by many blood vessels and cranial nerves. Basilar skull fractures are associated with hemorrhage into the surrounding brainstem.

Injuries caused by sudden blows to the head cause a positive-pressure wave on the impact side and a negative wave on the opposite side; this results in direct compression and vacuum forces being exerted on brain parenchyma, respectively. Both of these effects are observed in severe closed blunt trauma to the head. Lesions produced include coup and contrecoup intraparenchymal contusion and hemorrhage. The vacuum produced on the opposite side may produce gas bubbles from dissolved blood gases, and the extravascular release of these bubbles produces contrecoup cavitation. Intraparenchymal hemorrhage is the major feature of severe head injury. Neurologic deficits depend on the amount of involvement. The determining factor for survival with this injury is the location of the hemorrhage. The prognosis is not necessarily grave, if the brainstem is not involved, and there is a chance for recovery.[91]

Following the injury the brain begins to swell within minutes. Initially, the vessels in the brain dilate, so more blood flows into the injured area. Edema occurs as a result of impaired autoregulation of blood flow and reaches a peak 24 to 48 hours after the injury. Progressively rising intracerebral pressure can cause herniation of brain substance through openings at normal dividing membranes (e.g., at the falx cerebri or tentorium).[91]

Clinical signs. Hypotension or hypoxia must be aggressively treated, as either greatly reduces the prognosis of patients with head injuries. A "minineurologic" examination is performed on the unconscious patient, and all abnormalities are recorded as the results are observed. Resuscitative management is initiated as initial observations of breathing rate, rhythm, effort, and heart/pulse rate and strength are noted. The reactivity and size of the pupils to bright light are assessed. Ocular movements as well as oculovestibular and skeletal muscle motor responses are noted.

As the patient is manipulated, evidence of arousal or motor responses are noted. The level of consciousness is graded using a sliding scale much like the Glasgow Coma Scale used for human patients.[92] For further information on evaluation of the dog or cat with head injury, excellent reviews on the subject should be consulted (see Chapter 20).[91]

Management. Treatment initially involves tracheal intubation, oxygen supplementation, and hyperventilation.[87] As the endotracheal tube is passed, strength of jaw muscle tone, movement of the tongue, and the patient's gag reflex are noted; in deep coma no gag reflex is present. As intracerebral pressure elevations should be kept to a minimum, it is important when intubating to do it gently, without placing pressure on the patient's neck. The head should be kept elevated (up to 30 degrees), and absolutely no pressure should be placed on the patient's neck (e.g., no dressings around the neck and no compression of a jugular vein for blood sample collection). Ventilatory support should be continued to maintain mild hyperventilation ($Paco_2$, 25 torr). To control intracerebral pressure following severe head injury, assisting respiration is the most effective treatment.

If hypovolemic shock is present, 7.5% saline and 6% dextran are the infusion fluids of choice (5 ml/kg administered over 10 minutes). This treatment is followed by the use of colloids and blood, rather than crystalloids. During and after resuscitation, fluid administration should be limited to that which will keep the patient hydrated,[92] and excessive administration of crystalloids or dextrose and water should be avoided. In humans, 600 ml/m^2 of body-surface area per day is recommended for maintenance, and the fluid of choice is 2.5% dextrose and 0.45% normal saline.[92]

Monitoring of vital signs and neurologic function is continued in the intensive care unit, including level of consciousness, using a coma scale; breathing pattern and rate; pulse rate and systemic arterial blood pressure; size and reactivity of pupils; oculocephalic and oculovestibular responses; skeletal muscle responses; and temperature. To allow monitoring of intracerebral pressure an epidural "bolt" is placed into the calvarium using a technique that has been developed by

me and that is similar to an epidural technique used in humans.[93] A 5/32-in. drill bit fitted inside a plastic culture collection sleeve and adjusted to allow only its tip to project through the end is used to drill a hole through the skull at the level of the temporoparietal junction. A standard long intravenous catheter plug or a three-way stopcock, acting as the "bolt," is then inserted through the hole so that the end is flush with the dura. It will fit snugly into the hole and become tight as a small amount of pressure is put on the surface of the dura. The bolt is connected, via a saline-filled intravenous extension set to a calibrated electronic transducer (Statham) and pressure-recording system.[94] The sensitivity of the system is tested by briefly holding the lungs inflated. This maneuver should be associated with a rise in measured intracerebral pressure. A sterile dressing is applied carefully around the bolt to protect it, and intracerebral pressure is recorded. The mean intracerebral pressure on normal dogs under anesthesia has ranged from 5 to 15 mm Hg.[95] If pressures rise above 20 torr, intracranial hypertension is definitely present. In humans, sudden pressure increases up to 100 torr are associated with expanding hematomas or herniation due to severe unresponsive edema.[96]

Control of intracerebral pressure is paramount in the treatment of patients with severe head injuries. Failure to prevent increased intracerebral pressure is the most frequent physiologic cause of death in hospitalized patients with severe head injury.[87] Fortunately, epidural and subdural space occupation with expanding hematoma in both cats and dogs, following head injury, is not as common a clinical entity as it is in humans; therefore I highly recommend the use of mannitol and corticosteroids as initial treatment options (see Chapter 20). Clinicians must be able to perform decompressive surgery if bleeding does increase and intracerebral pressure rises.[92] Progression of increases in intracerebral pressure may be clinically evident by a deepening of the coma and decreased pupil reactivity. Sudden pupillary constriction or dilation are signs of catastrophic intracerebral pressure increase and the need for surgical intervention. If pressure cannot be controlled by the medical treatment described, then surgery is indicated to relieve the pressure by use of a wide unilateral or bilateral craniectomy, depending on clinical signs. The surgical procedure generally involves a lateral rostrotentorial approach.[97] Indications for surgical intervention also include open injuries from penetrating trauma or a severely depressed fracture that is evident on radiographs, physical examination, or computed tomographic scan.

Partial parenteral nutrition with a maintenance electrolyte solution, 3% amino acids, 3% glycerin (ProcalAmine), or 3% glucose (FreAmine plus dextrose) is initiated after ensuring normal hydration. After brain injury, patients are notoriously catabolic and should receive nutritional support through the period of coma and semicoma (recovery) when these animals are incapable of eating adequate amounts of food.

Prognosis. Any animal presented in an unconscious state following head trauma requires a guarded prognosis. Owners should be made aware of the uncertainty of the patient's course even if a neurologic examination suggests complete recovery is possible. Although a period of coma lasting 48 hours or longer demands a rather grave prognosis, some animals gradually recover sufficient neurologic function over a period of weeks to months to become an acceptable pet.

Certain clinical signs suggest irreversibility of neurologic lesions. These include progressive abnormal breathing patterns despite medical and surgical treatment (Cheyne-Stokes breathing, centroneurogenic hyperventilation, apneustic breathing, cluster breathing, and ataxic [terminal gasping] breathing); occurrence of bilateral dilated and fixed pupils that persist despite medical and surgical treatment; progressive bradycardia; and progression from decerebellate rigidity to a decerebrate rigidity.

Traumatic cardiac arrest

Definition. Cardiopulmonary collapse following a traumatic event in which no heartbeat or pulse is detectable.

Pathophysiology. Traumatic arrest is usually due to profound hypovolemic shock or major airway respiratory dysfunction caused by blunt or penetrating trauma. Massive hemorrhage involving 40% to 55% of blood volume is one of the most common causes of this form of cardiac arrest. Electrical mechanical dissociation, pulseless idioventricular rhythm, and ventricular asystole are common cardiac arrhythmias associated with traumatic arrest.[98] As closed-chest compressions are only one third as effective in generating forward blood flow as is open-chest cardiac massage, all animals suffering from traumatic arrest should be resuscitated with the latter method.[13,64]

Tension pneumothorax leading to profound cardiovascular collapse following blunt or penetrating trauma can be successfully resuscitated.[14,27] On opening the chest, immediate decompression takes place, with marked improvement in cardiovascular and pulmonary function often evident immediately.

Patients with profound hemorrhage within the chest or abdomen have been successfully resuscitated in some cases following resuscitative thoracotomy and/or celiotomy and cross clamping of the descending aorta, allowing significant improvement to heart and brain blood flow at a lifesaving point in time. At the same time, exposure allows definitive identification of the bleeding source(s) and immediate repair.

Resuscitative technique. On recognition of unconsciousness in the traumatized patient the airway is intubated. After airway intubation and the administration of positive-pressure ventilations (two to five), if there is no palpable pulse, the chest is opened at the fifth to sixth intercostal space.

The left thorax is entered unless injury to the right chest wall or thoracic inlet suggests that a right thoracotomy or parasternotomy should be performed. Skin incisions are performed with a scalpel blade, and the continued atraumatic dissection (exposure) is performed using a Mayo scissors in a pushing fashion.

With a parasternal approach, care must be taken not to injure the brachiocephalic vessels located in the thoracic inlet. The animal is placed in dorsal recumbency, and the tip of the Mayo scissors is inserted in the thoracic inlet and used to cut just alongside the sternum. The internal thoracic artery and vein may be cut and will require ligation following resuscitation.

As soon as the chest is opened, a Balfour retractor is inserted into the opened chest and the blades spread to provide exposure to the thoracic cavity. If a self-retaining retractor is not available, the ribs to either side of the incision can be cut at the costochondral junction and spread manually. These procedures allow enough room so the resuscitator's hand can be placed in the chest and cardiac massage performed. The pericardial-diaphragmatic ligament is isolated by a hooking motion with the middle finger of the nondominant hand and the pericardium opened at its apex using a Mayo scissors.

The aorta is cross clamped using a small feeding tube ($3\frac{1}{2}$ to 8 French). The tube is brought around the aorta using a curved hemostat at a level just caudal to the base of the heart. The same hemostat is then slid down on the loop of tubing to tighten it around the aorta. Time should be noted because after 5 minutes the tube must be loosened, at least temporarily.

Blood from the chest can be collected and reinfused if blood loss has been significant (35% to 50% of the patient's total blood volume) and homologous blood is not immediately available. Rapid blood replacement is mandatory in these patients. If blood is in short supply, plasma, hetastarch, or dextran can be used.[99] Potential future use of a blood substitute looks promising.[100] The least preferable choice for fluid resuscitation is a crystalloid, lactated Ringer's solution, infused at three to five times more than the volume lost. Animals that do receive this amount of fluid to maintain good perfusion will become edematous because of the expansion of the interstitial space by this fluid.[3]

All bleeding is controlled with pressure and suture, and the heart is squeezed at a rapid rate in order to propel the blood forward (see Chapter 32 for additional discussion of specific cardiopulmonary resuscitation guidelines). Definitive surgical treatments are performed if spontaneous cardiac activity can be reestablished. A broad-spectrum and bacteriocidal antibiotic and other agents useful for brain resuscitation (deferoxamine, mannitol) are administered (see section on Traumatic Shock above). The chest is irrigated copiously with saline or lactated Ringer's solution, and the closure is routine following placement of at least one chest tube.

Postoperative care. The animal is admitted to the intensive care unit, where close observation can be continued. Cardiac arrhythmias and respiratory depression can cause a recurrence of the arrest and must be aggressively treated if detected. Serial arterial blood gas measurements are recommended, and ventilatory support should be supplied as required to keep Pao_2 above 65 mm Hg (minimum) and $Paco_2$ between 25 and 30 mmHg. Chest tube care and chest physiotherapy are routine.

Within 12 hours, nutritional support should be started by nasoesophageal catheter feeding, using liquid meal or elemental diets infused through the catheter as a constant rate infusion at 1 to 2 ml/kg per day initially. Partial to total parenteral nutrition may also be used to supplement enteral feeding.

Prognosis. All patients in which a traumatic arrest has occurred have a poor chance of successful resuscitation, but the only alternative to not attempting cardiopulmonary resuscitation is certain death. Patients suffering from multiple system injury and those suffering arrest from blunt trauma have an extremely poor prognosis. Patients with some vital signs present at the time of admission have a much better chance of being successfully resuscitated.[26,30]

SECONDARY SURVEY
Complete history and physical examination

After the severely traumatized patient has undergone successful resuscitation for catastrophic life-threatening injuries, a thorough history and physical examination is performed. Following the mnemonic A CRASH PLAN can help remind the examiner and history taker to cover everything:

> A—airway (includes nose, larynx, neck, thoracic inlet)
> C—cardiovascular (includes heart, capillary refill time, pulse, blood pressure)
> R—respiratory (includes chest wall, lungs)
> A—abdomen (includes diaphragm, inguinal and flank areas)
> S—spine (includes entire spine)
> H—head (includes eyes, ears, teeth, mouth, tongue)
> P—pelvis (includes rectum, perineum, scrotum, vulva)
> L—limbs (includes bones and joints of all four limbs, feet)
> A—arteries and veins (includes all topical vessels)
> N—nerves (includes all cranial and peripheral nerves)

After a complete head-to-tail history and examination, special examination techniques are used to detect occult injuries as described below.

Radiographic assessment of the severely traumatized patient

Radiography of the chest and abdomen should be done on all patients that have been involved in a major traumatic incident, even though these animals may "look just fine." Many "silent" injuries are only exhibited by investigative imaging (Chapter 35). To perform the radiographic studies efficiently and rapidly, an automatic film processor is required. Capabilities of taking horizontal beam radiographs for the detection of free air in the chest or abdomen and for performing contrast studies of vessels, urinary tract, esophagus, bronchi, peritoneum, and spinal column (myelography) are also essential. Ultrasonographic examination can provide valuable diagnostic evaluations as well (see Chapter 35).

Laboratory assessment of the severely traumatized patient

All severely traumatized patients require a panel of laboratory evaluations. The tests are best performed on the samples initially collected at the beginning of treatment with serial evaluations as indicated (see Chapter 4). As a general rule, assessments of the following parameters are recommended:

Tests performed immediately: packed cell volume, total solids, glucose (stick), blood urea nitrogen (stick), urine specific gravity, blood gases (arterial, venous), cross match if blood transfusion anticipated.

Tests required within hours: complete blood count, microfilaria check, platelet count, white blood count differential, activated clotting time, urinalysis, serum electrolytes, and chemistry panel.

Special noninvasive tests required in severely injured

All severely injured patients should have their abdomen and chest carefully examined and reexamined. In long-haired animals, the removal of at least ventral abdominal hair is recommended in order to facilitate complete evaluations. If bruises are observed, the pattern of bruises often helps provide information about how the injury occurred and the forces that were applied to the different regions of the body. Penetrating injuries are also observed with this careful approach.

If red circular bruises are observed at the umbilicus, intraabdominal hemorrhage is likely.[31] Bruises in the inguinal regions suggest retroperitoneal hemorrhage (a common finding in pelvic fracture cases) or urogenital tract disruption. Subcutaneous emphysema suggests a pneumothorax if the accumulation is over the chest, and tracheal injury if located in the cervical region. Circumferential measurement of the abdomen can be used to help detect progressive expansion of the abdomen from blood, urine, and so forth.

Electrocardiography is important in the screening for cardiac arrhythmias commonly observed (ST-segment depression or elevation indicating myocardial ischemia, peaked T waves indicating hypoxemia or hyperkalemia, premature ventricular depolarizations and ventricular tachycardia indicative of myocardial contusion) following trauma.

Systemic arterial blood pressure assessments, measured with the assistance of a Doppler blood flow detector (Parks Medical Electronics, Aloah, OR) is helpful in determining cardiovascular function and should be serially performed routinely. The detector can also be used to investigate vascular integrity in limbs with fractures and in other injured areas (e.g., the kidney in the flank covered with a bruise or bruises).

Special invasive tests required in the severely injured

Thoracocentesis, abdominal paracentesis, and diagnostic peritoneal lavage are the three main invasive diagnostic tests performed in severely injured patients on a routine basis. Placement of multifenestrated catheters are preferred in many instances to enable a better opportunity to retrieve air or fluid accumulated in the chest or abdomen.

Repeated examination and maintaining a high index of suspicion

Careful monitoring and repeated examinations are a key to observing important changes that may indicate the presence of an occult injury. All traumatized patients should be hospitalized following the incident and observed for at least several hours. The animal should be placed in a cage and kept quiet. Vital signs should be checked frequently and preferably by the same person for a considerable period. The animal's level of consciousness, breathing effort and pattern, posture, pulse strength and rate, blood pressure, and heart, lung, and abdominal sounds are monitored. A flow sheet with the parameters monitored are recorded in columns that allow easy recognition of changes, alerting the team to problems.[101] Constant vigilance is necessary for early detection of problems, as early detection frequently determines success or failure in trauma management.

When major problems are detected: definitive care, referral

When major problems in the traumatized patient are detected following initial resuscitation, a decision must be made as to the timing of the definitive surgical or medical care required. Often the luxury of time is not possible to allow a second opinion. However, consultation is encouraged when time is available—that is, two heads are often better than one. Referral may be indicated with certain patients facing serious medical or surgical problems or complications. If time is not available for referral, it should be remembered that frequently there is only one opportunity from a financial and medical perspective to do the definitive repair. As surgical repair is performed, thoroughness and thoughtful approaches are more important than speed, as most severely injured animals will often tolerate prolonged surgical intervention better than a major postoperative complication. Major surgical intervention on a traumatized ill patient should not be performed by a team of any less than three fully equipped (instrumentation, supplies, knowledge, and skill) people—the veterinarian and two assistants. Ventilatory support and anesthesia monitoring is the major responsibility of one of these assistants. The second one can act as sterile assistant. Ideally, a fourth person to help the anesthetist and surgical team as the circulating nurse should be present.

REMARKS

The treatment of the seriously injured pet is one of the most difficult tasks the practicing veterinarian must accomplish. This situation is not only difficult from a medical and surgical standpoint, but also from a psychologic one. Owners are often upset and can be difficult to communicate with in the immediate postinjury period. The more serious the injury the more tense the situation. It is paramount that the patient and client be treated as a single unit. Compassion and genuine care given to both the patient and the client will be appreciated by both and will provide the framework for understanding, communication, and overall management of the animal's injuries. Trauma management takes a team effort and can stress this team of staff members as well. A staff that demonstrates a genuine caregiving and considerate attitude toward each other will be able to perform at their best and enjoy the work they do.

We are all practicing to be better diagnosticians, clinicians, and surgeons, and trauma management cases can be frustrating, challenging, and rewarding. The best treatment for the severely injured patient is prevention, but when we cannot deliver that approach we must act with assuredness and with team work.

REFERENCES

1. Cowley RA. Initial evaluation and management. In Cowley RA, ed. Shock Trauma/Critical Care Manual. Baltimore: University Park Press, 1982;3-5.
2. Trunky DD. Trauma care systems. Emerg Med Clin North Am 1984;2:913-919.
3. Shoemaker WC. Comparisons of the relative effectiveness of whole blood transfusions and various types of fluid therapy in resuscitation. Crit Care Med 1976;4:71-76.
4. Rackow EC, Fein IA, Siegel J. The relationships of colloid osmotic pressure pulmonary artery wedge pressure gradient to pulmonary edema and mortality in critically ill patients. Chest 1982;82:433-438.
5. Hafen BQ, Karren KJ. Prehospital Emergency Care, 3rd ed. Englewood, CO: Morton Publishing, 1989;9-15.
6. Veterinary Emergency and Critical Care Society Emergency Service Standards and Guidelines Committee. Recommended Definitions and Guidelines for Veterinary Emergency Service Standards in the United States. In Veterinary Emergency and Critical Care Society Director, Miami:VECCS, 1987;10-16.
7. Hafen BQ, Karren KJ. Prehospital Emergency Care, 3rd ed. Englewood, CO: Morton Publishing, 1989;101-103.
8. Clinton JE, Ruiz E. Emergency airway management procedures. In Roberts J, Hedges JR, eds. Clinical Procedures in Emergency Medicine. Philadelphia: WB Saunders, 1985;2-29.
9. Ruben H, Hansen E, MacNaughton FI. High capacity suction technique. Anesthesia 1979;34:349-353.
10. Anderson JH, Crowe DT. Teaching Critical Care to Law Enforcement Personnel. In Scientific Proceedings of the Second International Symposium of the Veterinary Emergency and Critical Care Society. San Antonio, TX: VECCS, 1990;671.
11. Crowe DT. Pet First Aid and Cardiopulmonary Resuscitation. Athens, GA: University of Georgia, 1988.
12. Halperin HR, Guerci AD, Chandra N, et al. Vest inflation without simultaneous ventilation during cardiac arrest in dogs: Improved survival from prolonged cardiopulmonary resuscitation. Circulation 1986;74:1407-1412.
13. Bircher N, Safar P. Comparison of standard and "new" closed-chest CPR and open-chest CPR in dogs. Crit Care Med 1981;9:384-391.
14. Robello CD, Crowe DT. Cardiopulmonary resuscitation: Current recommendations. Vet Clin North Am 1989;19:1127-1149.
15. Crowe DT, Downs MO. Physiological effects of abdominal binding in normal and intraabdominally bleeding dogs [abstract]. Vet Surg 1986;15:24.
16. Roth JA, Rutherford RB. Regional blood flow effects of G suit application during hemorrhagic shock. Surg Gynecol Obstet 1971;133:637-643.
17. Shoemaker WC. Shock states: Pathophysiology, monitoring, outcome prediction, and therapy. In Shoemaker WC, Ayres S, Grenvik A, Holbrook PR, Thompson WL, eds. Textbook of Critical Care. Philadelphia: WB Saunders, 1989;977-993.
18. Hafen BQ, Karen KJ. Prehospital Emergency Care, 3rd ed. Englewood, CO: Morton Publishing, 1989;101-103.
19. Kristoffersen MB, Rattenborg CC, Holaday DA. Asphyxial death: the roles of acute anoxia, hypercarbia, and acidosis. Anesthesiology 1967;28:488.
20. Allo MD, Miller CL. Airway management. In Zuidema GD, Rutherford RB, Ballinger WF, eds. The Management of Trauma. Philadelphia: WB Saunders, 1985;379-390.
21. Kelman GR, Nunn JF. Clinical recognition of hypoxemia under florescent lamps. Lancet 1966;1:1400-1404.
22. Fitzpatrick RK, Crowe DT. Nasal oxygen administration in dogs and cats: experimental and clinical investigations. J Am Anim Hosp Assoc 1986;10:293-300.
23. Heimlich HJ, Hoffman KA, Canestri FR. Food-choking and drowning deaths prevented by external subdiaphragmatic compression: Physiological. Ann Thorac Surg 1975;20:188-194.
24. Gordon AS, Belton MK, Ridolpho PF. Emergency management of foreign body airway obstruction. Comparison of artificial tough techniques, manual extraction maneuvers, and simple mechanical devices. In Safer P, Elam J, eds. Advances in Cardiopulmonary Resuscitation. New York: Springer-Verlag, 1977;58-59.
25. Hemingway A, Simmons DH. Respiratory response to acute progressive pneumothorax (in dogs). J Appl Physiol 1958;13:165-170.
26. Mattox K, Jordan G. The emergency center as a site for major surgery. J Am Coll Emerg Physicians 1974;3:372-378.
27. Rutherford RB, Hurt HH, Brickman RD, et al. The pathophysiology and treatment of progressive tension pneumothorax. J Trauma 1968;8:212-220.
28. Trunky DD, Sheldon GF, Collins JA. The treatment of shock. In Zuidema GD, Rutherford RB, Ballinger WF, eds. The Management of Trauma, 4th ed. Philadelphia: WB Saunders, 1985;105-125.
29. Hardaway RM. Expansion of the extravascular space in severe shock. Am J Surg 1964;142:258-264.
30. Jackimczykm K, Markovchick V, Rosen P. Traumatic cardiac arrest. In Harwood AL, ed. Cardiopulmonary Resuscitation. Baltimore: Williams & Wilkins, 1982;167-176.
31. Crowe DT, Todoroff RJ. Umbilical masses and discolorations as signs of intraabdominal disease. J Am Anim Hosp Assoc 1982;18:742-748.
32. Crowe DT. Internal and external abdominal counterpressure. Abstract presentations of the Advanced Session of the Veterinary Critical Care Society annual meeting, Las Vegas, NV, 1982.
33. Crowe DT. Diagnostic abdominal paracentesis techniques: clinical evaluation in 129 dogs and cats. J Am Anim Hosp Assoc 1984;20:223-230.
34. Ledgerwood A. The role of thoracic aorta occlusion for massive hemoperitoneum. J Trauma 1976;16:610-615.
35. Sankaran S. Thoracic aorta clamping for prophylaxis against sudden cardiac arrest during laparotomy for acute massive hemoperitoneum. J Trauma 1975;15:290-297.

36. Shane RA, Campbell GS. Protective effects of external counterpressure in acute hemorrhagic hypotension. Am J Surg 1965;110:355-359.

37. Eddy DM, Wangensteen SL, Ludewig RM. The kinetics of fluid loss from leaks in arteries tested by an experimental ex vivo preparation and external counterpressure. Surgery 1968;64:541-546.

38. Ludewig RM, Wangensteen SL. Aortic bleeding and the effect of external counterpressure. Surg Gynecol Obstet 1969;128:252-258.

39. Crowe DT, MacDonald M, Gaston J, Miller G, Wells M. The use of a pneumatic garment in the management of hemorrhage and hypovolemic shock in dogs and cats: a prospective clinical investigation. Sci Proc Second Int Vet Emerg Crit Care Symp 1990;2:650.

40. Crowe DT. Performing life-saving cardiovascular surgery. Vet Med 1989;84:77-96.

41. Maull KI, Krahwinkel DJ, Rozycki GS, Nelson HS. Cardiopulmonary effects of the pneumatic anti-shock garment on swine with diaphragmatic hernia. Surg Gynecol Obstet 1986;162:17-23.

42. Wilder RJ. Initial management of the critically injured patient. Prog Crit Care Med 1984;1:1-14.

43. Anderson JH, Crowe DT. An emergency cutdown procedure using the maxillary vein. Sci Proc Second Int Vet Emerg Crit Care Symp 1990;2:662.

44. Otto CM, Kaufman GM, Crowe DT. Intraosseous infusion of fluids and therapeutics. Comp Contin Educ Pract Vet Small Anim 1989;22:421-431.

45. Spivey WH, Lathers CM, Malone D, et al. Comparison of intraosseous, central and peripheral venous routes of administration of sodium bicarbonate during CPR in pigs. Ann Emerg Med 1985;14:1135-1140.

46. Otto CM, Crowe DT. Intraosseous catheters. In Kirk RW, ed. Current Veterinary Therapy XI. Philadelphia: WB Saunders, 1991 (in press).

47. Holcroft JW, Vasser MJ, Turner JE, et al. 3% NaCl and 7.5% NaCl/dextran 70 in the resuscitation of severely injured patients. Ann Surg 1987;206:279-288.

48. Maningas PA, DeGuzman LR, Tillman FJ, et al. Small-volume infusion of 7.5% NaCl in 6% dextran 70 for the treatment of severe hemorrhagic shock in swine. Ann Emerg Med 1986;15:1131-1137.

49. Baidsell EF, Cooley DA. The mechanism of paraplegia after temporary thoracic aortic occlusion. Surgery 1961; 51:351-355.

50. Markowitz J, Archibald J, Downie HG. Experimental Surgery Including Surgical Physiology, 5th ed. Baltimore: Williams & Wilkins, 1964;581-598.

51. Katz NM, Blackstone EH, Kirklin JW, Karp RB. Incremental risk factors for spinal cord injury following operation for acute traumatic aortic transection. J Thorac Cardiovasc Surg 1981;81;669-674.

52. LaRue SM, Withrow SJ, Wykes PM. Lung resection using surgical staples in dogs and cats. Vet Surg 1987; 16:238-240.

53. Blass CE, Moore RW. The tourniquet in surgery. Vet Surg 1984;13:111-114.

54. Heppenstall RB, Balderston R, Goodwin C. Pathophysiologic effects distal to a tourniquet in the dog. J Trauma 1979;19:234-238.

55. Crowe DT. The steps in arresting abdominal hemorrhage. Vet Med 1988;83:676-781.

56. Markowitz J, Archibald J, Downie HG. Experimental Surgery Including Surgical Physiology, 5th ed. Baltimore: Williams & Wilkins, 1964;529-533.

57. Whiting PM, Breznock EG, More P, et al. Partial hepatectomy with temporary hepatic vascular occlusion in dog with hepatic arteriovenous fistulas. Vet Surg 1986; 15:171-180.

58. Crowe DT. Autotransfusion in the trauma patient. Vet Clin North Am Small Anim Pract 1980;10:581-597.

59. Lewis DD, Bellenger CR, Lewis DT, et al. Hepatic lobectomy in the dog: a comparison of stapling and ligation techniques. Vet Surg 1990;19:221-225.

60. Hosgood G, Bone DL, Vorhees WD, et al. Splenectomy in the dog by ligation of the splenic and short gastric arteries. Vet Surg 1989;18:110-113.

61. Crowe DT. Surgery and surgical diseases of the spleen. Proceedings of the 14th Annual Veterinary Surgery Forum—Small Animal Digestive Systems. Chicago, IL: ACVS, 1986;73-78.

62. Abbott WM, Cooper JD, Austen WG. The effect of aortic clamping and declamping on renal blood flow distribution. J Surg Res 1973;14:385-392.

63. Cangiano JL, Kest L. Use of G-suite for uncontrollable bleeding after percutaneous renal biopsy. J Trauma 1972;107:360-361.

64. Safer P. The pathophysiology of dying and reanimation. In Schwartz GR, Safer P, Stone J, et al., eds. Principles and Practice of Emergency Medicine, 2nd ed. Philadelphia: WB Saunders, 1986;2-41.

65. Safer P, Caroline N. Acute respiratory insufficiency. In Schwartz GR, Safer P, Stone J, et al., eds. Principles and Practice of Emergency Medicine, 2nd ed. Philadelphia: WB Saunders, 1986;42-85.

66. Moore FD. The effects of hemorrhage on body composition. N Engl J Med 1965;273:567-572.

67. Falk JL, Rackow EC, Weil MH. Colloid and crystalloid fluid resuscitation. In Shoemaker WC, Ayres S, Grenvik A, Holbrook PR, Thompson WL, eds. Textbook of Critical Care. Philadelphia: WB Saunders, 1989;1055-1073.

68. Goodwin JK, Schaer M. Septic shock. Vet Clin North Am 1989;19:1239-1258.

69. Maejima K, Keitch E, Berg R. Promotion by burn stress of translocation of bacteria from the gastrointestinal tracts of mice. Arch Surg 1984;119:166-170.

70. Murtaugh RJ, Mason GD. Antibiotic pressure and nosocomial disease. Vet Clin North Am 1989;19:1259-1274.

71. United States Pharmacopeial Convention. Drug information for the health care professional, vol. IB, Rockville, MD: The United States Pharmacopeial Convention, Inc., 1990.

72. Anderson MD, Chernow B. Pharmacologic principles. In Civetta JM, Taylor RW, Kirby RR, eds. Critical Care. Philadelphia: LB Lippincott, 1988;483-500.

73. Shantney CH, Lillelehi RC. Pathophysiology and therapy of shock. In Zschoche DA, ed. Mosby's Comprehensive Review of Critical Care, 2nd ed. St. Louis: Mosby–Year Book, 1981.

74. Weil MH, Rackow EC. Cardiovascular system failure. In Schwartz GR, Safer P, Stone JH, et al., eds. Principles and Practice of Emergency Medicine. Philadelphia: WB Saunders, 1986;86-103.

75. White BC. Pharmacology of resuscitation. In Harwood AL, ed. Cardiopulmonary Resuscitation. Baltimore: Williams & Wilkins, 1982;79-88.

76. Haskins SH. Shock (The pathophysiology and management of the circulatory collapses states). In Kirk RW, ed. Current Veterinary Therapy VIII. Philadelphia: WB Saunders, 1983;2-27.

77. Hinshaw LB, et al. Prevention of death in endotoxic shock by glucose administration. Surg Gynec Obstet 1974;139;851-859.

78. Manny J, et al. Effect of glucose-insulin-potassium on survival in experimental endotoxic shock. Surg Gynecol Obstet 1978;147:405-407.

79. Markov AK. Increasing survival of dogs subjected to hemorrhagic shock by the administration of fructose 1-6 diphosphate. Surgery 1987;102:515-527.

80. Crowe DT. Nutrition in critical patients: administering the support therapies. Vet Med 1989;84:152-180.

81. Sori AJ, Rush BF Jr, Lysz TW, et al. The gut as a source of sepsis after hemorrhagic shock. Ann Surg 1988;155:187-192.

82. Ephgrave KS, Kleiman-Wexler RL, Adair CG. Enteral nutrients prevent stress ulceration and increase intragastric volume. Crit Care Med 1990;18:621-624.

83. Bednarski RM. Anesthesia and pain control. Vet Clin North Am 1989;19:1223-1237.

84. Muir WW. Brain hypoperfusion post resuscitation. Vet Clin North Am 1989;19:1151-1164.

85. Crowell JW, Jones CF, Smith EE. Effect of allopurinol on hemorrhagic in dogs. Am J Physiol 1969;216:744-748.

86. Coalson JJ. Pathophysiologic features of infant and adult respiratory distress syndrome. In Shoemaker WC, Ayres S, Grenvik A, Holbrook PR, Thompson WL, eds. Textbook of Critical Care. Philadelphia: WB Saunders, 1989;484-491.

87. Wilson RF. Accidental and surgical trauma. In Shoemaker WC, Ayres S, Grenvik A, Holbrook PR, Thompson WL, eds. Textbook of Critical Care. Philadelphia: WB Saunders, 1989;1230-1271.

88. Ayres SM. The structural basis of pulmonary function. In Shoemaker WC, Ayres S, Grenvik A, Holbrook PR, Thompson WL, eds. Textbook of Critical Care. Philadelphia: WB Saunders, 1989;464-478.

89. Braughler JM, et al. Evaluation of an intensive methylprednisolone sodium succinate dosing regimen in experimental spinal cord injury, J Neurol Surg 1987;67:102-105.

90. Crowe, DT. Traumatic pulmonary contusions, hematomas, pseudocysts, and acute respiratory distress syndrome: An update. Compend Contin Educ Pract Vet 1983;5:396-407.

91. Selcer RR. Trauma to the central nervous system. Vet Clin North Am Small Anim Pract 1980;10:619-639.

92. Bouzarth WF, Goldman HW. Emergency management of trauma: trauma to the head. In Schwartz GR, Safer P, Stone JH, et al., eds. Principles and Practice of Emergency Medicine. Philadelphia: WB Saunders, 1986; 1297-1308.

93. Koster WG, Kuypers MH. Epidural measurement of intracranial pressure. In Shulman K, Marmarou A, Miller LD, et al, eds. Intracranial Pressure IV. Berlin: Springer-Verlag 1980;371-376.

94. Becker D, Remondino RL. Intracranial pressure monitoring. In Shoemaker WC, Ayres, Grenvik A, Holbrook PR, Thompson WL, eds. Textbook of Critical Care. Philadelphia: WB Saunders 1989;291-295.

95. Jaggy A. Personal communication. Bern, Switzerland: University of Bern, School of Veterinary Medicine, Neurology Institute, October 1990.

96. Hoerlein BF, Oliver JE. Brain surgery. In Hoerlein BF, ed. Canine Neurology, 2nd ed. Philadelphia: WB Saunders, 1971;527-559.

97. Rosner MJ, Becker DP. Origin and evolution of plateau waves. J Neurosurg 1984;60;312-317.

98. Crowe DT. Cardiopulmonary resuscitation and advanced life support. In Zaslow IM, ed. Veterinary Trauma and Critical Care. Philadelphia: Lea & Febiger, 1984;507-539.

99. Kirby R. Clinical advantages of 6% hetastarch during fluid resuscitation. Scientific Proceedings of Second International Veterinary Emergency and Critical Care Symposium. San Antonio, TX:VECCS, 1990;331-332.

100. Ross JN. Future of blood substitutes. Scientific Proceedings of Second International Veterinary Emergency and Critical Care Symposium. San Antonio, TX:VECCS, 1990;333.

101. Davis H Jr. Monitoring the critical ill patient or how to tell when your patient is getting into trouble. Scientific Proceedings of Second International Veterinary Emergency and Critical Care Symposium. San Antonio, TX: VECCS, 1990;585-598.

11 Surgical Emergencies: Gastric Dilatation-Volvulus, Intervertebral Disk Disease, Spinal Trauma, and Fracture Management

John Berg and *Randy J. Boudrieau*

GASTRIC DILATATION-VOLVULUS

Gastric dilatation-volvulus (GDV) is an abnormal distention and displacement of the canine stomach. It is one of the most common animal diseases to require emergency surgery, and because it is often complicated by severe shock and other systemic problems, it is associated with a significant mortality rate.

Etiology

The precise cause of GDV is currently unknown. Although the condition is reported in cats and small breeds of dogs,[1] the vast majority of cases occur in large, deep-chested breeds of dogs. One current theory is that dogs with this body configuration are predisposed to GDV by domestic feeding patterns.[2] Commercial diets are lower in protein and roughage and higher in carbohydrates and caloric density than the diets of wild carnivores, and they tend to produce slow gastric emptying. In addition, commercial diets are highly processed to make them "readily digestible" and fermentable, so that these diets swell within the stomach postprandially when water or gastric secretions are added. These diets select for a characteristic gastric flora consisting principally of *Clostridium perfringens,* which is capable of fermenting the diets to produce large volumes of gastric gas. Finally, domesticated dogs are often fed only once daily for convenience, rather than in several smaller feedings as occurs in the wild. These factors produce a chronically enlarged, distended stomach and may lead to stretching of the ligaments supporting the stomach. If another factor is superimposed, such as heavy exercise or overconsumption of water, the stomach is prone to acute dilatation and volvulus.

Other researchers have suggested that dogs with GDV may have chronic elevations in the hormone gastrin.[3] Elevated gastrin levels may predispose to GDV by delaying gastric emptying, producing pyloric muscular and antral mucosal hypertrophy and increasing lower esophageal sphincter pressure.[3] Subsequent work, however, has shown normal fasting gastrin levels and normal lower esophageal sphincter pressures in dogs that had previously recovered from GDV.[4]

Pathophysiology

Gastric volvulus may occur in either a clockwise or a counterclockwise direction when viewed from behind the standing animal.[5] Clockwise rotation is by far the most common. The relatively undistended pylorus and pyloric antrum move downward, cross the midline from right to left, pass under the distended fundus of the stomach, and move upward along the left abdominal wall, coming to rest near the cardia of the stomach.[5] The greater curvature becomes positioned against the left abdominal wall and the dorsal border of the abdominal cavity, and the greater omentum follows the greater curvature or may tear near the splenic artery.[5] If the omentum remains intact, it will be found at surgery to cover the ventral aspect of the stomach.

In counterclockwise volvulus, which is extremely rare, the pylorus and pyloric antrum move upward along the right abdominal wall and come to rest near the cardia.[5] The greater curvature is minimally displaced.[5] At surgery, the ventral aspect of the stomach is not covered by omentum.

Regardless of the direction of gastric displacement, it is often complicated by dramatic systemic effects. Although the physiologic effects of GDV are complex and interrelated, most of them arise directly or indirectly from the severe circulatory shock that usually accompanies the condition. An understanding of these effects is crucial in providing proper emergency care.

Systemic manifestations of GDV

Two factors contribute to circulatory shock in GDV. The dilated stomach compresses the caudal vena cava and portal vein, causing blood pooling in the abdominal viscera and the caudal skeletal musculature.[1] Venous return to the heart decreases, leading to a fall in cardiac output and the development of systemic hypotension.[1,5,6] In addition, fluid sequestered in the dilated stomach is unavailable for intestinal absorption, contributing to hypovolemic shock. This combination of obstructive and hypovolemic shock is the first problem that should be addressed in treating GDV.

The acid-base status of dogs with GDV may be quite variable. In one series of patients, acid-base status at the time of admission to the hospital was most often normal.[7] It was hypothesized that two opposing metabolic processes may occur in GDV. Hydrogen ions are sequestered in the gastric lumen, resulting in an increase in plasma bicarbonate ion concentration and metabolic alkalosis. Meanwhile, circulatory shock decreases oxygenation of tissues, increasing lactic acid production and causing metabolic acidosis. The end result is no net change in arterial pH. A separate study found that although approximately 34% of dogs with GDV had a normal acid-base status, about 26% had metabolic acidosis.[8]

The most common electrolyte abnormality in GDV appears to be hypokalemia.[8] This tends to be a problem especially in the postoperative period, when anorexia, vomiting, and the administration of potassium-deficient fluids all may contribute to whole-body potassium depletion.

Severe cardiac arrhythmias occur in approximately 40% of dogs with GDV.[9] Most arrhythmias are ventricular in origin, although supraventricular arrhythmias may also be seen.[9] Arrhythmias usually have a delayed onset, commonly occurring between 12 and 36 hours after the onset of GDV.[9] Cardiac arrhythmias of delayed onset

are probably best explained by poor venous return to the heart during GDV, which in turn results in reduced coronary arterial blood flow.[9] Experimental ligation of the canine coronary arteries is typically followed by a 6- to 12-hour period of normal cardiac rhythm prior to the onset of ventricular tachycardia.[10] Myocardial ischemia has been demonstrated histologically in a significant proportion of dogs dying of GDV.[11] Other contributing factors may include autonomic imbalance,[9] acid-base and electrolyte abnormalities,[9] and circulating cardioactive substances such as catecholamines and myocardial depressant factor.[12]

The markedly distended stomach may mechanically restrict respiration, leading to a decreased minute volume and hypoventilation.[5] The cardiopulmonary system is further compromised in its ability to provide oxygenated blood by poor venous return and low cardiac output, compounding the problem of tissue hypoxia.

Two factors predispose dogs with GDV to septic shock. Occlusion of the portal vein and caudal vena cava decreases hepatic blood flow, compromising the ability of the reticuloendothelial system to neutralize endotoxins absorbed from the gastrointestinal tract.[1] In addition, circulatory damage to the gastric mucosa may allow systemic absorption of endotoxins that would not occur otherwise.[7]

Finally, the combination of severe systemic tissue injury resulting from hypoxia, sludging of blood flow due to circulatory shock, and sepsis makes dogs with GDV prone to disseminated intravascular coagulation.[13]

History and clinical signs

There are three distinct clinical presentations for GDV: acute gastric dilatation with volvulus, acute gastric dilatation without volvulus, and chronic GDV. Acute gastric dilatation with volvulus is by far the most common. The signs usually develop within 3 hours of feeding and are sometimes related to postprandial exercise.[5] The most characteristic signs noticed by owners are severe abdominal distention and tympany, retching with an inability to vomit, restlessness, and salivation. The severity of illness at the time of presentation can vary widely and depends in part on how long the condition has been present; while some dogs are ambulatory, bright, and alert, others are recumbent and moribund. Physical examination findings may include rapid, labored breathing; weak, rapid pulses; cardiac arrhythmias with or without pulse deficits; and pale mucous membranes with a prolonged capillary refill time.

It is important to recognize that acute GDV

may occasionally occur in patients that are boarding or are hospitalized for unrelated problems. It is likely that the change in diet and feeding patterns and the stress of hospitalization contribute to GDV in these dogs. It is recommended that large, deep-chested breeds of dogs, particularly those that appear anxious about being hospitalized, be fed several small meals daily and be monitored closely for signs of GDV.

Acute gastric dilatation without volvulus can be a confusing clinical presentation. It is most often caused by simple gluttony, and is therefore usually seen in immature dogs, although it can occur in older dogs.[14] Patients appear to be unable to relieve the gastric distention effectively by vomiting, probably because of the tremendous volume of material ingested. These dogs often have eaten something unusual, such as chicken skins or plastic bags, and the ingesta does not readily pass from the stomach. Clinical signs may closely resemble those of classic acute GDV, and an emergency gastrostomy is occasionally necessary to provide gastric decompression. A second cause of gastric dilatation without volvulus is classic GDV in which the stomach has returned to its normal position. This may occur spontaneously or may result from preoperative decompression of the stomach.[14] Occasionally, volvulus is documented radiographically, but at surgery the stomach is found to be in its normal position. It is often not possible to determine in cases of simple gastric dilatation whether a volvulus was initially present or not; however, this knowledge is not necessary to provide appropriate treatment.

A final clinical presentation that occurs very rarely is chronic GDV. Dogs with this condition have histories that may include chronic vomiting, weight loss, eructation, and intermittent episodes of mild bloating that resolves spontaneously.[14,15] Chronic GDV is diagnosed by contrast radiography and is treated by gastropexy.

Radiography

In the vast majority of cases, the diagnosis of acute GDV can be made based on clinical signs alone. Radiography is occasionally helpful, particularly in distinguishing simple gastric dilatation from gastric dilatation with volvulus. Radiographs should be obtained only after the patient has been appropriately treated for shock and the stomach has been decompressed.

Although on rare occasions positive contrast studies are necessary to determine whether gastric volvulus is present, the diagnosis can usually be based on plain radiographs. The radiographic view of choice for diagnosing gastric volvulus is the right lateral recumbent view.[16] In volvulus,

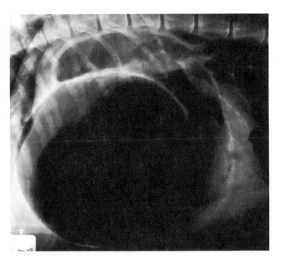

Fig. 11-1 Right lateral recumbent radiograph from a dog with gastric dilatation-volvulus. The pylorus and proximal small intestine are gas-filled and are positioned dorsal to the fundus of the stomach. A tissue-dense line representing a fold in the stomach separates the pylorus from the remainder of the stomach (compartmentalization).

the pylorus is usually positioned to the left of midline, dorsally and cranially to the fundus of the stomach. With the patient in right lateral recumbency, the pylorus will be appear gas-filled rather than fluid-filled (Fig. 11-1). In addition, the stomach may appear compartmentalized, with a tissue-dense line representing a fold in the stomach separating the compartments.[5] Radiographic findings may include gas within the wall of the stomach, (indicating gastric necrosis), an abnormal splenic location, and splenomegaly.

Emergency treatment

The first step in the emergency care of dogs with GDV is treatment of shock (Chapter 14). In addition to administration of intravenous fluids, successful treatment of shock in GDV requires immediate gastric decompression. During the treatment for shock, arterial blood gases and serum electrolyte levels should be determined, and continuous electrocardiographic monitoring should be initiated. The specific management of acid-base and electrolyte disturbances and cardiac arrhythmias are discussed elsewhere in this book (Chapters 17 and 38). It should be recognized that abnormalities in acid-base status often resolve following treatment of shock.[7,8] Several techniques may be used to provide and maintain decompression of the stomach.

Orogastric intubation. The most rapid method for decompressing the stomach is to pass an orogastric tube. Stomach tubes should be made of soft, pliable plastic and should be of large diameter (¼ in. to 1 in.). There should be several side holes in the distal end, and the distal tip should be smooth and lubricated so that it does not abrade the esophagus. With the animal in sternal or lateral recumbency and a mouth speculum in place, the tube is introduced slowly until the animal swallows it. The tip of the tube should then be palpable in the cervical esophagus. Once correct placement is ensured, the tube is advanced into the stomach. If the tube cannot be advanced past the cardia, repositioning the animal may help. When the tube is correctly placed, gastric gas will escape, and fluid gastric contents can be aspirated. Periodically flushing the tube with lukewarm water may allow more complete emptying of the stomach. If the volvulus is severe, it may be impossible to pass the tube through the cardia, and percutaneous gastrocentesis is indicated.

Percutaneous gastrocentesis. Gastrocentesis should be performed at a location where there is obvious tympany on percussion. The left abdominal wall caudal to the last rib is usually a safe site. Following a quick sterile preparation, one or two large-bore needles (e.g., 14-gauge) are passed into the stomach. Once the stomach is partially decompressed by gastrocentesis, it may be possible to pass an orogastric tube to complete the decompression.

Following decompression, a decision regarding the need for emergency surgery should be made. If an orogastric tube cannot be passed, or if only partial or temporary relief of gastric distention can be accomplished, immediate surgery is indicated. Radiographs are not essential in this situation, since they are unlikely to change the decision to operate or influence the choice of surgical procedures. If gastric decompression can be accomplished, radiographs should be taken to determine the position of the stomach. If the stomach is in an abnormal position, surgery should be performed as soon as possible, even if the stomach does not tend to redistend rapidly. Research has shown that severe gastric volvulus, even without dilatation, interferes with gastric venous drainage and may result in necrosis of the gastric wall.[17] If the stomach is in a normal position, the patient should be closely monitored, but emergency surgery is not necessary. However, prophylactic gastropexy may be elected at a later time.

In some practice situations, it may be necessary to refer patients for surgery once emergency care has been provided. If the owner must travel for a significant time (e.g., more than 30 minutes), steps should be taken to maintain gastric decompression during the trip. Possibilities include a percutaneous gastrostomy tube, a pharyngostomy tube, or a temporary gastrostomy. These techniques can be performed in 5 to 10 minutes using local anesthesia, and are described in standard textbooks of veterinary surgery.[18]

Surgery

The goals of surgery for GDV are correction of gastric displacement, evaluation of the integrity of the gastric wall, evaluation of the splenic vascular supply, and prevention of recurrence. Patients with severe systemic manifestations of GDV, particularly those in which septic shock is suspected, may be given broad-spectrum antibiotics perioperatively.

Correction of gastric displacement. Derotation of the stomach should be accomplished as quickly as possible. The vast majority of displacements occur in the clockwise direction and can be recognized by the presence of omentum covering the ventral surface of the stomach. With the surgeon standing on the dog's right side, the pyloric region is grasped by passing the right hand dorsally along the left body wall. The right hand then pulls the pylorus ventrally while the left hand pushes the fundus out of the way. Using the two hands, the stomach can be returned to its normal position. Occasionally, it is necessary to relieve distention by aspirating the stomach with a large-bore needle and suction before derotation can be accomplished. Once the stomach is returned to its normal position, an orogastric tube is passed and the stomach is emptied as completely as possible. Gastrostomy may be necessary if the stomach cannot be substantially emptied by orogastric intubation.

Evaluation of the integrity of the gastric wall. Necrosis of the gastric wall is a serious complication of GDV. Volvulus compromises venous drainage from the greater curvature of the stomach by producing kinking, stretching, or actual tearing of the short gastric veins.[17] Severe distention of the stomach compounds the venous stasis, as does the general hypotensive state of the patient. The gastric mucosa may become ulcerated and hemorrhagic, and ultimately, the entire gastric wall in the region of the greater curvature may become necrotic. Necrotic areas of gastric wall must be resected to prevent perforation and peritonitis or septic shock resulting from absorption of endotoxins.

Determination of the presence and extent of gastric necrosis can be extremely difficult. Damage to the short gastric vessels alone does not necessarily produce necrosis, because of the extensive collateral circulation to the gastric wall.[19] Although intravenous fluorescein dye may be used to evaluate gastric viability, standard clinical criteria are proven to be more reliable.[20] Pale green or gray serosal surfaces have lost arterial supply and should be resected.[19] Black or dark purple regions have severely compromised venous drainage and are usually resected. Dark red areas generally are not resected. Other observations, such as thinning of the gastric wall or lack of hemorrhage from a cut surface, may contribute to a decision to resect.

Techniques for partial gastrectomy have been described previously.[5] It may be necessary to resect large areas of the greater curvature, and resection can be particularly difficult if necrosis extends into the region of the cardia. Surgical stapling equipment can significantly simplify the resection, and does not require entering the gastric lumen.

The mortality rate for GDV is significantly higher if gastric necrosis is present.[18] In one study, 63% of dogs requiring partial gastrectomy died of postoperative complications including septic shock, peritonitis, and aspiration pneumonia.[19]

Evaluation of the splenic vascular supply. The spleen should be removed only if there is thrombosis of the splenic vein or its branches.[5] The splenic vein is inspected by creating a small opening in the greater omentum slightly to the left of midline.[5] Splenectomy is performed when indicated.[18]

Gastropexy techniques. Few topics have received as much attention in the veterinary literature as the relative merits of the various gastropexy techniques for prevention of recurrence of GDV. Although there are situations in which a certain type of gastropexy may be preferable, each of the commonly performed gastropexies is more than adequate to prevent recurrence and can work well for every case. The surgeon should use a gastropexy that he or she can perform quickly and securely. The most popular types of gastropexies include tube gastrostomy, simple gastropexy, circumcostal gastropexy, and belt-loop gastropexy.

A tube gastrostomy is created by passing an 18 to 24 French Foley catheter through a stab incision in the right abdominal wall, then into the stomach through a purse-string suture placed near the pyloric antrum. With the bulb inflated in the lumen of the stomach, the stomach is drawn to the abdominal wall by applying traction to the catheter and is then sutured to the abdominal musculature. Tube gastrostomies have resulted in a recurrence rate of 5% or lower, and complications are very unusual.[21,22] The technique is particularly useful when a partial gastrectomy has been performed, because by periodically aspirating the tube the stomach may be kept empty, thereby relieving tension on the suture line. Nutrition in this situation can be provided by needle-catheter jejunostomy.[23] Disadvantages of tube gastrostomy include the potential for leakage of gastric contents around the tube (cellulitis, peritonitis) and the need to leave the tube in place for 5 to 7 days so that a fistulous tract can form before it is removed, preventing leakage of gastric contents into the abdomen.

A simple gastropexy can be performed by suturing the pyloric antrum to the right abdominal wall.[24] The strength of a simple gastropexy can be improved if the abdominal wall and pyloric antrum are superficially incised or scarified prior to suturing.[25] Although some surgeons have questioned the strength of the simple gastropexy, the technique is very quick and easy to perform, and has never been proven to be inadequate for preventing recurrence of GDV. It has the additional advantage of not requiring entrance into the gastric lumen.

The circumcostal gastropexy was developed to provide a potentially stronger adhesion than the simple gastropexy while maintaining the advantage of not entering the gastric lumen.[26] In this technique, a flap of gastric muscularis and serosa is brought around one of the last four ribs to anchor the pyloric antrum to the right abdominal wall.[26] The reported postoperative recurrence rate is very similar to that for tube gastrostomy.[27,28] The technique is relatively simple to perform and is proven to provide a strong, permanent adhesion.[29]

The belt-loop gastropexy is performed by creating a "belt-loop" flap in the transversus abdominal muscle caudal to the right costal arch and a tongue-shaped seromuscular flap in the pyloric antrum.[30] The tongue-shaped flap is pulled through the belt-loop flap and reattached to the stomach.[30] This is a simple technique for creating a strong gastropexy without entering the gastric lumen, and it prevents potential complications of the circumcostal gastropexy such as iatrogenic rib fracture and iatrogenic pneumothorax.[30] Clinical results in a series of 20 patients were excellent.[30]

Postoperative care

If possible, dogs with GDV should be continuously monitored for the first 1 to 3 days following surgery. In uncomplicated cases, intravenous fluids are usually continued for the first 24 hours postoperatively. Small quantities of water can be offered orally 12 hours postoperatively, and by 24 hours postoperatively, intravenous fluids may be discontinued. Oral feeding can be initiated at this time.

In patients that have undergone partial gastrectomy, precautions should be taken to reduce the likelihood of gastric dehiscence. Ideally, oral feeding should be avoided for 3 to 5 days. Fluids can be provided intravenously, and nutritional support can be given through a needle-catheter jejunostomy placed at the time of surgery.[23] Commercially available polymeric diets are ideal for this purpose (Chapter 37).[31] Patients should be monitored closely for evidence of gastric dehiscence and peritonitis, particularly during Days 3 through 5 postoperatively. Signs of peritonitis may include an acute deterioration in clinical course, fever, abdominal discomfort, vomiting, and loss of appetite. A complete blood count may reveal neutrophilia with a marked left shift, and abdominocentesis will usually confirm the diagnosis. Immediate surgical exploration of the abdomen is indicated if gastric dehiscence is suspected.

All patients with GDV should be monitored closely for acid-base and electrolyte disturbances, cardiac arrhythmias, disseminated intravascular coagulation, and septic shock. In general, patients can be discharged from the hospital 3 to 5 days postoperatively if complications have not developed. Once at home, to help prevent recurrence, patients should be given 2 or 3 small meals daily and should be discouraged from exercising after eating.

Prognosis

The prognosis for dogs with GDV is extremely variable. With appropriate care, uncomplicated cases can have an excellent prognosis. On the other hand, dogs presenting with severe systemic problems, particularly shock or gastric necrosis, must be given a very guarded prognosis.

THORACOLUMBAR INTERVERTEBRAL DISK DISEASE

Herniation of canine thoracolumbar intervertebral disks is by far the most common neurologic condition requiring emergency surgery in animals. Herniation of cervical intervertebral disks is less common, and because it usually produces neck pain only or neck pain with mild, ambulatory tetraparesis, it is usually not considered a surgical emergency.[32]

Etiology and signalment

The intervertebral disks are resilient, shock-absorbing structures consisting of a central nucleus pulposus encircled by an annulus fibrosus. The nucleus pulposus is a gellike matrix of collagen fibrils and glycosaminoglycans, and the annulus fibrosus is formed by concentric fibrous lamellae that are attached to the vertebral body end plates.[33] The ventral aspect of the annulus is considerably thicker than the dorsal aspect, so disk herniations usually occur in the dorsal direction.[34]

Two different types of metaplastic degeneration of intervertebral discs were defined by Hansen in 1952.[35] The most common occurs in chondrodystrophic breeds of dogs, in which the disks undergo chondroid degeneration. The nucleus pulposus of each disk becomes progressively more cartilaginous and mineralized, and the annulus fibrosus degenerates concurrently. In chondrodystrophic breeds, these changes have occurred in the majority of the disks by 1 year of age. The disks lose their normal resiliency and are prone to the acute, massive rupture referred to as a Hansen Type I disk protrusion. This type of disk protrusion will be emphasized in this chapter.

Although Hansen Type I disk herniations are occasionally seen in large breeds of dogs, the vast majority occur in the small, chondrodystrophic breeds. Roughly one half to three fourths of affected animals are Dachshunds; however, the Beagle, Pekingese, Lhasa Apso, and other small breeds are also at significant risk.[36,37] Most patients are middle aged and older, and there does not appear to be a distinct sex predilection.

The second type of intervertebral disk degeneration is fibrous metaplasia, which occurs as part of the aging process in nonchondrodystrophic breeds of dogs.[35] This is a more insidious process that results in the slow, domelike bulging of the dorsal annulus referred to as a Hansen Type II disk protrusion. This condition is seen in older patients and generally produces mild neurologic signs that do not require emergency care.

History and clinical signs

The history and clinical signs of acute thoracolumbar disk herniations vary considerably. Many patients have episodes of chronic, intermittent lumbar pain prior to an acute, catastrophic disk herniation. Pain may arise from the damaged disk itself (diskogenic pain), or from irritation of the meninges or nerve roots (radicular pain). Herniations may be precipitated by trauma; however, most cases appear to occur spontaneously without any apparent inciting cause. Over 65% of thoracolumbar herniations occur between T11-12 and L1-2, with the T12-13 interspace being the single most common site of rupture.[33] Thoracic disk herniations above the level of T10-11 rarely occur, because they are prevented by the intercapital ligaments, which run between the heads of each pair of ribs. Herniations in the middle and lower lumbar spine involving the lumbar intumescence of the spinal cord are occasionally seen; however, the vast majority of herniations produce the neurologic deficits typical of compressive lesions between spinal cord segments T3 and L3. These deficits reflect damage to the ascending sensory neurons and descending upper motor neurons supplying the hindlimbs. Signs of upper motor neuron damage include spastic paresis of the hindlimbs, increased hindlimb muscle tone, and hyperactive hindlimb spinal reflexes.

Compressive spinal cord lesions usually cause major neurologic functions to be lost in a predictable sequence. With increasing severity of spinal cord compression, deficits in conscious proprioception are noted first, followed by a loss of voluntary motor movements, and finally loss of deep pain perception. This sequence allows patients with intervertebral disk herniations to be staged according to the severity of their neurologic deficits. The choice of treatment always depends at least in part on the patient's neurologic stage. One convenient staging system is as follows:

Stage 1—Pain only; no neurologic deficits
Stage 2—Mild to moderate ambulatory paresis
Stage 3—Nonambulatory paresis; some voluntary motor movements present
Stage 4—Nonambulatory paresis; no voluntary motor movements present; deep pain perception present
Stage 5—Loss of deep pain perception (paraplegia)

Dogs with neurologic signs compatible with a lesion between spinal cord segments T3 and L3 may have a disk herniation anywhere between interspaces T2-3 and L2-3, and it is important to be able to localize the lesion more accurately, particularly if surgery is planned. Further localization of the lesion can be made by evaluating the panniculus reflex, sensory level, and level of hyperpathia.

1. Panniculus reflex—This reflex is elicited by lightly pricking or squeezing the skin over the back, which should cause contraction of the cutaneous truncus muscle and quick movement of the skin. The reflex is mediated by segmental sensory neurons and passes cranially through the spinal cord to the C8 and T1 cord segments, which give rise to the lateral thoracic nerve.[38] The evaluation is begun in the lumbosacral area and proceeds cranially. In normal dogs, the reflex is absent caudal to the midlumbar spine; however, it may occasionally be present as far back as the lumbosacral junction.[38] In dogs with severe thoracolumbar spinal cord compression, the reflex may be absent caudal to the lesion.

2. Sensory level—The sensory level is determined by forcefully pinching the skin over the back with forceps, and observing for evidence that the animal feels the stimulus. Testing begins over the lower lumbar spine and proceeds cranially. Animals with severe spinal cord compression may be analgesic caudal to the lesion. Response to this test is extremely variable, as many animals are stoic and do not strongly object to the skin pinching.

3. Hyperpathia—Digital pressure on the dorsal spinous processes or transverse processes near the involved interspace may elicit a painful response. Occasionally, this response consists only of a subtle tensing of the abdominal musculature,[33] but it is often absent.

According to one study, these tests, in combination with neurologic examination, will allow determination of correct interspace only 40% of the time, but will allow localization within two interspaces 75% of the time.[39] In combination with radiographic evaluation, neurologic evaluation permits highly accurate localization of thoracolumbar disk herniations.

Approximately 15% of all disk herniations occur at interspaces L3-4, L4-5, or L5-6.[39] Clinical signs in these patients may include lower motor neuron involvement of the femoral and/or sciatic nerves (i.e., flaccid paresis of the hindlimbs, decreased hindlimb muscle tone, hypoactive hindlimb spinal reflexes, and possibly muscle atrophy). In animals that have lost deep pain perception due to a herniation in one of these locations, an important differential diagnosis is a severe disk herniation resulting in descending myelomalacia.[40] Myelomalacia is a spontaneous degeneration of the spinal cord that may ascend or descend from the site of the lesion. If myelomalacia ascends far enough, lower motor neuron involvement of the forelimbs may develop, and these patients often die of respiratory failure. If the condition descends into the lumbar intumescence, clinical signs may closely mimic a severe disk herniation in the same area. The conditions are important to differentiate because the prognosis in myelomalacia is grave. Clinical signs that may be present in myelomalacia but that will not be present in lower lumbar disk herniations are neurologic deficits in the forelimbs, loss of tone in the abdominal musculature, cranial migration of the sensory level with time, and respiratory difficulty. Myelomalacia is an indication for euthanasia.

Radiography

The presumptive diagnosis of an intervertebral disk herniation is confirmed by radiography. For

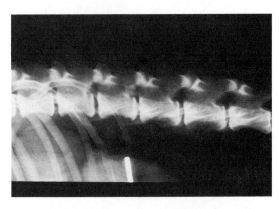

Fig. 11-2 Lateral radiograph from a dog with an intervertebral disk herniation at L2-3. There is mild narrowing of the intervertebral space, and calcified disk material is visible within the spinal canal.

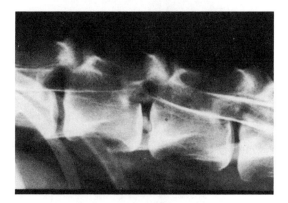

Fig. 11-3 Lateral myelogram from the dog shown in Fig. 11-2. A large, ventral extradural mass representing calcified disk material is present at L2-3.

patients presented during emergency hours, it is not necessary to obtain radiographs immediately unless surgery is being contemplated (see below). Plain radiographs are best obtained under general anesthesia unless the patient is extremely cooperative. In general, lateral views of the thoracolumbar spine are far more useful than dorsoventral views, although both views should be obtained in every case. The following radiographic findings strongly suggest an acute intervertebral disk herniation[41] (Fig. 11-2):

1. Narrowing and/or wedging of an intervertebral space. The primary x-ray beam should be directly centered over the interspace in question in order to evaluate the interspace properly.
2. Narrowing of an intervertebral foramen or narrowing of the space between adjacent articular processes.
3. A calcified mass within the spinal canal with corresponding narrowing of the intervertebral space or foramen. Calcification of an intervertebral disk in its normal position does not imply herniation and is frequently seen in chondrodystrophic breeds over 1 year of age.

After radiographs have been obtained, myelography may be necessary. Myelography is indicated only for patients that are considered to be candidates for surgery; if conservative management is planned for a patient with radiographic evidence of an acute disk herniation, myelography is very unlikely to alter the course of therapy. Although surgery can be performed based on radiographic findings alone, many surgeons prefer to obtain a myelogram for every surgical patient, since plain radiographic localization of disk herni-

ations is reported to have an accuracy of only about 75%.[39] Myelography is absolutely indicated when neurologic and radiographic localization are incompatible, when there are no visible radiographic lesions, when there is more than one suspicious radiographic lesion, or when the history or clinical findings are not highly suggestive of an intervertebral disk herniation.[33,39] Injection of the myelographic contrast medium may be made at either the cisternal or lumbar sites, although postmyelographic seizures are less common following lumbar injection.[42] Both lateral and dorsoventral views should be obtained to aid in planning the surgical approach. In acute intervertebral disk herniations, myelography will usually demonstrate a ventral or ventrolateral extradural mass (Fig. 11-3), unless local spinal cord swelling is severe enough to obliterate the subarachnoid space.

Treatment

The choice of treatment for dogs with acute thoracolumbar disk herniations is, and probably will remain, an area of great controversy. The following commonly used guidelines are recommended; however, many clinicians advocate other treatment protocols:

Stage 1—Conservative care with close at-home monitoring
Stage 2—Conservative care with close in-hospital monitoring
Stage 3—Surgical decompression
Stage 4—Surgical decompression
Stage 5—Surgical decompression

Conservative care. Conservative care for dogs in Stage 1 or 2 usually consists of strictly enforced rest and the administration of corticosteroids. Ideally, patients should be confined to a cage or small room, with exercise restricted to periodic short leash walks. Running or jumping should be absolutely forbidden. Even if the patient improves very quickly in response to rest and corticosteroid administration, confinement should be continued for at least 2 to 3 weeks. Corticosteroid administration will often make the patient feel much better, and if activity is unrestricted, an acute, severe disk herniation may be precipitated. Although a number of corticosteroid regimens are available, prednisolone (0.5 mg/kg every 12 hours for 3 to 5 days) is usually efficacious.

Surgery

Most surgeons would readily agree that patients with acute intervertebral disk herniations presenting in Stage 4 or 5 require decompressive surgery.[33,43] The need for surgery for acutely nonambulatory patients that retain some voluntary motor ability (Stage 3) is controversial; although conservative care is an option for these patients, many of them will ultimately require surgery. Occasionally, Stage 1 or 2 patients will fail to improve or will deteriorate neurologically despite appropriate conservative care, and will also require decompressive surgery.[43]

The timing of surgery is also controversial. At Tufts University School of Veterinary Medicine, patients presenting acutely in Stage 4 or 5 are considered candidates for emergency decompressive surgery performed immediately following radiography and/or myelography. Surgery is often delayed until regular office hours for patients in Stage 3. These patients are very closely monitored during the interval between presentation and surgery, and emergency surgery is performed if significant neurologic deterioration is noted. Decompressive surgery for patients with chronic Stage 1 or 2 signs is an elective procedure.

Prior to myelography and surgery, patients should be given corticosteroids. Steroids are known to benefit the acutely injured spinal cord through a number of mechanisms (Chapter 20) and will be most beneficial if administered before any intraoperative manipulation of the spinal cord.[44] Dexamethasone is usually used because of its potency and rapid onset of action.[44] Typically, 2 mg/kg is given intravenously preoperatively followed by 0.1 to 0.2 mg/kg subcutaneously or intramuscularly for 48 hours postoperatively.[33]

The two decompressive techniques most commonly performed in small animal surgery are dorsal laminectomy and hemilaminectomy.[33,40] These should be regarded as approaches rather than definitive surgical techniques. A significant body of research suggests that laminectomy or hemilaminectomy without mass removal provides very little decompression of the spinal cord.[43] If the ventral mass is not removed, only minor dorsal displacement occurs following laminectomy.[45] A ventral mass places marked axial tension on the cord that is especially severe on its dorsal surface, and laminectomy will not relieve this tension.[46] Finally, a ventral extradural mass significantly disturbs spinal cord blood supply, even following laminectomy.[33]

The decision to perform a dorsal laminectomy versus a hemilaminectomy is often determined by the surgeon's individual preference. Dorsal laminectomy is somewhat more versatile than hemilaminectomy, because it allows removal of ventrolateral disk extrusions on either side of the spinal cord. On the other hand, masses lying immediately beneath the spinal cord are difficult to remove through a dorsal laminectomy without manipulation of the cord. Hemilaminectomy is preferred for ventral extrusions and for ventrolateral extrusions if neurologic examination or myelography indicate that the disk is on one side. Hemilaminectomy will not permit removal of ventrolaterally extruded disks on the opposite side of the spinal cord.

Prophylactic fenestration

Fenestration is the removal of the nucleus pulposus of the intervertebral disks through a small incision in the annulus fibrosus. In the thoracolumbar spine, the T11-12 through L3-4 disks are usually fenestrated, and several surgical approaches have been described.[47-49] Thoracolumbar disk fenestration is not as commonly performed as the decompressive techniques, probably because the procedure is technically demanding and because of controversy regarding its value and indications. Fenestration should be regarded as a prophylactic measure designed to prevent future catastrophic disk herniations. It is unlikely to relieve either radicular pain or signs of spinal cord compression caused by extruded disk material lying within the spinal canal.[43] Fenestration is usually performed as an isolated procedure for dogs in Stage 1 or 2 or in conjunction with decompressive surgery for dogs in Stage 3, 4, or 5. In the latter patients, the need for fenestration has been questioned, since the incidence of a later disk extrusion at a second interspace is under 3%.[39] Other studies indicate a higher recurrence rate and support the prophylactic value of thoracolumbar disk fenestration[50]; controlled trials are needed.

Postoperative care

Extensive postoperative nursing care is essential for nonambulatory patients undergoing decompressive surgery. Major postoperative concerns include prevention and treatment of cystitis, decubital ulcers, and gastrointestinal ulceration and provision of physical therapy.

Many patients with severe intervertebral disk herniations (Stage 4 or 5) lose voluntary control of urination, and retain urine due to spasticity of the smooth and striated urethral musculature.[51] When the bladder becomes fully distended, small amounts of urine may drip from the penis or vulva, but a large residual volume remains.[38] The bladder is typically very difficult to express, particularly in male dogs. In order to prevent retention cystitis, the bladder should be emptied thoroughly by manual expression or catheterization at least three times daily. Drugs that relax the smooth and striated urethral musculature (phenoxybenzamine and diazepam, respectively) may occasionally be helpful.[51] Urine obtained by cystocentesis should be cultured periodically, and therapeutic antibiotics should be initiated if indicated. Most patients in Stage 4 or 5 will begin involuntary reflex urination mediated by the sacral segments of the spinal cord within 1 or 2 weeks postoperatively, even if there has been no improvement in overall neurologic status.[38] This type of urination can often be initiated by a small amount of abdominal pressure, but voiding is incomplete, and the risk of retention cystitis remains. At this stage, most owners are able to care for the patient at home, but should be made aware that the patient will have no voluntary control of urination until approximately the time of significant recovery of voluntary motor movements in the hind legs.

Decubital ulcers are chronic, full-thickness skin lesions that develop over pressure points in recumbent patients. They are most likely to occur over bony prominences such as the greater trochanter, ischial tuberosity, or acromion process. Although decubital ulcers can develop in any non-ambulatory patient, they are most likely to occur in large, heavy dogs. They are best prevented by keeping recumbent animals on a soft, padded surface and turning them every 3 to 4 hours. Waterbeds are ideal for this purpose. The patient should be kept clean and dry at all times; urine scalding in particular will rapidly promote the development of decubital ulcers. Rubberized racks are available that prevent urine and feces from collecting around the patient, while the holes in the rack protect the bony prominences from excessive pressure. Once decubital ulcers are allowed to develop, they are often difficult or impossible to treat successfully until the patient becomes ambulatory. One method of treatment is to place a doughnut-shaped bandage around the ulcer to pro-

tect it from pressure, while keeping the wound as clean as possible as it heals by second intention.

A potentially devastating complication in postoperative patients receiving corticosteroids is the development of gastrointestinal ulceration.[52,53] Although the pathogenesis of this syndrome is complex, it is known that either steroid administration or acute spinal cord injury may produce gastrointestinal complications; when the two are present in combination, the syndrome becomes very common.[52] In one large retrospective study, 2% of neurologic patients receiving corticosteroids died of gastrointestinal ulceration.[52] The syndrome has been most commonly associated with dexamethasone administration, and it appears that patients with severe neurologic deficits are most likely to be affected.[52,53] Clinical signs include diarrhea, melena, depression, anorexia, and vomiting; however, death due to peritonitis and sepsis may occur without prior signs.[52] Development of any of these signs dictates that steroid therapy be discontinued.

Physical therapy, in the form of passive or active exercise, is one of the simplest steps that can be taken to promote the recovery of paralyzed animals. Aside from the obvious benefits to circulation, muscle tone, and joint mobility, physical therapy often produces a marked improvement in the attitude of the patient. At minimum, physical therapy should consist of passive manipulation of the limbs. All joints should be repeatedly moved through a full range of motion for 5 to 10 minutes two or three times daily. Swimming is an ideal form of physical therapy, because it allows non-weight-bearing voluntary movement of the weakened limbs. Swimming also requires mass movement patterns, which facilitate neurologic improvement, and helps to keep the patient clean, which discourages the development of decubital ulcers.[54] Patients should be monitored constantly and supported if necessary during swimming, and the incision should be protected with a water-resistant petroleum jelly. Swimming in warm water for 20 minutes once daily is adequate for most patients.

Once at home, owners can walk the patient outside by providing support at the base of the tail or passing a sling under the belly. Carts are also available for paraplegic large and small dogs (K-9 Cart Co., Berwyn, PA). These carts allow the patient to become more mobile, and keep the patient out of the recumbent position without constant assistance from the owner. For dogs that are expected to recover, carts should be used only to assist in the general program of physical therapy. Dogs may become overly dependent on the cart, which will impede a complete recovery.[33] Constant use of a cart is recommended only for paraplegic patients with no hope of recovery.

Prognosis

Preoperatively, it is very difficult to establish an accurate prognosis for dogs with acute, severe disk herniations, and this fact should be conveyed to the owner. Although prognosis is definitely related to chronicity and neurologic stage,[33] it is often impossible to precisely categorize a patient prior to surgery, because it is difficult to know whether neurologic deterioration has peaked or will continue to progress. For this reason, an animal may be worse after surgery despite an atraumatic removal of disk material. Owners should understand that a more accurate prognosis can usually be given 1 to 2 days after surgery.

It is well recognized that the most important prognostic factor is the presence or absence of deep pain perception.[33,39,55] In general, nonambulatory patients that retain deep pain perception prior to surgery have a good prognosis.[33] It is reported that 40% to 90% of these patients will regain the ability to walk.[39,55] The time required for recovery is extremely variable and may range from less than a week to several months. Paraplegic patients must be given a guarded prognosis, and the prognosis becomes worse the longer deep pain perception has been absent prior to surgery. If decompressive surgery is performed early, these patients may have a fair prognosis; one study showed that 50% of paraplegic dogs operated on within 36 hours of losing the ability to walk eventually recovered.[55] Owners of these animals should understand that if recovery is to occur at all, it may require many months and will entail a major personal commitment.

SPINAL TRAUMA

Spinal fractures and luxations are usually caused by serious automobile trauma, and are commonly accompanied by other injuries. Patients with spinal trauma should be treated for shock and thoroughly evaluated for life-threatening problems before the spinal injury is treated. In most cases, an accurate assessment of neurologic deficits is impossible until shock has been resolved.

Biomechanics of spinal fractures and luxations

Spinal fractures and luxations usually occur at the junctions of mobile and immobile portions of the spinal column.[56,57] Although any region of the spine may be damaged, the majority of spinal injuries in dogs occur in the axis, in the lower thoracic or upper lumbar spine, and at the lumbosacral junction.

In humans, the decision to operate and the type of repair selected is often predicated on the specific skeletal and soft-tissue supporting elements of the spinal column that are damaged. The spinal column can be divided into two anatomic regions: a ventral compartment consisting of the vertebral body, intervertebral disk, dorsal and ventral longitudinal ligaments, and intertransverse ligaments; and a dorsal compartment consisting of the lamina, pedicles, dorsal spinous processes, articular processes, and supraspinous, interspinous, and interarcuate ligaments.[56] Injuries confined to a single compartment produce relatively minor instability and can often be treated conservatively.[56] Unfortunately, injuries to a single compartment are unusual in animals, and are very difficult to diagnose with confidence.[56] As discussed below, the decision to operate in animals is based on radiographic findings, neurologic status and trend, and a general impression of spinal stability.

Spinal injuries usually result from one or more of the following forces: flexion, extension, compression, and rotation. Most spinal trauma in animals involves some degree of hyperflexion of the spine. These forces produce fractures or luxations with predictable configurations, the most common of which are discussed below.

Transverse or oblique fractures. Transverse or oblique fractures most commonly involve the axis or the seventh lumbar vertebra. In the cervical spine, the skull, atlas, and body of the axis form a unit that is relatively stable during flexion of the neck.[58] Severe flexion and distraction forces in the neck are concentrated in the axis, and produce oblique or transverse fractures through the vertebral body or pedicles[57] (Fig. 11-4). The caudal

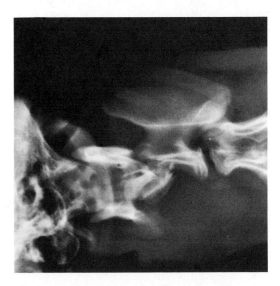

Fig. 11-4 Lateral radiographs from a dog with a transverse fracture through the body of the axis.

segment of these fractures often displaces cranially and dorsally.

In the lower lumbar spine, flexional forces often produce oblique fractures through the body of L7. If a significant rotary component is also present, a fracture-dislocation may result, with significant displacement of the lumbosacral junction.[57] The caudal segment is usually displaced cranially and ventrally by the weight and muscle action of the sacral and pelvic unit.[57]

Compression fractures. Compression fractures of the vertebral bodies may have either a bursting or a wedge configuration. In either case, the dorsal supporting structures remain intact to some extent, and may provide enough stability to allow conservative management.[57] Bursting compression fractures occur when compressive forces act along a straightened segment of vertebral bodies, while wedge compression fractures occur when compression is combined with flexion[57] (Fig. 11-5). In either case, bone fragments or an intervertebral disk may be driven dorsally into the spinal cord.

Luxations and fracture-luxations. A luxation or subluxation at an intervertebral space occurs when flexion is combined with simultaneous rotation[57] (Fig. 11-6). In the cervical spine, the articular facets may become interlocked unilaterally or bilaterally when luxations occur.[57] Bilateral interlocking of the facets usually implies severe spinal cord compression or transection.[57] Similar forces may also produce a fracture-luxation.[57] Typically, the caudoventral aspect of the vertebral body cranial to the luxated interspace will be fractured, and the caudal segment of the fracture luxation displaces ventrally (Fig. 11-7).

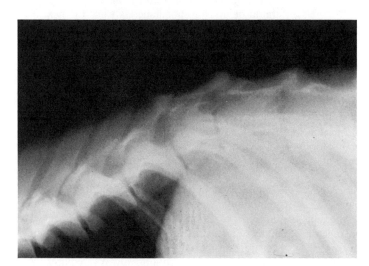

Fig. 11-5. Lateral radiograph from a dog with a wedge compression fracture of T11.

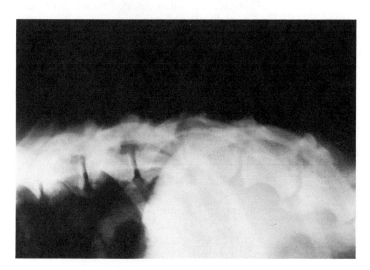

Fig. 11-6. Lateral radiograph from a dog with subluxation at T12-13.

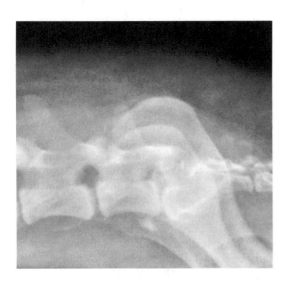

Fig. 11-7. Lateral radiograph from a dog with a fracture-luxation of the lumbosacral junction. There is a small fracture of the caudoventral aspect of the vertebral body of L7, and compression of the cauda equina is produced by ventral displacement of the caudal segment.

Clinical signs

Animals with spinal injuries are often in extreme pain. With fractures in the thoracolumbar region, obvious displacement of the fracture or luxation may be palpable. Neurologic evaluation should not be attempted until shock has been appropriately treated and the patient has been thoroughly evaluated for other life-threatening problems. Extreme care should be taken in performing the neurologic examination if there is suspicion that the spine is unstable. In some cases, it may not be possible to test postural reactions or voluntary motor movements without risking further injury to the patient.

Multiple fractures of the spine are quite common, and it is possible for the neurologic deficits produced by one lesion to mask those produced by a second lesion. For example, any lesion producing lower motor neuron deficits will mask an upper motor neuron lesion higher in the spinal cord. For this reason, radiographic evaluation of patients with spinal trauma should always include survey radiographs of the entire spinal column.

Some dogs with thoracolumbar spinal cord injuries may demonstrate Schiff-Sherrington syndrome. This syndrome is characterized by flaccid paraplegia of the pelvic limbs, extensor rigidity of the forelimbs, and intact spinal reflexes caudal to the lesion.[59] Extensor rigidity of the forelimbs is caused by damage to "border cells," which are neurons located in the lumbar spinal cord that are inhibitory to the motor neurons in the cervical intumescence responsible for forelimb extension.[59] Aside from the extensor hypertonia, the forelimbs exhibit a normal gait and postural reactions.[59] Although Schiff-Sherrington syndrome usually implies severe compression or transection of the spinal cord, some recovery may be possible.[57,59] Forelimb rigidity is often seen as a response to pain in animals with spinal injury, and can also result from upper motor neuron damage in animals with cervical lesions. These two situations should be differentiated from Schiff-Sherrington syndrome because of the grave prognosis usually associated with the latter.

Emergency care and radiographic evaluation

Patients with neurologic deficits resulting from acute injury to the spinal column should be given corticosteroids (dexamethasone, 2 mg/kg intravenously initially, followed by 0.1 to 0.2 mg/kg intramuscularly or subcutaneously for the next 3 to 4 days). The benefits and side effects of corticosteroids in acute spinal cord injury are discussed in the section on Thoracolumbar Intervertebral Disk Disease (above).

The goals of the radiographic evaluation are to localize the lesion specifically, to help decide whether surgery is indicated, to aid in the selection of a surgical procedure, and to assist in establishing the prognosis. If possible, general anesthesia should be avoided initially, so that normal muscle tone is maintained, which helps to stabilize the spinal column. Survey radiographs of the entire spine can be obtained in the awake animal, and if necessary, myelography or higher-detail films of a specific area can then be obtained under general anesthesia. Adequate radiographic evaluation of the spinal column always requires both dorsoventral and lateral views.

Although it is often not performed, myelography is probably indicated in most animals with spinal injuries. In any spinal fracture or luxation, fragments of bone or herniated disk material within the spinal canal may contribute to extradural compression of the spinal cord. While these fragments may not be visible on plain films, they may be demonstrated by myelography. Simple reduction of the fracture or luxation may not provide adequate decompression in these cases. Unfortunately, many spinal injuries produce spinal cord swelling severe enough to obliterate the subarachnoid space, so that contrast material is not visible in the area of the injury. Nevertheless, myelography is a diagnostic step that may occasionally provide crucial information.

The prognostic value of radiography in cases of spinal trauma is often limited. Severe vertebral displacement in the thoracic or lumbar spine implies a grave prognosis. In the cervical spine, severe displacement may be accompanied by relatively minor neurologic deficits, because the large epidural space often prevents significant compression of the cord. A radiograph provides no prognostic information for injuries that are minimally displaced, because it represents only the relative position of spinal segments at a point in time. Even fractures or luxations that are perfectly aligned may have completely transected the spinal cord at the time of injury. Prognosis is best based on results of neurologic evaluations of the animal (Chapter 20).

Nonsurgical management

The ideal candidate for nonsurgical management is a patient with a stable, minimally displaced fracture or luxation and relatively mild neurologic deficits. Nonsurgical management consists of strict confinement, close neurologic and radiographic monitoring, and, in some cases, application of an external splint.

Patients should be confined to a cage or a very small space at home. It is often difficult for owners to provide adequate exercise restriction, particularly for young, energetic dogs. Oral tranquilizers can be helpful in reducing the activity level of these patients; however, it is often advisable to hospitalize the animal for the first few weeks if the owner is not able to restrict activity. Neurologic status should be evaluated by the veterinarian at least weekly for the first 3 to 4 weeks. Survey lateral radiographs may be obtained at these reevaluations to ascertain that further displacement of the spinal segments has not occurred. Confinement should be continued until complete fracture healing is documented radiographically. This usually requires at least 6 to 8 weeks.

External coaptation may provide additional stability in certain cases of spinal fractures. A splint should be used only if it can be properly applied and is not resisted by the patient. The splint should be centered over the lesion; if the fracture or luxation is near the end of the splint, the splint will act as a fulcrum and increase the likelihood of further injury. An effective neck splint should extend from the midportion of the horizontal mandible to the midportion of the sternum, while splints for thoracolumbar injuries should cover the entire thoracic and lumbar spine. Splints are usually constructed from casting material or malleable aluminum bars, and should be heavily padded. Application of a snugly conforming splint requires heavy sedation or general anesthesia. If a splint is well tolerated, it should be left in place until the injury has healed completely. The owner should be aware that the splint provides only minimal additional stability, and does not decrease the need for exercise restriction.

Indications for surgery

The decision to operate in patients with spinal trauma is often extremely difficult. There are three major indications for surgery.

Stabilization of the spinal column. While human patients with spinal injuries are often placed in traction or simply confined to a bed, animals often require surgical stabilization because it is difficult to restrict their activity adequately. Surgical stabilization is definitely indicated for injuries that are palpably unstable or significantly displaced. Some injuries, for example, nondisplaced compression fractures in which the dorsal compartment is intact, are inherently stable and may be managed nonsurgically. It can be very difficult to assess accurately the stability of a spinal injury, and the decision to provide surgical stabilization is often an empirical clinical judgment. When there is doubt, surgical stabilization should be considered the appropriate approach, since catastrophic damage to the spinal cord may occur if surgery is not performed.

Decompression of the spinal cord. The decision to provide decompression of the spinal cord is based on both the radiographic and neurologic assessment. Surgical decompression is indicated if ongoing compression of the spinal cord, either by displaced spinal segments or fragments of bone or intervertebral disk, is demonstrated by radiography or myelography. Although the indications for decompression are very controversial, it is most often considered for patients with nonambulatory paresis, while ambulatory patients are candidates for nonsurgical management.[56,57] As discussed in the section on thoracolumbar disk herniations, decompressive surgery is usually considered an emergency procedure. In patients treated nonsurgically, the neurologic status should be closely monitored, and surgery should be considered if deterioration is noted.

Exploratory laminectomy and durotomy. Exploratory laminectomy and durotomy may be elected for patients that have lost deep pain perception. In general, loss of deep pain perception following spinal trauma is an extremely poor prognostic sign. If durotomy reveals either transection or advanced malacia of the spinal cord, there is no chance for recovery and euthanasia is indicated. In patients with less severe neurologic deficits, direct observation of the spinal cord will not provide prognostic information, and laminectomy is considered only as a decompressive measure.

Surgical management

Decompression of the spinal cord is accomplished by laminectomy if fragments of bone or disk material are producing compression, or by reduction of the fracture or luxation if compression is caused by displaced spinal segments. Hemilaminectomy is preferred over dorsal laminectomy because it spares the dorsal spinous processes and causes less destabilization of the dorsal compartment.[56] Removal of ventrally located bone fragments or disk material is more easily accomplished through a hemilaminectomy. If the compressive mass cannot be adequately removed by hemilaminectomy, bilateral hemilaminectomies can be performed. Surgical stabilization should be provided following laminectomy to compensate for lost stability, even in patients with relatively stable injuries.

Several techniques are available for the stabilization of spinal injuries. The choice of technique depends on the nature and location of the injury, the size of the patient, and the degree of instability. The precise indications for each technique have not been defined, and the choice is often a matter of individual preference. Advantages and disadvantages of the commonly used techniques are described below.

Dorsal spinous process plating. Both metal (Auburn Spinal Plate, Richards Manufacturing Co., Memphis, TN) and plastic (Lubra Plate, Lubra Co., Fort Collins, CO) plates are available for stabilization using the dorsal spinous processes. The metal plates are placed on either side of the dorsal spinous processes and are connected by bolts that run through the processes. Two pro-cesses on either side of the fracture are included. The plastic plates are applied similarly, but are designed to "sandwich" the dorsal spinous processes by placing the bolts between rather than through the processes (Fig. 11-8). Three or four processes on either side of the injury are included. Whereas the metal plates are completely rigid, the plastic plates permit bending laterally.

Dorsal spinous process plating is used only for injuries involving the thoracic or lumbar spine. The plates are rapidly and easily applied, and can be combined with vertebral body plates or vertebral body cross pinning to improve stability.[60] The plates are not applicable if the dorsal spinous processes are fractured, and they may be difficult to apply securely in the lower thoracic and lower lumbar regions, where the dorsal spinous processes are small. They may not provide adequate stabilization of vertebral-body compression fractures, which usually require stabilization of the ventral compartment. Postoperative fracture of the dorsal spinous processes has been observed occasionally, but it is not caused by compromise of vascular supply to the processes by the plates.[61]

Vertebral-body plating. Vertebral-body plates are applied to the dorsolateral aspects of the vertebral bodies immediately dorsal to the transverse processes (Fig. 11-9). They are used for thoracic and cranial lumbar fractures and luxations, and are an extremely stable means of fixation.[60] The approach is the same as that used for hemilaminectomy, and the plates can easily be applied beneath a hemilaminectomy site. Spinal nerves emerging from the intervertebral foramina in the region are severed to prevent entrapment by the

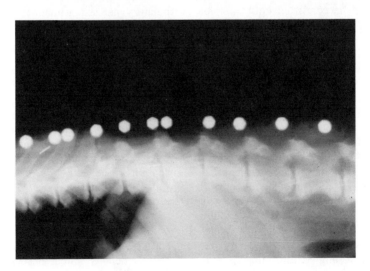

Fig. 11-8.. Postoperative lateral radiograph of the dog shown in Fig. 11-6, demonstrating the use of plastic dorsal spinous plates. Bolts are placed between the dorsal spinous processes to "sandwich" the processes between the plates.

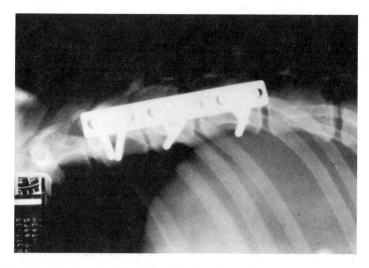

Fig. 11-9. Postoperative lateral radiograph of the dog shown in Fig. 11-5, demonstrating the use of vertebral-body plates. Vertebral-body plates are often used to repair compression fractures because they provide stabilization of the ventral compartment.

plate. In vertebral-body compression fractures, the plates can be used to span the fracture site, with screws placed in the vertebral bodies cranial and caudal to the lesion. The plates can be difficult to apply in the thoracic region without disarticulation or removal of the costovertebral junctions and cannot be applied caudally to L3 because this would require severing spinal nerves contributing to the lumbosacral plexus.

Pins and methylmethacrylate. In this technique, two or more pins are driven perpendicularly into the vertebral bodies cranial and caudal to the fracture or luxation, and the ends of the pins are covered with methylmethacrylate bone cement.[62] This is an extremely versatile technique that may be used in any area of the spine and in patients of any size. A ventral approach is used in the cervical spine, and a dorsal approach in the thoracic or lumbar spine. Fractures of the axis can be very rigidly stabilized with this technique[63] (Fig. 11-10), and it is applicable in the caudal lumbar region, where the lumbosacral plexus and small dorsal spinous processes limit the use of other techniques. It is also useful in the thoracic region, because disarticulation of the costovertebral junctions is not necessary. The technique is easily modified to allow repair of various types of injuries; for example, vertebral-body compression fractures may be repaired by spanning the damaged vertebra. Uncommon complications include wound infection and pin migration.[62]

Dorsal spinous process "stapling." Dorsal spinous process "stapling" is accomplished by secur-

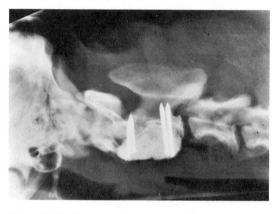

Fig. 11-10. Postoperative lateral radiographs of the dog shown in Fig. 11-4, demonstrating the use of pins and methylmethacrylate. The pins are placed at an angle to avoid the spinal canal.

ing a pin to two dorsal spinous processes cranial to the lesion and two processes caudal to the lesion.[64] The ends of the pin are bent to pass through the most cranial and caudal processes, and the intervening processes are secured to the pin with orthopedic wire. This technique provides adequate stabilization of thoracic and lumbar injuries in small dogs and cats.[56,57,64] Fractures or luxations in larger animals may be repaired with a modification of the technique in which two or more pins are used.[65]

Vertebral-body pinning. Thoracic and lumbar fractures and luxations may be repaired by placing cross pins through adjacent vertebral bodies. This technique is most useful for luxations and epiphyseal fractures, because the vertebral bodies are not damaged in these injuries. It is probably the weakest of the fixation techniques,[60] and it is generally used only when other methods are not applicable. The presence of the ribs in the thoracic region limits this technique to the lumbar spine.

Lumbosacral fracture-luxations

Lumbosacral injuries are generally difficult to repair using the techniques described above because of the extremely small dorsal spinous processes in the region, the presence of the lumbosacral plexus, and the presence of the ilial wings, which severely limit lateral exposure. A common fixation technique is the use of a transilial pin to prevent cranioventral displacement of the caudal segment. The pin is placed through the wings of the ilium and dorsocaudal to the base of the dorsal spinous process of L7 (Fig. 11-11). This technique can be combined with dorsal spinous process plating[56] or spinal "stapling"[65] to increase the stability of the repair.

Postoperative care

Postoperative care of patients with spinal injuries is very similar to that described in the section on intervertebral disk disease. These patients should be very strictly confined until healing is complete. Neurologic status should be closely monitored. Radiographs are usually obtained at approximately 1 and 2 months postoperatively to ascertain that healing is progressing and that the implants are stable.

Prognosis

The prognosis for patients with spinal trauma depends on the severity and duration of neurologic

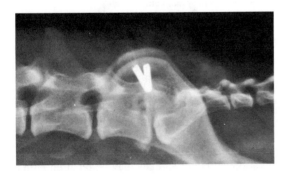

Fig. 11-11. Postoperative lateral and dorsoventral radiographs of the dog shown in Fig. 11-7, demonstrating the use of a transilial pin. The pin prevents cranioventral displacement of the caudal segment.

deficits prior to treatment. While clinical studies of large numbers of patients have not been conducted, the prognosis for spinal trauma is usually assumed to be similar to that for other conditions causing acute spinal cord compression. Any animal that retains voluntary motor ability has a good chance for a full recovery. Patients that have lost deep pain perception have an extremely guarded prognosis, particularly if marked displacement of spinal segments is demonstrated radiographically. Euthanasia should be strongly considered for these animals.

EMERGENCY FRACTURE MANAGEMENT

A fracture is not life threatening, and the overall status and subsequent stabilization of the patient is paramount (Chapter 10). This discussion is limited to the appendicular skeleton and the appropriate handling of the fractured part in order to optimize a favorable outcome and avoid predictable complications. The goal of fracture management is to avoid "functional limb failure": fracture disease (muscle atrophy, tissue adhesions, joint stiffness, osteoporosis), infection, and delayed union or nonunion, with the possible end result of loss of limb function and amputation.

First aid

First aid provided by owners or bystanders is an important, but overlooked area of patient treatment. First aid administration "at the scene" (local wound management, splinting of fractures, and expedient transport to the appropriate medical facility) has significantly decreased both morbidity and mortality in humans.[66] Similar results would be expected in animals. An injured pet, however, is often frightened, painful, and aggressive. Appropriate measures (muzzle) should be undertaken to ensure owner safety prior to first aid administration.

First aid for open wounds and fractures involves control of bleeding, prevention of further contamination, immobilization of the part, and keeping the patient quiet.[66,67] Hemorrhage is best controlled by direct pressure to the wounds with clean materials (avoid cotton or materials that "shed" fibers). Tourniquets should be avoided. Foreign material on the surface of the wound should be removed; however, removal of embedded particles may cause severe bleeding or further damage nerves and muscles and thus is not recommended. Immobilizing the fractured part will help prevent further injury. Splinting the affected part may be easily performed with a number of objects, such as magazines, the folded side of a cardboard box, a large stick, or a pillow.

Primary survey

Following presentation of the animal to the hospital, the overall hemodynamic status of the patient is assessed and any abnormalities appropriately treated. A complete musculoskeletal and neurologic examination is performed. A single broken bone may be obvious; however, other musculoskeletal and neurologic injuries must not be overlooked. A simple and rapid assessment for other musculoskeletal and neurologic injuries can be made by determining the ambulatory status of the animal. Care needs to be exercised in handling and supporting the patient; providing stable and secure footing (carpet) is usually sufficient. Three-legged ambulation is expected with a single fracture. Evaluation of the involved limb includes assessment of any wounds (see below), assessment of the soft-tissue (crush) injury, and evaluation of neurologic and vascular compromise. These latter parameters are difficult to assess. Abnormalities of motor function may simply reflect the mechanical situation. Crude estimations of neurologic function can be made by determining presence or absence of pain sensation in the corresponding dermatomes. Warmth of the digits or active capillary bleeding from a cut nail bed may provide information concerning the arterial blood supply. Swelling and edema of the limb may reflect venous and lymphatic obstruction.

A new sterile dressing is applied to the wound following removal of any temporary bandage. The wound should remain covered in the hospital environment. This procedure decreases the risk of bacterial contamination and hospital-acquired infection.[66-69] Further wound treatment is undertaken following patient stabilization (see below).

The basic premise of fracture management in the emergency patient is immobilization of the limb to prevent further injury and the appropriate treatment of open wounds. With rare exception, definitive repair is not undertaken as an emergency procedure. Immediate repair should be considered only in certain open (Grade 3) fractures. In this instance, immobilization of the fracture fragments and proper soft-tissue management (not perfect anatomic realignment) are the primary goals. This immediate intervention is considered only when the patient is physiologically uncompromised. In these cases, the clinician must delicately balance delayed intervention with the possibility of patient death with early intervention versus infection, loss of limb function, or loss of limb.

Sedation

Many patients are inappropriately "sedated" with various barbiturates or phenothiazine tranquilizers, shortly following presentation, for the purpose of keeping the patient quiet or to obtain radiographs of the fracture. The fracture patient has sustained major trauma and although many animals may appear "healthy" at the time of presentation, the administration of cardiovascular or respiratory depressant drugs within hours of the injury may severely compromise and destabilize the patient. Radiographs of the fracture are rarely, if ever, necessary for the initial evaluation. Chemical restraint should be used only in the unmanageable patient in order to prevent self-induced injury.

If sedation is necessary, hypotensive agents (phenothiazine tranquilizers or barbiturates) are avoided. Narcotics are recommended, as their effects may be reversed and their cardiovascular and respiratory depressant properties are less pronounced. General anesthesia is contraindicated until complete evaluation (thorough physical examination, complete blood count, serum biochemical profile, urinalysis, thoracic and abdominal radiographs) and stabilization of the animal has been accomplished.

Recommendations for analgesic use may be found in Chapter 12.

Splints—introduction

Temporary immobilization of the fracture is undertaken to prevent motion of the bone fragments that could damage muscles, nerves, and blood vessels, or cause skin laceration (allowing a closed fracture to become open); to control excessive bleeding; and to minimize pain.[66,70] Fractures distal to the elbow and stifle joints are most amenable to temporary immobilization due to the anatomic configuration of the limbs. These fractures also have a greater likelihood of causing additional soft-tissue trauma if not properly immobilized. Fractures proximal to the elbow and stifle joints may be managed with cage rest because greater soft-tissue covering (muscle) is present, the animal can successfully guard these injuries, and proper immobilization is difficult to apply to these areas.

Splints—specific applications

Soft-tissue wounds need to be appropriately treated before applying any type of splint. If definitive management of the wound cannot be performed due to patient compromise, the hair surrounding the wound should be clipped and the wound washed and then covered with a nonadherent dressing.[67-69]

***Robert Jones bandages*[70] (Fig. 11-12).** Robert Jones bandages are heavily padded support bandages for immobilization of fractures below the

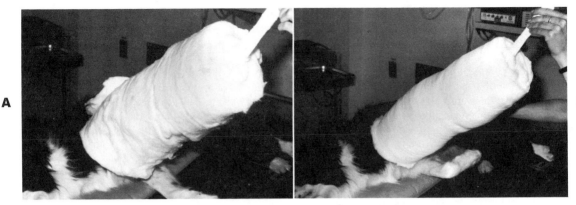

Fig. 11-12 A, Robert Jones bandage. Stirrups (supporting and anchoring distal limb) and roll cotton have been applied. Note the bulkiness and size of bandage before the cotton is compressed. **B,** Cotton layer has been compressed (Fig. 11-12, *A*) by application of the first layer of outer wrap (gauze roll). The remaining layers of the bandage are subsequently applied (Fig. 11-13).

stifle and elbow joints. These bandages are comfortable, soft, compressive bandages that cover the wound, control edema and hemorrhage, and immobilize the fracture. Approximately 2 lb of cotton are used for a 20- to 25-kg animal. The need for "bulkiness" of this bandage cannot be overemphasized. This "bulkiness" is required to avoid ischemia, as the outer layers are compressed tightly to achieve fracture immobilization and support. This bandage is ideal for radial-ulnar and tibial-fibular fractures due to its ability to provide comfortable support, prevent additional soft-tissue trauma in areas of minimal soft-tissue coverage, and due to the ease of its application.

To apply the bandage, two 1-in.-wide tape strips ("stirrups") are applied either on the cranial and caudal or medial and lateral surface of the metacarpal-metatarsal region and extended approximately 6 in. beyond the digits. A cotton roll is applied to the limb. The roll is split lengthwise (providing two 6-in.-wide rolls instead of a single 12-in.-wide roll) to allow greater ease of application. The cotton is applied distally (leaving P_3 of digits III and IV exposed) to proximally (axillary-inguinal area). The bandage is applied snugly and as evenly as possible, attempting to maintain a uniform cylindrical shape. Following application of sufficient quantity of cotton, conforming gauze roll (Kling, Johnson & Johnson, New Brunswick, NJ) (6 in.) is secured around the cotton and wrapped as tightly as possible from distal to proximal. The tape "stirrups" are folded back and secured to the gauze. Finally, an elastic (Vetrap, Animal Care Products/3M, St. Paul, MN) or adhesive elastic (Elasticon, Johnson & Johnson,

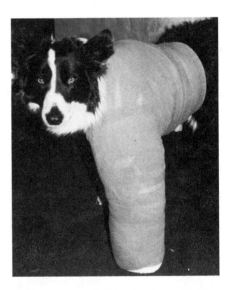

Fig. 11-13. Completed Spica bandage. Similar to the Robert Jones bandage (Fig. 11-12) but the padding has been carried proximally encircling the trunk. Additional rigid support has been added (fiberglass splint).

New Brunswick, NJ) wrap is applied covering the entire bandage (leaving the central two digits exposed for evaluation).

Spica splint[70] (Fig. 11-13). A Spica splint is a proximal extension of the Robert Jones bandage over the shoulder or hip joint. This bandage is additionally supported with a lateral splint (aluminum rod, plaster, fiberglass). This bandage effectively immobilizes the shoulder or hip joints and allows stabilization of femoral or humeral fractures. This splint is a difficult bandage to apply,

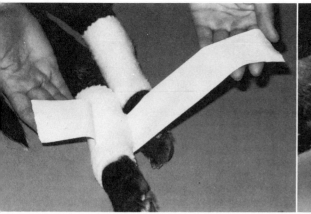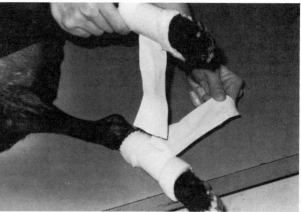

B

Fig. 11-14.. **A,** Hobbles. Cast padding (2 to 3 layers) encircles the metatarsal bones and 2-in. tape is applied without fully encircling the limb. (Taped right limb shown.) **B,** The same procedure is repeated on the left limb (direction of adhesive reversed), and both tapes are secured to each other.

especially in the recumbent animal, as the bandage encircles the trunk. Hobbles are easier to apply and may be adequate for immobilization of fractures of the long bones of the upper extremities. If the animal is quiet and appropriately "guards" the fractured part, cage rest may be sufficient.

Hobbles (Fig. 11-14). This bandage secures either the front or rear limbs a maximum distance apart to prevent "splaying" or "splits." It is used for proximal limb fractures or pelvic fractures in animals not inclined to rest quietly.

To apply this bandage, the metacarpal-metatarsal area is encircled with two to three layers of cast padding. Tape (2 in. wide) is subsequently applied, adhering to itself medial to both limbs (and not encircling the metacarpal-metatarsal bones). The two tapes are then fixed together the maximum distance desired (generally the width of the animal's torso).

Open fractures—emergency management

Open fractures are a special case requiring the additional considerations of appropriate wound management. This discussion centers on a rational and practical approach to the fracture patient with an open wound. (See Chapters 16 and 31 for specific comments on open wound management and debridement). All open fractures are considered to be contaminated. The degree of contamination and soft-tissue injury surrounding the fracture form the basis for the classification and treatment rationale for open fractures (see the following boxes).

The goal in treating open fractures is the prevention of osteomyelitis. This goal may be ac-

---

**OPEN FRACTURE
CLASSIFICATION[69,71,72]**

Grade 1   A small wound with minimal soft-tissue trauma, without obvious contamination, and no skin loss. The wound has occurred from within (the fracture fragment has penetrated the skin and has usually returned to the depth of the wound).

Grade 2   A wound inflicted from the exterior with moderate contusion of skin (minimal skin loss), underlying subcutaneous tissue and muscle, and bone may be exposed or lost (the degree of soft-tissue contamination may vary from mild to severe)

Grade 3   A large to massive wound due to large external forces with extensive skin, muscle, and possibly neurovascular damage. There is obvious skin loss, obvious gross contamination of bone and soft tissues, exposed bone, and usually bone loss.

---

complished by adhering to the following basic principles: avoidance of additional wound contamination, appropriate soft-tissue management (debridement) to reduce the possibility of infection, and stabilization of the fracture in a manner that allows continued treatment of the soft tissues.[68,69,71-74] Treatment of the soft tissues in addition to appropriate skeletal fixation is paramount: preservation of blood supply is as important as fracture stabilization to successful fracture healing. Antibiotics are not a substitute for proper wound management, as they only aid host defense

---

OPEN FRACTURE TREATMENT[68,69,75]

Grade 1   General cleansing of the wound and temporary limb immobilization is performed. Treatment is similar to closed fractures. Antibiotics are not generally administered, although perioperative prophylaxis is considered. Bacterial cultures and sensitivities (aerobic and anaerobic) may be obtained at surgery. Culturing the wound tract often yields disappointing and unreliable results. Definitive fracture management is performed following stabilization of the animal.

Grade 2   General cleansing of the wound with "superficial" debridement (removal of gross contamination) under aseptic conditions in wound areas of easy accessibility (no deep probing, as the animal is awake and not generally sedated) is recommended. Bacterial cultures from within the wound are obtained, and empirical antibiotic therapy (cephalothin sodium [Keflin, Eli Lilly, Indianapolis, IN] 40 mg/kg subcutaneously every 8 hours) is initiated pending culture results. Wet-to-dry gauze dressings are applied and changed daily. Temporary limb immobilization is performed followed by definitive fracture management and further debridement following stabilization of the animal. Primary skin closure is considered. If any question exists regarding the degree of contamination or viability of the soft tissues, the wound is left open and wet-to-dry dressings continue to be used. Secondary closure is considered following establishment of a healthy granulation-tissue bed.

Grade 3   General cleansing of the wound is performed: "superficial" debridement as in Grade 2 cases, immediately followed by a more aggressive "deep" debridement, provided the animal can be safely sedated/anesthetized. The "deep" debridement is performed in the operating room under aseptic conditions. Bacterial cultures are obtained and empirical antibiotic therapy instituted. Definitive fracture repair is performed. Reculturing the wound is considered at the termination of the surgical procedure. The wound is left open to heal secondarily, and wet-to-dry bandage changes are continued. An autogenous cancellous graft to fill areas of bony defects is considered once a healthy granulation-tissue bed has formed, provided soft-tissue coverage of the graft can be safely performed. Secondary wound closure may be considered; however, these wounds are generally left to heal by second intention.

---

mechanisms. General treatment guidelines are based on the fracture classification (see box above).

The need for copious lavage (>10 L) and adequate debridement of Grade 2 and Grade 3 open fractures cannot be overemphasized.[68,69,73,74] Isotonic solutions are preferred for use in lavage; however, a practical alternative in early wound debridement is to use tap water from a showerhead nozzle. The primary objective is removal of foreign material and dilution of bacteria in the wound. The potential cytotoxic effects of using hypotonic solution (tap water) in appropriate quantities is weighed against insufficient lavage using physiologic solution. All devitalized tissue and dirt must be removed. This is a slow, tedious, and time-consuming process when performed properly. The Grade 3 open fracture is a special case and is the only instance in which "emergency" surgery is considered. This consideration is warranted due to the high probability of complications (osteomyelitis, fracture disease) and the likelihood of a functional failure with delayed fracture repair. Immediate intervention lessens the chance for these possibilities, but the

prognosis still remains guarded. Anesthesia and surgery shortly after admission in these individuals must be used judiciously as patient death may be the end result of inappropriate intervention.

Numerous forms of fracture stabilization have been utilized for reduction of open fractures. It is important to note that fractures will heal in the presence of infection if properly (rigidly) stabilized.[71,72] A main objective is preservation of the fragile capillary network (granulation tissue) that is forming during the healing process. Intramedullary pins can be used to repair open fractures; however, it has been stated that this method will spread contamination into the medullary canal.[76] Substantiation that this complication has actually occurred is currently lacking. Bone plating provides excellent long-term stability; however, plating requires larger surgical exposures and longer duration of surgery. These factors increase the potential for wound contamination and contribute to further soft-tissue devitalization due to increased dissection.[76]

External skeletal fixation (Kirschner-Ehmer) has many advantages.[69,76] The foremost advantage is avoidance of the traumatized area in applying the fixation. Surgical trauma and potential devascularization are avoided at the wound/fracture site. Surgery within the wound margins is confined to care of the soft tissues (debridement). External skeletal fixation also requires minimal application time and allows continued postoperative access to all areas of the wound. This form of fixation is often considered "ideal" for Grade 3 open fractures. With this method, "perfect" anatomical alignment/reduction of the fracture need not be attained. Skeletal stability is maintained, and preservation of the soft-tissue structures ensures optimal conditions for fracture healing.

REFERENCES

1. Wingfield WE. The stomach. In Bojrab MJ, ed. Pathophysiology in Small Animal Surgery. Philadelphia: Lea & Febiger, 1981;101-111.
2. Van Kruiningen HJ, Wojan LD, Stake PE, Lord PF. The influence of diet and feeding frequency on gastric function in the dog. J Am Anim Hosp Assoc 1987;23:145-153.
3. Leib MS, Wingfield WE, Twedt DC, Bottoms GD. Plasma gastrin immunoreactivity in dogs with acute gastric dilatation-volvulus. J Am Vet Med Assoc 1984;185:205-208.
4. Hall JA, Twedt DC. Comparative study of lower esophageal sphincter pressure and endogenous gastrin activity in normal dogs and dogs with prior gastric dilatation-volvulus syndromes (Abstract). Proc Am Coll Vet Int Med 1986;4(2):14-57.
5. Van Sluijs FJ, Happe RP. Surgical diseases of the stomach. In Slatter DH, ed. Textbook of Small Animal Surgery. Philadelphia: WB Saunders, 1985;685-717.
6. Orton EC, Muir WW. Hemodynamics during experimental gastric dilation-volvulus in dogs. J Vet Res 1983;44:1512-1515.
7. Wingfield WE, Twedt DC, Moore RW, et al. Acid-base and electrolyte values in dogs with acute gastric dilatation-volvulus. J Am Vet Med Assoc 1982;180:1070-1072.
8. Muir WW. Acid-base and electrolyte disturbances in dogs with gastric dilatation-volvulus. J Am Vet Med Assoc 1982;181:229-232.
9. Muir WW. Gastric dilatation-volvulus in the dog, with emphasis on cardiac arrhythmias. J Am Vet Med Assoc 1982;180:739-742.
10. Harris AS. Delayed development of ventricular ectopic rhythms following experimental coronary occlusion. Circulation 1950;1:1316-1328.
11. Muir WW, Weisbrode SE. Myocardial ischemia in dogs with gastric dilatation-volvulus. J Am Vet Med Assoc 1982;181:363-366.
12. Orton EC, Muir WW. Isovolumetric indices and humoral cardioactive substance bioassay during clinical and experimentally induced gastric dilatation-volvulus in dogs. J Vet Res 1983;44:1516-1520.
13. Feldman BF. Disseminated intravascular coagulation. Compend Contin Educ Prac Vet 1981;3:46-54.
14. Leib MS, Blass LE. Acute gastric dilatation in the dog: Various clinical presentations. Compend Contin Educ Prac Vet 1984;6:707-712.
15. Leib MS, Monroe WE, Martin RA. Suspected chronic gastric volvulus in a dog with normal gastric emptying of liquids. J Am Vet Med Assoc 1987;191:699-700.
16. Hathcock JR. Radiographic view of choice for the diagnosis of gastric volvulus: the right lateral recumbent view. J Am Anim Hosp Assoc 1984;20:967-969.
17. Lantz GC, Bottoms GD, Carlton WW, Newman S, Cantwell HD. The effect of 360° gastric volvulus on the blood supply of the nondistended normal dog stomach. J Vet Surg 1984;13:189-195.
18. Bojrab MJ, ed. Current Techniques in Small Animal Surgery, 2nd ed. Philadelphia: Lea & Febiger, 1983.
19. Matthiesen DT. Partial gastrectomy as treatment of gastric volvulus: Results in 30 dogs. J Vet Surg 1985;14:185-193.
20. Wheaton LG, Tacker HL, Caldwell S. Intravenous fluorescein as an indicator of gastric viability in gastric dilatation-volvulus. J Am Anim Hosp Assoc 1986;22:197-204.
21. Flanders JA, Harvey HJ. Results of tube gastrostomy as treatment for gastric volvulus in the dog. J Am Vet Med Assoc 1984;185:74-77.
22. Johnson RG, Barrus J, Greene RW. Gastric dilatation-volvulus: recurrence rate following tube gastrostomy. J Am Anim Hosp Assoc 1984;20:33-37.
23. Delaney HM, Carnevale N, Garvey JW, Moss CM. Postoperative nutritional support using needle catheter feeding jejunostomy. Ann Surg 1977;186:165-170.
24. Levine SH, Caywood DD. Biomechanical evaluation of gastropexy techniques in the dog. J Vet Surg 1983;12:166-169.
25. MacCoy DM, Sykes GP, Hoffer RE, Harvey HJ. A gastropexy technique for permanent fixation of the pyloric antrum. J Am Anim Hosp Assoc 1982;18:763-768.
26. Fallah AM, Lumb WV, Nelson AW, Frandson RD, Withrow SJ. Circumcostal gastropexy in the dog: a preliminary study. J Vet Surg 1982;11:9-12.
27. Woolfson JM, Kostolich M. Circumcostal gastropexy: clinical use of the technique in 34 dogs with gastric dilatation-volvulus. J Am Anim Hosp Assoc 1986;22:825-830.
28. Leib MS, Konde LJ, Wingfield WE, Twedt DC. Circumcostal gastropexy for preventing recurrence of gastric dilatation-volvulus in the dog: an evaluation of 30 cases. J Am Vet Med Assoc 1985;187:245-248.
29. Fox SM, McCoy CP, Cooper RC, Baine JC. Circumcostal gastropexy versus tube gastrostomy: histological comparison of gastropexy adhesions. J Am Anim Hosp Assoc 1988;24:273-279.
30. Whitney WO, Scavelli TD, Matthiesen DT, Burk RL. Belt-loop gastropexy: technique and surgical results in 20 dogs. J Am Anim Hosp Assoc 1989;25:75-83.
31. Crowe DT. Enteral nutrition for critically ill or injured patients, part III. Compend Contin Educ Pract Vet 1986;8:826-836.
32. Seim HB, Prata RG. Ventral decompression for the treatment of cervical disc disease in the dog: a review of 54 cases. J Am Anim Hosp Assoc 1982;18:233-240.
33. Walker TL, Betts CW. Intervertebral disc disease. In Slatter DH, ed. Textbook of Small Animal Surgery. Philadelphia: WB Saunders, 1985;685-717.
34. Horlein BF. Intervertebral discs. In Hoerlein BF, ed. Canine neurology: Diagnosis and treatment. 3rd ed. Philadelphia: WB Saunders, 1978;470-560.
35. Hansen HJ. A pathologic-anatomical study on disc degeneration in dogs. Acta Orthop Scand 1952;Suppl II.
36. Gage ED. Incidence of clinical disc disease in the dog. J Am Anim Hosp Assoc 1975;11:135.
37. Priester WA. Canine intervertebral disc disease-occurrence by age, breed, and sex among 8,117 cases. Theriogenology 1976;6:293.
38. DeLahunta A. Veterinary Neuroanatomy and Clinical Neurology, 2nd ed. Philadelphia: WB Saunders, 1983.

39. Brown NO, Helphrey ML, Prata RG. Thoracolumbar disc disease in the dog: a retrospective analysis of 187 cases. J Am Anim Hosp Assoc 1977;13:665-672.
40. Trotter EJ. Thoracolumbar disc disease. In Bojrab MH, ed. Current Techniques in Small Animal Surgery, 2nd ed. Philadelphia: Lea & Febiger, 1983;562-574.
41. Bartels JE. Intervertebral disc disease. In Thrall DE, ed. Textbook of Veterinary Diagnostic Radiology. Philadelphia: WB Saunders, 1983;51-56.
42. Adams WM, Stowater JL. Complications of metrizamide myelography in the dog: a summary of 107 case histories. J Vet Radiol 1981;22:27-34.
43. Prata RG. Neurosurgical treatment of thoracolumbar disks: the rationale and value of laminectomy with concomitant disk removal. J Am Anim Hosp Assoc 1981; 17:17-26.
44. Berg RJ. Pathophysiology and medical management of acute spinal cord injury. Compend Contin Educ Pract Vet 1985;7:646-654.
45. Doppman JL, Girton M. Angiographic study of the effect of laminectomy in the presence of acute anterior epidural masses. J Neurosurg 1976;45(2):195-202.
46. Patterson RH, Arbit E. A surgical approach through the pedicle to protruded thoracic discs. J Neurosurg 1978; 48:768.
47. Flo GL, Brinker WO. Lateral fenestration of thoracolumbar discs. J Am Anim Hosp Assoc 1975;11:619.
48. Yturraspe DH, Lumb WV. A dorsolateral muscle-splitting approach for thoracolumbar disk fenestration in the dog. J Am Vet Med Assoc 1973;162:1037.
49. Bojrab MJ. Prophylactic thoracolumbar disk fenestration. In Current Techniques in Small Animal Surgery, 2nd ed. Philadelphia: Lea and Febiger, 1983;575-576.
50. Levine SH, Caywood DD. Recurrence of neurologic deficits in dogs treated for thoracolumbar disk disease. J Am Anim Hosp Assoc 1984;20:899-894.
51. Rosin AH, Ross L. Diagnosis and pharmacological management of disorders of urinary continence in the dog. Compend Contin Educ Prac Vet 1981;3:601-608.
52. Moore RW, Withrow SJ. Gastrointestinal hemorrhage and pancreatitis associated with intervertebral disk disease in the dog. J Am Vet Med Assoc 1982;180:1443-1447.
53. Toombs JP, Collins LG, Graves GM, et al. Colonic perforation in corticosteroid treated dogs. J Am Vet Med Assoc 1986;188:145-150.
54. Tangner CH. Physical therapy in small animal patients: basic principles and application. Compend Contin Educ Prac Vet 1984;6:933-936.
55. Gambardella PC. Dorsal decompressive laminectomy for treatment of thoracolumbar disc disease in dogs: a retrospective study of 98 cases. J Vet Surg 1980;1:24-26.
56. Matthieson DT. Thoracolumbar spinal fractures/luxations: surgical management. Compend Contin Educ Prac Vet 1983;5:867-878.
57. Walker TL, Tomlinson J, Sorjonen D, Kornegay JN. Diseases of the spinal column. In Slatter DH, ed. Textbook of Small Animal Surgery. Philadelphia: WB Saunders, 1985;1367-1395.

58. Stone EA, Betts CW, Chambers JN. Cervical fractures in the dog: a literature and case review. J Am Anim Hosp Assoc 1979;15:463.
59. DeLahunta A. Small animal spinal cord disease. In Veterinary Neuroanatomy and Clinical Neurology, 2nd ed. Philadelphia: WB Saunders, 1983;175-214.
60. Walter MC, Smith GK, Newton CD. Canine lumbar spinal internal fixation techniques: A comparative biomechanical study. J Vet Surg 1986;15:191-198.
61. Rischen CG, Wilson JW, Swain CA. Effect of application of polyvinilidine plates on the dorsal spinous processes of dogs. J Vet Surg 1987;16:294-298.
62. Blass CE, Seim HB. Spinal fixation in dogs using Steinmann pins and methylmethacrylate. J Vet Surg 1984; 13:203-210.
63. Blass CE, Waldron DR, van Ee RT. Cervical stabilization in three dogs using Steinmann pins and methylmethacrylate. J Am Anim Hosp Assoc 1988;24:61-68.
64. Gage ED. Surgical repair of spinal fractures in small breeds. Vet Med Small Anim Clin 1971;66:1095-1101.
65. McAnulty JF, Lenehan TM, Maletz LM. Modified segmental spinal instrumentation in repair of spinal fractures and luxations in dogs. Vet Surg 1986;15:143-149.
66. The Committee on Injuries, American Academy of Orthopedic Surgeons. Emergency Care and Transportation of the Sick and Injured. Menasha, WI: George Banta, 1971.
67. Nunamaker DM. Treatment of open fractures in small animals. Compend Contin Educ Pract Vet 1979;1:66-74.
68. Aron DN. Management of open musculoskeletal injuries. Semin Vet Med Surg Small Anim 1988;3:290-301.
69. Swaim SF, Pope ER Early management of limb degloving injuries. Semin Vet Med Surg Small Anim 1988; 3:274-281.
70. Arnoczky SP, Blass CE, McCoy L: External coaptation and bandaging. In Slatter DH, ed. Textbook of Small Animal Surgery. Philadelphia: WB Saunders, 1985;1988-2003.
71. Muller ME, Allgower M, Schneider R, et al. Manual of Internal Fixation: Techniques Recommended by the A-O group, 2nd ed. Berlin: Springer-Verlag, 1979.
72. Brinker WO, Hohn RB, Prieur WD. Manual of Internal Fixation in Small Animals. Berlin: Springer-Verlag, 1984.
73. Gustilo RB, Anderson JR. Prevention of infection in the treatment of one thousand and twenty-five open fractures of long bones. Retrospective and prospective analysis. J Bone Joint Surg [Am] 1976;58:453-458.
74. Gustilo RB, Mendoza RM, Williams DN. Problem in the management of type III (severe) open fractures: a new classification of type III open fractures. J Trauma 1984; 24:742-746.
75. Swaim SF, Wilhaf D. The physic, physiology, and chemistry of bandaging open wounds. Compend Contin Educ Pract Vet 1985;7:146-156.
76. Etter C, Burri C, Claes HL, et al. Treatment by external fixation of open fractures associated with severe soft tissue damage of the leg: biomechanical principles and clinical experience. Clin Orthop Relat Res 1983;178:80-88.

12 Preoperative and Postoperative Management of the Emergency Surgical Patient

Marc R. Raffe

PREOPERATIVE CONSIDERATIONS FOR THE CRITICAL PATIENT

Preoperative evaluation of the critical patient requires rapid, accurate assessment of systemic abnormalities that have an impact on patient homeostasis during anesthesia. Physical examination should be carried out in a rapid, organized manner so that identification of all problems can be completed in a brief period. Diagnostic data such as clinical laboratory and radiographic evaluation will aid in confirming clinical impressions. Prioritizing the identified problems into life threatening, primary treatment, and delayed treatment will aid the clinician in focusing on issues that may affect the outcome of the anesthetic procedure. Following identification, the clinician can rank problems based on their potential consequences during anesthesia. The problems that can be managed and stabilized in a reasonable time frame are treated prior to anesthesia; those that require intense support or aggressive correction constitute reason to delay anesthesia. It is important that the clinician objectively evaluate and categorize each problem identified so that accurate treatment and stabilization can occur prior to anesthesia.

Metabolic response to trauma

In the presence of injury, a coordinated physiologic response occurs. Following injury, release of neurohumoral substances, such as adrenocorticotropic hormone, cortisol, catecholamines, glucagon, renin-angiotensin-aldosterone, antidiuretic hormone, endorphins, enkephalins, and somatotropic hormone, stabilize an animal that otherwise would succumb to the primary insult.[1] This fact must be kept in mind when evaluating the patient for anesthesia because many anesthetic drugs will block this neurohumoral response. In an injured patient that has been compensated homeostatically by neurohumoral activation, inhibiting the response during anesthesia may decompensate the patient, resulting in a life-threatening episode.

Cardiovascular response to trauma

Cardiovascular homeostasis is central to the successful outcome of anesthesia in the compromised patient. Cardiovascular insult may be the result of primary cardiac injury, electrical rhythm disturbance (dysrhythmia), suboptimal mechanical activity secondary to electrolyte and acid-base abnormalities, and loss or sequestration of circulating blood volume. All these factors result in reduced tissue perfusion and oxygen delivery to critical organs. The neuroendocrine response described above is integrated with the cardiovascular response.[1] Initially, the cardiovascular response in injured states is vasoconstriction to nonessential regions of the body while preserving blood flow to the brain, heart, and kidney. Heart rate and cardiac output will initially rise, but may be unable to keep up with demand and ultimately may fall below normal levels. If the initial response is inadequate, reduction in cardiovascular performance will occur, stimulating further redistribution of blood to critical organs and evoking extensive compensatory responses to conserve fluid balance. If these compensatory responses are unsuccessful in stabilizing the patient, a cascade of destabilizing responses occurs, culminating in complete cardiovascular collapse and death.

Blood loss or fluid translocation will exacerbate the cycle described above by further reducing perfusion to critical tissues and evoking a global pressor response modulated through baroreceptors in the carotid and aortic bodies. Redistribution of regional blood flow cannot occur in cases with significant blood loss.[1] Only increased extraction of oxygen at the tissue beds maintains homeostasis during acute hypovolemia. Ultimately, this increased extraction may create a substantial oxygen deficit, jeopardizing the animal. In cases of severe blood loss or cardiovascular embarrassment, clinical signs of shock may be noted during initial evaluation. Shock is the culmination of inadequate compensation for reduced cardac output and tissue perfusion. Inadequate circulating fluid volume, coupled with compromised cardiac function, is the main defect that requires treatment prior to anesthesia.

Respiratory response to trauma

Respiratory compromise may result from primary injury to the respiratory tree or in response to systemic disturbances such as shock. The major concern associated with respiratory system injury is inadequate oxygen transfer to the cardiovascular system. Initial examination should include evaluation of the upper respiratory system and lung as well as assessment of the integrity of the thorax. Facial injuries, laryngeal lacerations, and tracheal wounds impair transport of oxygen from the external environment to the lung. These lesions can be life threatening and are managed by establishing a patent airway. Lower respiratory tract injuries associated with the thoracic wall, diaphragm, and pulmonary tissue present a challenge to patient stabilization prior to anesthesia. Once the lesions have been identified, corrective or supportive therapy can be initiated prior to anesthesia. Primary pulmonary injury can easily be overlooked in the initial evaluation period. The time course of anatomic changes noted on radiography is delayed as compared with the physiologic disturbance.[2] For this reason, the patient's respiratory rate and pattern and mucous membrane color should be evaluated during initial examination. Any indication of increased respiratory rate, breathing effort, or cyanosis in the absence of upper airway or thoracic wall injury indicates primary pulmonary injury. In these cases, surgery should be deferred and the patient stabilized for a minimum of 24 hours. An initial evaluation of stable cardiovascular and pulmonary function in a patient with diaphragmatic hernia dictates that corrective surgery should be performed. Decompensation of the hernia produced by further visceral entrapment or herniation is possible if repair is unnecessarily delayed. Thoracic-wall injury can be asymptomatic or life threatening in magnitude. The patient with flail chest represents the most serious class of injury. Stabilization of the flail seg-

ment is important, but requires anesthesia in many cases.

Renal response to trauma

Hypovolemia is associated with trauma in many cases. As a result, the kidney will try to conserve water, thus reducing urine production. Water conservation is modulated by liberation of antidiuretic hormone and activation of renin-angiotensin-aldosterone pathway in response to hypotension. Prerenal azotemia may be associated with hypovolemia and reduced renal perfusion. If long-term hypotension occurs, there is a risk of acute renal failure. As time progresses, cortical ischemia occurs, resulting in "vasomotor nephropathy."[3] This is reversible with therapy, but left untreated, it can produce irreversible renal damage. Myoglobinuria associated with soft-tissue injury may interplay to induce or exacerbate tubular injury.[1] Precipitation of myoglobin in tubules inhibits urine production and contributes to azotemia.

Following resuscitation, fluid mobilization from injured tissues occurs. This redistribution, in conjunction with the intravenous fluids administered during the resuscitation period, may result in "fluid overload syndrome." It is important to monitor urine output and hydration status (skin turgor, body weight, total serum solids) during and following the resuscitation period to guard against this complication.

Gastrointestinal response to trauma

Injury to the gastrointestinal tract and liver can be subtle but life threatening. Hepatic injury is a common feature of trauma. Direct contusion and ischemic damage from poor perfusion are common causes of hepatic injury. Acute injury commonly results in elevation of serum alanine transaminase, alkaline phosphatase, and bilirubin concentrations. The increase in serum enzyme levels occur early after injury and decrease toward normal in 2 to 4 days. Continued elevation in these enzyme levels suggests ongoing injury that may be related to primary disease states.

Gastrointestinal problems following trauma may include ileus, bowel ischemia secondary to hypoperfusion, gastric distention, vomiting, and hemorrhage. Many of these conditions may result in compromised bowel with release of endotoxins and sequestration of water and electrolytes. These factors may contribute to secondary complications represented by shock and endotoxemia.[4] Clinical signs range from subtle (pyrexia, leukophilia) to overt (pyrexia, leukopenia, tachycardia, hyperpnea, injection of mucous membranes, hypoglycemia) depending on the individual case. Identification and correction are recommended prior to anesthesia to reduce morbidity and mortality from anesthesia and surgery.

Nervous system response

Evaluation of mental status, cranial nerve function, symmetry of the face and head, and integrity of senses provides a summary of the overall central nervous system function in the trauma patient. Spinal cord and peripheral nerve integrity can be evaluated by neurologic evaluation with particular reference to integrative functions such as posture, pain, and motor function. Detection of deficits in these parameters can help to localize the level and extent of the lesion, allowing formulation of an anesthetic plan that minimizes potential for exacerbation of any neurologic dysfunction.

Immunologic response

Although immunocompetence cannot be evaluated easily or specifically, one should anticipate that stress and injury induce changes in immune status. Increased morbidity and mortality occur following exposure to infectious agents when an animal is in an immunocompromised state. All traumatized or debilitated animals should be considered at risk for immunoincompetence and supported by appropriate therapy, including nutrition, fluids, acid-base correction, and antimicrobial therapy as indicated.[1]

PREOPERATIVE SUPPORT OF THE CRITICAL PATIENT

Once the systemic disturbances are identified, initial management is directed at stabilizing and treating the causative problems. It is imperative that the patient undergo preoperative stabilization prior to anesthetic drug exposure. Preoperative stabilization is directed at four fundamental goals: support of cardiovascular and pulmonary function, correcting fluid and electrolyte deficits, correcting acid-base disturbances, and support and therapy of secondary organ systems. Without stabilization, increased morbidity and mortality of the critical patient can be expected during the anesthetic period.[5]

Support of cardiopulmonary function is central to a successful anesthetic episode. Circulating fluid volume support by administration of crystalloid, colloid, or blood products is central to stabilization. Inotropic agents may be indicated once circulating volume is stabilized to maintain or restore perfusion to critical tissues. Therapy for shock as outlined in Chapter 14 is important to ensure perfusion. Assurance of upper airway patency and unrestricted airflow is critical prior to anesthesia. If upper airway integrity is in doubt, intervention to ensure patency is mandatory

(Chapters 10 and 25). Abnormalities in chest wall, diaphragm, and pulmonary function must be identified and corrective measures taken to stabilize the patient prior to anesthesia (Chapters 25 and 36).

Electrolyte and acid-base balance should be evaluated and abnormalities noted should be treated prior to anesthesia. These issues are critical to successful treatment of the patient as derangements in those parameters may contribute to cardiovascular compromise or collapse. The parameters that are critical to evaluate are serum potassium and bicarbonate ion concentrations. Generally, the two major disturbances that are encountered are hyperkalemia and metabolic acidosis. Hyperkalemia is noted with many conditions, including massive soft-tissue injury, gastrointestinal disease, and renal disease. If potassium levels exceed plasma levels of 5.5 mEq/L, an increased morbidity and mortality may be noted.[6] In many cases, hyperkalemia is associated with metabolic acidosis, through translocation of potassium into the extracellular compartment in exchange for hydrogen ions. Therapy for acidosis will concurrently reduce the potassium level.

Adequate splanchnic organ function is critical for anesthetic management. Stabilizing hepatic and renal function ensures fluid, electrolyte, and acid-base regulation. Both organ systems are involved in biotransformation and excretion of many anesthetic drugs. Compromise of hepatic or renal function may result in delayed emergence from anesthesia, acid-base and electrolyte abnormalities, and reduced cardiovascular function.[7]

Neurologic injuries should be stabilized prior to anesthesia. Cranial injuries are associated with increased risk based on elevated intracranial pressure and compromised perfusion. Medical management and stabilization should be initiated prior to anesthesia. Spinal and peripheral neurologic injuries are less serious; however, autonomic nervous system volatility reflected in oscillations of heart rate, cardiac rhythm and blood pressure may be noted in the acute phase following trauma.

FORMULATING THE ANESTHETIC PLAN

Once initial evaluation and stabilization has been completed, decisions regarding anesthetic drug selection and support during the perioperative period must be made. Drug selection should be made on the basis of minimizing further impairment in physiologic function. Anesthetic agents whose effects can be pharmacologically reversed are preferred, permitting additional control of the patient in emergency situations. The unstable emergency patient poses significant risk during anesthesia. Acute destabilization can occur in cardiopulmonary, splanchnic organ, and central nervous system function. Important anesthetic considerations during the perioperative period include hypotension, shock, respiratory arrest, cardiac arrest, acute renal failure, elevated intracranial pressure, and autonomic nervous system volatility. Anesthetic agents and techniques that minimize these complications should be selected. For this reason, the use of long-acting tranquilizers and sedative-hypnotics should be avoided in emergency anesthesia protocols. Drug classes that are preferred for general anesthesia include opioids, neuroleptanalgesics, benzodiazepine-class tranquilizers, and inhalant agents. The use of local or regional analgesia may be all that is required to accomplish surgical goals.

The availability of resuscitation drugs and equipment is essential. The most serious complication associated with anesthesia is cardiopulmonary dysfunction. Despite preoperative stabilization, hypotension, shock, respiratory arrest, and total cardiovascular collapse may present formidable challenges during anesthesia. The high incidence of these intraoperative complications dictates that all patients be stabilized prior to anesthesia, that patent airway be provided in all patients, that supplemental oxygen be administered, and that multiple venous accesses be established for fluid and drug administration. To minimize secondary complications associated with splanchnic organ dysfunction, isotonic fluids are routinely administered perioperatively. Correction of acid-base and electrolyte disturbances is continued throughout the perioperative period (Chapter 38). Colloids or blood components are administered as needed (Chapters 34 and 38).

All critical patients are monitored intraoperatively with an electrocardiographic monitor, esophageal stethoscope, and indirect blood pressure (using Doppler or oscillometric principle) monitors. Auscultation can be used to indirectly determine the strength of myocardial contractility by evaluating heart sound intensity. Changes in respiratory rate and pattern, as well as heart rate and pattern can also be determined by observation and auscultation. Bradyarrhythmias may be treated with anticholinergic drugs (atropine) or chronotropic agents (dopamine). Reduced mechanical activity should be treated with inotropic support drugs (dopamine or dobutamine). A portable "crash box" should be available with the critical patient (Chapter 3).

TRANSITION FROM ANESTHESIA TO AN AWAKE CONDITION

Anesthetic recovery should be timed so that it occurs shortly following completion of the surgical procedure. When inhalation anesthesia is used for maintainence of anesthesia, the anesthetic agent concentration is reduced by 25% at the start of wound closure, and progressively reduced until agent is discontinued approximately 5 minutes prior to completion of surgery. The timing is based on considerations for maintaining orotracheal intubation or placing a tracheostomy tube following completion of the surgical procedure and whether recovery should be delayed until external bandaging and splinting is completed. If supplemental oxygen is required in the postoperative period, a nasal oxygen catheter is placed at this time (Chapter 25).

Continuous monitoring is maintained during recovery, as emergence from anesthesia can be associated with significant alterations in physiologic stability. The recovery room should be a quiet, dim, warm area to minimize unnecessary patient stimulation. External rewarming by use of recirculating water pads and radiant heat lamps is provided. The patient is dried so that water evaporation does not cause further reduction in body temperature.

Recovery period

The recovery period is one of the most important times during anesthesia in the critical patient. Transition from anesthesia to awake state is a critical, but frequently overlooked period during anesthesia. Arousal evokes significant physiologic responses that may place the critical patient in jeopardy until recovery is complete. Anesthetic recovery is the reverse of induction in that return of protective neurohumoral reflexes occurs as anesthetic drugs are metabolized or excreted. Until these reflexes are restored, the patient cannot protect itself physiologically from potential sequelae associated with anesthetic recovery. The presence of cardiopulmonary, thermoregulatory, and splanchnic organ compromise may interact to further jeopardize the critical patient. The critical patient requires intense monitoring and observation during the recovery period to prevent further complications. The overall goal of the recovery period is to restabilize the patient from the effects of drugs administered for anesthesia.[8,9]

Cardiovascular complications during recovery. Several complications related to the cardiovascular system can be noted following surgery.[8,9] Blood loss may be associated with the surgical repair and needs to be quickly recognized and stabilized. Clinical signs associated with hemorrhage in the recovering patient are no different from those seen in the awake patient, but progressive blood loss may contribute to delayed or incomplete emergence from anesthesia in addition to causing signs of hypovolemia. Serial monitoring of membrane color, capillary refill time, hematocrit, total solids, heart rate, and blood pressure are parameters that can be used to determine the severity of blood loss.

Blood pressure monitoring is helpful in assessing the overall cardiovascular performance of the patient. Frequently, significant changes in blood pressure occur during the period of emergence from anesthesia. Because of overall activation of the sympathetic nervous system, hypertension is frequently noted as the patient passes through Stage 2 anesthesia. The development of hypertension reflects increased levels of circulating catecholamines, resulting in tachycardia and vasoconstriction. Recognition of pain by the animal may also contribute to this response. Reduced blood oxygen levels may also stimulate the cardiovascular response, producing hypertension.

Hypotension may be noted as a result of residual effects of anesthetic drugs, vasodilatation related to anesthetic drugs, hypovolemia, sepsis, cardiac tamponade, sudden positional changes, acidosis, and hyperkalemia. Therapy is directed at identifying the underlying problem and correcting the imbalance.[8]

High-risk or critical patients should be monitored for dysrhythmias during the recovery period. Potential causes for dysrhythmias include hypoxemia, hypercapnia, acid-base and/or electrolyte disturbance, high levels of circulating catecholamines, and primary cardiac disease. Physical monitoring techniques such as simultaneous auscultation and pulse palpation are valuable in detecting rhythm disturbances. Further characterization can be accomplished with an electrocardiographic monitor. One study indicates that up to 30% of all recovering patients demonstrate transient dysrhythmias.[10]

Changes in heart rate may be noted during recovery. Tachycardia is commonly noted during emergence from anesthesia. Tachycardia can be related to anesthetic drug effects, catecholamines, hypoxemia, hypercarbia, and pain. Tachycardia may be detrimental to the critical patient because it increases myocardial work and oxygen consumption. In the debilitated patient, this may create physiologic instability during recovery. Bradycardia may be a reflection of hypothermia, residual effects of anesthetic drugs, high vagal tone, late-stage hypoxemia or hypercapnia, increased intracranial pressure, or primary cardiac disease. Supportive care related to thermal balance, reversal or compensation for drug effect, and therapy for underlying causes of bradycardia are indicated to reestablish normal heart rate.

Pulmonary complications during recovery.

Respiratory compromise occurs following anesthetic drug administration.[8,9] Drug interaction with regulatory mechanisms, compromise of gas exchange, and postural changes all contribute to reduced ventilation during anesthesia. The recovery period ideally reverses or attenuates the respiratory compromise that exists. However, the critical patient may not be capable of responding to the challenges presented during the restabilization process. Preexisting injury or disease to the head, face, trachea, and chest may produce compromise in regulation of breathing or gas exchange. Upper airway patency must be maintained following extubation and may require tracheostomy to bypass upper airway obstruction. Support of gas exchange by manual or mechanical ventilation may be necessary until the patient can support its own breathing. Supplemental oxygen administration by face mask, nasal catheter, or cricothyroid catheter may be indicated. Adequate respiratory function must be assessed by observing blood gas data, respiratory rate, respiratory effort, and deep breathing or "sigh" capability. Support or control of ventilation must be present until spontaneous ventilation is adequate.

Less frequent, but life-threatening complications must be recognized should they occur during recovery.[9] It is imperative that a clear, unobstructed airway be present during recovery, as the increased respiratory effort associated with airway obstruction is detrimental to the patient. Airway obstruction can follow upper airway surgery, be secondary to massive facial injury, or may be breed-related in brachycephalic dogs and cats. Hypoxemia, pneumothorax, pneumomediastinum, cor pulmonale, pulmonary edema, and death can occur following airway obstruction. Irrespective of cause, treatment is directed at reestablishing a patent airway by clearing upper respiratory structures or introduction of an artificial airway. Aspiration of blood or ingesta can also produce life-threatening consequences. The critical patient may have an incomplete history that can include a meal prior to injury. One must assume this to be a possibility in all patients. Aspiration usually occurs immediately following induction of anesthesia or removal of an artificial airway.[9] Aspiration can produce blockage of the airway, as well as initiating a series of reflexes that reduces gas exchange and affects cardiac performance. Aspiration must be immediately recognized and treated by postural drainage, lavage and suction of the airway (normal saline or Ringer's lactate solution to clear particulate debris), and treatment for secondary pulmonary edema. Bacterial bronchopneumonia can occur secondarily to aspiration, and should this occur, initiation of antibiotic therapy is recommended.[9] Failure to treat aspiration pneumonitis will initiate a series of reflexes that can result in diminished gas exchange, hypoxemia, and death.

Restrictive bandaging around the thorax or abdomen can significantly impair ventilation during recovery. Bandages should be applied such that a hand can be comfortably slid between the bandage and skin surface. Bandage materials that have elastic fibers incorporated within should not be used unless bandage tension is prereleased by unwinding the material and rewinding in a neutral position. This approach avoids the potential for progressive constriction following application.

Central nervous system complications during recovery. Complications following anesthesia may be related to drug interaction in the central nervous system. Delayed emergence from anesthesia is the most common complication encountered. Numerous causes may contribute to this problem, including hypothermia, hypoglycemia, drug metabolism, and shock. Therapy directed at the underlying cause will assist in hastening recovery. Application of warm-water pads and heat lamps should be used during recovery to restore core body temperature. This will increase metabolism and facilitate drug detoxification and elimination. Hypoglycemia is common in young debilitated patients. Blood glucose levels should be monitored and glucose supplemented as needed. The shivering reflex occurs during emergence and acts to generate heat and restore normothermia. Increased glucose and oxygen availability is required during this period to generate heat. Glucose is essential to act as an energy substrate during this time.

Drug pharmacokinetics and metabolism are major issues in emergence from anesthesia. In the critical patient, drug classes with central nervous system effects that can be pharmacologically reversed are preferred. Opioids are the prototype class of drugs that have specific reversal drugs. Antagonists such as yohimbine and derivatives, as well as benzodiazepine antagonists hold promise to reverse the central nervous system effects of alpha$_2$ agonists and benzodiazepine tranquilizers. Their future availability may favor use of these agents in the critical patient.

Pain will be a factor in all critical patients. Supplemental systemic analgesics such as opioids or local nerve blocks to inhibit pain are two commonly used techniques to ameliorate pain. The patient should be frequently assessed for evidence of pain during emergence from anesthesia. If the surgical technique permits, local nerve blocks with long-acting agents such as 0.5% bupivacane are performed prior to recovery. Supplemental an-

Table 12-1 Postoperative analgesia

| Agent | Route | Dosage (mg/kg) | |
		Dog	Cat
Opioids			
Morphine	IM	1-2	0.1-0.5
Oxymorphone	IM, IV	0.05-0.2	0.05-0.1
Butorphanol	IM, SC	0.4-0.8	0.2-0.4
Meperidine	IM	3-5	3-5
Buprenorphine	IM	0.01	0.01
Dissociatives			
Ketamine	IM	1-2	1-2
Nonsteroidal antiinflammatory drugs			
Flunixin meglumine	IV	0.5-1	0.5-1
Adjunct drugs used with above classes*			
Diazepam	IV	0.1	0.1
Midazolam	IM, IV	0.05-0.1	0.05-0.1
Pentobarbital	IV	2-4	2-4
Acepromazine	IV	0.01	0.01

IM = intramuscular; IV = intravenous; SC = subcutaneous.
*These drugs are not analgesics, but provide sedation in combination with analgesic drugs

algesics such as butorphanol, meperidine, oxymorphone, pentazocine, and buprenorphine are considered during recovery (Table 12-1).

Emergence agitation (delirium) is a common complication following anesthesia. Selection of rapidly excreted drugs and the use of anesthetic reversal agents can be accompanied by delirium during recovery. This delirium is the "mirror image" of Stage 2 anesthesia. Usually, gentle restraint and a quiet environment will be all that is necessary until recovery is complete and somnolence returns. If protracted delirum is noted, small doses of tranquilizers to block this behavior may be administered. Use of 0.25 to 1.0 mg acepromazine intravenously or 2.5 mg diazepam intravenously is suggested in these cases.

Splanchnic organ complications during recovery. Splanchnic organ dysfunction is subtle and not easily noted during recovery. The principal complication is renal failure. Oliguria can be associated with many factors, including anesthesia. Urine output should be monitored in critical patients to ensure that 1.0 to 2.0 ml/kg/per hour of urine is produced. To maintain urine production (renal perfusion), polyionic fluid therapy is initiated at 10 ml/kg/per hour during anesthesia and maintained during recovery. If oliguria is noted, furosemide (0.5 mg/kg intravenously) is administered. Furosemide administration may be repeated at 15-minute intervals for a maximum of four times. If oliguria persists, an infusion of dopamine (1 to 3 μg/kg/min) is instituted. This combined therapy usually restores urine production.

Acute hepatitis is rare following anesthesia. The disease does not manifest itself for 24 to 48 hours after emergence from anesthesia, placing it outside the immediate postanesthetic period.

Gastrointestinal motility is impaired for a variable period following anesthesia. Specific therapy to enhance gastrointestinal motility is not administered following anesthesia. If opioids have been selected in the anesthetic protocol, use of opioid antagonists will reverse opioid-induced gut stasis.

Fluid therapy during recovery. Fluid therapy (Ringer's lactate or Hartmann's solution) initiated during the preoperative and intraoperative periods should be continued during recovery. Because of autonomic imbalance associated with the effects of anesthetic drugs and reflex autoregulation of the vascular capacitance, circulating fluid volume is suboptimal during recovery. Fluid support should be continued to minimize the risk of hypovolemia that may contribute to hypotension, shock, and oliguric renal failure. Studies in man indicate that polyionic fluid administration maintains postoperative urine production better than administration of hypotonic or dextrose-containing fluids.[11] Generally, supplemental diuretic therapy is not necessary to maintain urine output during recovery.

Acid-base management during recovery. Preexisting disturbances in acid-base balance should be treated during the perioperative period and continued in the recovery period. Metabolic acidosis is the most common disturbance encountered in the critical patient. Supplemental buffer base such as sodium bicarbonate may be administered to aid in correction of base deficit (Chapter 38). A total base deficit is calculated based on a standard formula. We initiate replacement with one third the calculated deficit by bolus infusion, with the remaining two-thirds administered over the next 12 to 24 hours. Overshoot of correction and resultant metabolic alkalosis is avoided by using this approach. In patients with critical deficits (base deficit of −10 or greater), the clinician may elect to replace one half the calculated deficit during the acute period with the remaining half administered over the next 12 hours.

THE NEXT 12 HOURS

Emergence from anesthesia does not "guarantee" that a successful outcome will follow. Many physiologic disturbances created by the combination of presenting disease and anesthetic drugs are not quickly restored to normal base-line conditions. For this reason, vigilance should be maintained for the first 12 hours following anesthesia in any critical patient. Constant monitoring of physical parameters and specified laboratory data are done in a critical care environment.

Good nursing care, a supportive environment, and vigilance are important factors in successful outcome. Critical patients cannot be left unattended and unmonitored in general wards. A warm, dry, quiet environment is helpful in the stabilization period. A facility that permits continuation of fluids or supplemental drugs, as well as monitoring capability, is mandatory. Trained personnel, who are capable of noting trends and have the "intuition" to recognize when the patient is deteriorating, are essential. An intensive care approach is required for anesthetic recoveries and continued postoperative management in critical patients.

Once recovery is complete, the patient reverts to treatment protocols devised during the preoperative period and revised during the postoperative time. The overall goal is to have restabilization by 24 hours postanesthesia.

SUMMARY

The critical patient requires vigilance during all phases of anesthesia. The preoperative period is critical for stabilizing cardiopulmonary and splanchnic organ function prior to administration of anesthetic drugs. The recovery period has the additional risk of combining the preexisting disease or injury with physiologic change inherent with anesthetic drug administration. The patient must be closely supervised and supported until it has the capability to support its own reflexes, physiologic control mechanisms, and maintain normal organ function. Until the clinician is convinced of the patient's capability to provide these functions, continuous monitoring and treatment are mandatory for successful outcome.

REFERENCES

1. Stamp G. Metabolic response to trauma. In Zaslow IM, ed. Veterinary Trauma and Critical Care. Philadelphia: Lea & Febiger, 1984;25-63.
2. Blasidell FW, Lewis FR. Respiratory Distress Syndrome of Shock and Trauma: Posttraumatic Respiratory Failure. Philadelphia: WB Saunders, 1977.
3. Danielson RA. Differential diagnosis and treatment of oliguria in posttraumatic and postoperative patients. Surg Clin North Am 1975;55:697-702.
4. Saik RP, Chadwick C, Katz J. Gastrointestinal disorders. In Katz J, Benumof J, Kadis LB, eds. Anesthesia and Uncommon Diseases. Philadelphia: WB Saunders, 1981;384-449.
5. Hubbell JAE. Anesthesia for the emergency surgical patient. In Bright RM, ed. Surgical Emergencies. New York: Churchill Livingstone, 1986;45-60.

6. Deutsch S. Effects of anesthetics on the kidney. Surg Clin North Am 1975;55:775-786.

7. Sturnin L. The Liver and Anesthesia. Philadelphia: WB Saunders, 1977.

8. Webb AI. Postoperative care and oxygen therapy. In Short CE, ed. Principles and Practice in Veterinary Anesthesia. Baltimore: Williams & Wilkins, 1987;547-557.

9. Dripps RD, Eckenhoff JE, Vandam LD, eds. Introduction to Anesthesia: The Principles of Safe Practice, 6th ed. Philadelphia: WB Saunders, 1982.

10. Buss DD, Hess RE, Webb AI, Spencer KR. Incidence of postanesthetic arrhythmias in the dog. J Small Anim Pract 1982;23:399-404.

11. Engquist A. Fluid and electrolyte therapy in association with uncomplicated surgical procedures. Acta Anesthesiol Scand 1969;29:13-16.

13 Acute Abdomen

Deborah J. Davenport and Robert A. Martin

By definition, an acute abdomen is the sudden onset of abdominal pain or discomfort. The condition is often characterized by inappetence, lethargy, weakness, collapse, abdominal distention, vomiting, or other gastrointestinal signs. Prompt diagnosis of conditions causing acute abdominal pain is necessary in order to avoid irreversible disease progression, surgical delay, or unnecessary surgery. A list of gastrointestinal, hepatopancreatic, urogenital, and miscellaneous disorders that may present as an acute abdomen is presented below.

Disorders that may present as an acute abdomen

Gastrointestinal
  Gastric dilatation-volvulus
  Gastric ulceration, perforation, or rupture
  Bacterial or viral gastroenteritis
  Hemorrhagic gastroenteritis
  Intestinal obstruction by foreign body or tumor
  Intestinal volvulus
  Intestinal ulceration, perforation, or rupture
  Intestinal intussusception
  Mesenteric avulsion
  Mesenteric volvulus
  Mesenteric lymphadenitis
  Cecal inversion
  Colonic perforation or rupture
  Obstipation
  Umbilical, inguinal, diaphragmatic, scrotal or abdominal wall hernia with strangulated viscera
Hepatopancreatic
  Acute hepatitis—toxic, infectious
  Hepatic abscess
  Hepatic rupture
  Hepatic neoplasia
  Cholecystitis
  Cholangiohepatitis
  Gallbladder rupture
  Common bile duct obstruction
  Bile duct rupture
  Acute pancreatitis
  Pancreatic neoplasia
Urogenital
  Acute nephritis
  Pyelonephritis
  Ureteral obstruction or rupture
  Urethral obstruction or rupture
  Bladder rupture
  Acute bacterial prostatitis
  Prostatic abscess
  Metritis
  Pyometra
  Testicular or uterine torsion
Miscellaneous
  Peritonitis
  Splenic torsion
  Splenic rupture—tumor, trauma
  Intervertebral disk herniation
  Poisonings—arsenicals, zinc
  Tumor necrosis, abscess, hemorrhage
  Abdominal-wall hematoma

A systematic approach to the diagnosis and treatment of patients presenting with an acute abdomen is required due to the insidious nature and variable presentations of many abdominal disorders. Diagnostic tools include history taking, physical examination, laboratory testing, radiography, abdominocentesis, ultrasound, abdominal lavage, and surgical exploration.

The astute clinician must first recognize and treat any immediate threats to life in patients with abdominal pain or trauma. These may include airway obstruction, hemorrhage, sepsis, shock, cardiac arrhythmias, severe acid-base disorders, myocardial hypoxia, pulmonary compromise, and severe anemia.

153

HISTORY

The most readily available, least expensive, and least invasive tools for evaluation of dogs or cats presenting with an acute abdomen are anamnesis and physical examination. Accurate history taking is very important for assessment of such animals. In addition to routine anamnestic questions regarding length of illness and changes in appetite, water consumption, urination, and defecation, the owner should be questioned about vomiting and diarrhea. If episodes of vomiting or diarrhea are occurring, they should be characterized as to frequency, presence of blood, volume, and relationship to meals. Owners should be queried about the possibility of their pet's exposure to toxins, foreign-body ingestion, automobile accidents, fight wounds, and other traumatic injury. Treatments administered by owners or other veterinarians and the response of the animal to such treatments should be ascertained. The veterinarian must remember that the history may be misleading when the animal's injury is owner-induced, whether accidentally or maliciously.

PHYSICAL EXAMINATION

Physical examination should be thorough, but accomplished with minimal manipulation and stress to the animal. If life-threatening conditions are detected during this portion of the examination, they should be addressed immediately. Supportive treatment can be administered while history taking and physical examination are performed. Examinations should be interspersed with frequent determinations of vital signs and assessments of response to emergency therapy. A complete examination will assess all body systems and consist of inspection, palpation, auscultation and percussion. All information gathered from physical examinations should be serially recorded, as sequential examinations performed over a 1- to 12-hour period may give evidence of a progressively deteriorating or improving condition. Flow sheets for the recording of data should be formulated. Basic physiologic monitoring should include assessment of body temperature, pulse rate, respiratory rate, capillary refill time, packed cell volume, plasma protein, and urine output. A decreasing packed cell volume on serial examination is an indication for abdominocentesis, thoracocentesis, or diagnostic peritoneal lavage. Parameters such as central venous pressure and arterial blood pressure should also be monitored when possible. The animal's response to supportive care offers important diagnostic information. Progressive deterioration in the patient's condition despite appropriate medical treatment should spur the veterinarian to consider additional diagnostic and therapeutic procedures.

A general patient assessment should include gait, attitude, strength, and posture. This information may serve to give the clinician an idea of both the location and severity of a disorder or injury. Certain postures are characteristic of certain disorders. For example, a "praying" or kneeling posture is often adopted by dogs and cats with gastric or duodenal ulceration.

The cardiovascular and respiratory systems should receive particular attention in the patient with acute abdominal pain. Capillary refill time, mucous membrane color, pulse rate, pulse rhythm and quality, and respiratory rate and character should be assessed. Shock in animals with acute abdominal pain usually indicates severe hemorrhage or sepsis. Icteric mucous membranes are suggestive of hepatic, biliary, or hemolytic disease.

Examination of the abdomen is often the key to diagnosis of acute abdominal disorders. A complete abdominal examination includes inspection, superficial and deep palpation, auscultation, and percussion. In a systematic fashion, the abdomen should be evaluated for body-wall hernias, organ displacement, pain, fluid, and masses.

Visualization of abdominal skin and abdominal size and shape can offer important diagnostic information. The patient's haircoat should be clipped to visualize better the skin of the abdomen, inguinal, and perineal regions. Abdominal distention and effusions may be more evident when the hair is removed. The clinician should be alert for evidence of bruising, localized swelling, puncture wounds, umbilical or inguinal discoloration, herniation of abdominal organs, or intraabdominal masses. Small puncture wounds may seal and be difficult to detect, even with clipping of the hair. The "iceberg" principle of small puncture wounds, caused by animal bites or projectiles should be remembered. The entry wound may appear insignificant as compared with the damage caused to deeper tissues. Circular red discolorations of the umbilicus have been associated with marked intraabdominal hemorrhage.[1] The perineal and inguinal areas should be closely examined for evidence of discoloration and irritation, which might herald urethral rupture and urine leakage.

Superficial abdominal palpation is very helpful in detection of pain (splinting, guarding, or nausea). Repeatable muscle splinting on abdominal palpation is evidence of serious abdominal disease. Abdominal muscle guarding, especially when coupled with vomiting, usually indicates peritoneal irritation.

Deeper palpation of the abdomen allows evaluation of the size and character of intraabdominal organs and detection of abdominal fluid. Using gentle compression, the clinician should perform ballottement on the abdomen to detect intraabdominal fluid and attempt to isolate and characterize individual abdominal organs. Deep palpation should be performed regionally, as localization of abdominal pain may be helpful in identification of the disease process.

Deep palpation of the cranial abdomen can provide information regarding the pancreas, liver, duodenum, biliary structures, and the stomach. Assessment of these structures can be difficult, particularly in the dog, as they are often contained within the rib cage. Elevation of the forequarters and/or light sedation of the patient may facilitate palpation of these structures.

Palpation of the midabdomen may reveal changes in the character and size of the kidneys, bowel, mesentery, mesenteric lymph nodes, adrenal glands, uterus, and spleen. Progressively enlarging masses in the region of the kidneys suggest retroperitoneal blood or urine accumulations.

Examination of the caudal abdomen can provide information regarding the colon, rectum, prostate, uterus, urinary bladder, and inguinal rings. With urinary bladder rupture, the patient may exhibit systemic signs of uremia in addition to abdominal pain and distention. A rigid, painful, distended urinary bladder suggests lower urinary tract obstruction from urolithiasis, trauma, foreign bodies, or neoplasia (Chapter 21). Occasionally, severe prostatic disease may also result in urethral obstruction in dogs.

Auscultation of the abdomen, while not performed as part of many routine physical examinations, may give valuable information regarding gas-filled viscera and gastrointestinal motility in patients with acute abdomens. Auscultation is best performed over a clipped body surface using the diaphragm of the stethoscope. If clipping of the abdomen has not been performed, the use of lubricants (such as K-Y jelly) will dampen sounds attributable to hair rubbing. If bowel sounds are absent, the presence of abdominal fluid or generalized ileus is suggested. The absence of bowel sounds is often indicative of paralytic ileus in association with peritonitis. Normal bowel sounds may be present immediately following trauma, as ileus or ascites may not develop for several hours to days postinjury. Therefore, the clinician should auscultate the abdomen serially. "Ectopic" bowel sounds associated with swellings of the abdominal wall should lead the clinician to suspect body-wall or diaphragmatic hernias.

Percussion during abdominal auscultation can reveal tympany of gas-filled viscera. If tympanic sounds are present, gastric or small-intestinal obstruction, dilatation, or volvulus should be suspected. Percussion can aid in detection of abdominal fluid. With the animal in a standing position, a fluid line can be percussed between areas of dullness and resonance. This finding on abdominal percussion has been termed the "puddle" sign.[2]

Rectal examination is important for evaluation of the character and color of stools, detection of melena or hematochezia, and assessment of the sublumbar lymph nodes, prostate, pelvis, and pelvic urethra. The urinary bladder and urethra are commonly damaged with fractures of the pubis and ischium. Fracture fragments may sever or pierce the urinary bladder or urethra. Detection of pelvic fractures should lead the clinician to suspect possible organ damage.

The accuracy of the physical examination in assessing patients with acute abdomen has been questioned. Much of the controversy centers on physical examination in cases of abdominal trauma. In previous reports,[3-5] physical examination and history were successful in predicting the presence or absence of serious visceral injury in only 50% to 60% of patients with abdominal trauma. Significant errors in diagnosis may occur during the initial physical examination of acute abdomen cases, but serial physical examinations improve accuracy. False negative findings have the potential to be life threatening for the patient. The clinician should maintain a high index of suspicion for occult injury in abdominal trauma cases. The clinician should not overlook subtle clinical findings and should suspect the worst.

Based on historical data and serial physical examination findings, the clinician should select additional tests (complete blood count, platelet count, coagulation screen, serum biochemical profile, urinalysis, radiography, ultrasonography, diagnostic peritoneal lavage) to assist in achieving a diagnosis. The time involved in performing serial examinations and waiting for test results can be detrimental if the patient is deteriorating rapidly. The clinician must be astute and achieve a balance in which both unnecessary delay in surgical intervention and unnecessary exploratory surgery are avoided.

CLINICAL PATHOLOGY

Laboratory tests are useful diagnostic tools in the evaluation of patients presenting with an acute abdomen. Laboratory results may provide a definitive diagnosis or may offer confirmatory data. The hemogram may serve to characterize an anemia, if present. The leukogram (white blood cell number and distribution) are helpful in assessing the patient for disease associated with inflammation and/or infection. Leukopenia and degenerative shifts in white blood cell number and distribution (neutrophils) are indicative of severe disease. The plasma protein concentration can be useful in assessing hydration, hemorrhage, and exogenous protein losses. If the platelet count is low or if the patient exhibits excessive hemorrhage, the clinician should consider further tests of coagulation. Thrombocytopenia can be associated with disseminated intravascular coagulation, platelet sequestration within an enlarged liver or spleen, and/or consumption due to hemorrhage.

The serum biochemical profile results can be very helpful in localization of the cause of acute abdominal pain (kidney, liver, pancreas, bowel). Increased blood urea nitrogen and serum creatinine concentrations suggest urinary tract involvement, either primary or secondary. Increased serum amylase and lipase activities support pancreatic disease, but must be interpreted in conjunction with results of renal function tests. Hypoglycemia suggests the potential of pancreatic or hepatic neoplasia and/or sepsis. Increased serum bilirubin concentration and gamma-glutamyl transferase and alkaline phosphatase activities (with or without elevations in alanine aminotransferase and aspartate aminotransferase activities) support a diagnosis of biliary tract disease or obstruction. Hepatocellular diseases may exhibit similar elevations in bilirubin, gamma-glutamyl transferase and alkaline phosphatase as well as consistent increases in serum alanine aminotransferase and aspartate aminotransferase activities.

The serum biochemical profile also provides important information regarding acid-base and electrolyte balance. Serial determinations of electrolytes are recommended in the monitoring of these critical patients, particularly those receiving fluid therapy. Abnormal total carbon dioxide values indicate the need for arterial blood gas determinations.

A urinalysis is mandatory in the evaluation of patients with acute abdominal discomfort. The urinalysis can provide localizing information or may give evidence of renal dysfunction. Elevations in urine specific gravity suggest hemoconcentration. Isosthenuria, especially if coupled with azotemia, cylindriuria, glycosuria, and proteinuria is indicative of renal insufficiency. Pyuria, hematuria, and crystalluria should lead the clinician to suspect lower and upper urinary tract disease.

RADIOLOGY

Radiographic assessment of the abdominal cavity is a standard diagnostic procedure in all acute ab-

domen cases. Radiographic evidence of organ distention or displacement, free peritoneal fluid or gas, the presence of gastrointestinal foreign bodies, and/or the loss of diaphragmatic or abdominal-wall integrity may provide a definitive diagnosis or aid in the final decision to explore the abdomen surgically. Contrast radiography can be used to document gastrointestinal obstruction or perforation.

With gastrointestinal obstruction, bowel loops are usually segmentally enlarged to a diameter two times normal. Intestinal volvulus is often characterized by lateral displacement and folding of markedly distended bowel loops. Adynamic ileus associated with drug therapy or infectious causes usually demonstrates a more generalized and less severe distention of bowel loops.

In the absence of prior abdominal surgery or trocarization, free peritoneal gas is diagnostic for a penetrating abdominal wound or a ruptured hollow viscus. Both conditions are indications for immediate surgical exploration. Free peritoneal gas is seen most easily on the caudal dorsal surface of the diaphragm (Fig. 13-1).

Loss of radiographic detail in the retroperitoneal space is indicative of renal or ureteral trauma (hemorrhage or urine leakage). Further definition of these radiographic findings requires ultrasonographic evaluation and positive contrast urography.

Loss of serosal surface detail throughout the abdominal cavity indicates generalized free peritoneal fluid (Fig. 13-2). This finding is nonspecific and requires further diagnostic evaluation (ultrasonographic evaluation, abdominocentesis, diagnostic peritoneal lavage) to identify the character and origin of the ascitic fluid.

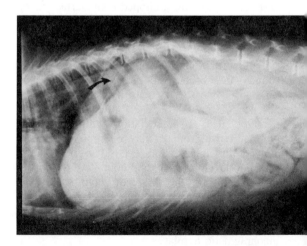

Fig. 13-1 Free peritoneal gas *(arrow)* present in a dog postoperatively.

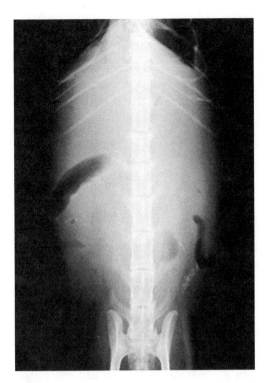

Fig. 13-2 Free peritoneal fluid in a cat as evidenced by loss of serosal detail.

Radiographic evaluations may need to be repeated in order to detect conditions that may not be apparent on initial radiographic evaluation.[6] For example, peritonitis associated with focal intestinal perforation or compromised blood supply to a segment of bowel may take days to manifest radiographic signs. Serial radiography is useful in monitoring a patient's progress and response to treatment.

Contrast studies of urogenital and gastrointestinal tract may be indicated to define abnormalities identified on survey abdominal films. Positive contrast cystourethrography is the definitive diagnostic procedure for detection of a ruptured urinary bladder or urethra. Intravenous urography is indicated if inguinal bruising, macroscopic hematuria, or loss of radiographic detail of the retroperitoneal space is recognized. If gastrointestinal perforation is suspected, aqueous iodine contrast agents are recommended for contrast radiography to avoid the peritoneal irritation associated with free barium in the abdomen.

Ultrasound evaluation of the abdomen may provide information that supports radiographic findings, or sonograms may contribute diagnostic information not provided by survey or contrast abdominal radiographs. In our experience, ultrasonography is of greatest use in evaluating the liver, biliary tract, spleen, prostate, kidneys, and ureters. Normal and abnormal pancreatic features (pancreatitis) may be difficult to identify ultrasonographically.

ABDOMINOCENTESIS

Abdominocentesis using a multifenestrated catheter such as a peritoneal dialysis catheter (Travenol Laboratories, Deerfield, IL) coupled with peritoneal lavage has become the diagnostic "bottom line" in acute abdomen cases when other diagnostic criteria are equivocal (Fig. 13-3).[4] Diagnostic peritoneal lavage is a valuable adjunct to anamnesis, physical examination, and survey radiography. Diagnostic peritoneal lavage is very helpful in determining the severity of abdominal injuries. For that reason, this procedure is often warranted before the results of other tests are available. Abdominocentesis and diagnostic peritoneal lavage are not indicated, however, when there is good historical, physical, or radiographic evidence of the need for exploratory laparotomy.[7]

The sensitivity of diagnostic peritoneal lavage techniques provides the clinician with greater than 90% assurance of rendering a correct decision regarding surgical exploration in the patient with acute abdomen.[5] False negative diagnostic peritoneal lavage findings occur primarily with retroperitoneal injury and diaphragmatic hernias. False positive results are rare, but may occur secondary to iatrogenic hemorrhage or viscus perforation from prior needle abdominocentesis.

To perform diagnostic peritoneal lavage, the patient is placed in dorsal recumbency and an area of skin 1 to 2 cm caudal to the umbilicus is aseptically prepared. The urinary bladder should be emptied via manual expression or catheterization. The body wall is locally anesthetized with 2% lidocaine, and an incision is made through the skin, subcutaneous tissues and superficial abdominal fascia. Meticulous control of hemorrhage is necessary to avoid bleeding into the peritoneal cavity that may result in erroneous diagnostic peritoneal lavage results.

The lavage catheter should be directed caudally and dorsally through the body wall until the fenestrated component is entirely within the abdominal cavity. Abdominal fluid may flow freely from the catheter following its insertion. If not, the animal is rolled gently from side to side before attempting dependent drainage through the open catheter tip. If these manipulations do not yield fluid, diagnostic peritoneal lavage is indicated.

To perform diagnostic peritoneal lavage, administer 22 mL/kg of body weight of warmed 0.9% sodium chloride or lactated Ringer's solution through the multifenestrated catheter by grav-

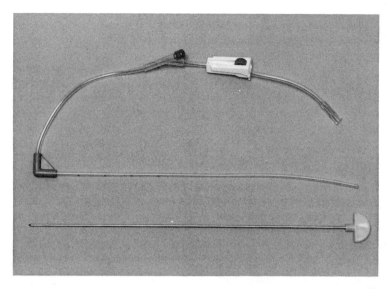

Fig. 13-3 A multifenestrated catheter (Trocath, Kendall-McGaw, Santa Ana, CA) suitable for diagnostic peritoneal lavage.

ity flow. Gently roll the patient from side to side to distribute the lavage fluid within the abdomen. Connect an empty bottle to the setup and place it below the level of the abdomen. If the fluid is clear, remove the dialysis catheter and suture both the linea alba and the skin appropriately. If the aliquot of collected fluid is pink or grossly red, remove the infusion set, cap the dialysis catheter in a sterile manner, and fix it in place pending packed cell volume determination. The catheter may be sutured in place and bandaged. If the packed cell volume of the lavage effluent is greater than 2 to 5%, another lavage sample should be collected by gravity flow 20 to 30 minutes later and compared to the first to assess for continued hemorrhage. In animals with acute injuries that may require repeated reassessments, the catheter may be left in place for up to 3 hours.

Diagnostic peritoneal lavage fluid should be analyzed as outlined in Table 13-1. Analysis should include an assessment of fluid color and turbidity, hematocrit, red and white blood cell counts, biochemical tests, and cytologic examination. A clear fluid indicates normalcy. Exceptions to this generalization include retroperitoneal injuries and recent peritoneal (<3 hours) contamination. Clear, but slightly turbid fluid mandates a cytologic examination. A pink fluid suggests mild hemorrhage, while a dark red fluid is indicative of major abdominal hemorrhage. If the hematocrit of the fluid is <1% and the red cell count is <100,000 μL, mild hemorrhage is suggested. If the packed cell volume is >5% or the red cell

count is >100,000 to 200,000/μL, major abdominal hemorrhage has occurred.[3]

A white blood cell count of 1000/μL indicates a major peritoneal inflammatory response. The presence of degenerative or toxic neutrophils implies that a suppurative, potentially serious condition exists. The presence of a mixed population of bacteria, particularly if intracellular bacteria are identified, confirms sepsis and peritonitis.

The presence of vegetable fibers implies gastrointestinal rupture or contamination from a penetrating abdominal wound. Neoplastic cells indicate the presence of an intraabdominal tumor.

Biochemical analysis of diagnostic peritoneal lavage fluid should include tests for the detection of bilirubin, creatinine, and amylase. A positive Icotest (Ames, Elkhart, IN) indicates leakage of bile from the hepatobiliary tree or a proximal gastrointestinal tract rupture. If the lavage effluent creatinine concentration exceeds serum creatinine concentration, then leakage of urine from the bladder, ureters, or kidneys has occurred. The presence of effluent amylase activity in concentrations greater than those of serum is considered indicative of pancreatic inflammation or intestinal ischemia.[8]

One must evaluate the results of diagnostic peritoneal lavage fluid analysis in conjunction with the patient's clinical manifestations. Overzealous interpretation of cytologic and biochemical findings can result in false positive findings and injudicious surgery.[9]

Reported complications of diagnostic peritoneal

Table 13-1 Assessment of diagnostic peritoneal lavage fluid

	Hemorrhage	Bowel rupture	Bile peritonitis	Bladder rupture
Color	Pink to red	Variable	Clear to yellow	Variable
Turbidity	N to ↑	↑	↑	N to ↑
Hematocrit	↑	N	N	N
Red blood cell count	↑	N	N	N
White blood cell count	↑	↑↑↑	↑↑	↑↑
Cytologic examination	Mixed WBC	Neutrophils	Neutrophils	Neutrophils
Biochemical tests				
Bilirubin	N	N	↑↑	N
Creatinine	N	N	N	↑↑
Amylase	N	N to ↑	N	N

N = normal; ↑ = increased; WBC = white blood cells.

lavage include subcutaneous hematoma formation, subcutaneous leakage of lavage fluid, and visceral perforation.[5] In addition, the technique must be used cautiously in the presence of dyspnea, organomegaly (gravid uterus, enlarged spleen, dilated bowel loops), suspected body-wall adhesions, or suspected diaphragmatic hernia.[10] The minilaparotomy approach to catheter placement may be safely implemented in such patients.

The technique of needle abdominocentesis is best reserved for patients with a palpable accumulation of free peritoneal fluid. However, because of the ease and safety of the procedure, needle abdominocentesis using an 18- to 20-gauge needle is often performed prior to diagnostic peritoneal lavage. The sensitivity of the technique is only about 50%, but specificity is sufficiently high to warrant its application.[4,5] A four-quadrant needle abdominocentesis using an open-needle technique is recommended. Ideally, the patient should remain standing while needle abdominocentesis is performed. Following aseptic preparation, the needle should be placed through the body wall at a 30- to 45-degree angle in order to avoid perforation of abdominal viscera. The finding of frank blood, gastrointestinal contents, or elevated creatinine content on a single needle abdominocentesis sample can be misleading.[11] Significant findings will be repeatable. Negative results of needle abdominocentesis are an indication to proceed with diagnostic peritoneal lavage in animals with an acute abdomen.

EXPLORATORY SURGERY

To pursue abdominal exploration in patients with acute abdomen means the clinician has confirmed a diagnosis of a surgical disease or has strong evidence that a surgical disease exists, although the diagnosis remains open (see list below).

Indications for exploratory abdominal surgery

Penetrating abdominal injury
Presence of bacteria on diagnostic peritoneal lavage
Presence of >2000/μL white blood cells in lavage effluent
Presence of >500/μL white blood cells in lavage effluent if degenerative neutrophils are present
Presence of vegetable fibers in the lavage effluent
Presence of a lavage effluent creatinine greater than serum creatinine
Presence of bilirubin in the lavage effluent
Hemoperitoneum not responsive to volume replacement
Free air in the peritoneal cavity
Abdominal hernia
Continuing evidence of peritoneal irritation

When the generally accepted surgical indications are not met, but clinical judgment supports an abdominal exploration, the risk/benefit ratio of surgery must be less than one to proceed. The clinician should consider the following questions:

Is surgery urgently needed or is additional supportive therapy indicated? Is the diagnosis accurate or are additional diagnostic tests and a longer observation period indicated? Should prophylactic antibiotics be given? What are the anesthetic hazards?[11]

When the benefits of surgery outweigh the risks following a thorough serial patient evaluation as described previously, then surgery should be performed. If exploratory surgery is not elected, proper treatment of the patient with an acute abdomen should include careful surveillance and repeated risk-benefit assessments.

As a diagnostic tool, exploratory surgery provides a quick means of ruling in or ruling out serious abdominal disease that could result in patient deterioration. Exploration provides for therapeutic measures when a surgically correctable disease exists. The goal of the clinician is to minimize needless abdominal exploration. Negative findings must be expected on occasion. In these situations, appropriate collection of biopsy specimens may add significantly to case management.

Penetrating abdominal wounds represent a select group of acute abdomen cases. Following stab wounds in human patients, wound exploration under local anesthesia is recommended as the preferred technique to determine whether the peritoneum has been entered.[12] If the peritoneal cavity has been violated, then visceral damage is assessed by diagnostic peritoneal lavage. A similar approach could be followed in veterinary medicine. Bite and gunshot wounds do not fit the category of "stablike" wounds and one should assume severe internal injuries until proven otherwise.[10]

The timing of surgery is another difficult decision, even after a diagnosis of surgical disease has been reached. The urgency of surgical exploration depends on whether survival of the patient will be adversely influenced by a delay in surgical intervention. Most patients will benefit from conservative medical management and surgery can and should be postponed until patient stabilization has been attempted and achieved. Patients with uroperitoneum and bile peritonitis are better anesthetic risks after 24 hours of aggressive fluid therapy and peritoneal lavage and drainage.[11] Patient homeostasis cannot always be reestablished without eliminating the primary disease process. The time required (1 to 2 hours) to prepare the patient for abdominal exploration is usually adequate for volume expansion and correction of acid-base and electrolyte disturbances.

Whether as a diagnostic or therapeutic tool, exploratory surgery should be undertaken in a thorough, systematic manner. Prior to surgery, the patient should be clipped and the skin aseptically prepared from the cranial thorax to the perineal region. The surgical incision should extend from the xiphoid cartilage caudally to the pubic brim. After placement of self-retaining abdominal retractors, the ventral aspect and lesser curvature of the stomach should be examined, including palpation for the potential intraluminal foreign bodies or mural masses. The pylorus, cardia, and esophageal hiatus should be examined and palpated. Examination should include the gastric fundus, greater curvature, the left portion of the diaphragm (including its crus attachment), and palpation for retroperitoneal masses and abscesses.

The surgeon should also examine the left lateral, medial, quadrate, and right medial lobes of the liver. The central tendon of the diaphragm and the caudal vena cava and hiatus should also be assessed. The gallbladder and the hepatic, cystic, and common bile ducts should be examined. The gallbladder may be digitally expressed to confirm the patency of the common bile duct. The portal vein, common hepatic artery, and common bile duct can be palpated by placing a finger through the epiploic foramen. Examination should proceed to the right lateral and caudate liver lobes, the right diaphragm and crus, the right adrenal gland, and the right kidney. By elevating the duodenum ventrally and to the left, the mesoduodenum will contain the small intestines, facilitating this inspection.

In the midabdomen, the descending duodenum, the right limb of the pancreas, the portal vein, caudal vena cava, the right ovary and uterine horn in the female, and the right ureter are visualized and palpated. The retroperitoneal space can be palpated at this point. The entire small bowel should be traced to the ileocolic junction. Both sides of the bowel should be inspected and palpated while fanning out the attached mesentery to inspect the jejunal arteries, veins, and associated lymph nodes. Following evaluation of the small bowel, the ascending and transverse colon, the mesocolon, and associated blood supply are examined. The omentum is then reflected cranioventrally and examined, and the angle and left limb of the pancreas, the dorsal aspect of the stomach, the spleen and the mesenteric root (celiac and cranial mesenteric arteries) and the abdominal aorta are evaluated. The descending colon, the left adrenal gland and kidney, the left ovary and uterine horn in the female, the left ureter, the associated retroperitoneal space, and the caudal mesenteric artery are examined and palpated. Elevating the descending colon ventrally and to the right allows the mesocolon to contain the small intestines facilitating examination of these areas.

In the caudal abdomen the colorectal junction, the urinary bladder, the uterine body and cervix in the female, the inguinal rings bilaterally, and the prostate gland in the male are inspected. If adequate examination of the entire abdominal body wall has not been accomplished during these maneuvers, then this evaluation (including palpation of the prepubic tendon attachment to the pubis) will complete the exploration.

In animals with abdominal hemorrhage requiring exploration, the systematic examination should begin with the liver and spleen, as these organs are the most likely sources of severe, ongoing hemorrhage.

On the rare occasions when the patient's condition is so critical that any prolongation of intraoperative time could be detrimental, rapid identification and therapy of the surgical lesion may be followed by abdominal closure. This approach assumes a calculated risk that additional lesions may be overlooked. In the vast majority of cases, a truncated exploratory procedure is unwarranted and considered poor surgical management.

Localized or generalized peritonitis may be encountered surgically in the patient with acute abdomen. Generalized peritonitis secondary to leakage of gastrointestinal contents into the peritoneal cavity is most often seen in the dog as a result of surgical complication or trauma.[13-15] Other common causes of peritonitis include traumatic rupture of the biliary and urinary tracts and pancreatic disease.

Initial surgical management requires identification and correction of the inciting cause, copious abdominal lavage with warm, sterile physiologic saline solution, and an accurate determination of the need for continued abdominal drainage. Localized peritonitis or gross contamination may be managed by thorough lavage alone or by intraoperative lavage in combination with tube drainage of the abdominal cavity postoperatively. Tube drainage of the abdominal cavity often is only partially effective, as adhesions may seal the tube after abdominal closure. Triple-lumen sump drains are more effective than simple-lumen drains, and they can be connected to a low-pressure suction device to improve drainage.[16] An "ingress" tube into the abdominal cavity may be installed surgically to provide intermittent abdominal lavage in conjunction with suction drainage to treat peritonitis. Careful management of tube abdominal drains is necessary to prevent ascending bacterial contamination.

Generalized peritonitis or gross peritoneal soilage is best managed by open abdominal drainage. Patient care is intensive, but the efficacy of drainage is superior to other methods. The incised linea alba is loosely laced together with a monofilament nonabsorbable suture material (nylon, polypropylene) of appropriate size (0 to 00), leaving a 1- to 6-cm gap, depending on patient size.[13] In the male dog, the paraprepucial incision is closed routinely in three layers, leaving only the incision cranial to the prepuce open for drainage. Subcutaneous tissues and skin are not closed and sterile bandages are used to contain the abdominal viscera, collect and quantitate drainage, and keep the peritoneal cavity clean.[13] Bandage changes are frequent in the initial 24 to 48 hours as bandages become soaked by drainage fluids or soiled with urine or feces. A minimum of once-daily bandage changes is required. The abdominal cavity is closed usually by 3 to 4 days after sur-

gery. If drainage continues for 5 to 6 days, reexploration is indicated.[13] Other indications for reexploration include a sudden change in the character of the drainage or identification of gross contamination of the drainage with bile or intestinal contents.

Abdominal closure following open abdominal drainage involves breaking down granulation tissue that has formed on the open wound margins and lacing the linea alba together with preplaced loose continuous suture, beginning at either end of the incision. Subcutaneous and skin closure are routine.

Potential complications of open abdominal drainage include loss of body fluids (hypoproteinemia, dehydration, weight loss), further contamination of the peritoneal cavity, adhesions to the bandages, evisceration, and inability to achieve complete peritoneal drainage.[13,14,16] Animals surviving until complete abdominal closure is undertaken have a good prognosis for overall survival.[13,14]

CONCLUSION

Most patients with acute abdomen require surgical intervention. A surgical decision should be favored when the results of diagnostic evaluations are equivocal. If diagnostic or therapeutic surgery is not performed, proper management includes careful surveillance and repeated physical examinations for at least 48 hours. The value of consultation with associates cannot be overlooked in the evaluation of patients presenting with acute abdominal pain. Second opinions from clinicians with different areas of expertise and perspectives are invaluable in providing the best possible patient care.

REFERENCES

1. Crowe DT, Todoroff RJ. Umbilical masses and discolorations as signs of intra-abdominal disease. J Am Anim Hosp Assoc 1982;18:295-298.
2. Lawson JO, Weissbein AS. The puddle sign—as an aid in the diagnosis of minimal ascites. N Engl J Med 1959; 260:652.
3. Bjorling DE, Crowe DT, Kolata RJ, Rawlings CA. Penetrating abdominal wounds in dogs and cats. J Am Anim Hosp Assoc 1982;18:742-748.
4. Crowe DT, Crane SW. Diagnostic abdominal paracentesis and lavage in the evaluation of abdominal injuries in dogs and cats: clinical and experimental investigations. J Am Vet Med Assoc 1976;168:700-705.
5. Crowe DT. Diagnostic abdominal paracentesis techniques: clinical evaluation in 129 dogs and cats. J Am Anim Hosp Assoc 1984;20:223-230.
6. Burt JK, Roat CR. Radiographic manifestations of abdominal trauma. J Am Anim Hosp Assoc 1971;7:328.
7. Crowe DT. Abdominocentesis and diagnostic peritoneal lavage in small animals. Mod Vet Pract 1984;65:877-882.

8. Dillon AR, Spano JS. The acute abdomen. Vet Clin North Am Small Anim Pract 1983;13:461-476.

9. Hunt CA. Diagnostic peritoneal paracentesis and lavage. Compend Contin Educ Pract Vet 1980;2:449-455.

10. Crane SW. Evaluation and management of adbominal trauma in the dog and cat. Vet Clin North Am 1980; 10:655-689.

11. Knecht CD. Emergency surgery: the patient versus the disease. J Am Vet Med Assoc 1981;179:1372-1375.

12. Moore EE, Marx JA. Penetrating abdominal wounds: rationale for exploratory laparotomy. JAMA 1985;253: 2705-2708.

13. Greenfield CL, Walshaw R. Open peritoneal drainage for treatment of contaminated peritoneal cavity and septic peritonitis in dogs and cats: 24 cases (1980-1986). J Am Vet Med Assoc 1987;191:100-105.

14. Woolfson JM, Dulish ML. Open abdominal drainage in the treatment of generalized peritonitis in 25 dogs and cats. Vet Surg 1986;15:27-32.

15. Hosgood G, Salisbury SK. Generalized peritonitis in dogs: 50 cases (1975-1986). J Am Vet Med Assoc 1988; 193:1448-1450.

16. Donner GS, Ellison GW. The use and misuse of abdominal drains in small animal surgery. Compend Contin Educ Pract Vet 1986;8:705-714.

14 Shock

Wendy A. Ware

Shock is generally regarded as a state of acute, severe circulatory failure. Blood transport does not meet the oxygen and nutrient requirements of vital organs or remove accumulated metabolites at a sufficient rate. This causes progressive and eventually fatal derangement of physiologic processes. A reduction in total cardiac output, often the result of massive intravascular volume loss, or a maldistribution of blood flow can lead to the clinical entity known as shock.

There are many causes of shock (see box, p. 164). Four general categories have been described: hypovolemic (oligemic), distributive (vasculogenic), cardiogenic, and obstructive.[1,2] Hypovolemic shock can result from the external or internal loss of blood, plasma or fluid and electrolytes. The category of distributive shock includes septic shock as well as other insults that cause maldistribution of blood flow and inadequate perfusion of vital organs. Cardiogenic shock results from profound impairment of cardiac function. Obstructive shock, sometimes considered a subdivision of cardiogenic shock, is caused by such impediments to blood flow as massive pulmonary embolism or cardiac tamponade. Components of more than one cause are often present in the same patient. Relative or absolute hypovolemia is a common accompaniment to all forms of shock.

The first clinical evidence of shock is usually arterial hypotension, with its associated changes. These clinical signs can include tachycardia, weak arterial pulses, pallor, peripheral cyanosis, hyperventilation, oliguria, and mental depression. However, shock is not simply characterized as a state of hypotension, with low blood flow and high peripheral resistance; many physiologic changes occur before hypotension develops. The clinical syndrome may vary depending on the time course of shock development and the presence of complicating factors such as compartmental fluid shifts and disseminated intravascular coagulation. Multiple pathophysiologic mechanisms become involved as shock progresses, and the dominant abnormality may change as a function of time and treatment. In the early stages of shock, most physiologic alterations relate to the underlying events causing the shock. Later, as tissue and microcirculatory abnormalities develop, the release of various metabolites contributes to the development of advanced shock, in which the distinction between types of shock fades.[3] Although the metabolic responses to shock can differ in certain ways depending on its cause, there are underlying similarities. The final common pathway is inadequate or inappropriate tissue perfusion, which then results in cellular hypoxia.[3] Reduced substrate supplies and accumulation of cell metabolites are contributing factors.

PATHOPHYSIOLOGIC CHANGES

Various compensatory changes are activated as shock develops and arterial pressure declines. In the initial phases these compensations may be sufficient to allow reversal of shock. However, as time passes and further derangements of circulation and cellular function occur the shock becomes irreversible, even with aggressive therapy. Indeed, with time the compensatory mechanisms can contribute to worsening peripheral perfusion and organ function.[4]

The body's response to acute injury, including fluid loss, is initiated by the central nervous system. Multiple afferent stimuli, including arterial and venous pressure and volume, osmolality, pH, hypoxia, pain and anxiety, tissue damage, and sepsis, are integrated by the hypothalamus.[5] Signals are sent to the sympathetic nervous system and adrenal medulla to release catecholamines. At the same time the anterior pituitary initiates a cas-

CAUSES OF SHOCK

Hypovolemic
  Hemorrhage (internal or external)
  Plasma loss or sequestration (e.g., burns, ascites,
    peritonitis, pancreatitis)
  Fluid and electrolyte loss (e.g., dehydration,
    vomiting, diarrhea, diabetes insipidus or mellitus,
    adrenocortical insufficiency)
Distributive
  Sepsis and endotoxemia
  Metabolic (e.g., renal or hepatic failure, severe
    acidosis or alkalosis)
  Toxic (e.g., sedative or anesthetic overdose, heavy
    metal toxicosis)
  Endocrinologic (e.g., uncontrolled diabetes mellitus,
    adrenocortical insufficiency)
  Neurogenic (cerebral or spinal disease)
  Anaphylactic
  Hyperviscosity syndromes
Cardiogenic
  Myopathic (cardiomyopathy, myocarditis,
    myocardial infarction)
  Intracardiac disease (e.g., ruptured chordae
    tendineae, acute aortic regurgitation, aortic
    stenosis, hypertrophic obstructive
    cardiomyopathy, intracardiac tumor)
  Arrhythmias (severe bradyarrhythmias or
    tachyarrhythmias)
  Drugs (overdose of vasodilator, beta-adrenergic
    blocker, calcium entry blocker)
Obstructive
  Pericardial tamponade
  Pulmonary hypertension (e.g., heartworm disease,
    pulmonary embolism)

cade of hormones in response to the injury. Catecholamine release and production of angiotensin are accompanied by release of other hormones such as cortisol, growth hormone, aldosterone, and antidiuretic hormone (vasopressin). The combined effect of these substances is to mobilize energy reserves, support blood pressure, and conserve salt and water. Initially their effects are protective; later they can lead to breakdown of cellular integrity.

Increases in heart rate and myocardial contractility along with peripheral vasoconstriction result from sympathetic activation. These effects serve to maintain blood pressure and increase vital organ perfusion by redistributing flow away from skin, skeletal muscle, and renal and splanchnic beds. The rich alpha-adrenergic innervation of these tissues is largely responsible for this blood flow redistribution. Plasma catecholamine levels have been shown to be elevated in shock and may be an index of severity and/or prognosis.[5]

Renal arterial hypotension and increases in renal sympathetic traffic contribute to peripheral vasoconstriction and retention of salt and water by stimulating renin release from the juxtaglomerular cells. Renin catalyzes the conversion of the peptide angiotensinogen to angiotensin I, which is then converted to the active angiotensin II by angiotensin-converting enzyme, located in the lung and elsewhere. The effects of angiotensin II are multiple, but potent vasoconstriction and stimulation of aldosterone release from the adrenal cortex are two of its major effects. Aldosterone promotes the renal retention of sodium (accompanied by water) and thereby serves to increase vascular volume. Angiotensin II and catecholamines facilitate each other's actions and release. Angiotensin II has been incriminated as a cause of heart failure after prolonged, severe hemorrhage in humans.[5]

Epinephrine, along with antidiuretic hormone and glucagon, also facilitates hepatic glycogenolysis, lipolysis, and the release of nonesterified fatty acids, which are an important fuel source in shock. Glycogenolysis also results in lactate production in skeletal muscles. Increased catecholamine as well as cortisol and glucagon levels contribute to peripheral insulin resistance.

Antidiuretic hormone and adrenocorticotropic hormone (ACTH) are also important "stress" hormones. Increased production follows from several stimuli, such as increased blood osmolality (detected by hypothalamic osmoreceptors), decreased arterial pressure and volume (detected by vascular mechanoreceptors), and psychologic stress (relayed via the limbic system). Angiotensin II is also thought to stimulate the release of antidiuretic hormone as well.[5] The effects of antidiuretic hormone include vasoconstriction and retention of water by the kidneys.

Corticotropin-releasing hormone, antidiuretic hormone, epinephrine, and other hormones stimulate the release of ACTH.[6] Consequently, cortisol and corticosterone, which have a major role in protecting the animal from the effects of hypovolemia, are produced. The release of ACTH in response to acute hemorrhage is rapid; cortisol levels quickly parallel the rise in ACTH. Glucocorticoid release in response to hemorrhage and other stresses has an important role in the metabolic response. Glucocorticoids may act to dampen the endogenous defense reactions originally activated by the stressors.[6] Glucocorticoids are also thought to facilitate an adequate cardiovascular response to surgical and other stresses, mediated by permissive support for the vascular effects of catecholamines and other hormones.[6] Increased cortisol secretion also appears to play an important part in the restitution of blood volume after hemorrhage by somehow inducing a rise in plasma osmolality. Intracellular water is then drawn to the interstitial space, which increases interstitial pressure and enhances the transfer of preformed protein to the vascular system through routes such as lymphovenous shunts.[6] Restoration of plasma protein is accompanied by replacement of blood volume. This can occur within 24 hours for a 10% blood loss. Other adrenal and pituitary factors probably also are important in this regard.[6]

The release of endorphins from the pituitary gland also occurs with stress. These endogenous opiates are thought to mediate longer-term neuronal and endocrine changes. Various autacoids such as serotonin, histamine, and kinins are also influential in shock. Plasma kinins (such as bradykinin) are vasodilator polypeptides that increase capillary permeability. They are released by both hypoxia and endotoxemia from inactive precursors (kininogens) present in plasma.[5] Initiation of the process is thought to result from activation of Hageman factor (XII). This leads to conversion of kininogen to kinin by the proteolytic enzymes kallikreins, which are released from leukocytes and injured tissues. Activation of Hageman factor also promotes complement activation; resulting substances appear to cause leukocyte aggregation and endothelial cell damage.[5] Kinins and the substances described below may not be important in uncomplicated hypovolemia, but occur in the presence of shock compounded by trauma and sepsis.[7]

Local mediators of microvascular injury include the arachidonic acid metabolites, as well as platelet activating factor, plasma or phagocyte-derived proteases, fibrinogen degradation products, and toxic oxygen radicals released by activated white blood cells.[8] The arachidonate metabolites (prostaglandins, prostacyclin, thromboxane A_2, and leukotrienes) are associated with changes in platelet aggregability and reductions in blood pressure, which may occur in terminal shock with disseminated intravascular coagulation. These cyclooxygenase and lipoxygenase metabolites are produced in large amounts in septic shock. Macrophages, platelets, neutrophils, and mast cells are all involved in the production of these metabolites, which cause significant hemodynamic effects, including pulmonary vasoconstriction, systemic vasodilation, and increased pulmonary capillary permeability.[9,10] Thromboxane A_2, cysteinyl-leukotrienes, and platelet activating factor by themselves can produce shock and death in intact animals.[8] The E and F groups of prostaglandins have opposing physiologic effects on the microcirculation; thus, their relative concentration

rather than absolute level is most important. The same is true for the thromboxane:prostacyclin ratio. Inconclusive early pharmacologic attempts to block the adverse effects of prostaglandins in shock using nonselective blocking drugs such as aspirin or indomethacin probably are related to this; in septic shock nonsteroidal antiinflammatory agents may modify the hemodynamic derangements.[5] Glucocorticoids inhibit the common arachidonate precursor, phospholipase A_2, and thus block both pathways. Leukotrienes are potent chemotactic factors that also cause bronchoconstriction, vasoconstriction, and microvascular exudation of protein.[5,8] It is probable that arachidonate metabolites have a causative role in acute respiratory distress syndrome, one of the major complications of shock. Production of arachidonate metabolites is stimulated by hypoxia, damage from lysosomal enzymes, and neurohumoral agents or metabolites.[8,11] In hypovolemia complicated by tissue injury or sepsis, macrophages may produce interleukin 1. This lymphokine appears to depend on arachidonate metabolism for its capacity to induce fever and regulate immune function.[5]

Histamine has been thought to play a part in the cause of shock, but it is not believed to be important in initiating hypovolemic shock. Histamine causes vasodilation and is derived mainly from mast-cell granules; its production is increased by endotoxin.[5] Histamine and serotonin may play a secondary part in the pulmonary vascular response to shock. Both histamine and serotonin are important in anaphylactic shock.

Myocardial depressant factor, released from hypoxic pancreatic acinar cells, is thought to be another extracardiac cause of heart failure in shock. This substance produces a negative inotropic effect, constricts splanchnic vessels, and depresses phagocytosis in the fixed macrophages of the reticuloendothelial system.[1,12] A substance called reticuloendothelial depressant factor, which reduces the cellular immune response during shock, has also been described.[1]

MICROCIRCULATORY DISTURBANCES

Because the early catecholamine-induced vasoconstrictor response to hypovolemia is not uniform, resulting in redistribution of blood flow in favor of certain "vital" organs, microcirculatory changes tend to occur in less perfused tissues first. Impaired perfusion may have far-reaching effects on organ function. Normal hemodynamic measurements do not necessarily reflect the magnitude of flow reduction to nonvital areas. For example, a 10% reduction in blood volume produced little change in heart rate and arterial pressure, but an almost 30% reduction in colon blood flow and oxygen availability in one study.[5] The significant reduction in splanchnic blood flow has a great impact on liver function, since about 70% of liver blood flow is from the portal vein. Although the liver cells themselves are relatively resistant to hypoxia, disturbances in reticuloendothelial and hepatocellular function may occur early.

In the early stages of shock, there is fairly normal autoregulation of the microcirculation although generalized vasoconstriction is present because of sympathetic nervous activation. This autoregulation serves to keep microvascular blood flow relatively constant over a wide range of arterial pressures. As shock progresses and ischemia worsens, the accumulation of locally vasoactive metabolites such as lysosomal enzymes, kinins, histamine, and various prostaglandins cause loss of autoregulation, making flow to the microcirculation dependent on arterial perfusion pressure. These substances also promote increased capillary permeability, depression of myocardial contractility, development of intravascular coagulation, and ultimately, death.[3]

Autoregulation of microvascular blood flow can be adversely affected by pathologic changes in vessel walls. Although this can be quite important in humans with hypertension or atherosclerosis, administration of general anesthetics or sedatives may also disturb the normal vasoconstrictor responses to hypovolemia in other species as well. Even when overall blood flow to an organ or region seems adequate, the flow may be traversing "preferred" route capillaries rather than nutrient vessels. Shunting through arteriovenous anastomoses can also occur.[5] Maldistribution of tissue perfusion is the result.

Increases in blood viscosity also impair microcirculatory flow by leading to rouleau formation, with aggregation of red blood cells and platelets in low-flow vessels. Many factors can enhance platelet aggregation, including adenosine diphosphate, thrombin, collagen fragments, hydrogen ions, epinephrine, and endotoxin. Endotoxemia readily results from trauma, pancreatitis, and splanchnic ischemia; the severity of peripheral circulatory failure associated with these conditions is partly due to the effects of endotoxemia on the complement, coagulation, and fibrinolytic cascades. In low-flow states, therefore, a degree of hemodilution (packed cell volume about 30%) is thought to improve tissue oxygen delivery, assuming arterial oxygen tension and cardiac output are normal.

The fluid volume within the interstitial compartment is almost four times the plasma volume.

Most of this is found in the skin, viscera, and skeletal muscle. With sustained hemorrhage, much of this fluid is transferred to the vascular compartment. Later, as microvascular pressure relationships change, transport of fluid from the vascular to interstitial compartments occurs; some of this fluid enters hypoxic cells to a degree dependent on the severity and duration of shock. The gastrointestinal tract appears most vulnerable to this cell swelling. Ultimately, the fate of the animal may be largely influenced by the absorption of gut toxins through a damaged mucosa.

An early consequence of decreased oxygen availability is a reduction in cellular adenosine triphosphate (ATP) content. When tissue oxygen tension decreases to a critical level, oxidative phosphorylation is uncoupled and ATP production gradually ceases.[5] This results in mitochondrial swelling, cell membrane deterioration, abnormalities in calcium flux within the cell, intracellular accumulation of Na^+, Ca^{++}, water, and lactic acidosis. Anoxic damage and high intracellular Ca^{++} interfere with plasma membrane adenylate cyclase activity; this prevents normal catecholamine responsiveness and may explain why precapillary arterioles do not respond to adrenergic agents during late shock.[11] Energy depletion is probably not the only factor in cell membrane dysfunction, however, since this has also occurred despite normal tissue ATP concentrations.[13] In severe shock, lactate accumulation can increase fivefold or so. High plasma lactate levels have been correlated with a poor prognosis.[11]

Lysosomal disruption is believed to follow rather than cause cell death. Significant structural changes occur in other cell organelles late in the ischemic process also. The susceptibility of cells to hypoxia and ischemia varies. For example, astrocytes survive for only seconds, skeletal muscle functions anaerobically for about 30 minutes, and hepatic cells can function for several hours.[5] Plasma membrane and early mitochondrial changes may be reversible if prompt therapy is given. Experimentally, several agents have been shown to attenuate or reverse some adverse metabolic effects: $ATP\text{-}MgCl_2$,[5] glucose-insulin-K^+,[5,14] calcium channel blockers,[5,14] and corticosteroids.[5] As yet the clinical value of these agents remains unproven.

With progression of the shock state marked decreases in systemic arterial pressure and cardiac output occur. More and more tissues are forced into anaerobic glycolysis as ischemia and hypoxia develop in vital organs. The resulting lactic acidosis is potentiated by reduced liver metabolism and reduced renal excretion of circulating lactate. Hyperglycemia may result from catecholamine-stimulated glycogenolysis, inhibition of insulin release and peripheral insulin resistance. Eventually, though, glycogen stores are depleted and hypoglycemia ensues.

The development of disseminated intravascular coagulation may potentiate regional ischemia. Activation of the coagulation and platelet cascades, followed by the fibrinolytic plasmin cascade is initiated by endothelial and tissue damage from hypoxia, endotoxins, exotoxins, and immune complexes; collagen is exposed and tissue thromboplastins are released into the circulation, triggering these cascades. Hypercoagulability (mediated by platelet and coagulation cascades) with microvasculature thrombosis and tissue ischemia, or hypocoagulability (mediated by plasmin cascade) with abnormal bleeding may predominate. Hypercoagulability is accentuated by poor capillary blood flow and increased viscosity, acidosis, high fibrinogen levels, increased platelet adhesiveness and catecholamines.[16] Eventually, coagulation precursors are depleted and the fibrinolytic process predominates.

EFFECTS ON VARIOUS ORGAN SYSTEMS
Heart

The effects of shock on different organ systems may be profound. In the heart, prolonged shock of any cause leads to a decrease in cardiac function associated with poor coronary perfusion, hypoxia, reduced cellular ATP, and metabolic acidosis. Persistence of high intracellular Ca^{++} in the heart interferes with diastolic and systolic function and eventually can lead to asystole.[5] Circulating myocardial depressant factors can contribute to decreased cardiac performance. As myocardial function and compliance decline and end diastolic pressures rise, coronary perfusion is further compromised. Sympathetic activation of the heart increases oxygen demands in the face of reduced oxygen delivery. Peripheral vasoconstriction further increases left ventricular outflow impedance, oxygen demand, and myocardial ischemia. Arrhythmias may result and can intensify shock by further decreasing cardiac output. Unless the shock is effectively treated, the downward spiral of events progresses until cardiac dysfunction becomes irreversible and the animal dies.[1,4]

Lung

In the lung, hyperventilation (with respiratory alkalosis) occurs early, possibly in response to the effects of vasoactive substances on pulmonary receptors. Later, hyperventilation is an attempt to compensate for the progressive metabolic acidosis that develops.[3] Poor pulmonary blood flow predisposes to atelectasis and infection. Respiratory failure in untreated shock may result from respiratory muscle fatigue secondary to ischemia, failure of the respiratory center, development of "shock lung," or a combination.[3,4] Acute respiratory distress syndrome (ARDS) or "shock lung" often follows shock of any cause, in man within 24 to 72 hours. Multiple pathologic factors may cause the interstitial and alveolar edema that occurs, including increased alveolar capillary membrane permeability, high capillary hydrostatic pressure (from left ventricular failure), reduced plasma oncotic pressure, reduced pulmonary lymphatic function, deficient surfactant production (secondary to hypoxia), loss of alveolar type I cells, and replacement by proliferating type II cells (resulting in thickening of the alveolar septa).[3,4] Onset of widespread lung injury has been attributed to complement activation and white-cell aggregation, release of superoxides from neutrophil phagocytosis, proteases causing destruction of collagen and fibronectin, and platelet aggregation.[4] Prostaglandins and thromboxane are thought to be involved, especially in endotoxic shock.[4] Compromised reticuloendothelial system function causes reduced clearance of bacterial components, fibrin and fibrin degradation products, and injured platelets, all of which can contribute to pulmonary edema. Extravasated protein raises pulmonary interstitial oncotic pressure and facilitates edema formation. Infiltration of the pulmonary interstitium with mesenchymal, inflammatory, and other cells can lead to capillary and alveolar obliteration with interstitial fibrosis.[3] Clinically, these pulmonary changes are characterized by tachypnea, inspiratory crackles, and potentially severe hypoxemia. Reduced pulmonary compliance, and ventilation-perfusion mismatch leading to venous admixture, and intrapulmonary right to left shunts develop as pulmonary edema worsens. Pulmonary edema in shock is potentiated by excess intravenous fluid administration and bacterial exposure. Dogs appear to be less susceptible to ARDS than humans and cats.

Kidney

In the kidney, initial compensation for reduced blood flow is provided by increased efferent arteriolar tone, which helps maintain glomerular filtration rate, and redistribution of intrarenal blood flow to nephrons deep within the cortex. However, oliguria and acute renal failure develop with worsening renal ischemia. It is thought that abnormalities of intrarenal blood flow distribution as well as diminishing glomerular filtration rate caused by afferent arteriolar constriction are involved. Structural factors contributing to renal embarrassment include leakage of filtrate through injured tubular endothelium, which causes interstitial edema and tubular collapse, tubular obstruction with casts and debris, and tubular necrosis.[4] With supportive care, possibly including dialysis, adequate renal function usually returns.[4]

Gastrointestinal

With hypoxia and ischemia resulting from vasoconstriction, the liver may develop isolated areas of centrilobular necrosis followed later by widespread hepatic necrosis. Reticuloendothelial cell function becomes compromised and may allow entry of intestinal bacteria into the circulation.[4] This may depend partly on declines in circulating opsonins such as fibronectin.[3]

The bowel is subject to hemorrhagic necrosis, especially of the gastric mucosal layer, secondary to severe vasoconstriction and ischemia.[3,4,13] Mucosal cell damage and necrosis lead to erosions and hemorrhage. With extensive submucosal hemorrhage significant sequestration of blood can occur. Bowel injury can lead to pooling of fluid in the gut and absorption of bacteria and toxins,[4] both of which can worsen the shock state. The effects of endotoxin, vasoactive substances (such as histamine and lysosomal hydrolases) and depressant factors further insult the tissue.

Intense vasoconstriction also occurs in the pancreas. Release of vasoactive and cardiodepressant polypeptides from the hypoxic pancreas may further the development and severity of shock.[3]

Central nervous system

The brain responds to hypoxia by vasodilation. To some degree this is opposed by hypocapnia resulting from hyperventilation. However, cerebral blood flow remains relatively constant until mean systemic arterial pressure falls below 60 mm Hg, when cerebral perfusion becomes progressively compromised.[4]

THERAPY

Therapy for an animal in shock should occur at several levels (see the following box). The initial aim is to restore organ perfusion in order to provide adequate oxygen for tissue needs. Restoration of arterial blood pressure, vascular volume, and cardiac output is of paramount importance in supporting tissue oxygenation. In addition, controlling or reversing the initiating cause of the shock, if possible, is obviously very important. Third, complications of shock such as acute renal failure, metabolic acidosis, coagulopathies, or ARDS must be prevented or managed (see box, p. 169). Delay in instituting therapy increases the likelihood that the shock state will become nonre-

---

GENERAL GUIDE TO SHOCK TREATMENT

Shock detected
  Place intravenous line
  Rapid fluid administration (isotonic with or without hypertonic crystalloid)
  Search for and treat cause of shock
Begin monitoring
  Capillary refill time
  Pulse rate and quality
  Respirations
  Rectal and toe web temperature
  Urine output
  Hematocrit
  Serum protein
  Arterial blood pressure
  Central venous pressure or pulmonary wedge pressure
  Blood gases
If hemodilution (packed cell volume <25-30%)
  Whole-blood transfusion
If hypoproteinemia (serum protein <3.5 or albumin <1.5 g/dL)
  Plasma transfusion or synthetic colloid administration
Packed cell volume/serum proteins at acceptable levels
  Continue isotonic crystalloid fluids
Continued poor peripheral perfusion, with high central venous pressure or pulmonary capillary wedge pressure
  Inotropic support (dopamine, dobutamine)
  Bicarbonate
  Careful fluid administration
  Consider glucocorticoid
  Consider antimicrobials
  Consider respiratory support
  Watch for and treat complications
Continued poor peripheral perfusion, with normal central venous pressure or pulmonary capillary wedge pressure
  Continued fluid push
  Bicarbonate
  Consider glucocorticoid
  Consider antimicrobials
  Watch for and treat complications
Return of acceptable perfusion
  Maintenance fluids
  Watch for and treat complications

---

versible, with development of multiple-organ failure, refractory and widespread microvascular and subcellular disturbances, and death.

Fluid administration

Blood volume expansion is considered the most important element of therapy. Adequate cardiac

COMPLICATIONS OF SHOCK

Oliguric acute renal failure
Metabolic acidosis
Gastrointestinal hemorrhage and ulceration
Endotoxemia/sepsis
Disseminated intravascular coagulopathy
Cardiac arrhythmias
Heart failure
Acute respiratory distress syndrome
Hyperglycemia (peripheral insulin resistance)
Hypoglycemia (septic or refractory shock)

output and systemic blood pressure, highly important to tissue perfusion, are dependent on blood volume. The degree of volume replacement needed by the animal in shock is variable. In general, dogs require 40 to 90 ml/kg and cats 20 to 60 ml/kg of initial (crystalloid) volume replacement.[10] Severe shock states, especially when accompanied by peripheral vasodilation (nonresponsive peripheral vasculature) such as septic shock, require much more volume replacement to achieve satisfactory cardiac filling pressures. The types of fluids used include both crystalloids and colloids. A crystalloid solution is one with particles with molecular weights less than 30,000, whereas colloid particles are larger and will not pass through a semipermeable membrane.

Crystalloids. Usually the initial fluid of choice is a crystalloid solution with a fairly normal sodium concentration (130 to 154 mEq/L). These fluids are inexpensive and can be given rapidly. When underlying cardiopulmonary or brain disease is present, however, careful monitoring is necessary to avoid pulmonary or cerebral edema while still restoring acceptable organ perfusion. Such large fluid replacement volumes are needed since only about 25% to 30% of a crystalloid solution remains in the vascular space 30 minutes after administration, the rest having diffused into the interstitial compartment.[10] Because of this rapid diffusion from the vascular space, further fluid administration in the form of colloids or whole blood may be needed if the animal again shows evidence of hypotension or vasoconstriction. Complicating interstitial edema may develop as fluid leaves the vascular space and can cause disturbances in organ function, especially of the pulmonary, cerebral, or gastrointestinal systems.[4] Administration of plasma, whole blood or synthetic colloids should help ameliorate this.

Rapid intravenous fluid administration is critical. Use of fluids relatively high in sodium such as normal (0.9%) saline or lactated Ringer's solution are recommended. The sodium in these fluids stays mostly in the extracellular and intravascular spaces, thus holding water here also. Because the vascular space is only about 30% of the volume of the extracellular fluid compartment, the volume of these replacement crystalloids needs to be three to four times the volume lost. This will compensate for redistribution of this fluid to the extravascular, extracellular space. Crystalloid fluids with only small concentrations of sodium tend to move into the intracellular space to a greater degree. Thus, they have lesser volume expansion power and cause greater interstitial edema. Therefore, 5% dextrose in water and low sodium maintenance solutions are not recommended in the treatment of shock.[4]

Hypertonic saline. The use of hypertonic saline solutions (4% to 7.5%) has strong effects on extracellular and vascular volume expansion.[17,18] Small volumes of hypertonic saline (such as 4 to 5 ml/kg of 2400 mOsm [7.5%] solution) have had significant effects on resuscitation in hemorrhagic and septic shock.[13,17,19-21] The osmotic load "steals" fluid from the intracellular space to augment extracellular and circulating volume. Other effects also occur including a fall in peripheral vascular resistance (possibly from a direct vasodilating effect of the hypertonic solution) and improved cardiac contractility and performance. The administration of 6% dextran along with hypertonic saline increases the vascular volume expanding effect.[22]

In untreated hemorrhagic shock there is an endogenously generated increase in plasma osmolality that facilitates the expansion of blood volume early in shock. Several studies have shown that plasma osmolality can rise by 31 mOsm/L in just over an hour after hemorrhage.[23] This is primarily due to hyperglycemia, the degree of which depends on the extent of hemorrhage. The spontaneous rise in plasma osmolality will cause restoration of 5 to 10 ml of lost volume per kilogram of body weight over the course of 1 to 2 hours of hemorrhage.[23] The greatest source of added glucose and osmolality has been shown to be the hepatosplanchnic and renal vascular beds. The most important source of added vascular water was skin and skeletal muscle.[21,23] Sympathetic-mediated pancreatic release of glucagon, systemic catecholamine release and hepatic adrenergic activation are involved in sustaining the hepatic glucogenic response and increase in plasma osmolality that occurs in hemorrhagic shock.[23] Some studies have shown an estimate of two thirds of shed blood volume being replaced by intracellular and interstitial fluid in 1 hour.[23] It is believed that neurohumoral effects on the microvasculature are important, in addition to the osmotic changes contributing to increases in blood volume. In skeletal muscle capillary beds, early alpha-adrenergic and angiotensin II-mediated constriction of venous capacitance vessels, arteriolar resistance vessels, and precapillary sphincters reduces the size of the intravascular space relative to the circulating volume. Later, beta$_2$- and hypoxia-induced precapillary sphincter relaxation results in resetting of pericapillary resistance vessels and greater postcapillary vessel dilation; the net result is greater flow at lower pressure. This, along with increased plasma osmolality, favors Starling's forces for transfer of interstitial to vascular fluid. It is speculated that infusion of exogenous hypertonic fluid might be synergistic with this.[23]

Some experimental studies have shown a temporary improvement with one bolus of hypertonic saline, while others have produced a permanent resuscitative effect.[11,17,18,21,24] Some have suggested that the presence of a reflex involving the lungs is required for the effect.[21] There is debate as to whether it is the hypertonicity or the total sodium load that confers the beneficial circulatory effect. It is thought that the transient hemodynamic improvement after 7.5% sodium chloride could prevent or slow development of cellular damage and metabolic dysfunction during severe hypovolemia so that after volume repletion the shock is reversible.[11] The initial administration of small volumes of hypertonic saline has increased the response to subsequent infusions of isotonic fluids,[18] and it may be especially valuable when large amounts of isotonic fluid cannot be given fast enough. Adverse side effects from use of hypertonic saline appear to be minimal. Further information on the use of hypertonic saline is found in Chapter 38.

Colloids and blood. Hemodilution may result from excessively aggressive fluid therapy, especially after hemorrhage. Hypoproteinemia can allow fluid to seep into the interstitial space from the vascular space more easily, because of reduced intravascular colloid oncotic pressure. The ability to achieve adequate volume expansion is impaired and interstitial edema is increased, to the potential detriment of organ function. These are more likely to be significant clinical problems when total serum protein is less than 3.5 to 4 g/dL or albumin is less than 1.5 g/dL. Plasma or plasma substitutes should be administered when such a hypoproteinemic animal is still in need of volume expansion. These colloid volume expanders help counteract the effects of reduced plasma colloid oncotic pressure and can keep more fluid in the intravascular space. Plasma is the most effective colloid. Its effects are long lasting; for example, the half-life of canine albumin is about 15 days.[2]

The hemoglobin concentration of circulating blood is important because of its crucial role in oxygen transport. In severe shock, especially from sepsis or trauma, blood loss and hemodilution may cause a significant drop in oxygen-carrying capacity in the face of increased oxygen demands. In these instances, a hematocrit below 30% may be insufficient to meet tissue oxygen needs. In less severe cases of shock, the animal may tolerate a packed cell volume in the 20% to 25% range. When excessive hemodilution has occurred, especially if the packed cell volume is near or below 20%, and further volume loading is indicated, whole blood should be given. Fresh blood or plasma will also provide platelets and clotting factors, which may be needed if disseminated intravascular coagulation is occurring. Fresh frozen plasma also will supply clotting factors. Further information on transfusions is found in Chapter 34.

Dextrans or other synthetic colloid volume expanders are helpful in the absence of suitable plasma or whole blood. Dextrans are high-molecular-weight polysaccharides available in two forms. Dextran 70 (a 6% solution) is similar to albumin in that it has an average molecular weight of 70,000. Dextran 40 (a 10% solution) has an average molecular weight of 40,000. The dextran 70 has a longer half-life (about 24 hours), whereas dextran 40 is rapidly excreted in the urine and has a half-life of only about 3 hours.[16] Dextran 40 has been used mainly to augment blood volume and tissue perfusion during the early phases of therapy and to decrease microvascular sludging. Another synthetic colloid is hydroxyethyl starch (hetastarch), available as a 400,000 molecular weight, 6% solution. This substance is effective for 12 to 48 hours.[16] The dosage for these synthetic colloids is 10 to 20 mL/kg per day. Infusion rates should be limited to 2 to 5 ml/kg/hr. Adverse effects of colloids include hypervolemia, hyperviscosity, and hemorrhagic diathesis (usually as a result of too rapid or excessive administration). Rarely, allergic reactions to the synthetic colloids can occur. If capillary damage is present, colloids may leak from the vasculature; with ARDS this potentiates pulmonary edema.[4]

Other high-osmolality solutions include hypertonic glucose and mannitol. Because these have very short durations of action they are not recommended for volume expansion in hypoproteinemic states.

Cardiovascular support

In most cases, underlying cardiac function in the early stages of shock is adequate and the patient responds well to aggressive fluid therapy and restoration of venous return. Cardiac output and myocardial perfusion increase, and blood pressure usually returns to normal. However, with cardiogenic shock, or the late stages of other types of shock when the heart and blood vessels become unresponsive to volume replacement, the use of inotropic or vasoactive drugs can be important. When there is evidence of poor peripheral perfusion and low cardiac output despite vigorous fluid therapy, along with an elevated central venous pressure, positive inotropic therapy should be initiated.

The drugs most often used for inotropic support are dopamine and dobutamine. In addition to having positive inotropic effects mediated by beta receptors, in low dosages (2 to 5 μg/kg per minute) dopamine can improve renal and splanchnic perfusion by its vasodilatory effects via dopaminergic receptor activation. Higher dosages of dopamine can cause tachycardia and vasoconstriction by stimulation of alpha receptors. Dobutamine is a synthetic catecholamine with mainly $beta_1$ effects. It has minimal effects on heart rate and peripheral vascular resistance except at high dosages. Recommended infusion rates are 3 to 10 μg/kg per minute. Isoproterenol has strong vasodilating properties and should not be used in shock. Epinephrine is arrhythmogenic and has vasoconstrictor effects; it is not used on a sustained basis in shock.

Drugs that have strong alpha-adrenergic effects such as norepinephrine, phenylephrine, or methoxamine are generally not indicated. These drugs have powerful vasoconstrictive effects and thus can further impair tissue perfusion. However, such a drug could be useful in late shock, in which persistent hypotension and low systemic vascular resistance are unresponsive to aggressive volume expansion (see Chapter 15).

Cardiac rhythm disturbances occur frequently in some types of shock, especially that caused by trauma. Antiarrhythmic therapy may be indicated depending on the severity of the arrhythmia and the animal's hemodynamic status. For ventricular tachyarrhythmias, lidocaine is the first drug of choice. This intravenous agent has minimal cardiodepressant and hypotensive effects. Boluses of up to a total of 8 mg/kg can be give initially to dogs. Cats are much more sensitive to the neurotoxic effects of this drug. Initial doses of 0.25 mg/kg up to 1 mg/kg slowly intravenously can be used. Lidocaine can be given by intravenous constant rate infusion at 25 to 80 μg/kg per minute

for dogs. Further information on this and other antiarrhythmic therapy can be found in Chapter 17.

Glucocorticoids

After many years of study, the use of glucocorticoids in shock is still controversial. Some studies suggest their use in septic shock is advantageous,[25-27] while others show no beneficial effect in reversing shock or reducing overall mortality.[3,28] Postulated beneficial effects, especially in septic shock, include restoration of the phagocytic function of the reticuloendothelial system, reduced platelet and neutrophil aggregation, stabilization of lysosomal membranes, inhibition of the release of vasoactive peptides, interference with the arachidonic acid cascade by inhibiting phospholipase A_2, promotion of increased oxygen delivery to peripheral tissues, elevation of blood glucose levels, and reduction of cerebral edema.[29] Their inhibitory effects on leukocyte margination and perivascular leukocyte degeneration are thought to be especially important in septic shock, since secondary pulmonary insufficiency appears to be in large part caused by pericapillary sequestration of leukocytes.[30] Corticosteroids may also reduce the absorption of endotoxin from the gut.[31] Detrimental effects can include gastrointestinal hemorrhage and ulceration, immunosuppression, delayed wound healing, adrenal suppression, hepatopathy, and exacerbation of the severity of acute pancreatitis. If a glucocorticoid is selected as part of therapy, it should be given as early as possible in the course of the shock state and in large doses. Studies have shown that an aqueous salt is needed for optimal effects.[26] Suggested intravenous shock doses are hydrocortisone (sodium phosphate or sodium succinate esters) 300 mg/kg every 4 hours, prednisolone (sodium phosphate or sodium succinate esters) 10 to 30 mg/kg every 8 hours, and dexamethasone (sodium phosphate or sodium succinate esters) 6 to 15 mg/kg every 12 hours.

Acid-base balance

Use of a crystalloid solution containing a bicarbonatelike anion for initial volume replacement helps prevent dilutional acidosis that can occur with normal saline or plain Ringer's solution. The addition of 24 mEq/L of sodium bicarbonate to 0.9% saline will counteract its acidifying tendency.[16] Lactate (as in lactated Ringer's solution) is adequate, although hepatic metabolism is required for it to be effective. Concern that use of lactated Ringer's solution would aggravate existing lactic acidosis has not been borne out experimentally.[4] Acetate and gluconate are metabolized by other tissues as well and may be preferable to lactate.[32] Bicarbonate does not need to be metabolized to be effective.

Severe metabolic acidosis secondary to anaerobic metabolism may develop in shock. Ideally, arterial or venous blood gases should be used to measure the degree of acidosis. In this way the animal's base deficit can be determined and calculation of replacement sodium bicarbonate made by multiplying base deficit times 0.3 times kilograms of body weight. Slow intravenous bicarbonate administration (over 30 minutes) can then be initiated if necessary (see Chapter 38). When blood gas analysis is unavailable, measurement of venous bicarbonate or total carbon dioxide can give an estimate of acid-base status as long as pulmonary function is relatively normal. Clinical estimation of the adequacy of peripheral perfusion can help guide bicarbonate therapy in the absence of the above methods. Empirical doses of 1.0, 3.0, and 5.0 mg/kg of intravenous sodium bicarbonate have been recommended for mild, moderate, and severe malperfusion, respectively.[2] Bicarbonate, if given too rapidly or in excessive amounts, can cause alkalosis, severe hypotension, paradoxical cerebrospinal fluid acidosis, cerebral edema, hypercapnia, and vomiting. The need for bicarbonate therapy should be reassessed every 30 minutes initially, since its effects can be transient in the face of ongoing metabolic disturbances.

Renal support

Restoration of blood volume and arterial pressure are most important to renal perfusion. If urine output does not improve sufficiently once vascular volume and pressure have been adequately restored, diuretic therapy is indicated. Placement of an indwelling urinary catheter is helpful for monitoring urine flow rate. Furosemide (4 to 5 mg/kg intravenously) promotes renal vasodilation and has potent diuretic effects. A second dose may be given if the first has had no effect after 10 to 15 minutes. Alternatively, mannitol or glucose (0.5 g/kg intravenously over 20 to 30 minutes) acts as an osmotic diuretic by increasing blood volume and renal perfusion. If this is ineffective or contraindicated for any reason (e.g., congestive heart failure), dopamine (2 to 5 μg/kg per minute intravenously) should be tried. This drug promotes renal vasodilation through stimulation of dopaminergic receptors. The initial infusion dose should be low, then titrated slowly upward to effect. The dose should be decreased if the adverse effect of alpha-mediated peripheral vasoconstriction occurs. Sometimes the combination of furosemide and dopamine along with fluid therapy is effec-

tive. However, aggressive diuretic use may not improve glomerular filtration rate or prevent acute renal failure.[3] The potential of these drugs to aggravate hypovolemia and electrolyte disturbances should be recognized.

Respiratory support

Providing supplemental oxygen may be advantageous to patients in shock. Assisted ventilation, possibly with positive end-expiratory pressure, may be required as shock becomes more severe and pulmonary complications develop or if derangement of the respiratory center occurs. Chapter 36 contains specific information regarding respiratory support therapy.

Antibacterial therapy

The use of appropriate antibacterial therapy is critical in septic shock. When shock therapy is initiated, appropriate samples should be obtained for culture. Until these results are available, the initial antibiotic agents chosen should possess broad-spectrum activity. An in-depth discussion of septic shock and its treatment is found in Chapter 15.

Other therapies

Experimentally, antiprostaglandin antiinflammatory agents have been associated with hemodynamic improvement and increased survival in septic shock, especially when used in conjunction with fluids, antibiotics, and corticosteroids.[16] Important adverse side effects can include gastrointestinal ulceration and hemorrhage[16] and possibly renal damage (especially in the face of decreased renal perfusion). Further information on antiprostaglandins in septic shock is found in Chapter 15.

The development of disseminated intravascular coagulation is an important complication of shock. The patient's coagulation status and platelet numbers should be evaluated, especially if bleeding from multiple sites, petechiae, or abnormal clotting time is observed. Again, treatment of the underlying condition, vigorous fluid therapy to improve the microcirculation, and appropriate antibiotic therapy are important. In the hypercoagulable state, heparin is used. The effective dose is variable (see Chapter 23). A recommended starting dosage is 5 to 10 units/kg subcutaneously every 8 to 12 hours.[33] Several hours may be needed for effect because of heparin's dependence on antithrombin III. Since heparin can stimulate platelet aggregation,[15] aspirin administration (25 mg/kg, repeated if necessary once every 3 days) may counteract this. Depletion of clotting factors or their inhibition by fibrin and fibrin degradation products may require the use of fresh plasma transfusion with heparin treatment.

Use of cimetidine or ranitidine to decrease gastric acid secretion may help protect against mucosal ulceration. Sucralfate may prevent worsening of existing ulcers or perforation by its coating action (see Chapter 22). Nutritional support is important, especially in septic patients (see Chapter 37).

In shock, the use of such experimental treatments as naloxone,[16,34] fibronectin,[35] and granulocyte transfusion has been described. The development of lipopolysaccharide core or multivalent oligosaccharide antisera and other innovative therapies should expand the treatment arsenal in the future. In several laboratory models of shock, naloxone has had variable beneficial effects in reversing hypotension[34,36-38]; however, clinical trials in humans have not been encouraging.[39] Agents such as thyrotropin-releasing hormone and triiodothyronine are also being investigated for possible beneficial effects in septic and other types of shock.[3,40,41] Other experimental therapies include infusion of fructose-1, 6-diphosphate,[42] and administration of converting enzyme or thromboxane synthetase inhibitors.[43]

ASSESSING PATIENT STATUS

Because the hemodynamic and metabolic sequelae of the shock state are continually changing, it is important to assess clinical status frequently as well as taking objective measurements and adjusting therapy accordingly. Rapid fluid administration should proceed until there is evidence of adequate pulse quality and reversal of severe peripheral vasoconstriction. Objective measures of hemodynamic status include central venous pressure in the high normal range (5 to 10 or 12 cm H_2O), pulmonary capillary wedge pressure in the high normal range (10 to 15 mm Hg), or arterial blood pressure greater than 60 mm Hg (mean), and greater than 80 mm Hg (systolic). Return of these hemodynamic variables to acceptable levels does not ensure adequate regional blood flow and organ perfusion, however. Because of the profound vasoconstrictive response, especially in the early stages of shock, arterial blood pressure or femoral pulse pressure may be misleading measures of the adequacy of volume replacement. Use of central venous pressure gives an indication of right ventricular filling pressures, and in the absence of cardiopulmonary disease it may approximate left ventricular filling pressure; however, it does not necessarily reflect circulating blood volume.[3,4] If widespread venoconstriction or reduced right ventricular function is present, or if mechanical ventilatory support is used, central venous pressure may not decrease with hypovolemia. Thus, use of central venous pressure alone to guide fluid therapy may be misleading. The placement of a Swan-Ganz catheter into the pulmonary artery allows measurement of pulmonary arterial pressures and pulmonary capillary wedge pressures (which reflect left atrial and, thus, left ventricular filling pressures), as well as providing access for mixed venous blood samples. Indirect measures of organ perfusion such as capillary refill time, mucous membrane color, urine output, toe-web temperature, and improved mentation are also important in assessing therapy.[44]

Electrolyte balance should be monitored as therapy progresses. Once the initial fluid loading has been accomplished, adjustments in the electrolyte composition of the administered fluid may be necessary. Blood glucose must also be monitored, especially in septic shock, where high glucose utilization can result in significant hypoglycemia.

SPECIFIC SHOCK SYNDROMES
Hemorrhagic shock

The effects of hemorrhage vary depending on the amount and rapidity of blood loss, the patient's age and underlying health, and the speed and adequacy of resuscitation. In general, the rapid loss of about 30% or more of blood volume results in hemorrhagic shock. Initial therapy is aimed at preventing further blood loss and rapid replacement of blood volume. Secondary goals of treatment include reducing the consequences of decreased blood volume, such as low arterial pressure, poor cardiac output, and increased sympathetic nervous response.

Nonhemorrhagic hypovolemic shock

Loss of fluid from the body or third-space sequestration of fluid can result in shock. Examples include severe burns, obstructive or adynamic ileus, pancreatitis, protracted vomiting or diarrhea, diabetes insipidus, excess renal sodium and water loss, ascites, peritonitis, trauma to skeletal muscle, and excessive diuretic use. With severe thermal injury the amount of fluid lost is proportional to the area burned; increased capillary permeability leads to fluid sequestration in the extravascular space, with tissue edema and hemoconcentration (see Chapter 16).

Clinical features of hypovolemic shock include arterial vasoconstriction, hypotension, reduced venous pressure, hemoconcentration, tachycardia, and oliguria. Rapid fluid replacement is obviously important, along with correction of the underlying cause.

Distributive shock

This category includes shock states caused by sepsis, neurologic disturbance, anaphylaxis, or metabolic, toxic or endocrinologic depression of vasomotor tone. The common feature is inappropriate vasodilation leading to maldistribution of vascular volume and impaired organ perfusion. Cardiac output may be increased, decreased, or normal. Refer to Chapter 15 for further information regarding septic shock and endotoxemia.

On occasion, neurogenic shock results from primary central nervous system disease, toxic depression of the nervous system, heat stroke, or other causes. Disturbances in autonomic regulation are thought to be involved, with sudden loss of sympathetic tone.[3] The features of neurogenic shock include relative hypovolemia from reduced sympathetic tone, and increased vagal tone with vasodilation and bradycardia. If possible, the underlying cause should be addressed and fluids, positive inotropic support, and pressor agents given.

Anaphylactic shock

Exposure to a natural antigen or drug in a sensitized individual can induce a peracute systemic hypersensitivity reaction (anaphylaxis), which may progress to anaphylactic shock. The combination of specific antigen and reaginic (usually IgE) antibody on mast cells and basophils results in cell degranulation and release of vasoactive mediators. Histamine, leukotrienes, platelet-activating factor, and other substances, including prostaglandins, thromboxane, kinins, and catecholamines are involved in anaphylaxis.[8,45] These mediators cause widespread vasodilation, increases in capillary permeability, bronchoconstriction, and changes in the coagulation system. It is thought that leukotrienes C4, D4, and E4 (slow-reacting substances of anaphylaxis) and histamine are the major mediators in dogs and cats.[45] Although IgE-mediated mast-cell degranulation is the most common cause of anaphylaxis, mast-cell and basophil degranulation can also be triggered by complement components (C3a, C5a) generated by the alternate complement pathway. Some bacterial and fungal cell walls, polysaccharides, enzymes, tumor cells, and other substances may activate the alternate complement pathway.[45] Clinical signs occur within minutes of exposure. Hypotension is the hallmark of anaphylactic shock. Angioedema, urticaria, laryngeal edema, gastrointestinal inflammation, and bronchospasm may also occur. In dogs there is marked constriction of hepatic veins accompanied by portal hypertension and splanchnic congestion; decreased venous return to the heart, signs of plasma vol-

ume depletion with hemoconcentration, and shock result.[3,45] Pallor, tachycardia, vomiting, diarrhea, respiratory distress, and collapse are the clinical signs, along with angioedema and urticaria. In cats, the respiratory as well as intestinal tracts are severely affected. Cutaneous signs and pruritus are more common in cats than in dogs.[45]

Therapy involves removal of antigen exposure, epinephrine, antihistamines, glucocorticoids, and intravenous fluids. Epinephrine (0.01 ml/kg of 1:1000 dilution intramuscularly) reduces bronchoconstriction and splanchnic blood pooling. With severe hypotension, the 1:10,000 dilution of epinephrine can be given intravenously in 0.5- to 1.0-mL boluses up to a maximum of 5.0 mL. Epinephrine may be repeated within 15 to 30 minutes if needed. The antihistamine diphenhydramine can be administered intramuscularly or slowly intravenously (1.0 to 2.0 mg/kg). Glucocorticoids may be helpful in suppressing the hypersensitivity response although their efficacy in reducing mortality in shock is controversial. Suggested doses of water-soluble glucocorticoids are listed above. Rapid intravenous fluid administration is important in anaphylactic shock as in other types of shock. Respiratory support and bronchodilators are given as needed.

Cardiogenic and obstructive shock

Cardiogenic shock occurs when the pumping function of the heart is severely impaired, leading to circulatory failure. Along with clinical signs of reduced cardiac output, arterial hypotension, and high sympathetic tone there may be evidence of cardiac arrhythmias, acute pulmonary edema, rapid and shallow respirations, decreased-intensity heart sounds, and systemic venous distention (if right heart failure is present). The underlying pathophysiologic abnormality must be identified for optimal treatment of cardiogenic or obstructive shock. For example, inotropic support, along with diuretic, fluid, and other therapies is required for cardiomyopathy (cardiogenic shock), whereas pericardiocentesis is needed if the cause is pericardial tamponade (obstructive shock). Further information on cardiologic emergencies is found in Chapter 17.

REFERENCES

1. Sobel BE. Cardiac and noncardiac forms of acute circulatory failure (shock). In Braunwald E, ed. Heart Diease: A Textbook of Cardiovascular Medicine. Philadelphia: WB Saunders, 1984;578-604.
2. Schertel ER, Muir WW. Shock: Pathophysiology, monitoring, and therapy. In Kirk RW, ed. Current Veterinary Therapy X. Philadelphia: WB Saunders, 1989;316-330.
3. Skowronski GA. The pathophysiology of shock. Med J Aust 1988;148:576-583.

4. Billhardt RA, Rosenbusch SW. Cardiogenic and hypovolemic shock. Med Clin North Am 1986;70:853-876.
5. Ledingham IM, Ramsay G. Hypovolaemic shock. Br J Anaesth 1986;58:169-189.
6. Kemppainen RJ. Pituitary-adrenal responses to hemorrhage. ACVIM Forum Proc 1987;5:84-86.
7. Whaley K, Yee Khong T, McCartney AC, Ledingham IM. Alternate pathway complement activation and its control in gram-negative endotoxin shock. J Clin Lab Immun 1979;2:117.
8. Feuerstein G, Hallenbeck JM. Prostaglandins, leukotrienes, and platelet-activating factor in shock. Annu Rev Pharmacol Toxicol 1987;27:301-313.
9. Fletcher JR, Ramwell PW, Herman CM. Prostaglandins and the hemodynamic course of endotoxin shock. J Surg Res 1976;20:589-594.
10. Haskins SC. Shock. In Fox PR, ed. Canine and Feline Cardiology. New York; Churchill Livingstone, 1988;229-254.
11. Ferguson DC. Metabolic and endocrine alterations in shock. ACVIM Forum Proc 1987;5:80-83.
12. Bitterman H, Triolo J, Lefer AM. Use of hypertonic saline in the treatment of hemorrhagic shock. Circ Shock 1987;21:271-283.
13. Bailey RW, Bulkley GB, Hamilton SR, et al. The fundamental hemodynamic mechanism underlying gastric "stress ulceration" in cardiogenic shock. Ann Surg 1987; 205:597-612.
14. Luypaert P, Vincent JL, Domb M, et al. Fluid resuscitation with hypertonic saline in endotoxic shock. Circ Shock 1986;20:311-320.
15. Lee HC, Lum BKB. Protective action of calcium entry blockers in endotoxin shock. Circ Shock 1986;18:193-203.
16. Hardaway RM. Pathology and pathophysiology of disseminated intravascular coagulation. In Cowley RA, Trump BF, eds. Pathophysiology of Shock, Anoxia, and Ischemia. Baltimore: Williams & Wilkins, 1982;186-197.
17. Nakayama S, Sibley L, Gunther RA, et al. Small-volume resuscitation with hypertonic saline (2400 mOsm/L) during hemorrhagic shock. Circ Shock 1984;13:149-159.
18. Kramer GC, Perron PR, Lindsey DC, et al. Small volume resuscitation with hypertonic saline dextran solution. Surgery 1986;100:239-245.
19. Layon J, Duncan D, Gallagher TJ, et al. Hypertonic saline as a resuscitation solution in hemorrhagic shock: effects on extravascular lung water and cardiopulmonary function. Anesth Analg 1987;66:154-158.
20. Peters RM, Shackford SR, Hogan JS, et al. Comparison of isotonic and hypertonic fluids in resuscitation from hypovolemic shock. Surg Gynecol Obstet 1986;163:219-224.
21. Rocha-e-Silva M, Negraes GA, Soares AM, et al. Hypertonic resuscitation from severe hemorrhagic shock: patterns of regional circulation. Circ Shock 1986;19:165-175.
22. Smith GJ, Kramer GC, Perron P. A comparison of several hypertonic solutions for resuscitation of bled sheep. J Surg Res 1985;39:517-528.
23. Fettman MJ. Hypertonic crystalloid solution for treating hemorrhagic shock. Compend Contin Educ 1985;7:915-920.
24. Velasco IT, Pontieri V, Rocha-e-Silva M, et al. Hyperosmotic NaCl and severe hemorrhagic shock. Am J Physiol 1980;239:H664-H673.
25. Schumer W. Steroids in the treatment of clinical septic shock. Ann Surg 1976;184:333.
26. White GL, White GS, Kosanke SD, et al. Therapeutic effects of prednisolone sodium succinate vs dexamethasone in dogs subjected to E. coli septic shock. J Am Anim Hosp Assoc 1982;18:639-648.
27. Hardaway RM, Williams CH, Dozier SE. Influence of steroids on hemorrhagic and traumatic shock. J Trauma 1987;27:667-670.
28. Sprung CL, Caralis PV, Marcial EH, et al. The effects of high-dose corticosteroids in patients with septic shock. N Engl J Med 1984;311:1137-1143.
29. Hubbard JD, Janssen HF. Effects of methylprednisolone upon vascular permeability changes in endotoxic shock. Circ Shock 1986;18:179-192.
30. Shasby DM, Hunninghake GW. Endotoxin-induced pulmonary leukostasis. In Hinshaw LB, ed. Handbook of Endotoxin, vol. 2: Pathophysiology of Endotoxin. New York: Elsevier Science, 1985;105-128.
31. Gaffin SL, Gathiram P, Wells MT. Effect of corticosteroid prophylaxis on lipopolysaccharide levels associated with intestinal ischemia in cats. Crit Care Med 1986; 14:889-891.
32. Hartsfield SM, Thurmon JC, Corbin JE. Effects of sodium acetate, bicarbonate and lactate on acid-base status in anaesthetized dogs. J Vet Pharmacol Ther 1981;4:51-61.
33. Ruehl W, Mills C, Feldman BF. Rational therapy in disseminated intravascular coagulation. J Am Vet Med Assoc 1982;181:76-78.
34. Vargish T, Beamer K. Hemodynamic effects of naloxone in early canine hypovolemic shock. Circ Shock 1985; 17:45-57.
35. Saba TM, Jaffe E. Plasma fibronectin (opsonic glycoprotein): its synthesis by vascular endothelial cells and role in cardiopulmonary integrity after trauma as related to reticuloendothelial function. Am J Med 1980;68:577.
36. Beamer KC, Vargish T. Effect of methylprednisolone on naloxone's hemodynamic response in canine hypovolemic shock. Crit Care Med 1986;14:115-119.
37. Van der Meer K, Valkenburg PW, Bastiaans AC, et al. Effect of naloxone on blood pressure and survival in different shock models in rats. Eur J Pharmacol 1986; 124:299-308.
38. Lechner RB, Gurll NJ, Reynolds DG. Naloxone potentiates the cardiovascular effects of catecholamines in canine hemorrhagic shock. Circ Shock 1985;16:347-361.
39. McIntosh TK, Palter M, Grasberger R, et al. Endorphins in primate hemorrhagic shock: beneficial action of opiate antagonists. J Surg Res 1986;40:265-275.
40. Teba L, Zakaria M, Dedhia HV, et al. Beneficial effect of thyrotropin-releasing hormone in canine hemorrhagic shock. Circ Shock 1987;21:51-57.
41. Long JB, Lake CR, Reed AA, et al. Effects of naloxone and thyrotropin releasing hormone on plasma catecholamines, corticosterone and arterial pressure in normal and endotoxemic rats. Circ Shock 1986;18:1-10.
42. Markov AK, Terry J, White TZ, et al. Increasing survival of dogs subjected to hemorrhagic shock by administration of fructose 1-6 diphosphate. Surgery 1987;102:515-527.
43. Bitterman H, Phillips GR, Dragon G, et al. Potentiation of the protective effects of a converting enzyme inhibitor and a thromboxane synthetase inhibitor in hemorrhagic shock. J Pharmacol Exp Ther 1987;242:8-14.
44. Haskins SC. Fluid, electrolyte and acid-base considerations in shock. ACVIM Forum Proc 1987;5:72-75.
45. Degen MA. Acute hypersensitivity reactions. In Kirk RW, ed. Current Veterinary Therapy X. Philadelphia: WB Saunders, 1989;537-543.

15 Sepsis Versus Septic Shock

Elizabeth M. Hardie

Sepsis and septic shock are conditions familiar to all clinicians treating critically ill animals. Precise definitions of the various terms relating to sepsis, such as bacteremia, septicemia, endotoxemia, sepsis, septic shock, warm shock, cold shock, sepsis syndrome, multiple organ failure, etc., have been lacking. Recently, the following definitions have been proposed[1]:

Bacteremia—Positive blood cultures indicating the presence of viable bacteria in the circulating blood.

Sepsis—Clinical evidence of infection (tachypnea, tachycardia, fever or hypothermia) is present in the patient.

Sepsis syndrome—Sepsis with evidence of altered organ perfusion. Tachycardia, fever or hypothermia, tachypnea, and one or more of the following: respiratory dysfunction (partial pressure of arterial oxygen/fractional inspired oxygen concentration <280), elevated blood lactate concentration, or oliguria (output <0.5 mL/kg body weight for at least 1 hour). Positive or negative blood cultures may be present.

Septic shock—Sepsis syndrome with hypotension (systolic blood pressure <90 mm Hg or decrease from base line >40 mm Hg) that is responsive to intravenous fluids or pharmacologic intervention.

Refractory shock—Septic shock that does not respond to conventional therapy within a specific time interval (1 hour). The terms "septic shock" and "refractory shock" would replace the terms "warm shock" and "cold shock." The latter term is particularly confusing, since it is used to designate both reversible septic shock with increased systemic resistance (as in acute peritonitis) and irreversible end-stage shock.

The above terminology was designed for use in human patients, in whom respiratory insufficiency is an early and predictable marker of sepsis. These definitions will probably be appropriate for the cat, a species that develops similar respiratory dysfunction in response to sepsis. The dog is notoriously resistant to respiratory dysfunction in sepsis; the liver and gastrointestinal tract fail first in this species. For dogs then, the definition of sepsis syndrome would be:

Sepsis with evidence of altered organ perfusion. Tachycardia, fever or hypothermia, and tachypnea with one or more of the following: liver dysfunction, elevated lactate level, or oliguria (output <0.5 ml/kg body weight for at least 1 hour). Positive or negative blood cultures may be present.

Use of the revised terminology emphasizes that bacteremia and sepsis are not synonymous, that clinical signs of sepsis occur in response to a wide variety of organisms and conditions, that organ failure and shock are separate but associated conditions, and that shock may be reversible or irreversible. This terminology more precisely defines the entire spectrum and progression of sepsis than older terminology and should be adopted. The term "septicemia," which has been used for "bacteremia," "endotoxemia," and "sepsis" should be dropped. The term "endotoxemia" should be reserved to mean "the presence of gram-negative endotoxin in the blood."

The exact relations between organism type, bacteremia, endotoxemia, sepsis, and shock have not been well defined, but there is clearly a balance between the invading microorganism and the host response. Both organism and host factors can tip the balance, resulting in the familiar progression to shock and death. Organism characteristics that affect the balance include organism type, organism virulence, and organism numbers. Organism type was once thought to be of primary importance, with higher mortality being related to

I would like to acknowledge the assistance of Drs. Bernard D. Hansen, Kris Krus-Elliott, John Dodam, and Peter Hellyer in the preparation of this manuscript.

infection with gram-negative organisms. Human intensive care unit (ICU) clinicians today place little importance on the exact organism, because gram-negative bacteremia, gram-positive bacteremia, and fungemia all result in similar clinical signs and produce equivalent mortality.[2] In a prospective study of bacteremia in canine and feline patients in the ICU, no difference in mortality was found between patients with gram-positive, gram-negative, and polymicrobial bacteremia.[3] Organism virulence is determined by such things as the presence of cell capsules, which isolate cell-wall antigens from host inflammatory cells, and the production of enzymes, which allow the microbe to move rapidly through tissue.[4] Organism numbers are positively correlated with mortality.[5] Intravenous infusion of 0.4×10^{10} *Escherichia coli* organisms per kilogram of body weight in baboons caused signs of inflammation, but no deaths. Infusion of only 10 times more organisms (4×10^{10} organisms per kilogram) resulted in the progression from inflammation to hypercoagulation to hypoxic cell injury and death. Infusion of the lethal dose was associated with the appearance of endotoxin, tumor necrosis factor, interleukin-1B, and interleukin-6 in the blood. No endotoxin and only minor amounts of cytokines were detected with the sublethal infusion.

Host factors that affect the balance between organism and host include the immune status of the host and the presence of concurrent disease. The immune system is of primary importance in the response to sepsis. Organisms and endotoxin are neutralized and destroyed by the immune system, but once a critical threshold is reached, the immune system is also responsible for the excessive release of mediators that causes progression to shock and death. Decreased function of the immune system (immunosuppression) increases the risk of death due to overwhelming infection.[6,7] Conversely, nonspecific stimulation of the immune system can also lead to increased risk of death due to increased mediator release.[8] Specific immunity (high levels of specific neutralizing antibody to the pathogen involved or high levels of antibodies to the core antigen shared by all gram-negative organism) results in decreased risk of death, presumably because organisms and endotoxin are destroyed prior to interacting with cells that release shock mediators.[9,10] Concurrent diseases that have been identified as placing the patient at increased risk of bacteremia include urinary tract infection, leukemia, portosystemic shunt, and diabetes mellitus.[3] Any concurrent serious disease increases the risk of death due to bacteremia.[3]

Treatment affects the outcome of the organism-

host interaction only if it is begun prior to the onset of irreversible changes.[11,12] The first irreversible change is the release of shock mediators. Hundreds of experiments have proven that blocking the release of these mediators can prevent death. Once the mediators have been released, however, even optimal treatment fails to increase survival rates above 50%. The second irreversible change is the occurrence of refractory hypotension. This stage is terminal, and treatment is essentially futile. In a study of human patients, the mortality rate was 12% if treatment was begun when fever and leukocytosis were present, 65% if treatment was initiated when either organ failure or shock was present, and 88% if shock and organ failure were present.[12] This study did not distinguish between septic shock and refractory shock, but one presumes that most patients in the 88% mortality group were in refractory shock. Assuming that sepsis in most veterinary patients is recognized after mediator release and prior to onset of refractory shock, a reasonable goal would be a 50% survival rate. As demonstrated in a lethal canine peritonitis model, two aspects of treatment are needed to achieve this goal.[2] Treatment with appropriate antibiotics increased the survival rate to 13%. Similarly, appropriate cardiovascular support increased the survival rate to 13%. A survival rate of 50% was reached only when both antibiotics and cardiovascular support were provided.

At present, survival rates above 50% are reached by preventing bacteremia and sepsis through meticulous and aggressive management of high-risk patients and by early recognition of sepsis.[13,14] The goal for the future is to increase the survival rate for the sepsis syndrome and septic shock above 50%. Intensive research into the interactions between organisms, endotoxin, and host cells is being conducted to meet this objective. Whether or not refractory shock will ever be treatable is not known. For now, clinicians should learn to recognize refractory shock in order to limit the suffering of the animal and the expense to the owner.

CLINICAL PRESENTATIONS OF SEPSIS

Historical findings associated with sepsis depend on the site of infection, the rapidity with which organisms are being disseminated, and the speed with which shock is developing.[15-17] Diseases that cause sepsis syndrome and shock (e.g., pyothorax, pyometra) will be associated with different histories than diseases associated with bacteremia. Diseases known to produce overt clinical signs of sepsis are listed in Table 15-1. Animals with these diseases are usually presented to the

Table 15-1 Diseases that usually result in overt clinical signs of sepsis

Disease	Typical organisms
Pyothorax	Mixed anaerobic infection
Peritonitis	Anaerobes, enteric gram-negative organisms
Pyometra	*E. coli*, anaerobes, Streptococcus spp., Staphylococcus spp.
Prostatic abscess	*E. coli*, other gram-negative enteric organisms, Staphylococcus spp., Streptococcus spp.
Liver abscess, biliary tract infection	Anaerobes, enteric gram-negative organisms
Renal abscess	*E. coli*, other gram-negative enteric organisms, Staphylococcus spp., Streptococcus spp.
Epididymitis and orchitis	Studies lacking; probably similar to urinary tract
Mastitis	Anaerobes, enteric gram-negative organisms
Wound infections	*Staph. intermedius*, nosocomial pathogens, Pseudomonas spp.

Table 15-2 Diseases associated with bacteremia

Disease	Typical organisms
Diskospondylitis*	*Staph. intermedius*
Bacterial endocarditis	*Staph. intermedius*, Streptococcus spp., *E. coli*, *Erysipelothrix rhusiopathiae*, Corynebacterium spp.
Urinary tract infection	*Staph. intermedius*, Streptococcus spp., *E. coli*, other gram-negative enteric organisms
Pyoderma	*Staph. intermedius*, Streptococcus spp.
Severe enteritis	*E. coli*
Severe gingivitis	Anaerobes, gram-negative organisms
Neoplasia	Enterobacteriaceae
Patients in ICU with urinary tract infection, leukemia, diabetes mellitus, portosystemic shunts	46% gram-negative bacilli, 30% gram-positive cocci, 31% anaerobes, 15% polymicrobial
Diseases listed in Table 15-1	See Table 15-1

*Not usually associated with sepsis.

clinician for treatment of the septic process. Diseases associated with bacteremia are listed in Table 15-2.[3,18,19] Animals with these diseases may or not be presented for treatment of a septic process. When these diseases are present, however, clinicians should maintain a high index of suspicion for bacteremia, since its presence usually adversely affects prognosis. Treatment with immunosuppressive drugs also increases the risk of bacteremia and sepsis, thus a thorough drug history should also be taken.[7]

Physical examination findings associated with sepsis can be vague.[3,17,18] As stated in the definition of sepsis, fever or hypothermia, tachycardia, and tachypnea are the hallmarks of this syndrome. The frequency with which each sign is present varies. In a study of dogs with bacteremia,[18] 75% had fever, while in a study of dogs with surgically confirmed sepsis, 40% had fever and 3% had hypothermia.[17] In a prospective study of patients in an ICU, Dow et al.[3] found that fever was most likely to be present with gram-positive or polymicrobial bacteremia, and least likely to be present with anaerobic bacteremia. Tachycardia and tachypnea can be difficult to define in the canine population due to the wide variation in normal values. For example, overt tachycardia (heart rate >160 beats per minute) was found in only 21% of dogs in whom postsurgical sepsis developed, but 47% had rate increases of 20% or more from hospital admission values. Tachypnea has not been documented in clinical studies of canine or feline sepsis, but it is always present in experimental models, suggesting that it is simply being missed in clinical patients. Additional clinical signs of sepsis include lethargy, depression, anorexia, vomiting and/or diarrhea, pain associated with the site of infection, or generalized pain.

Shock is often present. The manifestations of shock will differ, depending on the stage of sepsis and the volume status of the animal.[2,16,17,20] Animals with sepsis who have adequate intravascular volume and have not yet progressed to refractory shock will have what has classically been defined as "warm shock" or "hyperdynamic shock." This condition is associated with brick-red mucous membranes, tachycardia, high cardiac output, normal or low systemic arterial blood pressure, and low systemic vascular resistance. Animals with sepsis and inadequate intravascular volume (usually due to massive fluid shifts into the peritoneum or interstitium) have what has been called "cold shock" or "hypodynamic shock." This condition is characterized by pale mucous membranes, cold extremities, tachycardia, low cardiac output, low systemic arterial blood pressure, and high systemic vascular resistance. Unless the animal with hypodynamic shock has progressed to refractory shock, the provision of adequate amounts of intravenous fluids will convert hypodynamic shock to hyperdynamic shock. A small group of patients with hypodynamic shock will have overt myocardial depression and will require therapy with inotropes in addition to volume support.[21,22] Animals with refractory shock resemble those with cold or hypodynamic shock in that low systemic arterial blood pressure, cold extremities, and pale mucous membranes are usually present.[20] Systemic vascular resistance may be high or low, and cardiac output may be normal or low. Hypotension in these patients cannot be reversed because massive fluid leakage through the vascular endothelium prevents expansion of intravascular volume,[5] generalized vasodilation unresponsive to pressor therapy is present,[1,2,21] and/or myocardial depression limits cardiac output.[21,22]

The order of organ failure associated with sepsis varies with species. In the dog, the order is usually gastrointestinal tract, liver, kidney, then lung.[20,23] Clinical signs of gastrointestinal failure include anorexia, vomiting, diarrhea, and mucosal sloughing (manifested by vomitus or diarrhea containing blood and obvious mucosal remnants). Liver failure leads to anorexia, vomiting, and icterus. Anuria due to renal failure is rare. Anuria is usually associated with hypotension and shock, and correction of the animal's hemodynamic status resolves the problem. Lung failure rarely occurs prior to refractory shock and is associated with the development of pulmonary edema (pink-tinged frothy fluid is seen coming from the mouth and nostrils) and hypoxemia. Hyperpnea in the early stages of canine sepsis is due to respiratory compensation for metabolic acidosis, but true dyspnea is rarely seen. If persistent tachypnea and dyspnea are noted prior to refractory shock, the clinician should exclude pneumonia and pulmonary thromboembolism as causes, rather than suspecting ventilation failure.[24] In cats, the pattern of organ failure is different, and respiratory failure occurs early in the course of sepsis.[25] Tachypnea in cats should thus be presumed to be associated with hypoxemia from pulmonary failure.

Depression of cardiac function occurs early in the course of sepsis, but unless highly sensitive measures of cardiac function are used, overt failure will not be noticed until the later stages.[26,27] In dogs with cecal ligation peritonitis treated with continuous high-volume support, heart rate, stroke volume, and cardiac output increase over a 4-day period. During the same period, progressive left ventricular dysfunction occurs, as manifested by progressive dilation of the ventricle, decreased ventricular compliance, and a fall in the end-systolic pressure-volume index of function (E_{max}).[27] Studies of septic human patients have shown that similar changes occur in the right ventricle.[28,29] In a subgroup of human patients, myocardial failure is severe enough to affect cardiac output even early in the course of sepsis.[22]

Laboratory findings in sepsis

The primary laboratory finding associated with bacteremia or confirmed bacterial infection is an abnormal leukogram.[3,18,19] Dogs with bacteremia have either leukocytosis or leukopenia, an increased concentration of immature neutrophils (left-shift), and monocytosis. Platelet counts tend to be decreased.[3,30] The presence of toxic changes in the neutrophils has been associated with gram-negative infection.[19]

Hemoconcentration occurs following fluid losses from the intravascular space. The packed cell volume may increase to as high as 60% to 65% in acute overwhelming sepsis.[31] Total serum solids decrease due to movement of protein from blood to the tissues. The degree of hemoconcentration has prognostic value in that higher values are seen in animals dying within 7 to 10 hours of the onset of sepsis as compared with those dying after 25 hours or surviving.[32]

Serum biochemical abnormalities associated with sepsis reflect vascular leakage and organ dysfunction.[17,18,20] Hypoalbuminemia, hypoglycemia or hyperglycemia, and increased serum alkaline phosphatase activity are seen most often. Bilirubinemia and increased serum alanine aminotransferase concentration indicate liver failure. Not surprisingly, the presence of two or more serum biochemical abnormalities has been shown to be correlated with increased mortality.[18]

The clotting status of patients with sepsis can range from a hypercoagulable state to overt disseminated intravascular coagulation (DIC).[20,24,33]

In an experimental baboon model of sepsis,[5] fibrinogen concentrations increased in response to a sublethal injection of organisms, but rapidly decreased in response to a lethal injection. The fall in fibrinogen preceded the development of hypoxic cell injury and cardiovascular collapse by several hours. Evidence of DIC (low fibrinogen, prolonged prothrombin and activated partial thromboplastin times, increased fibrin degradation products) should thus be regarded as indicating a rapidly fatal infection. If organ failure and/or cardiovascular collapse are also present, irreversible shock is likely. The presence of low platelet numbers alone should not be used as evidence of DIC, because thrombocytopenia can occur independently from DIC in sepsis.[30]

Blood gas analysis in dogs with sepsis often indicates metabolic acidosis with respiratory compensation. The partial pressure of arterial carbon dioxide can decrease as low as 18 to 20 mm Hg in dogs to compensate for marked acidemia, and an arterial blood pH in the 7.3 to 7.4 range can be maintained in the face of plasma bicarbonate concentrations as low as 12 mEq/L.[31] Reduction of arterial blood pH to the 7.2 to 7.3 range is not seen in awake dogs with experimental sepsis until the late stage of irreversible shock.[31] Hypoxemia is also not seen in awake dogs with sepsis,[31] but may become apparent in sedated or anesthetized dogs that cannot control the depth and rate of respiration.[34] Blood gas changes have been measured in cats with endotoxemia but not sepsis.[25] Hypoxemia, hypercarbia, and metabolic acidosis develop rapidly.

Blood lactate concentrations are increased in sepsis for many reasons. Firstly, hemoconcentration and shock result in poor oxygen delivery to the tissues, resulting in anaerobic metabolism.[11,13,35] Secondly, endotoxin (or a mediator released very early in endotoxemia) causes impaired cellular oxidative respiration.[36] Thirdly, septic patients are usually hypermetabolic,[37] thus even when oxygen delivery to the tissues is restored, the metabolic needs of the patient may not be met. Blood lactate concentrations are early accurate predictors of ultimate survival in human surgical intensive care units, probably because they indicate the degree of metabolic insult suffered by the patient.[6] Survivors have lactate levels of 1.1 ± 0.2 mg/dL, while nonsurvivors have levels of 3.4 ± 0.7 mg/dL on their second day in the ICU. Further increases in lactate levels despite high cardiac output and normal or increased oxygen consumption predict the transition from compensated sepsis to end-stage septic multiple organ failure.[11] If lactate values are not available, dogs in endotoxic shock with high-anion-gap metabolic acidosis due to lactic acidosis have been shown to have the following approximate relationship between anion gap (AG) and lactic acid concentration[38]:

$$\text{lactate} = (0.27 \times \text{AG}) - 1.46.$$

PATHOPHYSIOLOGY OF SEPSIS
Microbial factors

Sepsis syndrome and shock can occur with numerous types of organisms, but septic shock due to gram-negative organisms is the most well studied.[39] Endotoxin, a component of the gram-negative bacterial cell wall appears to be the factor responsible for producing shock associated with gram-negative bacteremia. Endotoxin is composed of lipid, polyaccharide, and protein portions. The lipid portion (lipid A) is the most highly conserved portion of the molecule and is responsible for toxicity. The polysaccharide portion varies with each strain of bacteria and is responsible for the antigenicity of the molecule.

Interactions between microbes and cellular components

Endotoxin interacts directly with macrophages, neutrophils, and vascular endothelium.[40,41] Specific endotoxin receptors have been identified on macrophages,[42] and will probably be isolated from other cell types. Endotoxin binds to these receptors, resulting in release of mediators,[43] or "priming" of the cell to react more vigorously to other activating agents.[41] Below a critical dosage of endotoxin, the reaction incited by the interaction between endotoxin and cells is controlled.[5,41] Once a critical dosage is reached, however, malignant amplification of mediator release occurs, resulting in organ dysfunction and shock.[5,41] The "trigger" dosage varies among species, and also varies according to the responsiveness of the macrophages and neutrophils.

Mediator release

The list of mediators released during septic and endotoxic shock continues to grow.[39,41] Mediators can be grouped into three major categories: cytokines, lipid mediators, and secondary mediators. Cytokines are small polypeptide hormones released from inflammatory cells (chiefly macrophages).[5] Endotoxemia stimulates release of numerous cytokines, of which tumor necrosis factor[44] and interleukin-1[45] are the best understood. Lipid mediators are thought to arise mainly from neutrophils, platelets, vascular endothelium, and vascular smooth muscle.[39] Platelet-activating factor,[41] prostaglandins,[46] and leukotrienes[47] are lipid mediators. In the normal regulation of inflammation, cytokines and lipid mediators act as messengers between inflammatory cells, vascular endothelium, and platelets, resulting in modulation of immune function.[41] The mediators can stimulate production or inhibit release of each other and amplify or inhibit each others' actions. If the positive-feedback loops overwhelm the inhibitory loops, malignant amplification occurs.[41]

Each mediator has specific actions, in addition to potentiating effects of other mediators. Tumor necrosis factor has been shown to cause hypotension, respiratory dysfunction, bowel ischemia, metabolic abnormalities, anorexia, and when chronically infused, cachexia and wasting.[44] Interleukin-1 causes fever, neutropenia followed by neutrophilia, and sequestration of granulocytes in the pulmonary vasculature.[45] Platelet activating factor is known to cause platelet activation and aggregation; neutrophil activation, aggregation, and chemotaxis; increased activity of plasma proteases; vasodilation and severe hypotension; vasoconstriction in selected vascular beds, such as the heart and lungs; increased vascular permeability; and severe gastrointestinal ulceration.[41,48] Thromboxane, a product of the prostaglandin cascade, causes vasoconstriction and platelet aggregation, while prostaglandins I_2 and E_2 are associated with vasodilation and hypotension.[39,46] Leukotrienes cause vasoconstriction of specific vascular beds, increases in vascular permeability, and increased neutrophil chemotaxis.[46]

In response to liberated cytokines and lipid mediators, a host of secondary mediators are released as the animal responds to generalized activation of shock, clotting, and vascular endothelial damage. Plasma concentrations of histamine, serotonin, vasopressin, angiotensin II, catecholamines, and endogenous opiates all may be released in increased amounts.[39]

Mediator release leads to organ failure

The mix of mediators present at a given stage of sepsis is responsible for the clinical signs associated with that stage. For example, in porcine endotoxin-induced respiratory failure, early vasoconstriction has been associated with marked increases in plasma concentrations of tumor nerosis factor, platelet activating factor, and thromboxane. Later, development of pulmonary edema has been associated with release of platelet activating factor and leukotriene B_4.[48] The hyperdynamic state (high cardiac output, low peripheral vascular resistance) has been associated with increases in interleukin-1, tumor nerosis factor, and prostaglandin E.[6] Although the initial target organ in sepsis varies between species, multiple organs eventually fail because of accumulated hypoxic damage, oxygen radical and lysosomal enzyme damage, thrombosis, and metabolic derangements.[6,39] No matter what the initiating cause, multiple-organ failure represents the "final common pathway to death."[49]

THERAPY OF SEPSIS
Instrumentation

In the patient with sepsis syndrome or septic shock, several intravenous lines (including one central line) are placed to supply fluids, administer drugs, and withdraw blood samples. If venous access cannot be rapidly accomplished in the severely hypotensive patient, a bone marrow needle is used to administer fluids into the marrow cavity of the humerus or femur.[50] An indwelling urinary catheter is placed to monitor urine output. Systemic arterial blood pressure is initially measured using indirect methods, but ideally a direct arterial line is placed to monitor more accurately the systemic arterial blood pressure. Core and toe-web thermometers are placed to assess peripheral vasoconstriction and flow.[51] In order to assess the progress of treatment and watch for the development of multiple-organ failure, numerous variables (Table 15-3) must be monitored. Pretreatment values for these variables should be obtained, unless urgent resuscitation precludes this occurrence. A sterile urine sample should be saved to allow for culture if evidence of infection is present on urinalysis.

Antibiotics

Antibiotic therapy (Table 15-4) is initiated early. If oral antibiotics can be used, enrofloxacin, a quinolone with a wide spectrum of activity, is recommended.[52] Intravenous antibiotics are usually required because of the presence of shock and/or gastrointestinal failure. The organism(s) responsible for infection and their antibiotic sensitivity pattern will not be known at this time, thus therapy must effective against a broad range of pathogens. For dogs, therapy should be effective against gram-negative organisms (particularly *Escherichia coli* and *Klebsiella pneumoniae*), gram-positive organisms (*Staphylococcus intermedius*, Streptococcus spp., and Enterococcus spp.), and anaerobes (particularly *Clostridium perfringens*).[7,53] For cats, therapy should be particularly effective against gram-negative organisms (*E. coli, K. pneumoniae,* and Salmonella) and resistant anaerobes (*Propionibacterium acnes* and Bacteroides spp.).[3]

For dogs, a combination of amikacin and ampicillin is a recommended approach providing renal function is normal.[54] This recommendation is based on knowledge that virtually 100% of *E.*

Table 15-3 Monitoring variables for animals with sepsis

Parameter (frequency of monitoring)	Possible interpretation
Core temperature (every 3 hours)	<38°C: hypovolemic shock, bacteremia >40°C: bacteremia
Toe web temperature (every 3 hours)	>5.5°C lower than core: shock
Pulse rate (every hour, more if critical)	>150-200 beats per minute based on body size: shock
Respiratory rate (every hour)	Steady increase: metabolic acidosis, pulmonary thromboembolism, lung failure
Capillary refill time (every hour)	>2 seconds: shock
Mucous membrane color (every hour)	Pale: anemia, hypodynamic shock
Systemic arterial blood pressure (continuous or every hour)	<90 mm Hg or undetectable: shock
Central venous pressure (continuous or every hour)	<1-2 cm H_2O: hypovolemia >15 cm H_2O: intravascular volume overload, heart failure
Urine output (every hour)	<0.5 ml/kg per hour: shock, renal failure
Blood glucose concentration (every 6-8 hours)	<70 mg/dL: sepsis, replacement therapy needed
Packed cell volume (every 6-8 hours)	<20%: hemorrhage, volume overload dilution, replacement therapy needed >50%: severe hemoconcentration, volume loss
Total serum solids (every 6-8 hours)	<3.5 g/dL: third-space loss, volume-overload dilution
Albumin (if total solids <5 g/dL)	<1 g/dL: replacement therapy needed
Serum electrolytes (every 24 hours)	Potassium <3.5 mEq/L: replacement therapy needed Calcium decreasing: continued sepsis, continued albumin loss
Blood urea nitrogen (every 24 hours)	>30 mg/dL: hypovolemia or renal failure
Serum bilirubin concentration, alkaline phosphatase, alanine aminotransferase activities (every 48 hours)	Increasing values: sepsis
Arterial blood gases (as needed)	Metabolic acidosis: shock or sepsis; hypoxemia: lung failure, pulmonary thromboembolism, pneumonia

coli, *K. pneumoniae* and *Staph. intermedius* isolated from dogs remain sensitive to amikacin, while 95% to 99% of Streptococcus spp., 75% to 80% of Enterococcus spp., and all Clostridium are sensitive to ampicillin. (Sensitivity data from the microbiology laboratories of North Carolina State University and Colorado State University, Courtesy of Drs. David Aucoin and Robert L. Jones.) Most Proteus, Pseudomonas, and Salmonella spp. isolated from animals also remain sensitive to amikacin. The obvious "holes" in this combination are resistant enterococci and anaerobes. Thus, in cats and in dogs with known intraabdominal sepsis, a more effective antianaerobic drug such as clindamycin or metronidazole may be added to the aforementioned regimen.[55]

If renal function is known to be compromised, the clinician must decide if gram-positive or gram-negative/anaerobe infection is most likely. If gram-positive infection is likely, a first-generation cephalosporin, cefazolin,[56,57] is recommended. Approximately 95% to 99% of Staphylococcus and nonenterococcal Streptococcus spp. are sensitive to cefazolin, but activity against enterococci is limited. Activity against gram-nega-

tive organisms is unpredictable, and limited activity against anaerobes is present. If gram-negative/anaerobic infection is suspected, a second-generation cephalosporin, cefoxitin, is recommended. Despite good activity against gram-negative and anaerobic organisms, cefoxitin has very limited activity against gram-positive organisms.[56,57] Imipenem, a carbepenem, has the widest spectrum of any beta-lactam antibiotic and is my drug of choice for the compromised patient with sepsis with a documented resistant infection.[56,57]

Regardless of the initial antibiotic choice, rapid identification of the causal organism(s) and antibiotic sensitivities is necessary.[3] In a study of bacteremic canine and feline patients in the ICU, knowledge of organism type and antibiotic sensitivities resulted in a change of therapy in 37% of the animals.[3] Samples for culture should be obtained after initial resuscitation of the animal, even if antibiotic therapy has been initiated. The presence of antibiotics may not affect the recovery of organisms from blood cultures, and antibiotics rarely penetrate into accumulations of pus and exudate.[3]

Samples for blood culture should be taken di-

Table 15-4 Antibiotic drugs used to treat sepsis

Drug	Dosage (dog [D] or cat [C])	Daily cost* (20-kg dog)
Enrofloxacin	2.5-5 mg/kg PO every 12 hours (D) 2.5-5 mg/kg PO every 24 hours (C)	$ 1.00
Gentamicin	2-4 mg/kg IV every 8 hours	$ 0.60
Amikacin	7-10 mg/kg IV every 8 hours	$ 3.04
Tobramycin	2-4 mg/kg IV every 8 hours	$16.38
Ampicillin	20-40 mg/kg IV every 8 hours	$ 1.22
Clindamycin	5-15 mg/kg IV every hour	$ 6.60
Metronidazole	10 mg/kg IV every 8 hours	$14.00
Cefazolin	20 mg/kg IV every 8 hours	$ 1.98
Cefoxitin	20 mg/kg IV every 8 hours	$ 8.18
Imipenem	2-5 mg/kg IV every 8 hours	$ 8.59

PO = by mouth; IV = intravenously.
*1991 North Carolina State University pharmacy cost.

rectly from a vein after sterile preparation of the skin overlying the vein.[7] If necessary, cultures can be taken aseptically from a catheter that was recently placed using aseptic technique. Depending on the size of the animal, 5 to 10 ml of blood is drawn into the syringe and directly inoculated into the culture bottle. If smaller samples are taken, broth must be removed from the blood culture bottle such that the ratio of blood to broth remains 1:10. The cultures should be processed for isolation of both aerobic and anaerobic bacteria, because up to 30% of pathogens causing bacteremia may be anaerobes.[3] Ideally, two to three blood samples, taken at least 1 hour apart, should be obtained for culture. If fever is following a known pattern, blood samples should be drawn just prior to predicted fever spikes.

Cardiovascular support

Goals. The goal of resuscitation in septic shock is rapid restoration of tissue oxygen delivery, so that a lethal oxygen debt does not develop.[11] The most common mistake in our ICU is administration of too little fluids too slowly. The initial goal of fluid therapy should be to increase the animal's central venous pressure 2 to 5 cm H_2O within 15 minutes.

The goal of ongoing cardiovascular support during sepsis is supranormal oxygen delivery to the tissues, sufficient to meet the needs of the stressed hypermetabolic patient.[11,13,14] Oxygen delivery and consumption can be directly measured if a pulmonary arterial catheter is in place,[13] or if an indirect calorimeter is available.[11] In the absence of direct measurements of oxygen delivery and consumption, goals must be set using indirect measurements of cardiovascular function, tissue blood flow, oxygen delivery, and oxygen extraction[11,13,14,35,58] (Table 15-5).

Volume. Resuscitation can be accomplished using crystalloid fluids, colloid-crystalloid mixtures, or hypertonic solutions[59-67] (Table 15-6). Crystalloid fluid volumes needed to restore intravascular volume in sepsis are high (90 to 270 ml/kg), but can be reduced by coadministration of colloids. The choice of colloid depends on the patient's plasma albumin concentration, cost, and availability of colloid products. Species-matched plasma will directly replace fluid and protein losses to extravascular spaces (see Table 15-6), but adequate amounts are rarely available. The two major synthetic colloids in use are hetastarch 120 and dextran 70.[68] Hetastarch is a polymer made from a waxy starch consisting mainly of amylopectin, while dextran 70 is a glucose polymer with an average molecular weight of 70,000. Hetastarch has no antigenic properties, does not interfere with blood typing or cross matching, and is stable at widely fluctuating temperatures. Dextran 70 is antigenic, may rarely cause anaphylaxis, interferes with blood typing and cross matching due to rouleaux formation, interferes with blood glucose measurements, and must be stored at stable temperatures (25°C) or precipitates will form. The two solutions are equally effective at producing blood volume expansion.[69] At high dosages (20 ml/kg) both solutions result in increased clotting times due to decreased platelet function and altered fibrin clot structure. The limiting dosages for the two solutions are the same (20 ml/kg for the first 24 hours, 10 ml/kg per 24 hours thereafter). The cost of a 500-ml bag of hetastarch is $63.10, while the cost of a 500 ml bag of dextran 70 is $9.00. Synthetic colloids should be used with caution if the albumin level is <1gm/dl. Human albumin can be administered to maintain plasma protein levels without affecting clotting function.[62,70] Disadvantages of albumin administration are its high cost and the potential for antigenic reactions following repeated administration.

The two hypertonic solutions used most often are hypertonic saline[60,63,64] and glucose-insulin-

Table 15-5 Optimal cardiovascular therapeutic goals for animals with sepsis

If central venous catheter in place		If pulmonary artery catheter in place	
Blood pressure (mm Hg)	>120/80	Mixed venous oxygen tension (torr)	>40
Central venous pressure (cm saline)	>5 and <15	Pulmonary artery pressure (mm Hg)	>25/10
Hematocrit (%)	30-35	Pulmonary wedge pressure (mm Hg)	<18
Total solids (mg/dL)	>3.5 and <5.0		
Heart rate (beats per minute)	>70 and <150, dog >150 and <210, cat	Systemic vascular resistance (dyn × second/ cm^5 × m^2)	>1450
Temperature (°C)	>38 and <40		
Core-toe web temperature differential (°C)	<4	Pulmonary vascular resistance (dyn × second/ cm^5 × m^2)	45-250
Urine output (ml/kg per hour)	>2		
Arterial oxygen tension (torr)	>70	Oxygen extraction (%)	22-30
pH	>7.3 and <7.5	Cardiac index (L per minute × m^2)	>4.5
Base excess (mM/L)	−2 to +2	Oxygen delivery (ml per minute × m^2)	>600
Central venous oxygen saturation (%)	>70	Oxygen consumption (ml per minute × m^2)	>170
D(a − v)O$_2$* (ml/dL)	3		
P(a − v)co$_2$* (torr)	<6		

*D(a − v)o$_2$ is calculated by subtracting venous oxygen content from arterial oxygen content. Oxygen content = (hemoglobin concentration × 1.34 × oxygen saturation) + (0.003 × oxygen tension). P(a − v)co$_2$ is calculated by subtracting venous carbon dioxide tension from arterial carbon dioxide tension. Values obtained from blood drawn through a central venous catheter can be used for these calculations, but mixed venous blood drawn from a pulmonary artery catheter is preferred.

Table 15-6 Drugs used to treat animals with sepsis

Drug	Dosage	Frequency
Volume agents		
Hypertonic crystalloids, 7.5% sodium chloride solution (70 ml 23.4% sodium chloride in 180 ml 0.9% sodium chloride or 6% dextran 70)	4 ml/kg intravenously	Once
GIK solution (3 g glucose, 1-2 U insulin, 0.5 mEq potassium/kg in 250 mL lactated Ringer's)	Intravenously, 10% volume bolus, remainder infused over 4-5 hours	As needed
Colloids		
Plasma	Maximum: 20 mL/kg per 24 hours intravenously	As needed
Hetastarch 120 Dextran 70	Maximum: 20 ml/kg during first 24 hours, then 10 ml/kg per 24 hours intravenously	Slow infusion
3% albumin (12 ml 25% human albumin in 488 ml lactated Ringer's)	20 ml/kg intravenously	Resuscitation
Isotonic crystalloids		
Lactated Ringers	90-270 ml/kg intravenously 5-10 ml/kg/per hour intravenously	Resuscitation Ongoing needs in sepsis

Table 15-6 Drugs used to treat animals with sepsis—cont'd

Drug	Dosage	Frequency
Inotropes and pressor agents		
Dopamine	1-30 µg/kg/per minute intravenously	As needed (see text): monitor closely and titrate to obtain optimal oxygen delivery
Dobutamine	5-20 µg/kg/per minute intravenously	
Norepinephrine	0.01-0.4 µg/kg per minute intravenously	
Drugs for altered clotting function		
Heparin (low dosage)	75-100 units/kg subcutaneously	Every 6-8 hours
Heparin-activated plasma (incubate 5-10 units/kg heparin with 1 unit fresh plasma for 30 minutes)	10 ml/kg intravenously	Every 3 hours based on clotting function
Drugs for metabolic therapy		
Potassium chloride	0.125-0.25 mEq/kg per hour intravenously; do not exceed 0.5 mEq/kg per hour	
Glucose	50-500 mg/kg per hour intravenously	
Sodium bicarbonate	base excess $\times$ 0.3 $\times$ body weight in kg = mEq needed to correct deficit, slow intravenous drip	
Drugs for gastrointestinal tract failure		
Cimetidine	5-10 mg/kg intravenously, intramuscularly, or by mouth	Every 6-8 hours
Ranitidine	2 mg/kg intravenously, intramuscularly, or by mouth	Every 8-12 hours
Omeprazole	0.7 mg/kg by mouth	Every 24 hours
Misoprostol	3 µg/kg by mouth	Every 8-24 hours
Sucralfate	250 mg (cat) 500 mg (dog <20 kg) 1 gram (dog >20kg) by mouth	Every 8-12 hours
Kaolin/pectin	1-2 ml/kg by mouth	Every 6-8 hours
Metoclopramide	0.2-0.5 mg/kg subcutaneously	Every 6-8 hours
Drugs for renal failure		
Mannitol	0.25-1 g/kg intravenously	Once, slow bolus
Furosemide	1-2 mg/kg intravenously	Once, if no effect, repeat in 2 hours, increase dose 1 mg/kg
Dopamine	1-3 µg/kg per minute intravenously	Until urine production consistently >2 ml/kg per hour
Corticosteroids		
Methylprednisolone, sodium succinate	30 mg/kg intravenously	Once, before or early in shock
Dexamethasone, sodium phosphate	3-5 mg/kg intravenously	Once, before or early in shock

potassium (GIK).[61,64] Administration of hypertonic saline or a hypertonic saline-colloid mixture resulted in rapid cardiovascular improvement in dogs with induced endotoxic shock, but the effect was more transient than in hemorrhagic shock models. Administration of GIK will help treat hypoglycemia and have cardiovascular effects similar to hypertonic saline. The GIK solution must be continuously infused, and cardiovascular effects diminish with prolonged administration. Since there are no studies examining the effects of combining hypertonic saline and GIK, the clinician should probably choose between the two solutions.

I routinely resuscitate animals with sepsis by administering 7 ml/kg of dextran 70 and 15 ml/kg of lactated Ringer's solution. Bolus administration of the combination is repeated until therapeutic goals (see Table 15-5) are met. If the limiting dosage of dextran (20 ml/kg) occurs prior to restoration of circulatory function, additional amounts of lactated Ringer's solution are administered until goals are met, or until fluid administration is limited by central venous pressure (>15 cm H_2O), or hemodilution (packed cell volume <20%, total solids <3.5).

Once initial resuscitation is accomplished, ongoing fluid requirements of the animal remain high (5-10 ml/kg/per hour), particularly if peritonitis is present.[70,71] Administration of massive fluid volumes contributes to the development of hypoproteinemia, hypokalemia, and anemia.[72] Peripheral edema is to be expected in dogs with sepsis treated with adequate amounts of crystalloid fluids.[27,71] Colloids have been shown to be superior to crystalloids in maintaining hemodynamic function in several endotoxic shock models, and coadministration of colloids reduces the amounts of crystalloids needed.[59,62] If crystalloid fluids alone must be used, the clinician should be aware that no matter how much fluid is administered, the improvements in oxygen delivery and consumption obtained will not equal that achieved by administration of colloid-crystalloid mixtures.[69]

After resuscitation, packed cell volume and total solids are measured to assess the degree of hemodilution that has occurred. If packed cell volume is below 20%, or total solids are below 3.5 mg/dL, blood, plasma, or albumin are administered as needed to raise values to acceptable levels. Unless maximal doses of dextran 70 were used during resuscitation, the dextran administration rate is set to deliver 20 ml/kg in the first 24 hours. On subsequent days, the dextran rate is set to deliver 10 ml/kg per 24 hours. The lactated Ringer's administration rate is set at 5 to 10 ml/kg per hour, with the lower value being used if there is evidence of fluid overload. The lactated Ringer's solution should be supplemented with approximately 30 mEq/L of potassium chloride to maintain serum potassium levels. If hypoglycemia is present, glucose (often with insulin and potassium) is added to the lactated Ringer's solution. The rate of glucose and potassium administration are set to maintain serum values (see Table 15-6) (see Chapters 18 and 38).

Inotropes and pressors. Inotropic support and pressor agents (see Table 15-6) should be used only if therapeutic goals cannot be met with administration of fluid therapy.[14] If used without adequate knowledge and monitoring (heart rate and rhythm, core/toe-web temperature, central venous pressure, urine output, direct arterial blood pressure), these agents have the potential to do more harm than good and should be avoided. The most widely used drugs are dopamine, dobutamine, and norepinephrine.[21,72,73] At low dosages (0.5 to 5 µg/kg per minute), dopamine acts as a dopaminergic receptor agonist, producing renal and mesenteric vasodilation. At moderate dosages (5 to 10 µg/kg/per minute) dopamine mainly acts as a β_1 receptor agonist, resulting in increased heart rate and positive inotropism. Mild arteriolar and venous constriction occurs. At high dosages (>10 µg/kg per minute), dopamine acts as both a β_1 and α_1 receptor agonist, resulting in positive chronotropism, positive inotropism, and marked arteriolar and venous constriction. Dobutamine acts mainly as a β_1 agonist, resulting in positive chronotropism and inotropism. For a given dosage, however, dobutamine produces less chronotropism than dopamine. Dobutamine has no direct pressor effects, and may actually produce weak β_2-mediated arterial vasodilation. Norepinephrine is a strong α_1 and moderate β_1 agonist, and is used to produce arteriolar and venous constriction. Norepinephrine and dopamine have synergistic pressor effects, and administration of combinations of the two may raise blood pressure when one alone is ineffective.[72]

I use dobutamine for inotropic support in sepsis because in experimental studies increased oxygen delivery and consumption resulted from dobutamine as compared with dopamine therapy.[73] However, to maintain a given cardiac filling pressure, more fluids must be given with dobutamine than with dopamine.[73] Clinicians who are less aggressive with fluid therapy may thus wish to use dopamine in moderate dosages. Low dosages of dopamine are used to increase urine output if acceptable values are not reached with fluid and dobutamine administration.[72] Titrated dosages of norepinephrine can be used to raise blood pressure in patients with extreme hypotension.[72]

Since the goal of raising blood pressure is to improve oxygen delivery and consumption, pressure should only be raised until evidence of improved tissue blood flow (increased urine output, decreased core/toe-web temperature difference) is seen.[72] Stimulation of arteriolar vasoconstriction beyond that point will result in organ hypoxia. High-dose dopamine has been the pressor therapy of choice in human surgical ICU units in the past, but recent studies have shown little difference between norepinephrine and dopamine.[21,74]

Cardiovascular prognostic factors. Helpful prognostic indicators include the magnitude of weight gain of the animal over the first 24 hours, the need for pressor support, and heart rate.[71] Surviving dogs with experimental sepsis gained less weight (10 vs. 17%) despite being given similar amounts of fluids, had less need for pressors (22% of patients versus 75% of patients), and had lower heart rates (136 beats per minute versus 152 beats per minute) than nonsurvivors.

Prevention of thromboembolism

Dogs with sepsis are at high risk for clotting abnormalities.[7,24,33] If clotting times and platelet counts are normal at the time of presentation, preventive measures should be taken to prevent activation of intravascular clotting. If synthetic colloids are administered, these agents will serve this purpose.[68,75] If crystalloid fluids alone are used, low-dose heparin administration (see Table 15-6) may be indicated to prevent activation of clotting cascades and to maintain blood flow in the microcirculation.[76-78] If platelet counts are low and clotting times are prolonged, replacement therapy with heparin-activated or nonheparinized platelet-rich plasma can be used to treat DIC.[4,77] Care must be exercised if heparin therapy is combined with colloid administration because both therapies decrease clotting function.[75] It should be noted that most human ICU clinicians will not use heparin in sepsis or multiple-organ failure because of the risk of bleeding, choosing instead to replace clotting factors and platelets.[4]

Surgical treatment

As soon as the animal has received resuscitative treatment, a search should be made for any surgically correctable source of sepsis.[17,54] Physical examination will reveal superficial disease, but peritoneal aspiration or lavage, pleural aspiration, urinalysis, radiography, and/or ultrasonography may be needed to identify sources within body cavities. The criteria for the diagnosis of significant intraabdominal disease using peritoneal lavage have been determined[79,80] (Table 15-7), but it should be remembered that intraabdominal leukocyte counts do not increase until 2 to 3 hours after peritoneal contamination.

The principles of surgical therapy of sepsis are straightforward.[54] The source of the infection should be removed if possible, accumulations of exudate should be removed or drained, and adjuvant substances such as bile, blood, and fluid should be removed. If sepsis syndrome or shock is present and the source of sepsis is within the abdomen, a jejunal feeding tube should be placed, because patients with sepsis will tolerate jejunal feeding long before these individuals tolerate gastric feeding.[37] If the need for parenteral nutritional support is anticipated, a large-gauge central catheter is aseptically placed (see Chapter 37).

Anesthetic treatment of patients with sepsis is similar to that of any critical patient (see Chapters 12 and 33). Anesthetic regimens that can be quickly adjusted and that require minimal hepatic metabolism of drugs by the animal should be used. Dopamine or dobutamine infusions (see Table 15-6) may be needed to support cardiac function, even if they were not needed prior to surgery. Packed cell volume, total solids, and blood glucose concentrations should be monitored frequently during the intraoperative period, as these parameters may decrease rapidly in association with ongoing hemorrhage, release of endotoxin, and rapid fluid administration. Urine production should be monitored closely and anuria avoided. If hypertonic solutions have not been recently ad-

Table 15-7 Criteria for deciding if peritonitis is present on a peritoneal lavage sample (abdomen infused with isotonic crystalloid, 20 ml/kg)

	Before surgery	Two days after surgery
Color	Turbid or cloudy indicates peritonitis	Expect turbid fluid
White-cell count	>1000/μL = mild to moderate irritation	7000/μL normal
	>2000/μL = marked peritonitis	>9000/μL abnormal
Cytology	Toxic neutrophils, bacteria, vegetable fibers, organic debris indicate peritonitis	Toxic neutrophils, bacteria, vegetable fibers, organic debris present

ministered, a renal-protectant dose of mannitol (see Table 15-6) should be administered.

If samples of infected material have not been collected previously, these samples are collected during surgical treatment of the animal. Samples are submitted for Gram staining, cytologic evaluation, aerobic and anaerobic cultures, and antibiotic sensitivity testing. Gram-stain results are used to guide antibiotic therapy, particularly when unsuspected organisms are seen.

Postoperatively, the patient is closely monitored for expected complications, such as anemia, hypoglycemia, hypoproteinemia, hypokalemia, and shock.[17,81] Therapy is instituted to correct developing abnormalities as soon as a downward trend in a parameter is noted, rather than waiting until minimally acceptable values are reached.

Specific organ system therapy

Respiratory therapy. Respiratory support should be provided if the animal cannot maintain a partial pressure of arterial oxygen >70 mm Hg on room air or is showing obvious signs of respiratory distress.[11,13,14] Hypoxemia can often be corrected by increasing the inspired oxygen concentration with administration of nasal oxygen or by placing the animal in an oxygen cage. If equipment for measurement of blood gases is not available, oxygen supplementation should be supplied as soon as sepsis is suspected. If hypoxemia and/or respiratory distress do not resolve with oxygen therapy, the animal should be placed on a respirator (see Chapter 36). Adequate oxygen delivery to the tissues cannot be achieved if respiratory failure limits oxygen uptake into the blood.

Gastrointestinal tract therapy. Gastrointestinal protectants and drugs to reduce gastric acid production (see Table 15-6) are given to decrease the risk of life-threatening gastric and duodenal ulceration.[82] Loss of gastrointestinal mucosa routinely occurs due to villous hypoxia in the early stages of canine septic shock.[40] During the repair phase, ileus and intolerance of gastric feeding are common.[37] Ileus can be managed by correcting serum electrolytes, supplying small quantities of food through a jejunal feeding tube, and drug therapy with metoclopramide. Once ileus begins to resolve, small amounts of gastric or oral food may be tolerated, but large amounts usually induce vomiting. Early in the course of recovery from sepsis, canine patients usually tolerate jejunal infusion rates of 5 to 10 ml per hour. Gastric or oral feeding is usually tolerated once jejunal infusion rates are up to 25 to 30 ml per hour. Every attempt should be made to maintain some degree of gastrointestinal feeding, since food is needed to maintain and repair the gastrointestinal tract.[83,84]

The choice of solutions for optimal feeding is the subject of intense current research. I currently uses a commercial polymeric casein-based liquid diet (Clinicare Canine or Feline) for jejunal and nasogastric feeding, with a switch to a water/cat food slurry[85] for gastric feeding, unless tube-clogging problems are evident. The transition to oral feeding is made by offering the animal its choice of the liquid diet, pureed meat baby food, or a commercial canned high-protein diet (Hill's Feline or Canine p/d). Feeding is continued despite the occurrence of diarrhea, but foods that are lower in fat and higher in fiber are fed.[37]

Liver failure. There is no direct therapy for liver failure in sepsis beyond the provision of adequate oxygen delivery and optimal nutritional support. Decrease in liver enzyme activities and serum bilirubin concentration will occur as recovery progresses. Continuing increases in serum liver enzyme activities and serum bilirubin concentrations are a poor prognostic sign.[6,17,20]

Renal failure. Anuria during sepsis syndrome or septic shock is initially treated with aggressive cardiovascular resuscitation. If anuria persists despite adequate intravascular volume expansion, low-dose dopamine infusion and furosemide (see Table 15-6) are administered.[83] Hypertonic solutions of glucose, saline, or mannitol may be administered if hypertonic solutions have not already been used in resuscitation. Once urine flow is established, it should be maintained through optimal maintenance of hemodynamic status. Polyuria and hyposthenuria may continue for days after restoration of urine flow. Clinicians should also be aware that animals that have been adequately resuscitated often have extremely high urine flow rates (3 to 5 ml/kg/per hour).

Metabolic support. After a single life-threatening shock episode, patients undergo a period of hypermetabolism and catabolism of skeletal muscle protein lasting 7 to 10 days.[37] The magnitude of the response depends on the age of the patient (it is more pronounced in younger patients) and the severity of the oxygen debt.[6,11] The purpose of the hypermetabolic phase is to repair damaged tissues and to provide fuel to the liver for the synthesis of acute-phase proteins. If there is continuing injury or inflammation (such as a source of sepsis that cannot be eliminated), hypermetabolism will progress to metabolic failure. During the hypermetabolism stage, there is carbohydrate intolerance, and caloric needs must be met by supplying a mix of carbohydrate, fat, and protein. Progression to metabolic failure is associated with an increased reliance on amino acids as an oxidative fuel source and a decreasing tolerance of lipid.[37]

Healthy, well-nourished animals that undergo an acute episode of septic shock can tolerate starvation for 5 to 7 days without adverse effects.[37] Malnourished patients, patients with coexistent disease, and patients in whom resolution of sepsis is likely to be prolonged should be fed from the onset of sepsis (see Chapter 37). The caloric requirements of septic patients are 1.5 to 1.8 times the basal metabolic rate.[37,86] Mixtures for parenteral nutrition should provide 6 g/kg of protein unless hepatic or renal failure is present.[87] Amino acid mixtures containing 45% branched chain amino acids are optimal for patients with sepsis.[88] The rest of the calories are supplied by giving dextrose and lipid.[87] The current recommendations for therapy in people are to supply 20% to 30% of the nonprotein calories as lipids, and to monitor lipid clearance.[37] If lipid clearance decreases, metabolic failure should be suspected and the proportion of calories supplied as protein increased. Veterinary investigators have suggested supplying 50% of the nonprotein calories as lipids, particularly in cats.[87] Most lipid emulsions are made of long-chain fatty acid triglycerides, although there may be some benefit to using medium chain triglycerides and fish oil (omega-3 fatty acids) during sepsis.[37]

Enteral feeding should begin as soon as possible because early enteral feeding (within 6 hours of injury or surgery) is associated with decreased prevalence of gastrointestinal ulceration, maintenance of gastrointestinal barrier function, and decreased translocation of bacteria.[83] Optimal enteral feeding formulations for hypermetabolic and septic patients are under development.[83,84,89] Current formulations for human hypermetabolic patients contain approximately 20% to 25% of the total calories as protein, and 14% to 40% of nonprotein calories as fat.[84] The protein source may be whey, casein, or soy protein. The carbohydrate source may be cornstarch, maltodextrin, corn syrup, and/or sucrose. Lipids are usually a mixture of vegetable oils, with 0% to 50% being medium-chain triglycerides. Fish oil has recently been added to several products in an attempt to modify lipid mediator release.[84] Glutamine is often added because it is trophic for intestinal cells.[83]

Acid-base status. Acid-base abnormalities are due to poor tissue oxygen delivery and/or respiratory failure in sepsis.[4] They should be initially corrected by cardiovascular resuscitation and provision of respiratory support, if indicated. Persistent severe metabolic acidosis (pH <7.2, base excess less than −10 mM/L) despite optimal therapy is a very poor prognostic sign, and the clinician should begin to make decisions about when

to stop therapy.[6,11] Sodium bicarbonate therapy is controversial, but may be given if life-threatening acidemia (pH <7.1) is present.[90,91]

Controversial therapies

Glucocorticoids. High doses of glucocorticoids (see Table 15-6) have been consistently shown to improve survival in acute lethal septic shock models in numerous species.[92] The problem for clinicians, however, is that glucocorticoids must be given prior to or within the first 2 hours of the onset of sepsis to be effective.[92] In canine models, glucocorticoids must be given within the first 15 minutes of septic shock because severe mesenteric vasoconstriction rapidly leads to irreversible shock.[92] Septic disease in clinical patients is routinely not recognized until after the administration of glucorticoids is effective. In several well-controlled human trials, glucocorticoids given at the onset of septic shock did not improve survival rates and actually led to an increase in the incidence of secondary infections.[93,94] In a study of canine endocarditis patients, treatment with glucocorticoids had an adverse effect on survival.[18] Proper use of glucocorticoids would thus appear to be restricted to administration within the first 2 hours of a known contaminating incident or as prophylaxis in patients undergoing a surgical procedure associated with release of organisms.

Mediator blockers. A large number of compounds have been identified that block the mediators released early in the course of experimentally induced septic or endotoxic shock. The chief use of these drugs has been to elucidate the role of various mediators and their interactions rather than to improve survival in clinical patients. As these blockers ameliorate clinical signs and sometimes lead to increased survival, it is tempting to try using them in clinical patients.[95] Unfortunately, the same cautions that apply to glucocorticoids also apply to mediator blockers. Clinicians will rarely be able to recognize sepsis prior to the release of key mediators, and administration of blockers after mediator release is not likely to have much effect. Side effects and drug interactions that are not apparent in experimental models become evident once blockers are given to patients with sepsis. The mediator blocker being used most often by veterinary clinicians is flunixin meglumine, a potent nonsteroidal antiinflammatory agent that blocks prostaglandin release.[31,34] Prostaglandin release peaks in the first 2 hours of canine septic shock and flunixin meglumine is unlikely to have beneficial effects if administered past that time.[39] Clinical problems associated with the use of flunixin meglumine include gastrointestinal ulceration, particularly when used in association with glucocorticoids, and potentiation of methoxyflurane-induced renal failure.[96,97]

In the future, modulation of lipid mediator release is likely to take the form of modifications of dietary lipids in high-risk patients such that reduced substrate is available for release of lipid mediators.[84] Safe methods of moderating release of cytokines without causing immunosuppression have yet to be identified.

Opiate antagonists. Cardiovascular decompensation in sepsis, particularly unresponsive hypotension, appears to be partially mediated by endogenous opiates.[98] Infusions of high doses of naloxone, an opiate antagonist, initially showed promise as an agent to improve cardiovascular status in experimental sepsis.[4,95] When naloxone was tested in a variety of bacteremia and endotoxemia models, however, extremely confusing results were obtained. Naloxone led to increased, decreased, or no improvement in survival, depending on the model and the species. The improvements in cardiovascular status seen with naloxone administration can be achieved with administration of fluids, inotropes, and pressors. Naloxone is now rarely used in human ICUs. Naloxone is obviously contraindicated in patients in whom opiates are being used to relieve pain and decrease postoperative stress.

Antioxidants and oxygen radical scavengers. Oxygen radicals occur in sepsis secondary to activation of neutrophils and reperfusion of previously hypoxic tissues.[4,39,95] Agents that prevent oxidation or scavenge oxygen radicals reduce tissue damage in experimental sepsis models, but are most effective in models in which hypoxia and reperfusion are a major part of the model (bowel ischemia). The most commonly used antioxidant is alpha-tocopherol (vitamin E), while common scavenging agents include superoxide dismutase and catalase. These agents are relatively nontoxic, and administration may limit tissue damage in patients with sepsis. Patients being fed with intravenous lipid emulsions should routinely be given antioxidants.

Immunotherapy. The most promising new treatment for gram-negative bacteremia is passive immunization of patients using hyperimmune serum or monoclonal antibodies made against the core region of endotoxin.[4,9,10,95] Specific antibodies against given strains of gram-negative bacteria react mainly with the polysaccharide component of endotoxin. Specific antibodies have long been known to be protective against lethal bacteremia, but this protection could not be extended to clinical patients because it was impossible to predict which strain of bacteria would cause bacteremia.

All gram-negative bacteria share a common core region, which is usually covered by the outer polysaccharide tail. In certain mutant strains, however, the core region is exposed. Immunization with these mutant bacteria (J5 *Escherichia coli, Salmonella minnesota* Re 595) induces antibody formation against the core region. Serum containing high levels of antibodies to the core region can be given to patients in septic shock and results in improved survival. Antibodies against the core region are probably protective because during bacterial growth the core region is made before the outer sugars are added to the endotoxin molecule.

Once protection with anticore antibodies was demonstrated, major research efforts were launched to find anticore monoclonal antibodies that provided similar protection to serum. Protective monoclonal antibodies were found, and a recent clinical trial demonstrated improved survival (63% versus 45%) in treated patients with gram-negative bacteremia, but not in patients with suspected sepsis who did not prove to have gram-negative bacteremia.[10] The cost of treatment with the monoclonal preparations will probably be around $1,000 to $2,000, which will put it out of the range of most veterinary patients. Affordable serum products may eventually be developed for the veterinary market. Alternatively, prophylactic vaccination of high-risk patients has been proposed.

PREVENTION OF SEPSIS

The best approach to treating sepsis is to prevent its occurrence, if possible.[13,14] The approach taken by human researchers has been to closely define the high-risk patient, determine what variables separate survivors from nonsurvivors, and to then treat all high-risk patients to match the supranormal oxygen delivery and consumption values found in survivors. In a prospective clinical study of surgical patients, the mortality rate of patients treated to meet supranormal therapeutic goals was 21% versus 38% in patients treated to meet normal values. In a second study, high-risk surgical patients were randomized to a central venous catheter group (23% mortality), a pulmonary artery catheter group treated to meet normal values (33% mortality), or a pulmonary catheter artery group treated to meet supranormal values (4% mortality). The highest mortality rates occurred in patients who met all criteria for being a high-risk patient, but who were not entered into the study due to the need for immediate surgical intervention (40% mortality) or because the surgeon did not think that the patient was "sick enough" to warrant the risk of placing a pulmonary artery catheter (38% mortality). No episodes of sepsis occurred in the pulmonary catheter artery group treated to meet supranormal values.

Veterinary clinicians can rarely provide the intensive monitoring used in human intensive care units. They can treat trauma and surgical patients with the knowledge that therapeutic goals should aim for cardiac indices that are 120% to 150% of normal, and blood volumes that are 110% to 120% of normal. In the process, veterinary clinicians are likely to decrease the incidence of preventable sepsis and shock in their critical care patients.

REFERENCES

1. Bone RC. Sepsis, the sepsis syndrome, multi-organ failure: A plea for comparable definitions. Ann Intern Med 1991;114:332-333.
2. Natanson C. A canine model of septic shock. In Parillo JE, moderator. Septic shock in humans: advances in the understanding of pathogenesis, cardiovascular dysfunction, and therapy. Ann Intern Med 1990;113:227-242.
3. Dow SW, et al. Bacterial culture of blood from critically ill dogs and cats: 100 cases (1985-1987). J Am Vet Med Assoc 1989;195:113-117.
4. Sheagren JN. Mechanism-oriented therapy for multiple systems organ failure. Crit Care Clin 1989;5:393-409.
5. Creasey AA, et al. Endotoxin and cytokine profile in plasma of baboons challenged with lethal and sublethal Escherichia coli. Circ Shock 1991;33:84-91.
6. Cerra FB. The systemic septic response: concepts of pathogenesis. J Trauma 1990;30:S169-S174.
7. Calvert CA, Dow SW. Cardiovascular infections. In Greene CE, ed. Infectious Diseases of the Dog and Cat. Philadelphia: WB Saunders 1990;97-113.
8. McCuskey RS, et al. Kupffer cell function in host defense. Rev Infect Dis 1987;9:S616-S619.
9. Nys M, et al. Protective effect of polyclonal sera and of monoclonal antibodies active to Salmonella minnesota Re595 liposaccharide during experimental endotoxemia. J Inf Dis 1990;162:1087-1094.
10. Zeigler EJ, et al. Treatment of gram-negative bacteremia and septic shock with HA-1A human monoclonal antibody against endotoxin. N Engl J Med 1991;324:429-436.
11. Seigel JH. Through a glass darkly: the lung as a window to monitor oxygen consumption, energy metabolism, and severity of critical illness. Clin Chem 1990;36:1585-1593.
12. Macheido GW, Suval WD. Detection of sepsis in the postoperative patient. Surg Clin North Am 1988;68:215-228.
13. Shoemaker WC, et al. Prospective trial of supranormal values of survivors as therapeutic goals in high-risk surgical patients, Chest 1988;94:1176-1186.
14. Shoemaker WC, Kram HB, Appel PL. Therapy of shock based on pathophysiology, monitoring, and outcome prediction. Crit Care Med 1990;18:S19-S24.
15. Greene CE, ed. Infectious Diseases of the Dog and Cat. Philadelphia: WB Saunders, 1990.
16. Goodwin JK, Shauer M. Septic shock. Vet Clin North Am Small Anim Pract 1989;19:1239-1258.
17. Hardie EM, Rawlings CA, Calvert CA. Severe sepsis in selected surgical patients. J Am Anim Hosp Assoc 1986; 22:33-41.
18. Calvert CA, Greene CE, Hardie EM. Cardiovascular infections in dogs: epizootiology, clinical manifestations, and prognosis. J Am Vet Med Assoc 1985;187:612-616.
19. Hirsch DC, Spencer SJ, Biberstein EL. Blood culture of the canine patient. J Am Vet Med Assoc 1984;184:175-178.
20. Sugarman HJ, et al. Hemodynamics, oxygen consumption and serum catecholamine changes in progressive, lethal peritonitis in the dog. Surg Gynecol Obstet 1982;154:8-12.
21. Martin C, et al. Septic shock: a goal-directed therapy using volume loading, dobutamine and/or norepinephrine. Acta Anaesthesiol Scand 1990;34:413-417.
22. Jardin F et al. Sepsis-related cardiogenic shock. Crit Care Med 1990;18:1055-1060.
23. Gilbert RP. Mechanisms of the hemodynamic effects of endotoxin, Physiol Rev 1960;40:245-279.
24. LaRue MJ, Murtaugh RJ. Pulmonary thromboembolism in dogs: 47 cases, J Am Vet Med Assoc 1990;1978:1368-1372.
25. Parratt JR, Sturgess RM. The effects of the repeated administration of sodium meclofenamate, an inhibitor of prostaglandin synthetase, in feline endotoxin shock. Circ Shock 1975;2:301-310.
26. Guntheroth WG, et al. Left ventricular performance in endotoxin shock in dogs. Am J Physiol 1982;242:H172-H176.
27. Stahl TJ, et al. Sepsis-induced diastolic dysfunction in chronic canine peritonitis. Am J Physiol 1990;258:H625-H633.
28. Parillo JE. Opening remarks. In Parillo JE, moderator. Septic shock in humans: advances in the understanding of pathogenesis, cardiovascular dysfunction, and therapy. Ann Intern Med 1990;113:227-242.
29. Parker MM. Right ventricular dysfunction and dilatation, similar to left ventricular changes, characterize the cardiac depression of septic shock in humans. Chest 1990; 97:126-131.
30. Sugarman HJ, et al. Thrombocytopenia in progressive lethal canine peritonitis. Surg Gynecol Obstet 1982; 154:193-196.
31. Hardie EM, et al. Canine septic peritonitis: treatment with flunixin meglumine. Circ Shock 1983;11:159-173.
32. Chung TW, et al. Survival factors in a canine septic shock model. Circ Shock 1991;33:178-182.
33. Feldman BF. Disseminated intravascular coagulation. Compend Contin Educ Pract Vet 1981;3:46-54.
34. Hardie EM, et al. Escherichia coli-induced lung and liver dysfunction in dogs: effects of flunixin treatment. Am J Vet Res 1987;48:56-62.
35. Schertel ER, Muir WW. Shock: pathophysiology, monitoring, and therapy. In RW Kirk, ed. Current Veterinary Therapy X. Philadelphia: WB Saunders, 1989;316-330.
36. Schaefer CF, Lerner MR, Biber B. Dose-related reduction of intestinal cytochrome a,a3 induced by endotoxin in rats. Circ Shock 1991;33:17-25.
37. Cerra FB. Metabolic manifestations of multiple systems organ failure. Crit Care Clin 1989;5:119-129.
38. Hauptman JG, Tvedlen H. Osmolal and anion gaps in dogs with acute endotoxic shock. Am J Vet Res 1986; 487:1617-1673.
39. Hardie EM, Krus-Elliott K. Endotoxic shock. Part I. A review of causes. J Vet Intern Med 1990;4:258-266.
40. Brigham KL, Meyrick B. Endotoxin and lung injury. Am Rev Respir Dis 1985;113:913-927.
41. Braquet P, et al. PAF/cytokine auto-generated feedback networks in microvascular immune injury: consequences in shock, ischemia, and graft rejection, J Lipid Mediators 1989;1:75-112.

42. Morrison DC, et al. Monoclonal antibody to mouse lipopolysaccharide receptor protects mice against the lethal effects of endotoxin. J Infect Dis 1990;162:1063-1068.

43. Morris DD, Moore JN. Endotoxin-induced production of thromboxane and prostacylin by equine peritoneal macrophages. Circ Shock 1987;23:192-197.

44. Beutler B. Cachetin in tissue injury, shock, and related states. Crit Care Clin 1989;5:353-367.

45. Dinorello CA. Interleukin-1 and interleukin-1 antagonism. Blood 1991;77:1627-1652.

46. Petrak RA, Balk RA, Bone RC. Prostaglandins, cyclooxygenase inhibitors, and thromboxane synthetase inhibitors in the pathogenesis of multiple systems organ failure. Crit Care Clin 1989;5:303-314.

47. Sprague RS, et al. Proposed role for leukotrienes in the pathophysiology of multiple systems organ failure. Crit Care Clin 1989;5:315-329.

48. Olson NC, Joyce PB, Fleisher LN. Role of platelet-activating factor and eicosanoids during endotoxin-induced lung injury in pigs. Am J Physiol 1990;258:H1674-H1686.

49. Knaus WA, Wagner DP. Multiple systems organ failure: epidemiology and prognosis. Crit Care Clin 1989;5:221-232.

50. Otto CM, Kaufmann GM, Crowe DT. Intraosseus infusion of fluids and therapeutics. Compend Contin Educ Pract Vet 1989;11:421-431.

51. Kolata RJ. The clinical management of circulatory shock based on pathophysiological patterns. Compend Contin Educ Pract Vet 1980;2:314-322.

52. Peacock JE, et al. Prospective, randomized comparison sequential, intravenous followed by oral ciprofloxicin with intravenous ceftazidime in the treatment of serious infections. Am J Med 1989;87(Suppl 5A):185S-190S.

53. Garvey MS, Aucoin DP. Therapeutic strategies involving antimicrobial treatment of disseminated bacterial infection in small animals. J Am Vet Med Assoc 1984;185:1185-1190.

54. Hardie EM. Peritonitis from urogenital conditions. Prob Vet Med 1989;1:36-49.

55. Dow SW, Jones RL, Adney WS. Anaerobic bacterial infections and response to treatment in dogs and cats: 36 cases (1983-1985). J Am Vet Med Assoc 1986;189:930-934.

56. Donowitz GR, Mandell GL. Beta-lactam antibiotics. N Engl J Med 1988;318:490-500.

57. Thornsberry C. Review of in vitro activity of third-generation cephlosporins and other newer beta-lactam antibiotics against clinically important bacteria. Am J Med 1985;79(Suppl 2A):14-20.

58. Mecher CE, et al. Venous hypercarbia associated with severe sepsis and systemic hypoperfusion. Crit Care Med 1990;18:585-589.

59. Allen D, Kvievtys P, Granger N. Crystalloids versus colloids: implications in fluid therapy of dogs with intestinal obstruction. Am J Vet Res 1986;47:1751-1755.

60. Armistead CW, et al. Hypertonic saline solution-hetastarch for fluid resuscitation in experimental septic shock. Anesth Analg 1989;69:714-720.

61. Bornsveld W, et al. Ventricular function, hemodynamics, and oxygen consumption during infusions of blood, and glucose-insulin-potassium (GIK) in canine endotoxin shock. Circ Shock 1982;9:145-156.

62. Dawidson I, Ottoson J, Reisch JS. Infusion volumes of Ringer's lactate and 3% albumin solution as they relate to survival after resuscitation of a lethal intestinal shock. Circ Shock 1986;18:277-288.

63. Luypaert P, et al. Fluid resuscitation with hypertonic saline in endotoxic shock. Circ Shock 1986;20:311-320.

64. Manny J, Rabinovici N, Manny N. Effect of glucose-insulin-potassium on survival in experimental endotoxic shock. Surg Gynecol Obstet 1978;147:405-409.

65. Muir WW, et al. Small-volume resuscitation with hypertonic saline solution in hypovolemic cats. Am J Vet Res 1989;50:1883-1888.

66. Mullins RJ, Hudgens RW. Hypertonic saline resuscitates dogs in endotoxic shock. J Surg Res 1985;43:37-44.

67. Rocha-e-Silva M, et al. Hypertonic resuscitation from severe hemorrhagic shock: patterns of regional circulation. Circ Shock 1986;19:165-175.

68. Rocha-e-Silva M, et al. Replacement preparations. In McEvoy GK, ed. AHFS Drug Information 91. Bethesda, MD: American Society of Hospital Pharmacists, 1991;1500-1516.

69. Linko K, Makelainen A. Cardiorespiratory function after replacement of blood loss with hydroxyethyl starch 120, dextran 70, and Ringer's acetate in pigs. Crit Care Med 1989;17:1031-1035.

70. Emerson TE. Unique features of albumin: a brief review. Crit Care Med 1989;17:690-694.

71. Natanson C, et al. Antibiotics versus cardiovascular support in a canine model of human septic shock. Am J Physiol 1990;259:H1440-H1447.

72. Lawson N. Therapeutic combinations of vasopressors and inotropic agents. Semin Anesth 1990;9:270-287.

73. Vincent JL, et al. Dopamine compared with dobutamine in experimental septic shock: relevance to fluid administration. Anesth Analg 1987;66:565-571.

74. Schreuder WO. Effect of dopamine vs norepinephrine on hemodynamics in septic shock. Chest 1989;95:1282-1288.

75. Garvey MS. Fluid and electrolyte balance in critical patients. Vet Clin North Am Small Anim Pract 1989;19:1021-1057.

76. Perry MO. Anticoagulation: a surgical perspective. Am J Surg 1988;155:268-276.

77. Ruehl W, Mills C, Feldman BF. Rational therapy in disseminated intravascular coagulation. J Am Vet Med Assoc 1982;181:76-78.

78. Rana MW, et al. Heparin administration before or after hemorrhagic shock protects microvascular patency. Circ Shock 1990;13:59.

79. Hunt CA. Diagnostic peritoneal paracentesis and lavage. Compend Contin Educ Pract Vet 1980;6:449-453.

80. Bjorling DE, et al. Diagnostic peritoneal lavage before and after abdominal surgery in dogs. Am J Vet Res 1983;44:816-820.

81. Matthiesen DT, Manfra MS. Complications associated with the surgical treatment of prostatic abscessation. Prob Vet Med 1989;1:63-73.

82. Papich MG. Antiulcer therapy. Vet Med Rep 1989;1:309-320.

83. Barber AF, et al. Glutamine or fiber supplementation of a defined formula diet: impact on bacterial translocation, tissue composition, and response to endotoxin. J Parenter Enteral Nutr 1990;14:335-343.

84. Gottschlich MM, Jenkins M, Warden GD. Differential effects of three enteral dietary regimens on selected outcome variables in burn patients. J Parenter Enteral Nutr 1990;14:225-236.

85. Lewis LD, Morris ML. Hand MS. Small Animal Clinical Nutrition III. Topeka, KS: Mark Morris, 1987.

86. Linder A, Culter RE, Goodman WG. Synergism of dopamine plus forosemide in preventing acute renal failure in the dog. Kidney Int 1979;16:158-166.

87. Lippert AC, Armstrong PJ. Parenteral nutritional support. In Kirk RW, ed. Current Veterinary Therapy X. Philadelphia: WB Saunders, 1989;25-30.

88. Kawamura I, et al. Optimum branched-chain amino acid concentration for improving protein catabolism in severely stressed rats. J Parenter Enteral Nutr 1990;14:398-403.

89. Wheeler SL, McGuire BH. Enteral nutritional support. In Kirk RW, ed. Current Veterinary Therapy X. Philadelphia: WB Saunders, 1989;30-37.

90. Biebuyck JF. Sodium bicarbonate in the treatment of subtypes of acute lactic acidosis: physiologic considerations. Anesthesiology 1990;72:1064-1076.

91. Cooper DJ, et al. Bicarbonate does not improve hemodynamics in critically ill patients who have lactic acidosis. Ann Intern Med 1990;112:492-498.

92. Hinshaw LB, Beller-Todd BK, Archer LT. Current management of the septic shock patient: experimental basis for treatment. Circ Shock 1982;9:543-553.

93. Bone RC, et al. A controlled clinical trial of high-dose methylprednisolone in the treatment of severe sepsis and septic shock. N Engl J Med 1987;317:653-658.

94. Veterans Administration Systemic Sepsis Cooperative study group. Effect of high-dose glucocorticoid therapy on mortality in patients with clinical signs of systemic sepsis. N Engl J Med 1987;317:659-665.

95. Hardie EM, Krus-Elliott R. Endotoxic shock. Part II. A review of treatment. J Vet Intern Med 1990;4:306-314.

96. Dow SW, et al. Effects of flunixin and flunixin plus prednisone on the gastrointestinal tract of dogs. Am J Vet Res 1990;51:1131-1138.

97. Mathews K, et al. Renal failure in dogs associated with flunixin meglumine and methoxyflurane anesthesia. Vet Surg 1987;16:323.

98. Baker CH, et al. Reduced microvascular adrenergic receptor activity due to opiods in endotoxin shock. Circ Shock 1990;32:101-112.

16 Physical and Chemical Injuries: Heatstroke, Hypothermia, Burns, and Frostbite

David E. Lee-Parritz and Michael M. Pavletic

HEATSTROKE AND HYPERTHERMIA

Definition

Heatstroke is defined as marked pyrexia (40.5°C to 43.0°C) following exposure to elevated ambient temperatures. Nonexertional heatstroke is the most common presentation and develops when animals are confined in overheated automobiles or are chained outdoors on hot, sunny days. Exertional heatstroke is rare and occurs when nonacclimated animals are exercised in warm, humid weather. Heatstroke is a polysystemic disorder that results from the direct toxic effect of heat on cellular function.

Physiology

Normal dogs and cats maintain core normothermia over a wide range of environmental temperature. Heatstroke results when normal animals are exposed to extreme heat or when normal protective mechanisms are impaired through metabolic or anatomic disease. Heat is acquired from and lost to the environment through the interaction of radiation, convection, conduction, and evaporation. Evaporation and conduction are the principal mechanisms by which dogs and cats lose heat to the environment. Panting and the spreading of saliva on the fur by a cat during grooming are examples of heat loss by evaporation. Cooling occurs through conduction when animals prostrate themselves on cool surfaces, facilitating heat loss from the relatively hairless skin of the ventral abdomen.[1]

With mild heat stress, reflex vasoactivity maintains normothermia at low metabolic cost. Warm blood is shunted from large muscle masses and visceral organs to the relatively hairless, highly vascular skin of the feet, face, and ears. Peripheral vasodilation then allows heat loss by radiation and convection. Paradoxically, the insulating properties of fur protect against a hot environment. Fur, and the air it traps next to the skin, restricts the amount of heat absorbed by the body from the sun (radiation) and from warm surfaces (conduction).

Panting supplements reflex vasoactivity to increase heat loss during moderate heat stress. Panting is the primary method of heat loss at environmental temperatures >35°C. The panting animal directs large volumes of air across the mucosa of the tongue, oropharynx, and trachea. Vasodilation and fluid secretion from these tissues results in heat loss from the evaporation of water (0.6 kcal/g of water).[1]

Panting differs physiologically from sweating in several ways. Minute ventilation may increase up to 25-fold. Respiratory muscle activity produces heat.[1] Metabolic acidosis may develop as a consequence of respiratory muscle fatigue.[2] The efficiency of evaporative heat loss by panting may be reduced by high environmental humidity, limiting the absorptive capacity of the air or by anatomic defects of the larynx or trachea impairing breathing.

Despite the metabolic costs of panting as compared with sweating, clinically relevant advantages are evident. Because panting allows heat loss by evaporation of water from the respiratory tract, heat gain by radiation from exposed skin surfaces is limited. Animals that control body temperature through panting conserve sodium and are better able to maintain adequate circulatory volume during heat stress as compared with animals that sweat. As a result, severe electrolyte abnormalities are less common in dogs than in people with heatstroke.[1,3,4]

Pathophysiology

Neurologic damage is common with heatstroke. Neuronal death occurs as a direct result of thermal injury. In fatal heatstroke in humans, Purkinje cell dropout and multiple periventricular, cerebellar, and diencephalic hemorrhages are seen.[5] Hemoconcentration associated with dehydration may impair cerebral blood flow and cause thrombosis. In addition, cerebral metabolism is impaired because hepatic production of nucleotides required for cerebral glucose transport is impaired.[6] Neurologic impairment and impaired heat tolerance may persist after resolution of heatstroke.[4]

Hypovolemia and shock account for other clinical signs in heatstroke. Myocardial necrosis is seen histologically in fatal cases.[6] Thermal injury to endothelial cells and toxemia associated with metabolic stress may cause disseminated intravascular coagulation (DIC).[7] Acute renal failure may arise from hypotension, thermal injury to renal tubular epithelium, and myoglobinuria associated with rhabdomyolysis.[5]

Diagnosis

History and physical examination. The diagnosis of heatstroke is straightforward when extremely elevated rectal temperatures are encountered in an animal exposed to high environmental temperature. The history may offer valuable clues to diagnosis (see the following box).[8,9] Infant animals lack effective thermoregulatory ability until approximately 45 days of age.[10] Aged animals may have occult cardiac or respiratory disease that impairs heat tolerance.

PREDISPOSING FACTORS FOR HEATSTROKE

Impaired heat loss
   Obesity
   Respiratory disease
   Cardiac disease
   Dehydration
   Age extremes
   Lack of acclimatization
   Dehydration
Increased heat production
   Exercise
   Fever
   Hyperthyroidism
   Malignant hyperthermia
Toxicosis
   Strychnine
   Organophosphate

Depending on the history and physical examination findings, other differential diagnoses for pyrexia that should be considered include infection, neoplasia, and toxicosis. Panting will usually be seen in an animal with heatstroke unless severe neurologic damage has abolished the panting reflex. Fever associated with infectious agents will not result in panting because the hypothalamic set point is increased. It is possible, however, that infection may predispose an animal to heatstroke because normal protective mechanisms for heat loss may not be activated until the body temperature has increased beyond physiologic limits.[8]

Neurologic, respiratory, cardiovascular, and renal function should be assessed. Stupor is an early sign of neurologic dysfunction that may progress to involuntary paddling, coarse tremors, and seizures. Coma and loss of the menace and panting reflexes often signify the presence of severe cerebral edema and warrant a poor prognosis. Cyanosis, excessive respiratory effort or respiratory stridor should alert the clinician to the possible presence of complicating upper airway disease or secondary laryngeal and pharyngeal edema from prolonged panting. Concurrent upper airway disease (laryngeal paralysis, everted laryngeal saccules, or excess soft palate) is a potentially serious complicating factor, as panting is compromised. Respiratory collapse and cyanosis commonly occur in these cases. The presence of concomitant cardiac disease is suggested by weak or irregular pulses and/or jugular venous distention.

Laboratory diagnosis. Laboratory testing is indicated to exclude other causes of pyrexia and to evaluate vital organ function. The minimum data base in patients suspected of having heatstroke consists of a complete blood count, serum biochemistry profile, and urinalysis. Blood gas analysis provides valuable diagnostic information and allows more accurate monitoring. Hematochezia, development of petechiae, and prolonged bleeding from venipuncture sites indicate the possibility of DIC. These findings should prompt evaluation of the hemostatic pathways.

Hemoconcentration is a common finding in heatstroke.[4,7] Azotemia, proteinuria, and cylindruria indicate the presence of acute renal failure associated with hyperpyrexia and hypovolemia.[4] Serum liver enzyme activities may be moderately elevated due to hepatocyte damage.[4] Hypokalemia and hypophosphatemia may occur as a consequence of respiratory alkalosis. Hyperkalemia has been reported in experimentally induced heatstroke in dogs,[7] but not in clinical cases.[4] Mixed acid-base disturbances occur. Respiratory alkalosis from panting is complicated by metabolic acidosis associated with respiratory muscle fatigue and shock.

Management

The animal's body temperature should be normalized as quickly as possible. In man, mortality from heatstroke is proportional to the time required to achieve normal body temperature.[11] Clients should be advised to begin to cool their pets prior to transport if the emergency facility is further than a few minutes away. A stream of cool water from a garden hose or immersion of the animal in a large tub of cool water is the most physiologic method of temperature normalization. Directing an electric fan on the wet haircoat increases heat loss by evaporation and convection.[3]

Cooling of small animals occurs quickly; most dogs and cats will cool in a matter of minutes. An animal's body temperature is likely to fall further when active cooling is halted as cool blood from the periphery reaches the core. For this reason, active cooling of the animal should be stopped when the body temperature reaches 38.5°C. The rectal temperature should be monitored frequently after temperature normalization, as impaired thermoregulation may be a temporary or permanent consequence of heatstroke.[4] The use of ice baths is discouraged. Ice baths produce peripheral vasoconstriction, reducing heat loss and induce shivering, which increases heat formation.[3]

Laryngeal paralysis, laryngeal edema, or tracheal stenosis, if present, will impair heat loss through the respiratory system. These conditions may need to be temporarily corrected through emergency tracheostomy or endotracheal intubation.

Fluid therapy is crucial. Prolonged panting results in dehydration. Hypovolemia is exacerbated in heatstroke when decreased cardiac output reduces effective circulating volume. Water is lost in excess of sodium in panting. For this reason, resuscitation fluids are 0.45% saline or half-strength lactated Ringer's solution with 2.5% dextrose. Initial fluid administration rates are 50 to 80 ml/kg in the first hour, with additional fluids administered according to the animal's hemodynamic status and the results of laboratory testing. Thoracic auscultation, evaluation of jugular veins and capillary refill time and measurement of central venous, systemic arterial, and capillary wedge pressure can be useful in monitoring the hemodynamic status of heatstroke victims.

In exertional heatstroke, sodium bicarbonate (2 to 3 mEq/kg) added to intravenous fluids will alkalinize the urine and minimize renal tubular damage from myoglobin precipitation.[5] Bicarbon-

ate therapy should be guided by periodic determination of blood pH, blood bicarbonate concentration, and urine pH. Sodium bicarbonate should not be added to lactated Ringer's solution or other calcium-containing fluid.

Corticosteroids (dexamethasone sodium phosphate 1 mg/kg intravenously or prednisolone sodium succinate 5 to 11 mg/kg intravenously) may be given to decrease cerebral edema if signs of central nervous system dysfunction are present. Mannitol administration should be avoided initially because of the risk of inducing circulatory collapse.

Acepromazine (0.05 to 0.1 mg/kg intravenously) or diazepam (1 mg/kg intravenously) may be administered if severe shivering occurs. The alpha-blocking effect of acepromazine will also counteract peripheral vasoconstriction associated with aggressive cooling. Fluid therapy must be titrated to counteract possible drug-induced hypotension.

Additional drugs should be administered with caution. Antipyretics will not be useful in heatstroke because pyrexia in these animals does not result from resetting of the hypothalamic temperature regulation mechanism. In particular, nonsteroidal antiinflammatory drugs such as aspirin or flunixin meglumine are contraindicated because their effects may promote gastric bleeding, inhibit platelet function, and impair renal function. These drug effects must be avoided in a setting in which DIC might occur.

If present, DIC should resolve as the patient stabilizes. Additional therapy such as fresh or fresh frozen plasma or whole blood transfusions and heparin administration may be required in some cases.[5]

Monitoring and prognosis

Following initial resuscitation for heatstroke, animals should be monitored to ensure that possible sequelae of heatstroke are recognized and treated appropriately. Water consumption and urine output should be monitored, as nephrogenic diabetes insipidus is common in dogs recovering from severe heatstroke, and this condition may persist for many weeks.[4,5] Clients should be instructed to prevent future episodes of heatstroke and to treat underlying medical conditions that may be present.

ACCIDENTAL HYPOTHERMIA
Definition

Hypothermia occurs when an animal with a normal body temperature of 37°C develops a core temperature less than 35°C. Severe hypothermia is present when the core body temperature drops below 28°C. Accidental hypothermia occurs when a conscious animal is unable to maintain thermal homeostasis when exposed to extreme environmental cold. Accidental hypothermia may also be an unintended consequence of drug therapy, anesthesia, or surgery.

Pathophysiology

Animals maintain normal body temperature in cold environments by increasing endogenous heat production while minimizing heat loss to the environment. Heat production occurs through voluntary muscle activity and through increased muscle tone or shivering. Heat conservation occurs through behavioral means (shelter seeking) and by reflex physiologic responses. Piloerection traps an insulating layer of air next to the skin and peripheral vasoconstriction shunts warm blood away from the exposed skin of the feet, ears, and face. Acclimated animals are better able to endure cold than unacclimated animals for three reasons: (1) a thick fur coat minimizes heat lost by conduction and convection; (2) increased subcutaneous fat stores contribute to whole body insulation and provide an energy substrate for muscular activity; and (3) increased vasomotor control improves the ability to modulate blood flow and metabolic rate in response to environmental extremes.[1]

Hypothermia can develop in any animal exposed to cold conditions and may occur at relatively moderate temperatures in animals with impaired abilities for heat production or conservation. Cold-water immersion predisposes animals to hypothermia through massive heat loss from conduction. Evaporation induces progressive hypothermia until the animal is dry. Small dogs and cats are especially susceptible to hypothermia because of their greater surface area: mass ratio. Young animals have increased susceptibility because they may be behaviorally and physically unable to reach shelter and lack the glycogen, muscle, and fat reserves required to withstand cold.[10]

Diagnosis

History. Hypothermia may occur in any animal after exposure to extreme cold. Hypothermia may follow moderate exposure in unacclimated or highly susceptible individuals. Hypothermia associated with depression or other vague clinical signs in the absence of cold exposure may indicate the presence of hypothyroidism, cardiac disease, or toxicosis (see the following box).[9,12] Because standard clinical mercury thermometers record a range of only 34.5°C to 41°C, low-temperature thermometers are required to properly diagnose and treat hypothermic patients. Suitable

---

PREDISPOSING FACTORS FOR HYPOTHERMIA

Increased heat loss
    Trauma
    Cold-water immersion or wetting
    Exposure
    Surgery
Impaired heat production
    Hypothyroidism
    Cachexia
    Trauma
    Cardiac disease
Toxicosis
    Alcohol
    Ethylene glycol
    Anesthetics

---

inexpensive thermometers may be obtained from scientific supply houses.

Acquired illness may reduce cold tolerance. Traumatized animals and those with metabolic or infectious diseases are prone to hypothermia because of impaired reserves and inability to reach shelter. Severe burns predispose to hypothermia through fluid exudation and heat loss from damaged tissue.[13] Hypothyroidism is the most important metabolic disorder associated with accidental hypothermia in dogs because this common endocrinopathy may produce vague clinical signs that elude diagnosis or do not prompt owner concern.[14-17] Hypothyroidism impairs thermoregulation by reducing the hypothalamic set point and by blocking endogenous heat production. Shivering responses may be absent in hypothyroid animals with hypothermia.

Iatrogenic accidental hypothermia may result from anesthesia and surgery. General anesthesia impairs endogenous heat production through impaired thermoregulation, direct depression of metabolism and by eliminating muscle activity. Surgical preparation, exposure of body cavities, and breathing of cold, dry anesthetic gases all increase heat loss. Severe hypothermia delays recovery from anesthesia and may induce fatal cardiac arrhythmias. Alcohol used in surgical preparation increases evaporative heat loss. Minimizing surgical time, limiting surgical exposure, and providing supplemental heat to anesthetized animals reduce the incidence of hypothermia. Circulating-warm-water blankets are safe and effective supplemental heat sources. Radiant heat lamps may be useful in recovery or intensive care units. These lamps must be carefully used in order to prevent burns.[18]

Physical examination. Mild hypothermia (rectal temperature, 32°C to 35°C) may cause lethargy, incoordination, stupor, and increased muscle tone or shivering. Unconsciousness and loss of the shivering reflex occurs with moderate hypothermia (rectal temperature, 28°C to 32°C). Animals with severe hypothermia (rectal temperature, <28°C) may be presented in a state of collapse or may appear agonal with fixed dilated pupils and shallow, infrequent respirations.[19] Peripheral and facial edema has been reported in humans and may be confused with myxedema.[20] Poor skin turgor, sunken eyes, and dry or pale mucous membranes signify the presence of hypovolemia and shock.

Laboratory testing. A minimum data base consisting of complete blood count, total serum protein, and electrocardiography is indicated to determine the degree of dehydration and the presence of cardiac abnormalities. A serum biochemistry profile, urinalysis, and blood gas analysis allows for more accurate monitoring and may aid in the diagnosis of underlying illness. In suspected severe hypothyroidism and myxedema requiring emergency thyroxine administration, a blood sample for submission of basal thyroid hormone levels should be obtained.[21]

Clinical signs and metabolic disturbances in hypothermia result from hypovolemia and the direct effect of cold on renal, neurologic, and cardiac function. "Cold diuresis" is the chief cause of dehydration in hypothermic animals. This phenomenon results when peripheral vasoconstriction increases the glomerular filtration rate and when cold reduces tubular sensitivity to antidiuretic hormone and impairs tubular reabsorption of sodium and glucose. As dehydration progresses, hematocrit and hemoglobin concentrations increase, although serum electrolyte concentrations often remain normal. Pancreatic necrosis has been reported in 50% of cases of fatal hypothermia in man. Moderate hyperglycemia, hyperamylasemia, and increased serum activities of the hepatic enzymes may occur.[19,20]

Heart rate, arterial blood pressure, and respiratory rate increase in mild hypothermia but eventually these parameters decline as hypovolemia and progressive hypothermia worsen cardiac and brainstem function. Electrocardiographic changes accompanying mild hypothermia include prolongation of the P-R, Q-T, and QRS intervals, atrial ectopy, and T-wave inversion. Osborne, or J, waves are extra deflections at the QRS-ST junction that are pathognomonic of hypothermia when present. Osborne waves have only rarely been reported in the dog.[14,16] Atropine-resistant bradycardia and ventricular ectopy may develop as hy-

pothermia progresses. Cardiac arrest associated with ventricular fibrillation or asystole will often be present in severe hypothermia (rectal temperature below 28°C).[19]

Respiratory function is impaired because increased alveolar and interstitial lung water limits oxygen diffusion. Oxygen delivery is further impaired because of a left shift of the oxygen-hemoglobin dissociation curve. Hyperventilation and poor oxygenation resulting from pulmonary edema accompanies hypovolemia and poor tissue perfusion to produce mixed respiratory alkalosis and metabolic acidosis. Bronchial secretions may become thick and tenacious.[20] Edema fluid and thickened bronchial secretions may predispose the animal to the development of bacterial bronchopneumonia following recovery from hypothermia.[19]

Management

Vigorous resuscitation efforts are indicated for all hypothermic animals. Cardiac rhythm may be restored in an apparently lifeless animal if the circulation can be supported until core temperature exceeds 28°C. Hypothermic animals may withstand prolonged periods of cardiac arrest as a result of the cytoprotective effect of low temperature and lowered metabolic rate. These observations have led to the dictum in human medicine that "no one is dead until warm and dead."[21]

Mild hypothermia. Animals with mild hypothermia will recover if they are dried, wrapped in blankets, removed to a warm environment, and observed carefully until they are normothermic. Clinically evident dehydration warrants the administration of warmed parenteral fluids. Electrocardiographic monitoring allows detection and treatment of dangerous cardiac arrhythmias. Active core rewarming of these patients may be detrimental if the metabolic needs of major organ systems are raised before normal circulatory status has been achieved.[19]

Severe hypothermia. Respiratory and cardiovascular support is crucial to successful resuscitation of moderately to severely hypothermic animals. If endotracheal intubation is required, mask preoxygenation will lower the likelihood of ventricular fibrillation.[12,19] A large-bore jugular catheter should be quickly placed for administration of warmed 0.9% saline and for central venous pressure monitoring. Care should be taken to avoid contact with the endocardium by the catheter tip. Closed-chest cardiac compression should be instituted if asystole, ventricular fibrillation or pulseless cardiac rhythms are present. Once instituted, cardiac compression should be maintained until the body temperature exceeds 28°C. Drug therapy or electric cardioversion is likely to be futile until this temperature is reached. Bretyllium tosylate administration decreased the occurrence of ventricular fibrillation in experimentally hypothermic dogs, but has not been shown to be of clinical benefit in the treatment of hypothermia in people.[12]

Metabolic acidosis, if present, should be treated cautiously because the right shift of the oxygen-hemoglobin dissociation curve from metabolic acidosis partially compensates for the left shift in the dissociation curve from hypothermia. Blood gas values obtained should be corrected for the animal's actual body temperature, or falsely low pH and falsely elevated oxygen pressure may be obtained.[19] If severe shivering occurs, phenothiazines (acepromazine 0.05 to 0.1 mg/kg intravenously) or diazepam (1 mg/kg intravenously) should be judiciously given to prevent worsening of metabolic acidosis, which may precipitate ventricular fibrillation.[20]

Rewarming. Active rewarming of the moderate to severely hopothermic animal should begin after cardiovascular support and monitoring is initiated. Surface rewarming by circulating-warm-water blankets may be adequate for animals with stable cardiovascular function and core temperatures >30°C. Electric heating pads and heat lamps may readily cause cutaneous burns in hypothermic patients because vasoconstriction in these patients blocks dissipation of heat from surface tissues. These devices should be employed cautiously and used only when they are the only warming devices available.

Core rewarming is indicated for animals with core temperature <30°C or with unstable cardiovascular function. Peritoneal dialysis is the core rewarming method of choice. Colonic or gastric lavage with warm water is ineffective and potentially hazardous and should be avoided.[19] Warming inspired air to 45°C limits further heat loss, but does not contribute substantially to core rewarming and requires specialized equipment.[13] In man, active surface rewarming techniques raise body temperature at the rate of approximately 1°C per hour. Core rewarming techniques raise body temperature at 3 to 5°C per hour.[19]

Peritoneal dialysis is performed in the following manner. Two peritoneal dialysis catheters are inserted and the dialysate infused and removed repeatedly. Foley catheters and lactated Ringer's solution may be employed if specialized dialysis catheters and solutions are not available. Catheters may be placed intraoperatively if severe hypothermia is detected during a surgical procedure. Dialysis fluids should be warmed to 45°C. Fluids may be conveniently warmed by passing the administration line through a blood warming coil. If a blood warming coil is not available, bags or bottles of fluids should be warmed to 55°C in a microwave oven, incubator, or water bath, since a temperature drop of approximately 10°C may be expected as the fluid passes through a standard administration set.[19] Careful monitoring must continue until recovery is complete. Acid-base status, cardiac rhythm, and blood pressure may worsen during resuscitation as cold, acidemic blood from the periphery returns to the circulation in a phenomenon known as "after-drop."

BURNS
Definition

Burns result when intense heat damages skin and subcutaneous tissues. Accidental thermal burns result from exposure to scalding liquids or flames. Iatrogenic thermal burns result from misuse of grooming clippers, electric heating pads, and infrared heating lamps. Animals surviving electrocution develop burns at the site of electrical contact. Caustic materials inflict chemical burns that resemble thermal burns in their effect on the skin, although the systemic effects of the material must be considered during the initial phase of treatment.

The nature of the heat source and the duration of exposure determine the severity of the burn.[22] Sunburn is an example of a superficial burn characterized by erythema and reversible epidermal injury. Superficial partial-thickness burns destroy the epidermis and upper dermis. These burns retain pain sensation and blood supply and heal by epithelial regeneration in approximately 3 weeks.

Deep partial-thickness burns destroy the deeper layers of the dermis. Healing is slow, and extensive scar formation occurs because reepithelialization occurs primarily from the wound margins and from adnexal epithelium in the upper hypodermis. Scalds and heating pads inflict partial-thickness burns. Flames may cause partial or full-thickness burns.

Full-thickness burns involve all layers of the skin as well as subcutaneous tissues and heal only from the wound margins (Fig. 16-1). Partial-thickness burns may result in greater fluid and hemodynamic alterations than full-thickness burns because coagulation necrosis and vascular thrombosis associated with full-thickness burns limit local edema formation.[22] Deep partial-thickness and full-thickness wounds are anesthetic and bloodless. Full-thickness wounds may be charred or leathery in appearance or may be a bloodless "pearl" white in color. A "halo" of lightly burned skin may surround a full-thickness injury. A fissure commonly forms within 7 to 10 days after

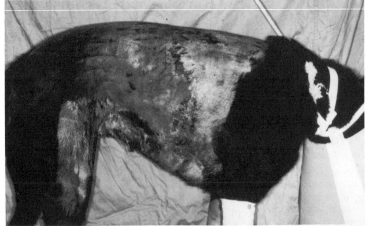

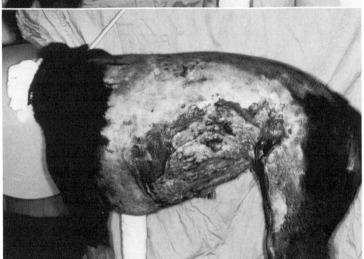

Fig. 16-1 A, Right and **B,** left lateral views of an extensive burn encircling the caudal trunk of a Labrador-cross dog. This injury resulted when the dog was maliciously set afire after being dowsed with lighter fluid. Surprisingly, the dog displayed no significant physiologic or biochemical abnormalities despite burn involvement estimated at 30% total body-surface area.

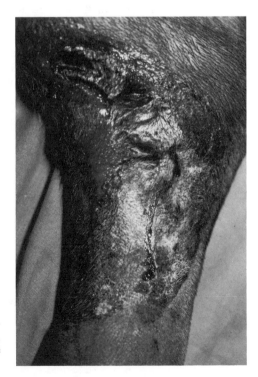

Fig. 16-2 Burn eschar of the lateral aspect of the distal hindlimb of a dog, resulting from a road pavement friction burn. Note the area of full-thickness injury at the center of the wound. A partial-thickness burn is present at the periphery.

Table 16-1 Injurious chemical agents*†

Agent	Clinical presentation	Mechanism of systemic toxicity	Immediate cleansing	Neutralization
Common acids				
Sulfuric, nitric, hydrochloric trichloracetic	Yellow, brown gray, or black eschar	Vapor	Water and soap	Magnesium hydroxide or sodium bicarbonate solution
Hydrofluoric	Erythema with central necrosis	None	Water	Calcium gluconate (10%) subcutaneously
Oxalic	Chalky white indolent ulcers	Ingestion only	Water	Calcium gluconate (10%)
Phenol (carbolic) and analogues	Painless, white or brown skin burn	Skin absorption	Water	Ethyl alcohol (10%) or glycerol
Chromic	Ulceration, blisters	Vapor	Water	Sodium hyposulfite
Hypochlorous (Clorox)	Second-degree	None	Water	Sodium thiosulfate (1%)
Other acids				
Tungstic, picric, tannic, cresylic, formic	Hard eschar	Skin absorption	Water	Cover with oil
Lyes (alkali)				
Sodium hydroxide, potassium hydroxide, calcium hydroxide, barium hydroxide, lithium hydroxide	Bullous erythema or slimy or slick eschar	Ingestion only	Water	Weak (0.5% to 5.0%) acetic acid; lemon juice
Ammonia	Bullous erythema or slimy or slick eschar	Vapor	Water	Weak (0.5% to 5.0%) acetic acid, lemon juice
Lime	Bullous erythema or slimy or slick eschar	Ingestion only	Brush off lime in water	Weak (0.5% to 5.0%) acetic acid; lemon juice
Alkyl mercury salts	Erythema, blisters	Skin absorption from blisters	Water and remove blisters	Copious irrigation
Sodium metal	Painful deep burns	None	Cover with oil	None except excision
Vesicants				
Mustard gas	Painful bullae	Vapor	Water; open vesicles during copious lavage	British antilewisite (BAL)
Tear gas	Erythema, ulcers	Vapor	Water	No specific agent
Phosphorus	Erythema to third-degree burn	Tissue absorption	Water; cold water packs	Copper sulfate for identification only
Ethylene oxide	Erythema to third-degree burn	None	Allow to vaporize; then water lavage	No specific agent

*For a complete discussion of chemicals and antidotes see Jelenko C. Chemicals that burn. *J Trauma* 1974;14:65-73.
†A complete listing and description of injurious chemical agents may be found in the *Fire Protection Guide on Hazardous Materials,* 7th ed. National Fire Protection Association, 470 Atlantic Ave., Boston, MA 02210.

full-thickness injury at the interface between viable and nonviable tissue[23-25] (Fig. 16-2).

Caustic agents destroy skin by denaturing skin proteins and causing coagulation necrosis. Cellular dehydration or intercellular edema may occur. Prolonged exposure may result in vascular thrombosis. Strong alkaline agents cause particularly deep tissue destruction because cellular dehydration, protein precipitation, and soap formation facilitate the passage of hydroxyl ions to deeper layers.[25] The extent of the injury associated with accidental or malicious exposure depends on the chemical, its concentration, the duration of contact, the degree of tissue penetration, and the compound's mechanism of action (Table 16-1). In general, caustic agents can be divided into strong acids and strong alkalis. Solvents used for painting, furniture strippers and concentrated flea dip solutions are chemical agents also capable of causing partial-thickness burns with prolonged contact.

Skilled intensive therapy may allow successful treatment of very extensive burns. It is instructive that human burn care units experience less than 10% mortality in patients with burns covering 50% total body-surface area (TBSA). Survival from burns covering 70% to 80% TBSA is common.[26] Dogs and cats may be able to tolerate burns more readily than humans. Fur limits skin damage by dissipating heat and burned canine and feline skin blisters less readily than human skin, limiting fluid shifts in the immediate postburn period. In addition, healing is facilitated by the large amount of pliable elastic skin on the neck and trunk of dogs and cats. Several case reports in dogs describe recovery from burns estimated to cover 40% to 60% TBSA.[27,28] In many cases, successful outcomes occurred despite limited initial resuscitation, suggesting that the grave prognosis traditionally given for veterinary burn patients[20,23] should be revised.[24] The prolonged hospitalization and home care required to manage infection, maintain normal function, and obtain acceptable appearance of the injured area may be extremely costly. This matter should be clarified with the owner before intensive therapy begins.

Pathophysiology

The skin is the organ most visibly affected in burns; however, cardiac, respiratory, and immune function are severely impaired in burns affecting greater than approximately 20% to 25% TBSA. The acute phase of burn injury lasts approximately 7 days. During this time, pathophysiologic changes and therapeutic requirements are similar to those seen in other severely traumatized individuals and primarily involve the cardiovascular and respiratory systems. The chronic phase of burn injury begins when cardiovascular and respiratory function has stabilized (7 to 10 days postinjury) and lasts until complete recovery has occurred. Wound healing occurs during this period and may be complicated by wound sepsis, cardiovascular and respiratory compromise, and excessive catabolism of body proteins.

Acute phase. The systemic response to burned skin determines the acute pathophysiologic changes that occur. Local edema occurs in partial-thickness burns. This edema results from capillary damage and the release of prostaglandins and oxygen free radicals. Generalized soft-tissue edema is seen in patients with burns greater than 25% TBSA. This edema results primarily from hypoalbuminemia, which follows the leakage of large amounts of plasma proteins into the burn, and from the systemic effects of inflammatory mediators released from the burn. Anemia is common, resulting from direct heat injury to erythrocytes and from increased erythrocyte fragility associated with the action of oxygen free radicals on erythrocyte wall lipids. Impaired erythropoiesis may persist until wound healing is complete. Circulating factors associated with burned skin may impair immune system function by altering lymphocyte and neutrophil function. The burned patient is very susceptible to hypothermia, as damaged skin allows heat loss by evaporation, conduction, convection, and radiation.[29]

Cardiac output falls 25% to 50% within minutes of a severe injury. This decrease in cardiac output results from hypovolemia and shock. High circulating catecholamine levels increase peripheral resistance and further reduce cardiac output. Myocardial contractility is directly impaired by carbon monoxide poisoning, if present. Myocardial depressant factors have been postulated in patients with burns greater than 40% TBSA.[29]

The sequelae of cardiac insufficiency in the immediate postburn period may be life threatening. Cutaneous vasoconstriction associated with shock may convert a partial-thickness burn to a full-thickness injury. Acute renal failure associated with hypovolemic shock is the most common cause of death in improperly resuscitated burn victims.[29,30]

Pulmonary function may be seriously impaired in the burned animal. Severe burns to the trunk impair respiration if pain or burn eschar restrict ventilation. The systemic effects of severe burns complicate smoke inhalation injuries (Chapter 25). Smoke inhalation produces hypoxemia directly from the low oxygen tension of inspired air and indirectly when carbon monoxide displaces oxygen from the hemoglobin molecule. Toxic components of smoke paralyze respiratory cilia and cause mucosal edema or ulceration, predisposing to retention of respiratory secretions and respiratory infection.[29,31]

The large absorptive surface of the upper respiratory tract usually limits thermal damage to the nasal and oral cavities or larynx unless live steam is inhaled. Laryngeal and pharyngeal edema may not occur for several hours following burn injury. If singed facial hair or oral mucosa is apparent when the animal is first examined, early endotracheal intubation may be indicated to facilitate oxygen delivery and reduce the risk of later emergency intubation.[29-31]

Chronic phase. Macrophages and neutrophils in the wound release cytokines and other soluble factors that mobilize additional inflammatory cells. This process induces a systemic hypermetabolic state in concert with catecholamines and cortisol released in response to pain and injury. Body temperature may rise up to 1°C during this period even in the absence of wound sepsis. Rapid catabolism of muscle protein occurs unless aggressive nutritional support is provided (Chapter 37). Wound infection often complicates burn healing and imposes additional metabolic stress. Early wound debridement and closure or grafting of the burn wound accompanied by meticulous antisepsis limits wound infection and speeds recovery.[29]

Cardiovascular, pulmonary, and renal function may be compromised during the chronic phase of wound healing. Cardiac output increases twofold to threefold in response to metabolic demands during the wound healing period. Hypermetabolism may cause cardiac failure in animals with compensated or asymptomatic cardiac disease. Ventilation increases in response to increased oxygen requirements and carbon dioxide production by tissues. Bacterial bronchopneumonia commonly occurs approximately 4 to 7 days after smoke inhalation as necrotic tracheobronchial epithelium sloughs and colonization by upper respiratory pathogens occurs. Polyuria results from urinary excretion of urea, solutes from the wound eschar, and sodium loading provided during resuscitation.[29]

Diagnosis

History and physical examination. The history and initial physical examination alert the clinician to the nature of the burn and possible pre-existing or concurrent injury. A detailed physical examination is required to assess all regional structures including the eyes, ears, oral cavity, respiratory tract, urogenital tract, anus, and footpads. Injuries below the cutaneous surface must be determined. Neurologic injuries, fractures, and other internal injuries are common in severely traumatized animals and should not be overlooked. Fur often protects the underlying skin from thermal burns, but it may also mask injuries. Careful clipping of hair from injured areas allows estimation of burn area and facilitates cleaning and debridement. Fur is readily plucked from the skin with partial-thickness or full-thickness burns.

Visual examination of the mouth and pharynx should be supplemented by examination of the sputum for carbonaceous material. Laryngoscopy or bronchoscopy may be indicated in some cases (including those of consumption or inhalation of caustic compounds). The animal's body temperature should be carefully monitored frequently throughout treatment. Hypothermia is common during the resuscitation phase with loss of the protective function of the skin. Fever is common as wound healing begins. Increased body temperature may result from hypermetabolism or wound sepsis.

The amount of burned skin relative to TBSA should be determined in order to calculate initial fluid therapy requirements and establish a prognosis. The extent of the burn may be accurately determined by measuring the burn area and calculating TBSA from the body weight. Alternatively, the burn area may be estimated according to the amount of skin damaged in a region of the body, knowing the approximate percentage TBSA contributed by each region. The Rule of 9s is a simple mnemonic developed for estimating burn area in man. In this rule, the head and neck and forelimbs each represent 9% TBSA, each rear limb 18% and the trunk 36%. The Rule of 9s underestimates the proportion of TBSA of the trunk and overestimates the proportion of TBSA of the limbs of dogs and cats; more accurate estimates of TBSA can be made using the values in Table 16-2.[1,29] The large amount of excess skin in breeds with prominent skin folds may limit the accuracy of these estimation methods.

Table 16-2 Regional body-surface area

	Cats	Man (Rule of 9s)
Head and neck	16%	9%
Chest	22%	36%
Flank	19%	
Forelimbs	15%	18%
Hindlimbs	20%	36%
Tail	4%	

Laboratory diagnosis. The minimum hematologic and serum biochemical database in burned patients should consist of complete blood count, total serum proteins, blood urea nitrogen, and serum glucose concentration. Anemia and hypoalbuminemia may be clinically significant within hours of a severe burn and will complicate resuscitation efforts. Alternatively, azotemia and hemoconcentration may signify dehydration associated with delayed or insufficient emergency therapy. Hyperglycemia related to increased catecholamine production is common immediately after severe burns. The complete serum biochemistry profile will aid in the detection of concurrent or preexisting disease.

Blood gas analysis should be obtained on patients with smoke inhalation or extensive injuries to the chest wall. Hypoxemia and hypercarbia may result from pulmonary parenchymal disease or reduced ventilation. Care should be taken when interpreting blood gas analyses from animals suffering from smoke inhalation. Arterial blood gas concentrations (partial pressures of arterial oxygen and carbon dioxide) may be within normal limits in carbon monoxide poisoning, yet oxygen delivery is severely impaired because the oxygen-carrying capacity of the hemoglobin molecule is reduced.[31]

Management

Initial wound care and resuscitation. Meticulous nursing care prevents infection and expedites burn wound healing. Prevention of wound sepsis requires containment and control of bacteria colonizing the burn wound; prompt removal of purulent exudates; limiting environmental contamination; avoiding additional injury of burned tissues; promoting an environment conducive to healing; and removing all nonviable tissue as early as is feasible. In the case of full-thickness injury, early eschar removal is crucial to control infection and promote a viable vascular bed suitable for closure. Excision is not routinely required in superficial and partial-thickness burns. In these injuries, topical management effectively controls infection, debrides nonviable tissue, and promotes reepithelialization of denuded areas.

Prudent initial therapy maximizes viability of burned skin. Skin has low thermal conductance and releases retained heat slowly, allowing thermal damage to continue after the initial injury. Application of chilled saline or water (3°C to 17°C) to the wound within 2 hours after injury expedites temperature normalization and may reduce the ultimate depth of the injury. The injured part should be cooled by immersion or application of compresses for at least 30 minutes. Care must be employed to avoid hypothermia when treating a large burn. Ice packs should not be employed, since excessive cold may further compromise injured tissues. Water baths or sprays are also useful for removing caustic materials from skin.[25]

Special care is required for injuries inflicted by hot tar. Hot tar may cause serious burns because it is tenacious and is applied at high temperature. Liberal application of an emulsifying agent facilitates removal of the tar during immersion. Neosporin ointment (Burroughs) contains the nonionic surface-acting emulsifying agent polyoxyethyelene sorbitan (Tween-80) and is a practical emulsifying agent for veterinary clinicians. Tween-80 or polysorbate, another emulsifying agent, may also be purchased in bulk from chemical supply firms.[32]

Most chemical burns encountered should be lavaged with large volumes of water (Table 16-1). Eyes are best lavaged copiously with sterile saline when available. Under experimental conditions, the results of chemical burn treatment required to return skin pH to normal, varied between acid and alkali burns. While lavage of 30% acid burns for 2 hours returned the skin pH to normal, it took over 12 hours of lavage with 50% sodium hydroxide burns. Deep chemical burns, especially those caused by alkali compounds, may require deep surgical excision when prolonged contact occurs.

Neutralizing agents are occasionally useful in limiting the extent of injury. They are not a substitute for copious lavage and should never be placed directly in contact with the undiluted chemical. If used following copious lavage, they can be applied to the wound in the form of gauze sponges loosely wrapped over the area for 20 minutes. This application may be repeated if necessary.

Analgesic administration is an integral part of the treatment of animals with burn injury. Administration of sedatives or general anesthesia to these animals may also be required during painful dressing changes or debridement procedures.

Aggressive fluid therapy is crucial to resuscitation of severely burned animals. Edema in burned and unburned tissue dramatically increases the fluid requirements of burn patients. Very large volumes of fluid may be required. In man, crystalloid fluids are administered at the rate of approximately 2 to 4 ml/kg × %TBSA. This fluid is given in addition to volumes required to treat shock and the estimated daily maintenance fluid requirement of 60 to 80 ml/kg. The flow rate is adjusted to provide half the resuscitation fluid in the first 8 hours after the injury and the remainder in the next 16 hours.[29,33]

To illustrate fluid requirements in veterinary burn patients, consider the case of a 30-kg dog with burns covering 30% TBSA. This animal requires 3600 to 6000 ml of fluid on the first day after injury (1800 to 3600 for burn compensation and 1800 to 2400 ml maintenance). Approximately 250 ml per hour are administered for the first 8 hours, and 150 ml per hour are administered for the next 16 hours.

Urine output is monitored and fluid administration is adjusted as necessary to maintain the urine flow rate higher than 0.5 ml/kg per hour. Dogs and cats may require less fluid than predicted by this formula because of the greater resistance of canine and feline skin to blistering and edema formation. Care should be taken to avoid iatrogenic infection from indwelling urinary catheters.

Isotonic crystalloid fluids such as lactated Ringer's solution or normal saline are satisfactory for fluid therapy during the resuscitation phase. Hypertonic saline and hypertonic lactated Ringer's solution (250 mEq/L sodium) administration have been reported to reduce fluid requirements and limit edema formation in humans.[29,34,35] Colloid solution (fresh frozen plasma, 2 to 3 ml/kg) administration reduces edema formation and may be beneficial during resuscitation.[34] Administration of glucose-containing solutions contributes to dehydration through inducing osmotic diuresis. Overhydration should be avoided, since increased tissue edema results.[29]

Fluids should be administered through a peripheral venous catheter inserted through unburned tissue. Central lines should be avoided unless indicated for monitoring purposes since thrombosis and infection may result.[29] Intraosseous fluids may be given if venous access cannot be achieved. Appropriate sites for intraosseous fluid administration include the femur via the trochanteric fossa, the tibia via the tibial crest, and the humerus via the greater tubercle.[36]

Pulmonary function must be ensured. Oxygen (100%) should be given to animals exposed to carbon monoxide to encourage carbon monoxide-hemoglobin dissociation (Chapter 25). Animals with oral or pharyngeal burns may require endotracheal intubation or maintenance of a tracheostomy for 4 to 5 days until edema resolves. Bronchodilator administration and mechanical ventilation with positive end-expiratory pressure (PEEP) may be required to maintain respiratory function in animals with burn injury and smoke inhalation, pulmonary edema, pneumonia, or airway compromise.[29]

Following initial resuscitation efforts, parenteral fluid administration is required primarily to replace free water lost from the wound by evaporation. The use of occlusive wound dressings reduces free water loss. In most cases fluids should be changed to 5% dextrose in 0.45% saline by 24 hours after the injury to minimize sodium loading. Parenteral fluids should be administered until oral consumption is sufficient to maintain hydration and renal function. If the animal is not eating normally, partial parenteral nutrition may be provided by giving the calculated fluid requirement in the form of a solution containing 10% dextrose, 3% amino acids, and 10% fat emulsion.[34] Whole blood or blood components should be given as required to correct severe anemia or hypoalbuminemia (Chapter 34).

Overhydration must be avoided during this period. The syndrome of inappropriate antidiuretic hormone secretion (SIADH) complicates fluid balance in some recovering human burn patients. SIADH may prevent the proper excretion of water resulting in hyponatremia and seizures. Periodic determination of serum sodium concentration and body weight allows detection and management of SIADH.[30]

Proper nutrition is required to limit excess protein catabolism and promote wound healing in animals with burn injury. Oral intake should be encouraged when possible to minimize cost and complications associated with enteral or parenteral nutritional support. Oral intake may not be possible for several days in burn patients, especially those with oral injuries. Parenteral or enteral support must be provided early in the management of these cases (Chapter 37). Proper dietary protein-carbohydrate balance should be ensured to minimize carbon dioxide and urea production. Water-soluble vitamins should be administered to replace the increased losses occurring through burn wounds.[29]

Antibiotic therapy. Rational antibiotic therapy controls infection and minimizes complications and cost in the burn patient. Endogenous cutaneous and enteric bacteria colonize the wound within the first several days after the injury. Antibiotics should be employed that reach therapeutic levels in burned tissue and are effective against *Staphylococcus aureus* and *Escherichia coli,* the predominant organisms in burned tissue.[29]

Topical antibiotics are preferred for treatment of burn wounds because the relatively poor circulation in burn eschar limits penetration by systemic antibiotics. Topical agents must not be irritating or toxic and should have minimal systemic effects. Although costly, silver sulfadiazine ointment (Silvadene, Marion) fulfills most of these criteria and is the most appropriate choice for empirical burn wound treatment.[25,37] Other topical agents such as gentamicin or polymyxin-bacitracin may be required if bacterial resistance or cutaneous hypersensitivity occurs. Transient leukopenia is the most common complication associated with silver sulfadiazine therapy in man and often resolves spontaneously despite continued administration of the drug.[29]

Systemic antibiotics should be administered to burn patients only when clearly indicated. Prophylactic antibiotics may be indicated to protect against transient bacteremia prior to surgical burn wound excision. Septicemia may occur if bacteria in the wound surface invade underlying tissues. Purulent exudates, wound biopsies, and blood should be cultured when systemic infection is suspected or when empirically chosen topical antibiotics do not control wound sepsis. Antibiotic sensitivity testing ensures appropriate antibiotic selection. Increased antibiotic dosage and frequency of administration along with periodic determination of serum antibiotic concentrations may be required to ensure adequate antibiotic therapy, since rapid antibiotic clearance occurs in many burn patients.[29]

Escharotomy and debridement

Escharotomy. Circumferential deep burns on the limbs may form a biologic tourniquet that compromises circulation to distal tissues. Extensive or deep burns on the thorax may physically restrict respiration. Early surgical incision of the burn tissue, or escharotomy, is indicated in these cases.[25]

Debridement of devitalized tissue controls burn sepsis and promotes the development of a viable vascular bed suitable for surgical closure. Several methods of debridement are available and may be employed according to the size and severity of the injury.

Conservative debridement. Conservative debridement employs immersion or wet dressings to soften the eschar and facilitate separation of necrotic tissue from surrounding and underlying viable tissue. Conservative debridement is indicated for all superficial or partial-thickness injuries. Full-thickness injuries for which conservative debridement is appropriate include small burns or burns adherent to tendons, ligaments, or underlying body structures in which the lack of a clear fascial plane hinders accurate excision.

Hydrotherapy is performed by immersion (sterile tub) of the injured part in warm tap water or saline solution for 20 to 30 minutes two or three times a day. Hydrotherapy is most appropriate for extensive burns involving the limbs or trunk. Water sprays may be more practical than immersion in large dogs. Small injuries may be treated with wet-to-wet dressings. Sterile gauze is moistened with sterile saline or lactated Ringer's solution and applied to the wound. Additional layers of sterile gauze are applied, secured with an adhesive bandage, and left in place for several hours. Additional fluids are applied periodically as the bandage dries. Following immersion or removal of the wet dressing, loose necrotic tissue is removed with thumb forceps and scissors. Finally, a suitable broad-spectrum antibiotic ointment is applied under an occlusive bandage. Antibiotic ointments may be "buttered" onto burned skin using a sterile glove or applicator.

Chemical debridement. Chemical debridement may facilitate removal of necrotic tissue in some burn patients. Enzymatic or chemical agents may be applied to open wounds or under occlusive dressings. Granulex-V (trypsin, balsam of peru, and castor oil) is an enzymatic debridement agent commonly used in veterinary practice. Other preparations contain proteases, ribonucleases, or collagenases in a nonirritating vehicle that may also contain antibiotics.

An economical agent for chemical debridement is buffered sodium hypochlorite (Dakin's) solution. Dakin's solution chemically dissolves necrotic tissue while preventing infection through the antibacterial action of chlorine and oxygen. Dakin's solution may be easily prepared in bulk quantities according to the following formula[37]:

Dakin's solution (0.25%) =
400 ml sodium hypochlorite 5% (bleach) +237 g sodium bicarbonate + 8000 ml (or a sufficient quantity) sterile distilled water.

If application of 0.25% Dakins solution causes pain, 0.125% Dakin's solution may be employed. Dakin's solution should be stored in dark glass containers and unused mixtures discarded after 3 days.

Aggressive debridement. Aggressive surgical debridement or "wound excision" is the removal of the entire burn wound followed by temporary or permanent closure.[25] Surgical debridement is indicated for large full-thickness burns because the presence of wound eschar impedes granulation-bed formation and increases the risk of infection. Surgical excision under general anesthesia eliminates the necrotic wound in a single stage. Grafting knives facilitate tangential excision of the nonviable tissue at the level of the hypodermis. A healthy granulation bed suitable for flap or graft closure forms within 5 to 7 days. Considerable hemorrhage may occur during excision, requiring electrocautery or ligatures for hemostatis.

Wound closure. Once a viable vascular wound bed is free of necrotic tissue and infection, definitive wound closure must be planned. Superficial and superficial partial-thickness burns frequently heal without complication. Deep partial-thickness

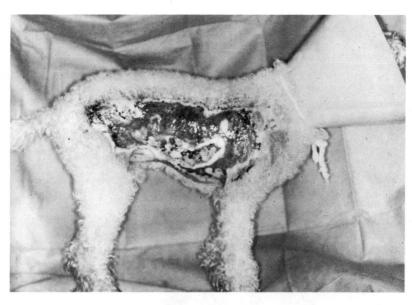

Fig. 16-3. Despite the ominous appearance, this electrical heating pad injury healed by second intention. Loose skin around the wound allowed maximal wound contraction. Retained islands of viable epithelium in the wound and healthy skin at the periphery provided ample donor sources for epithelialization.

and full-thickness injuries may require months for healing by contraction and epithelialization from neighboring skin (Fig. 16-3). Extensive burns usually require closure with skin grafts or skin flaps (Fig. 16-4).

Autogenous free grafts are often required for permanent coverage of large full-thickness burns. Allografts and xenografts may be used for temporary coverage of extensive partial-thickness injuries. Axial pattern flaps may be used alone or in combination with free grafts or local flap techniques. Partial-thickness grafts harvested with an electric or pneumatic dermatome and meshed with a 3:1 ratio are the most appropriate means of grafting large wounds (Fig. 16-5). Punch grafts and strip grafts may be suitable for smaller wounds.

Neglect of the burn wound may result in excessive scarring and wound contracture. Flexion surfaces and other areas subject to constant motion are especially susceptible to excessive wound contracture following major cutaneous losses. Z-plasty, pedicle grafts, and free grafts with scar division may be required if these complications occur.

Cosmetic results depend on the extent and severity of the burn. In contrast to human patients, cosmetic healing in veterinary patients requires normal hair growth. Most hair follicles are preserved in superficial and superficial partial-thickness burns. Normal hair growth is less likely fol-

lowing full-thickness burns because large numbers of hair follicles are lost. In these cases, skin flaps and full-thickness grafts may allow an adequate hair coat to develop (Figs. 16-6 and 16-7). Partial thickness skin grafts, result in a sparse hair coat and may not be as durable as full-thickness grafts. On occasion a satisfactory outcome may occur without skin grafting if wound contraction and overlapping of hair from healthy skin conceals a prominent burn scar. Owners should be informed that abnormal hair growth may be a permanent consequence of a severe burn.

Electrical injuries

Electricity may cause very severe injuries. Damage may vary according to the pathway and intensity of the current, duration of exposure, and tissue resistance. Electrical current generates heat as it passes through tissue. Thermal injury is severe at the point of contact, where current density is greatest. If high-intensity electrical current is applied over a small area, extensive coagulation necrosis may occur deep to the injury. Additional thermal injury may occur if arcing occurs between the source and conductor, or if hair or other tissue is ignited during contact. Electrical contact over a large surface such as wet skin decreases the current density. No burns may be evident in these cases, although ventricular fibrillation may occur.[25,38,39]

Most electrical injuries of small animals result

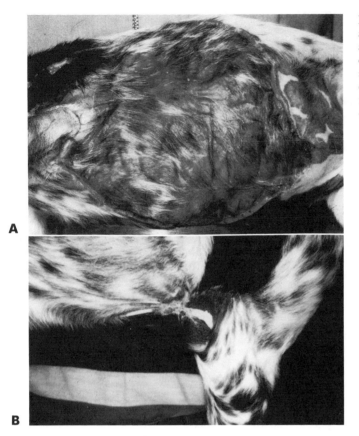

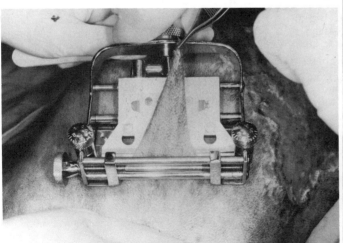

Fig. 16-4 A, Extensive thermal injury from an electrical heating pad on the ventrolateral abdomen and thorax in a young Setter-cross dog. **B,** Surprisingly, the wound healed by second intention after debridement and topical application of silver sulfadiazine ointment. The scar is small because of wound contraction and epithelialization.

Fig. 16-5 A, A Brown electric dermatome is used to harvest a split-thickness skin graft. **B,** Strips of harvested skin were meshed (3:1 expansion ratio) to maximize coverage of this extensive electrical heating pad injury.

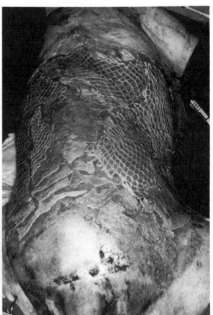

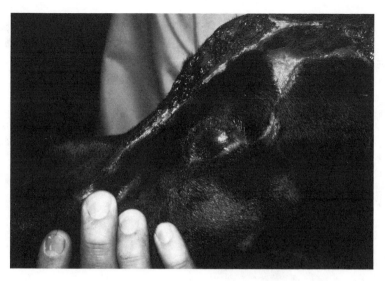

Fig. 16-6 Acid burn to the face and left eye of a Doberman Pinscher. Primary closure occurred following deep debridement. The scarred eyelids were restored using a mucocutaneous subdermal plexus flap from the upper lip.

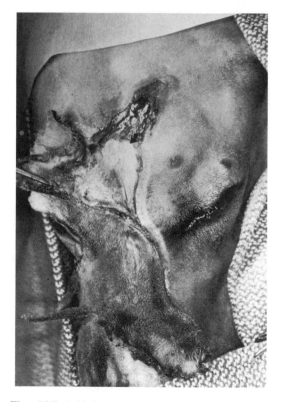

Fig. 16-7 Acid burn on the head of a Golden Retriever. Following debridement, closure was effected with skin flaps. Note the complete destruction of the skin, revealing the periosteum (arrow).

when dogs and cats bite electrical cords carrying low-voltage household alternating current (120 V, 60 Hz). Seizures, respiratory arrest or ventricular fibrillation may occur. Cardiopulmonary resuscitation may be necessary once the patient is separated from the electrical source.[25,38,39] Fulminating pulmonary edema may occur secondary to a neurogenic increase in peripheral vascular resistance[39]; aggressive treatment with oxygen, corticosteroids and diuretics is indicated in these circumstances (Fig. 16-8). Paralytic ileus and bowel infarction have been reported in humans[40] and should be suspected in dogs or cats that vomit or exhibit abdominal pain after electrical injury.

Electrical burns to the oral cavity may be pale yellow, tan, or gray in color. These burns usually heal within 3 weeks without surgical intervention, although oronasal fistulas may occur in some animals (Fig. 16-9). These injuries require closure with mucosal flaps, libial advancement flaps, or skin flaps. Large electrical burns on the extremities or trunk should be treated as any other thermal burn.

High-voltage electrical injuries are uncommon in dogs and cats and are usually fatal. The contact or entry point is usually depressed, charred, and leathery while the exit wound at the ground point may be explosive. Arcing may occur instead of grounding. In addition to obvious cutaneous injury, internal damage may involve the organs of the digestive, respiratory, musculoskeletal, or nervous systems.[25,38,41]

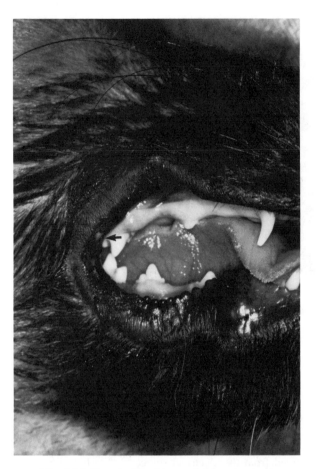

Fig. 16-8 Electrical cord burn of the oral commissure. This patient died from fulminating pulmonary edema.

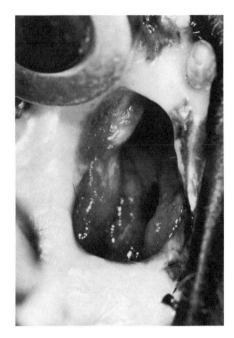

Fig. 16-9 Large oronasal fistula adjacent to the left canine tooth secondary to biting an electrical cord. A full-thickness labial advancement flap achieved partial closure of the fistula.

FROSTBITE
Definition

Frostbite is the freezing or effect of freezing a part of the body. Contact with metal, or other conductive or volatile liquids may rapidly accelerate the freezing process.[25,42] Hypothermic animals are prone to frostbite as peripheral vasoconstriction shunts blood from the periphery to vital core tissues.

Several mechanisms interact to produce tissue injury and death in frostbite. Ischemia results when peripheral vasoconstriction diverts oxygen, nutrients and heat to core tissue. In addition extracellular and intracellular ice may form, causing cell lysis. Vascular wall injury and hyperviscosity of blood may precipitate thrombosis.[25,42]

Animals are most susceptible to frostbite when exposed to high winds on very cold days. The ears, tail, and digits are the areas most often affected. Injury to these areas is often inapparent until the damaged tissue sloughs several days after exposure. Superficial frostbite results when the epidermis and dermis are affected. Deep frostbite results from freezing of subcutaneous tissues and underlying structures. Further classification of frostbitten tissue may be made after initial therapy is given: "first degree," erythema after warming; "second degree," blistering; "third degree," skin necrosis; and "fourth degree," gangrene. A good prognosis may be offered for first- and second-degree injuries, while third- and fourth-degree injuries are more susceptible to infection and possible tissue loss. Since mild and severe injuries may be indistinguishable for several days, a guarded prognosis and conservative therapy should be given until the severity of the injury is apparent[25,42] (Fig. 16-10).

Management

Frostbitten tissues should be rapidly rewarmed once the animal is in an environment where refreezing will not occur. The affected area should

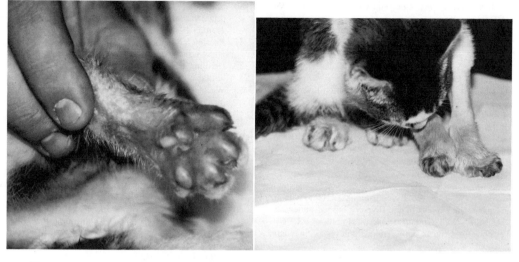

A **B**

Fig. 16-10. A, This kitten was accidentally shut in a refrigerator for several hours. Extensive swelling of the feet was evident on presentation. **B,** Necrosis and separation of the digits occurred after several days. The wounds eventually healed and the cat adapted adequately to a sedentary indoor lifestyle. Blankets and pillows on the floor provided comfortable areas for jumping.

be immersed in warm water in a receptacle of sufficient volume to maintain a temperature of 104 to 108°F (40 to 42°C) for at least 20 minutes or until thawing is complete. Tissues should never be rubbed or massaged. Soft, dry protective bandages should be applied to protect frostbitten tissues after thawing. Cage rest reduces pain and encourages healing of frostbitten feet. Topical antiseptics and careful debridement help prevent infection of necrotic tissue or ruptured blisters. Systemic infection may occur, requiring treatment with appropriate antibiotics. Analgesic administration is often required.[25]

Additional therapy for extensively frostbitten tissue may be indicated. Hypothermia, if present, requires treatment as previously discussed. "Chemical sympathectomy" with alpha-adrenergic blocking agents has maintained circulation in frostbitten limbs of a small number of human patients between 2 and 10 days after injury. Larger clinical trials in man and animals have not yet been performed. Heparin or low-molecular-weight dextran was advised at one time for treatment of vascular stasis; however, no consistent benefit has been shown in clinical trials.[25]

In many instances, mild frostbite is not noticed initially. Owners may present animals to the veterinarian after signs of necrosis are evident. Surgical debridement or amputation of the affected area may be necessary if natural separation has not occurred.

REFERENCES

1. Adams T. Carnivores. In Whittow GC, ed. Comparative Physiology of Thermoregulation, vol 2. New York: Academic Press, 1971;152-189.
2. Maskrey M. Metabolic and acid-base implications of thermal panting. In: Hales JRS, ed. Thermal Physiology. New York: Raven Press, 1984;347-352.
3. Graham BS, Lichtenstein MJ, Hinson JM, Theil GB. Nonexertional heatstroke: physiologic management and cooling in 14 patients. Arch Intern Med 1986;146:87-90.
4. Krum SH, Osborne CA. Heatstroke in the dog: a polysystemic disorder. J Am Vet Med Assoc 1977;170:531-535.
5. Jackson DL. Critical care neurology. In Shoemaker WC, Thompson WL, Holbrook PR, eds. Textbook of Critical Care Philadelphia: WB Saunders, 1984;944-947.
6. Larson RL, Carithers RW. A review of heat stroke and its complications in the canine. N Z Vet J 1985;33:202-206.
7. Schall WD. Heat stroke (heat stress, hyperpyrexia). In Kirk RW, ed. Current Veterinary Therapy VII. Philadelphia: WB Saunders, 1980;195-197.
8. Danzl DF. Hyperthermic syndromes. Am Fam Physician 1988;37:157-162.
9. Osweiler GD. Common poisonings in small animal practice. In Kirk RW, ed. Current Veterinary Therapy VII. Philadelphia: WB Saunders, 1980;122-129.
10. Olmstead CE, Villablanca JR, Torbiner M, Rhodes D. Development of thermoregulation in the kitten. Physiol Behav 1979;23:489-496.
11. Vicario SJ, Okabajue R, Haltom T. Rapid cooling in classic heatstroke: effect on mortality rates. Am J Emerg Med 1986;4:394-398.
12. Dean NC. Hypothermia—lifesaving procedures. Postgrad Med 1987;82:48-58.
13. Elder PT. Accidental hypothermia. In Shoemaker WC, Thompson WL, Holbrook PR, eds. Textbook of Critical Care. Philadelphia: WB Saunders, 1984;85-93.
14. Chastain CB, Graham CL, Riley MG. Myxedema coma in two dogs. Canine Pract 1982;9:20-34.

15. Smith M, Hypotermia. Compend Contin Educ Pract Vet 1985;7:321-326.
16. Bussadori C, Vercelli C. The Osborn wave in a dog with hypothermia. Boll Assoc Ital Vet Piccoli Anim 1987; 26:97-100.
17. Noxon JO. Accidental hypothermia associated with hypothyroidism. Canine Pract 1983;10:17-22.
18. Haskins SC. Hypothermia and its prevention during general anesthesia in cats. Am J Vet Res 1981;42:856-861.
19. Moss J. Accidental severe hypothermia. Surg Gynecol Obstet 1986;162:501-513.
20. Lonning PE, Skulberg A, Abyholm F. Accidental hypothermia. Acta Anaesthesiol Scand 1986;30:601-613.
21. Reuler JB. Hypothermia: pathophysiology, clinical settings, and management. Ann Intern Med 1978;89:519-527.
22. Monafo WW, Crabtree JH, Galster AD. Hemodynamic and metabolic support of the severely burned patient. In Shoemaker WC, Thompson WL, Holbrook PR, eds. Textbook of Critical Care. Philadelphia: WB Saunders, 1984;936-942.
23. Fox SM. Management of thermal burns I. Compend Contin Educ Pract Vet 1985;7:631-639.
24. Pavletic MM. Unpublished data.
25. Hummel RP. Clinical Burn Therapy. Boston: John Wright/PSG, 1982.
26. Demling RH. Burns. N Engl J Med 1985;313:1389-1398.
27. Fox SM. Management of thermal burns II. Compend Contin Educ Pract Vet 1986;8:439-444.
28. Probst CW, Peyton LC, Raymond LB. The surgical management of a large thermal burn in a dog. J Am Anim Hosp Assoc 1984;20:45-49.
29. Demling RH. Management of the burn patient. In Shoemaker WC, Thompson WL, Holbrook PR, eds. Textbook of Critical Care. Philadelphia: WB Saunders. 1989;1301-1316.
30. Shirani KZ, Vaughan GM, Robertson GL, et al. Inappropriate vasopressin secretion (SIADH) in burned patients. J Trauma 1983;23:217-224.
31. Beasley VR. Smoke inhalation. Vet Clin North Am 1990; 20:545-556.
32. Demling RN, Buerstatte RPH, Perea A. Management of hot tar burns. J Trauma 1980;20:242.
33. Wachtel TL, Frank HA, Fortune JB, Inansci W. Initial management of major burns. In Wachtel TL, Kahn V, Frank HA, eds. Current Topics in Burn Care. Rockville, MD: Aspens Systems, 1983;25-30.
34. Demling RH. Improved survival after massive burns. J Trauma 1983;23:179-184.
35. Gunn ML, Hansbrough JF, Davis JW, Furst SR, Field TO. Prospective, randomized trial of hypertonic sodium lactate versus lactated Ringer's solution for burn shock resuscitation. J Trauma 1989;29:1261-1267.
36. Otto CM, Kaufmann GM. Intraosseous infusion of fluids and therapeutics. Compend Contin Educ Pract Vet 1989; 11:421-430.
37. Rudolph R, Noe JM. Chronic Problem Wounds. Boston: Little, Brown, 1983.
38. Baxter CR. Present concepts in the management of major electrical injury. Surg Clin North Am 1970;50:1401-1418.
39. Kolata RJ, Burrows CF. The clinical features of injury by chewing electrical cords in dogs and cats. J Am Anim Hosp Assoc 1981;17:219-222.
40. Williams DB, Karl RC. Intestinal injury associated with low voltage electrocution. J Trauma 1981;21:246-250.
41. Waumett JD. Delayed neurologic injury secondary to high voltage current, with recovery. J Trauma 1980; 20:166-168.
42. Washburn B. Frostbite. Boston: Museum of Science, 1975.

17 Cardiac Emergencies

Robin E. Wall and *John E. Rush*

Acute myocardial infarction resulting from coronary atherosclerosis is one of the most common diseases requiring emergency management and critical care in humans, yet this disease is rare in veterinary patients. Despite this fact, many dogs and cats presented for emergency care or requiring intensive therapy and monitoring have either primary cardiovascular diseases or disorders that secondarily affect the cardiovascular system. Some of the most common cardiovascular emergencies are heart failure, cardiac tamponade, complications of heartworm disease, arterial thromboembolism, and serious cardiac arrhythmias. Successful treatment of these patients depends on an understanding of the disease processes as well as a working knowledge of the cardiovascular system and its compensatory responses.

THE CARDIOVASCULAR SYSTEM— PRINCIPLES AND COMPENSATORY RESPONSES

Cardiac output, the amount of blood pumped forward by the heart during a given period, is a function of stroke volume and heart rate. The determinants of stroke volume are afterload, preload, myocardial contractility, and synergy of ventricular contraction. Over a wide range, increases in heart rate are directly related to increases in cardiac output. Abnormalities in any of these factors (preload, afterload, contractility, heart rate, or dyssynergy of contraction due to arrhythmias) can lead to adverse hemodynamic consequences.

The relationship between ventricular performance and preload was initially demonstrated by Frank in 1898 and again by Starling in 1914. Preload, defined as the myocardial fiber length at the onset of contraction, is related to the end diastolic ventricular volume or pressure.[1,2] Increases in preload, caused by more "stretching" and interdigitation of myofibrils in the sarcomere, result in increased force of contraction and increased stroke volume. The detrimental aspects of increased preload include increased myocardial work and myocardial oxygen demand. Excessive increases in preload cause decompensation and signs of congestive heart failure. Clinical correlates of excessive preload include pulmonary edema, ascites, pleural effusion, and jugular-vein distention.

Afterload can be defined as the sum total of the forces impeding ventricular ejection of blood. Factors that contribute to afterload include systemic arteriolar vascular resistance, aortic impedance, blood viscosity, ventricular wall thickness, and the radius of the ventricle at the onset of systole.[2] The tension generated by the ventricle is a function of the afterload, and like preload, afterload contributes to the myocardial workload. Increased left ventricular wall thickness and increased systemic arteriolar resistance, common compensatory responses by the cardiovascular system, result in greater myocardial oxygen demand. If afterload is significantly increased, not only will the myocardial workload increase, but stroke volume may decrease as well. Afterload is difficult to measure, and although arterial blood pressure has been used as a clinical correlate, it is at best a crude indicator of afterload. Given the number of compensatory responses that act to increase afterload, it is probably safe to assume that most veterinary patients with congestive heart failure have increased afterload.

The contractility of the myocardium, or inotropic state, can be defined as the vigor of contraction. Contractility is an intrinsic property of the heart muscle that is independent of preload and afterload, yet loading conditions can directly increase or decrease contractility.[3] Stimulation of

213

alpha, and beta, myocardial receptors by cate-cholamines leads to a faster and more forceful contraction in addition to enhanced relaxation and diastolic recoil of the ventricle ("diastolic suc-tion"). While contractility is usually considered to be an indicator of systolic function, its effects on diastolic function must not be ignored. Contractil-ity is very difficult to measure, as changes in pre-load and afterload alter most of the clinically use-ful tests. In spite of the knowledge that these tests might be altered by loading conditions, clinical correlates of contractility include the force of the apex beat on the thorax, the character of the arte-rial pulse, and echocardiographic indices such as percent shortening fraction and velocity of cir-cumferential fiber shortening.

Heart rate and rhythm, the final contributors to cardiac performance, are easily assessed clinically using electrocardiography. Heart rate is influ-enced by numerous cardiac and extracardiac con-ditions affecting neural input to the heart. Para-sympathetic (vagal) stimulation leads to cardiac slowing and sympathetic stimulation increases heart rate. In general, increases in heart rate result in beneficial increases in cardiac output. The ex-ception is excessively high heart rates (above 200 beats per minute in the dog and 240 beats per minute in the cat), which compromise diastolic filling and coronary artery perfusion. Cardiac dys-rhythmias may cause excessively low heart rates, deleteriously high heart rates, or dyssynergy of ventricular contraction, all of which can diminish cardiac output.

An understanding of the compensatory mecha-nisms invoked by the animal with heart failure is required for appropriate management. The body employs many compensatory mechanisms in an attempt to maintain cardiac output and normal perfusion to vital organ systems. Activation of the sympathetic nervous system, stimulation of the renin-angiotensin-aldosterone system, increased secretion of antidiuretic hormone and atrial natri-uretic peptide, and increased sodium and water retention by the kidneys are but a few of these compensatory mechanisms.[4-6] Activation of the sympathetic nervous system helps maintain arte-rial blood pressure by vasoconstriction, increases cardiac output by increasing heart rate and con-tractility, and improves venous return (i.e., pre-load) as a result of venoconstriction.[7] In response to diminished renal perfusion, the renin-angioten-sin-aldosterone system is activated.[8,9] Angioten-sin II is a potent arterial and venous vasoconstric-tor, thus returning arterial blood pressure, and re-nal perfusion, toward normal. Preload is aug-mented by the combination of venoconstriction mediated by angiotensin II, the actions of aldoste-rone on the kidney to retain sodium and water, and changes in renal filtration fraction.

HEART FAILURE

The compensatory changes described above can allow an animal with heart disease to remain free of clinical signs for long periods. In chronic heart failure, the body must choose between maintain-ing arterial blood pressure, maintaining normal tissue perfusion, and maintaining normal cardiac filling pressures.[10] The most important of these three parameters is the maintenance of arterial blood pressure, which usually remains normal un-til the terminal stages of heart failure. Tissue per-fusion has the next priority, which means that cardiac filling pressures receive the lowest priority and are the first hemodynamic abnormality in most patients. In other words, most patients ini-tially present with signs of congestion (pulmonary edema, pleural effusion, ascites, jugular-vein dis-tention) and are able to maintain normal forward cardiac output. Arterial blood pressure and tissue perfusion are normal in patients with early heart failure. When heart failure becomes more severe, tissue perfusion is compromised, leading to poor capillary refill, prerenal azotemia, and peripheral vasoconstriction, causing extremities to become cold. At this stage, the tissues extract more oxy-

Table 17-1 Precipitating events in acute heart failure

Progression of under-lying heart disease	Systemic disease
Myocardial failure	Hypertension
Arterial thrombo-embolism	Hyperthyroidism
	Liver disease
Arrhythmias	Anemia
Pericardial disease (tamponade)	Septicemia
	Renal failure
Left atrial rupture	Pulmonary disease
Chordae tendineae rupture	Asthma
Failure of compensa-tory mechanisms	Chronic obstruc-tive pulmonary disease
Anesthesia	Chronic bronchi-tis
Trauma	
Fluid overload	Tracheobronchial collapse
Dehydration	
Exercise	
Excessive dietary salt	
Drugs	
Toxicity (e.g., digi-talis)	
Inadequate dosage/failure to admin-ister	

gen from the blood than they do normally. In the final stages of heart failure, maintenance of blood pressure is no longer possible and death is imminent.

Most animals with fulminant heart failure have a chronic disease and may have a previous history of exercise intolerance, coughing, weakness, or previously documented heart disease. The abrupt decline in the animal's hemodynamic status is often due to an additional cardiovascular "stressor" that takes an animal from a state of compensated heart failure to an uncompensated state (Table 17-1). Such stressors include cardiac arrhythmias, sodium overload from a salt-laden treat, fluid overload from excessive fluid therapy, and ruptured chordae tendineae. Systemic disease, such as hyperthyroidism, anemia, or hypertension, can also overwhelm the animal's compensatory mechanisms and precipitate fulminant heart failure.

Causes of heart failure

Endomyocardial diseases (Table 17-2) are the most common causes of heart disease in dogs and cats. Mitral-valve insufficiency secondary to endocardiosis, dilated cardiomyopathy in dogs, and the various forms of cardiomyopathy in cats are the most frequent causes of heart failure in companion animals. Mitral- and/or tricuspid-valve insufficiency due to endocardiosis is the most common heart disease in dogs.[11] Middle-aged to el-

Table 17-2 Acquired heart disease in the dog and cat

Dogs	Cats
Mitral-valve endocardiosis	Hypertrophic cardiomyopathy
Dilated cardiomyopathy	Idiopathic Hyperthyroidism Hypertension
Myocarditis Infective (e.g., viral) Infiltrative	Dilated cardiomyopathy
Valvular endocarditis	Restrictive or intermediate cardiomyopathy
Hypertrophic cardiomyopathy	Myocarditis (e.g., feline infectious peritonitis)
Cor pulmonale Heartworm disease Chronic obstructive pulmonary disease	Valvular disease (endocardiosis, endocarditis)
Pericardial disease	Heartworm disease Pericardial disease

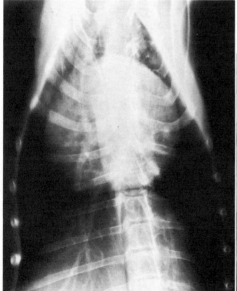 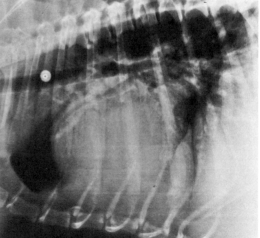

Fig. 17-1. **A** and **B**, Lateral and dorsoventral thoracic radiographic views of dilated cardiomyopathy in a 5-year-old Neapolitan mastiff with biventricular enlargement and biventricular failure radiographically characterized by pulmonary edema and distention of the caudal vena cava.

derly small-breed, male dogs are predisposed to heart disease. Many dogs remain asymptomatic for years. Decompensation may be due to progression of the disease with atrial enlargement and arrhythmias, ventricular myocardial failure, left atrial rupture with cardiac tamponade, or fulminant pulmonary edema secondary to rupture of the chordae tendineae.

Dilated cardiomyopathy is the second most frequently encountered cardiac disease in dogs. Middle-aged to older large-breed dogs are commonly affected, but the condition is rare in small dogs. Commonly affected breeds include Irish wolfhounds, Great Danes, German shepherds, St. Bernards, Doberman pinschers, and boxers, and the disease has been recently recognized in American cocker spaniels.[12] These patients characteristically have generalized cardiomegaly, with dilation of all cardiac chambers and the development of left ventricular or biventricular heart failure (Fig. 17-1). Atrial fibrillation is common in giant-breed dogs, while severe ventricular arrhythmias commonly develop in boxers and Doberman pinschers.[13] Ventricular arrhythmias increase the risk of sudden death in these breeds, and the ventricular arrhythmias in boxers are often refractory to treatment with conventional antiarrhythmic drugs. Doberman pinschers often present acutely with fulminant pulmonary edema and cardiogenic shock.[14,15] The prognosis for these patients is grave and their treatment can be difficult.

Myocardial disease, both idiopathic and secondary to systemic disease, is the most common cause of heart disease in cats.[16] Valvular diseases are less frequently encountered in cats. Since the recognition of the association between dilated cardiomyopathy and dietary taurine deficiency,[17] the incidence of dilated cardiomyopathy in cats has significantly decreased. Hypertrophic cardiomyopathy, intermediate forms of cardiomyopathy, and myocardial disease secondary to systemic disease such as hypertension and hyperthyroidism remain common conditions in cats.[16] Cats afflicted with hypertrophic cardiomyopathy suffer a diastolic (ventricular filling) dysfunction due to thickened, stiff ventricles. Tachycardia contributes to heart failure by shortening the duration of diastole and leading to diminished myocardial perfusion, further stiffening the ventricle and predisposing the animal to arrhythmias.[18] Impaired left ventricular outflow may result in animals with asymmetrical hypertrophy of the interventricular septum. Cats with cardiomyopathy frequently present acutely with respiratory distress due to pulmonary edema (Fig. 17-2) or pleural effusion. Arterial thromboembolism (discussed at the end of this chapter) provides an additional stress to

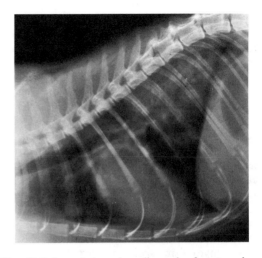

Fig. 17-2 Lateral thoracic radiograph of acute pulmonary edema in a cat with hypertrophic cardiomyopathy. Cardiomegaly and pulmonary venous congestion are also apparent.

Table 17-3 Clinical signs of heart failure

Venous congestion	Low output
Pulmonary edema	Hypothermia
Cyanotic membranes	Cold extremities
Tachypnea, dyspnea	Poor arterial pulses
Jugular-vein distention	Collapse, weakness
Pale, muddy mucous	Tachycardia
membranes	Prolonged capillary
Ascites	refill time
Hepatosplenomegaly	

these cats and often precipitates congestive heart failure.

Heart failure syndromes

The clinical signs associated with heart failure states in veterinary patients result from venous congestion or impaired cardiac output (Table 17-3). The distinction between these two syndromes assists in tailoring therapy to the individual patient's needs. In emergency, life-threatening situations, it can be difficult to ascertain the underlying cardiac disease. Therefore, treatment strategies designed according to the predominant clinical signs (venous congestion versus low cardiac output) and/or underlying mechanical dysfunction (increased afterload, impaired diastolic filling, or poor contractility) are useful in the emergency setting.

Although drug therapy will be directed on the basis of clinical signs, the importance of general therapies cannot be overemphasized. Patients with heart failure benefit from oxygen therapy, which can be administered using a number of techniques (Chapters 25 and 36). Cage rest and exercise restriction are essential—a short walk outside for a Doberman pinscher with severe heart failure may prove fatal. Free access to water, dietary sodium restriction (Hill's H/D or K/D diet or Purina Heart Diet), and treatment of concurrent cardiac arrhythmias is indicated. Centesis of thoracic or abdominal effusions is also indicated. When pleural effusion is present, as much fluid as possible should be removed. Some cats with severe heart failure may resist thoracocentesis and mild sedation should be administered to facilitate this procedure. Judicious removal of ascitic fluid is indicated in dogs with enough effusion to compress the diaphragm and hinder respiration. Mobilization of ascites with diuretic therapy is preferred to repeated abdominocentesis.

Heart failure with venous congestion. As previously discussed, maintenance of normal cardiac filling pressures is the lowest priority for the cardiovascular system. For this reason, the earliest signs of heart failure usually result from venous congestion. Venous congestion results from excessive increases in preload leading to increased ventricular filling pressures. Venous congestion may occur as isolated left ventricular "backward" heart failure (identified by pulmonary edema), right ventricular "backward" heart failure (recognized by ascites, jugular-vein distention, and in some cases pleural effusion), or biventricular "backward" failure in patients with both pulmonary edema and signs of right heart failure.

Clinical signs of heart failure in animals with venous congestion include tachypnea or dyspnea due to pulmonary edema, pleural effusion, hypoxia, or cardiac "asthma," pulmonary crackles due to pulmonary edema, and diminished intensity of airway and lung sounds due to pleural effusion. Systemic venous congestion is characterized by jugular venous distention, ascites, pleural and/or pericardial effusion, and hepatosplenomegaly. Cyanosis may result from poor oxygenation of hemoglobin in animals with severe pulmonary edema or pleural effusion. The presence of a S_3 or S_4 cardiac gallop is a strong predictor of present or imminent heart failure.

Treatment of venous congestion

Furosemide is the most commonly used diuretic in the treatment of the patient with acute or severe heart failure. It is a potent diuretic and can rapidly reduce cardiogenic pulmonary edema in most instances by decreasing intravascular volume and hence preload. The intravenous route of administration is preferred in the acute management of

heart failure as this route promotes venodilation[19] and a more rapid diuresis than intramuscular or oral administration.[20] Dosages up to 5 mg/kg every 2 hours are administered in the management of fulminant pulmonary edema (Table 17-4). However, once life-threatening pulmonary edema is controlled, the dosage is markedly reduced. Furosemide has a steep dose-response curve, such that low doses cause a mild diuresis and high doses lead to a profound diuresis. Typical maintenance doses for dogs are 2 to 4 mg/kg two to three times a day. Cats can often be treated with lower doses of furosemide, with maintenance doses commonly between 1 mg/kg once daily to 3 mg/kg twice a day. Excessive diuresis can lead to hypotension and prerenal azotemia. High doses of furosemide can also cause profound hypokalemia, which can further complicate cardiac function and contribute to generalized muscle weakness.[20] In spite of the potential for hypokalemia, this problem is a rare occurrence in animals who maintain a normal appetite; therefore potassium supplements are infrequently required.

Excessive increases in preload can be blunted by promoting venodilation (e.g., with nitroglycerin) and decreasing the pressor effect of angiotensin II (with angiotensin-converting enzyme [ACE] inhibitors). These drugs promote venous pooling of blood in the capacitance vessels, effectively decreasing preload on both ventricles and moving blood away from the lungs.[21,22] Administration of ACE inhibitors are also beneficial in decreasing aldosterone production and decreasing sodium and water retention, thereby decreasing intravascular volume.

Nitroglycerin, which primarily dilates systemic veins, is routinely used in the management of fulminant cardiogenic pulmonary edema. This drug acts directly on venous smooth muscle, promoting venodilation and venous pooling. Nitroglycerin paste (¼ in. to 1 in. of 2% nitroglycerin paste every 4 to 6 hours) is readily absorbed transcutaneously and can be applied on the ear pinna, axilla, flank, or sublingually. Newer transdermal adhesive patches (Nitro-Dur, Key Pharmaceuticals) are available, providing sustained release for 24 hours (2.5-mg patches; small dogs: ¼ of a patch; large dogs: 1 patch once daily). Tolerance to nitrates can develop in animals,[23] and for this reason, nitroglycerin is typically used for 2 or 3 days until additional therapies (ACE inhibitors, digoxin, other vasodilators) take effect. Nitroglycerin may be useful in the long-term management of heart failure by limiting use of the sustained release patches to 12 hours per day, with a 12-hour nitroglycerin-free interval.

Angiotensin-converting enzyme inhibitors (cap-

Table 17-4 Drug therapy in acute heart failure

Drug	Action	Dosage	Complications
Furosemide	Diuretic, decrease pre-load	1-5 mg/kg IV every 2 hours until pulmonary edema controlled Maintenance Dogs: 2 mg/kg per day to 4 mg/kg tid Cats: 1 mg/kg once daily to 3 mg/kg bid	Azotemia Hypotension Hypokalemia
Nitroglycerin (2% ointment)	Venodilator, preload reducer	Dogs: ¼ in. - 1 in. trans-cutaneously tid/qid Cats: ¼ in. tid/qid	Hypotension Azotemia Nausea Vomiting Tolerance
Sodium nitroprusside	Mixed vasodilator, decrease preload, after-load	Dogs: 1 μg/kg per minute, up to 3-10 μg/kg per minute CRI	Hypotension Prerenal azotemia Nausea
Hydralazine	Arterial dilator, decrease afterload	1 mg/kg, titrated up to 3 mg/kg po bid/tid	Hypotension Anorexia Reflex tachycardia Vomiting
Angiotensin-converting enzyme inhibitors	Decrease preload-venodilation and decrease blood volume and Decrease afterload-arterial dilation	Captopril: 0.5-1.5 mg/kg po bid/tid Enalapril: 0.5 mg/kg po sid/bid	Anorexia Vomiting Azotemia Diarrhea Hyperkalemia Hypotension
Morphine	Sedation, mild venodila-tion, decrease heart rate	Dogs: 0.25-1.0 mg/kg IM/SQ Cats: 0.05-0.1 mg kg IM/SQ	Tachypnea Excitation (cats) Vomition/defecation
Digoxin	Positive inotrope, im-proves systolic func-tion; antiarrhythmic (supraventricular tachy-cardia, atrial fibrilla-tion)	Dogs: 5-10 μg/kg IV every hour (maximum, 20-40 μg/kg); 0.22 mg/m^2 po divided bid (maintenance) Cats: 7-10 μg/kg every 12-48 hours	Nausea Vomiting Arrhythmias Conduction disorders Anorexia
Dopamine	Positive inotrope, im-prove perfusion and blood pressure	Dogs: 1-3 μg/kg per minute CRI up to 5-20 μg/kg per minute	Arrhythmias Tachycardia
Dobutamine	Positive inotrope improve cardiac output	Dogs: 2.5-10 μg/kg per minute Cats: 0.5-3.0 μg/kg per minute	Arrhythmias Seizures (cats) Vomiting

IV = intravenously; tid = three times a day; qid = four times a day; bid = twice a day; CRI = constant-rate intravenous infusion; po = orally; sid = once a day; IM = intramuscularly; SQ = subcutaneously.

topril, 0.5 to 1.5 mg/kg orally three times a day; enalapril 0.5 mg/kg orally once or twice daily) are also of benefit in patients with severe heart failure.[24] Vasodilation ensues due to ablation of the pressor effects of angiotensin II, and secondary inhibition of aldosterone release reduces sodium and water retention, thereby decreasing intravascular volume and venous congestion. Arteriolar dilation decreases afterload, thereby decreasing myocardial work and improving forward stroke volume. Administration of ACE inhibitors to animals with fulminant pulmonary edema is hindered by the fact that these drugs are available only in oral formulation. Nevertheless, they have a rapid onset of action following oral administration, often within 2 to 4 hours.[25] Of potential additional benefit is the knowledge that in humans with heart failure, ACE inhibitors have been shown to slow the progression of heart disease and prolong patient survival.[26] Hypotension, anorexia, and vomiting have been reported following administration of ACE inhibitors, although anorexia and gastrointestinal upset are less commonly noted with enalapril than with captopril. Azotemia has been observed following the administration of ACE inhibitors and can usually be attributed to prerenal causes. Reduction of the dosage of the concurrently administered diuretic furosemide usually results in resolution of the azotemia.

Sodium nitroprusside (1 to 10 μg/kg per minute intravenously, diluted in 500 ml of 5% dextrose in water) has been used in the management of fulminant pulmonary edema in patients who are refractory to conventional therapy. This drug causes both systemic venous and arterial dilation, markedly reducing right atrial and pulmonary capillary wedge pressure.[27] Sodium nitroprusside is a potent hypotensive agent and should be administered only when electrocardiographic, systemic arterial blood pressure, and close patient monitoring are possible. Side effects of sodium nitroprusside include hypotension, lethargy, and nausea. As with nitroglycerin, tolerance to sodium nitroprusside can develop in animals. Because of concerns of toxicity, the need for continuous infusion, and the potential for development of tolerance to drug effects, sodium nitroprusside is usually discontinued after 2 to 3 days of administration, as other medications are taking full effect.

An alternative afterload-reducing agent is the direct-acting arteriolar vasodilator hydralazine. Hydralazine is rapidly absorbed from the gastrointestinal tract, demonstrating an onset of action within an hour and maximum improvement in cardiac function 3 to 5 hours following administration.[28,29] The most frequent setting in which this drug is used is in the animal with chronic mitral regurgitation and congestive heart failure. The development of ACE inhibitors has led to a reduction in the number of animals receiving hydralazine. The dosage is titrated to obtain the desired effects of decreased pulmonary edema and a mean systemic arterial pressure of 70 to 80 mm Hg. The initial oral dosage is 1 mg/kg, which can be increased in 1-mg/kg increments to a maximum of 3 mg/kg.[28] The most frequently reported side effects of hydralazine include hypotension, anorexia, persistent vomiting, and reflex tachycardia.[21]

Morphine is commonly used in patients with acute heart failure who are anxious and dyspneic. The sedative effects associated with the administration of morphine (dogs: 0.25 to 1 mg/kg; cats: 0.05 to 0.1 mg/kg) may alleviate some of the animal's anxiety, decrease myocardial oxygen demand, and may convert a rapid, shallow respiratory pattern to slower, deeper breaths.[30] Occasionally, as with most narcotics, the animal may pant following administration and, in cats, excitability may be noted. Morphine administration may slow the heart rate and act as a mild venodilator, decreasing preload and assisting in the management of pulmonary edema.[31,32]

Treatment of heart failure with low cardiac output

As heart failure progresses, animals are no longer able to maintain adequate tissue perfusion, which results in weakness, cold extremities, and weak arterial pulses. In these animals, low cardiac output is usually present in conjunction with signs of venous congestion. The mucous membrane color may be pale due to sympathetically mediated vasoconstriction or cyanotic due to either severe hypoxemia from poor respiratory gas exchange or as a result of increased tissue extraction of oxygen. As cardiac output continues to worsen and there is peripheral sludging of blood, the mucous membranes become muddy. Capillary refill time is often prolonged due to poor tissue perfusion. In the preterminal animal, blood pressure can no longer be maintained in the normal range and cardiogenic shock results (collapse, poor arterial pulses, tachycardia, hypothermia). In addition to the previously discussed therapies for congestion, administration of positive inotropic agents is beneficial in the treatment of patients with acute or severe heart failure and evidence of low cardiac output.[33] The drugs of choice in the initial management of severe heart failure are the sympathomimetic amines dopamine and dobutamine.[34] Both of these agents have a short plasma half-life, undergoing extensive first-pass hepatic metabolism, and must be administered intravenously as a constant rate infusion. These drugs are used only in the initial treatment of animals with fulminating or refractory heart failure due to potential for development of "down-regulation" of β-adrenergic receptors associated with long-term use.[35] These catecholamines are also potentially arrhythmogenic and ECG monitoring is indicated.

Dopamine has numerous applications in the critically ill patient.[36-38] At low dosages (1 to 7.5 μg/kg/per minute) specific dopaminergic receptors within the renal, mesenteric, coronary, and cerebral vascular beds are affected. Stimulation of these receptors causes vasodilation and increased blood flow to the respective vascular bed.[36] At these doses, mild stimulation of β₁ receptors increases cardiac output without significant increases in heart rate or systemic vascular resistance. At higher infusion rates, α, β_1 and β_2 adrenergic receptors are stimulated,[37] leading to more significant increases in heart rate and inotropy (contractility) due to stimulation of β_1 receptors. β_2 receptors are located primarily on vascular and bronchial smooth muscle, causing vasodilation and bronchodilation when stimulated. Vasoconstriction and increased chronotropy result from stimulation of the α_1 receptors in vascular smooth muscle and in the myocardium, respectively. Therefore, at higher infusion rates, increased heart rate, contractility, and systemic arterial blood pressure result. Higher infusion rates are more arrhythmogenic and can substantially increase myocardial oxygen demand and workload.

The usual dosage of dopamine in a constant rate infusion for cardiovascular support in the heart failure patient is 2.5 to 10 μg/kg per minute.[30,39] Dopamine infusion is usually initiated at 1 to 3 μg/kg per minute. The patient should be closely monitored for the development of arrhythmias, increase in heart rate, or changes in systemic arterial blood pressure. The infusion rate can be cautiously increased in 3- to 5-μg/kg per minute increments until the desired effects are achieved or signs of toxicity develop.

Dobutamine is the sympathomimetic of choice in the management of acute heart failure.[40] It is significantly more expensive than dopamine but has less α_1 and β_2 effects. Dobutamine acts primarily as a β_1 agonist, increasing contractility, cardiac output, and coronary blood flow without significantly affecting systemic arterial blood pressure and heart rate. The undesirable side effects associated with dopamine infusion, such as cardiac arrhythmias, including sinus tachycardia, are less frequently encountered with dobutamine. As with dopamine, the initial infusion rate in dogs is low (1 to 3 μg/kg per minute) and is in-

crementally increased until the desired effects are obtained or until evidence of toxicity is observed. A beneficial response is usually noted in dogs at infusion rates between 2.5 and 7.5 μg/kg per minute. Dobutamine has been associated with adverse reactions in cats, such as vomiting, seizures and sudden death.[16] Most of these side effects are seen when infusions are administered for longer than 24 hours. Therefore, the infusion rate is much lower (0.5 to 3 μg/kg per minute) in cats, and close monitoring is imperative.

A positive clinical response to dobutamine or dopamine infusion is evidenced by improvement in arterial pulse quality, warming of extremities, and improved urine output. The animal's mucous membrane color and capillary refill time also improve in response to increased peripheral tissue perfusion. Central venous pressure and pulmonary capillary wedge pressure (indicators of preload) should decrease in response to therapy. Cardiac arrhythmias, increased heart rate, vomiting, and, in cats, seizures are evidence of an adverse reaction to catecholamine administration. Catecholamine infusion is discontinued for 20 to 30 minutes and restarted at a lower infusion rate if signs of toxicity develop or heart rate increases by 10% to 20%. These infusions may enhance atrioventricular nodal conduction. In animals with supraventricular tachycardia or atrial fibrillation who are dependent on a functional atrioventricular node to maintain a reasonable ventricular rate, the ventricular response rate may be excessively increased, resulting in a decreased diastolic filling period and compromised coronary blood flow. These patients should be digitalized prior to catecholamine infusion and closely monitored.

Occasionally, digitalis is employed in the treatment of an animal with acute heart failure.[41,42] The use of this drug is usually reserved for patients with supraventricular arrhythmias producing severe hemodynamic compromise; however, digitalis can also be used for its positive inotropic effects. Through its vagomimetic action, digitalis slows the ventricular response in atrial fibrillation and supraventricular tachycardias, as well as blocking reentrant atrial or AV nodal tachycardia. Digitalis can be administered intravenously if immediate digitalization is indicated. The recommended intravenous dosage of digoxin is 0.02 to 0.04 mg/kg, administering one fourth of this dose every hour for 4 hours until adequate reduction in heart rate is achieved or signs of toxicity occur.[41] If the patient's heart failure is less severe (e.g., dilated cardiomyopathy with atrial fibrillation and mild pulmonary edema), oral digoxin therapy is recommended to minimize toxicity (0.22 mg/m² divided twice daily or 0.022 mg/kg divided twice daily). Digitalis administration is contraindicated in patients with severe ventricular arrhythmias, especially ventricular arrhythmias that increase in severity or frequency following digitalization.

Patient monitoring

Following initial stabilization, the patient with heart failure requires frequent reevaluation. Continuous monitoring allows therapy to be tailored to meet the changing needs of the patient. Repeated physical examinations and assessing parameters such as mucous membrane color, body temperature, and pulse quality can aid in monitoring response to therapy and alert the clinician to patient deterioration. Improvement in peripheral tissue perfusion will be evidenced by normalization of body temperature, warming of the animal's extremities and ear pinna, improved capillary refill time, and improved arterial pulse quality. Increased depth of respiration, decreased respiratory rate, and decreased effort of breathing as well as resolution of crackles on thoracic auscultation are indicative of decreased pulmonary edema. Body weight should also be serially monitored and is useful in evaluating the balance between administered fluid therapy and diuresis.

Monitoring the patient with heart failure also involves assessment of clinical laboratory parameters. Hematocrit and total plasma protein, in conjunction with body weight and skin turgor, are indicators of hydration status. Serum urea nitrogen and/or creatinine are measures of hydration as well as cardiac output and renal perfusion. Serum creatinine and blood urea nitrogen concentrations are measured every 2 to 3 days during initial treatment of the critically ill animal. If these values are increasing, reduction in diuretic dosage is indicated, especially if clinical signs of heart failure is resolving and ACE inhibitors are being administered concurrently.

Serum electrolytes should be routinely evaluated, usually every 2 to 3 days, especially if therapy includes administration of high doses of furosemide. Hypokalemia is a common cause of patient deterioration, particularly in critically ill, anorectic patients. Hypokalemia can predispose the animal to cardiac arrhythmias, increase the risk of digitalis intoxication, and decrease the effectiveness of antiarrhythmic drugs.[43] If hypokalemia is present, potassium can be supplemented in intravenous fluids as potassium chloride, or orally in less critically ill patients using supplements such as potassium gluconate or potassium chloride (see Chapter 38).

Thoracic radiography should be performed as soon as possible following emergency treatment and stabilization of the animal. Radiographs of the animal can provide the clinician with confirmation of heart disease, assist in formulating a definitive diagnosis, and allow assessment of the extent of pulmonary edema or pleural effusion. Serial radiography allows evaluation of response or lack of response to treatment. If treatment is effective, pulmonary edema or pleural effusion will show substantial radiographic improvement within 2 to 3 days. It is also useful to repeat thoracic radiography following drainage of effusions by thoracocentesis or pericardiocentesis to assess the heart and pleural cavity more completely.

A multiple-lead electrocardiogram should be obtained at admission on all animals with heart disease. Electrocardiography permits accurate diagnosis and assessment of arrhythmias and may contribute further information toward the final diagnosis (e.g., ventricular enlargement patterns). All animals with severe, acute heart failure should be monitored by electrocardiography. Ideally, the patient should be continuously monitored, but if this is not possible, an electrocardiogram can be recorded every 4 to 6 hours. Intermittent monitoring is less desirable because some cardiac arrhythmias may not be detected and significant trends may not be appreciated. In animals who are at risk for cardiopulmonary arrest, bradyarrhythmias or other changes in cardiac rate or rhythm may indicate impending deterioration. Electrocardiography permits close monitoring of the response of an animal with a cardiac arrhythmia to therapy and monitoring for dopamine- or dobutamine-induced tachycardias or arrhythmias, enabling the clinician to adjust drug dosages or institute additional therapy.

Fluid therapy for the patient with heart failure is controversial and can be counterproductive if not monitored closely. Overzealous fluid administration can worsen venous congestion and pulmonary edema. However, administration of intravenous fluids may benefit the patient who has azotemia, whether due to volume depletion or impaired renal perfusion attributable to low cardiac output. Maintaining renal perfusion decreases the risk of intoxication by drugs dependent on the kidneys for excretion. Intravenous fluid therapy is also indicated if the patient is receiving infusions of drugs such as dobutamine. If fluid therapy is required, sodium-poor fluids (5% dextrose or 2.5% dextrose in 0.45% saline with potassium supplementation) are routinely administered at 50% to 75% (30 to 45 ml/kg per day) of the recommended maintenance requirements. If fluid therapy is initiated, central venous pressure (CVP) should be followed as an indicator of right heart filling pressures and excessive fluid administration. CVP measurements also permit assessment of the efficacy of therapy on reducing right ventricular filling pressures (i.e., preload reduction). Trends in central venous pressure tend to be more useful than a single measurement. However, CVP measurement is of limited value in assessing left ventricular filling pressures in patients with pulmonary edema due to left heart failure. If CVP increases by more than 5 cm H_2O following fluid administration, the infusion rate should be reduced.

Systemic arterial blood pressure measurements are useful in the treatment of patients with low cardiac output or severe heart failure.[44] In hypotensive patients, systemic arterial blood pressure measurements can be used to monitor response to the administration of dopamine or dobutamine infusions. Similarly, systemic arterial blood pressure measurements can confirm iatrogenic hypotension secondary to the administration of vasodilator therapy as well as confirm hypertension as an underlying contributor to the development of cardiac disease. Systemic arterial blood pressure can be measured through direct and indirect methods, yet because of complications and difficulties associated with direct arterial catheterization (arterial thrombosis, catheter-related sepsis and thrombophlebitis, patient discomfort), the indirect methods are more routinely employed (Dinamap). This oscillometric technique is quite useful in larger dogs with heart rates less than 200 beats per minute. In patients with elevated heart rates and in smaller dogs and cats, the Doppler technique of blood pressure measurement is more accurate for systolic blood pressure, although accurate diastolic pressures are more difficult to obtain.

Less commonly used techniques in the monitoring of the patient with acute heart failure are blood gas analysis and pulmonary artery catheterization. Serial blood gas analysis, both arterial and venous, allows tailoring of therapy to meet individual needs. An arterial oxygen partial pressure less than 65 mm Hg dictates a need for oxygen supplementation.[45] If the patient's partial pressure of arterial oxygen (Pao_2) remains less than 60 mm Hg despite oxygen supplementation or if the partial pressure of arterial carbon dioxide ($Paco_2$) is markedly elevated (greater than 50 mm Hg), mechanical ventilation should be considered (see Chapter 36). The partial pressure of oxygen in venous blood (Pvo_2) can be used as an indicator of peripheral tissue perfusion. As blood flow to the periphery is diminished, oxygen extraction by the tissues is increased in an attempt to meet metabolic demands. Therefore, it is reasonable to assume that if Pao_2 is normal, a decreased Pvo_2 indicates poor perfusion. An increase in $Pvco_2$ is also suggestive of increased anaerobic metabolism and poor oxygen supply to peripheral tissues. In light of these findings, appropriate therapy to improve oxygen delivery and peripheral tissue perfusion, such as intravenous fluids and positive inotropes, should be instituted.

Cardiac catheterization (see Chapter 4) with a specialized balloon-tipped catheter (Arrow Balloon Thermodilution Catheter, Arrow International, Inc.) can provide significant additional information regarding the patient's response to therapeutic interventions, particularly in the animal experiencing left heart failure. The Swan-Ganz catheter is inserted through the jugular vein and advanced into the pulmonary artery. The catheter has two ports positioned on either side of a small balloon. The proximal port, when properly positioned in the right atrium, permits CVP measurement. The distal port lies in the pulmonary artery, thereby measuring pulmonary artery pressure and, when the balloon is inflated, pulmonary capillary wedge pressure (PCWP). When the balloon is inflated, the recorded pressure is the pressure transmitted through the capillaries and is an indirect measure of left atrial filling pressure. In animals with elevated left ventricular diastolic pressure and left-sided heart failure, PCWP is routinely elevated. Changes in PCWP are a sensitive indicator of changes in cardiac function. In animals with severe pulmonary edema, PCWP consistently decreases following institution of appropriate therapy—preceding clinical and radiographic evidence of improvement. The Swan-Ganz catheter can also be used to measure cardiac output when coupled with a cardiac output computer. Catheterization of the heart provides valuable information, especially for the treatment of severely ill animals. However, due to the expense of the catheter and potential complications associated with its placement and maintenance, this technique is infrequently employed and underused.

CARDIAC ARRHYTHMIAS

Cardiac arrhythmias are defined as abnormalities of rate, rhythm, or conduction of electrical activity due to abnormal impulse formation or conduction. Arrhythmias are classified by the origin of the impulse (sinus node, atrial, junctional, ventricular) and the deviation of the rate from the normal sinus rate (tachycardia, bradycardia). The significance of an arrhythmia is dependant on two major factors: the type of arrhythmia (timing, frequency) and the associated clinical condition of the affected animal. Many arrhythmias do not require specific treatment and are self-limiting with treatment of the underlying disease. Serious arrhythmias, however, can significantly impair cardiac output, decrease coronary perfusion, and cause venous congestion leading to pulmonary edema. Hypotension, syncope and impaired myocardial performance can result from the presence of cardiac arrhythmias, leading to congestive heart failure, progression of the arrhythmia, systemic hypoperfusion, shock, and sudden death. Electrocardiographic evaluation should be performed in animals with suspected heart disease (e.g., overt heart failure, arrhythmias, murmur or gallop), animals with episodic clinical signs of syncope, weakness, or cyanosis, and animals with electrolyte disturbances (see box). Electrocardiographic evaluation is indicated for the detection and characterization of arrhythmias, monitoring an animal's response to therapy, evaluation of pacemaker function, and in the monitoring of unstable patients with cardiac and noncardiac disease. The presence or potential for development of arrhythmias should be suspected in patients with conditions resulting in poor tissue perfusion, hypoxemia, multiple trauma, ischemic injury to specific organs (e.g., gastric dilatation-volvulus complex, splenic masses), serum electrolyte ab-

---

CARDIAC ARRHYTHMIA EVALUATION IN THE SMALL ANIMAL PATIENT

The electrocardiogram—defining the arrhythmia
  Determine atrial rate
  Determine ventricular rate
  Atrioventricular synchronization
  Ectopic beats
    Timing (premature versus escape)
    Frequency/duration
    Effect on rhythm
Hemodynamics—defining any significant disturbance
  Weakness, syncope, lethargy
  Systemic arterial blood pressure, peripheral pulse
    quality
  Capillary refill time
  Urine output
  Chest radiography (venous congestion, pulmonary
    edema)
  Central venous pressure
Serum chemistries and acid-base status—defining
    contributing factors
  pH, bicarbonate concentration
  Electrolyte concentrations (sodium, potassium,
    calcium, chloride)
  Renal parameters (blood urea nitrogen, creatinine)
Pharmaceuticals—defining role in etiology or
    treatment
  Current medications, dose, frequency
  Previous response to therapy
  Side effects associated with therapy
  Renal, hepatic metabolism
  Potential drug interactions

---

normalities, and primary cardiac disease (Table 17-5).

The normal heart beat is initiated by the spontaneous depolarization of pacemaker cells in the sinoatrial node. The impulse is rapidly distributed through the atria and into the ventricles by an elaborate conduction system comprised of specialized myocardial cells. The electrocardiogram, a recording of the sum of the electrical potential generated by the heart during impulse formation and propagation, is the definitive tool for evaluating most cardiac arrhythmias (Table 17-6). There are several proposed mechanisms for the genesis of arrhythmias; however, the underlying mechanism usually cannot be determined from the surface electrocardiogram. The interested reader is directed to the available references on impulse formation, the conduction system, and mechanism of arrhythmia formation.[46-49]

Bradyarrhythmias

Sinus bradycardia. Sinus bradycardia is characterized by a normal sinus rhythm conducted at a rate of less than 60 beats per minute in dogs and 150 beats per minute in cats.[50] Sinus bradycardia may be physiologic or pathologic in origin. Physiologic bradycardia (e.g., hypothermia) rarely results in hemodynamic embarrassment. Increases in vagal tone lead to slowing of the discharge rate of the sinus node and are commonly associated with sinus bradycardia. Pathologic causes can cause weakness and on rare occasion syncope due to low cardiac output. Increased intracranial pressure, hypothyroidism, ocular or pharyngeal stimulation, and administration of certain anesthetic agents are common causes of bradyarrhythmias.[49,51] In many cases, the bradyarrhythmia is self-limiting with treatment of the underlying disease. Treatment of the underlying disease is especially important with sinus bradycardia secondary to hypothermia, anesthesia, and in animals at risk of cardiopulmonary arrest, as these conditions may be unresponsive to atropine and glycopyrrolate administration.

Treatment of most patients that are symptomatic for a sinus bradycardia involves administration of a parasympatholytic, such as atropine or glycopyrrolate, and intravascular volume expansion to increase preload and cardiac output. The intravenous route of administration should be avoided because of the potential for an initial increase in vagotonia and atrioventricular block resulting from the initial autonomic effects.[52] The subcutaneous or intramuscular route of administration is preferred in nonurgent situations. Alternatively, sympathomimetics (e.g., epinephrine, dopamine, isoproterenol) can be administered to

Table 17-5 Common clinical associations of cardiac arrhythmias

Supraventricular arrhythmias	
Sinus bradycardia	Increased vagal tone: increased intracranial pressure (brainstem lesions, head trauma), hypothermia, hypothyroidism, gastrointestinal disease; physiologic in young, athletic dogs
Sinus tachycardia	Increased sympathetic tone: excitement, fear, anxiety, hypotension, hypovolemia; hyperthyroidism; anemia
Supraventricular (atrial and junctional) premature complexes	Chronic valvular insufficiency (especially mitral); cardiomyopathy; chronic obstructive pulmonary disease; digitalis intoxication; anemia; hypoxia; atrial tumors; hypokalemia; anesthesia
Supraventricular tachycardia	As for supraventricular premature complexes; atrial septal defects; hyperthyroidism; cardiac catheterization; tricuspid valve dysplasia; accessory atrioventricular pathway (reentrant); heartworm disease; feline hypertrophic cardiomyopathy; trauma; electrocution
Atrial flutter and fibrillation	Atrial dilatation: cardiomyopathy, atrioventricular valve insufficiency, congenital heart disease; trauma; anesthesia
Ventricular arrhythmias	
Ventricular premature complexes and ventricular tachycardia	Cardiac disease: chronic valvular disease, congenital heart disease, pericardial disease, endomyocarditis; hypoxia; anemia; trauma; gastric dilatation-volvulus; sepsis; pulmonary disease; anesthetics; parasympatholytics; hyperthyroidism; acidosis; hypokalemia; autonomic imbalance; digitalis intoxication; pyometra
Ventricular flutter and fibrillation	As for ventricular tachycardia; severe underlying cardiac or metabolic disease
Conduction disturbances	
Sinoatrial arrest and sick sinus syndrome	High vagal tone; digitalis intoxication; surgical manipulation; breed predisposition includes dachshunds, pugs, cocker spaniels, and miniature schnauzers; can be associated with atrioventricular nodal and other conduction pathway disturbances
Atrial standstill	Hyperkalemia (acute renal failure, hypoadrenocorticism); atrial muscle dystrophy or myocarditis; dilated cardiomyopathy
Incomplete atrioventricular block (first-degree, second-degree)	Increased vagal tone; atrioventricular nodal disease; digitalis toxicity; narcotics; xylazine; cardiomyopathy; doxorubicin intoxication
Complete atrioventricular block (third-degree)	Atrioventricular nodal disease (infarct, neoplasia, fibrosis); severe drug toxicity (doxorubicin, digitalis); aortic-valve bacterial endocarditis; Lyme disease

increase the heart rate. These agents can have significant extracardiac effects, but are most useful in sinus bradycardia that is unresponsive to anticholinergic drugs and in the setting of sinus bradycardia and impending cardiac arrest. Pacemaker therapy is an option if the animal's bradycardia is unresponsive to medical therapy (see Chapter 41).

Atrial standstill. Atrial standstill results from inexcitability of the atrial musculature. The most common underlying causes are hyperkalemia and atrial muscular dystrophy of springer spaniels.[51] In the emergency setting, the most common causes of atrial standstill are hyperkalemia resulting from hypoadrenocorticism (Addison's disease) or acute renal failure, such as urinary tract obstruction. Hyperkalemia results in a variety of electrocardiographic abnormalities.[49] The early effects of hyperkalemia include peaked T waves and slowing of the sinus rate. Progressive elevations in serum potassium lead to diminished amplitude of the P wave and eventually total loss of the P wave and atrial activity (atrial standstill). At this point, the ventricular rhythm is usually still controlled by the sinus node, despite the lack of atrial activity, and the correct electrocardiographic (ECG) diagnosis is a sinoventricular rhythm. Terminally, intraventricular conduction is prolonged resulting in wide QRS complexes (sine-wave appearance) and a slowed ventricular response rate.

Table 17-6 Normal electrocardiographic parameters in the dog and cat (Lead II)

		Dog	Cat
Heart rate (beats per minute)		0-140 in adults; up to 180 in toy breeds; up to 220 in puppies	160-240
P wave	Width	Max: 4 msec	Max: 4 msec
	Height	Max: 0.4 mV	Max: 0.2 mV
P-R interval		6-13 msec	5-9 msec
QRS complex	Width	Max: 5 msec in small breeds; 6 msec in large breeds	4 msec
	Height (R wave)	Max: 2.5 mV in small breeds; 3.0 mV in large breeds	Max: 0.9 mV
	Depth (S wave)	Max: 0.35 mV	
ST segment	Depression	Max: 0.2 mV	Max: 0.1 mV
	Elevation	Max: 0.15 mV	Max: 0.1 mV
T wave		Less than ¼ R-wave amplitude	Max: 0.3 mV
Q-T interval	Width	15-25 msec; varies with heart rate	12-18 msec at normal heart rate (range, 7-20 msec)

Immediate therapeutic intervention is aimed at decreasing serum potassium concentration and improving the animal's hemodynamic status. Infusion of isotonic sodium chloride, sodium bicarbonate administration (1 mEq/kg over 3 to 4 minutes), and dextrose infusion promote movement of potassium into cells. Calcium gluconate administration (1 ml of a 10% solution per 10 kg of body weight) antagonizes the effect of potassium on the heart. Once the heart rhythm has been stabilized, treatment of the underlying cause of the hyperkalemia is pursued. A more complete discussion of the treatment of hyperkalemia is found is Chapters 18, 21, and 38.

Sinus arrest. Sinus arrest is characterized by failure of the sinus node to initiate impulse formation for a period of 2 P-P intervals or longer. If the pause in sinus node activity is regular or exactly 2 or 3 P-P intervals, sinoatrial block (blockage of the impulse prior to exiting the sinoatrial node) is present. Sinus arrest may occur with diseases of the sinoatrial node or secondary to high vagal tone, electrolyte disturbances, or drug intoxication (e.g., digitalis). This electrocardiographic finding may be an incidental finding in brachycephalic dogs, or it may be one of many ECG abnormalities in dogs with sick sinus syndrome. The clinical signs associated with sinus arrest include collapse, syncope, and sudden death if the subsidiary pacemakers fail to initiate an escape rhythm. Initial treatment of this arrhythmia is directed at resolution of the underlying cause. When drug therapy is required, anticholinergic agents or sympathomimetic drugs can be administered to increase the sinus rate and, if these drugs are ineffective, pacemaker therapy is indicated.

Sick sinus syndrome, the most common cause of sinus arrest in dogs, is a disease that results in failure of impulse formation by the sinus node and subsidiary pacemakers. The sinoatrial node is most commonly affected, although dysfunction of the atrioventricular node and disturbances of intraventricular conduction may accompany the disease. Paroxysmal supraventricular tachycardia is also commonly present, and in some animals it is difficult to determine whether clinical signs result from tachycardia or bradycardia. In fact, some recent information suggests that the long periods of sinus arrest are precipitated by the tachycardia, and treatment of the tachycardia may alleviate sinus arrest.[50] Common ECG abnormalities include irregular and inconsistent P-wave configurations, sinus arrest, junctional and ventricular escape complexes, and supraventricular tachycardias. Sick sinus syndrome disposes the animal to syncope, weakness, and, on very rare occasion, sudden death.

If clinical signs are manifest, medical management and artificial pacing are the therapeutic options. An atropine response test is useful to help determine which patients might respond to medical therapy and which might require cardiac pacing. Atropine (0.04 mg/kg intramuscularly) is administered after a baseline electrocardiogram is obtained and another is obtained 15 to 30 minutes following atropine administration. If the animal's heart rate increases in response to atropine, the animal might be successfully treated with oral anticholinergic therapy (propantheline, one-fourth to one or more 7.5 mg tablets orally two or three times a day). If the patient fails to respond or is intolerant of medical therapy, cardiac pacing should be employed (Chapter 41). With pacemaker therapy, the prognosis for animals with sick sinus syndrome is good to excellent.

Atrioventricular block. Atrioventricular (AV) block can be classified as incomplete (first- or second-degree) or complete (third-degree) and can result from high vagal tone, primary myocardial disease (e.g., cardiac neoplasia, Lyme disease), electrolyte disturbances, and drug administration. Incomplete AV block, especially first-degree or second-degree AV block Type I (Wenckebach) is often self-limiting with treatment of the underlying cause. High-grade second-degree AV block Type II (P:QRS > 3:1) and complete AV block are often associated with severe cardiac conduction pathway disease or drug intoxication. Patients with high-grade, type II (constant P-R interval) AV block with a widened QRS complex are at increased risk for progression to complete AV block. High-grade or complete AV block can result in clinical signs of weakness, syncope, and congestive heart failure in affected animals.

Therapy of animals with clinical signs of AV blockade involves addressing the underlying cause, such as withdrawal of drug therapy (e.g., digitalis, xylazine) and administration of sympathomimetic agents (isoproterenol, 0.4 mg in 250 ml of 5% dextrose, slow intravenous infusion to effect) or vagolytics (atropine, 0.04 mg/kg intramuscularly or subcutaneously). High-grade AV block and complete AV block are usually refractory to drug therapy; however, administration of sympathomimetic agents (terbutaline, 0.625 to 2.5 mg/orally three times a day) may increase the animal's ventricular escape rate and temporarily improve cardiac output.[51] Pacemaker therapy (Chapter 41) provides the most definitive therapy as long as the animal does not have concomitant myocardial failure. The median survival of these patients following pacemaker implantation approaches 1.5 years, with some patients surviving for longer than 3 years.

Tachyarrhythmias
Sinus tachycardia. Sinus tachycardia is a frequently encountered arrhythmia, usually representing a physiologic response in an effort to increase cardiac output. Elevated sympathetic tone, due to factors such as fear, anxiety, pain, and stress, commonly cause sinus tachycardia. Conditions such as heart failure, hypotension, anemia, and hypoxia in animals are also associated with a compensatory increase in sinus node discharge rate. Sinus tachycardia rarely results in hemodynamic embarrassment to an animal; however, myocardial workload and oxygen demand are increased. Administration of specific antiarrhythmic therapy is rarely indicated, and the sinus tachycardia will usually resolve spontaneously if the underlying cause is alleviated. However, if the arrhythmia is accompanied by congestive heart failure or hyperthyroidism, digitalis and beta-blockers, respectively, may be useful in slowing the heart rate (Table 17-7).

Supraventricular arrhythmias
Supraventricular tachycardia. Sinus tachycardia must be differentiated from supraventricular tachycardia since animals with sustained supraventricular tachycardias routinely require specific antiarrhythmic therapy. Supraventricular tachycardias originate from the atrial or junctional tissue, occurring as sustained or paroxysmal arrhythmias, often at heart rates greater than 300 per minute (Fig. 17-3). In humans, the majority of patients in whom supraventricular tachyarrhythmias develop have been diagnosed with pulmonary disease.[53] In addition to chronic obstructive pulmonary diseases and hypoxia, common associations in veterinary patients include cardiac diseases that result in atrial dilation, systemic diseases such as hyperthyroidism, and trauma.[54] These arrhythmias are associated with abnormal, irregular, or absent P-wave configuration and, unlike sinus tachycardia, may be abruptly terminated by a vagal maneuver. The most common mechanism causing sustained or paroxysmal supraventricular tachycardia is reentry via a circuit involving the AV node.[53]

Rapid or sustained supraventricular tachyarrhythmias can be life-threatening, requiring immediate intervention. A vagal maneuver, performed by applying firm pressure to the carotid sinus or eyes of an affected animal, can successfully terminate the arrhythmia. The carotid sinus is located at the bifurcation of the carotid artery immediately caudal to the angle of the mandible alongside the trachea. The carotid sinus is compressed against the transverse process of the cervical vertebrae and massaged in a cranial to caudal direction. The ocular vagal maneuver is performed by firmly applying direct pressure to both globes. If a vagal maneuver is ineffective, administration of intravenous drugs is warranted.

Table 17-7 Recommended dosages and effects associated with various antiarrhythmic drugs

Drug	Administration	Clinical uses	Side effects
Quinidine	D: 5-15 mg/kg po qid 5-10 mg/kg IV, IM	Ventricular arrhythmias Supraventricular arrhythmias	Bradycardia, atrioventricular block, hypotension, skeletal muscle weakness, nausea, vomiting
Procainamide	D: 3-6 mg/kg IV bolus 6-10 mg/kg IM 10-30 μg/kg per minute CRI 15-30 mg/kg po tid/qid C: ¼ of 250 mg tablet po per cat every 8 to 12 hours	Ventricular arrhythmias Supraventricular tachycardia	Similar to quinidine, but less hypotensive
Lidocaine	D: 2-3 mg/kg IV boluses; max., 8 mg/kg 40-100 μg/kg per minute CRI C: 0.25 mg/kg bolus 10 μg/kg per minute CRI	Ventricular arrhythmias Digitalis-induced arrhythmias	Tremors, seizures, nausea, ataxia especially in cats
Tocainide	D: 5-20 mg/kg po tid	Ventricular arrhythmias	See first three drugs
Propantheline	D: 2.5-30 mg po bid/tid	Supraventricular bradyarrhythmias Atrioventricular block responsive to parasympatholytic agents	Gastrointestinal disturbances
Propranolol	D: 0.1-1 mg/kg po tid 0.02 mg/kg IV bolus; max., 0.2 mg/kg C: 2.5-5 mg po bid/tid	Supraventricular tachycardia Ventricular tachycardia Hypertrophic cardiomyopathy Thyrotoxicosis	Bradycardia, hypotension, negative inotrope
Diltiazem	D: 0.5-1.0 mg/kg po tid C: 7.5 mg po bid/tid	Slow ventricular response in atrial fibrillation Hypertrophic cardiomyopathy	Negative inotrope, hypotension
Verapamil	D: 50 μg/kg IV bolus every 10 minutes, max., 150 μg/kg 1-2 mg/kg po tid/qid	Supraventricular tachycardia Hypertrophic cardiomyopathy	Negative inotrope, hypotension, bradycardia, atrioventricular block, nausea, vomiting, heart failure
Digoxin	D: 0.5-1 μg/kg every hour; max., 2-4 μg/kg IV 0.22 mg/m^2 divided bid C: 0.7-1 μg/kg every 12-48 hours	Supraventricular tachycardia Myocardial failure	Nausea, vomiting, arrhythmias, conduction disturbances

D = dog dosage; C = cat dosage; po = orally; qid = four times a day; IV = intravenously; IM = intramuscularly; CRI = constant-rate intravenous infusion; tid = three times a day; bid = twice a day.

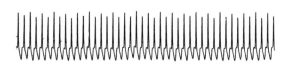

Fig. 17-3 Supraventricular tachycardia in a 3-year-old Labrador retriever presenting for vomiting and diarrhea with no evidence of heart disease. Heart rate approximately 350 beats per minute (paper speed 12.5 mm/per second).

Digoxin, the drug of choice in animals with concurrent congestive heart failure, is slowly administered intravenously at a dosage of 0.5 to 1.0 µg/kg every hour to a maximum dosage of 2 to 4 µg/kg. If myocardial function is unimpaired, propranolol or verapamil can be administered intravenously (Table 17-7). Propranolol, a nonspecific beta-adrenergic antagonist, inhibits sympathetic stimulation of the heart and has direct cardiac depressant effects on automaticity and conduction. Verapamil is currently the drug of choice to treat sustained supraventricular tachycardia in dogs without concurrent heart failure.[55] By blocking the slow calcium channels, verapamil decreases the automaticity of the sinus node, AV node, and ischemic myocardium, all of which depend on the slow channels for spontaneous depolarization. Calcium-channel blockers decrease the rate of conduction through the AV node, and this explains most of the success achieved in using these drugs to break reentrant supraventricular tachycardias.[55,56] Propranolol and verapamil are both negative inotropes and chronotropes and should not be administered sequentially due to potentially additive effects. When vagal maneuvers and drug therapy are ineffective in treating severe, life-threatening supraventricular tachycardia, electrical cardioversion is indicated if an ECG synchronized defibrillator is available.

Atrial fibrillation. Although atrial flutter and fibrillation can be differentiated electrocardiographically, the causes and treatment requirements are nearly identical. Atrial flutter is uncommon in veterinary medical patients and is often the transient predecessor to the development of atrial fibrillation. Atrial fibrillation is characterized by random, rapid, and chaotic atrial activity with an irregular ventricular response due to varying AV nodal conduction of atrial impulses (Fig. 17-4). The ventricular response to atrial fibrillation is usually quite rapid, with rates between 220 and 280 beats per minute in untreated dogs and rates often in excess of 300 beats per minute in untreated cats. The rapid ventricular rate results in decreased diastolic filling time, and because of ineffectual atrial activity, the atrial contribution to ventricular filling is eliminated. Under normal circumstances, the atrial contraction contributes 15% to 30% of the stroke volume.

Most small animal patients with atrial fibrillation have organic heart disease with associated dilated atria.[57] Chronic AV valve insufficiency, cardiomyopathy, and some congenital heart disease are common underlying conditions in the dog. The most common cause of atrial fibrillation in the cat is hypertrophic cardiomyopathy.[58] Since

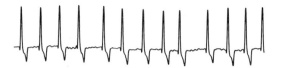

Fig. 17-4 Atrial fibrillation in a Great Dane with dilated cardiomyopathy, while on digoxin to slow the ventricular response rate. Heart rate 140 beats per minute with an irregular rhythm and fibrillation waves present (paper speed 25 mm/per second).

most animals have chronic, progressive heart disease, pharmacologic or electrical direct current conversion to normal sinus rhythm are rarely attempted. Even when conversion to sinus rhythm is successful in these patients, it is usually transient, and rapid reversion back to atrial fibrillation is common. Therefore, the goals of therapy are to decrease the ventricular response to a more physiologic heart rate and to control congestive heart failure when present.

In animals with significant atrial dilation, digitalis is administered with the goal of slowing the ventricular response to 160 beats per minute or less (see Table 17-7). Digitalis slows conduction of the atrial impulse through the AV node and also increases myocardial contractility, making this drug well suited for the patient with impaired systolic function. If the ventricular rate has not adequately slowed after 3 to 5 days of oral digitalis administration, additional drugs, such as a beta-adrenergic blocker or calcium-channel blocker, can be administered. Propranolol, diltiazem, and verapamil are commonly administered as adjunctive therapies to digitalis for slowing the ventricular response to atrial fibrillation. These drugs are negative inotropes, and the patient should be monitored for exacerbation of congestive heart failure.

Less frequently, anesthesia, digitalis intoxication, myocardial ischemia, and trauma can lead to atrial fibrillation in animals without underlying cardiac disease. If concurrent atrial dilation is not present, conversion to sinus rhythm can be attempted. Initially, dogs are treated with quinidine (5 to 15 mg/kg intramuscularly or 5 to 15 mg/kg orally four times a day for 48 to 72 hours). Diltiazem may also result in conversion in selected patients.[59] If atrial fibrillation persists, ECG-synchronized cardioversion or conventional drug therapies (digitalis, beta-blockers, calcium-channel blockers) can be used.

The prognosis with atrial fibrillation is guarded in animals with underlying cardiac disease. Some giant-breed dogs have survival times of nearly 2 years, whereas most animals die within the first year following diagnosis.

Ventricular arrhythmias

Ventricular premature depolarization and ventricular tachycardia. Ventricular premature depolarizations or ventricular premature complexes (VPCs) are ectopic impulses arising from the ventricles. Ventricular arrhythmias are characterized by wide, bizarre QRST deflections that come at a rate faster than the underlying cardiac rhythm. VPCs must be differentiated from ventricular escape complexes, which are morphologically identical but occur only after a pause in the rhythm, because escape beats function as a rescue mechanism to maintain cardiac output. Ventricular tachycardia is a series of repetitive ventricular complexes (Fig. 17-5), either sustained or paroxysmal, with a ventricular rate in excess of 140 beats per minute.

Ventricular arrhythmias are the most common rhythm disturbance in the dog. Many causes and associations are recognized for ventricular arrhythmias, including endomyocardial diseases, pericardial disease, and extracardiac conditions such as gastric-dilatation volvulus, anemia, trauma, and sepsis.[60] Ventricular tachycardia often results in impaired cardiac output, myocardial ischemia, and occasionally progresses to ventricular flutter or fibrillation. Clinical signs include weakness, collapse, syncope, and sudden death.

Isolated, infrequent VPCs are rarely treated; however, rapid ventricular tachycardia (rates >200 beats per minute) is almost always treated. There is considerable debate over the management of arrhythmias that fall in the "gray zone" between isolated VPCs and rapid ventricular tachycardia.[61-63] Proarrhythmic effects of antiarrhythmic drugs may lead to worsening of these arrhythmias in approximately 5% to 15% of human patients.[64,65] Additional side effects from antiarrhythmic drugs are fairly common, and most antiarrhythmic drugs are expensive. Arguments in favor of using antiarrhythmic drugs are that they might prevent sudden death and they might improve the quality of life in animals that are symptomatic due to ventricular arrhythmias.

General guidelines to follow when considering initiation of antiarrhythmic drugs include the following (see box). First, animals that are symptomatic (weakness, syncope, worsening heart failure) due to ventricular arrhythmias should be treated. Secondly, animals with ventricular arrhythmias who are recognized to be at increased risk for sudden death (i.e., boxers and Doberman pinschers with dilated cardiomyopathy) should be treated. Animals with severe systemic diseases and ventricular tachycardia at rates in excess of 160 beats per minute should be treated. Finally, animals with multiform (multifocal) VPCs, those with repetitive patterns, and those with close coupling of the premature VPC to the previous T wave (R-on-T phenomenon) may require treatment, especially if they have cardiac enlargement or underlying myocardial disease.

Intravenous lidocaine administration is initially employed in the treatment of ventricular tachycardia in dogs requiring immediate therapy. Lidocaine administration decreases cardiac automaticity and conduction velocity, causing minimal adverse hemodynamic side effects. A lidocaine bolus (2 to 4 mg/kg) is administered intravenously, and if a good response is noted, then lidocaine is continued as a constant-rate intravenous infusion (dogs: 40 to 80 μg/kg per minute). Lidocaine must be given by continuous infusion because of its short plasma half-life and rapid redistribution. The effects of a lidocaine constant-rate infusion can take up to 5 hours to be realized if additional

---

RECOMMENDATIONS FOR THE TREATMENT OF VENTRICULAR ARRHYTHMIAS IN DOGS

Greater than 20 isolated premature ventricular depolarizations per minute

Ventricular arrhythmias in breeds predisposed to sudden death (Doberman pinschers, boxers)

Clinical signs of weakness, syncope, or collapse attributable to ectopic ventricular activity

Frequent couplets, triplets, bigeminy, sustained ventricular tachycardia

Close coupling of the QRS complex to the T wave of the preceding complex (R-on-T phenomenon); predisposes to ventricular tachycardia or ventricular fibrillation

Multiform ventricular complexes suggesting multiple ectopic foci within the ventricles

---

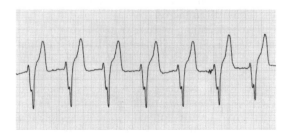

Fig. 17-5 Ventricular tachycardia secondary to traumatic myocarditis in a young dog hit by a car 24 hours before. Heart rate 160 beats per minute (paper speed 50 mm/per second).

boluses are not administered when the infusion is initiated. At high dosages, lidocaine administration does cause neurologic side effects, such as depression, tremors, vomiting, and seizures. Lidocaine-induced seizure activity in animals should be treated with diazepam (0.5 mg/kg intravenously). Cats are more susceptible to the neurotoxic side effects of lidocaine and should be treated cautiously and at a markedly reduced dosage (see Table 17-7). Hemodynamic alterations attributable to ventricular arrhythmias are rarely severe enough to require lidocaine infusion in cats as treatment of heart failure or the primary disorder usually leads to resolution of the dysrrhythmia. In animals that need continued antiarrhythmic therapy, procainamide, quinidine, mexiletine, or tocainide is initiated as the patient is weaned off the lidocaine infusion, usually over a 24-hour period.

If lidocaine is ineffective, intravenous procainamide is probably the second choice. An intravenous bolus of 3 to 6 mg/kg is followed by a continuous-rate infusion of 10 to 40 μg/kg per minute. Oral procainamide is substituted for injectable formulations when the patient is stable, or oral drug using the sustained release preparation can be started immediately in asymptomatic dogs that do not require initial rapid treatment. Some clinical experience indicates that procainamide may be safe in cats at a dose of 62.5 mg three times a day.

Propranolol has been recommended for the initial treatment of ventricular tachycardia in cats, and is commonly used as an additional drug when the first antiarrhythmic (e.g., lidocaine, procainamide) fails to control the ventricular arrhythmia in dogs. Some dogs with ventricular arrhythmias resulting from trauma or observed in association with gastric dilation and volvulus seem to respond better to a combination of propranolol and analgesics (butorphanol, 0.2 mg/kg four times a day) than to conventional Class I antiarrhythmics.

Little information is available on the appropriate time to discontinue antiarrhythmic therapy and the therapeutic end point that indicates successful antiarrhythmic therapy. Animals with underlying myocardial disease or cardiac dilation should continue to receive antiarrhythmic therapy for life. Patients with "normal" hearts and transient arrhythmias associated with systemic, metabolic, or acid-base disorders may require therapy for several days to several weeks, but these arrhythmias are usually transient. Of greater concern is determination of a desirable therapeutic end point. It is unlikely that an antiarrhythmic drug will suppress all ventricular ectopic activity, so total elimination of the arrhythmia is an unrealistic end point.

Suppression of repetitive forms, alleviation of clinical signs, or a reduction in the rate of ventricular tachycardia to less than 140 beats per minute may be more realistic goals or therapeutic end points.

Ventricular fibrillation and flutter. Ventricular flutter and fibrillation are often terminal arrhythmias (see Chapter 32). Ventricular fibrillation is characterized by random cardiac electrical and mechanical activity. Effective cardiac output drops to zero. Ventricular flutter is more organized than ventricular fibrillation, often resembling a rapid sine wave. Ventricular fibrillation can be described as either coarse or fine, with coarse ventricular fibrillation having a higher amplitude. Rapid intervention is imperative in animals with ventricular fibrillation in order to prevent irreversible cell damage due to hypoxia and acidosis.

Electrical defibrillation is the treatment of choice for ventricular fibrillation. A precordial thump, on rare occasion, has proven effective in converting the random ventricular activity to a sinus rhythm. Chemical defibrillation can be attempted using potassium chloride (1 mEq/kg intravenously) and acetylcholine (6 mg/kg intravenously) administration or bretylium tosylate. Anecdotal reports on the use of bretylium tosylate in dogs have described mixed results; however, it seems that this drug might be most useful to prevent ventricular fibrillation, or to be used in conjunction with electrical defibrillation.

PERICARDIAL DISEASE

Although the pericardium is not essential for life, diseases of the pericardium and pericardial space can result in physiologic aberrations that can be dramatic and life threatening. However, the clinical signs of pericardial disease are often nonspecific, presenting a diagnostic challenge. Pericardial disease has been estimated to represent 1% of canine cardiovascular disease and is one of the most common causes of right-sided heart failure.[66] Clinically apparent pericardial disease is less common in the cat.[67]

The pericardium consists of two layers of tissue that form a sac containing a small volume of transudate. The fibrous, outer layer extends onto the origins of the great vessels, attaching dorsally. It is the fibrous pericardium that is responsible for the poor distensibility of the pericardium. The inner, serous layer is formed by the invagination of the heart such that one surface is adherent to the fibrous pericardium (parietal layer) and the other to the heart (visceral layer). The cavity formed between the two layers of the serous pericardium is the pericardial cavity. The pericardial sac maintains the heart in an optimal functional position within the thoracic cavity, minimizes friction by serving as a lubricated sac, and protects against infectious processes. The most important physiologic effects of the pericardium are limiting diastolic ventricular volume (thus preventing acute overload) and limiting ventricular compliance. The normal pericardium provides little resistance to ventricular diastolic filling unless the ventricles are dilated. The pericardium maintains optimal transmural pressure, coupling right and left ventricular diastolic pressures, and balancing stroke volume, especially at elevated right ventricular filling pressure.[68]

Congenital pericardial disease

Pericardial cysts, partial or complete absence of the pericardium, and peritoneopericardial diaphragmatic hernia are congenital pericardial anomalies that have been reported in dogs and cats.[67,69] Pericardial cysts are quite rare, resulting from abnormal development of mesenchymal tissue or incarceration of omentum during fetal development. The clinical signs are primarily related to the respiratory system, and surgical resection of the cyst with or without subtotal pericardiectomy results in resolution of the clinical signs. Absence of the pericardium has been reported as an incidental finding, without any associated clinical signs.

The most frequently encountered congenital defect of the pericardium in both dogs and cats is a peritoneopericardial diaphragmatic hernia (PPDH).[69,70] The formation of the hernia is attributed to failure of fusion of the transverse septum with the pleuroperitoneal folds during fetal development, resulting in incomplete division of the coelom into abdominal and thoracic cavities. Prenatal

A
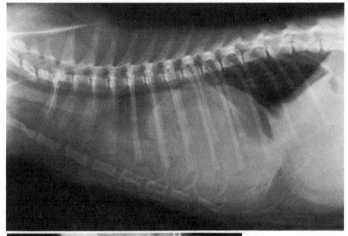

B
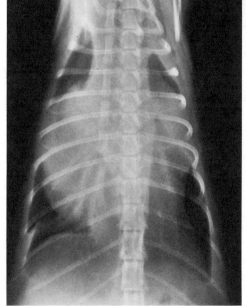

Fig. 17-6 **A** and **B**, Ventrodorsal and lateral thoracic radiographs obtained from a 10-month-old male domestic shorthaired cat with congenital peritoneopericardial diaphragmatic hernia. A small amount of pleural fluid is present. Note the markedly enlarged and globoid cardiac shape along with the continuity of the cardiac silhouette and diaphragm on both radiographs.

trauma or injury can also result in formation of PPDH. Sternal deformities, pectus excavatum, and ventral abdominal wall defects often accompany PPDH.[69] Multiple cardiac defects have also been reported in a litter of collies with PPDH.[71]

Peritoneopericardial diaphragmatic hernias are presumed to be present from birth; however, clinical signs may become apparent at any age or the patient may remain asymptomatic throughout its life. The persistent communication between the peritoneal and pericardial cavities permits herniation of abdominal contents into the pericardial cavity, resulting in clinical signs of gastrointestinal disease (vomiting, anorexia, weight loss). Clinical signs of respiratory dysfunction (dyspnea, cough) are less common, and cardiovascular complications, such as congestive heart failure are rarely associated with PPDH.

Physical examination of animals with PPDH often reveals muffled heart sounds and displacement of the precordial impulse. Sternal defects, borborygmus on auscultation of the thoracic cavity, and a relative absence of organs on abdominal palpation are occasionally detected with physical examination.

Thoracic radiography is a valuable tool for the diagnosis of PPDH. The cardiac silhouette is dramatically enlarged and often globoid, with elevation of the trachea (Fig. 17-6). Abnormal fat or gas densities may overlie the heart. Abdominal radiography may indicate an absence or cranial displacement of abdominal contents. Electrocardiographic findings are more variable, occasionally revealing low-amplitude QRS complexes or electrical axis deviation.

The preferred diagnostic test is echocardiography. Ultrasound evaluation of the thorax permits noninvasive evaluation of discontinuity of the diaphragm as well as detection of abdominal contents within the pericardial cavity with apposition of liver or other organs and the heart. Positive or negative contrast peritoneographic examination, radiographic contrast studies of the gastrointestinal tract, fluoroscopic evaluation, and nonselective angiography can be used to confirm the diagnosis of PPDH.

Surgical reduction of the herniated abdominal contents with closure of the defect is the treatment of choice. Adhesions between the parietal pericardium and visceral peritoneum and incarceration or strangulation of abdominal organs can on rare occasion complicate surgical intervention. There is risk of a pneumothorax developing postoperatively if the thoracic cavity is entered. Compromise of the animal's respiratory and cardiovascular systems can present an anesthetic risk, and the anesthetist should be prepared for rapid application of supportive measures (intubation during anesthetic induction, thoracocentesis, ventilation, intravenous fluid administration). The prognosis for resolution of clinical signs is excellent in uncomplicated cases.

Acquired pericardial disease

The major acquired pathophysiologic processes affecting the pericardium are pericardial effusion and constrictive pericarditis. The conditions reported to cause pericardial disease in dogs and cats are listed in Table 17-8. Pericardial effusion accounts for more than 90% of clinically apparent acquired pericardial disease in small animals.[67] Pericardial effusion has been recognized in cats, although it is rarely associated with the development of cardiac tamponade.[72]

Pericardial effusion and cardiac tamponade. Pericardial effusion is defined as the excessive accumulation of fluid within the pericardial cavity. The clinical presentation of a patient with pericardial effusion depends on the rate of fluid accumulation and the ability of the pericardium to expand to accommodate the fluid. Clinical signs of cardiac tamponade do not develop until the accumulated fluid reaches a critical volume and pressure, exceeding the elastic limit of the pericardium.[73] When this limit is reached, the intrapericardial pressure becomes greater than the intrapleural pressure. Due to the poor elasticity of the pericardium, the majority of the increased intrapericardial pressure is absorbed by the cardiac wall. The intraatrial and intraventricular pressures increase, leading to an increased end-diastolic filling pressure and eventually impaired ventricular filling. Therefore, with progressive pericardial effusion resulting in tamponade, there is a decrease in stroke volume and cardiac output without alteration in contractility.[74]

In addition to the primary hemodynamic effect of tamponade (decreased stroke volume), there are compensatory hemodynamic changes that contribute to the clinical findings. Initial response to a decrease in stroke volume includes increased peripheral systemic vascular resistance, central venous pressure, and heart rate. The increase in peripheral vascular resistance is an attempt to maintain arterial pressure as cardiac output declines. Central venous pressure is increased due to the transference of intrapericardial pressure across the cardiac wall, causing increased atrial filling pressures, as well as increased venous return to the heart secondary to vasoconstriction. In an attempt to maintain cardiac output and restore blood flow, the heart rate is elevated.

Clinical signs of right-sided heart failure (ascites, hepatomegaly, jugular venous distention) usually predominate with chronic pericardial disease due to the collapse of the right atrium and

Table 17-8 Pericardial diseases of dogs and cats

	Dogs	Cats
Congenital disorders	Peritoneopericardial diaphragmatic hernia	Peritoneopericardial diaphragmatic hernia
	Pericardial defects	Pericardial defects
	Pericardial cyst	Pericardial cyst
Acquired disorders		
Pericardial effusion		
Infectious	Canine distemper virus	Feline infectious peritonitis
	Actinomyces	*Pasteurella*
	Nocardia	Botryomycosis
	Leptospirosis	Toxoplasmosis
	Coccidioides immitis	
Inflammatory	Idiopathic	
Neoplastic	Hemangiosarcoma	Lymphosarcoma
	Chemodectoma	Metastatic carcinoma
	Mesothelioma	Hemangiosarcoma
	Thyroid carcinoma	Mesothelioma
	Metastatic neoplasia	
Metabolic	Hypoproteinemia	Hypoproteinemia
	Uremia	Hyperthyroidism
		Uremia
Cardiac	Congestive heart failure	Congestive heart failure
	Cardiomyopathy	Cardiomyopathy
	Chronic valvular disease	
	Congenital defects	
	Rupture	Rupture
	Left atrial tear	Left atrial tear
	Trauma	Trauma
	Catheterization	Catheterization
	Endomyocardial biopsy	
Coagulopathies	Anticoagulant rodenticides	Anticoagulant rodenticides
Constrictive	Idiopathic	Idiopathic
pericarditis	Infectious/inflammatory	Infectious/inflammatory
	Neoplasia	Neoplasia

ventricle attributable to the lower filling pressures in the right heart.[75,76] With progression of the disease, venous return to the left side of the heart is impaired and signs of low cardiac output to the systemic arterial circulation (syncope, hypotension, azotemia) result. With acute pericardial effusion, the clinical signs are usually associated with forward failure (shock, collapse).[76] Therefore, markedly variable volumes of fluid can accumulate before a significant increase in intrapericardial pressure and ventricular compression is observed. Clinical signs of cardiac tamponade accompanying acute, rapidly developing effusions and effusions complicated by pericardial fibrosis occur with accumulation of smaller fluid volumes (25 to 100 ml). In contrast, the volume of fluid required to produce clinical signs of cardiac tamponade in animals with chronic, slowly progressive pericardial effusions can be up to 1 L in some cases.[66]

The most common causes of acquired pericar-

dial effusion in dogs are idiopathic ("benign") pericardial effusion and effusion resulting from cardiac neoplasia.[77] Hemangiosarcoma of the right atrial appendage or atrial-wall and heart-base tumors are the most commonly reported neoplastic processes associated with the development of pericardial effusion in dogs.[70,78] Ectopic thyroid carcinoma, mesothelioma, lymphoid neoplasia, and ectopic parathyroid carcinoma represent less common causes of acquired pericardial disease in dogs.[67,77] Left atrial rupture, chronic uremia, infectious pericarditis, and congestive heart failure also can be associated with the development of pericardial effusion. Transudative effusions, related to conditions such as congestive heart failure and hypoproteinemia, are common but rarely cause cardiac tamponade or other clinical signs because of the small volume of fluid that accumulates. In cats, feline infectious peritonitis, chronic uremia, toxoplasmosis, congestive heart failure, and a variety of other diseases have been reported to affect the pericardial cavity.[72] Primary cardiac tumors are rare in the cat, and idiopathic pericardial effusion has not been reported.

Diagnosis. Pericardial disease is most frequently diagnosed in large-breed, male dogs older than 6 years of age. Idiopathic pericardial effusion occurs most frequently in medium to large male dogs, with the age of onset ranging from 1 to 14 years (average, 6 years). Middle-aged to older large-breed dogs have a higher prevalence of neoplastic effusions. German shepherds and golden retrievers appear to be predisposed to both idiopathic and hemangiosarcoma-related pericardial effusion.[77,79] Brachycephalic breeds, such as English bulldogs and boxers have been reported to be predisposed to the development of aortic body tumors.[80]

Clinical signs of pericardial disease are related to decreased cardiac output and systemic venous congestion. Historical findings include weakness, syncope, dyspnea, weight loss, abdominal distention, and occasionally gastrointestinal signs such as anorexia and vomiting. Right-sided heart failure often predominates due to the chronic onset and the compensatory hemodynamic changes that occur. Animals with acutely developing effusions caused by left atrial rupture secondary to chronic mitral insufficiency, sudden hemorrhage from a cardiac neoplasm (especially hemangiosarcoma), or traumatic rupture of the right atrium, often present with acute hypotension and cardiogenic shock or sudden death.[74]

The triad of decreased heart sounds, decreased arterial pulse quality, and jugular-vein distention is highly suggestive of pericardial effusion with tamponade. Pallor, weight loss, pericardial friction rub, and cardiac arrhythmias can also be detected; however, most patients have no auscultatable murmur, arrhythmia, or gallop. Pulsus paradoxus, although not specific for pericardial disease, may also be present. This condition is characterized by an exaggerated decrease (>10 mm Hg) in systolic arterial blood pressure accompanying inspiration. During inspiration, the filling of the right ventricle is enhanced, resulting in exaggerated shifts of the intraventricular septum. Consequently, left ventricular filling is impaired and systolic arterial blood pressure decreases with the attendant decrease in stroke volume.

The results of routine laboratory tests are unlikely to provide definitive information regarding the diagnosis of pericardial disease. Nonspecific changes such as hypoproteinemia, neutrophilic leukocytosis, and anemia might be evident.[81] The serum biochemical profile may reveal nonspecific changes associated with hepatic congestion or mild azotemia if renal perfusion is impaired.

Hemangiosarcoma has been associated with erythrocyte abnormalities such as anemia, circulating nucleated red blood cells, schistocytes, and spherocytes. Thrombocytopenia and other coagulation disorders are also reported with hemangiosarcoma.[82] Analysis of fluid aspirated from the thoracic or abdominal cavity of animals with pericardial effusion usually reveals a modified transudate, compatible with heart failure. Cats with pericardial disease due to feline infectious peritonitis (FIP) may have high serum FIP titers, and centesis of the abdomen or thorax often reveals fluid more suggestive of FIP than heart failure. Lymphosarcoma in cats with pericardial disease is often associated with a positive result on feline leukemia virus tests or evidence of lymphosarcoma elsewhere in the body.

Thoracic radiography is of diagnostic value in animals with chronic pericardial effusion; however, the findings may be less remarkable if the effusion develops acutely. Chronic pericardial disease results in stretching of the fibrous component of the pericardium evidenced by generalized cardiomegaly with loss of cardiac chamber definition (Fig. 17-7). Typically, the cardiac silhouette is slightly enlarged, within normal limits, or may suggest longstanding mitral-valve insufficiency in patients in whom acute pericardial effusion develops. Radiographic findings often include mild pleural effusion and substantial distention of the caudal vena cava. These radiographic findings are often compatible with chronic AV valve insufficiency, primary myocardial disease, and congeni-

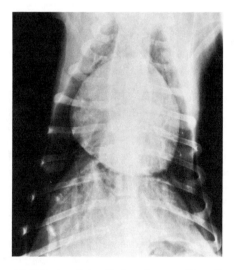

Fig. 17-7 Pericardial effusion in an older German shepherd. The globoid silhouette is not pathognomonic for pericardial effusion and can be difficult to differentiate from other causes of congestive heart failure, such as dilated cardiomyopathy (see Fig. 17-1).

tal disorders, thereby limiting the usefulness of survey thoracic radiography. If the pericardial effusion is due to a heart-base tumor, there may be increased soft-tissue density in the anterior mediastinum or dorsal displacement of the trachea in this region.

Electrocardiographic findings supportive of the diagnosis of pericardial disease include low-amplitude QRS complexes, electrical alternans, *p-mitrale,* and nonspecific ST-segment deviation or elevation. Diminished-amplitude QRS complexes, the most frequently observed ECG abnormality, are defined in the dog as being less than 1.0 mV in all leads.[70,81] In the cat it is more difficult to define low-amplitude QRS complexes; however, the finding of QRS complexes less than 0.15 mV in all leads or a significant decrease in complex size as compared with a previous electrocardiogram is suggestive of pericardial disease in the cat. Electrical alternans is characterized by the regular beat-to-beat variation of QRS complex size and/or morphology. This ECG finding results from changes in the position of the heart within the pericardial cavity attributable to the accumulation of fluid. Electrical alternans tends to be a more common finding with large-volume effusions and, when present, is highly suggestive of pericardial effusion.[83] Supraventricular and ventricular arrhythmias have also been reported in association with pericardial disease; however, the most common rhythm diagnoses are normal sinus rhythm and sinus tachycardia.

The most specific and sensitive means for confirming and characterizing pericardial effusion is echocardiographic evaluation.[84,85] Echocardiography demonstrates an echo-free space, or fluid space, encircling the heart between the epicardium and parietal pericardium[86] (Fig. 17-8). In extreme situations, the intraventricular septum

flattens and displaces toward the left ventricle. Cardiac tamponade is evidenced by diastolic collapse of the right atrium and ventricle. Mass lesions can be visualized, usually associated with the right atrium, right atrial appendage, or the heart base. These findings provide important therapeutic and prognostic information. Concomitant cardiac disorders (e.g., feline cardiomyopathy) can also be detected and characterized.

Contrast pneumopericardiographic techniques can assist in the determination of the underlying cause for pericardial effusion (Fig. 17-9).[87] However, the technique is more invasive than and is inferior to ultrasonographic evaluation for the localization of an intrapericardial mass lesion.

Angiographic procedures in animals with pericardial effusion can be used to support the presumed diagnosis of pericardial effusion and to define etiology. These procedures have been used primarily to outline heart-base or intracardiac (typically within the auricular wall) tumors, or to demonstrate displacement of cardiac structures by a mass lesion.[88] The presence of pericardial effusion is suggested by elevation of the cardiac chambers away from the sternum and increased separation of the contrast-defined endocardium and the outer border of the pericardial shadow.

Pericardiocentesis can be performed to confirm the diagnosis of pericardial effusion as well as to obtain fluid for cytologic evaluation and culture if indicated. Pericardial effusions are classified as hemorrhagic, transudative, or exudative. Congestive heart failure and hypoproteinemia result in transudates, whereas exudates are suggestive of infectious causes. Hemorrhagic effusions are found in the majority of dogs with pericardial effusion. These effusions are usually of a sterile, noninflammatory character, and macroscopic or cytologic evaluation of the fluid does not tend to

Fig. 17-8 Echocardiographic demonstration of pericardial effusion characterized as an echo-free space surrounding the heart between the epicardium and the parietal pericardium *(arrows).*

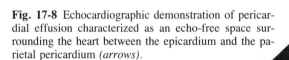

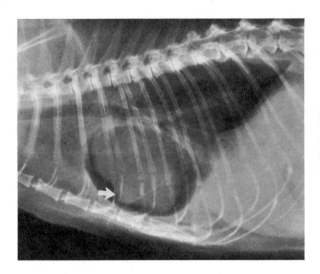

Fig. 17-9 Contrast pneumopericardiogram in a cat with pericardial effusion secondary to a right ventricular mass *(arrow)*. Pleural effusion due to cardiac tamponade and right-sided heart failure is also present.

discriminate between the different neoplastic causes and idiopathic effusion.[89] Blood gas analysis may prove useful in discriminating between neoplastic and inflammatory effusions.[84] The pH of the fluid removed by pericardiocentesis in dogs with neoplastic effusions is usually above 7.2, and the pH in cases of idiopathic or inflammatory diseases is often less than 7.1.[90] Unless the cause is bacteria or fungi, fluid analysis rarely provides the definitive diagnosis.

Treatment. The underlying disease and the clinical complications associated with the pericardial effusion are the major determinants of case management. Pericardial effusion due to systemic disease—such as hypoproteinemia, congestive heart failure, and uremia—or due to peritoneopericardial diaphragmatic hernia resolve with correction of the underlying problem. If there is evidence of cardiac tamponade, without ongoing hemorrhage, pericardiocentesis is indicated.[81,91] Pericardiocentesis provides rapid relief of clinical signs in animals with cardiac tamponade by correcting the underlying cause of the reduced cardiac output—restriction of diastolic filling. This procedure can be performed with minimal risk to the patient, using mild sedation if necessary for fractious or anxious animals. The patient should be in either left lateral or sternal recumbency. The right hemithorax, between the third and eighth intercostal space, extending from above the costochondral junction to the sternum, is clipped and the skin is aseptically prepared. The skin and muscles of the fourth or fifth intercostal space are infiltrated with lidocaine. A variety of catheters can be used to access the pericardial space. The catheter must be of sufficient length to reach the pericardial cavity (at least 3 cm) and have a diameter large enough to permit easy removal of fluid.

The catheter preferred by us is an over-the-needle, 16-gauge catheter. With the patient being monitored continuously by electrocardiography, the catheter is carefully advanced through the skin and intercostal muscles, directed toward the heart. Once pericardial fluid is obtained, the catheter is advanced over the stylet, and it is then attached to extension tubing, a three-way stopcock, and a large syringe (35 or 60 ml). Gentle suction is applied, removing as much fluid as possible. The catheter can also be inserted while suction is being applied, advancing the catheter until pericardial fluid is obtained. If there is concern as to the origin of the fluid, the fluid can be evaluated for clot formation and centrifuged in a microhematocrit tube. Chronic effusions rarely clot, frequently exhibit xanthochromia of the supernatant, and usually have a packed cell volume that differs from that of blood. The presence of clots and a packed cell volume comparable to blood is suggestive of active, acute pericardial hemorrhage and cannot be differentiated from a cardiac puncture by appearance.

The potential complications of pericardiocentesis include laceration of a coronary vessel, ventricular arrhythmias, and exacerbation of hemorrhage.[91] The risk of lacerating a coronary vessel can be reduced significantly by approaching the pericardial space from the right hemithorax. Ventricular arrhythmias are not uncommon and are due to contact of the needle with the myocardium. If arrhythmias are observed, the catheter should be retracted a short distance. The patient should also be monitored in the period following pericardiocentesis for cardiac arrhythmias attributable to reperfusion of previously ischemic myocardium. Hemorrhage into the pleural or pericardial cavity is an uncommon, albeit life-threatening, complication. Close monitoring of the animal's mucous membrane color, pulse rate and quality, hematocrit, and total plasma protein concentration can aid in the detection of life-threatening hemorrhage. If such a complication should arise, the attending clinician should be prepared to provide emergency treatment such as intravenous fluids or whole-blood transfusion and, potentially, resuscitative thoracotomy if the hemorrhage continues (see Chapter 10).

If the pericardial effusion is due to ongoing hemorrhage, there is risk of exacerbating the hemorrhage with pericardiocentesis and/or lacerating the pericardium resulting in exsanguination into the thoracic cavity. If the patient is stable and there is suspected active pericardial hemorrhage, it is recommended to monitor the patient carefully, delaying or completely avoiding pericardiocentesis. If pericardial hemorrhage secondary to trauma or congestive heart failure (ruptured left atrium) is suspected, pericardiocentesis should be avoided unless life-threatening tamponade is imminent. If pericardiocentesis must be performed, the attending clinician should be prepared for recurrence of cardiac tamponade or life-threatening hemorrhage into the thoracic cavity. If cardiac tamponade is not resulting from the pericardial hemorrhage and the patient is hemodynamically stable, pericardiocentesis can be avoided and the patient treated conservatively. Cage rest, frequent patient monitoring, and moderate expansion of the intravascular volume to maintain cardiac output and peripheral perfusion are often the only interventions indicated. Hemorrhage due to cardiac trauma or left atrial tear usually subsides as a fibrin clot forms over the rent. Pericardial hemorrhage can also occur secondary to coagulopathies, such as anticoagulant rodenticide intoxication. In these cases, vitamin K and replacement of clotting factors with fresh frozen plasma or whole-blood transfusion are indicated as adjunctive therapies.

The long-term prognosis for a patient with pericardial hemorrhage is good in successfully treated cases of anticoagulant rodenticide intoxication and trauma but guarded to poor if the underlying cause of the hemorrhage is left atrial rupture secondary to primary cardiac disease.

The pathophysiologic aspects of pericardial effusion limit the usefulness of medical treatments. The minimal lymphatic and venous drainage of the pericardium, as well as reactive inflammation of the pericardium, limit the benefit of diuretic administration in reducing the volume of most pericardial effusions. Pericardial effusion secondary to congestive heart failure and hypoproteinemia are exceptions to this generalization and these patients may benefit from diuretic administration. Overzealous use of diuretics can lead to the development of azotemia, hypotension, and weakness in the animal because of additional decreases in cardiac output. The administration of digitalis and other positive inotropes are usually not indicated, since most patients have normal myocardial function. Digitalis glycosides are indicated only if the animal demonstrates supraventricular tachycardias or myocardial failure accompanying the pericardial effusion. The administration of afterload- and preload-reducing agents (e.g., ACE inhibitors) should be avoided or used very cautiously, as these drugs cause vasodilation and aggravate hypotension, resulting in exacerbation of collapse and weakness in the animal.

If the patient is suspected of having idiopathic pericardial effusion, the effusion will resolve following one or two pericardiocenteses in approximately 50% of dogs.[77] Recurrences have been described within a few days or may require years to manifest. Intrapericardial and/or systemic administration of antiinflammatory agents have been recommended to limit recurrences.[90,92] However, there have been no controlled studies documenting benefit of this therapeutic approach. If the patient requires repeated pericardiocenteses, subtotal pericardectomy is recommended.

Surgical intervention is recommended following the first or second recurrence of the effusion in an animal. Surgical exploration of the chest following the initial diagnosis could be advocated, as this approach would allow early detection of small, potentially resectable masses not previously identified, avoid the potential for the development of acute cardiac tamponade, and provide the opportunity to biopsy the pericardium. Surgical treatment involves resection of the pericardium ventral to the phrenic nerve.[93] Partial pericardiectomy (pericardial window technique) has provided unsatisfactory results and is not recommended. Subtotal pericardiectomy has provided excellent results in dogs with idiopathic pericardial effusion, and most dogs remain asymptomatic following this treatment. Occasionally, hemorrhagic pleural effusions will develop in dogs, and these may require repeated thoracocentesis or surgical placement of pleuroperitoneal shunts.

If the cause of the pericardial effusion has been identified as a mass lesion, the patient can be treated with either repeated pericardiocentesis or surgical intervention. Pericardial cysts, abscesses, and some small neoplastic lesions can be resected. Hemangiosarcomas tend to be aggressive, incurable tumors, and surgical intervention is probably ineffective in improving survival.[94] Attempts to resect many right atrial hemangiosarcomas surgically has resulted in a high postoperative mortality rate. The potential for sudden hemorrhage in these cases precludes the routine use of pericardiectomy. There are anectodal reports of suturing the pericardium around the unresectable mass lesion with the goal of preventing tamponade and exsanguination. Heart-base tumors tend to be slow growing and less likely to metastasize; however, these tumors are usually unresectable due to the location and invasive nature of the mass. Nevertheless, pericardiectomy can alleviate the clinical signs of tamponade and the patient can remain comfortable for months to years.

Infectious pericardial disease with bacterial or fungal organisms should be treated with antimicrobial agents directed by culture and sensitivity testing. Placement of an indwelling pericardial catheter for several days allows pericardial drainage and lavage. Constrictive pericardial disease may eventually develop in animals with infectious pericarditis. Cats with FIP involving the pericardium have a poor prognosis.

Constrictive pericarditis. Constrictive pericarditis is an uncommon disease resulting from fibrosis and thickening of the pericardium.[95] The parietal and/or visceral pericardia may be involved. The development of constrictive pericarditis has been associated with the presence of penetrating foreign bodies, infection, and neoplasia as well as subsequent to chronic, idiopathic pericardial effusion. In most cases, however, the cause is not determined. Large-breed dogs generally older than 4 years tend to be the most commonly affected. In the cat, constrictive pericarditis is rare. Physical examination findings in patients with constrictive pericarditis include weakness, dyspnea, diminished arterial pulses, decreased heart sounds, ascites, and venous congestion.

The clinical signs of constrictive pericarditis, as with cardiac tamponade associated with pericardial effusion, are the result of impaired ventricular diastolic function. The most frequent historic complaints are abdominal distention, weakness, and dyspnea. Early diastolic filling is not impaired; however, once the limit of the noncompliant and fibrotic pericardium is reached, the ventricular pressure increases rapidly. When the ventricular pressure equals atrial pressure, cardiac filling ceases prematurely, leading to decreased stroke volume and cardiac output. In humans with constrictive pericarditis, the abrupt cessation of ventricular filling has been associated with a mid-diastolic "knock," an infrequent auscultatory finding in dogs. The x and y descent of the jugular pulse tend to be sharper, and pulsus paradoxus

is usually absent. Compensatory mechanisms evident in an attempt to improve the animal's cardiac output include increased heart rate and elevated atrial and venous filling pressure. Since the onset is usually gradual, right-sided heart failure (ascites, hepatomegaly, jugular vein distention) develops in most patients, and these patients rarely present with clinical signs of shock.

The findings on thoracic radiography are usually unremarkable, with occasional evidence of mild to moderate cardiomegaly, distention of the caudal vena cava, and pleural effusion. Electrocardiographic abnormalities include low-amplitude QRS complexes, supraventricular arrhythmias (supraventricular tachycardia, atrial fibrillation), and, most consistently, *p-mitrale* (width of P wave >0.04 msec).

Pericardial thickening and impaired left ventricular diastolic function are reported echocardiographic abnormalities in humans with constrictive pericardial disease.[96] However, echocardiographic examination has also been reported to be nondiagnostic in humans due to nonspecificity of the echocardiographic findings. There are no descriptions reported of the echocardiographic features of constrictive pericarditis in dogs and cats.

Cardiac catheterization is probably the best diagnostic tool, short of exploratory thoracotomy. Catheterization of the heart reveals equalization of end-diastolic pressures within the right atrium and ventricle, increased central venous pressure (often greater than 10 mm Hg), and decreased stroke volume.[96] The diagnosis of constrictive pericarditis is a difficult one to make, but should be suspected in patients with evidence of right-sided heart failure in the absence of radiographic and physical examination findings compatible with other forms of heart disease.

Constrictive pericarditis appears to be progressive in nature, usually responding poorly to conservative, medical management. Subtotal pericardiectomy is the treatment of choice if the disease is limited to the parietal pericardium, and this treatment often provides a favorable outcome. If the visceral pericardium becomes fibrotic and thickened, epicardial stripping is required. This procedure is associated with a high prevalence of complications, including intramyocardial hemorrhage and pulmonary thromboembolism. Medical therapy, such as exercise, diuretic administration, and salt restriction, may be used as adjuncts to surgical treatment in these instances; however, the prognosis is less favorable.

HEARTWORM DISEASE

Heartworm disease (HWD) is a common clinical problem in endemic regions, with an infection rate approaching 45% of the canine population in some areas.[97] Heartworm disease can be associated with numerous clinical manifestations. Most commonly, it presents as a chronic disorder of the heart and lungs. However, some of the consequences of HWD, such as pulmonary thromboembolism and caval syndrome, can be life threatening and present as acute, fulminating disorders.

Heartworm caval syndrome

Caval syndrome is an acute life-threatening complication of HWD, characterized by hemolytic anemia, impaired hemodynamics, and multisystem dysfunction.[98] The syndrome occurs in 16% to 20% of dogs with HWD, commonly manifesting itself in the spring or early summer, and is associated with a high mortality rate.[99] As with uncomplicated HWD, the frequency is related to geographic factors and nonuse of prophylactic therapy. The predisposing factors for HWD also apply to caval syndrome as evidenced by the common signalment: large, male, sporting breed dogs, 1.5 to 10 years of age. Seventy-five percent to 90% of animals with caval syndrome are male. It is suggested that either male dogs have a facilitating factor or females possess a protective factor. Caval syndrome has been reported in cats,[100] albeit rarely.

Pathophysiology. Caval syndrome is characterized by a heavy infestation of *Dirofilaria immitis,* often with adult worm burdens greater than 60 per dog. Fifty-five percent to 84% of the worm burden is located in the venae cavae and right atrium.[97,98] Retrograde migration of adult worms into the right atrium and venae cavae can occur 5 to 17 months after infection. This produces a partial inflow obstruction and tricuspid insufficiency due to mechanical interference with valve function. Tricuspid insufficiency is worsened by the pulmonary hypertension associated with chronic HWD. These factors contribute to decreasing the left ventricular preload, resulting in impaired left ventricular filling and cardiac output. Occasionally, arrhythmias can occur and further compromise cardiac function and impair tissue perfusion. Death is usually due to cardiogenic shock, often within the first 24 to 72 hours following onset of clinical signs.

The pathogenesis of caval syndrome in dogs is not entirely understood. The development of clinical signs of caval syndrome cannot be attributed simply to the total worm burden or worms per kilogram of body weight.[99] In dogs with similar worm burdens, those with caval syndrome had significantly higher pulmonary arterial blood pressure.[98] The marked elevations in pulmonary arterial blood pressures in these animals is not com-

pletely understood; however, it appears to be a significant contributing factor to the pathogenesis of caval syndrome and associated clinical signs.

The clinical picture of caval syndrome often involves hemolysis, hepatic and renal dysfunction, and disseminated intravascular coagulation (DIC).[97-99,101] Hemolytic anemia occurs as a result of erythrocyte trauma associated with the passage of these red blood cells through a "sieve of adult heartworms" in the right atrium and venae cavae as well as fibrin strands within capillary beds associated with DIC (microangiopathic anemia). Intravascular hemolysis, in addition to causing anemia, produces hemoglobinuria and hemoglobinemia. Hemoglobinemia may be a contributing factor in the development of hepatorenal dysfunction; however, the cause of these manifestations is unclear, with passive congestion secondary to right heart failure, DIC, and hypoperfusion representing possible contributing factors. Hepatomegaly, cavernous dilation of hepatic vessels, venous thrombosis, centrilobular necrosis, and fibrosis are common pathologic features associated with hepatic dysfunction.[102] The kidneys demonstrate histopathologic changes compatible with pigment nephropathy such as tubular necrosis, hemoglobin casts, and hemosiderosis. Impaired hepatic function results in decreased removal of procoagulants from the circulation, and this occurrence coupled with intravascular hemolysis contributes to the development of DIC.

Diagnosis. Animals with caval syndrome usually present acutely anorectic, depressed, and weak. Occasionally, clients complain that their animals are demonstrating dyspnea, coughing, and, less often, hemoptysis. Physical examination shows low cardiac output (weakness, prolonged capillary refill time) and right-sided heart failure (jugular-vein distention, jugular pulsation). Increased intensity of lung sounds and a right apical systolic murmur of tricuspid insufficiency are commonly auscultated. Hepatosplenomegaly, a loud split second heart sound and/or gallop, ascites, and jaundice are common clinical findings in the animal with caval syndrome.

The initial data base in an animal with suspected caval syndrome should entail a complete blood count, serum biochemical profile, urinalysis, coagulation screen, and complete cardiovascular evaluation. Hemoglobinemia and microfilaremia are hallmark findings, occurring in approximately 85% of dogs with caval syndrome. A complete blood count often reveals moderate anemia, usually regenerative, with nucleated erythrocytes, target cells, and red blood cell fragments (schistocytes, spherocytes, spur cells). A leukocytosis with neutrophilia, eosinophilia, and a variable left shift is often present. Disseminated intravascular coagulation is evidenced by decreased platelet numbers, decreased fibrinogen concentration, and increases in other coagulation parameters, such as fibrin degradation products, one-stage prothrombin time, activated partial thromboplastin time, and activated clotting time. Moderate increases in serum liver enzyme activities, including aspartate aminotransferase, alanine aminotransferase, and lactic dehydrogenase; elevated blood urea nitrogen concentration with a normal serum creatinine concentration; and hyperbilirubinemia are common findings on serum biochemical analysis. Hypoalbuminemia with hyperglobulinemia (increased alpha- and gamma-globulins) occurs routinely in animals with caval syndrome. Urinalysis reveals hemoglobinuria in over 50% of patients.[101]

Electrocardiographic evaluation occasionally reveals evidence of right-sided heart disease, such as deviation of the mean electrical axis to the right (average, + 129) and deep S waves in V_5 (S >0.8 mV). Less commonly, sinus tachycardia and premature atrial and ventricular complexes will be present.[101]

Tortuous pulmonary arteries, an enlarged main pulmonary artery segment, right atrial enlargement, and distention of the caudal vena cava are routinely visualized with thoracic radiography. Occasionally, there is evidence of right ventricular enlargement and pleural effusion.[103]

Central venous pressure is increased in 80% to 90% of patients and should be routinely measured and monitored through the course of therapy. Although rarely used, cardiac catheterization routinely demonstrates increased pulmonary artery, right atrial, and right ventricular pressures and impaired cardiac output.

Echocardiographic evidence of massive right atrial worm infestation that is observed to move into the right ventricle during diastole is pathognomonic for caval syndrome. Echocardiographic abnormalities can include enlargement of the right ventricular lumen and paradoxical septal motion due to increased right ventricular volume and pressure.[104] Left ventricular function is usually normal, but the diastolic diameter of the left ventricle is often decreased as a result of pulmonary hypertension, causing decreased left ventricular preload.

Management. The complex pathophysiologic derangements with caval syndrome require intensive management and careful monitoring. The prognosis for survival is poor if removal of the adult heartworms from the venae cavae and right atrium is not undertaken. Even with successful removal of the worms, the mortality rate in animals with caval syndrome can approach 40%.[97,101] The extent of the effect of the caval syndrome on vital organ function and the severity of cardiac involvement must be established rapidly in these affected animals. Central venous pressure should be measured to assess the degree of heart failure as well as to monitor the administration of intravenous fluid therapy. Arterial and venous blood gases are useful in assessing hypoperfusion of tissues (decreased pH and bicarbonate due to lactic acidosis, decreased Pvo_2 from increased oxygen extraction) and monitoring for the development of pulmonary thromboembolism.

Intravenous fluid administration is beneficial in improving cardiac output and tissue perfusion. The administration of fluid therapy improves renal blood flow, decreases the potential for pigment nephropathy secondary to hemoglobinemia, and limits the development of DIC by correcting metabolic acidosis and preventing capillary sludging of blood. Intravenous fluids must be administered judiciously, since intravenous fluid overload will exacerbate congestive heart failure. Ideally, an indwelling jugular catheter should be placed to permit CVP measurements and should be placed in a manner so as not to interfere with removal of the adult heartworms (i.e., not into the right atrium). The rate of fluid administration depends on the animal's hemodynamic status. If the patient appears to be hemodynamically compromised, fluids should be administered as rapidly as possible without increasing the CVP to greater than 10 to 15 cm H_2O. If the CVP is normal (-3 to 5 cm H_2O), intravenous fluids can be administered aggressively at rates as high as 60 to 90 ml/kg per hour (shock dose). Administration of whole blood and blood products are rarely needed for the treatment of the anemia and hypoproteinemia associated with caval syndrome.

When the blood pH decreases to less than 7.2, endogenous buffer systems inadequately compensate. The dosage of sodium bicarbonate to be administered can be calculated from the base excess multiplied by body weight in kilograms times 0.3 or empirically administered at 1 mEq/kg intravenously (see Chapters 21 and 38). If the calculated dose is based on blood gas analysis, half of the determined dose is administered slowly intravenously as a bolus, then the remainder is administered over the next 6 to 12 hours with the intravenous fluids.

Strict cage rest is imperative to minimize the workload on the heart, prevent onset or exacerbation of heart failure, and minimize complications. Appropriate therapy is indicated if hemodynamics and cardiac output are impaired by sepsis and endotoxemia or cardiac arrhythmias. Since myocardial function is not impaired, digitalis administration is rarely, if ever, indicated.

Aspirin administration has been shown to improve survival in animals with congestive heart failure and severe pulmonary arteritis complicating HWD, therefore this treatment should be routinely used in the treatment of the animal with caval syndrome.[105] Aspirin administration decreases platelet adhesiveness and release of platelet-derived growth factors, thereby decreasing myointimal proliferation of the pulmonary arteries, even in face of persistent dirofilariasis. Pulmonary blood flow is improved, as is left ventricular filling and the prevalence of thromboembolic complications, and DIC is decreased as a result of aspirin administration.

Surgical removal of the adult heartworms (worm embolectomy) should be performed as soon as is practical.[106] The patient is placed in left lateral recumbency using mild sedation and local anesthesia. The ventral cervical region is clipped and aseptically cleansed. The right jugular vein is surgically isolated and ligated cranially. Straight alligator forceps (20 to 40 cm in length) are inserted into the jugular vein through a small incision made caudal to the ligature. The forceps are carefully guided down the vein to the level of the fourth or fifth intercostal space. Occasionally, difficulty is encountered as the forceps pass through the thoracic inlet. This problem is resolved by gentle manipulation and extension of the patient's neck by an assistant. The forceps may need to be directed medially at the base of the heart. Once positioned, the jaws of the forceps are opened and closed to grasp the worms, and then retracted out of the vein. The procedure is repeated until five or six successive attempts fail to produce worms. After completion, the jugular vein is ligated and the incision closed routinely. In addition to straight alligator forceps, flexible alligator forceps[107] and endoscopic baskets have been used for worm retrieval.

Following worm removal, the animal's CVP usually decreases by 40%, as does the intensity of the murmur and the jugular pulses. Hemoglobinemia and hemoglobinuria rapidly clear, biochemical aberrations normalize over a short period, and as long as 2 to 4 weeks may be required for the anemia to resolve sufficiently. Immediate and gradual continued improvement in hemodynamics can be expected over the next 24 hours. However, worm removal does not improve right ventricular afterload because pulmonary vascular resistance is unaffected. Therefore, right-sided heart failure is still possible, and continued fluid administration should be monitored. After the animal has been stabilized for 2 or 3 weeks therapy to

kill adult worms (adulticide) can be instituted. However, blood urea nitrogen concentrations and serum liver enzyme activity should be carefully monitored. During this period, strict cage rest and aspirin therapy should be continued unless significant complications related to aspirin therapy are encountered. In general, the prognosis for patients with caval syndrome is guarded to poor. Despite successful worm embolectomy, 15% to 40% of patients die.[97,99,101] If hypothermia, DIC, or CVP measurements greater than 20 cm H_2O are present, the prognosis is grave.

Pulmonary thromboembolism

Pulmonary thromboembolism can occur naturally or secondary to adulticide therapy in animals with HWD. Pulmonary thromboembolism is the most common and potentially life-threatening complication of adulticide therapy in dogs.[108] Dead and/or dying adults cause regional pulmonary artery thrombosis, complicated by severe vascular endothelial damage, inflammation, and edema of the pulmonary interstitium and alveoli associated with HWD. Most clinical signs and deaths due to complications of adulticide heartworm therapy usually occur 5 to 21 days after treatment.[99,109] Severe, life-threatening pulmonary thromboembolism should not be unexpected if the animal's routine data base and radiographs have been adequately assessed.

The pathophysiologic effects of pulmonary thromboembolism include ventilation-perfusion mismatching and exacerbation of pulmonary hypertension with progressive increases in right ventricular afterload. Acute pulmonary thromboembolism can result in morbidity or fatalities due to fulminating heart failure, exsanguination, or DIC.

The most common clinical signs in animals with HWD and pulmonary thromboembolism include lethargy, weakness, anorexia, fever, and cough. Occasionally, hemoptysis or other overt evidence of bleeding is noted. Physical examination of the animal usually reveals an elevated body temperature, tachycardia, and abnormal lung sounds. Evidence of right-sided heart failure (jugular-vein distention and pulses, ascites) and hemorrhage (pale mucous membranes) may be present.

Radiographic evidence of severely enlarged, tortuous pulmonary arteries and preexisting pulmonary thromboembolism appears to be associated with an increased risk of thromboembolic complications following adulticide therapy.[97] Radiographic changes associated with pulmonary thromboembolism are variable. The caudal and accessory lung lobes are the most commonly affected. Periarterial granulomas may be visualized as poorly defined, coalescing interstitial and alveolar infiltrates near the affected vessels.

Nonregenerative anemia and neutrophilic leukocytosis with eosinophilia and basophilia are common abnormalities detected on a complete blood count in animals with HWD and pulmonary thromboembolism. The presence of thrombocytopenia suggests concomitant DIC. Prerenal azotemia and moderate serum liver enzyme elevations are frequently noted abnormalities of serum biochemical analysis.

If the patient's clinical signs are mild, conservative therapy with strict cage rest accompanying aspirin (0.5 mg/kg orally twice a day to 5 mg/kg orally once a day) and corticosteroid (prednisone 1 to 2 mg/kg orally once a day) administration is indicated. If severe dyspnea, cough, and hemoptysis are present, the patient should be hospitalized. In addition to strict cage rest and corticosteroid treatment, supplemental oxygen, heparin (50 to 100 IU/kg subcutaneously three or four times a day), and possibly bronchodilators (e.g., aminophylline, 4 to 6 mg/kg orally or intravenously three times a day) should be administered. If hemoptysis or DIC is present or if the animal's platelet count is less than 50,000/μl, aspirin therapy should be discontinued. The animal usually exhibits marked improvement within 1 to 2 days after initiation of therapy.

FELINE ARTERIAL THROMBOEMBOLISM

Arterial thromboembolism is a frequently recognized clinical problem in cats and is a common complication of myocardial disease. The majority of cats diagnosed with arterial thromboembolism also have an underlying cardiomyopathy, with the reported prevalence as high as 50% in cats with hypertrophic cardiomyopathy.[110] The thrombus commonly arises in the dilated left atrium; however, it may arise from the left ventricle or, on rare occasion, in the right side of the heart. Some cats have no detectable underlying cardiac disease; however, absence of an underlying cause such as cardiomyopathy, bacterial endocarditis, excessive left ventricular moderator bands, or neoplasia is uncommon.[111]

Pathophysiology

The pathophysiologic factors that predispose to thrombus formation are endothelial injury, altered blood flow, and altered coagulation.[112] Trauma induced by turbulence of the blood flow within the left ventricle and "jet lesions" in the left atria due to mitral insufficiency expose the vascular subendothelium, thereby activating the intrinsic coagulation cascade. There are variable degrees of endothelial inflammation associated with feline cardiomyopathies, and endocardial fibrosis may also affect the atrial and ventricular endocardial surfaces.[113] Stasis and abnormal flow of blood, as is present in dilated cardiac chambers, promote platelet aggregation and adhesion with subsequent activation of the intrinsic clotting pathways.[112] Alterations in intracavitary blood flow can also result secondary to left ventricular outflow obstruction (e.g., hypertrophic cardiomyopathy). The presence of excessive moderator bands may alter ventricular architecture, creating turbulence of blood. The cat appears to have a greater platelet number relative to body size as compared with other species as well as an increased platelet reactivity and serotonin concentration.[114] Disseminated intravascular coagulation, due to consumptive coagulopathies, liver-mediated coagulopathy, or the effects of thromboembolism, is often present in cats with cardiomyopathy and, if present, further contributes to hypercoagulability.

The physical presence of an arterial obstruction is not sufficient to produce the clinical signs associated with arterial thromboembolism in cats. Experimental studies obstructing the distal aorta of cats with ligatures have failed to produce clinical signs due to the persistence of collateral circulation.[115] However, if a thrombus is produced at the site of occlusion, collateral blood flow becomes impaired.[116] Vasoactive substances, including serotonin and prostaglandins, are presumed to be released from activated platelets, resulting in vasoconstriction of collateral vasculature. Experimentally, administration of serotonin antagonists[117] or inhibitors of prostaglandin synthesis[118] have been shown to prevent collateral vasoconstriction.

Diagnosis

The clinical signs of arterial thromboembolism are dependent on the tissue affected and the degree of ischemic injury. The terminal aorta (aortic trifurcation) and forelimb vessels are the most common sites in which an embolus can lodge, and this condition is easily recognized clinically. However, the occlusion of vessels of the heart, kidney, brain, or gastrointestinal tract with smaller emboli can be more difficult to diagnose. Clinical signs of thromboembolism are associated with abrupt occlusion of blood flow and ischemic injury to the tissues distal to the occlusion. Occlusion of the distal aorta is associated with acute onset of hindlimb paresis, pain, absence of femoral pulses, and cold, firm musculature. The nailbeds are often cyanotic and do not bleed when cut. Microemboli causing intermittent claudication often appear clinically insignificant; however, these occurrences may often precede extensive thromboembolism. Ischemic neuropathy and myopathy result in hyporeflexia or areflexia, absence of pain sensation, flaccid paralysis, and with partial, microembolization, mild deficits such as dropped hocks and hindlimb ataxia. The clinical signs of thromboembolization to the forelimbs or hindlimbs can be unilateral or bilateral. Signs referable to acute oliguric or anuric renal failure will develop if the renal arteries are occluded. Embolization of the gastrointestinal tract can produce mild signs, including diarrhea and vomiting, or severe problems attributable to intestinal necrosis and perforation.

The majority of cats presenting with arterial thromboembolism will have clinical signs associated with an underlying cardiomyopathy, often decompensated.[119] Murmurs, gallop rhythms, arrhythmias, and tachypnea are common findings on physical examination of these animals. There may be evidence of congestive heart failure, including jugular-vein distention, muffled heart sounds due to pleural effusion, and, less commonly, pulmonary edema.

Routine laboratory evaluation of cats with thromboembolism usually reveals nonspecific changes. Nonregenerative anemia and a neutrophilic leukocytosis compatible with a stress response are common hematologic findings. Elevations in serum creatine kinase, aspartate aminotransferase, and alanine aminotransferase activities and blood glucose concentration may also be noted. Hyperkalemia often develops secondary to reperfusion of the ischemic tissue or impaired renal perfusion. Impaired renal blood flow, whether due to occlusion of renal arteries or poor cardiac output, also results in azotemia. Metabolic acidosis, usually due to lactic acid, results from reperfusion of ischemic regions or poor perfusion of tissues secondary to cardiac disease.

Thoracic radiography, electrocardiography, and echocardiography are indicated to determine and define the underlying cause of the arterial thromboembolism. If bacterial endocarditis is suspected, blood cultures should be obtained. An activated clotting time or complete coagulation screen is helpful in detecting DIC as a predisposing or complicating factor in these cats, as well as providing base-line data prior to institution of anticoagulant therapy.

Nonselective contrast angiography is a useful diagnostic tool for evaluating an underlying cardiomyopathy, determining the anatomic extent of the embolus, and assessing collateral blood flow. Angiographic evaluations performed in cats with aortic thromboembolism and treated for heart failure, demonstrated evidence of collateral flow in 60% of the afflicted cats at 24 hours and 70% after 5 days. Angiograms are especially useful in the detection of renal artery occlusion, since rapid clinical recognition of this occurrence is often difficult. Regional blood flow can also be determined using Doppler ultrasound techniques and nuclear tracers.[120] Imaging of the affected regional vasculature by one of these methods permits definitive diagnostic evaluation. Nevertheless, the patient must be the primary consideration, and the patient should be adequately stabilized prior to attempting invasive diagnostic procedures.

Medical treatment

If left untreated, the outcome of arterial thromboembolism depends on the extent of the occlusion, the affected organ systems, and time to reperfusion.[111] Affected limbs may be lost due to ischemic necrosis, these limbs may remain paralyzed due to peripheral nerve and muscle damage, or some degree of function may return. The patient may die from toxemia or septicemia associated with necrosis of a limb or from complications related to reperfusion injury. Overall, the response to currently employed therapies, both medical and surgical, has been poor.

The stress of embolization can lead to severe cardiac decompensation in cats with cardiomyopathy. Pulmonary edema, hypothermia, and shock may be present, indicating a need for oxygen therapy, judicious fluid and diuretic administration, and application of external warmth. Pain secondary to the ischemic neuromyopathy can be alleviated by administration of morphine (0.1 mg/kg subcutaneously every 4 hours) and by minimizing patient manipulation and muscle palpation.

Short-term management of arterial occlusion is directed at preventing propagation of the thromboembolus and promoting collateral circulation. Medical therapy in cats with thromboembolic disease consists of administration of vasodilators, anticoagulants, and thrombolytics. Acepromazine (0.2 to 0.4 mg/kg subcutaneously three times a day) and hydralazine (0.5 to 0.8 mg/kg orally three times a day) have been administered in attempt to promote collateral blood flow (Table 17–9). Acepromazine promotes arteriolar vasodilation through alpha-adrenergic antagonism, and the drug also provides some sedation for the patient. Hydralazine is a direct-acting arterial smooth-muscle relaxant. Although some cats have shown improvement following administration of vasodilator therapy, the clinical efficacy of these agents remains to be proven. Calcium-channel blockers such as verapamil or diltiazem may have a role in

Table 17-9 Pharmacologic therapy of feline arterial thromboembolism

Anticoagulants	
Heparin	50-75U/kg SQ tid/qid
Coumadin	0.1 mg/kg po sid
Aspirin	1.25 grains po every 3 days
Vasodilators	
Hydralazine	0.5-0.8 mg/kg po tid
Acepromazine	0.2-0.4 mg/kg SQ tid
Analgesics	
Morphine	0.1 mg/kg SQ every 4-6 hours
Butorphanol	0.1-0.2 mg/kg IM/SQ every 4-6 hours
Thrombolytics	
Streptokinase	90,000 IU over 20-30 minutes, then 45,000 IU per hour × 3 hours
Tissue plasminogen activator	1-10 mg/kg IV at 0.25-1 mg/kg per hour

SQ = subcutaneously; tid = three times a day; qid = four times a day; po = orally; sid = once a day; IM = intramuscularly; IV = intravenously.

the therapy of feline[111,121] arterial thromboembolism (Table 17-7). Calcium-channel blockers produce vasodilation by inhibiting the calcium-dependent contraction of vascular smooth muscle. However, the most beneficial effect of the administration of calcium-channel blockers may be inhibition of platelet aggregation. Inhibition of calcium uptake by activated platelets prevents the release of vasoactive and platelet-aggregating factors.[121] Calcium-channel blockers, which promote vasodilation, decrease platelet aggregation, and have potentially beneficial cardiac effects, warrant further investigation.

Anticoagulant administration is useful in preventing propagation of the initial thromboembolus and in reducing formation of new thrombi; however, these drugs are ineffective in causing clot lysis.[111] Heparin and warfarin are often used in the initial treatment of cats with arterial thromboembolism. Heparin administration may prevent embolus enlargement by inhibiting further clot formation. Minimizing clot mass may assist in the maintenance of collateral circulation. The patient should be monitored for evidence of spontaneous hemorrhage by serial evaluation of hematocrit and total plasma protein concentration, heart rate, mucous membrane color, and capillary refill time. Anticoagulant therapy is adjusted as needed to maintain an activated clotting time or prothrombin time to 1.25 to 2 times the base-line level.

Aspirin administration may be of benefit prophylactically and as a treatment following a thromboembolic event. When administered prior to experimental aortic obstruction, collateral circulation was promoted.[116] Aspirin alters platelet function and reduces aggregation by irreversibly inhibiting thromboxane A_2 synthesis. Thromboxane A_2 promotes vasoconstriction and platelet aggregation by release of ADP. Aspirin administration following a thromboembolic event may serve to minimize clot formation and to blunt the vasoconstrictive response of the collateral vasculature attributed in part to thromboxane A_2. However, aspirin administration also inhibits vascular endothelial prostacyclin synthesis.[122] Prostacyclin inhibits platelet aggregation and promotes vasodilation. Dosage of aspirin that selectively inhibits thromboxane A_2 production yet spares prostacyclin synthesis has not been demonstrated. These conflicting actions may contribute to the failure of aspirin therapy to prevent thrombus formation.

Thrombolytic therapy represents a new and promising method for resolution of arterial thromboembolism. Early clinical trials in cats have demonstrated promising results[123,124]; however, these therapies are not without certain risks. In a normal physiologic state, as intravascular thrombi occur and hemostatic processes are activated, naturally occurring thrombolytic agents are activated. This fibrinolytic system is comprised of plasminogen and plasminogen activators and inhibitors. Plasminogen activators catalyze the conversion of plasminogen to plasmin, which in turn hydrolyzes fibrin and fibrinogen. The result is limitation or dissolution of existing thrombi and prevention of additional thrombus formation.

Plasminogen activators used in fibrinolytic therapy are urokinase, streptokinase, and tissue plasminogen activator (t-PA). These agents require adequate circulating quantities of plasminogen to be effective. The conventional activators (urokinase and streptokinase) have minimal affinity for fibrin, thereby activating circulating and fibrin-bound plasminogen indiscriminately. A systemic fibrinolytic state is produced, due to the activation of circulating plasminogen, formation of fibrin degradation products, and degradation of coagulation factors, predisposing the patient to spontaneous hemorrhage. Unfortunately, the adverse and desired effects cannot be dissociated, presenting a substantial risk for the patient. There have been attempts to infuse these nonselective plasminogen activators locally (intraarterially) in human patients with acute myocardial infarction, at doses below those associated with systemic fibrinolysis.

Newer fibrinolytic agents, particularly t-PA, may present fewer risks to the patient. Tissue plasminogen activator is an intrinsic protein present in all mammals. Recombinant DNA techniques and recent approval by the Food and Drug Administration have made its use possible, despite significant expense. There are numerous reports of treatment with t-PA of humans with acute myocardial infarcts, pulmonary thromboembolism, and peripheral occlusive vascular disease.[125,126] Tissue plasminogen activator has been shown to have a lower affinity for circulating plasminogen as compared with its affinity for fibrin-bound plasminogen. Like plasminogen, t-PA has a high affinity for fibrin within a clot, and the two proteins appear to bind in close proximity, potentiating the conversion of plasminogen catalyzed by t-PA at the primary target site. The potential for systemic fibrinolysis is minimized at dosages administered effective for thrombolysis.

In cats, a shortened time to reperfusion and ambulation has been demonstrated in clinical trials with administration of 0.25 to 1.0 mg/kg of t-PA per hour for a total of 1 to 10 mg/kg intravenously.[124] Of the cats that survived therapy, all were walking within 48 hours. Unfortunately, many others died as a result of acidosis and hyperkalemia associated with reperfusion.

For thrombolytic therapy to be maximally effective it should be administered within 6 hours of vascular occlusion.[127] In humans, another factor affecting thrombolysis is the location of the thrombus. Thrombi that are located in small vessels or that completely occlude a vessel are difficult to lyse.

In addition to the potential for producing a systemic fibrinolytic state, administration of thrombolytic therapy is associated with additional complications that accompany reperfusion of ischemic tissues. Reperfusion injury occurs when blood flow and oxygen supply is returned to ischemic tissues. During the hypoxic episode, the tissue depletes its adenosine triphosphate (ATP) stores and depends on anaerobic metabolism, producing lactic acid. The depletion of and inability to re-form ATP results in accumulation of degradation products such as hypoxanthine. On reperfusion of the tissues, hypoxanthine is converted to xanthine in the presence of oxygen, leading to the formation of toxic oxygen radicals and subsequently to cellular damage. Death due to acute reperfusion is presumed to be related to the release of metabolic toxins into the systemic circulation.

The optimal dosage of thrombolytic agents has not been determined in the cat, and approximately 30% to 50% of patients will have return of nearly normal function after 6 weeks of aspirin therapy alone. These factors, as well as the risks and costs associated with the administration of plasminogen activators, have raised questions about the benefit to the patient of early reperfusion.

Surgical intervention

Surgical embolectomy has not been associated with a positive outcome in many cats with arterial thromboembolism, probably due in part to delayed intervention. The presence of cardiac arrhythmias, DIC, congestive heart failure, and other physiologic derangements result in a patient that is a poor anesthetic risk. Many patients present for treatment after the ischemic neuromyopathy has become advanced. Nevertheless, early surgical intervention may provide a rapid return to function as well as spare the patient's life in the instance of occlusion of the renal arteries.

Surgical removal of a distal aortic thromboembolus involves approaching the caudal abdominal aorta via a ventral abdominal incision.[128] The area of the aortic trifurcation is isolated and the aorta, internal and external iliac arteries, and the sacral artery are temporarily occluded. A longitudinal incision is then made into the aorta over the thrombus, using fine forceps to remove the clot. The ligatures are briefly loosened, flushing the site of residual clots through the arteriotomy. If the renal or mesenteric arteries are involved, the thrombus is milked toward the incision. The arteriotomy is closed with 5-0 nonabsorbable suture material and the abdomen closed routinely. This procedure has been abandoned for the treatment of human patients with thromboembolic disease because of a mortality rate approaching 50% attributed to the stress of anesthesia on an already compromised cardiovascular system.[129] Similar results have been recorded in feline patients.

The current method of embolectomy in humans involves the use of Fogarty catheters (Fogarty Arterial Embolectomy Catheter, American Hospital Supply) introduced through a femoral arteriotomy.[130] Using moderate sedation and local anesthesia, the deflated balloon at the catheter tip is passed through and proximal to the thrombus. The balloon is inflated and the catheter pulled distally, dislodging the obstruction. The thrombus is removed through the arteriotomy with fine forceps and the ligatures briefly loosened to permit flushing of residual clots through the arteriotomy. Continued medical management to prevent recurrence is recommended postoperatively. In humans, complications unrelated to anesthesia have been reported in embolectomized patients, and the mortality rate appears to be 10% to 25%. Unfortunately, surgery must be performed in tissue that is devoid of blood supply, increasing the likelihood of infection and poor wound healing.

Reperfusion injury

The reperfusion of ischemic tissue, as occurs with the administration of plasminogen activators or surgical embolectomy, results in mobilization of sequestered toxic metabolites, including potassium and lactic acid. Activated clotting factors and other thrombi that have formed in the veins of the ischemic limb are also released into the circulation, predisposing to pulmonary thromboembolism. After restoration of blood flow, myoglobinuria and myoglobinemia have been observed, which can lead to acute renal failure attributable to pigment nephropathy. In human patients with rigor and cyanosis of the affected limbs, the development of complications associated with medical or surgical embolectomy are common, with an associated mortality rate approaching 81%. Unfortunately, these features characterize many occurrences of arterial thromboembolism in cats and additional investigations are definitely required.

Prognosis

The most important factor in predicting outcome is the patient's underlying cardiac disease. Cats that develop arterial thromboemboli often die during the crisis due to the additional stresses placed on an already compromised heart. Ischemia sufficient to cause gangrenous necrosis also indicates a poor prognosis. Cats surviving the initial thromboembolic event have a guarded prognosis due to their underlying cardiomyopathy.

The time from onset of clinical signs to presentation can be a factor if thrombolytic agents or embolectomy are to be employed. The effects on the clot size appear to be maximized and the risk of complications appear to be minimized if these treatments are applied early in the course of the disease. These treatment methods are ideally used within 6 hours of the thromboembolic episode.

With successful and uncomplicated management, motor function will gradually return to the affected limbs over 2 to 4 weeks, while proprioceptive deficits may persist for months.[131] Nevertheless, successful treatment of the thromboembolism and appropriate management of the cardiomyopathy does not necessarily prevent recurrence, which may be seen in up to 90% of cats surviving the first episode of thromboembolism.

REFERENCES

1. Calvin JE, Sibbald WJ. Applied cardiovascular physiology in the critically ill with special reference to diastole and ventricular interaction. In Shoemaker WC, Ayres S, et al., eds. Textbook of critical care medicine. Philadelphia: WB Saunders, 1989;312-325.
2. Milnor WR. Cardiac dynamics. In Hemodynamics. Baltimore: Williams & Wilkins, 1982;244-271.
3. Weber K, Janicki JS, et al. The contractile behavior of the heart and its functional coupling to the circulation. Prog Cardiovasc Dis 1982;24:375.
4. Francis GS. Neuroendocrine manifestations of congestive heart failure. Am J Cardiol 1988;62:9.
5. Uretsky BF, Verbalis JG, et al. Control of atrial natriuretic peptide secretion in patients with severe congestive heart failure. J Clin Endocrinol Metab 1990;71:146.
6. Cody RJ, Atlas SA, et al. Atrial natriuretic factor in normal subjects and heart failure patients. J Clin Invest 1986;78:1362.
7. Ware WW, Lund DD, et al. Sympathetic activation in dogs with congestive heart failure caused by chronic mitral valve disease and dilated cardiomyopathy. J Am Vet Med Assoc 1990;197:1475.
8. Ayers CR, Bowden RE, Schrank JP. Mechanisms of sodium retention in congestive heart failure. Adv Exp Med Biol 1972;17:227.
9. Knowlen GG, Kittleson MD. Captopril therapy in dogs with heart failure. In: Kirk RW, ed. Current veterinary therapy IX. Philadelphia: WB Saunders, 1986; 334-339.
10. Kittleson MD. Management of heart failure: concepts, strategies, and drug pharmacology. In Fox PR, ed. Canine and feline cardiology. New York: Churchill Livingstone, 1988;171-204.
11. Rubin GJ. Chronic atrial-ventricular valvular insufficiency. Proc Acad Vet Cardiol 1991;2:49-55.
12. Kittleson MD, Pion PD, et al. Dilated cardiomyopathy in American cocker spaniels: taurine deficiency and preliminary results of response to supplementation [abstract]. Proc Am Coll Vet Intern Med 1991;9:879.
13. Ware WA, Bonagura JD. Canine myocardial disease. In Kirk RW, ed. Current Veterinary Therapy IX. Philadelphia: WB Saunders, 1986;370-380
14. Calvert CA, Chapman WL, Toal RL. Congestive cardiomyopathy in Doberman pinscher dogs. J Am Vet Med Assoc 1982;181:598.
15. Calvert CA. Dilated cardiomyopathy in Doberman pinschers. Compend Contin Educ Pract Vet 1986;8:417.
16. Atkins CE, Snyder PS. Feline cardiovascular disease: Epidemiology, pathophysiology, and therapy. Proc Am Coll Vet Intern Med 1991;9:215-221.
17. Pion PD, Kittleson MD, et al. Myocardial failure in cats associated with low plasma taurine: a reversible cardiomyopathy. Science 1987;237:764.
18. Grossman W, Barry WH. Diastolic pressure-volume relationship in the diseased heart. Fed Proc 1980;39:18.
19. Brater DC, Chennavasin P, Dehner GJ. Prolonged hemodynamic effect of furosemide in congestive heart failure. Am Heart J 1985;108:1031.
20. Dikshit K, Vyden JK, et al. Renal and extrarenal effects of furosemide in congestive heart failure after acute myocardial infarction. N Engl J Med 1973;288:1087.
21. Bonagura JD, Muir WW. Vasodilator therapy. In Kirk RW, ed. Current Veterinary Therapy IX. Philadelphia: WB Saunders, 1986;329-333.
22. Miller RR, Fennell WH, et al. Differential systemic arterial and venous actions and consequent cardiac effects of vasodilator drugs. Prog Cardiovasc Dis 1982;24:353.
23. Barron JT, Parrillo JE. Congestive heart failure: Vasodilator therapy. In Parillo JE, ed. Current Therapy in Critical Care Medicine. Philadelphia: BC Decker, 1991;87-92.
24. Kostis JB. Angiotensin converting enzyme inhibitors, Part II: Clinical use. Am Heart J 1988;116:1591.
25. Benitz AM, Hamlin RL, Ericsson GF. Titration of enalapril dose for dogs with induced heart failure [abstract]. Proc Am Coll Vet Intern Med 1991;9:879.
26. The CONSENSUS Trial Study Group. Effects of enalapril on mortality in severe congestive heart failure: Results of the Cooperative North Scandinavian Enalapril Survival Study (CONSENSUS). N Engl J Med 1987;316:1429.

27. Mason DT, ed. Symposium on vasodilator and inotropic therapy of heart failure. Am J Med 1978;65:101.

28. Kittleson MD, Eyster GE, et al. Oral hydralazine therapy for chronic mitral regurgitation in the dog. J Am Vet Med Assoc 1983;182:1205.

29. Kittleson MD, Johnson LE, Oliver NB. Acute hemodynamic effects of hydralazine in dogs with chronic mitral regurgitation. J Am Vet Med Assoc 1985;187:258.

30. Rush JE. Emergency therapy of heart failure. Proc Am Coll Vet Intern Med 1991;9:223-226.

31. Vismara LA, Leaman DM, Zelis R. Effects of morphine on venous tone in patients with acute pulmonary edema. Circulation 1976;54:335.

32. Zelis R, Mansour EJ, et al. The cardiovascular effects of morphine: the peripheral capacitance and resistance vessels in human subjects. J Clin Invest 1974;54:1247.

33. Leier CV, Heban PT, et al. Comparative systemic and renal hemodynamic effects of dopamine and dobutamine in patients with cardiomyopathy and heart failure. Circulation 1978;588:466.

34. Goldstein RA, Passamani ER, Roberts R. A comparison of dopamine and dobutamine in patients with acute infarction and cardiac failure. N Engl J Med 1980;303:846.

35. Bristow MR, Ginsburg R, et al. Decreased catecholemine sensitivity and betaadrenergic receptor density in failing human hearts. N Engl J Med 1982;307:205.

36. Dasta JF, Kirby MG. Pharmacology and therapeutic uses of low-dose dopamine. Pharmacology 1986;6:304.

37. Chernow B, Rainey TG, Lake CR. Endogenous and exogenous catecholemines in critical care medicine. Crit Care Med 1982;10:409.

38. Goldberg LI. Cardiovascular and renal actions of dopamine: potential clinical applications. Pharmacol Rev 1972;24:1.

39. Beregovich J, Bianchi C, et al. Dose related hemodynamic and renal effects of dopamine in congestive heart failure. Am Heart J 1974;87:550.

40. Sonnenblick EH, Frishman WH, LeJemtel TH. Dobutamine: a new synthetic cardioactive sympathetic amine. N Engl J Med 1979;300:17.

41. Kittleson MD, Eyster GE, et al. Efficacy of digoxin administration in dogs with idiopathic congestive cardiomyopathy. J Am Vet Med Assoc 1985;186:162.

42. Miller MS. Practical selected therapeutic concepts for congestive heart failure and cardiac arrhythmias. Proc Am Coll Vet Intern Med 1991;9:667-669.

43. Freedman BI, Burkart JM. Hypokalemia. Crit Care Clin 1991;1:145.

44. Schertel ER, Muir MW. Shock: Pathophysiology, monitoring, and therapy. In Kirk RW, ed. Current veterinary therapy X. Philadelphia: WB Saunders, 1989;316-330.

45. Shapiro BA, Cane RD. Interpretation of blood gases. In Shoemaker WC, Ayres S, et al, eds. Textbook of critical care. Philadelphia: WB Saunders, 1989;305-311.

46. Tilley LP, ed. Essentials of canine and feline electrocardiography, ed 2. Philadelphia: Lea & Febiger, 1985.

47. Braunwald E, ed. Heart disease: A textbook of cardiovascular medicine, ed 3. Philadelphia: WB Saunders, 1988.

48. Zipes DP, Jalife J, eds. Cardiac electrophysiology: From cell to bedside. Philadelphia: WB Saunders, 1990.

49. Rakita L, Vrobel TR. Electrocardiography in critical care medicine. In: Shoemaker WD, Ayres S, et al. eds. In: Textbook of critical care medicine. Philadelphia: WB Saunders, 1991;353-376.

50. Hamlin RL. Function of the SA node in health and disease. Proc Acad Vet Cardiol 1991;2:31-34.

51. Sisson DD. Bradyarrhythmias and cardiac pacing. In: Kirk RW, ed. Current veterinary therapy X. Philadelphia: WB Saunders, 1989;286-294.

52. Fox PR, Papich MG. Complications of cardiopulmonary drug therapy. In Kirk RW, ed. Current veterinary therapy X. Philadelphia, WB Saunders, 1989;308-315.

53. Kastor JA. Multifocal atrial tachycardia. N Engl J Med 1990;322:1713.

54. Tilley LP, Miller MS. Antiarrhythmic drugs and management of cardiac arrhythmias. In Kirk RW, ed. Current veterinary therapy IX. Philadelphia: WB Saunders, 1986;346-360.

55. Kittleson M, Keene B, et al. Verapamil for acute termination of supraventricular tachycardia in dogs. J Am Vet Med Assoc 1988;193:1525.

56. Allert JA, Adams HR. New perspectives in cardiovascular medicine: the calcium channel blocking drugs. J Am Vet Med Assoc 1987;190:573.

57. Bonagura JD, Ware WW. Atrial fibrillation in the dog: clinical findings in 81 cases. J Am Anim Hosp Assoc 1986;22:111.

58. Fox PR. Feline myocardial disease. In Fox PR, ed. Canine and feline cardiology. New York: Churchill Livingstone, 1988;435-466.

59. Colucci WS, Fifer XX, et al. Calcium channel blockers in congestive heart failure: theoretic considerations and clinical experience. Am J Med 1985;78(suppl 2B):9.

60. Ware WA, Hamlin RL. Therapy for ventricular arrhythmias. In Kirk RW, ed. Current veterinary therapy X. Philadelphia: WB Saunders, 1989;278-286.

61. Hamlin RL. To treat or not to treat ventricular arrhythmias in dogs. Proc Am Coll Vet Intern Med 1991;9:685-687.

62. Tilley LP. Pro-con: Should ventricular arrhythmias be treated in dogs? Proc Am Coll Vet Intern Med 1991;9:681-683.

63. Lown B, Graboys TB. Evaluation and management of the patient with ventricular arrhythmia. Cardiac Impulse 1985;6:1.

64. Goldstein RE, Tibbits PA, Oetgen WJ. Proarrhythmic effects of antiarrhythmic drugs. In Greenberg HM, et al. eds. Clinical aspects of life-threatening arrhythmias. Ann N Y Acad Sci 1844;427:94.

65. Torres V, Flowers D, Somberg JC. The arrhythmogenicity of antiarrhythmic agents. Am Heart J 1985;109:1090.

66. Bouvy BM, Bjorling DE. Pericardial effusion in dogs and cats, Part 1. Compend Contin Educ Pract Vet 1991;13:417.

67. Reed JR. Pericardial disease of the dog and cat. In Bonagura JD, ed. Contemporary issues in small animal practice: Cardiology. New York: Churchill Livingstone, 1987;177-218.

68. Holt JP. The normal pericardium. Am J Cardiol 1970;26:455.

69. Evans SM, Biery DN. Congenital peritoneapericardial diaphragmatic hernia in the dog and cat: a literature review and 17 additional case histories. J Am Vet Radiol Soc 1980;21:108.

70. Ettinger SJ, Suter PF. Canine cardiology. Philadelphia: WB Saunders, 1970.

71. Eyster GE, Evans AT, et al. Congenital pericardial diaphragmatic hernia and multiple cardiac defects in a litter of collies. J Am Vet Med Assoc 1977;170:516.

72. Rush JR, Keene BW, Fox PR. Pericardial disease in the cat: a retrospective evaluation of 66 cases. J Am Anim Hosp Assoc 1990;26:39.

73. Thomas WP. Pericardial disease. In Ettinger S, ed. Textbook of small animal internal medicine, ed. 2. Philadelphia: WB Saunders, 1985;1080-1097.

74. Sharp JT, Bunnell IL, Holland JF, et al. Hemodynamics induced during cardiac tamponade in man. Am J Med 1960;29:640-648.

75. Reddy PS, Curtis SE et al. Cardiac tamponade: hemodynamic observations in man. Circulation 1978;58:265.

76. Shabetai R. The pathophysiology of cardiac tamponade and constriction. Cardiovasc Clin 1976;7:67.

77. Berg RJ, Wingfield WE. Pericardial effusion in the dog: review of 42 cases. J Am Anim Hosp Assoc 1984;20:721-730.

78. Jones CL. Pericardial effusion in the dog. Compend Contin Educ Pract Vet 1979;1:680.

79. Berg RJ, Wingfield WE, Hoopes PJ. Idiopathic pericardial effusion in eight dogs. J Am Vet Med Assoc 1984;185:988.

80. Johnson KH. Aortic body tumors in the dog. J Am Vet Med Assoc 1968;152:154.

81. Rush JR, Atkins CE. Pericardial disease. In Allen DG, ed. Small animal medicine. Philadelphia: JB Lippincott, 1991;309-321.

82. Hammer AS, Couto CG, et al. Hemostatic abnormalities in dogs with hemangiosarcoma. J Vet Intern Med 1991;5:11.

83. Bonagura JD. Electrical alternans associated with pericardial effusion in the dog. J Am Vet Med Assoc 1981;178:574.

84. Christensen EE, Bonte FJ. The relative accuracy of echocardiography, intravenous carbon dioxide studies, and blood-pool scanning in detecting pericardial effusion. Radiology 1968;91:265.

85. Feigenbaum H, ed. Echocardiography, ed. 3. Philadelphia: Lea & Febiger, 1981.

86. Bonagura JD, Pipers FS. Echocardiographic features of pericardial effusion in dogs. J Am Vet Med Assoc 1981;179:49.

87. Thomas WP, Reed JR, et al. Diagnostic pneumopericardiography in dogs with spontaneous pericardial effusion. Vet Radiol 1984;25:2.

88. Buchanan JW. Selective angiography and angiocardiography in dogs with acquired cardiovascular disease. J Am Vet Radiol Soc 1965;6:5.

89. Sisson D, Thomas WP, et al. Diagnostic value of pericardial fluid analysis in the dog. J Am Vet Med Assoc 1984;184:51.

90. Edwards NJ. Pericardial disease. Proc Acad Vet Cardiol 1991;2:39-40.

91. Krikorian JG, Hancock EW. Pericardiocentesis. Am J Med 1978;65:808-814.

92. Lorell BH, Braunwald E. Pericardial disease. In Braunwald E, ed. Heart disease: a textbook of cardiovascular medicine. Philadelphia; WB Saunders, 1984;1470-1527.

93. Eyster GE, Probst M. Basic cardiac procedures. In Slatter DH, ed. Textbook of small animal surgery. Philadelphia: WB Saunders, 1985;1107-1131.

94. Aronsohn M. Cardiac hemangiosarcoma in the dog: a review of 38 cases. J Am Vet Med Assoc 1985;187:922.

95. Thomas W, Reed R. Constrictive pericardial disease in the dog. J Am Vet Med Assoc 1984;184:546.

96. Thomas JD, LeWinter MM. Pericardial disease in the intensive care setting. J Intern Care Med 1987;2:33.

97. Atkins CE. Heartworm disease. In Allen DG, ed. Small animal medicine. Philadelphia: JB Lippincott, 1991;341-363.

98. Atkins CE. Caval syndrome in the dog. Semin Vet Med Surg 1977;2:64.

99. Hribernik TN. Canine and feline heartworm disease. In Kirk RW, ed. Current veterinary therapy X. Philadelphia: WB Saunders, 1989;263-270.

100. Takehashi N, Matsui A, et al. Feline caval syndrome: A case report. J Am Anim Hosp Assoc 1988;24:245.

101. Rawlings CA. Heartworm disease in dogs and cats. Philadelphia: WB Saunders, 1986.

102. vonLichtenberg F, Jackson RF, Otto GF. Hepatic lesions in dogs with dirofilariasis. J Am Vet Med Assoc 1962;141:121.

103. Losonsky JM, Thrall DE, Lewis RE. Thoracic radiographic abnormalities in 200 dogs with spontaneous heartworm infections. Vet Radiol 1983;24:120.

104. Atkins CE, Keene BW, McGuirk SM. Pathophysiology of cardiac dysfunction in an experimental model of heartworm caval syndrome in the dog: An echocardiographic study. Am J Vet Radiol 1988;49:403.

105. Calvert CA. Treatment of heartworm disease with associated severe pulmonary artery disease. In Otto GF, ed. Proceedings of the Heartworm Symposium. The American Heartworm Society, Washington, DC, 1986;125-129.

106. Jackson RF, Seymore WG, et al. Surgical treatment of the caval syndrome of canine heartworm disease. J Am Vet Med Assoc 1977;171:1065.

107. Ishihara K, Kitagwa H, Sisaki Y. Efficacy of heartworm removal in dogs with dirofilarial hemoglobinuria using flexible alligator forceps. Jpn J Vet Sci 1988;50:739.

108. Knight DH. Heartworm disease. In Ettinger SJ, ed. Textbook of veterinary internal medicine, ed. 2. Philadelphia: WB Saunders, 1983;1097-1124.

109. Rawlings CA, Calvert CA. Heartworm disease. In Ettinger SJ, ed. Textbook of veterinary internal medicine, ed 3. Philadelphia: WB Saunders, 1989;1163-1184.

110. Liu S-K, Tilley LP, Lod DF. Feline cardiomyopathy. In Roy G, Dona G, eds. Recent advances in studies on cardiac structure and metabolism, vol. 10. Baltimore: University Park Press, 1975;627-640.

111. Flanders JA. Feline arterial thromboembolism. Compend Contin Educ Pract Vet 1986;8:473.

112. Mustard JF, Packham MA. Thromboembolism, a manifestation of the response of blood to injury. Circulation 1970;62:1.

113. Liu SK, Tilley LP. Animal models of primary myocardial disease. Yale J Biol Med 1980;53:191.

114. Dodds WJ. Platelet function in animals: Species specificities. In Gaetano G, Garrattini S, eds. Platelets: a multidisciplinary approach. New York: Raven Press, 1978;45-59.

115. Imhoff RK. Production of aortic occlusion resembling acute aortic embolism syndrome in cats. Nature 1961;192:979.

116. Schaub RG, Meyers KM, et al. Inhibition of feline collateral vessel development following experimental thromboembolic occlusion. Circ Res 1976;39:736.

117. Olmstead ML, Butler HC. Five-hydroxytryptamine antagonists and feline aortic thromboembolism. J Small Anim Pract 1977;18:247.

118. Schaub RG, Gates KA, Roberts RE. Effect of aspirin on collateral blood flow following experimental arterial thrombosis. Am J Vet Radiol 1982;43:1647.

119. Tilley LP, Liu S-K, Fox PR. Myocardial disease. In Ettinger SJ, ed. Textbook of veterinary internal medicine, ed 2. Philadelphia: WB Saunders, 1982;1029-1051.

120. Daniel GB, Wantschek L, et al. Diagnosis of arterial thromboembolism in 2 dogs with radionuclide angiography. Vet Radiol 1990;31:182.

121. Schmunk GA, Lefer AM. Antiaggregatory actions of calcium channel blockers in cat platelets. Res Commun Chem Pathol Pharmacol 1982;35:179.

122. Kelton JG, Hirsch J, et al. Thrombogenic effect of high dose aspirin in rabbits. J Clin Invest 1978;62:892.

123. Killingsworth CR, Eyster GE. Streptokinase treatment of cats with experimentally induced arterial thromboembolism. Am J Vet Res 1986;47:1351.

124. Pion PD, Kittleson MD. Thrombolysis of arterial thromboembolism in cats using tissue plasminogen activator [abstract]. Proc Am Coll Vet Intern Med 1987;5:925.

125. Yasuda T, Gold HK. Acute myocardial infarction and thrombolytic therapy. Thromb Res 1990;Suppl 10: 73-79.

126. Hyers TM. New diagnostic and therapeutic strategies in venous thromboembolic disease. In Taylor RW, Shoemaker WC, eds. Critical care state of the art XII. Society of Critical Care Medicine 1991;12:255-292.

127. Bell WR, Meek AG. Guidelines for use of thrombolytic agents. N Engl J Med 1979;301:1266.

128. DeHoff WD, Greene RW, Greiner TP. Surgical management of abdominal emergencies. Vet Clin North Am 1972;2:328.

129. Schein CJ, Hoffert PW, Hurwitt ES. Aortic embolectomy: a critical evaluation of eleven consecutive cases. Surgery 1956;39:950.

130. Fogarty TJ, Cranley JJ, et al. A method for extraction of arterial emboli and thrombi. Surg Gynecol Obstet 1963;116:241.

131. Holzworth J, Simpson R, Hind A. Aortic thrombosis with posterior paralysis in the cat. Cornell Vet 1955;44:468.

18 Metabolic and Endocrine Emergencies

Michael Schaer and *Joseph Taboada*

Metabolic and endocrine emergencies can be difficult to diagnose because their clinical signs mimic other common medical disorders. An accurate diagnosis depends on the clinician's index of suspicion and familiarity with the clinical features of these disorders. The metabolic and endocrinologic disorders that will be discussed in this section include diabetic ketoacidosis and the nonketotic hyperosmolar syndrome, hypoglycemia, hypoadrenocorticism, hypothyroid myxedema coma, feline thyrotoxicosis, water deprivation in diabetes insipidus, pheochromocytoma, hypercalcemia, hypocalcemia, and hepatic encephalopathy. The discussion of each disorder will include a brief review of applied pathophysiology, history and physical examination findings, diagnosis, treatment objectives, and patient monitoring.

DIABETIC KETOACIDOSIS
Pathophysiology

Hyperglycemia and ketoacidosis occur when there is an absolute or relative deficiency of insulin. These abnormalities are exaggerated by concomitant hyperglucagonemia. The insulin deficiency causes decreased peripheral tissue glucose utilization, glycogenolysis, gluconeogenesis, lipolysis, and proteolysis that result in marked tissue catabolism and persistent hyperglycemia. The increase in the blood glucose concentration creates an osmotic gradient that causes cellular dehydration and an osmotic diuresis with resultant urinary losses of glucose, water and several electrolytes (including Na^+, K^+, Cl^-, $HPO_4^=$, $H_2PO_4^-$).

Ketogenesis begins with peripheral lipolysis and the subsequent delivery of fatty acids to the liver. Insulinopenia and hyperglucagonemia stimulate increased hepatic carnitine and acylcarnitine transferase activity, which stimulates the hepatic ketogenic pathway.[1] The organic ketoacids that are released into the bloodstream are poorly metabolized and incompletely buffered, resulting in an elevated anion gap metabolic acidosis.

History and physical examination findings and diagnosis

Historical findings include polydipsia, polyuria, polyphagia, and weight loss. Lethargy, weakness, anorexia, and vomiting ensue. The onset of acute decompensation can range from a few days to months following the onset of clinical signs.

The decompensated ketoacidotic diabetic is dehydrated, weak, and depressed. Scleral injection and palpable hepatomegaly may be evident. Diabetes may be complicated by renal insufficiency, acute pancreatitis, and infections.

The diagnosis depends on the demonstration of hyperglycemia, hyperketonemia, glycosuria, and ketonuria. Coexisting serum biochemical abnormalities often include azotemia, hypokalemia, hyponatremia, hypophosphatemia, liver enzyme elevation, and decreased total carbon dioxide (metabolic acidosis). Anemia, hemoconcentration, or leukocytosis may occur. Upper or lower urinary tract infection, as evidenced by pyuria and bacteriuria, is often present.

Treatment

The therapeutic objectives for diabetic ketoacidosis include rehydration with isotonic parenteral fluids, replenishment of depleted electrolytes (especially sodium and potassium), correction of severe acidosis (arterial pH <7.1), and normalization of blood glucose.

Fluid replacement. Replacement and maintenance fluid needs should be calculated as described in Chapter 38. Severe dehydration (>8%) requires that approximately half the calculated fluid deficit be replaced over the first 2 to 4 hours, with the remaining volume given over the subsequent 20-to-22-hour period. Lactated Ringer's solution is usually the fluid of choice. The lactate is not accompanied by [H^+] and will not promote lactic acidosis. Saline (0.9%) is the fluid of choice when the patient is hyponatremic (serum sodium <132 mEq/L). In order to avoid hypernatremia, 0.9% saline should not be used as a maintenance fluid. Acetated Ringer's solution should not be used to treat ketoacidosis. The acetate anions can act as a substrate for acetoacetate formation. Dextrose (2.5% in 0.45% saline) should be administered once the patient's blood glucose level decreases below 250 mg/dl, allowing for the maintenance of euglycemia with the continued use of insulin.

Following rehydration, fluid administration rates for oliguric patients should equal the volume of urine output added to the estimated insensible water loss (15 ml/kg per day). The use of closed-system indwelling urethral catheters should be restricted to the patient with oliguria.

Potassium replacement. Hypokalemia is the most important electrolyte disturbance encountered in the patient with diabetic ketoacidosis.[1] Some patients are initially normokalemic. Hypokalemia, associated with treatment, is inevitable due to serum dilution from rehydration, continued urinary losses, and the cellular influx of potassium accompanying the correction of metabolic acidosis and the use of insulin.

Potassium supplementation is provided with potassium chloride solution added to the parenteral fluids. Potassium phosphate solution can be used if the animal is hypophosphatemic. Potassium supplementation should be delayed until hydration, blood pressure, and urine output are improved (see Chapter 38). Potassium could be added to the initial fluid infusion, but the rate of potassium infusion should not exceed 0.5 mEq/kg per hour.

Correction of acidosis

The use of sodium bicarbonate solution should be restricted to patients with a blood pH of less than 7.1[2] Bicarbonate treatment should be discontinued when the blood pH is restored to a level of 7.25 to avoid oversupplementation. The amount (in milliequivalents) of bicarbonate required for extracellular replacement = 0.3 × kilograms of body weight × base deficit. Ketogenesis will cease and ketoacids will be metabolized to bicarbonate after fluid and insulin treatment. The lactate in lactated Ringer's solution will be converted to bicarbonate (over a period of several hours) following correction of hypovolemia. In our experience, most dogs and cats with ketoacidosis do not require sodium bicarbonate treatment.

Insulin. Regular crystalline insulin should be used when the patient has signs of depression, dehydration, anorexia, and vomiting. The various routes of administration (intravenous, intramuscular, subcutaneous) and rapid onset and short duration of action allow the clinician to adjust treatment according to the patient's needs.[3-6]

To avoid the problems associated with insulin overdosage, a continuous low-dose insulin infusion can be used.[6] One successful technique in the dog involves the addition of regular insulin to lactated Ringer's solution following the first 2 hours of rehydration. A pediatric infusion set (or fluid infusion pump) should be used to deliver 0.5 to 1.0 unit per hour. Varying the concentration of the insulin infusion may help avoid fluid overload. The amount of insulin adhering to the tubing and the bottle is negligible. Blood glucose determinations and appropriate insulin dosage adjustments should be made every 1 to 2 hours. When laboratory facilities are unavailable, blood glucose reagent strips (Chemstrip bG, Biodynamics or Dextrostix, Ames) can be used for approximate blood glucose measurements.[7] Several reflectance colorimeters are now commercially available to enhance the accuracy of these reagent strips. The possibility of hypokalemia with intravenous insulin administration necessitates frequent serum potassium determinations.

Low doses of regular insulin can also be administered intramuscularly in the dehydrated patient.[3,4] Initially, 2 units are administered intramuscularly to cats and dogs weighing less than 10 kg. For dogs weighing more than 10 kg, the initial dose is 0.25 unit/kg. Hourly injections of 1 unit for cats and small dogs and 0.1 unit/kg for larger dogs are administered until hourly blood glucose determinations are less than 250 mg/dl. The subcutaneous route can then be used every 6 to 8 hours (Table 18-1). The use of low-dose syringes (Lo-dose Insulin Syringes, Becton Dickson) is recommended.

The subcutaneous route of insulin administration is especially important when intensive care facilities are unavailable. The initial dose is 0.5 unit/kg of body weight, followed by doses every 6 to 8 hours (see Table 18-1). This regimen allows for a gradual reduction of blood glucose levels, thus lessening the chance of iatrogenic hypoglycemia and hypokalemia. Subcutaneously administered insulin will not be absorbed effectively when the patient is markedly hypotensive.

Monitoring

Frequent reexamination of the patient and serial biochemical testing is required during initial stabilization (24 to 48 hours). Clinical signs of im-

Table 18-1 Sliding scale technique for subcutaneous regular insulin administration in the ketoacidotic cat and dog—blood monitoring

Blood glucose	Units of regular insulin every 6 hours*	Intravenous drip supplement
>400 mg/dl	Increase 1-2 units above the previous dose (cat and small dog)	—
	Increase 2-4 units above the previous dose (medium to large dogs, respectively)	—
240-400 mg/dl	Repeat previous dose (cat and small dog)	2.5% dextrose when blood glucose <250 mg/dl
	Increase 1-2 units above previous dose (medium to large dogs, respectively)	2.5% dextrose when blood glucose <250 mg/dl
180-240 mg/dl	Decrease 2 units from previous dose (cat and small dog)	2.5% dextrose
	Decrease 4 units from previous dose (medium and large dogs)	2.5% dextrose
<180 mg/dl	Omit insulin for 4-6 hours	2.5% dextrose

*These insulin dosages are only empirical recommendations. The clinician should adjust subsequent doses according to each individual patient's response.

provement include improved mentation, hydration, and muscular strength. A sudden onset or worsening of mental depression might reflect the occurrence of cerebral edema caused by a rapid fall in blood glucose levels.[8] Following stabilization, the animal should have thorough physical examinations and serum biochemical determinations daily. Treatment adjustments should be made as appropriate.

Persistent ketonuria during the first 72 hours in the setting of a clinically improved patient is common. Ketonuria often persists as the other biochemical parameters improve, especially when betahydroxybutyrate was the initially predominant ketoacid. Betahydroxybutyrate is converted to acetoacetate prior to metabolic conversion to bicarbonate.[1] The nitroprusside (ketone-detecting) reagent test results will be positive with acetoacetate and acetone but negative with betahydroxybutyrate.

NONKETOTIC HYPEROSMOLAR DIABETIC SYNDROME (NKHDS)
Pathophysiology

Two concepts have been advanced to explain the pathophysiology of the nonketotic hyperosmolar diabetic syndrome.[9] The first hypothesis suggests that small amounts of insulin are available for the liver (reflecting residual beta-cell secretory activity) while there is an insufficient amount of insulin for the uptake of glucose and inhibition of lipolysis in peripheral tissues. Intrahepatic oxidation of incoming free fatty acids is inactivated and those fatty acids are directed along nonketogenic metabolic pathways such as triglyceride synthesis.

This concept could account for the absence of hyperketonemia. The second hypothesis suggests that enhanced gluconeogenesis occurs in the liver due to the prevailing portal vein ratio of glucagon to insulin. This effect is responsible for the development of massive hyperglycemia.

Severe hyperglycemia can establish an osmotic gradient between the extracellular and intracellular compartments of the brain, resulting in neuronal cellular dehydration and dysfunction. The brain counteracts this osmotic gradient by forming "idiogenic osmoles." As the extracellular hyperosmolality increases, water leaves the cells. A marked decrease in consciousness and other neurologic abnormalities ensue.[10-13]

History and physical examination findings

Polydipsia, polyuria, weakness, and vomiting occur early in NKHDS. Thirst may diminish despite mounting levels of hyperglycemia.

Physical examination reveals marked dehydration, hypotension, and mental depression.[13-15] Neurologic signs can include grand mal seizures, hemiparesis, hyperreflexia, muscle fasciculations, and nystagmus suggestive of diffuse cortical or subcortical damage.[12,13]

Diagnosis

Several clinicopathologic abnormalities characterize NKHDS. The blood glucose levels are often elevated above 800 mg/dl. Serum osmolality is elevated (normal serum osmolality, 290 to 310 mOsm/kg body water) and best determined by the freezing-point-depression method utilizing an osmometer. It can also be calculated by the following formula:

$$mOsm/kg = 2 \text{ (serum Na}^+ + K^+) \text{ (mEq/L)}$$
$$+ \frac{\text{blood glucose (mg/dl)}}{18} + \frac{\text{BUN (mg/dl)}}{2.8}$$

where BUN denotes blood urea nitrogen. Most patients with NKHDS will have a serum osmolality of greater than 350 mOsm. The majority of patients have renal or prerenal azotemia. Serum sodium and potassium levels are variable. Normokalemia is associated with depleted total body potassium stores. If the patient is hypokalemic, this value reflects a profound total body potassium deficit.

Some patients with NKHDS have a metabolic acidosis despite the absence of detectable blood and urinary ketones.[10] This might be attributed to lactic acid accumulation, renal insufficiency, and unidentified organic acids.

Treatment

The treatment objectives include reestablishing euhydration and adequate urine output, using regular crystalline insulin judiciously to avoid a precipitous decline in blood glucose levels, and providing appropriate potassium supplementation. Patience is the key to treating this type of patient. A brisk lowering of serum osmolality (hyperglycemia) can cause cerebral edema due to the presence of idiogenic osmoles in the brain.[8] Remember, go slowly.

Fluid therapy should proceed at the usual recommended rates for volume repletion and maintenance (Chapter 38). It should consist of 0.9% saline if the patient is hypotensive or hyponatremic. Treatment is changed to 0.45% saline when blood pressure and hydration are restored to normal.

The regular insulin requirement for the nonketotic hyperosmolar diabetic is often less than that required for the diabetic ketoacidotic patient.[13] Close monitoring of the blood glucose levels is essential. Ideally, the blood glucose should be gradually decreased to 250 to 300 mg/dl after 6 to 8 hours of treatment. Parenteral fluids should be switched to 2.5% or 5% dextrose in 0.45% saline when the blood glucose declines to 250 mg/dl.

HYPOGLYCEMIA
Pathophysiology

The most common causes of hypoglycemia include pancreatic beta-cell adenocarcinoma (insulinoma),[16] insulin overdosage, sepsis,[17,18] extrapancreatic neoplasia,[19,20] adrenocortical insufficiency, glycogen storage diseases,[21,22] congenital portosystemic shunts, malnutrition, and pediatric metabolic enzyme immaturity.[21,22] The hypoglycemia of sepsis is thought to be due to decreased hepatic glucose production with or without increased peripheral utilization.[17,18] Hypoglycemia of malignancy is thought to be due to the production of nonsuppressible insulin-like peptides or insulin-like growth factors by the tumor.[19,20] The neoplasms most frequently involved include hepatomas, lymphoreticular tumors, large mesenchymal tumors, and certain carcinomas.

In small animals, clinical signs of hypoglycemia usually occur when blood glucose levels drop below 50 mg/dl. The clinical effects of hypoglycemia are directly related to both the rapidity and the degree of the blood glucose decline. Compensatory hormonal regulatory mechanisms provide for the hypersecretion of glucagon, epinephrine, cortisol, and growth hormone.[23] Their combined effects serve to inhibit the peripheral actions of insulin and to stimulate glycogenolysis and gluconeogenesis. Adrenal medullary responses cause hyperepinephrinemia, resulting in some of the initial signs of hypoglycemia (anxiety, tachycardia, pallor, and hypothermia). A continued decline in blood glucose causes cerebral cortical dysfunction. The impaired cerebral metabolic activity promotes decreased brain oxygen utilization and eventual neuronal destruction. This process proceeds to involve the midbrain and medullary structures.

History and physical examination findings

The history will vary with the cause of hypoglycemia. The stress of a new environment or an illness and anorexia in puppies and kittens might exceed their metabolic capacity to meet energy needs, causing them to lapse into an acute hypoglycemic coma. Insulinomas, on the other hand, characteristically cause a chronic waxing and waning pattern of clinical signs in an older patient.

The signs of hypoglycemia will depend on the cause, the rate and duration of blood glucose decline, and the capacity of the animal's compensatory counterregulatory hormonal mechanisms. The initial signs of catecholamine excess are soon followed by signs of cerebral cortical dysfunction that include behavioral changes, dementia, weakness, muscle twitching, seizures, and coma. Hypoglycemia may be subclinical. Clinical signs related to the predisposing cause (sepsis, adrenocortical insufficiency) may accompany or mask the signs of hypoglycemia.

Diagnosis

When hypoglycemia arises from insulin overdose, the history provides for neuroglycopenia within an anticipated time following the insulin injection. Furthermore, in the diabetic animal receiving morning insulin injections the finding of marked glycosuria in the early morning and minimal or absent glycosuria in the late morning or early afternoon is suspicious for a transient effect of insulin or posthypoglycemic hyperglycemia (Somogyi reaction).

In the middle-aged and geriatric animal not receiving exogenous insulin, hypoglycemia should warrant the investigation for a pancreatic beta-cell tumor or extrapancreatic cancer.[16,20,24,25]

The diagnostic workup should include chest and abdominal radiographs, complete blood count, serum biochemical profile, and urinalysis.

When an islet-cell tumor is suspected, the diagnosis depends on the demonstration of hypoglycemia with coexisting inappropriate hyperinsulinemia. The amended insulin:glucose ratio (I:G) is helpful in making the diagnosis. Values >50 are suspicious for insulinomas:

$$\text{Amended I:G} = \frac{\text{serum insulin (units/ml)} \times 100}{\text{blood glucose (mg/dl)} - 30}$$

Ordinarily, paired fasting serum samples for glucose and insulin determinations will suffice for diagnosing insulinoma. Fasting should be done under close observation. When the test results are equivocal, provocative tests such as the glucagon or leucine tolerance tests can be done.

Treatment

Hypoglycemia is a metabolic emergency requiring prompt recognition and immediate treatment. Intravenous dextrose solution should be administered to hospitalized patients with signs of neuroglycopenia. *The emergency dose of 50% dextrose solution is 1 ml/kg (0.5 gm/kg body weight) by intravenous bolus administration.* Depending on the suspected cause of hypoglycemia, a constant in-

travenous infusion of 5% to 10% dextrose solution may be necessary.

Injectable glucagon (Glucagon, Lilly; 0.03 mg/kg body weight intravenously, subcutaneously, or intramuscularly) will elevate blood glucose levels for approximately 30 minutes.[23] Glucagon can be used to help treat severe hypoglycemia, especially when intravenous access is difficult.

Clients with diabetic pets should be instructed about signs of hypoglycemia, and they should always keep an oral carbohydrate (Karo syrup) supplement available, to administer until further medical therapy can be provided. It should not be given to the unconscious patient, however.

Animals with severe hypoglycemia (<40 mg/dl) associated with hyperinsulinism or extrapancreatic neoplasia should have surgery after acceptable blood glucose levels (>60 mg/dl) are restored.[16,20,24] Blood glucose levels in preoperative hypoglycemic animals and those with metastatic pancreatic beta-cell carcinomas can be temporarily maintained (in most cases) with the drugs listed in Table 18-2.[26-28] Diazoxide and prednisone are the initial drugs of choice in the dog.

The postoperative complications associated with the surgical resection of insulinoma include acute pancreatitis, transient or permanent insulin-dependent diabetes mellitus, and recurrent hypoglycemia associated with metastatic disease.[16,24] The prognosis is guarded in dogs because most tumors are adenocarcinomas.

ACUTE ADRENOCORTICAL INSUFFICIENCY (ADDISON'S DISEASE)

Adrenocortical insufficiency can result from the following causes: idiopathic adrenal atrophy and immune-mediated adrenocortical destruction, glu-

Table 18-2 Drugs used to maintain adequate blood glucose levels in dogs with metastatic insulinoma

Drug	Dosage	Mechanism
Diazoxide	10 mg/kg per day divided into two doses; can be gradually increased to 30 mg/kg per day	Inhibits beta-cell insulin secretion Raises blood glucose by an extrapancreatic effect
Thiazide diuretics	Chlorothiazide, 20 mg/kg sid/bid; hydrochlorothiazide 2 mg/kg sid/bid	Limits sodium retention and potentiates the action of diazoxide
Propranolol	0.2-1.0 mg/kg tid	Inhibits beta-cell insulin secretion by beta-adrenergic blockade, uncommonly used
Phenytoin	50-80 mg/kg orally tid (in dogs)	Inhibits beta-cell insulin release, uncommonly used and of minimal benefit
Glucocorticoids	0.25-0.50 mg/kg per day divided bid	Promotes gluconeogenesis and peripheral insulin resistance

sid = once a day; bid = twice a day; tid = three times a day.

cocorticoid administration causing iatrogenic adrenocortical atrophy, *o, p′* - DDD-induced adrenocortical destruction, hemorrhage or infarction of the adrenal glands, mycotic or other granulomatous disease, neoplastic involvement, surgical adrenalectomy, and anterior pituitary gland insufficiency.

Pathophysiology

The pathophysiologic consequences of primary adrenocortical insufficiency are a direct result of glucocorticoid and mineralocorticoid deficiencies.[4,10] Glucocorticoid depletion causes impaired gluconeogenesis and glycogenolysis, decreased sensitization of blood vessels to catecholamines, impaired renal water excretion, and decreased vitality as characterized by poor appetite, lethargy, and impaired mentation.

Aldosterone is a mineralocorticoid hormone that plays an important part in sodium and potassium homeostasis. Hypoaldosteronism causes excessive renal sodium and chloride ion excretion and potassium and hydrogen ion retention. The clinical and pathophysiologic effects of the resultant hyponatremia include lethargy, mental depression, nausea, hypotension, impaired cardiac output, poor renal perfusion, and hypovolemic shock. Hyperkalemia causes muscle weakness, hyporeflexia, and impaired cardiac conduction. Moderate to marked hyponatremia (serum sodium <132 mEq/L) and hyperkalemia (serum potassium >7.0 mEq/L) are usually present in the addisonian crisis.

History and physical examination findings and diagnosis

Historical complaints include thin body condition, periodic vomiting and/or diarrhea, and lethargy. Polydipsia and polyuria may be present.[29] The chronicity of signs can vary from weeks to months; suddenly culminating in an acute hypotensive collapse. Alternatively, the addisonian crisis may be acutely triggered by stress without prior signs.

The critically ill patient with Addison's disease typically shows hypothermia, dehydration, depressed mentation, weak pulses, and marked muscle weakness. Additional clinical findings can include shallow respirations, pale mucous membranes, slow capillary refill time, and cardiac arrhythmias.[29-31]

The electrocardiogram can be used to detect hyperkalemia. The most common electrocardiographic abnormalities include flattened P waves, increased P-R interval, increased positive or negative deflection in the T waves, broadened QRS complexes, bradycardia, sinoventricular complexes, and atrial standstill (Figs. 18-1 and 18-2).[32,33]

The usual clinicopathologic findings include hyperkalemia and hyponatremia (sodium:potassium, <20:1), mild to moderate hypochloremia, azotemia, hyperphosphatemia, and metabolic acidosis. Mild hypercalcemia is often present, but hypoglycemia is rarely seen.[30-33]

Confirmation of the diagnosis depends on the demonstration of absent or minimal adrenocor-

A

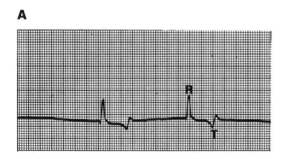

B

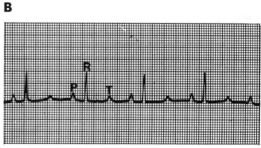

Fig. 18-1 A, This electrocardiographic tracing is a lead II rhythm strip from a 3-year-old male poodle in addisonian crisis (serum sodium = 110 mEq/L; serum potassium = 8.2 mEq/L). Depicted is atrial standstill (bradycardia with no P waves) with a sinoventricular rhythm. The T waves are biphasic and large in amplitude and the R-wave amplitude is small. **B,** Lead II electrocardiogram from the same dog 2 hours after treatment, illustrating restored sinus rhythm, decreased Q-T interval, decreased T-wave amplitude, and normal R wave. (From Schaer M. Hypoadrenocorticism. In Kirk RW ed. Current veterinary therapy VII—Small animal practice. Philadelphia: WB Saunders, 1980;986-987.)

A

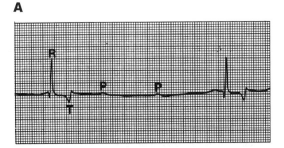

B

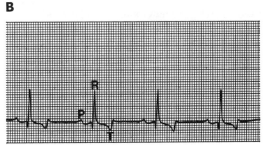

Fig. 18-2 A, This electrocardiographic tracing is a lead II rhythm strip from an 8-year-old female mixed-breed dog in addisonian crisis (serum sodium = 122 mEq/L;serum potassium = 8.5 mEq/L). Depicted is complete heart block (more P waves than QRS complexes with no association). **B,** Lead II electrocardiogram from the same dog three hours after treatment with desoxycorticosterone acetate, intravenous saline, calcium gluconate, bicarbonate, and insulin-dextrose, illustrating return of normal sinus rhythm. (From Schaer M. Hypoadrenocorticism. In Kirk RW, ed. Current veterinary therapy VII—Small animal practice. Philadelphia: WB Saunders, 1980;986-987.)

tical response to an injection of corticotropin (ACTH).[34,35] In order to avoid an unnecessary delay of therapy, it is recommended that the following procedure be performed soon after the patient's admission:

1. Draw blood for hemogram, serum biochemistry profile, and basal plasma or serum cortisol determinations.
2. Begin intravenous fluids (0.9% saline) and give 2 to 5 mg/kg of dexamethasone intravenously (prednisolone and prednisone will interfere with cortisol assays).
3. Administer 0.25 mg of α-1, 24-corticotropin (Cortrosyn, Organon) intramuscularly or intravenously.
4. One hour later, obtain a second blood sample for plasma or serum cortisol determination.

Treatment

The therapeutic objectives include intravascular volume repletion, reversal of the hyponatremia and hyperkalemia, providing glucocorticoid replacement and recognizing and reversing any life-threatening cardiac arrhythmias.[29-31,35]

The fluid of choice is 0.9% sodium chloride, and it should be administered intravenously. If the dog is markedly hypotensive, the saline should be infused at a rate of 40 to 80 ml/kg body weight (20-40 ml/kg for a cat) during the first 1 to 2 hours of treatment. Isotonic saline should be evenly infused at a maintenance rate of approximately 60 to 70 ml/kg for the remainder of the 24-hour period. Central venous pressure monitoring may be useful in preventing iatrogenic fluid overload. The administration of intravenous fluids

is discontinued when hydration, urine output, serum electrolytes, and the serum creatinine levels are restored to normal (usually after 48 to 72 hours of treatment).

Mineralocorticoid hormone supplementation is also necessary to enhance renal distal tubular sodium reabsorption and potassium excretion. Deoxycorticosterone pivilate (Ciba) 2.0 mg/kg given intramuscularly every 3 weeks and Florinef (fludrocortisone; Squibb) 0.1 to 0.8 mg daily are used for mineralocorticoid supplementation. Periodic reassessment of the serum electrolyte levels will serve as a helpful treatment guide.

The glucocorticoid deficiency is corrected with rapid-acting drugs such as prednisolone sodium succinate (Solu-Delta-Cortef, Upjohn), or dexamethasone or hydrocortisone. Prednisone and hydrocortisone should not be given until the ACTH stimulation test is completed. The initial intravenous doses of prednisolone sodium succinate and dexamethasone are 5 to 10 mg/kg and 2 to 5 mg/kg body weight, respectively. Subsequent glucocorticoid requirements are fulfilled by administering 1 mg/kg of prednisolone orally, intramuscularly, or intravenously every 12 hours for 48 hours. The dose is then reduced to 0.25 to 0.5 mg/kg every 12 hours for the duration of hospitalization. Cortisone acetate (0.5 mg/kg/day) can be used in place of prednisone for added mineralocorticoid effect.

Serum potassium concentrations greater than 7.0 mEq/L cause progressive depressions of the excitability and conduction velocity of the myocardium.[32] Treatment entails the administration of drugs that will either antagonize the effects of potassium or lower its serum level by displacing it intracellularly. The emergency measures for the

Table 18-3 Emergency treatment of the addisonian crisis

Problem	Treatment
Hypovolemia	Sodium chloride 0.9%: 40-80 ml/kg IV (20-40 ml/kg for a cat) over first 1-2 hours; maintain at 60-70 ml/kg/24 hours
Hyponatremia and hyperkalemia	Sodium chloride solution: see above; desoxycorticosterone acetate: 1-5 mg in proportion to body weight IM sid or fludrocortisone acetate 0.1 mg/5 to 10 kg po sid
Hyperkalemic myocardial toxicity	1. Sodium bicarbonate: 1-2 mEq/kg IV 2. Regular crystalline insulin: 0.25 unit/kg with 2-3 g dextrose per unit of insulin IV 3. Calcium gluconate 10%: 1-1.5 ml/kg IV over 10-20 minutes
Hypocortisolemia	Prednisolone sodium succinate[*]: 5-10 mg/kg IV; dexamethasone 2-5 mg/kg IV; or hydrocortisone succinate[a] 25-50 mg/kg IV
Hypoglycemia	Dextrose 50%: 1 ml/kg IV bolus initially; maintain on 2.5% dextrose and 0.9% saline solution IV

IV = intravenously; IM = intramuscularly; sid = once a day; po = orally.
[*]Following completion of ACTH stimulation test.

treatment of myocardial toxicity usually are required once and need not be repeated. A summary of the emergency treatment of an addisonian crisis is shown in Table 18-3.

HYPOTHYROID MYXEDEMA COMA
Pathophysiology

This is a rare condition in the dog. Clinical recognition is important because of its severe consequences. Hypothyroid myxedema rests on markedly depleted thyroid hormone levels. The signs are a dramatic extension of those characteristic of hypothyroidism.[36]

History and physical examination findings and diagnosis

The history describes decreased exercise, cold intolerance, mental apathy, lethargy, and constipation. The more common signs of hypothyroidism (obesity, "pathetic faces," alopecia, and other dermatologic changes) are usually of a prolonged duration.[36,37] Signs associated with myxedema represent an acute decline in the patient's condition. Patients often present after being in a cold or stressful environment. This condition is characterized by profound mental depression, hypothermia, hypotension, hyporeflexia, hypoventilation, bradycardia and myxedema.[36-39] The clinicopathologic signs include normochromic normocytic anemia, hypercholesterolemia, and low serum concentrations of triiodothyronine and thyroxine. In humans, hyponatremia, low serum osmolality and high urine osmolality have been reported.[36,39]

Treatment

Carbon dioxide retention and hypoxia due to hypoventilation should be treated with assisted ventilation and oxygen.[38] Hypotension and hyponatremia are treated with intravenous isotonic saline solution. Hypotonic fluids and overhydration should be avoided.[38,39] External rewarming for hypothermia is contraindicated since already diminished cardiac output may be diverted from vital organs and cardiovascular collapse can ensue.[38]

In humans, thyroid hormone replacement is initiated with a single intravenous dose of 0.2 to 0.5 mg of sodium levothyroxine and followed by 0.1 mg once daily until oral l-thyroxine treatment is instituted.[38,39] Since most veterinary practices do not have parenteral l-thyroxine available, the oral tablet form will be the preferred method for thyroid hormone replacement.[40] l-Thyroxine treatment should commence with low dosages (0.0015 mg/kg orally twice a day) and gradually be increased over the next several weeks to 0.02 mg/kg per day. Prednisolone sodium succinate or dexamethasone should be given in order to counteract any degree of transient glucocorticoid deficiency that might arise with the initial doses of l-thyroxine.

FELINE THYROTOXICOSIS
Pathophysiology

Feline hyperthyroidism is a disorder of the older cat (5 to 22 years old) that is usually due to thyroid adenomatous hyperplasia. The clinical consequences are due to the hypermetabolic effects of excess thyroid hormone secretion. The most dramatic effect is cardiac disease that can progress to fulminant congestive heart failure and the patient's death.

History and physical examination findings

The most common historical signs include weight loss, polyphagia, hyperactivity, polyuria and polydipsia, diarrhea, and vomiting.[41] Signs of cardiac dysfunction (exercise intolerance, inappetence, dyspnea, and weakness) can occur as the disease progresses.[41,42] Some cats present with "apathetic" hyperthyroidism (moribund patient in heart failure without any premonitory signs).

Cats with advanced stages of hyperthyroidism demonstrate severe sinus tachycardia, cardiac arrhythmias, unilateral or bilateral palpable thyroid gland enlargement, marked weight loss, mental depression, and weakness.[41-43] Cardiac auscultation often detects a gallop rhythm. Dyspnea due to pleural effusion or pulmonary edema may be present.

Diagnosis

The history and physical examination findings are strongly suggestive in cats that have palpable thyroid gland enlargement. In other cats, the diagnosis is not as obvious and depends on evaluation of other clinical findings.

The electrocardiographic (ECG) signs include sinus tachycardia, increased R-wave amplitudes (normal lead II, 0.9 mV), atrial and ventricular arrhythmias, prolonged QRS duration, shortened Q-T intervals and intraventricular conduction disturbances.[41]

Fifty percent of cats with hyperthyroidism have cardiomegaly on thoracic radiography.[43] Cats in heart failure will have pulmonary edema and/or pleural effusion.

Echocardiography is the most useful diagnostic method for assessing cardiac muscle abnormalities.[42] Echocardiographic changes include left ventricular hypertrophy, aortic root and left atrial enlargement, increased shortening fraction, and hyperkinetic septal- and free-wall motion.

Serum biochemical abnormalities include elevations in concentrations of alanine aminotransferase, aspartate aminotransferase, and alkaline phosphatase.[41] Serum thyroid hormone concentrations are characteristically elevated (the normal values in our laboratory are thyroxine 0.8 to 3.5 μg/dl and triiodothyronine, 15 to 104 ng/dl).

Thyroid nuclear imaging (^{99m}Tc) is a diagnostic radioisotope procedure that accurately locates hyperactive gland(s) and aids in detection of metastatic thyroid neoplasia and ectopic hyperactive thyroid tissue.[41] Bilateral glandular involvement occurs in 70% of hyperthyroid cats.

Treatment

The cat with hyperthyroid-induced heart failure and/or severe cardiac conduction abnormalities constitutes a medical emergency. Those with congestive heart failure and pulmonary edema should receive furosemide (Lasix, Hoechst-Roussel) at a dosage of 1 to 2 mg/kg divided twice daily. Oxygen therapy and thoracocentesis (when indicated) are quite helpful. Echocardiographic evaluation will define the presence of systolic (dilatation) or diastolic (hypertrophic) dysfunction. In the presence of systolic dysfunction, digoxin treatment may be indicated. Propranolol (Inderal, Ayerst) is a beta-adrenergic blocking drug that is used to counteract tachycardia and to improve diastolic filling in hypertrophic cardiac disease. Propranolol should not be used until the congestive heart failure signs have abated. The recommended oral dose ranges from 2.5 mg to 5.0 mg two to three times daily in proportion to the animal's size and treatment response.

Methimazole (Tapazole, Lilly) is the antithyroid drug of choice for cats. It prevents the organification of iodide in the thyroid gland but will not inhibit the secretion of preformed stored hormone. The loading dose is 5 mg two to three times daily. This drug is given until a euthyroid state is achieved and until other forms of treatment with more lasting effects (thyroidectomy, iodine-131) can be accomplished.

Hypocalcemia can occur as a postoperative complication to bilateral thyroidectomy. This results from inadvertent surgical removal of all four parathyroid glands or from ischemic injury to the remaining parathyroid tissue. When hypocalcemia occurs the following treatment is recommended:

1. Immediately after surgery give 10% calcium gluconate at a dosage of 5 ml/kg distributed slowly over 24 hours. This is best administered through the intravenous fluids. Begin oral vitamin D (dihydrotachysterol) supplementation at a dosage of 0.03 mg/kg per day (see section on Hypocalcemia below, for further treatment recommendations).
2. Determine the serum calcium level every 24 hours and discontinue the calcium infusion as serum calcium levels normalize.

PITUITARY AND NEPHROGENIC DIABETES INSIPIDUS
Pathophysiology

Diabetes insipidus becomes a medical emergency when the animal loses access to water or the ability to consume it (vomiting). Continued water loss through diuresis (lack of antidiuretic hormone [ADH] secretion or renal response to it) results in a severe water deficit. The consequences include marked dehydration, hypotension, impaired renal perfusion, hypernatremic encephalopathy, and death.[44,45]

History and physical examination findings

Historical findings most commonly include polydipsia and polyuria. Following water deprivation lethargy, weakness, vomiting, and grand mal seizures may occur.

Decompensated patients with diabetes insipidus have profound mental depression and dehydration. Signs of interstitial fluid deficits will not occur until late in the course of fluid restriction because the hypertonic extracellular fluid space will attract water from the intracellular space, thereby providing for adequate interstitial water. Cellular dehydration will be profound. This becomes clinically apparent with brain dysfunction including seizures.[45,46] In severe cases, the animal will become anuric as a result of ischemic renal tubular disease.

Diagnosis

The clinicopathologic signs include hypernatremia, hyperchloremia, serum hyperosmolality (>310 mOsm/L) with hypoosmolar urine (<400 mOsm/L), elevated serum liver enzyme activities (due to hypovolemia), and azotemia. Severe brain dysfunction occurs when the serum sodium concentration acutely exceeds 160 mEq/L. The rapidity of rise of serum sodium concentration as well as the extent of rise contribute to onset of seizures.[45] The hemogram reflects severe hemoconcentration and a stress leukocytosis. Measured serum ADH levels (if available) are inappropriately low in pituitary diabetes insipidus, but might be elevated or normal in nephrogenic diabetes insipidus.

Treatment

The main treatment objectives in these severely hypernatremic patients include the correction of hypotension, the gradual reversal of hypernatremia, and the cessation of the water diuresis.

Severe circulatory impairment (marked dehydration, prolonged capillary refill time, palpably weak pulses, and oliguria) should be corrected with rapid intravenous administration of isotonic saline. The remaining water deficit should be corrected with 5% dextrose in water or hypotonic (0.45%) saline solutions.

Rapid replacement of the water deficits can cause seizures and cerebral edema because of an osmotic disequilibrium created between the brain

and the cerebrospinal fluid.[45-48] Therefore, half the calculated water deficit should be administered in the first 24 hours, followed by correction of the remaining deficit over the next 1 to 2 days.[47] The free water deficit can be calculated using the following formula:

Free water deficit $= 0.6 \times BW$
$$\times \left(1 - \frac{\text{normal serum Na}^+}{\text{current serum Na}^+} \right)$$

where BW denotes body weight in kilograms.

With pituitary-dependent diabetes insipidus, water diuresis is initially treated by administering vasopression tannate in oil (2.5 to 10 units intramuscularly). The patient can be maintained with the conjunctival or nasal application of desmopressin (DDAVP, pivopril), a synthetic ADH analog.[49] Patients with nephrogenic diabetes insipidus should be maintained with chlorothiazide (20 to 40 mg/kg per day orally).

PHEOCHROMOCYTOMA
Pathophysiology

Pheochromocytoma in the dog is a rare tumor arising from the adrenal medulla. The pathophysiologic effects are due to hypersecretion of norepinephrine and epinephrine resulting in hypertension, dyspnea and, cardiac tachyarrhythmias.[50] Some tumors are nonfunctional and may remain occult or can cause clinical signs by invading adjacent structures.

History and physical examination findings

Common historical signs in the dog include paroxysms of panting, anxiety, depression, restlessness, weakness, tremors, cerebral dysfunction, dyspnea, polyuria and polydipsia, and cutaneous flushing.[51-53]

The physical examination findings will depend on whether the tumor is hypersecreting catecholamines or whether it has invaded the posterior vena cava.[51-53] The former situation constitutes an endocrinologic emergency, with presence of hypertension, tachycardia, tachyarrhythmias, and congestive heart failure. The clinical signs associated with postcaval invasion include ascites, impaired venous return, and inadequate cardiac output. These two syndromes may occur concomitantly.

Diagnosis

Paramount to making this diagnosis is the clinician's suspicion for its presence and the detection of systemic hypertension. Radiographic techniques such as pyelography, arteriography, venography, computed tomography (CT scan), and ultrasonography might confirm the tumor's presence.[53]

Quantitating levels of plasma catecholamine and urine catecholamine metabolites is a useful diagnostic tool in human medicine.[54] These tests are not widely used in veterinary medicine because of their expense and the lack of established normal and abnormal levels.

Treatment

The main objective is to remove the pheochromocytoma surgically. Prior to surgery or in cases with metastatic disease, the preferred antihypertensive drug is phenoxybenzamine hydrochloride (Dibenzyline, Smith Kline & French), an alpha-adrenergic blocking drug (0.2 to 1.5 mg/kg orally twice a day).[50,53] The phenoxybenzamine dosage should begin low and be increased according to the patient's tolerance and response.

The beta-adrenergic blocking drug propranolol (Inderal, Ayerst; 0.2 to 2 mg/kg orally three times a day) can be used to counteract tachyarrhythmias and hypertension. *Phenoxybenzamine must be given before the propranolol in order to avoid a hypertensive crisis.*[50] When given in the absence of alpha-adrenergic blockade, propranolol can cause a paradoxical increase in blood pressure by blocking beta-receptor-mediated vasodilation in skeletal muscle.[50]

The animal should be closely monitored during surgery for changes in blood pressure and cardiac tachyarrhythmias. A hypertensive crisis can be treated by intravenous administration of the short-acting alpha-adrenergic blocking drug, phentolamine (Regitine, Ciba; 0.02 to 0.1 mg/kg).[53] Tachyarrhythmias can be treated with intravenous propranolol (0.03 to 0.06 mg/kg). *Remember to give phentolamine prior to the propranolol.*

HYPERCALCEMIA
Pathophysiology

The clinical signs of hypercalcemia are vague. Serum calcium concentrations greater than 15 to 20 mg/dl constitute a serious medical emergency and warrant prompt therapeutic intervention.

Calcium is an important component of every body tissue. Calcium homeostasis involves the interplay of parathyroid hormone (PTH), calcitonin, and vitamin D on skeletal, intestinal, and renal fluxes of calcium and phosphorus ions.[55] Serum ionized calcium is maintained within a narrow physiologic range (4.5 to 6 mg/dl). Immature animals have slightly higher normal serum calcium values than adults.

Animals with mild hypercalcemia are asymptomatic or have minimal clinical manifestations.[55] Complications and clinical signs are more likely to occur when the serum calcium concentration remains high for extended periods, when serum calcium values exceed 15 mg/dl, or when hypercalcemia is accompanied by hyperphosphatemia.[55]

Hypercalcemia can be caused by a variety of disorders affecting the dog and cat (Table 18-4).[56-63] The most common reason for symptomatic hypercalcemia is malignancy. The mechanisms are varied and, in most cases, have not been completely defined. Tumor-cell production of PTH-like polypeptides, lymphokines, bone resorbing factors, vitamin D-like sterols, and polypeptide growth factors are probably important mediators.[55,60-64] Prostaglandin E_2 and direct resorption of bone by cancer cells probably play a less important role. Lymphoma is the most common tumor causing hypercalcemia in the dog (10% to 40% prevalence).[61,65] Hypercalcemia is rarely associated with lymphoma in cats. Hypercalcemia associated with renal failure presents a difficult diagnostic dilemma.[59] Renal failure can be a cause or effect of the increased serum calcium concentration.

Primary hyperparathyroidism is a condition in which one or more of the parathyroid glands produce excess PTH. The disease is becoming more commonly recognized in the dog.[55,56,66] It is

Table 18-4 Possible causes of hypercalcemia in the dog

Primary hyperparathyroidism
    Adenoma*
    Adenocarcinoma
    Hyperplasia*
    Familial hyperplasia (German shepherd)
    Multiple endocrine neoplasia type 2
Malignancy
    Lymphoma*
    Apocrine gland adenocarcinoma of the anal
      sac
    Multiple myeloma
    Mammary gland adenocarcinoma
    Myeloproliferative disease*
    Tumors involving lung, thyroid, pancreas,
      testicle, nasal cavity
    Metastatic bone tumors
Adrenocortical insufficiency
Renal failure*
Vitamin D toxicosis*
    Cestrum diurnum (day-blooming jasmine)*
    Rodenticides*
Granulomatous disease
    Blastomycosis
    Schistosomiasis
Septic osteomyelitis
Disuse osteoporosis
Hypothermia*

*Reported cause of hypercalcemia in the cat.

rarely reported in the cat. A solitary parathyroid adenoma is usually the underlying source of excessive PTH production, but hyperplasia of one or more glands and functional parathyroid adenocarcinoma have been reported.

One of the body's adaptive mechanisms to hypercalcemia is deposition of calcium phosphate salts in the soft tissues. Nephrocalcinosis can lead to irreversible renal failure. The lungs, stomach, blood vessels, heart, and skin are often affected but clinically silent sites of mineralization. Soft-tissue mineralization starts to occur when the product of the calcium (mg/dl) and phosphorus (mg/dl) exceeds 70.

History and physical examination findings

The mean age of dogs with primary hyperparathyroidism and anal sac tumors is 10 years.[55,56,60] A sex predilection is not apparent except in anal sac adenocarcinomas in which there is a 90% predilection in females. When hypercalcemia develops in a young dog (less than 2 years old), iatrogenic hypervitaminosis D, renal failure, Addison's disease, or lymphoma should be suspected. Familial parathyroid hyperplasia has been reported in a pair of 2-week-old German shepherd pups.[55,66] There may be an increased prevalence of primary hyperparathyroidism in Keeshond dogs.[55,66]

Historical complaints are generally nonspecific and often reflect the underlying disease. The clinical signs of hypercalcemia are intermittent weakness, inappetence, listlessness, exercise intolerance, and polyuria with secondary polydipsia (caused by calcium interference with and damage to renal ADH receptors).[55] Polyuria and polydipsia occur in more than half the cases of primary hyperparathyroidism. Gastrointestinal signs (vomiting, constipation, diarrhea) and neurologic abnormalities (twitching, seizures, coma, stupor) are less common clinical signs of hypercalcemia.

Excessive vitamin/mineral supplementation and possible exposure to day-blooming jasmine or vitamin D-based rodenticides should be explored in the history. This approach may provide the only clue to diagnosing these potential causes of hypercalcemia.

The animal should be examined for evidence of lymphosarcoma and mammary or anal sac adenocarcinomas. A thorough perineal and rectal examination should be performed, as apocrine gland adenocarcinomas of the anal sacs can be a centimeter or less in diameter. A completely normal physical examination heightens the possible diagnosis of primary hyperparathyroidism.

Diagnosis

Hypercalcemia should be a consistent finding, as spuriously elevated calcium values are commonly encountered. It is important to note that lipemia will falsely increase serum calcium values if spectrophotometric methods of measurement are used. Blood collected in tubes containing ethylenediamine tetraacetic acid (EDTA) or washed with detergents can also give falsely elevated values.[67]

The medical workup for hypercalcemia is first directed at ruling out extraparathyroidal neoplasia. The initial data base should include radiographic examination of the chest and abdomen, hemogram, urinalysis, and serum biochemistry panel (Table 18-5). The urine specific gravity is usually within the isosthenuric range. Ultrasonography may supplement radiology in searching for occult neoplasia or granulomatous disease.

Concurrent or secondary renal failure can elevate the serum phosphorus, making the differentiation between hypercalcemic conditions difficult.[55] Renal failure is not as common in patients with primary hyperparathyroidism as with other causes of hypercalcemia, because the low phosphorus values decrease the likelihood of nephrocalcinosis. Serum phosphorus values are variable in nonazotemic patients with hypercalcemia of malignancy. Hyperchloremic metabolic acidosis may be associated with canine primary hyperparathyroidism. A chloride:phosphorus ratio greater than 33 is suggestive of primary hyperparathyroidism in man, but this measurement has not been adequately assessed in the dog.[55]

Lymph node and bone marrow aspirates or biopsies are used to rule out lymphoma as a cause of hypercalcemia. A PTH assay, if available, may show increased levels of serum immunoreactive PTH in primary hyperparathyroidism and renal failure.[55]

When a complete diagnostic evaluation reveals no definitive cause of the hypercalcemia, the clinician should surgically explore the patient's neck to visualize and biopsy or excise any enlarged parathyroid gland.

A short drug trial with an agent effective in treating lymphoma can be tried when occult lymphoma is still suspected or if cervical exploration is unrevealing. Prednisone (2 mg/kg orally twice a day) will usually decrease serum calcium in 48 to 72 hours. This decrease in serum calcium following prednisone treatment may be nonspecific. Some authors have recommended use of a single dose of L-asparaginase (20,000 IU/m^2 intravenously). The serum calcium should decrease in 72 hours in cases of lymphoma.

Treatment

Primary therapeutic efforts should be focused on correcting the underlying disease process. However, serum calcium levels >14 mg/dl often require immediate symptomatic treatment (Table 18-6).[58,65,67,68]

Table 18-5 The significance of diagnostic test results associated with hypercalcemia

Diagnostic Test	Diagnostic Consideration
Hemogram	
Eosinophilia	Hypoadrenocorticism
Normocytic-normochromic anemia	Neoplasia, chronic renal disease, chronic disease
Thrombocytopenia	Lymphoma with bone marrow involvement, myelo-proliferative disease, multiple myeloma
Leukocytosis	Granulomatous disease, infection
Serum chemistry	
Hyperphosphatemia	Renal failure, hypoadrenocorticism, vitamin D toxicity
Hypophosphatemia	Primary hyperparathyroidism, neoplasia
Azotemia (increased blood urea nitrogen, creatinine)	Renal failure, hypoadrenocorticism, dehydration
Increased serum alkaline phosphatase activity	Neoplasia (primary or metastatic to liver or bone); primary hyperparathyroidism
Increased transaminase activity	Neoplasia
Hyperglobulinemia	Multiple myeloma, lymphoma
Radiographs	
Hepatomegaly	Lymphoma
Splenomegaly	Lymphoma
Mediastinal mass	Lymphoma
Iliac lymphadenopathy	Lymphoma, metastatic anal sac tumor
Hilar lymphadenopathy	Lymphoma, blastomycosis
Osteolytic lesions	Multiple myeloma, bone metastasis, systemic mycosis

Osteopenia
  Soft-tissue calcification
  Pathologic fractures
  Nephrolithiasis
  Cystic calculi
	Primary hyperparathyroidism (late in disease course)

Electrocardiogram	Shortened Q-T interval

Table 18-6 Recommended treatment of hypercalcemia[65,67,68]

Item	Indication	Special Comments
Intravenous 0.9% sodium chloride	Rehydration To impair renal Ca^{++} reabsorption and to promote calciuresis	1. Replace dehydration deficit over 3-4 hours 2. Maintain fluid administration at 2-3 times maintenance 3. Supplement with potassium as needed
Furosemide	Calciuresis	1. 2 mg/kg IV every 12 hours; if no response give 5 mg/kg IV every hour 2. Thiazide diuretics contraindicated
Prednisone	Hypercalcemia secondary to neoplasia	2 mg/kg bid
Calcitonin	Life threatening, unresponsive hypercalcemia	4 U/kg IV, then 4 to 8 units/kg SC bid/tid
Plicamycin (mithramycin)	Unresponsive hypercalcemia	Side effects make it less desirable
Diphosphonates	Chronic hypercalcemia of malignancy	Inhibits hydroxyapatite crystal formation and dissolution

IV = intravenously; bid= twice a day; SC= subcutaneously; tid= three times a day.

HYPOCALCEMIA
Pathophysiology

Symptomatic hypocalcemia (caused by decreases in the serum ionized calcium) is uncommon and constitutes a medical emergency. Ionized calcium is essential for nerve cell membrane stabilization, acetylcholine release, and muscle contraction. The nervous system is particularly sensitive to decreases in serum ionized calcium levels. Hypocalcemia causes peripheral nerves to become progressively excitable and to discharge spontaneously. The resultant tetany is the hallmark of hypocalcemia in small animals. Spontaneous neuronal discharges within the central nervous system can lead to seizures. Diseases that decrease or interfere with PTH and vitamin D production or action, increase serum phosphorus concentration, or drain calcium reserves can be associated with hypocalcemia (Table 18-7).

Asymptomatic hypocalcemia is common in dogs.[69] It is less common in cats. Hypoalbuminemia is the most common cause of hypocalcemia. This is due to a decrease in the protein-bound portion of serum calcium. Despite the low total serum calcium the serum ionized calcium remains unchanged and clinical signs are absent. Abnormalities in serum calcium due to decreased protein or albumin concentrations can be adjusted for by using one of the following formulas[69,70]:

Adjusted Ca (mg/dl) = measured Ca (mg/dl)
$$- \text{albumin (g/dl)} + 3.5$$

Adjusted Ca (mg/dl) = measured Ca (mg/dl)
$$- [0.4 \times \text{total protein (g/dl)}] + 3.3$$

Renal failure is a common cause of hypocalcemia in dogs.[70] Hyperphosphatemia, decreased activation of 25-hydroxyvitamin D_3, peripheral PTH resistance, increased renal calcium excretion, and decreased intestinal absorption of calcium contribute to the development of hypocalcemia. Clinical signs of hypocalcemia occur less frequently with renal failure than with other causes of hypocalcemia. The metabolic acidosis that accompanies renal disease increases the serum ionized fraction of calcium.

Primary hypoparathyroidism is an uncommon cause of hypocalcemia.[69,71-73] Decreased PTH production associated with immune-mediated destruction of the parathyroid glands is thought to exist in most naturally occurring cases. Iatrogenic hypoparathyroidism following thyroidectomy is the most common cause of symptomatic hypocalcemia in cats.[74]

Postparturient hypocalcemia (eclampsia) is seen in lactating bitches (and, rarely, queens) and usually occurs during the first 21 days after whelping (range, 20 days prepartum to 45 days postpar-

Table 18-7 Causes of hypocalcemia

Hypoalbuminemia (ionized calcium normal)
Eclampsia
Hypoparathyroidism
  Iatrogenic
  Post-bilateral thyroidectomy
  Post-removal of a parathyroid adenoma
  Lymphocytic parathyroiditis
  Idiopathic parathyroid atrophy
  Parathyroid destruction via tumor
  Infarct of a parathyroid adenoma
  Peripheral PTH resistance
  Canine-distemper-virus associated
Chronic renal failure
Acute renal failure
Ethylene glycol toxicity
Urethral obstruction
Acute pancreatitis
Nutritional secondary hyperparathyroidism
Intestinal malabsorption syndromes
Phosphate-containing-enema toxicity
Hypercalcitoninism (medullary carcinoma of the thyroid)
Miscellaneous causes
  Laboratory error
  Transfusion using citrated blood
  Soft-tissue trauma
  Sepsis
  Vitamin D deficiency
  Hypomagnesemia

tum).[75] Hypocalcemia is probably the result of an imbalance between the rates of inflow and outflow from the extracellular calcium pool.

Rapid increases in the serum phosphorus concentration caused by acute renal failure, urethral obstruction, and phosphate-containing enemas can precipitate a hypocalcemic crisis.[69] Binding of available calcium ions and soft-tissue mineralization are important in the pathogenesis. Acute pancreatitis can also lead to binding of calcium in insoluble soaps formed from saponification of peripancreatic fat.[76] Hypocalcemia associated with acute pancreatitis is rarely of clinical significance.

History and physical examination findings

Clinical signs of hypocalcemia include nervousness, mental depression, muscle twitching, tetany, seizures, stiff gait, tachycardia, panting, pyrexia, and face rubbing.[71] Signs usually occur when total serum calcium is less than 6.5 mg/dl. Hyperthermia commonly accompanies the excessive neuromuscular activity associated with sustained tetany or seizure activity.

The history should differentiate eclampsia, enema-induced hyperphosphatemia, or postsurgical hypoparathyroidism. Eclampsia usually is seen in small or medium-sized bitches nursing large litters. Signs occur suddenly, and hyperthermia is usually present. Phosphate intoxication following administration of phosphate enema is more common in cats or small dogs, especially when colonic obstructive disease or renal insufficiency is also present. Hypocalcemia following bilateral thyroidectomy in cats most commonly occurs within 1 to 3 days postoperatively. Hypocalcemia can occur following removal of a functional parathyroid adenoma due to chronic feedback inhibition of the function of remaining parathyroid glands.

Renal disease and primary hypoparathyroidism should be considered when the history and physical examination fail to reveal a cause. Small-breed (toy poodle, miniature schnauzer) adult females and Saint Bernards may be predisposed to primary hypoparathyroidism.[69,72] Clinical signs may be sudden in onset or chronic and intermittent, often being brought on by excitement or stress. Cataracts are occasionally seen as a sequela to hypoparathyroidism in the dog.

Diagnosis

Hypocalcemia should be considered in any animal presented for sudden onset of tetany or seizures. Chronic hypocalcemia is often a serendipitous finding when a routine data base is generated in the diagnostic approach to an animal with a neuromuscular disease. Hypocalcemia should be verified by repeated measurement, especially when consistent clinical signs are lacking. The serum albumin should be assessed when considering the significance of hypocalcemia.

The diagnosis of primary hypoparathyroidism is made by ruling out other causes of hypocalcemia. Azotemia with isosthenuria would be expected with hypocalcemia accompanying renal failure. Hyperphosphatemia is seen with renal failure, urethral obstruction, phosphate-containing-enema administration, and primary hypoparathyroidism. Hypernatremia is commonly associated with phosphate-enema-induced disease. Serum lipase and amylase activities may be increased in pancreatitis or renal failure. Hypomagnesemia has been noted in some dogs with primary hypoparathyroidism; it may be a cause or effect of hypoparathyroidism.

The electrocardiogram can show tachycardia and a prolonged Q-T interval with hypocalcemia.[69] These changes are inconsistent and electrocardiography is insensitive in assessing serum calcium levels.

Measurements of serum immunoreactive parathyroid hormone (iPTH) levels are considered essential for the diagnosis of hypoparathyroidism in humans. The scarcity of reported canine cases in which iPTH has been measured and the concerns about the validity of assays used in dogs makes measurement of iPTH of questionable value at this time. Fortunately, most of the other causes of hypocalcemia can be ruled out by the historical and clinicopathologic data.

Emergency treatment

Hypocalcemic tetany or seizures require immediate intravenous calcium treatment.[73,74,77] Calcium gluconate is preferable to calcium chloride because the former is not irritating if inadvertently administered perivascularly. The initial dose is given to effect, usually 5 to 15 mg/kg of elemental calcium (0.5 to 1.5 ml/kg 10% calcium gluconate), slowly intravenously over a 10- to 30-minute period. The heart rate should be monitored by auscultation or by electrocardiography. If bradycardia or shortening of the Q-T interval occurs, treatment should be temporarily discontinued. A maintenance 10% calcium gluconate intravenous infusion can be given at a rate of 2 ml/kg over each subsequent 6- to 8-hour period. Maintenance calcium infusion is rarely needed when eclampsia is the underlying cause of hypocalcemia. A blood glucose determination should be done, especially if tetany or seizures have been longstanding. Hypoglycemia should be treated with intravenous 50% dextrose solution (1 ml/kg).

Hyperthermia may result from the excessive muscle contraction of hypocalcemic tetany. Cool water soaks and the use of a fan will help decrease body temperature in severe cases. Treatment of the underlying hypocalcemia will usually alleviate any hyperthermia. Hypothermia is a common complication of overzealous attempts to decrease body temperature.

Maintenance therapy

Long-term maintenance treatment with oral calcium and/or vitamin D will be needed in hypoparathyroidism.[71] Oral calcium salts should be dosed according to the elemental calcium content (Table 18-8); 50 to 100 mg of elemental calcium per kilogram per day is recommended (about 500 to 1000 mg/kg per day of calcium gluconate or 400 to 800 mg/kg per day of calcium lactate).[74] Oral vitamin D should be initiated along with the calcium supplementation (Table 18-9). Vitamin D_2 is the least expensive form available but has a slow onset of action as compared with some of the more potent hydroxylated forms of vitamin D. Ideally, the serum calcium should be maintained in the low normal range (8.0 to 9.0 mg/dl). Hypercalcemia is a common problem associated with oversupplementation and can be detrimental (see section on Hypercalcemia, above). Oral calcium

Table 18-8 Commercially available calcium sources

Source	Dosage Forms		Elemental Calcium Content (%)	Elemental Calcium (mg)
Calcium gluconate	Tablet:	325 mg	9.2	30 mg
		500 mg		45 mg
		650 mg		45 mg
		1000 mg		90 mg
Calcium lactate	Tablet:	325 mg	13	42 mg
		650 mg		85 mg
Calcium carbonate	Tablet:	625 mg	40	250 mg
		650 mg		260 mg
		667 mg		267 mg
		750 mg		300 mg
		1250 mg		500 mg
Calcium citrate	Tablet:	950 mg	21	200 mg
Dibasic calcium phosphate	Tablet:	486 mg	23	112 mg
Calcium glubionate	Syrup:	1800 mg/5 ml	6.5	115 mg/5 ml
Cottage cheese		1 tablespoon		25 mg
Macaroni and cheese		1 cup		400 mg
Milk		8 oz		300 mg

Table 18-9 Vitamin D preparations and dosages

Preparation	Relative Potency	Trade Name (Manufacturer)	Dosage Form	Daily Dose*
Vitamin D_2 (ergocalciferol)	1	Calciferol (Schwarz Pharma)	50,000 U tablet	Initial: 4000-6000 U/kg per day
			500,000 U/ml injection	Maintenance: 1000-2000 U/kg per day
		Calciferol drops (Schwartz Pharma)	8,000 U/ml	
		Drisdol (Sterling)	50,000 U capsule	
		Vitamin D (various)	50,000 U capsule	
		Deltalin (Lilly)	50,000 U capsule	
Vitamin D_3 (cholecalciferol)	1	Vitamin D_3 (Freeda)	1,000 U capsule	
		Delta D (Freeda)	400 U tablet	
Calcifediol (25-hydroxycholecalciferol)	15	Calderol (Organon)	20 μg capsule	
			50 μg capsule	
Calcitriol (1,25-dihydroxycholecalciferol)	2000	Rocaltrol (Hoffmann-LaRoche)	0.25 μg	0.03-0.06 μg/kg per day
			0.5 μg	
Dihydrotachysterol	3	DHT (Roxane)	0.125 mg tablet	Initial: 0.02-0.03 mg/kg per day
			0.2 mg tablet	
			0.4 mg tablet	Maintenance: 0.01-0.02 mg/kg per day every 24-48 hours
			0.2 mg/ml solution	
			0.2 mg/5 ml solution	
		Hytakerol (Sterling)	0.125 mg capsule	
			0.25 mg/ml solution	

*Adjustments should be made in each animal based on frequent serum calcium monitoring. (Serum calcium concentrations should be maintained in the low normal range.)

and vitamin D should be decreased if hypercalcemia is noted. Animals fed a high-quality pet-food diet can usually be weaned off calcium supplementation over the first 4 to 6 months, but continued vitamin D supplementation will be needed.

Iatrogenically induced hypoparathyroidism

Postsurgical hypoparathyroidism is a common occurrence in cats following bilateral thyroidectomy (10% to 35% prevalence).[69] Ablation of parathyroid tissue and disruption of the parathyroid blood supply due to dissection are the primary reasons for development of this complication. In addition, removal of a functional parathyroid adenoma of-

ten results in postoperative hypocalcemia due to atrophy of the remaining parathyroid glands associated with the chronic hypercalcemia. Serum calcium levels should be measured following surgery until stable values are obtained.

Animals should be monitored closely for 24 to 72 hours postoperatively for signs of hypocalcemia. Cats frequently have slightly low serum calcium values the day after thyroidectomy. In cats especially, severe clinical signs may not be seen despite low serum calcium concentrations unless the patient is stressed. Symptomatic hypocalcemia should be treated immediately. Cats with serum calcium levels less than 6.5 mg/dl should be

Table 18-10 Clinicopathologic findings associated with hepatoencephalopathy

		Comment
Hematology		
Packed cell volume (%)	Normal or low	Microcytosis is a consistent finding
Mean corpuscular volume	Usually low	but is not always associated with
Mean corpuscular hemoglobin concentration	Normal	anemia; the cause is unknown
White blood cell count	Usually normal	
Serum chemistry		
Albumin	Low or normal	Severe liver dysfunction is necessary
Total protein	Low or normal	before albumin values decline
BUN	Usually low	Dehydration or gastrointestinal bleeding may falsely elevate the blood urea nitrogen (bringing it into the normal range)
Transaminases	Normal or high	Values are often normal with portosystemic shunts or cirrhosis; serum enzymes activities are markedly increased in acute hepatitis or toxic hepatocellular degeneration
Alkaline phosphatase	Normal or high	Increased if cholestasis or sepsis is
Total bilirubin	Usually normal	present
Glucose	Variable	Hypoglycemia potentiates hepatoencephalopathy; hyperglycemia may occur in cats with hepatic lipidosis
Potassium	Low to normal	Hypokalemia will enhance hepatoencephalopathy
Bile acids	Markedly increased	
Ammonia	Increased	Fasting blood ammonia values may be normal, but results of ammonia tolerance testing will be abnormal
Coagulogram		
One stage prothrombin time	Normal to prolonged	The liver is involved in the synthesis
Activated partial thromboplastin time	Normal to prolonged	of clotting factors (I, II, V, VII, IX, X); a coagulogram should be
Activated clotting time	Normal to prolonged	performed before considering a liver biopsy or laparotomy
Urinalysis	Ammonium biurate crystals	Most frequently seen with portosystemic shunts
Cerebrospinal fluid	Normal	
Electroencephalogram	Slowing of cerebral electrical activity	This is a nonspecific finding compatible with metabolically induced central nervous system disease

Table 18-11 Predisposing factors to development of hepatic encephalopathy or coma

Factor	Comments
High-protein meal	The patient should be kept npo until the initial CNS signs have been controlled
Gastrointestinal bleeding	Bleeding secondary to ulceration should be treated with cimetidine (5-10 mg/kg po, IV qid) and sucralfate (0.5-1 g po tid); bleeding from concurrent parasitism, coagulopathy, or gastrointestinal neoplasia should be considered
Blood transfusion	Fresh whole blood should be used; stored blood contains high levels of ammonia
Azotemia	Fluid therapy should be instituted to correct azotemia; volume expansion will improve renal and hepatic blood flow and dilute circulating toxins
Systemic infections	Liver failure predisposes animals to systemic infections; the catabolic state induced will contribute to the endogenous nitrogen load
Sedatives, tranquilizers, anesthetics, organophosphates	Recommended doses of CNS depressant drugs are often poorly tolerated (especially acepromazine); diazepam at half the normally recommended dose can be used to control seizures
Diuretics	Care should be used when using diuretics to treat concurrent ascites; hypokalemia and azotemia induced by overzealous diuretic therapy can induce hepatic coma
Methionine	Methionine is converted to mercaptans by gut bacteria; its use in liver failure should be avoided
Arginine deficiency	Arginine is an essential amino acid for cats; dietary therapy in cats must include enough protein to meet this requirement

npo = nothing by mouth; CNS = central nervous system; po = orally; IV = intravenously; qid = four times a day; tid = three times a day.

placed on a maintenance calcium infusion (2 ml 10% calcium gluconate/kg every 6 to 8 hours). Oral calcium and vitamin D supplementation should be instituted in these cases and the calcium-containing infusion should be discontinued when the serum calcium is maintained within the low normal range. Dihydrotachysterol is recommended over vitamin D_2 because of its ability to raise serum calcium concentrations more rapidly.

HEPATIC ENCEPHALOPATHY
Pathophysiology

Hepatic encephalopathy is a complex metabolic disturbance resulting from decreased hepatic clearance of toxins produced by resident gastrointestinal microflora.[78] Increased levels of these toxic metabolites within the central nervous system cause the neurologic disturbances that characterize this syndrome.[78,79] Congenital portosystemic shunts and end-stage liver disease resulting in acquired portosystemic collateral circulation are the most common causes of hepatic encephalopathy.[79] Acute fulminant liver failure due to toxic or infectious causes and congenital deficiency of certain liver enzymes necessary to convert ammonia to urea are examples of less common causes.

Ammonia (derived from bacterial hydrolysis of urea and deamination of ingested and mucosal derived proteins), mercaptans, short-chain fatty acids, skatols, indoles, and gamma-aminobutyric acid are bacterial bioproducts absorbed from the gut that are potential mediators of hepatic encephalopathy. Increased serum concentrations of aromatic amino acids (phenylalanine, tyrosine; from decreased hepatic clearance) and decreased branched chain amino acid (valine, leucine, isoleucine; from increased utilization for energy) concentrations result in the production of false neurotransmitters that interfere with normal synaptic impulse transmission.[78-80] The central nervous system dysfunction initiated by these substances is not completely understood. The mechanisms appear to involve metabolic rather than structural alterations in the central nervous system. The effects are usually reversible, provided normal hepatic function or portal blood flow is restored.

History and physical examination findings and diagnosis

The clinical signs of hepatic encephalopathy are generally paroxysmal and variable in character. The primary neurologic abnormalities encountered include mental depression, stupor,

Table 18-12 Therapy of hepatic encephalopathy

	Product and Dosage	Comment
General supportive care		
Fluid therapy	0.9 or 0.45% sodium chloride + 2.5% dextrose	0.45% should be used after volume expansion to prevent sodium and water retention; lactated Ringer's solution should be avoided
Acid-base	Sodium bicarbonate	Sodium bicarbonate should be used if severe acidosis is present; alkalosis increases ammonia penetration across the blood-brain barrier so overzealous sodium bicarbonate administration should be avoided
Hypokalemia	Potassium chloride	Supplementation should be based on serum potassium values
Decreasing gastrointestinal toxin production and absorption		
Enemas	Warm water every 6 hours or Lactulose (20%) 50-200 ml total or Betadine solution diluted 1:10 to 1:100 with warm water	Enemas are important during treatment of hepatic coma
Antibiotics	Neomycin 20 mg/kg po bid/tid or Metronidazole 30-60 mg/kg po divided bid/tid	
Lactulose	5-30 ml po bid/qid so that 2-3 soft stools per day are maintained	This dissacharide is cleaved in the colon; the acidic environment created decreases the colonic microbial population and traps NH_4^+ within the bowel lumen. It also has an osmotic cathartic effect
Hepatic seizures		
Glucose	50% dextrose, 1 ml/kg IV	Dextrose should be used initially; careful use of diazepam is indicated if dextrose alone is insufficient to control the seizures; barbiturates should be avoided
Diazepam	0.25-0.5 mg/kg IV in increments of 2.5-5 mg; give to effect	

po = orally; bid = twice a day; tid = three times a day; qid = four times a day; IV = intravenously.

coma, behavioral abnormalities, ataxia, circling, pacing, panting, head pressing, amaurosis, and seizures.[78,79,81] Hypersalivation is a prominent sign in cats with hepatic encephalopathy.[82,83] Clinical signs may appear to worsen after a meal. Animals with hepatic encephalopathy may have a history of sensitivity to tranquilizers,

sedatives, anticonvulsants, or anesthetic agents.

Clinical signs related to the underlying hepatic disease (anorexia, weight loss, vomiting, diarrhea, polyuria, polydipsia, ascites, abdominal pain, icterus) might be observed.

Neurologic signs accompanying clinicopathologic evidence of liver disease is suggestive of hepatic encephalopathy (Table 18-10).[79,84,85] Patients with portosystemic shunts and end-stage liver disease may have normal serum alanine aminotransferase and alkaline phosphatase activities.[78,84-86] Measurement of serum bile acids (fasting and 2-hour postprandial) reveals moderately to markedly elevated levels in hepatic encephalopathy.[85] Sulfobromophthalein sodium retention is increased in acquired liver disease, but may be normal in portosystemic shunt.[78,87] Elevated fasting blood ammonia levels or a 3- to 4-fold increase in blood ammonia levels 30 minutes after an oral ammonium chloride challenge (100 mg/kg) confirms hepatic encephalopathy.[78,87] A liver biopsy is often necessary to determine the underlying hepatic disease. Contrast radiography, ultrasonography, or scintigraphy of the portal vasculature is necessary to demonstrate congenital portosystemic shunts.

Treatment

Treatment of life-threatening hepatic encephalopathy will frequently be required before a specific diagnosis can be obtained. Treatment requires aggressive attempts to lower blood levels of ammonia and other toxins. Diagnosis and correction of predisposing factors (Table 18-11), bowel "cleansing," control of the gastrointestinal microbial population, and supportive fluid therapy (Table 18-12) are important treatment considerations during short- and long-term treatment of animals with hepatic encephalopathy.[78-81,85,88]

Restriction of dietary protein and increasing dietary carbohydrate content are important factors in long-term treatment of animals with hepatic encephalopathy.[80] A protein intake of 1.4 to 2.2 g/kg per day is recommended in dogs with hepatic encephalopathy. Red meat should be avoided. Milk, cheese, and vegetable proteins are best used in diet formulations. Dietary fat should be restricted to minimize the production of short-chain fatty acids by colonic microflora. Frequent small feedings are recommended. Commercial protein-restricted prescription diets (K/D, Hills) are an alternative to home-made diets. An ample supply of dietary protein and arginine may be more important than protein restriction in resolving hepatic encephalopathy in cats with hepatic lipidosis.[83]

REFERENCES

1. Kreisberg RA. Diabetic ketoacidosis: New concepts and trends in pathogenesis and treatment. Ann Intern Med 1978;88:681-695.
2. Adrogue HJ, Wilson H, Boyd III AE, Suki WN, Eknoyan G. Plasma acid-base patterns in diabetic ketoacidosis. N Engl J Med 1982;307:1603-1610.
3. Chastain CB. Intensive care of dogs and cats with diabetic ketoacidosis. J Am Vet Med Assoc 1981;179:972-978.
4. Chastain CB, Nichols CE. Low-dose intramuscular insulin therapy for diabetic ketoacidosis in dogs. J Am Vet Med Assoc 1981;178:561-564.
5. Morgan RV. Endocrine and metabolic emergencies—Part I. Compend Contin Educ Pract Vet 1982;4:755-760.
6. Schall WD, Cornelius LM. Diabetic ketoacidosis. In Kirk RW, ed. Current veterinary therapy VII—Small animal practice. Philadelphia: WB Saunders, 1980;1016-1019.
7. Morris LR, McGee JA, Kitabchi AE. Correlation between plasma and urine glucose in diabetes. Ann Intern Med 1981;94(Part 1):469-471.
8. Arieff AI, Kleeman CR. Studies on mechanisms of cerebral edema in diabetic comas—effects of hyperglycemia and rapid lowering of plasma glucose in normal rabbits. J Clin Invest 1973;52:571-583.
9. Joffe BI, Krut LH, Goldberg RB, Sextel HC. Pathogenesis of nonketotic hyperosmolar diabetic coma. Lancet 1975;1:1069-1071.
10. Gerich JE, Martin MM, Recant L. Clinical and metabolic characteristics of hyperosmolar nonketotic coma. Diabetes 1971;20:228-238.
11. Kozak GP, Rolla AR. Diabetic comas. In Kozak GP, ed. Clinical diabetes mellitus. Philadelphia: WB Saunders, 1982;109-145.
12. Maccario M. Neurological dysfunction associated with nonketotic hyperglycemia. Arch Neurol 1968;19:525-534.
13. Podolsky S. Hyperosmolar nonketotic coma in the elderly diabetic. Med Clin North Am 1978;62:815-828.
14. Schaer M. Diabetic hyperosmolar nonketotic syndrome in a cat. J Am Anim Hosp Assoc 1975;11:42-46.
15. Schaer M, Scott R, Wilkens R, Kay W, Calvert C, Wolland M. Hyperosmolar syndrome in the non-ketoacidotic diabetic dog. J Am Anim Hosp Assoc 1974;10:357-361.
16. Leifer CE, Peterson ME, Matus RE. Insulin-secreting tumor: diagnosis and medical and surgical management in 55 dogs. J Am Vet Med Assoc 1986;188:60-64.
17. Breitschwerdt EB, Loar AS, Hribernik TN, McGrath RK. Hypoglycemia in four dogs with sepsis. J Am Vet Med Assoc 1981;178:1072-1076.
18. Miller S, Wallace RJ Jr, Musher DM, Septimus EJ, Kohl S, Baughn RE. Hypoglycemia as a manifestation of sepsis. Am J Med 1980;68:649-654.
19. Gorden P, Hendricks CM, Kahn CR, Megyesi K, Roth J. Hypoglycemia associated with non-islet-cell tumor and insulin-like growth factors. N Engl J Med 1981;305:1452-1455.
20. Leifer CE, Peterson ME, Matus RE, Patnaik AK. Hypoglycemia associated with nonislet cell tumor in 13 dogs. J Am Vet Med Assoc 1985;186:53-58.
21. Atkins CE. Disorders of glucose homeostasis in neonatal and juvenile dogs: hypoglycemia—Part I. Compend Contin Educ Pract Vet 1984;6:197-204.
22. Atkins CE. Disorders of glucose homeostasis in neonatal and juvenile dogs: hypoglycemia—Part II. Compend Contin Educ Pract Vet 1984;6:353-364.
23. Larner J. Insulin and oral hypoglycemic drugs; glucagon. In Gilman AG, Goodman LS, Rall TW, Murad F, eds. Goodman and Gilman's the pharmacological basis of therapeutics, ed. 7. New York: MacMillan, 1985;1490-1512.
24. Mehlhaff CJ, Peterson ME, Patnaik AK, Carrillo JM. Insulin-producing islet cell neoplasms: Surgical considerations and general management in 35 dogs. J Am Anim Hosp Assoc 1985;21:607-612.
25. Service FJ, Dale AJ, Elveback LR, Jiang N. Insulinoma—clinical and diagnostic features of 60 consecutive cases. Mayo Clin Proc 1976;51:417-429.
26. Blum I, Doron M, Laron Z, Atsmon A. Prevention of hypoglycemic attacks by propranolol in a patient suffering from insulinoma. Diabetes 1975;24:535-537.

27. Knopp RH, Sheinin JC, Freinkel N. Diphenylhydantoin and an insulin-secreting islet adenoma. Arch Intern Med 1972;130:904-908.

28. Nelson RW, Foodman MS. Medical management of canine hyperinsulinism. J Am Vet Med Assoc 1985;187:78-82.

29. Willard MD, Schall WD, McCaw DE, Nachreiner RF. Canine hypoadrenocorticism: Report of 37 cases and review of 39 previously reported cases. J Am Vet Med Assoc 1982;180:59-62.

30. Schaer M. Hypoadrenocorticism. In Kirk RW, ed. Current veterinary therapy—small animal practice VII. Philadelphia: WB Saunders, 1980;983-988.

31. Schrader LA. Hypoadrenocorticism. In Kirk RW, ed. Current veterinary therapy—Small animal practice IX. Philadelphia: WB Saunders, 1986;972-977.

32. Ettinger PO, Regan TJ, Oldewurtel HA. Hyperkalemia, cardiac conduction and the electrocardiogram: A review. Am Heart J 1974;88:360-371.

33. Tilley LP. Essentials of canine and feline electrocardiography. St Louis: CV Mosby, 1979;158.

34. Feldman EC, Tyrrell JB, Bohannon NV. The synthetic ACTH stimulation test and measurement of endogenous plasma ACTH levels: Useful diagnostic indicators for adrenal disease in dogs. J Am Anim Hosp Assoc 1978;14:524-531.

35. Gonzales RB. Selected emergency endocrinologic problems. In Schwartz GR, Safar P, Stone JH, Storey PB, Wagner DK, eds. Principles and practice of emergency medicine. Philadelphia: WB Saunders, 1986;1085-1093.

36. Bastenie PA, Bonnyns M, Vahaelst L. Natural history of primary myxedema. Am J Med 1985;79:91-100.

37. Bowen D, Schaer M, Riley W: Autoimmune polyglandular syndrome in a dog: A case report. J Am Anim Hosp Assoc 1986;22:649-654.

38. Gonzales RB: Selected emergency endocrinologic problems. In Schwartz GR, Safar P, Stone JH, Storey PB, Wagner DK, eds. Principles and practice of emergency medicine, ed. 2. Philadelphia: WB Saunders, 1986;1087-1089.

39. Saltman RJ. Thyroid and adrenal disorders. In Orland MJ, Saltman RJ, eds. Manual of medical therapeutics, ed. 25. Boston: Little, Brown, 1986;339-340.

40. Rosychuk R. Management of hypothyroidism. In Kirk RW, ed. Current veterinary therapy VIII—small animal practice. Philadelphia: WB Saunders, 1983;869-876.

41. Peterson ME, Turrel JM. Feline hyperthyroidism. In Kirk RW, ed. Current veterinary therapy IX—small animal practice. Philadelphia: WB Saunders, 1986;1026-1033.

42. Bond BR. Hyperthyroid heart disease in cats. In Kirk RW, ed. Current veterinary therapy IX—small animal practice. Philadelphia: WB Saunders, 1986;399-402.

43. Liu SL, Peterson ME, Fox PR. Hypertrophic cardiomyopathy and hyperthyroidism in the cat. J Am Vet Med Assoc 1984;185:52-57.

44. Culpepper RM, Hebert SC, Andreoli TE. The posterior pituitary and water metabolism. In Wilson JD, Foster DW, eds. Williams textbook of endocrinology. Philadelphia: WB Saunders, 1985;614-652.

45. Feig PU. Hypernatremia and hypertonic syndromes. Med Clin North Am 1981;65:271-290.

46. Snyder NA, Feigal DW, Arieff AI. Hypernatremia in elderly patients. Ann Intern Med 1987;107:309-319.

47. Windus DW. Fluid and electrolyte management. In Orland MJ, Saltman RJ, eds. Manual of medical therapeutics. Boston: Little, Brown, 1986;46-47.

48. Schrier RW, Berl T. Disorders of water metabolism. In Schrier RW, ed. Renal and electrolyte disorders, ed. 2. Boston: Little, Brown, 1976;32-38.

49. Feldman EC, Nelson RW, eds. Canine and feline endocrinology and reproduction. Philadelphia: WB Saunders, 1987;1-26.

50. Landsberg L, Young JB. Catecholamines and the adrenal medulla. In Wilson JD, Foster DW, eds. Williams textbook of endocrinology, ed. 7. Philadelphia: WB Saunders, 1985;891-965.

51. Schaer M. Pheochromocytoma in a dog: a case report. J Am Anim Hosp Assoc 1980;16:583-587.

52. Twedt DC: Pheochromocytoma in the canine. J Am Anim Hosp Assoc 1975;11:491-496.

53. Wheeler SL. Canine pheochromocytoma. In Kirk RW, ed. Current veterinary therapy IX—small animal practice. Philadelphia: WB Saunders, 1986;977-981.

54. Bravo EL, Tarazi RC, Gifford RW, Stewart BH. Circulating and urinary catecholamines in pheochromocytoma—diagnostic and pathophysiologic implications. N Engl J Med 1979;301:682-686.

55. Feldman EC, Nelson RW. The parathyroid gland-primary hyperparathyroidism. In Feldman EC, Nelson RW, eds. Canine and feline endocrinology and reproduction. Philadelphia: WB Saunders, 1987;328-356.

56. Berger B, Feldman E. Primary hyperparathyroidism in dogs: 21 cases (1976-1986). J Am Vet Med Assoc 1987;191:350-356.

57. Dow SW, Legendre AM, Stiff M, Green C. Hypercalcemia associated with blastomycosis in dogs. J Am Vet Med Assoc 1986;188:706-709.

58. Finco DR. Interpretation of serum calcium concentration in the dog. Compend Contin Educ Pract Vet 1983;5:778-786.

59. Finco DR, Rowland GN. Hypercalcemia secondary to chronic renal failure in the dog: a report of four cases. J Am Vet Med Assoc 1978;173:990-994.

60. Hause WR, Stevenson S, Meuten DJ, Capen CC. Pseudohyperparathyroidism associated with adenocarcinomas of anal sac origin in four dogs. J Am Anim Hosp Assoc 1981;17:373-379.

61. Meuten DJ, Capen CC, Kociba GJ, Chew DJ. Hypercalcemia associated with malignancy in dogs. Proc Sixth Kal Kan Symp 1982;6:95-100.

62. Mundy GR, Ibbotson KJ, D'Souza SM, et al. The hypercalcemia of cancer: clinical implications and pathogenic mechanisms. N Engl J Med 1984;310:1718-1727.

63. Troy GC, Forrester D, Cockburn C, et al. *Heterobilharzia americana* infection and hypercalcemia in a dog: a case report. J Am Anim Hosp Assoc 1987;23:35-40.

64. Strewler GJ, Nissenson RA. Nonparathyroid hypercalcemia. Adv Intern Med 1987;32:235-258.

65. Meuten DJ. Hypercalcemia. Vet Clin North Am 1984;14:891-910.

66. Capen CC. Diagnosis and management of parathyroid diseases in animals. Proc Sixth Kal Kan Symp 1982;6:67-79.

67. Kruger JM, Osborne CA, Polzin DJ. Treatment of hypercalcemia. In Kirk RW, ed. Current veterinary therapy IX. Philadelphia: WB Saunders, 1986;75-94.

68. Bilezikian JP. The medical management of primary hyperparathyroidism. Ann Intern Med 1982;96:198-202.

69. Feldman EC, Nelson RW. Hypocalcemia-hypoparathyroidism. In Feldman EC, Nelson RW, eds. Canine and feline endocrinology and reproduction. Philadelphia: WB Saunders, 1987;357-374.

70. Chew DJ, Meuten DJ. Disorders of calcium and phosphorus metabolism. Vet Clin North Am 1982;12:411-438.

71. Bruyette DS, Feldman EC. Primary hypoparathyroidism in the dog. J Vet Intern Med 1988;2:7-14.

72. Jones BR, Alley MR. Primary idiopathic hypoparathyroidism in St. Bernard dogs. N Z Vet J 1985;33:94-97.

73. Peterson ME. Hypoparathyroidism. In Kirk RW, ed. Current veterinary therapy IX. Philadelphia: WB Saunders, 1986;1039-1045.

74. Peterson ME. Treatment of canine and feline hypoparathyroidism. J Am Vet Med Assoc 1982;181:1434-1436.

75. Martin SL, Capen CC. Puerperal tetany. In Kirk RW, ed. Current veterinary therapy VII. Philadelphia: WB Saunders, 1980;1027-1029.

76. Schaer M. A clinicopathologic survey of acute pancreatitis in 30 dogs and 5 cats. J Am Anim Hosp Assoc 1979;15:681-687.

77. Russo EA, Lees GE. Treatment of hypocalcemia. In Kirk RW, ed. Current veterinary therapy IX. Philadelphia: WB Saunders, 1986;91-94.

78. Hardy RM. Diseases of the liver. In Ettinger SJ, ed. Textbook of veterinary internal medicine. Philadelphia: WB Saunders, 1983;1372-1434.

79. Sherding RG. Hepatic encephalopathy in the dog. Compend Contin Educ Pract Vet 1979;1:55-63.

80. Strombeck DR, Schaeffer MC, Rogers QR. Dietary therapy for dogs with chronic hepatic insufficiency. In Kirk RW, ed. Current veterinary therapy VIII—small animal practice. Philadelphia: WB Saunders, 1983;817-821.

81. Drazner FH. Hepatic encephalopathy in the dog. In Kirk RW, ed. Current veterinary therapy VIII—small animal practice. Philadelphia: WB Saunders, 1983;829-834.

82. Scavelli TD, Hornbuckle WE, Roth L, et al. Portosystemic shunts in cats: Seven cases (1976-1984). J Am Vet Med Assoc 1986;189:317-325.

83. Zawie DA, Garvey MS. Feline hepatic disease. Vet Clin North Am 1984;14:1201-1230.

84. Meyer DJ, Burrows CF. The liver part II. Biochemical diagnosis of hepatobiliary disorders in the dog. Compend Contin Educ Pract Vet 1982;4:706-714.

85. Twedt DC, ed. Symposium on liver diseases. Vet Clin North Am 1985;15:1.

86. Griffiths GL, Lumsden JH, Valli VEO. Hematologic and biochemical changes in dogs with portosystemic shunts. J Am Anim Hosp Assoc 1981;17:705-710.

87. Meyer DJ. The liver, part I. Biochemical tests for the evaluation of the hepatobiliary system. Compend Contin Educ Pract Vet 1982;4:663-673.

88. Johnson S. Medical emergencies of the digestive tract and abdomen. Contemp Issues Small Anim Pract 1985;1:213-254.

19 Ocular Emergencies

Alan Bachrach, Jr.

An ocular emergency is defined as any condition causing severe ocular pain or deformity or that threatens, or has already caused, loss of vision. Frequently, ocular emergencies occur secondarily to generalized trauma, and these ocular injuries are not often detected or treated immediately.

When clients call concerning a possible ophthalmic emergency, they should be advised to seek immediate veterinary evaluation and treatment. In the event of proptosis, the client should be instructed to keep the eye moist with a dampened cloth. Immediate irrigation is indicated following exposure of the eye to an irritating or caustic substance, as the degree of ocular damage is directly proportional to the length of time before neutralization of the chemical irritant.

ASSESSMENT OF OCULAR INJURIES
Anamnesis

As with emergencies involving other organ systems, it is important to obtain as complete a history as possible. The time of the onset and progression of the injury/disease should be noted, as well as the existence of prior ophthalmic problems. Was there a known exposure to a chemical irritant? Was there any indication of blunt or penetrating trauma? Are there other clinical signs present suggesting systemic disease; e.g., polydipsia and polyuria, as with diabetes mellitus?

Examination

Ocular examinations are best performed in a quiet room that can be darkened. Initially, the animal should be observed from a distance of several feet. This procedure is helpful in the evaluation of facial contour and symmetry. Facial hemorrhage or edema, muscle palsy, and ptosis, as well as the presence of a conjugate gaze, may be noted. The latter is the use of both eyes as a functional pair in the process of appropriately observing a visual stimulus. The position of the globe within the orbit should be observed. With exophthalmos, there may be a concomitant deviation of gaze, prolapse of the membrana nictitans, exposure keratitis and pain on attempting to open the mouth.

The orbital margins should be palpated for the presence of fractures, subcutaneous emphysema, edema, or pain. Subcutaneous emphysema may be indicative of a fracture permitting communication with the nasal cavity and/or a sinus. It is important to examine all ocular and adnexal structures, as the animal's condition permits.

The box below lists the requisite instruments and drugs for use in examination of ocular and adnexal structures.

INSTRUMENTS AND DRUGS NEEDED TO EXAMINE OCULAR AND ADNEXAL STRUCTURES

Penlight
Magnifying loupe
Direct ophthalmoscope or indirect ophthalmoscopic lens
Tissue forceps
Fine (conjunctival or corneal) forceps
Strabismus (eye muscle) hook or eyelid retractor
Eyelid speculum
Lacrimal cannula
Tonometer
Topical anesthetic; e.g., 0.5% proparacaine hydrochloride
Short-acting mydriatic; e.g., 1% tropicamide
Sterile eye wash solution
Fluorescein-impregnated sterile strips
Schirmer tear test strips

It is important to ascertain whether or not an animal is sighted. A simple method of evaluating vision is to observe if an animal follows a cotton ball dropped in front of each eye. The "menace reflex or reaction" also provides information regarding the presence of vision. The animal should retract the globe and blink in response to a threatening gesture, provided that cranial nerves II, VI, and VII are intact. Efferent responses induced by stimulation of tactile hairs may provide a false positive reaction, however. Observation of the animal in a "strange environment" is usually sufficient for determining the presence of vision. An attempt may be made to blindfold each eye if a unilateral visual deficit is suspected. It is helpful to occlude the blind eye first, and then to observe any difference when the sighted eye is covered. The animal will frequently tolerate bandaging of the blind eye.

GLOBE AND ORBIT
Proptosis

Proptosis (forward displacement of the globe from the orbit) is common in canine brachycephalic breeds due to the shallow orbit, associated exophthalmos and enlarged interpalpebral fissure (Fig. 19-1). Proptosis in these breeds can also be associated with aggressive restraint of the animal, and thus, care must be exercised in this regard.

Long duration of the proptosis and the persistence of a dilated pupil following replacement of the globe into the orbit, connotes a poor prognosis for preservation of vision.

Entrapment of the eyelids behind the globe, as well as retrobulbar hemorrhage and edema, prevents easy replacement of the globe into the orbit. Replacement is preferably performed under general anesthesia. Application of a sterile lubricant, e.g., saline, is helpful in decreasing further damage to the globe. Eye muscle hooks can be used to pull the eyelids out and away from the globe at the medial canthus (Fig. 19-2). This manipulation is followed by the application of gentle pressure to the globe. A lateral canthotomy may be needed to facilitate replacement of the globe; however, this procedure is frequently not necessary. Following replacement of the globe, a temporary tarsorrhaphy is used to keep the eye in the orbit. Posttraumatic lagophthalmos (inability to close the eyelids completely) is another indication for performing a tarsorrhaphy.

The procedure is performed as follows:

1. Two sections of a flat, soft, pliable material (rubber band) are cut to the length of the eyelids. These bands are to be used to prevent pressure necrosis of the thin skin of the eyelid by the suture.
2. Nonabsorbable suture (4-0) is placed through the rubber band and halfway through the superior or inferior eyelid, 6 to 8 mm from the free margin (edge of the eyelid).
3. The suture exits from a Meibomian duct opening on the free margin (edge) of the superior or inferior eyelid.
4. The suture needle is then placed into the free margin on the inferior or superior eyelid and exits the skin surface 6 to 8 mm from the free margin.

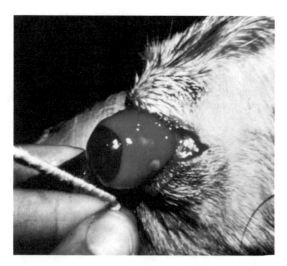

Fig. 19-1 Traumatic proptosis of left globe. (Courtesy of Dr. Milton Wyman.)

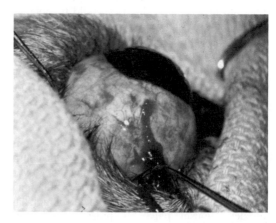

Fig. 19-2 Replacement of a globe with the use of an eye muscle hook.

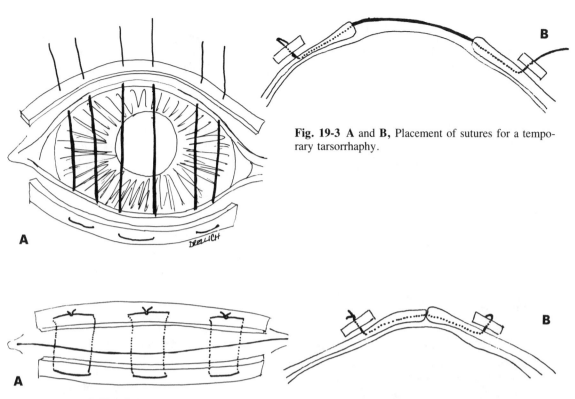

Fig. 19-3 **A** and **B,** Placement of sutures for a temporary tarsorrhaphy.

Fig 19-4. **A** and **B,** Completed temporary tarsorrhaphy with sutures knotted.

5. The suture needle is passed through a second rubber band placed on the inferior or superior eyelid.
6. The process of suture passage is reversed, maintaining equal distance between all structures through which the needle and suture pass (Fig. 19-3).
7. At least three horizontal mattress sutures are preplaced and then tied. (An opening should be left at the medial canthus to permit instillation of medication.) Sufficient tension should be applied so as to gently evert the eyelid margins, in order to prevent suture material from abrading the cornea (Fig. 19-4).

Postoperative medical treatment. Ice packs (or cold compresses) are used 4 to 6 times daily for the first 24 hours, followed by warm compresses thereafter. These applications are valuable in preventing and reducing accompanying periorbital edema.

Topical medication applied consists of the use of an antibiotic ointment four times a day or solution every 4 hours, in combination with an ocular corticosteroid preparation, if the corneal epithelium is intact. Since anterior uveitis is common with this type of injury, application of a 1% atro-

pine sulfate ointment or solution four times a day is advocated as well. Ointments are preferable to solutions in order to ensure intraocular penetration, with the tarsorrhaphy in place.

The use of an Elizabethan collar may be necessary to prevent additional trauma to the eye.

Complications occurring secondary to traumatic proptosis include the following:

1. Exotropia (lateral deviation of the globe) can be caused by avulsion of the medial rectus muscle. Avulsion of the inferior oblique and inferior rectus muscles may occur as well (Fig. 19-5).
2. Blindness can occur secondary to avulsion or compression of the optic nerve or as a sequel to intraocular damage.
3. Xerophthalmia (drying or desiccation of the eye) is related to the duration of the injury and is common with concomitant cranial nerve VII palsy.
4. Insensitive cornea predisposes the eye to xerophthalmia by inhibiting the blink response and distribution of the precorneal tear film.
5. Exposure keratitis and corneal necrosis occur with desiccation and injury of exposed cornea prior to replacement of a proptosed

globe and with persistent lagophthalmos following replacement of the globe.

6. Intraocular sequelae; including iritis, chorioretinitis, lens luxation, and retinal detachment.

Retrobulbar abscess

Retrobulbar abscesses are more common in hunting dogs, and the history usually includes apparent "anorexia"; i.e., the dog is interested in food, but has marked difficulty in prehension and chewing.

Clinical signs of a retrobulbar abscess include exophthalmos, pain on opening the mouth, incarceration and prolapse of the membrana nictitans, chemosis, conjunctival injection, and occasion-

ally, secondary anterior uveitis or glaucoma (Fig. 19-6). Invariably, there is pain on attempting to open the animal's mouth due to the forward movement of the vertical ramus of the mandible.

The cause of retrobulbar abscess is frequently unknown, but this condition can result from the following:

1. Migration of foreign body from oral cavity,
2. Migration of foreign body from conjunctiva,
3. Dental abscess (last upper molar),
4. Inflammation or neoplasia of zygomatic salivary gland, or
5. Eosinophilic myositis of the medial pterygoid muscles.

Treatment. Examination of the oral cavity of animals with retrobulbar abscess requires administration of analgesia and/or sedation; for treatment, these animals require general anesthesia. Frequently, a swollen, hyperemic area is present in the mouth, just caudal to the last upper molar. This area can initially be aspirated, especially if one anticipates submitting a specimen for microbiologic culture and antibiotic sensitivity testing or for cytologic examination. An incision is necessary to establish drainage ventrally into the mouth. The incision can be enlarged with a curved hemostat, if necessary. However, care should be exercised to avoid penetration of the globe and optic nerve or creation of excessive retrobulbar hemorrhage.

Following incision, drainage, and irrigation, soft compresses are beneficial in reducing periocular swelling. Oral or parenteral administration of a broad-spectrum antibiotic is advised, along with appropriate topical treatment of the affected eye (antibiotic or antibiotic/corticosteroid ointment to be applied four times a day). If there is accompa-

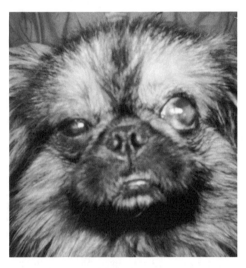

Fig. 19-5 Lateral deviation of left globe associated with extraocular (medial rectus) muscle avulsion accompanying proptosis.

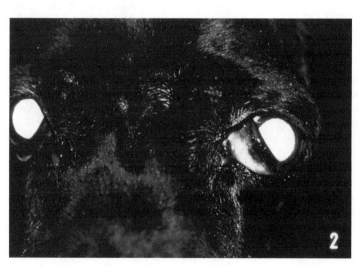

Fig. 19-6 Exophthalmos and incarceration of the membrana nictitans of left eye associated with retrobulbar abscess. (Courtesy of Dr. Milton Wyman.)

nying anterior uveitis, then atropine ointment is also applied to the eye four times a day. A soft diet is recommended until mastication can occur without pain.

Complications. Complications associated with retrobulbar abscesses can include exposure keratitis, anterior uveitis, and blindness. The globe should be observed for lagophthalmos, and if present, frequent topical application of a tear replacement (lubricant) is required. The tear replacement should be instilled at least six to eight times daily.

Perforating and penetrating ocular injuries

Conjunctival, corneal and scleral foreign bodies. Initially, attempts should be made to remove ocular foreign bodies by irrigation, following the instillation of a topical anesthetic. If extraction of the foreign body is required, fine surgical forceps or an ophthalmic needle holder may be used to grasp the foreign body. A small-gauge hypodermic needle (e.g., 25 or 26) can also be used to aid in the removal of a foreign body (Fig. 19-7).

Intraocular foreign bodies. Projectiles (B-B pellets, birdshot) and glass are the most common penetrating ocular foreign bodies of domestic animals. Foreign bodies may lodge in the cornea, anterior chamber, iris, lens, vitreous, or the posterior wall of the eye, with the trajectory dependent on the velocity and the angle of entry. Foreign bodies may pass through the globe and lodge within the orbit. (See section on Corneal Foreign Bodies below.)

Examination. Examination prior to the development of opacities in the clear media is preferable. Visualization of intraocular foreign bodies is enhanced with magnification and good illumination.

Direct visualization may require additional instrumentation; e.g., biomicroscopy (slit-lamp examination), indirect ophthalmoscopy, and gonioscopy. Indirect examination techniques include radiography and ultrasonography.

Surgical removal. The clinician must consider the risks of leaving a penetrating ocular foreign object alone versus the risk of additional injury to the eye associated with surgical intervention. Magnetic foreign bodies and foreign bodies within the anterior chamber are reasonable surgical options. Extremely poor results are frequently obtained with the attempted retrieval of a foreign object from the vitreous cavity.

Sequelae. The outcome associated with an intraocular foreign body is dependent on the chemical composition of the foreign body and its location within the eye. Foreign bodies composed of iron and steel may lead to the development of intraocular siderosis (i.e., the deposition of iron pigments in the cornea, iris, lens, and retina, with associated degenerative changes in these structures), which may culminate in phthisis bulbi or secondary glaucoma.

Copper and its alloys (bronze, brass) may lead to intraocular chalcosis, as manifest by inflammation, hypopyon, and localized abscess formation. The slow release of copper associated with degradation of the foreign body, results in copper deposition in Descemet's membrane and in the anterior lens capsule.

Intraocular foreign objects composed of mercury, aluminum, nickel, zinc, and lead cause intraocular inflammation, resulting in loss of function.

Precious metals, stone, carbon, glass, plaster, and rubber are usually inert within the eye; how-

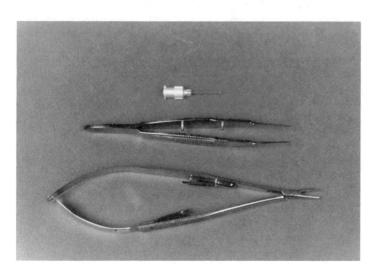

Fig. 19-7 Small-gauge hypodermic needle, ophthalmic surgical forceps, and needle holder, which can be used for removal of conjunctival or corneal foreign bodies.

ever, mechanical trauma associated with the entry or continued presence of these materials, may initiate serious sequelae.

Rupture and collapse of the globe

An attempt should be made to preserve the globe cosmetically, if not functionally, following rupture of an eye (see section on Corneal Laceration below). An enucleation can be performed at a later date, if necessary.

The sequelae of a ruptured, collapsed globe include anterior uveitis, panuveitis, endophthalmitis, panophthalmitis, secondary glaucoma, and phthisis bulbi.

It is important that the anterior chamber be reformed following the suturing of the defect in the cornea and/or sclera. Balanced salt solution (Alcon) or lactated Ringer's solution is injected at the limbus with a 25- or 26-gauge hypodermic needle. The addition of an air bubble allows for compression and aids in reestablishment of the anterior chamber depth. Care must be taken to avoid overdistention of the anterior chamber with fluid and air. The presence of the air bubble is reassuring postoperatively in demonstrating the integrity of the corneal closure.

EYELIDS
Ecchymosis

Bruising of the eyelids is usually the result of blunt trauma, and it develops because of the excellent vascular supply to these structures.

The eye should be thoroughly examined for the presence of associated injury. Treatment consists of application of cold compresses during the first 24 hours and warm compresses thereafter.

Edema

Acute, marked edema of the eyelids may accompany generalized edema of the head attributable to an allergic response (Fig. 19-8). This edema is usually nonpainful, but may be pruritic. The cause is usually unknown, but may be due to an insect or snake bite.

Frequently, the reaction is self-limiting, but treatment involving parenteral administration of a corticosteroid and/or epinephrine, may be required. This treatment is always indicated in the presence of concomitant laryngeal edema and dyspnea.

Lacerations

Eyelid lacerations are commonly associated with automobile injuries and bite wounds. These lacerations should be surgically repaired as soon as possible to preserve function and cosmetic appearance (Fig. 19-9).

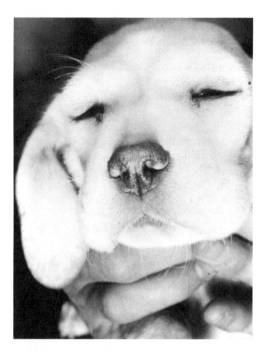

Fig. 19-8 Puppy with acute, generalized facial and eyelid edema.

Routine surgical preparation is performed, with particular attention to gentle cleansing and thorough irrigation of the lacerated tissue and the conjunctival sac. Debridement of wound margins or necrotic tissue is performed with care to remove as little tissue as possible. Minimal debridement is performed in order to minimize wound contracture and eyelid deformity. Complications such as infection, ischemia, and necrosis of the eyelids are seldom a problem because of the excellent vascular supply to the eyelids.

The eyelid is sutured in two layers, with the conjunctiva sutured first. Absorbable suture (6-0 or 7-0) is used for closure of the conjunctiva, with a simple continuous pattern. For lacerations through the eyelid margin, suturing is begun at the apex of the laceration (away from the free eyelid margin). The skin is sutured with 4-0 to 6-0 nonabsorbable suture in a simple continuous pattern beginning at the free eyelid margin. It is imperative that there be good apposition of the pigmented free margin of the eyelid. Suture removal is performed in a minimum of 10 days.

The use of an Elizabethan collar may be necessary to prevent additional trauma to the eye.

CONJUNCTIVA

No ocular emergency exists that involves only the conjunctiva. Involvement of the conjunctiva may

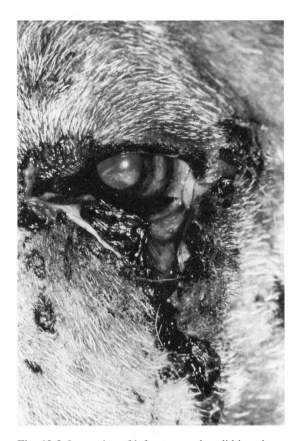

Fig. 19-9 Laceration of inferotemporal eyelid in a dog.

be associated with other ocular or systemic injury/disease.

Lacerations

Conjunctival lacerations usually will accompany eyelid lacerations. Surgical repair is performed so that the suture material is placed in the fibrous (deeper) aspect of the conjunctiva, using 6-0 or 7-0 absorbable suture material in a continuous pattern. A broad-spectrum ocular antibiotic solution or ointment is applied four times a day for 1 week.

Chemosis

Conjunctival edema may occur secondary to trauma to the globe or exposure of the conjunctiva to a topical irritant.

Medical therapy consists of thorough irrigation, if there has been exposure to a topical irritant, and treatment with a topical ocular corticosteroid preparation unless there is an accompanying ulceration of the cornea. If the latter is present, then a topical antibiotic preparation is used.

Subconjunctival hemorrhage

Subconjunctival hemorrhage is of little consequence, but its presence suggests traumatic injury, systemic disease (immune-mediated thrombocytopenia) or exposure to toxins (vitamin K antagonist rodenticides). In animals with subconjunctival hemorrhage it is important that both retinas and the entire animal be evaluated for signs of systemic disease.

Treatment consists of application of cold compresses initially for the primary ocular abnormality, and treatment as indicated for other ocular or systemic manifestations. Subconjunctival hemorrhage will resolve gradually, as the blood is resorbed over 1 to 2 weeks.

CORNEA
Simple superficial corneal ulcer

Superficial corneal ulcers may be caused by corneal contact with a mild irritant (soap), ocular trauma, or the presence of an ocular foreign body (Fig. 19-10). Clinical signs associated with corneal ulceration may include blepharospasm, epiphora, and pawing at the eye.

Fluorescein will be retained in the area of the ulcer and there may be an accompanying secondary anterior uveitis.

A thorough ocular examination is important and should include eversion of the eyelids and membrana nictitans, as foreign bodies may be embedded in the conjunctival lining of these structures. Any concomitant ocular problems should be evaluated and treated appropriately.

A broad-spectrum antibiotic ointment (or solution) is used for topical treatment; e.g., triple antibiotic (bacitracin, neomycin, polymixin B sulfate) every 2 to 6 hours. Topical atropine administration is not indicated unless there is an accompanying anterior uveitis. A collagen shield (Opti-Cor, Pitman-Moore) can be placed on the cornea to enhance epithelialization as well as comfort (Fig. 19-11). The collagen shield can be presoaked in the appropriate antibiotic, and will thus act as a drug delivery system.

Corneal ulcers should be reevaluated within 24 to 48 hours of initiating treatment. Healing generally occurs within 1 to 2 days of medical treatment, and surgical procedures are not indicated in the treatment of uncomplicated corneal ulcers.

Deep stromal ulcer and/or descemetocele

Deep corneal lesions may be secondary to corneal exposure and drying associated with lagophthalmos. This is a common occurrence in the brachycephalic breeds, which are normally exophthalmic due to the presence of a shallow orbit;

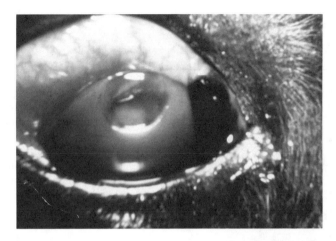

Fig. 19-10. Corneal ulceration of right eye with chemosis, injection of conjunctival vessels, corneal edema, and vascularization secondary to presence previously of an embedded corneal foreign body.

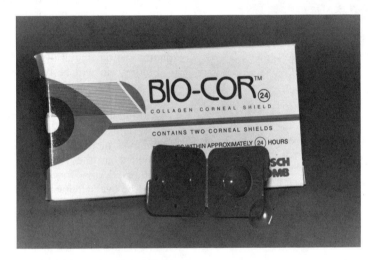

Fig. 19-11. Collagen corneal shield (Opti-Cor; Pitman-Moore).

e.g., Boston terrier, Pekingese, pug. Proptosis may result in cranial nerve V, VI, and VII damage leading to lagophthalmos. The trigeminal nerve (V) transmits sensation from the cornea, while the abducens (VI) innervates the retractor oculi muscle, and the facial nerve (VII) innervates the orbicularis muscle, responsible for the closure of the eyelids. A buphthalmic (enlarged) globe, secondary to glaucoma, will frequently have accompanying lagophthalmos.

Keratoconjunctivitis sicca will often result in deep corneal lesions. Keratoconjunctivitis associated with *Pseudomonas* and other coagulase-positive bacteria can cause stromal necrosis and release of collagenase; effecting a rapid destruction of the cornea (Fig. 19-12).

Paradoxically, animals with deep corneal ulcers

generally have less pain than those with a superficial corneal lesion, unless other accompanying ocular problems are present.

Descemet's membrane will not retain fluorescein, but the margins of the ulcer will, and Descemet's membrane may protrude anteriorly through the stroma.

Treatment involves addressing the cause (e.g., keratoconjunctivitis sicca) when identifiable. A broad-spectrum ocular antibiotic ointment or solution is applied every 1 to 2 hours. The use of collagen shields may be indicated (see section on Simple Superficial Corneal Ulceration above). If a collagenase ulcer is present, gentamicin or tobramycin is preferred for topical therapy.

Frequent topical instillation of an anticollagenase drug such as acetylcysteine (Mucomyst;

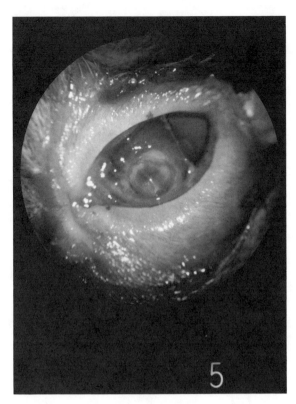

Fig. 19-12 Descemetocele secondary to a collagenase-mediated ulcer that occurred following penetrating ocular trauma in a cat.

Mead Johnson) is imperative for the treatment of suspected collagenase ulcers. The 10% or 20% acetylcysteine solution is diluted by half with a tear replacement, and is administered every hour initially. Aggressive medical treatment usually results in improvement in the condition within 24 to 48 hours.

Surgical treatment of deep corneal ulcers may involve debridement of the margins of the ulcer, if necrotic tissue is present. A conjunctival or membrana nictitans flap may then be performed to enhance healing, as well as to provide comfort and protection (Fig. 19-13).

Corneal laceration without a staphyloma or iris prolapse

Surgical treatment is usually necessary in treating this type of corneal wound. Including an analgesic and tranquilizer in the preanesthetic medication is helpful in ensuring a smooth recovery, and thus in preventing additional trauma to the eye (see Chapter 33). An alternative method would be the intravenous administration of a low dose of

either type of agent at the beginning of the recovery period. Following administration of general anesthesia and routine surgical preparation, the globe is irrigated with sterile saline. An ocular antibiotic solution, as well as atropine solution, are applied topically.

If the corneal laceration involves the limbus, the adjacent sclera should be inspected, as the laceration may extend into this tissue. An incision of the overlying bulbar conjunctiva may be required to examine the sclera adequately. If there is a laceration of the sclera, the surgical repair of the cornea is extended to include it.

The cornea (and sclera) is sutured with 6-0 or 7-0 absorbable suture, placed to a depth of the midstroma, in a simple interrupted pattern, with a cutting-edge needle. Nonabsorbable suture is less reactive and will result in less scarring; however, general anesthesia might be required for suture removal. The anterior chamber is re-formed with balanced salt solution or sterile saline injected at the limbus with a 25- or 26-gauge needle. Air bubbles that are concomitantly injected will be reabsorbed within a few hours to a few days. Removal of nonabsorbable sutures should occur in 10 to 14 days. A conjunctival flap may also be used to afford additional protection and comfort (Fig. 19-13). The conjunctival flap sutures are removed in 14 days.

Topical treatment consists of application of a broad-spectrum ocular antibiotic ointment (every 6 hours), or a solution (every 4 hours). Atropine ointment or solution (1%), is also used every 6 hours. Oral or parenteral administration of an antibiotic is recommended. Ultimately, a topical corticosteroid is used to treat the accompanying anterior uveitis and to reduce scarring of the cornea. This administration is initiated when one is certain that there is no intraocular or corneal infection, and that the laceration is healing. The use of an Elizabethan collar may be necessary to prevent additional trauma to the eye.

Corneal laceration with a staphyloma or iris prolapse

A staphyloma is a protrusion of the cornea or sclera with incorporation of the underlying uvea (iris, ciliary body, or posteriorly, the choroid). A staphyloma or iris prolapse is treated similarly to a corneal laceration, but initially the protruding tissue must be replaced to its normal location and/ or repaired.

A staphyloma may need to be incised in order to separate and reposition the underlying uveal tissue (usually iris). The cornea (and/or sclera) is sutured to prevent a recurrence of the protrusion of the fibrous (outer) layer of the globe. Applica-

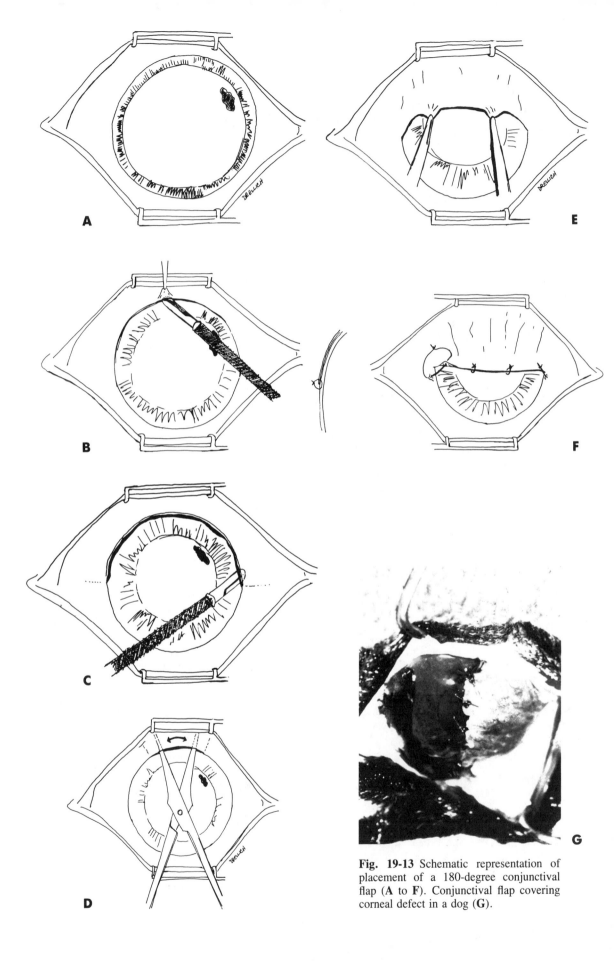

Fig. 19-13 Schematic representation of placement of a 180-degree conjunctival flap (**A** to **F**). Conjunctival flap covering corneal defect in a dog (**G**).

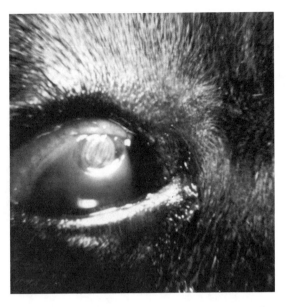

Fig. 19-14 Melon seed embedded in the cornea of a dog.

tion of a conjunctival flap might be beneficial in further strengthening the surgical site (Fig. 19-13).

An iris prolapse is invariably covered with a blood-fibrin clot, which must be gently removed. Fibrous adhesions between the cornea and iris are frequently present and must be broken down. If the prolapsed iris is viable, then it can be replaced into the anterior chamber. Any blood or fibrin clots can be removed from the anterior chamber at that time. If the prolapsed iris is necrotic, then a sector (wedge) iridectomy is performed using an ophthalmic electric cautery.

Corneal foreign bodies (Fig. 19-14)

Removal of a corneal stromal foreign body will require topical anesthesia, proper restraint, magnification, and good illumination. If necessary, sedation and/or general anesthesia may also be indicated. Following foreign-body removal, the eye is treated as for a deep corneal ulcer.

If there has been a penetrating foreign body, then a corneal limbal incision must be made for removal of the object. Both the corneal wound, created by the foreign body, and the limbal incision, are repaired as described for a corneal laceration.

UVEA

The uvea is the middle layer of the three concentric tunics (coats) of the globe. It is the vascular supply to the intraocular structures and is comprised of the iris, ciliary body, and choroid.

Hyphema

The most common cause of hyphema is trauma; however, hyphema may be secondary to a penetrating wound, an intraocular neoplasm, retinal detachment, glaucoma, or coagulopathy. Thus, careful physical diagnosis is required. Hyphema can result from anterior and/or posterior uveal bleeding. Simple hyphema will usually resolve spontaneously in 2 to 10 days, resulting in no long-term visual impairment.

The principles of therapy of hyphema include:

1. Arrest of continued bleeding and prevention of recurrent bleeding.
2. Enhancement of elimination of blood from the anterior chamber via the iridocorneal angle.
3. Monitoring for and control of secondary glaucoma, caused by occlusion of the iridocorneal angle by erythrocytes and fibrin.
4. Treatment of associated injuries.
5. Detection and treatment of nonglaucomatous complications of hyphema, such as synechia, dyscoria (irregular pupil), corectopia (eccentric pupil), and cataract formation.

Treatment of hyphema includes confinement of the animal in order to prevent rebleeding, which may occur within 5 days of the initial injury. Erythrocytes and/or macrophages may occlude the drainage angle, resulting in glaucoma. Thus, the intraocular tension (pressure) should be monitored closely by tonometry.

The medical treatment of hyphema is similar to the treatment of anterior uveitis:

1. Dilation of the pupil with application of 1% atropine sulfate ointment or solution four times a day to prevent posterior synechia and arrest ciliary muscle spasm, and
2. Topical corticosteroid administration every 4 to 6 hours; e.g., 0.1% dexamethasone, 1% prednisolone, to control anterior segment inflammation.

Evacuation of blood or blood clots from the anterior chamber is recommended only in the event of the development of secondary glaucoma. This procedure is performed via an anterior chamber paracentesis at the limbus, or via a surgical incision at the same site. These procedures would be futile if performed in situations with recurrent bleeding. Aspirin (prostaglandin inhibitor) administration for control of intraocular inflammation is contraindicated if there is evidence of ongoing or recurrent bleeding.

Uveitis

Uveitis may occur secondary to ocular trauma, even if there is no penetration of the globe, and may arise secondary to extension of disease from adjacent ocular tissues, systemic disease, antigenic protein exposure, or a resorbing cataract (lens-induced uveitis). The lens has a different embryologic tissue origin than the remainder of the eye, and lens development precedes that of the immune system. Thus, when there is a "leakage" of lens protein into the eye, it is recognized as "foreign" and stimulates an immune reaction.

Clinical signs of anterior uveitis include pain, as manifest by blepharospasm, epiphora, and photophobia. There is an associated congestion (injection) of conjunctival vasculature, as well as chemosis. Ciliary injection (deep corneal limbal vascularization) may be present. The anterior chamber may appear cloudy, "aqueous flare" cells may be noted, hypopyon (white blood cells in the anterior chamber), iridal changes (development of thickening or fluffiness), and miosis may be observed (Fig. 19-15). Keratic precipitates may be observed on the corneal endothelium, most commonly in an inferonasal location.

Treatment of uveitis is directed toward identification and treatment of the primary cause. The data base should include ocular examination, complete blood count, serum biochemical profile, and possibly specific serologic titers (e.g., toxoplasmosis, blastomycosis, etc.) and an immune profile. A topical corticosteroid ointment or solution (e.g., 0.1% dexamethasone or 1% prednisolone) is administered every 4 to 6 hours. If the pathogenesis is not known, a combination antibiotic-corticosteroid preparation is generally used. Hydrocortisone, present in many combined

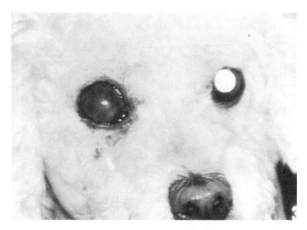

Fig. 19-16 Glaucoma secondary to anterior uveitis (buphthalmos, conjunctival hyperemia, chemosis, corneal edema, corneal neovascularization, and ciliary injection).

products, will not usually be effective as the sole corticosteroid in the treatment of most cases of anterior uveitis. Oral or parenteral corticosteroid administration is not indicated with therapy of anterior uveitis, but should be employed when there is choroidal involvement. Administration of systemic antibiotics may be indicated initially, especially if the cause is unknown or a concomitant infection is identified or suspected.

Administration of prostaglandin inhibitors (aspirin) may be beneficial as antiinflammatory and analgesic agents. The dosage of aspirin for a dog is 10 to 25 mg/kg divided two or three times a day; while that for a cat would be 80 mg (1.25 gr) every 48 to 72 hours.

The sequelae of uveitis include synechia (anterior and posterior), cyclitic (inflammatory) membranes, secondary glaucoma, cataract formation, and phthisis (atrophia) bulbi (Fig. 19-16).

GLAUCOMA

Glaucoma is defined as an increase in intraocular tension beyond the limits of health and function (Fig. 19-17). Canine breeds having a predisposition for primary glaucoma include the basset hound, beagle, cocker spaniel, miniature and toy poodle, Norwegian elkhound, fox terrier, Sealyham terrier, Samoyed, and Alaskan malamute. In addition, there are breeds (chow chow, Shar-Pei, Newfoundland, Great Dane) in which a congenitally compromised iridocorneal angle (goniodysgenesis) has been demonstrated. Primary glaucoma is not common in cats.

Many dogs with glaucoma present with a history of recurrent attacks of pain, epiphora, con-

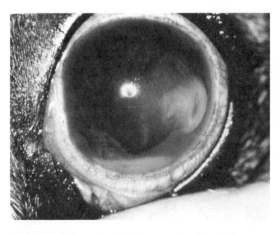

Fig. 19-15 Anterior uveitis associated with corneal perforation, conjunctival hyperemia, chemosis, hypopyon, iridal thickening, and miosis.

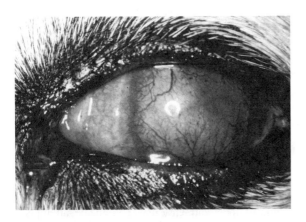

Fig. 19-17 Glaucoma.

junctivitis, and visual impairment. The cardinal signs of glaucoma include:

1. Pain (blepharospasm, enophthalmos, epiphora),
2. Marked conjunctival blood vessel injection (congestion) and hyperemia,
3. Corneal edema,
4. Insensitive cornea,
5. Dilated, fixed pupil, and
6. Visual deficit or blindness.

Classification

Primary glaucoma is an increase in intraocular pressure without previous disease, and secondary glaucoma is caused by a preceding disease condition (lens luxation, lens-induced uveitis, phacolytic glaucoma, and neoplasia).

Findings observed with chronic glaucoma include buphthalmos, episcleral venous congestion, "keratitis," and fundic lesions (attenuation of retinal vasculature, retinal atrophy, and cupping of the optic disk). The key to successful treatment of glaucoma is early diagnosis, prior to the development of the cardinal signs.

Acute glaucoma is a true ocular emergency occurring commonly in dogs, especially in breeds with a predilection for primary glaucoma, and uncommonly in cats. The condition is usually clinically manifest as a unilateral problem; however, the second eye generally is similarly affected.

The intraocular pressure in acute congestive glaucoma frequently exceeds 50 mm Hg. The affected eye is painful and the dog will frequently exhibit changes in behavior (lethargy, irritability, anorexia, hiding).

Diagnosis

The normal intraocular pressure is 15 to 27 mm Hg for a dog and 15 to 30 mm Hg for a cat. An increase in intraocular pressure, or a difference of 8 mm Hg or more between the two eyes is essential for the diagnosis of glaucoma. A Schiotz tonometer is used for the measurement of intraocular pressure. This tonometer was designed and calibrated for the human cornea; however, with practice and correct positioning on the center of the cornea, it can serve as an invaluable instrument for the diagnosis of glaucoma in dogs and cats. Application of topical anesthetic is essential prior to the use of any tonometer. Electronic applanation tonometers are most accurate and reliable, but are much more expensive.

Treatment

The goal of emergency therapy is to reduce the intraocular pressure as rapidly and safely as possible. Glaucoma therapy is dependent on identification and specific treatment of the underlying cause and administration of drugs to maintain the intraocular pressure within physiologic limits. Three types of drugs are used in the treatment of acute glaucoma: (1) those that reduce intraocular volume, (2) those that decrease aqueous production, and (3) those that increase the outflow of aqueous.

Hyperosmotic agents are used orally or intravenously to increase the osmolarity of plasma, resulting in subsequent dehydration of the vitreous and a decrease in intraocular volume. Two hyperosmotic agents are available for the treatment of acute glaucoma: glycerol (50%, 1 to 2 ml/kg orally) and mannitol (20%, 1 to 2 g/kg intravenously). Both hyperosmotic agents are administered slowly over a 20- to 30-minute period. Emesis, due to gastric irritation, is a frequent side effect following administration of glycerol. The maximum effect of the hyperosmotic agents occurs within 1 hour of administration, with a duration of effect of 4 to 8 hours. For these drugs to be effective, water must be withheld for 3 hours after administration.

Carbonic anhydrase inhibitors decrease intraocular pressure by reducing the production of aqueous by 20% to 30%. Acetazolamide (Diamox, Storz Pharmaceuticals) is more commonly prescribed for use in humans, but is poorly tolerated by dogs and cats because of its tendency to cause acidosis in these species. Dichlorphenamide (Daranide, Merck Sharp & Dohme) and methazolamide (Neptazane, Storz Pharmaceuticals) are better tolerated and are, therefore, frequently prescribed. The recommended dosages are as follows:

1. Dichlorphenamide—2.5 mg/lb orally divided two or three times a day.

2. Methazolamide—2.5 to 5 mg/lb orally divided two or three times a day.
3. Acetazolamide—10 to 15 mg/lb orally divided two or three times a day.

Beta-adrenergic blocking agents have been used successfully in recent years for topical therapy in the treatment of glaucoma. These drugs usually are not irritating when applied topically and also require less frequent administration as compared with miotics. The precise mechanism of action of this type of drug is not presently known. Three examples of beta blockers, and their concentrations are as follows:

1. Timolol maleate (Timoptic, Merck Sharp & Dohme)—0.25%, 0.5% 1 drop twice a day.
2. Betaxolol hydrochloride (Betoptic, Alcon Laboratories)—0.5% 1 drop twice a day.
3. Evobunalol (Betagan, Allergan Pharmaceuticals)—0.5% 1 drop twice a day.

Both direct- and indirect-acting parasympathomimetics (miotics) have long been used topically in the eye for the treatment of glaucoma. As mentioned, these drugs may cause ocular irritation, and should not be used to treat glaucoma secondary to anterior uveitis, as this application may potentiate the uveitis.

Pilocarpine is a direct-acting parasympathomimetic and produces miosis through contraction of the iris sphincter and also results in opening the trabecular meshwork spaces to facilitate the outflow of aqueous humor. Pilocarpine is available in concentrations from 1% to 6%, with 2% being the optical concentration for use in dogs. Pilocarpine is usually instilled three times a day.

Echothiophate (Phospholine Iodide, Wyeth-Ayerst), demecarium bromide (Humorsol, Merck Sharp & Dohme), and isoflurophate (Floropryl, Merck Sharp & Dohme) are cholinesterase inhibitors, and are examples of indirect-acting parasympathomimetics. Both agents are usually administered twice a day and are available in the following concentrations:

1. Echothiophate: 0.03% to 0.25%
2. Demecarium bromide: 0.125% and 0.25%
3. Isoflurophate: 0.025% ointment

Sympathomimetics can also be used topically for glaucoma therapy. These drugs lower intraocular tension by increasing the coefficient of aqueous humor outflow. Epinephrine is available in concentrations from 0.5% to 2%. Epinephrine should not be used if narrow drainage glaucoma is suspected, as the accompanying dilation of the pupil may further compromise the angle.

Combinations of epinephrine and pilocarpine are available at varying concentrations of both drugs, for example, P_2E_1 (Alcon Laboratories) and E-Pilo-2 (Iolab Pharmaceuticals). The numbers represent the percent concentration of the particular drug and administration of these drug combinations is usually three times a day.

If the glaucoma is secondary to anterior uveitis, then it is suggested that, in addition to the appropriate glaucoma therapy, the primary problem be treated aggressively. Thus, under these conditions, atropine ointment or solution and a topical corticosteroid should be administered four times a day. This approach is advocated even though some of the treatments may complicate attempts to decrease the intraocular pressure; for example, atropine administration causes mydriasis, which may further compromise the drainage angle.

Paracentesis of the anterior chamber is not used to decrease the intraocular pressure. This procedure predisposes the eye to intraocular hemorrhage and retinal detachment.

Various surgical procedures may be necessary to assist in control of the intraocular pressure. However, only a lens extraction would need to be performed on an emergency basis. The indication for an emergency lens extraction would be an anterior lens luxation resulting in "pupillary block" glaucoma.

Finally, it is imperative that the contralateral eye be evaluated, especially with measurement of intraocular pressure and gonioscopy. This examination of the iridocorneal angle would determine if there is a predisposition to the development of glaucoma in the "unaffected" eye. Gonioscopic examination of the uninvolved eye might provide retrospective information regarding the pathogenesis of the problem in the affected eye.

SUDDEN BLINDNESS

It is essential to obtain a complete history and perform a physical examination in addition to a thorough ocular examination. The latter would reveal causes of blindness such as anterior uveitis, cataract, glaucoma, papilledema, retinitis, and retinal detachment. If no abnormalities are observed, especially involving the fundus, then optic neuritis and sudden acquired retinal degeneration (SARD) should be considered. The latter is acute blindness occurring in middle-aged or older dogs, frequently with accompanying clinical signs of endocrine disease (polyphagia, polydipsia, and polyuria) possibly related to a neoplasm of the pituitary gland.

Optic neuritis is not common, but is a syndrome characterized by acute blindness associated with dilated pupils that are nonresponsive or minimally responsive to light, and normal retinal appearance on fundic evaluation. The various causes can include lead poisoning, peracute canine distemper infection, granulomatous meningoencephalitis (GME), cryptococcosis, and lymphosarcoma. Frequently, no definitive diagnosis is made and the cause is regarded as idiopathic.

A complete neurologic examination should be performed in animals with sudden-onset blindness. Neurologic deficits may be present with the various causes considered. A complete blood count and serum biochemical profile are advised. If neurologic abnormalities are noted, then a cerebrospinal fluid analysis is also indicated.

An electroretinogram is helpful in making the diagnosis of SARD, as it is flat (negative) before ophthalmoscopic signs of retinal atrophy develop.

Optic neuritis can be treated; however, there is no treatment for SARD-related blindness. An in-depth medical and endocrine evaluation are indicated, and it may be possible to ameliorate the endocrine-related signs. Optic neuritis and serous retinal detachments not associated with hypertension are treated with administration of corticosteroids (2 mg/kg divided twice a day, followed by tapering dosages over a 3- to 4-week period).

Apparent sudden blindness in older cats is frequently caused by retinal hemorrhage and detachment secondary to hypertension associated with renal disease. Measurement of systemic arterial blood pressure, in addition to evaluation of a serum biochemical profile, is helpful in arriving at the diagnosis of the underlying cause of the ocular changes. The treatment in these animals is directed toward medical management of the renal disease and hypertension. The prognosis for restoration of vision is guarded to poor for retinal hemorrhage and/or detachment.

SUGGESTED READINGS

Bistner SI, Aguirre G, Batik G. Atlas of veterinary ophthalmic surgery. Philadelphia: WB Saunders, 1977.

Gelatt KN. The canine glaucomas. In Gelatt KN, ed. Veterinary ophthalmology. Philadelphia: Lea & Febiger, 1981.

Havener WH. Ocular pharmacology. St. Louis: Mosby–Year Book, 1983.

Morgan RV. Ocular emergencies. Compend Contin Educ Pract Vet 1982;4:37-45.

Physician's desk reference for ophthalmology—1991. Oradell, NJ: Medical Economics Press, 1991.

Slatter DH. Fundamentals of veterinary ophthalmology. Philadelphia: WB Saunders, 1990.

Szymanski CJ. Ocular emergencies. Contemp Issues Small Anim Pract 1985;1:315-328.

van der Woerdt A. Sudden acquired retinal degeneration in the dog: clinical and laboratory findings in 36 cases. Prog Vet Comp Ophthalmol 1991;1:11-18.

Winston SM. Ocular emergencies. Vet Clin North Am 1981;11:59-76.

Wyman M. Manual of small animal ophthalmology. New York: Churchill Livingstone, 1986.

20 Neurologic Emergencies

Kenneth Lee Schunk

SPINAL CORD TRAUMA
Pathophysiology

Spinal cord trauma most commonly results from direct physical trauma and is usually accompanied by vertebral fracture, luxation, or intervertebral disk extrusion (Chapter 11). Occasionally, spinal cord injury occurs without visible trauma to supporting structures.

Despite extensive research, controversy exists concerning the pathophysiology of acute spinal cord injury. The most dramatic postinjury response is decreased spinal cord blood flow (SCBF), which is more pronounced in the central gray matter.[1] This ischemia can proceed without ongoing spinal cord compression. Normal autoregulation of SCBF is lost following spinal cord trauma, and systemic hypotension due to increased plasma endorphin activity has been postulated as causing ischemia in this setting.[2] Other causes of reduced SCBF include mechanical damage to the microvasculature, thrombosis of small vessels, small-vessel obstruction secondary to endothelial swelling, and increased interstitial fluid pressure due to vasogenic edema.[3] Vasospasm induced by vasoactive substances such as norepinephrine, serotonin, and histamine has been proposed as a cause of progressive myelomalacia following spinal cord trauma.[2,3] Ischemia with resultant hypoxia results in the production of oxygen-free radicals and subsequent peroxidation of unsaturated fatty acids within membranes.[4]

An early pathologic change found in the injured spinal cord is central gray matter hemorrhagic necrosis, which occurs within 60 minutes of the trauma. Progressive histologic changes are also seen in the white matter over the first several hours. The pathologic changes spread radially and longitudinally from the point of injury.

Clinical evaluation

Clinical signs are acute in onset and occur immediately following the trauma in most cases. Although the signs are generally nonprogressive, vertebral column instability or ongoing hemorrhage and myelomalacia may allow the symptoms to worsen over time.

Varying degrees of paresis and ataxia caudal to the site of the spinal cord injury are seen following the accident (Table 20-1). In addition, the animal often exhibits hyperesthesia localized at the site of the trauma.

On presentation, the animal should be placed in lateral recumbancy and evaluated for nonneurologic injuries. The neurologic examination should then be performed with minimal patient movement while the animal is in lateral recumbancy. Segmental spinal reflexes, muscle tone, and superficial and deep pain sensation are carefully evaluated. Palpation of the spinal column may reveal the presence of a vertebral fracture or luxation.

Radiographs should be evaluated following the neurologic examination. Prior to moving the animal, the spine should be immobilized by external support if possible. The vertebral column regions, which account for the neurologic symptoms, should be radiographed. The objectives of the radiographic evaluation are to identify the precise location of the lesion(s) and determine the type of spinal column injury in order to assess the need for surgical management. The possibility of multiple spinal column injuries should always be considered.

The majority of small animals with spinal cord trauma have radiographic evidence of vertebral fractures or luxations. Most vertebral injuries occur near the junction of a mobile and an immobile

288

Table 20-1 Regional neurologic signs following spinal cord trauma

Site of Injury	Symptoms
C1-C5	Tetraparesis/tetraplegia with upper motor neuron signs in all four limbs; cervical rigidity and pain; pain sensation normal to decreased caudal to injury; Horner's syndrome
C6-T2	Tetraparesis/tetraplegia with lower motor neuron signs in thoracic limbs and upper motor neuron signs in pelvic limbs; cervical rigidity and pain; pain sensation normal to decreased caudal to injury; Horner's syndrome
T3-L3	Paraparesis/paraplegia with upper motor neuron signs in pelvic limbs; pain sensation normal to decreased caudal to injury
L4-Cd5	Paraparesis/paraplegia with lower motor neuron signs in pelvic limbs; pain sensation normal to decreased caudal to injury; dilated anus, atonic bladder, and hypotonic tail

portion of the spine (e.g., thoracolumbar junction). Radiography determines only the degree of luxation present at the time of the examination, and the spinal cord injury is often worse than the radiographic appearance. It is important to examine the radiograph for the size of the intervertebral disk spaces, since acute disk extrusion may occur at the time of the injury. In some animals, there is no radiographic evidence of trauma, and myelography is required to detect the site of the lesion.

Treatment

Medical treatment. Initial therapy should be directed at life threatening nonneural injuries. Despite extensive research, controversy exists concerning which drugs and dosages are effective in the treatment of spinal cord trauma. If any drug is going to be beneficial, it must be administered as soon as possible following the injury.

Corticosteroids continue to be the most commonly used drugs for acute spinal cord trauma in veterinary medicine. In addition to their antiinflammatory effects and ability to stabilize cell membranes, corticosteroids may improve SCBF, decrease injury-induced oxygen-free radical formation and associated peroxidation of unsaturated fatty acids, increase activity of spinal cord so-

dium, potassium-ATPase, and prevent neurofilament degradation.[4] I currently use dexamethasone sodium phosphate (2 mg/kg, intravenously, initially followed by 0.2 mg/kg of dexamethasone two or three times a day for several days). Gastrointestinal ulceration and hemorrhage are common side effects of corticosteroids when used in patients with spinal cord injury.

Osmotic diuretics, such as mannitol, have been shown to be effective in the treatment of cytotoxic brain edema; however, there is little evidence to support their use in animals with spinal cord trauma. Despite the potential beneficial effects of dimethylsulfoxide, the drug has not been used extensively in veterinary medicine following acute spinal cord injury.[3] Naloxone, an opiate antagonist, and thyrotropin-releasing hormone act by blocking the effects of endogenous opioids (endorphins), which are released following spinal trauma.[2,5] Encouraging experimental studies with these drugs have led to clinical trials to determine their effectiveness in humans with spinal cord injury.[5,6]

Nursing care is critical to the successful treatment of animals with spinal injuries. Unnecessary movement should be avoided. Repositioning the animal every few hours and providing suitable bedding helps prevent decubital sores. The urinary bladder should be emptied three times a day by manual pressure or intermittent catheterization in order to prevent urine retention.

Surgical treatment. Surgery is indicated when it is necessary to stabilize an unstable vertebral column and to decompress the spinal cord (see Chapter 11). In general, surgery should be performed as soon as possible. In addition to stabilization and decompressive procedures, myelotomy and normothermic or hypothermic perfusion have been used for the treatment of spinal cord trauma.[7]

Prognosis

The prognosis is based primarily on the severity of the injury to the spinal cord as determined by neurologic examination. An animal who is ambulatory usually has a good prognosis. If the animal is nonambulatory but has voluntary movement and good sensation, the prognosis is fair. An animal who is nonambulatory with no voluntary movement but intact pain sensation has a guarded prognosis. A grave prognosis is warranted for an animal with no voluntary movement and no deep pain sensation. In addition, animals with significant lower motor neuron injuries of the spinal cord have a guarded to poor prognosis because of the severity of gray matter lesions.

Despite these guidelines, the prognosis for an

individual animal can be difficult to determine. The instability of certain fractures and the size of the animal can influence the outcome in some cases. In general, some improvement in neurologic function should be seen within the first 14 days, although there is no set time for this to occur.

BRAIN TRAUMA
Pathogenesis

Brain trauma may result in concussion (transient loss of consciousness without gross or microscopic brain lesions), contusion, laceration, and hemorrhage. Intracranial hemorrhage may be extradural, subdural, subarachnoid, or intraparenchymal. The clinical manifestations vary depending on the location and severity of the injury. Head injury may also result in linear, elevated, depressed, or compound (open) skull fractures. Basilar fractures may extend into the ear, orbit, or nasal cavity and provide portals for bacteria to enter the central nervous system.

The major sequelae to brain trauma are brain edema, hypoxia/ischemia, and increased intracranial pressure (ICP). Vasogenic edema is the accumulation of fluid in the extracellular space secondary to increased vascular permeability and is the principal type of edema following brain injury.[8] Increased arterial blood pressure potentiates the formation of vasogenic edema. This is important to consider since the increased ICP accompanying developing vasogenic edema results in further arterial hypertension. Intracellular edema associated with impaired cellular metabolism (cytotoxic edema) also occurs.

Hypoxic and ischemic changes are common neuropathologic findings following brain trauma. Autoregulation, which maintains cerebral blood flow in the normal range despite variations in systemic arterial blood pressure and blood gas composition, is often impaired following trauma. Hypotension and any decreased oxygen saturation of the blood result in tissue hypoxia. The associated brain edema and increased ICP will result in further reduction in cerebral blood flow.

Following head trauma, hemorrhage and brain edema often result in increased ICP. The magnitude of the increased ICP and the ability of the brain to accommodate is in part determined by the intracranial blood volume. Increased arterial carbon dioxide partial pressure, decreased oxygen content of the blood, and increased cerebral metabolic rate secondary to fever or seizures will increase cerebral blood volume. In addition, certain anesthetic agents such as methoxyflurane and halothane increase cerebral blood volume due to vasodilation. An increase in cerebral blood volume in an animal with brain trauma may increase ICP and result in herniation of the brain.

Clinical evaluation

A brief history is important in order to obtain information concerning the nature of the trauma and the onset and progression of the animal's neurologic signs.

Following a thorough physical examination, an initial neurologic assessment is done to establish a base line and to provide information regarding the localization and severity of the injury. The skull should be carefully palpated for fractures. Radiographs of the skull are useful in identifying fractures; however, sedation or anesthesia may be needed to position the animal properly.

Animals with brainstem injuries often have a worse prognosis than animals with cerebral injuries. Since pupil size and responsiveness, ocular movements, and posture and motor activity are helpful in differentiating cerebral and brainstem injuries, special attention should be given to these during the examination. Animals with cerebral injuries may have abnormally small pupils that are responsive to light. Midsized or dilated pupils that are unresponsive to light suggest midbrain involvement. Dilated, unresponsive pupils are also seen with oculomotor nerve lesions. Small, unresponsive pupils suggest the presence of a pontine injury. Unilateral lesions involving the cerebellar nuclei can also produce anisocoria.[9] Primary ocular trauma should be considered when evaluating pupillary size and responsiveness to light.

Normal oculocephalic nystagmus requires the functional integrity of the peripheral vestibular apparatus, brainstem vestibular structures and pathways, and cranial nerves III, IV and VI. Abnormal oculocephalic nystagmus in animals without bilateral peripheral vestibular injury implies the presence of brainstem trauma.

Decerebrate posturing often accompanied by opisthotonos, abnormal pupils, and semicoma or coma suggests severe midbrain trauma and signifies a grave prognosis. It is important not to confuse decerebrate posturing with posturing observed following cerebellar trauma. Animals with acute cerebellar lesions exhibit opisthotonos and forelimb rigidity; however, these animals have normal consciousness and intact vestibular nystagmus.

Animals with head trauma may also sustain injuries to their peripheral nervous system and exhibit cranial nerve paralyses. Despite the permanent nature of some of these injuries, they usually do not significantly alter the prognosis of the patient. The loss of cranial nerve function may also result from trauma to the brainstem; however, these animals will exhibit other symptoms of brainstem injury.

Vestibular symptoms, such as head tilt, abnormal nystagmus, and ataxia, following cranial trauma may result from inner ear injury or from involvement of the vestibular system within the medulla or cerebellum. Patients with central vestibular damage usually have additional symptoms of cerebellar ataxia, limb paresis or paralysis, altered consciousness, or "central" nystagmus (vertical, positional). Animals with injuries to the inner ear labyrinth often have fractures of the petrous temporal bone and hemorrhage from the external ear. In general, the prognosis is better for injuries involving the peripheral vestibular apparatus.

Serial neurologic examinations should be performed in the evaluation of animals with brain trauma. The determination of the location, extent, and progression of the injury is critical in formulating a prognosis and is based on sequential examinations.

Treatment

Initial supportive care. The cardiovascular and respiratory systems should be carefully evaluated since decreased cardiac and respiratory function will contribute to the progression of brain injury. Initial supportive care for animals with brain trauma include the following:

1. Establish a patent airway.
2. Ensure adequate ventilation and provide an oxygen-rich environment.
3. Elevate the patient's head and prevent compression of the jugular veins.
4. Prevent aspiration into airways.
5. Establish an intravenous line, but carefully monitor fluid administration, as overhydration will contribute to brain edema.

Specific medical therapy. The goal of therapy is to reduce brain edema, control intracranial pressure and to prevent hypoxia/ischemia. Despite the unproven role of glucocorticoids in the management of head trauma, I routinely use dexamethasone sodium phosphate (2 mg/kg intravenously initially; then 0.2 mg/kg three times a day for 36 to 48 hours; then taper slowly over the next 5 to 7 days) in order to reduce vasogenic edema.[9]

If the patient is semicomatose or comatose, hyperventilation with oxygen should be considered. This prevents hypercarbia, which causes vasodilation and increased intracranial pressure.

Hyperosmolar agents, such as mannitol, remove water from normal but not edematous brain tissue by creating an osmotic gradient across functionally intact cerebral vessels. Hypertonic solutions also decrease cerebrospinal fluid formation and cerebral vasodilation, effectively lowering ICP in the presence or absence of an intact blood-brain barrier.[10] Mannitol should not be given to an animal that is hypovolemic. When indicated, 0.25 to 1.0 gm/kg of 20% mannitol is given intravenously; the effective duration of action is 1 to 3 hours. Furosemide (2 mg/kg intravenously) can be administered with mannitol to enhance the reduction in ICP and to prolong mannitol's effect.[10] Serum electrolytes and urine output should be monitored when furosemide and mannitol are used repeatedly.

The animal should be evaluated every 15 to 30 minutes over the first 6 to 12 hours depending on the neurologic status. If improvement is observed within the first 4 to 6 hours, a favorable prognosis is indicated.

Surgical therapy. Surgical decompression is indicated when there is an open skull fracture or a depressed bone fragment. If the patient is neurologically stable, surgery to elevate a depressed skull fracture can be delayed for 24 to 48 hours.[11] Any animal whose signs continue to deteriorate from the initial neurologic examination despite aggressive medical therapy is a candidate for decompressive surgery. A unilateral craniectomy can be performed if a hematoma is suspected and can be localized based on neurologic examination or diagnostic imaging (CT scan); otherwise, a bilateral craniectomy is indicated.

A balanced anesthetic protocol should be used to limit the adverse anesthetic effects on cerebral blood flow and ICP (see Chapter 33). Preanesthetic drugs should be avoided in order to prevent respiratory depression. A narcotic-barbiturate combination is recommended for induction.[12] Ketamine should not be used since it increases cerebral blood flow.[12] Following intubation, intermittent positive-pressure ventilation is recommended. Maintenance of anesthesia can be accomplished by use of a narcotic-barbiturate combination or a low concentration of isoflurane. Since inhalation anesthetics increase cerebral blood flow, their use should be minimized.

ABNORMALITIES OF CONSCIOUSNESS

Animals are occasionally presented for evaluation because of an altered consciousness. Organic brain diseases (tumor, trauma, encephalitis, infarct, and hemorrhage) and several metabolic and toxic disorders commonly cause some alteration in consciousness.

The state of consciousness is regulated by the interaction between the brainstem and cerebrum. The ascending reticular activating system, which is located in the rostral brainstem, activates the cerebrum in response to various stimuli. Diseases capable of affecting the cerebrum diffusely or the rostral brainstem diffusely or focally may result in an abnormal consciousness. It should be emphasized that for cerebral disease to cause abnormal consciousness, the disease must be bilateral and diffuse, since the normal cerebral reserves are extensive and pleuripotential.[13]

Altered states of consciousness in animals may be described in terms of decreasing levels of awareness. Animals that are lethargic, sleepy, and less responsive to their environment are *depressed*. Disoriented, irritable, or fearful animals that respond to their environment in an inappropriate manner are in a state of *delirium*. *Semicoma* or *stupor* is characterized by deep sleep from which the animal can be aroused only with vigorous or painful stimuli. An unconscious and totally unresponsive animal is described as being *comatose*.

Pathogenesis

The box at right lists the causes of altered consciousness in small animals.

Patients with metabolic encephalopathy have normal pupils and oculocephalic responses and do not have lateralizing or focal abnormalities on their neurologic examinations. Except for an altered consciousness and depressed postural reactions, metabolic disorders do not usually produce any other neurologic abnormalities.

Patients with diffuse or multifocal central nervous system disease often have inflammatory brain disease. These animals usually have asymmetrical findings on the neurologic examination. Symptoms frequently seen include abnormal nystagmus, cranial nerve dysfunction, cerebellovestibular ataxia, and cervical pain. The diagnosis is usually confirmed by cerebrospinal fluid analysis.

Patients with focal central nervous system lesions usually have focal neurologic findings such as asymmetrical postural reactions. It is important to remember that animals with mass lesions resulting in altered consciousness often have increased ICP, which may result in brain herniation and a variety of neurologic signs. Transtentorial herniation (herniation of the cerebrum under the tentorium cerebelli) results in brainstem compression and pupillary dilation. Cerebellar herniation through the foramen magnum causes slowing of respiration, mucous membrane pallor, and bradycardia secondary to medullary compression.

The diagnosis is dependent on obtaining an adequate history concerning toxin exposure and metabolic disease, performing serial neurologic examinations, and evaluating the metabolic status of the animal. Cerebrospinal fluid analysis, skull

CAUSES OF ALTERED CONSCIOUSNESS IN SMALL ANIMALS

Metabolic or toxic encephalopathy
  Hypoglycemia
  Hepatic encephalopathy
  Diabetes mellitus
  Uremia
  Addisonian crisis
  Ethylene glycol toxicity
  Barbiturate overdose
  Other toxins[12]
  Severe systemic infections
Multifocal or diffuse disease
  Inflammatory brain disease
  Subarachnoid hemorrhage
  Trauma
Focal disease
  Neoplasia
  Focal encephalitis
  Hemorrhage/infarction
  Trauma

radiography, electroencephalography, brainstem auditory evoked responses, and computed tomography may be needed in the evaluation of patients with primary central nervous system disease.

Clinical evaluation

A complete and detailed history should be obtained when an animal is presented in an altered state of consciousness. In addition, a physical examination and serial neurologic evaluations should be performed.

The initial goal of the clinical evaluation is to determine if the animal has metabolic or toxic encephalopathy or organic brain disease. Neurologic abnormalities that are asymmetrical (deficits more pronounced on one side of the body) are strongly suggestive of structural brain disease. The neurologic findings often allow localization of the disease process within the nervous system. Animals with organic brain disease may have localizing signs characteristic of brainstem and/or cerebral involvement. On the other hand, metabolic disorders usually produce symmetrical, diffuse cerebral symptoms that often fluctuate in severity (see box above).

During the neurologic examination, special attention is given to the pupil size and responsiveness, ocular position and movement, and posture and motor activity of the limbs (refer to the section on Brain Trauma above). Alteration in pupil size, symmetry, and responsiveness to light may suggest involvement at different levels of the central nervous system. In animals with metabolic encephalopathy, the pupils are usually normal; occasionally, small, responsive pupils are observed. Cerebral disorders and metabolic encephalopathy do not alter the ability to elicit normal vestibular nystagmus; therefore, patients with absent or abnormal vestibular ocular movements usually have brainstem dysfunction.

Alterations in posture, muscle tone, and motor function may reveal significant information concerning the localization of the disease process in animals with altered consciousness. Decerebrate posturing in a comatose animal usually indicates a lesion in the midbrain. Diffuse cerebral disease, diencephalic lesions, and metabolic disorders result in tetraparesis with depressed or absent postural reactions; rhythmic walking movements may be elicited in these animals when the patient is supported in a normal standing position.

Although specific alterations in the breathing pattern are useful in the localization of lesions resulting in coma in humans, this has not been true in animals. Serious brainstem disease may result in ataxic respirations, hyperventilation, or hypoventilation. Animals with diffuse cerebral disease of an organic nature often have normal respiratory patterns. Cerebral dysfunction secondary to metabolic disorders may be accompanied by abnormal respiratory responses associated with the underlying metabolic changes.

Treatment

The proper treatment of an animal with altered consciousness depends on the underlying cause. Initial support of a semicomatose or comatose animal is similar to that given to animals with brain injury (refer to the section on Brain Trauma above).

Any animal suspected of having organic brain disease as the underlying cause may have cerebral edema and increased ICP and may require specific medical therapy including corticosteroids, mannitol, and ventilatory support (refer to the section on Brain Trauma above).

Following the determination of the specific cause and institution of appropriate therapy, the patient should begin to improve within 12 to 24 hours in most cases. Persistent coma over several days despite vigorous treatment warrants a poor prognosis.

SEIZURES

Animals that have repeated generalized motor seizures, without intervening periods of consciousness, have status epilepticus and are neurologic emergencies. Animals with cluster seizures have repeated seizures within a relatively short time

span but regain consciousness in between the seizures. These patients also require immediate attention.

Patients with status epilepticus undergo a variety of central nervous system and systemic derangements that dictate that the seizures be terminated as soon as possible. Repeated seizures cause an increased rate of oxidative metabolism in the central nervous system, resulting in an increase in carbon dioxide production that can potentiate central nervous system acidosis and edema.[14] The associated reduction in cerebral cortical partial pressure of oxygen leads to regional oxygen insufficiency.[15] Neuronal calcium concentrations increase, and toxic amounts of prostaglandins, leukotrienes, and arachidonic acid accumulate, leading to brain edema and cell death.[15] An increase in cerebrospinal fluid pressure may also occur. Permanent cell damage occurs in vulnerable neurons due to excessively increased metabolic demands.[15]

Systemic alterations include an initial hyperglycemia followed by hypoglycemia, hyperthermia, dehydration, and lactic acidosis. Cardiac arrhythmias and neurogenic pulmonary edema may occasionally be seen. These systemic sequelae are life threatening and require immediate and vigorous therapy (see Chapters 16-18, 25, and 38).

There are a variety of potential causes for multiple seizures in small animals, including hypoglycemia, hypocalcemia, toxins, encephalitis, cerebral neoplasia, trauma, vascular accidents, and idiopathic (functional) epilepsy. The final diagnosis is based on the results of the history, physical and neurologic examinations, and a variety of ancillary tests including a complete blood count, serum chemistry profile, blood lead determination, cerebrospinal fluid analysis, and computed tomography.

Treatment

The primary goals in the treatment of an animal having seizures is to stop the seizures and provide supportive care. An adequate airway needs to be maintained and, if necessary, oxygen should be administered to prevent hypoxemia. An intravenous line should be established and blood samples should be collected for a complete blood count, blood glucose concentration, serum chemistry profile, and blood lead level. If the history, clinical signs, and laboratory data suggest the presence of hypoglycemia, the animal should be treated with dextrose. A 50% dextrose solution (2 to 3 ml for toy breeds and up 30 to 50 ml for giant-breed dogs) is given as a slow bolus intravenously. If the patient responds, a continuous infusion of 5% dextrose solution is administered intravenously, and the blood glucose concentration is closely monitored. If hypocalcemia is suspected, 10% calcium gluconate should be administered slowly as an intravenous bolus while monitoring the animal's heart rate and electrocardiogram (Chapter 18).

The treatment of choice to control seizures not associated with hypoglycemia or hypocalcemia is diazepam administration (0.25 mg to 0.5 mg/kg intravenously slowly to effect). Since diazepam, as well as clonazepam, crosses the blood-brain barrier faster than other anticonvulsants, it is effective in the treatment of most animals with status epilepticus. The seizures should stop within 3 minutes but may recur within 10 to 20 minutes because of the rapid distribution of the drug to various tissues. The initial dose may be repeated every 5 minutes for a total of three treatments if the animal continues to seize. If the desired response is not achieved, phenobarbital is administered (2 to 4 mg/kg intravenously). This initial dose can be repeated until a total dose of 20 mg/kg has been administered; however, it will take approximately 15 minutes for phenobarbital to have its maximal effect.[16] If seizures continue, general anesthesia using a long-acting barbiturate (e.g., pentobarbital) is administered. General anesthesia with gas anesthetics potentiate or cause increased ICP and should be avoided. Ultra-short-acting barbituates and phenothiazine tranquilizers should not be used, because they potentiate seizure activity. Anticonvulsants will need to be continued after the seizures are controlled. Intramuscular phenobarbital can be used until the animal is able to swallow oral medication.

During the course of initial anticonvulsant therapy, the animal should receive an intravenous infusion of a balanced electrolyte solution (Chapter 38). Hyperthermia should be treated, but caution must be used to avoid overzealous cooling (see Chapter 16). In addition, vital signs and urine output should be monitored closely until the animal has recovered (Chapter 4).

Multiple seizures occurring in combination with treatment effects often result in depression, dementia, visual deficits, and symmetrical abnor- malities in the animal's gait for several days. Therefore, serial neurologic examinations are necessary to determine the significance of any deficits observed during the initial postictal period. Clinically manifested sequelae of status epilepticus that may persist include personality and behavioral changes, altered mental status, and visual deficits.

REFERENCES

1. Braund KG. Acute spinal cord traumatic compression. In Bojrab MJ, ed. Pathophysiology in small animal surgery. Philadelphia: Lea & Febiger, 1981:220-227.
2. Faden AI, Jacobs TP, Holaday JW. Opiate antagonist improves neurologic recovery after spinal injury. Science 1981;211:493-494.
3. Berg RJ, Rucker NC. Pathophysiology and medical management of acute spinal cord injury. Compend Contin Educ Pract Vet 1985;7:646-654.
4. Hall Ed, Wolf DL, Braughler JM. Effects of a single large dose of methylprednisolone sodium succinate on experimental posttraumatic spinal cord ischemia. J Neurosurg 1984;61:124-130.
5. Faden AI, Jacobs TP, Holaday JW. Thyrotropin-releasing hormone improves neurologic recovery after spinal trauma in cats. N Engl J Med 1981;305:1063-1067.
6. Flamm ES, Young W, Collins WF, Piepmier J, Clifton GL, Fischer B. A Phase I trial of naloxone treatment in acute spinal cord injury. J Neurosurg 1985;63:390-397.
7. Swaim SF. Vertebral and spinal cord surgery. In Oliver JE, Hoerlein BF, Mayhew IG, eds. Veterinary neurology. Philadelphia: WB Saunders, 1987;416-469.
8. Fishman AP. Brain edema. N Engl J Med 1975;293:706-712.
9. deLahunta A. Veterinary neuroanatomy and clinical neurology, ed. 2. Philadelphia: WB Saunders, 1983;13.
10. Pollay M, Fullenwider C, Roberts A, Stevens FA. Effect of mannitol and furosemide on blood-brain osmotic gradient and intracranial pressure. J Neurosurg 1983;59:945-950.
11. Shores A. Craniocorebral trauma. In Kirk RW, ed. Current veterinary therapy X. Philadelphia: WB Saunders, 1989;847-853.
12. Dayrell-Hart B, Klide AM. Intracranial dysfunctions: stupor and coma. Vet Clin North Am 1989;6:1209-1222.
13. Plum F, Posner JB. The diagnosis of stupor and coma, ed. 3. Philadelphia: FA Davis, 1982.
14. Brooks BR, Adams RD, Cerebrospinal fluid acid-base and lactate changes after seizures in unanesthetized man. Neurology 1975;25:935.
15. Delgado-Escueta AV, Wasterlain C, Treiman DM, Porter RJ. Management of status epilepticus. N Engl J Med 1982;306:1337-1340.
16. Brown SA. Anticonvulsant therapy in small animals. Vet Clin North Am 1988;6:1197-1216.

21 Urologic Emergencies

Mary Anna Labato

UPPER URINARY TRACT TRAUMA

The emergency management of urologic injuries is influenced by a multitude of factors, including type of trauma, site of trauma, confirmation or suspicion of associated injuries, and clinical status/stability of the patient. Associated injuries often demand priority attention with definitive management of urologic injury often delayed until the patient is stabilized and able to withstand operative procedures.[1]

Injuries to the urinary tract result from blunt trauma and penetrating wounds. Automobile accidents are the cause of most injuries to the kidney and urinary tract of dogs and cats. Blunt trauma to the kidneys and urinary tract commonly result from automobile accidents, falls ("high-rise" syndrome), and malicious beatings. Penetrating wounds involving the kidneys and urinary tract result from bite wounds and crushing injuries ("big animal-little animal" syndrome), gunshot, or stab wounds.[2-4] There is no age, sex, or breed predisposition in the occurrence of urinary tract trauma. There is often a history of unsupervised activity and trauma.

All animals with evidence of external abdominal trauma, pelvic injuries, and evidence of intraabdominal injury should be evaluated for urinary tract trauma. The prevalence of urinary tract trauma associated with pelvic trauma has not been well defined. Reported prevalences have varied, but a commonly used figure is that one third of animals injured by automobiles suffer trauma to the abdomen or pelvis, leading to involvement of some aspect of the urinary system.[5] In one study 100 dogs sustaining blunt pelvic trauma were evaluated as to urinary tract injury; of the 100 dogs, 39 had some abnormality.[6] There was no correlation between pelvic fracture severity and the presence or nature of urinary tract trauma.[6] The clinical signs associated with urologic injuries include shock, abdominal pain, lethargy, an enlarging abdominal mass, abdominal effusion, stranguria, hematuria, oliguria, and anuria. A detailed history and a complete physical examination of the patient are essential to diagnose trauma to the urinary tract correctly[2,7-9] (see box).

Renal trauma

Blunt. In the dog and cat the kidneys are well-protected organs, and severe blunt trauma is required to injure them. The kidneys are fairly mobile in the abdominal cavity, and they are surrounded by the vertebrae, ribs, lumbar musculature, fat, and a fibrous capsule.

Blunt abdominal trauma results in renal parenchymal damage that can vary from minor subcapsular bleeding to a ruptured kidney with hemorrhagic shock, acute renal failure, or exsanguination. Renal contusions are the most frequent injury. Contusions seldom cause organ dysfunction, may result in mild hematuria, and are usually self-limiting and asymptomatic. A hematoma may result in local ischemic injury to the parenchyma. Laceration of the capsule and parenchyma may heal without surgical intervention when only a small area of one kidney is involved. If the laceration is more severe it may lead to hemorrhage and leakage of urine through the parenchyma and capsule into the retroperitoneal space or peritoneal cavity, resulting in hypovolemic shock, anemia, and chemical (sterile) peritonitis. Blunt trauma may also cause a rupture of the abdominal wall musculature and herniation of the kidney into a subcutaneous position.

The most severe injury to the kidney is avulsion of the renal vascular pedicle with profuse hemorrhage into the abdominal cavity or retroperitoneal space. Animals with avulsion of the renal pedicle may not survive long enough to reach the

295

MANAGEMENT OF URINARY TRACT TRAUMA

Treat hypovolemic shock and other life-threatening injuries
Insert urinary catheter
    Assess patency of lower urinary tract
    Obtain urine sample for analysis and culture
Diagnostic procedures
    Serum creatinine and blood urea nitrogen levels
    Serum electrolyte and blood gas evaluation
    Complete blood count
    Abdominocentesis or peritoneal lavage for creatinine level, cytology, and culture
Radiographic examination
    Survey abdominal and pelvic radiograph
    Excretory urogram
    Positive contrast cystourethrogram
    Ultrasonography
Supportive care
    Intravenous fluid administration
    Correct electrolyte/acid-base abnormalities
    Treat concomitant injuries
    Broad-spectrum antibiotic administration as indicated
Surgical repair
Patient monitoring
    Serial determination of complete blood count and blood urea nitrogen, serum creatinine, and serum electrolyte levels
    Monitor urine production/catheter position and patency
    Monitor body temperature and signs of abdominal discomfort
    Repeat contrast radiography

emergency clinic. Damage to the vascular pedicle caused by crushing injuries or thrombosis can result in renal ischemic injury.

Laceration or avulsion of the renal pelvis or ureter is an uncommon but severe injury that allows urine and blood to escape into the retroperitoneal space, resulting in cellulitis.[2-4,10]

Penetrating. Differentiation must be made between low-velocity injuries (bite wounds, stab wounds) and high-velocity injuries. High-velocity bullet wounds usually are the most life threatening. Patients with high-velocity injuries are frequently presented in shock with abdominal muscle spasm and pain. Vascular injury is common, and the degree of parenchymal damage is often great because of the potential energy conveyed by the rapidly moving missile. Many nephrectomies and partial nephrectomies are performed in patients with high-velocity penetrating injuries because of the inability to define the extent of injury.[11]

Clinical signs. The most common clinical sign of renal trauma is hematuria (microscopic or macroscopic). Although hematuria reflects renal injury, the degree of hematuria at presentation correlates poorly with the extent of renal damage. In humans, renal injury unaccompanied by hematuria is reported as occurring with frequencies varying from 0.5% to 25% (parenchymal injury) and 24% to 40% (pedicle injuries).[1] There currently are no data describing these comparisons in veterinary medicine.

Localized pain in the sublumbar region or abdominal discomfort may be present, but is often difficult to ascertain in the traumatized patient. The history or physical examination should make note of any progressively enlarging retroperitoneal mass or free abdominal fluid. If urine or blood accumulates in the retroperitoneal space, a cellulitis causing fever and pain may be noted. If the peritoneum has been damaged, abdominal discomfort and effusion (peritonitis) may be noted. Soft-tissue trauma to the caudal ribs, lumbar vertebrae, and lumbar muscles may also produce pain in the general region of the kidneys.

Diagnosis. The diagnosis of renal trauma is not easily established. A major differential is trauma to another portion of the urinary tract. Localization of urinary tract injury is an important therapeutic consideration. Urinalysis is indicated, but may not localize the site of injury to the kidney. Microscopic hematuria and proteinuria is suggestive of urinary trauma and, depending on the clinical state of the patient, should be closely monitored (stable patient) or aggressively pursued (unstable patient). A study in human medicine has concluded that urinary dipstick testing is a safe, accurate, and reliable screening method for the presence or absence of hematuria in patients sustaining either blunt or penetrating abdominal trauma.[12] Serum creatinine and blood urea nitrogen levels may be normal or elevated due to prerenal (hypovolemia), renal, or postrenal (urinary tract disruption) causes. These values may be normal with mild or unilateral renal trauma. If there is an abdominal effusion present, an abdominal paracentesis should be performed. Any fluid obtained should be analyzed for the presence of blood, urea, creatinine, bacteria, white blood cells, and ingesta. If the fluid creatinine level is greater than the serum creatinine level, urinary tract rupture is demonstrated.[2,3]

Abdominal radiography is always indicated in the evaluation of patients with renal trauma. Radiography may be helpful in identifying unilateral renomegaly—the result of a hematoma. The presence of blood or urine in the retroperitoneal space may be suggested by asymmetry, displacement, or nonvisualization of renal shadow(s); displacement of the colon; or a hazy, streaking density in the sublumbar area. The accumulation of blood or urine in the abdominal cavity will cause reduction or loss of the normal intraabdominal detail on radiography.

Excretory urography is usually necessary to localize and define the nature of renal injury. Excretory urography will concurrently assess function of the contralateral (noninjured) kidney in cases of unilateral renal injury.[13] With a renal injury, the normal kidney may be excreting all the urine and the injured kidney could be completely nonfunctional.[2,3] The techniques for excretory urography have been discussed in detail elsewhere.[4,13-17] Rupture of the renal capsule/parenchyma or a laceration of the renal pelvis will cause extravasation of contrast material into the retroperitoneal space or abdominal cavity (Fig. 21-1). Contrast material may accumulate diffusely within the renal capsule if there is parenchymal injury with an intact capsule. With damage to or avulsion of the renal pedicle there may be nonvisualization of the affected kidney. Hematoma formation is suggested by irregularities in the renal pelvis. In a study of 127 human patients sustaining blunt renal trauma in which excretory urography was performed, it was demonstrated that when the intravenous pyelogram was reported as normal there was no renal damage other than contusion. Findings, of nonvisualization of the kidney or extravasation of the contrast material were associated with renal fractures, perforation, or pedicle injuries in all cases.[18] In penetrating trauma the intravenous pyelogram was unreliable in ruling out serious renal injury.[18] If the excretory urogram fails to visualize one or both kidneys, renal arteriography may be considered. This technique has the advantage of being able to delineate damage to the vascular pedicle.

Delayed contrast excretion and incomplete filling of the pelvis are nonspecific findings in all types of trauma and require further examinations: serial intravenous pyelography, arteriography, ul-

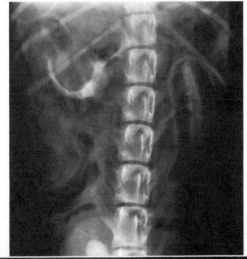

A

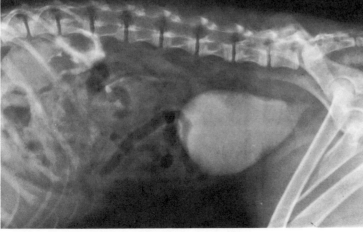

B

Fig. 21-1 **A,** Ventrodorsal, and **B,** lateral abdominal radiographs of an intravenous pyelogram in a dog, demonstrating subcapsular contrast around right kidney due to renal pelvic rupture.

trasonography, renal nuclear imaging, or computed tomography.[18,19] Ultrasonography can delineate renomegaly (hematoma) and retroperitoneal fluid. Computed tomography is comparable to excretory urography and is advocated for evaluation of the stable patient with blunt abdominal organ injury, the patient with multiple injuries, and for the patient suspected of having major traumatic injury.[1]

Treatment. Initial treatment is directed to stabilizing the traumatized patient with intravenous fluids and appropriate shock therapy (Chapters 10 and 14). Renal contusions, mild lacerations, and hematomas are generally self-limiting and are not treated. A hematoma or large contusion is not disturbed unless the lesion is expanding from continued hemorrhage. Severe lacerations of the renal capsule, parenchyma, or renal pelvis require laparotomy with debridement and suturing of the defect. With severe crushing or laceration of one pole of the kidney, treatment consists of partial nephrectomy. Generalized crushing (greater than 50% of the kidney) or avulsion of the vascular pedicle usually requires total nephrectomy. It is important first to ensure normal function of the contralateral kidney. Techniques for partial and total nephrectomy have been discussed elsewhere.[4,8,9,20] Broad-spectrum antibiotics are recommended perioperatively during nephrectomy and postoperatively for treatment in the case of peritonitis.

Whether the renal injury is handled by medical or surgical means, the patient should be closely monitored. Intravenous fluids should be administered at 88 to 110 ml/kg per day to maintain adequate renal perfusion and to provide a diuresis to prevent clot formation (obstruction). Urine output should be measured to assess adequate urine production and renal perfusion. The patient should be monitored for pyrexia and persistent abdominal pain or distention. Laboratory parameters that should be monitored are blood urea nitrogen, serum creatinine, and serum electrolyte levels. Urine should be monitored for persistence of hematuria. Repeat excretory urography should be performed in 10 to 21 days to assess renal blood flow and integrity.

Ureteral trauma

Injury to the ureters most commonly results from blunt trauma (automobile injury or a fall). Acute injury to the ureter(s) can be self-limiting and mild, or it may be serious (avulsion from the kidney or bladder). In the previously mentioned study of pelvic trauma,[6] four dogs (out of the 39 with urinary tract trauma) had an avulsed ureter as suggested by retroperitoneal density changes

on survey radiography. Three dogs had radiographic evidence of hydroureter/hydronephrosis on excretory urography. Hydroureter/hydronephrosis secondary to ureteral trauma is probably the result of clot (hematoma) formation within the ureteral wall lumen or temporarily decreased ureteral peristalsis.[6] Ureteral injury may occur due to penetrating wounds or poor surgical technique while performing an ovariohysterectomy or other abdominal surgical procedure. In human medicine, 90% of ureteral injuries are the consequence of gunshot wounds. Spinal hyperextension injuries in children are unique to the production of upper ureteral avulsion.[1]

Trauma to the ureter generally results in extravasation of urine into the retroperitoneal space, with or without extension into the peritoneal cavity. The retroperitoneal accumulation of urine may result in the development of cellulitis.[21] Leakage of urine into the peritoneal space will result in sterile peritonitis; if the urine contains bacteria, a septic peritonitis will develop. The development of peritonitis leading to systemic illness and dehydration will result in prerenal azotemia. In the event that a ureter is avulsed from the bladder and urine leakage occurs into the peritoneal cavity, the volume accumulating in the peritoneum may be significant enough to cause peritonitis and result in postrenal azotemia (even though voiding of urine is preserved).

Clinical signs. Clinical signs of a ruptured ureter are often vague and nonlocalizing, developing acutely or over several days. Hematuria is an inconsistent finding with ureteral trauma. The development of retroperitoneal cellulitis may cause localized pain or abdominal discomfort. Patients with peritonitis have evidence of abdominal discomfort and distention, pyrexia, vomiting, and ileus. Animals with ureteral calculi and neoplasms may also present with sublumbar pain. Uroabdomen associated with ureteral injury must be differentiated from other causes of abdominal effusion and acute abdomen. Hydroureter and hydronephrosis secondary to urethral stricture of obstruction may take weeks to months to develop. Typically, azotemia does not develop if there is unilateral ureteral obstruction.

Radiographic evaluation of the abdomen may demonstrate abdominal effusion and soft-tissue densities in the region of the kidney or trigone of the bladder, and sublumbar tissue fascial planes may be recognized if urine leakage has occurred retroperitoneally. The excretory urogram is the most useful diagnostic procedure to localize the site of rupture and urine leakage. Avulsion of a ureter may allow leakage of contrast medium into the peritoneal cavity. A partial tear close to the kidney will reveal contrast agent extravasation into the retroperitoneal space.[2,21,22] Ultrasonography is a useful diagnostic adjunct to excretory urography, in differentiating hematoma formation from urine leakage.[2,21]

Diagnostic procedures should include an urinalysis (hematuria), a complete blood count (leukocytosis if peritonitis is present), and a serum biochemical profile (azotemia, if significant reabsorption of urine has occurred). Abdominal paracentesis should be performed to evaluate the character of any abdominal effusion. The fluid should be analyzed for creatinine content and cultured for bacterial organisms if peritonitis is suspected.

Treatment. Ureteral trauma usually requires that an exploratory laparotomy be performed to assess and repair the damage. In humans, the most frequent ureteral injury associated with blunt trauma is avulsion at the ureteropelvic junction, and the procedure most frequently chosen is ureteral reimplantation.[23] In the dog and cat, the two most common sites of injury are at the renal pelvis or the trigone of the bladder.[5,21] Small ureteral tears may spontaneously heal, so the extravasation of a small amount of urine is not an absolute indication for immediate surgery. There is no information available in the veterinary literature as to how many of these tears that heal spontaneously progress to areas of strictures. For this reason, in animals, early exploratory surgery and definitive surgical repair is preferred over prolonged conservative medical management. Small lacerations of the ureter are debrided and sutured with absorbable suture material 5-0 to 7-0 (chromic cat gut, polyglycolic acid).[5] The suture line can be sealed with a thin film of a fluorinated tissue adhesive (fluoroalkyl cyanoacrylate). Larger, transecting lacerations of the ureter require reanastomosis. A polyethylene or polyvinyl catheter may be used as a stent at the site of ureteral reanastomosis (passed through the urinary bladder and out the urethra), to minimize postoperative stricture formation. These catheter stents are left in place for 5 to 7 days.[5] Damage to long portions of the ureter may necessitate replacement of the ureter with a segment of ileum.[22] If the ureteral avulsion or laceration is at the kidney, reanastomosis or closure may be possible by using a stenting catheter[5]; nephropexy to the abdominal wall may be required with this technique. Ureteral avulsion near the urinary bladder may allow for reimplantation of the ureter into the urinary bladder.[5,21,22] If the ureteral tissue is extensively devitalized or severe hydronephrosis is present, then nephrectomy is indicated.[2,5,21,23]

Regardless of the surgical repair performed, copious abdominal lavage should be performed during surgery. Broad-spectrum antibiotics are recommended perioperatively. If infection is suspected, cultures should be obtained and continued antibiotic therapy administered. If cultures are negative in 24 to 48 hours, antibiotic therapy is discontinued. Intravenous fluid therapy with a balanced electrolyte solution should be administered for 5 to 7 days to maintain adequate renal blood flow and urine flow through the repaired ureter. Parameters that should be monitored postoperatively include urine output, blood urea nitrogen and serum creatinine concentrations, serum electrolytes, white blood cell count, and body temperature. Excretory urography should be performed 3 to 5 days postoperatively to assess the patency of the ureter. Forty percent of damaged ureters develop early strictures (localized swelling, inflammation), and 50% of these strictures persist (devascularization injury). The integrity of the ureter should be reevaluated in 10 to 14 days in these cases to see if the stricture persists or has resolved spontaneously. Excretory urography should also be repeated routinely at 1 and 3 months after surgical repair to assess patency of the ureter.[2,5,21]

LOWER URINARY TRACT TRAUMA
Urinary bladder trauma

Trauma to the urinary bladder is very common. It may occur as the result of blunt abdominal trauma (automobile accident or a fall), penetrating wounds (animal bite, a gunshot or knife injury, or penetrating pelvic fractures), overaggressive abdominal palpation or forceful catheterization, urethral obstruction (calculi, tumors, idiopathic feline lower urinary tract disorders), and excessive straining at parturition.

In one study of 100 dogs with pelvic fractures from blunt trauma, 39 dogs had abnormalities in the urinary tract. Of these, 7 dogs had ruptured bladders, 15 others had bladder mucosal irregularities or clots, and 5 dogs had herniated or displaced bladders.[6] In most cases of blunt abdominal trauma, a contusion or mild self-limiting mucosal hemorrhage and hematuria is the most common bladder injury.[24,25] In another study, 29% of dogs with abdominal trauma secondary to automobile injury had ruptured bladders.[2,6,24-25] The most common site of bladder rupture is in the fundic region; rupture here is most likely to occur if the bladder is full prior to injury.

In a study of "high-rise syndrome" in cats, 132 cases were reviewed; nine cats had radiographic evidence of hydroperitoneum or hemoperitoneum. Three of these cats had ruptured urinary bladders. Hematuria without bladder rupture was documented in five cats; in all five the hematuria resolved spontaneously.[26] It is believed that some cats may partially void before impact, thus decreasing the chances for bladder rupture.[6,24-26]

Male dogs appear to be more prone to bladder rupture than female dogs; this may be due to a longer and narrower distal urethra, resulting in a greater resistance to urine flow than in the female.[24,25]

The bladder is almost impossible to injure when empty except when penetrated by a sharp object. When the urinary bladder is full, any pressure on the caudal abdomen is transmitted to the bladder and injury or rupture may occur. Lower urinary tract ruptures produce more dramatic early signs than do ruptures high in the urinary tract.[20,23] Urine accumulation within the peritoneal cavity will cause chemical peritonitis. Septic peritonitis will develop if there is a urinary tract infection present prior to urinary bladder rupture.

The presence of urine (hyperosmolar fluid) in large quantities in the peritoneal cavity will lead to osmotically induced shifts in fluid compartments. Because urine is hyperosmolar to plasma it will draw water from the extracellular space into the peritoneal cavity. Electrolytes are rapidly reabsorbed with equilibrium occurring between peritoneal fluid and plasma concentrations. The rate and degree of diffusion across the peritoneal membrane is dependent on the molecular size of the solute. Urea is a relatively small molecule that rapidly diffuses across the peritoneal membrane. Although urine has a higher concentration of urea than plasma, the concentration in plasma and the peritoneal cavity rapidly reach equilibrium. Creatinine is a larger molecule than urea, and it diffuses much more slowly across the peritoneum. Therefore, comparison of plasma to peritoneal fluid creatinine concentration is the best method of determining whether the peritoneal fluid is urine; the creatinine concentration of urine-contaminated peritoneal fluid is characteristically at least twice that of plasma.[9,24,25]

The development of azotemia, hyponatremia, hyperkalemia, hyperphosphatemia, and metabolic acidosis depends on the health of the animal prior to bladder rupture and the presence or absence of concurrent injuries, dehydration, and partial voiding.[2,9,24,25] Small tears in the bladder wall may quickly seal; any urine leaked into the peritoneal cavity is readily reabsorbed, and adverse effects do not occur. Essentially, this is what occurs each time a cystocentesis is performed.

Clinical signs. Clinical signs of bladder rupture vary greatly depending on the degree of damage and the duration of rupture. Clinical signs of shock or signs referable to damage of other organ systems may mask signs related to the urinary system in traumatized animals. The animal may initially respond to treatment for shock and other injuries, and then deteriorate over the next few days. Clinical signs caused by bladder rupture may take hours to days to manifest. If bladder rupture is left untreated, death may occur within 48 to 72 hours.

Animals with urinary bladder rupture may present acutely with abdominal pain, abdominal distention, and shock. Alternatively, these animals may manifest nonspecific and slowly progressive signs (anorexia, lethargy, fever, vomiting, dehydration) as azotemia develops. Peritonitis is suggested by abdominal pain or splinting, and a stiff or stilted gait. Vomiting may be associated with ileus, peritonitis, or postrenal uremia.[2,9,24,25]

Hematuria is a very common sign of bladder trauma. Hematuria usually resolves within a few days. In humans, more than 90% of patients with bladder trauma have hematuria.[2,23-25]

The ability to pass urine is variable and voiding of urine does not mean that the bladder is intact. If a urethral catheter is passed, it may enter the peritoneum through a tear in the bladder wall, and extravasated urine that is collected can give the false impression that the bladder is intact. An absence of urine may be found on passing a urethral catheter in an animal with bladder trauma. This is an unreliable sign of bladder rupture, as the patient may have voided or may be in shock.

A routine physical examination should be performed on all animals with a history or clinical signs of abdominal trauma. The caudal abdomen should be palpated prior to and following fluid therapy to detect the urinary bladder. Ballottement should be performed on the abdomen in order to detect free fluid. A rectal examination should be performed to evaluate the integrity of the pelvis and the pelvic urethra. Witnessing voluntary urination by the animal may be helpful, but observing urination or collecting urine via a catheter does not ensure an intact bladder wall. In the case of an iatrogenic rupture, the bladder may be distended one minute and small the next instant. While animals with traumatic bladder ruptures may go undetected and unattended for 24 hours, animals with bladder ruptures secondary to urethral obstruction deteriorate rapidly and must be attended to promptly as they are often uremic prior to bladder rupture.[24,25]

The laboratory findings of an animal with bladder rupture are nonspecific and dependent on the duration of the injury. A urinalysis often reveals hematuria, proteinuria, and pyuria. A complete blood count may demonstrate hemoconcentration and a leukocytosis (peritonitis). The results of a serum biochemistry profile may reveal azotemia, hyperkalemia, hyperphosphatemia, hyponatremia, and hypochloremia. Electrocardiography may be useful for detection of hyperkalemia (see Chapter 18). Blood gas analysis often reveals metabolic acidosis. Abdominal paracentesis or lavage should be performed when an abdominal effusion is detected or suspected (see Chapter 13).

Abdominal radiographs should be evaluated to determine if a bladder silhouette is visible; rupture should be considered if there is poor delineation of the bladder, if the bladder is greatly contracted, or if there is loss of the normal serosal detail of abdominal organs. Sterile saline (4 to 6 ml/kg) may be infused into the bladder to allow palpation of an intact bladder and improve its radiographic visualization. Positive contrast cystourethrography is the diagnostic test of choice in evaluating bladder trauma.[2,17] A water-soluble organic iodide contrast medium (meglumine 60% diluted to 10%) is recommended. Infuse the 10% solution of positive contrast media until the bladder is maximally distended as determined by digital palpation.[17] If bladder rupture is present, extravasation of contrast media will be observed in the peritoneal cavity (Fig. 21-2). Small ruptures may not be detected in this manner. Double-contrast cystography may reveal large blood clots in the bladder, a traumatic diverticulum, or mucosal separation in cases of bladder trauma without bladder rupture.[17] Excretory urography should also be performed to assess the upper urinary tract prior to surgery, especially in instances of blunt abdominal trauma.

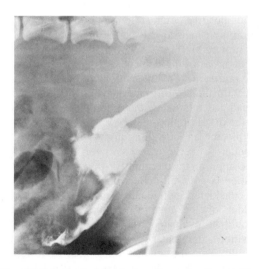

Fig. 21-2 Lateral abdominal radiograph of a positive contrast cystogram in a dog demonstrating a very irregular appearing bladder and extravasation of contrast medium into the caudoventral peritoneal cavity.

Treatment. Contusions, partial mucosal tears, and other injuries to the bladder that result in hematuria without bladder rupture should be treated conservatively. A broad-spectrum antibiotic should be administered for 7 to 10 days if concomitant or secondary urinary tract infection is present. If the hematuria is excessive, cold sterile saline should be infused into the bladder to reduce the hemorrhage and aid in removal of blood clots that may cause urethral obstruction or act as a nidus for infection. Intravenous fluid therapy is indicated to maintain urine flow in these cases.[24]

Patients with bladder rupture should be stabilized prior to surgical intervention. Intravenous fluid therapy should be instituted in order to maintain fluid balance and correct dehydration (Chapter 38). The electrolyte abnormalities associated with a ruptured bladder dictate the initial fluid of choice (normal saline). Sodium bicarbonate is administered as indicated based on blood gas analysis (administered when pH <7.2). As the animal's condition improves and the biochemical abnormalities resolve, the fluid administration may be changed to a balanced electrolyte solution (lactated Ringer's solution). An indwelling urinary catheter should be placed in the bladder to minimize continued urine leakage into the peritoneum. If the patient is in extremely critical condition (uremia or peritonitis), peritoneal dialysis (Chapter 39) should be instituted to remove urine from the peritoneal cavity and correct the uremia. Peritoneal dialysis may allow surgery to be delayed for a few days in order to stabilize any associated injuries (flail chest, pericardial tamponade, pneumothorax, arrhythmias) prior to surgical correction of a bladder rupture. Following patient stabilization, exploratory laparotomy should be performed. The techniques for surgical repair of the bladder wall have been discussed in detail.[27] The abdomen should be lavaged intraoperatively with copious amounts of sterile saline to remove urine and reduce peritonitis.[2,20,24,25,27] Appropriate cultures should be taken prior to or at the time of surgery.

Intravenous fluid therapy should be continued postoperatively to maintain hydration, correct any remaining electrolyte abnormalities, and to ensure urine production. Urine output and the degree of hematuria should be closely monitored for 2 to 5 days. Indwelling urinary catheter usage should be avoided at this point in order to reduce intravesicular trauma and risk of ascending infection, and intermittent catheterization should be employed as needed to assess urine production and assist in voiding. Antibiotic therapy should be administered for at least 7 to 10 days in cases with positive culture results. A ruptured bladder is an emergency that requires careful diagnosis and immediate treatment, including surgical intervention. With appropriate treatment, the patient's prognosis for recovery and return to normal function is good.

Urethral trauma

The causes of urethral trauma are similar to those of bladder trauma. Most commonly, urethral trauma or rupture is associated with pelvic fractures or fractures of the os penis in the dog, penetrating wounds (bites or lacerations), poor catheterization techniques, and urethral obstructions. The degree of trauma may vary from urethritis to perforation to complete severance. The most common site of urethral rupture is at the cysto-urethral junction. Urethral obstruction will be dealt with elsewhere in this chapter; this section will deal with the management of urethral trauma.[2,9,24,28,29]

Rupture of the urethra at the trigone allows urine to escape into the peritoneal cavity; the sequelae are consistent with that of bladder rupture. With urethral tears, urine will more commonly leak into the retroperitoneal soft tissues (perineal region), resulting in cellulitis. Postrenal azotemia may occur due to the reabsorption of urine by the tissues.

Clinical signs. The clinical signs depend on the site of urethral injury and whether or not urine outflow is affected. There is no age or breed predisposition. Male dogs are more commonly affected than female dogs or cats. A longer urethral length and an increased zone of resistance to urine outflow is the reason for the increased prevalence of urethral rupture following trauma in male dogs. If the urethral rupture has occurred at the trigone, the clinical signs that are produced in the animal are similar to a ruptured bladder. Animals with lacerations in the distal urethra present with local pain, cellulitis, dysuria, and hematuria. An animal with a complete urethral disruption may present "anuric" with a painful distended bladder. Progressive lethargy, vomiting, and anorexia are signs associated with the concurrent postrenal azotemia that may occur following urethral trauma in animals. Tissue necrosis at the site of urethral rupture is not uncommon following the extravasation of urine. Laboratory evaluation of the patient with urethral rupture results in data similar to that found in animals with a ruptured bladder, i.e., leukocytosis, dehydration, and azotemia.

Urethral laceration or rupture must be high on the list of differential diagnoses in trauma patients with multiple pelvic fractures, bite wounds of the perineum or penis, or stranguria and pain localized to the urethra. Differential diagnoses, de-

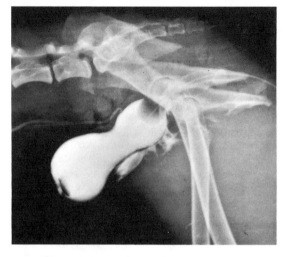

Fig. 21-3 Lateral abdominal radiograph of a cystourethrogram in a dog, demonstrating pelvic fractures and urethral rupture secondary to injury by an automobile. Extravasation of contrast material appears centered on the cranial portion of the pelvic urethra and has opacified the retroperitoneal tissues.

pending on the constellation of clinical signs, should include trauma to other portions of the urinary tract, soft-tissue damage in the perineal region, periurethral abscess, or neoplasia, and other causes of abdominal fluid accumulation. An attempt should be made to pass a urinary catheter. In cases of urethral trauma, it may not be possible to pass the catheter into the bladder, depending on the size and location of the tear. Radiographic evaluation may reveal soft-tissue swelling in the perineal region, loss of abdominal contrast, and concomitant pelvic fractures or fractures of the os penis. The definitive diagnostic test is the retrograde positive contrast urethrogram. Contrast medium is visualized outside the urethra at the point of rupture(s) (Fig. 21-3); small lacerations may show up as filling defects.

Treatment. Treatment of urethral trauma varies with the severity and location of the rupture. Small lacerations, without complete transection, of the distal urethra may be treated conservatively by placing an indwelling urinary catheter into the bladder (to serve as a stent) for 10 to 14 days. The appropriate duration for posttrauma catheterization is not well defined, and each patient must be considered individually based on the cause and extent of the urethral trauma.[30] The catheter should be evaluated frequently to ensure proper position and patency. An Elizabethan collar should be used to prevent the animal from removing the catheter. The catheter should not forcibly distend the urethra, as this situation may lead to increased stricture formation. Urethral ruptures caused by fractures of the os penis may be corrected with surgical stabilization of the os penis in conjunction with suturing of the urethra (accompanied by indwelling catheterization) or urethrostomy proximal to the fracture.[31] A prescrotal or perineal urethrostomy may be performed if there is extensive tissue damage accompanying distal urethral tears or when the urethral tear is proximal to the os penis. In cats, ruptured urethras are frequently associated with attempts at catheterization to relieve a urethral obstruction. The site is commonly in the penile urethra, and a perineal urethrostomy is often indicated for treatment of these urethral tears. Lacerations involving the pelvic urethra and separation of the urethra from the bladder at the trigone usually require surgical exploration (pelvic symphysiotomy) and urethral reanastomosis. The laceration should be sutured over an indwelling urinary catheter and the catheter is left in place for 10 to 14 days.

If the animal with a urethral rupture is initially unstable for anesthesia, and an indwelling urethral catheter into the bladder cannot be placed; a temporary tube cystotomy using a Foley catheter can be performed, under local anesthesia or reversible narcotic analgesia, to allow continued passage of urine. By using a temporary tube cystotomy, surgery can be delayed for 3 to 5 days while the patient is being stabilized.[30,32]

It is important to monitor the position and patency of the indwelling urethral catheter following surgical repair of urethral tears. The bladder should be kept as small as possible. Development of urinary tract infection should be anticipated when indwelling urinary catheterization is employed. Frequent urinalyses should be performed, and urine should be collected for bacteriologic culture at the first indication of infection. The most common complications following repair of urethral tears are continued urine leakage and dehiscence leading to stricture formation. Periurethral cellulitis should be treated with warm compresses. Perineal wound drainage and continued debridement may be necessary if tissue necrosis is extensive. A possible complication of intrapelvic urethral trauma is urinary incontinence from the primary injury or from surgical trauma.[30] A sympathetic alpha agonist such as phenylpropanolamine may be indicated (2.2 mg/kg divided twice a day).[33] A cystourethrogram should be performed 4 to 6 weeks after repair of urethral injuries to assess the patency of the urethra.[2,28-35]

Urethral prolapse

Urethral prolapse is uncommon and occurs most often in male dogs of the brachycephalic breeds as a result of excessive sexual excitement or masturbation. Urethral prolapse may also occur as the result of excessive stranguria secondary to urethral calculi or a genitourinary tract infection.

Clinical signs associated with urethral prolapse include excessive licking of the prepuce and bleeding from the prepucial orifice. Examination of the prepuce and penis reveals variable lengths of red or purple urethral mucosa protruding from the urethral orifice.

A urethral prolapse should be reduced as soon as possible, to avoid devitalization of the tissue. Urethral prolapses may reduce spontaneously, but often will recur. The treatment consists of anesthetizing the dog and manually reducing the prolapse with a urinary catheter. A purse-string suture should be placed around the penile orifice and left in place for 5 to 7 days. If the prolapsed portion can not be manually reduced, amputation of the redundant mucosa will be necessary.

Postoperatively, an Elizabethan collar and sedation are often required to prevent self-mutilation. Castration may be necessary to reduce the chances of recurrence. Affected animals should be evaluated and treated for any underlying urinary tract infections or uroliths.

URETHRAL OBSTRUCTION—DOG

Urethral obstruction is a common occurrence in dogs. Causes of urethral obstruction include urolithiasis, prostatic disease, neoplasia, and trauma to the urethra, pelvis, or os penis. Acute obstruction most often affects the male dog because of the anatomical configuration of the urethra. Urethral obstruction secondary to urolithiasis has the highest prevalence, with a frequency ranging from 0.4% to 2.8% of hospital admissions.[24]

Causes

The most common causes of urethral obstruction in the dog are uroliths and gelatinous urethral plugs. Urolithiasis has been reported in all ages of dogs. The most common age for affected dogs is between 3 and 7 years, with a mean age of 5.5 years. There are few reports in dogs under 8 weeks of age.[36] The most common site of urolith obstruction in the male dog is at the proximal aspect of the penis. Urolithiasis causing urethral obstruction in the female dog is rare. There are five common types of calculi based on composition: magnesium ammonium phosphate (struvite), calcium oxalate, urate, cysteine, and silica. Struvite uroliths are the most common form found in dogs (70%) and frequently occur in association with urinary tract infections. Further details on the topic of canine urolithiasis may be found elsewhere.[24,37-39]

Transitional-cell carcinoma at the bladder

trigone or along the urethra is frequently associated with complete or partial urethral obstruction. Urethral neoplasia develops predominantly in female dogs; 69% to 90% of those developing in the male are squamous-cell carcinomas.[40] There is one report of two cases of penile neoplasia (squamous-cell carcinoma of the penile urethra and mesenchymal chondrosarcoma of the os penis) causing complete urethral obstruction.[40]

Urethral obstruction can occur as a result of stricture formation during healing of fractures of the os penis,[41] as a result of foreign bodies lodging in the urethra, and in association with pelvic or urethral trauma, obstructive urethritis, or as a complication of dystocia.[42]

Clinical signs

The clinical signs associated with acute urethral obstruction include pain, stranguria, dysuria, "anuria," anxiousness, pacing, and licking at the penis or vulva. Commonly, the owner will mistakenly believe the patient has constipation. As the obstruction persists, post-renal uremia develops with metabolic acidosis, hyperkalemia, dehydration, hyperventilation, bradycardia, and hypothermia. An extremely uremic animal with an obstruction of long duration will often be presented in a comatose state. If the obstruction is not relieved, death usually occurs within 3 to 5 days. Prolonged overdistention of the bladder may result in necrosis and bladder-wall rupture.

There has been one report of a dog presenting with hyperammonemia following urethral obstruction.[43] In humans with normal hepatic function the most common cause of hyperammonemia is urinary stasis and infection with urea-splitting organisms.[43]

Urethral obstruction is diagnosed by history (stranguria or "anuria") and physical examination. Abdominal palpation usually reveals a large, turgid bladder that cannot be manually expressed. Attempts to pass a urinary catheter into the bladder are often unsuccessful. Abdominal and pelvic radiography may demonstrate radiodense calculi or a foreign body as the cause of the urethral obstruction. Radiographic contrast studies may be required to outline neoplasia and radiolucent calculi and to evaluate the integrity of the bladder. A complete blood count, urinalysis with microbiological culture and antibiotic sensitivity testing, serum biochemical profile, and an arterial blood gas are indicated to assess the extent of injury to the kidneys and the degree of electrolyte and metabolic imbalance resulting from the obstruction. Uroliths obtained during urethral catheterization procedures should be qualitatively and quantitatively analyzed and cultured.

Treatment

An animal presenting for a urinary tract obstruction should always be treated as an emergency. The primary goals are to relieve the obstruction, treat postrenal uremia, and eliminate the cause of the problem (see box on p. 305). Overzealous palpation of the urinary bladder should be avoided in animals with urethral obstruction, as this manipulation often leads to iatrogenic bladder rupture.

Relief of urethral obstruction. Administration of sedatives to the dog prior to attempting urethral catheterization is advisable in many cases in order to minimize iatrogenic complications and to decrease urethral spasms. Sedatives must be used with caution in uremic dogs. Barbiturates and dissociative drugs will have delayed clearance and are potentially toxic in uremic animals. Narcotic agents such as oxymorphone or butorphanol are preferable because the narcotic effect of these drugs is reversible. Promazine tranquilizers, inhalant anesthetics, and a topical anesthetic flushed into the urethra prior to catheterization may be used.

In the case of obstruction secondary to uroliths, the obstruction may be relieved by hydropulsion of the calculi out of the distal urethra and/or into the bladder. A urinary catheter is cautiously advanced into the urethra until the obstruction is encountered. Saline (12-ml aliquots) is injected into the catheter, as the urethral orifice is compressed around the catheter, in an attempt to flush the grit or urolith into the bladder. If this manipulation does not relieve the obstruction, then an assistant should compress the pelvic urethra against the pelvic floor by rectal manipulation while hydropulsion is repeated. Saline is reinjected to distend the urethra and the catheter is quickly withdrawn while digital pressure is released. Once the catheter is passed into the bladder, the bladder should be completely emptied and flushed with sterile crystalloid solution and the catheter sutured in place to maintain a patent lower urinary tract. The catheter should be connected to a closed collection system to minimize bacterial contamination of the urinary tract and subsequent infection (Fig. 21-4).

If hydropulsion cannot dislodge the calculi, or if the obstruction is due to a cause (neoplasia) that prohibits passage of a catheter into the bladder, then the bladder should be emptied by cystocentesis (22-gauge needle). These animals require an emergency surgical procedure to establish a patent lower urinary tract (urethrostomy, tube cystostomy in cases with extensive pelvic trauma or neoplasia).

Four types of urethrostomy are recommended:

MANAGEMENT OF URETHRAL OBSTRUCTIONS IN THE DOG

Relieve obstruction
  Insert urethral catheter past obstruction
  Hydropulsion (urolithiasis)
    Relieve urethral spasm with topical anesthetic
    Sedate patient using a narcotic analgesic
      Oxymorphone: 0.1 to 0.2 mg/kg intravenously
      Butorphanol: 0.4 to 0.8 mg/kg intravenously
    Backflush into bladder using normal saline
  Cystocentesis
  Emergency surgical procedures (if unable to relieve obstruction)
    Urethrostomy—temporary or permanent
    Tube cystostomy
Suture indwelling urinary or cystostomy catheter in place
  Ensures patency of lower urinary tract
  Measure urine production
Diagnostic procedures/laboratory data
  Complete blood count
  Serum biochemical profile
    Monitor serum electrolytes
    Monitor serum creatinine, blood urea nitrogen
    Determine anion gap
  Blood gases
  Urinalysis—culture and sensitivity
  Abdominal and pelvic radiographs
    Survey films
    Contrast studies
  Calculi
    Quantitative and qualitative analysis
    Culture and sensitivity
Fluid therapy
  Intravenous fluids
    Initially normal saline (correct for dehydration and promote diuresis): estimated milliliters of fluid for administration over 24 hours =

% dehydration × body weight (kg) × 1000 ml + 66 ml/kg × body weight (kg)
After correction of dehydration, electrolyte and acid-base imbalances, switch to balanced electrolyte solutions
Correct metabolic derangements
  Hyperkalemia
    Normal saline
    Sodium bicarbonate 1.0-2.0 mEq/kg intravenously
    Regular insulin 1.0 unit/kg followed by glucose at 2 g/unit of insulin, give 25% of glucose dosage over the initial 5 minutes, then place the remainder in intravenous fluids to make a 2.5% dextrose solution
    10% calcium gluconate or 10% calcium chloride, 10% calcium gluconate—1 ml/2.5 kg intravenously slowly, 10% calcium chloride—1 ml/10 kg intravenously slowly
Metabolic acidosis
  Sodium bicarbonate (mEq) = 0.3 × body weight (kg) × base deficit (mEq/L)
  Infection
    Antibiotics
Monitoring the patient post obstruction
  Urine production
  Packed cell volume, total serum solids
  Blood urea nitrogen, serum creatinine, serum electrolytes
  Electrocardiogram
Definitive treatment for cause of obstruction
  Cystotomy—uroliths
  Surgery, chemotherapy—neoplasia
  Internal fixation, ostectomy—fractured pelvis, os penis

---

prescrotal, scrotal, antepubic, and perineal. A scrotal urethrostomy is the preferred option, if possible. The advantages to the scrotal urethrostomy are that the urethra is wide and accessible at this location.[32] The surgical options may be used for temporary or permanent urethrostomies.[24,32] A permanent urethrostomy is preferred because it aids in prevention of further obstruction and will not result in stricture and narrowing of the urethra when the surgical site heals.

Postrenal uremia. Any urethral obstruction that is longer than 24 hours in duration will result in a postrenal azotemia and possibly in obstructive nephropathy or acute renal failure. The patient with severe uremia will require extensive fluid diuresis. The fluid of choice is normal saline

until electrolyte abnormalities are corrected; then a balanced electrolyte solution may be substituted. When fluid deficits, electrolyte, and acid-base imbalances are corrected, an osmotic diuresis may be instituted, if needed, using 5% dextrose in lactated Ringer's solution to improve renal function and reverse azotemia.[44]

The most serious electrolyte abnormality encountered with urethral obstruction is hyperkalemia. Hyperkalemia should be suspected when bradycardia and the electrocardiographic changes of peaked T waves, prolonged PR intervals, diminished P-wave amplitude, and atrial standstill are observed. If the serum potassium concentration is greater than 6.0 mEq/L, the relief of the obstruction and intravenous infusion of normal sa-

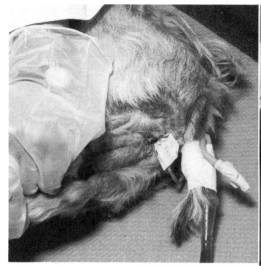

A

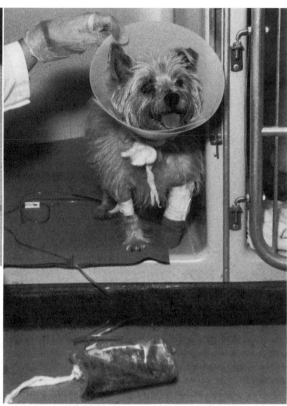

B

Fig. 21-4 A and **B**, An indwelling Foley urinary catheter sutured in place and attached to a closed collection system. Empty sterile fluid bags and administration sets may be substituted for prepackaged urinary collection systems.

line may not lower the serum potassium rapidly enough to obviate lethal cardiotoxicity. Sodium bicarbonate (1.0-2.0 mEq/kg) can be administered intravenously to temporarily translocate extracellular potassium into cells. Alternative treatment to manage the acute hyperkalemic crisis includes administration of regular insulin intravenously (1.0 unit/kg)[44] followed by a glucose bolus (2 g/unit of insulin administered) to translocate potassium intracellularly, or 10% calcium chloride/10% calcium gluconate as a slow intravenous infusion for direct cardioprotective effects.[42,44]

Metabolic acidosis is a frequent complication of total urethral obstruction. If the serum pH is below 7.1, then sodium bicarbonate should be administered until the pH has reached 7.2. The dose of bicarbonate required is calculated from the following equation:

$$mEq\ HCO_3^- = 0.3 \times BW \times base\ deficit\ (mEq/L)$$

where BW denotes body weight in kilograms.

Once the obstruction is relieved and dehydration corrected, a postobstructive polyuric phase is common. Determination of urine volume produced is helpful in determining fluid needs. Measuring intake and output will allow calculation of correct fluid volumes required to keep pace with urine production, prevent further dehydration, and resolve azotemia. The indwelling urethral or cystostomy catheter should be maintained until definitive treatment has been effected for the underlying cause of the urethral obstruction. Serial determination of total serum solids and serum electrolyte, creatinine, and blood urea nitrogen concentrations should be performed every 24 hours until values have stabilized or returned to normal.

Elimination of cause. Once the patient has been stabilized, the underlying cause of the obstruction should be treated. Calculi that have been hydropulsed into the bladder should be removed by cystotomy, analyzed, and cultured. Obstructive urethritis should be treated with an indwelling catheter, antibiotics, antiinflammatory agents, and antispasmodics.

Fractures of the os penis or pelvis should be stabilized by internal fixation. If the fracture of the os penis or pelvis is recent then urethral catheterization should be accompanied by internal orthopedic fixation. In the case of an old fracture, it is usually the healing process resulting in a fibrous or bony callus that causes the urethral obstruction. Surgical correction will require either a urethrostomy or a partial ostectomy.[41]

Neoplasia carries with it a poor prognosis, but

palliative measures include surgical excision, urethrostomy, and chemotherapy.

Underlying urinary tract infection associated with any cause of urethral obstruction should be treated with the appropriate antibiotic (based on culture and sensitivity testing) for a minimum of 7 to 10 days.

URETHRAL OBSTRUCTION—CAT

The most frequently seen urologic emergency in the male cat, and infrequently the female cat, is urethral obstruction, commonly a manifestation of feline idiopathic lower urinary tract disorders.[22,45-53] The inability to urinate leads to increased pressure within the urinary tract, postrenal azotemia, metabolic acidosis, and serum electrolyte changes. The seriousness of the problem is directly related to the length of time that the cat has had obstruction.

Causes

The most common cause of urethral obstruction in the male cat is a urethral plug. The plugs are composed of crystalline and cellular material with a proteinaceous matrix and are typically soft, pastelike, cylindrical structures.

The urethral lumen of male cats may occasionally become obstructed by tissue sloughed from the mucosal surface of the lower urinary tract; one report lists as causes a pseudomembranous cystitis and a transitional-cell carcinoma of the bladder.[45]

Urolithiasis may result in urethral obstruction of cats. Struvite urolithiasis comprises the most common form in the cat. Ammonium urate, uric acid, calcium phosphate, and calcium oxalate uroliths are less commonly reported. Cystine uroliths have not been reported in cats; there is one report of silica as a major constituent of a urolith in a cat.[45,54] Other causes of urethral obstruction in male and female cats include inflammatory diseases of the urethra (urethritis), neoplasia of the urethra or periurethral structures, and urethral strictures secondary to trauma.[53,55]

Clinical signs

Clinical signs of urethral obstruction in the cat are similar to those seen in the dog. Common clinical signs include pollakiuria, stranguria, hematuria, or an inability to urinate despite repeated attempts. The obstructed cat is frequently presented by the owner with the chief complaint that the cat has constipation and tenesmus; this is a common misinterpretation of the cat's frequent visits to the litter box. Inappropriate urination or attempts at urination, urinating outside of the litter box, licking at the genitals, pacing, vocalization, vomiting, anorexia, weakness, and dehydration are other common clinical signs.

Whereas dogs develop signs of postrenal uremia within 24 hours of obstruction, cats typically do not become severely uremic until 48 hours after complete obstruction. As the metabolic and electrolyte derangements worsen with the progression of uremia, hyperventilation secondary to acidosis and bradycardia secondary to hyperkalemia develop. As the cat becomes moribund it will become hypothermic and may be presented in a state of collapse. Death will occur within 3 to 5 days if the obstruction is not alleviated.[48] Prolonged overdistention of the bladder may result in necrosis of the bladder wall and rupture.

Diagnosis

The diagnosis of a urethral obstruction in cats is often apparent from the history and clinical signs. Physical examination reveals a distended, turgid bladder and painful caudal abdomen. Very often the penis of cats with urethral obstruction is swollen, inflamed, and protruded from the prepuce. A careful and gentle attempt at expressing the bladder manually is generally unsuccessful.

Abdominal and pelvic radiography is important in determining the causes of the urethral obstruction. Survey radiographs may be obtained immediately if the patient's condition is noncritical; otherwise radiographic evaluations should be postponed until the cat's urethral obstruction is relieved and the patient is stabilized.

Blood samples should be submitted for a complete blood count and serum biochemical profile. The hemogram usually demonstrates evidence of hemoconcentration secondary to dehydration. A stress leukogram may be present. The serum biochemical profile often reveals azotemia, mild hyponatremia, mild hypochloremia, hyperphosphatemia, hyperglycemia, and hypocalcemia. Metabolic acidosis will be seen in cats with complete obstruction of greater than 24 hours' duration.

Urinalysis reveals hematuria and often crystalluria. Pyuria and bacteriuria are inconsistent findings; only 10% of cats will have bacterial infections documented by urine culture.[48,55] Whenever urinary calculi are observed and recovered (during catheterization and hydropulsion, cystotomy/urethrostomy) they should be qualitatively and quantitatively analyzed and cultured.

Treatment of the cat with complicated obstruction

The immediate goal of treatment in the cat with obstruction is to relieve the obstruction. Proper restraint of the cat is an important consideration so that the obstruction can be relieved quickly and as atraumatically as possible. In severely ill patients physical restraint alone or in combination with a local anesthetic may be sufficient to allow urethral catheterization for relief of the obstruction. Wrapping the cat in a towel or placing in a cat restraint bag may help to protect the patient and medical staff. If local anesthetics are used to anesthetize the urethral mucosa during attempted catheterization, they should be administered in small quantities; topical anesthetic solutions should not be used as primary flushing solutions because these agents may induce systemic toxicity if absorbed. I commonly use 0.5 to 1.0 ml of 2% lidocaine. The topic of pharmacologic restraint in cats with obstructive uropathy has always prompted great controversy. Anesthetics must be given cautiously, as the patient with postrenal uremia often requires minimal dosages/concentrations. Administration of short-acting barbiturates that are metabolized by the liver or the use of inhalant anesthetic may be considered if general anesthesia is required. While the use of ketamine hydrochloride in cats with postrenal azotemia can be criticized, because the drug is excreted in active form by the kidneys, this drug has been used safely at low dosages (5 to 10 mg intravenously).[56]

Relief of urethral obstruction. The urethral plug occasionally can be removed from the urethra by gently rolling the penis between the thumb and forefinger. If this approach does not result in immediate relief of the urethral obstruction, it should be discontinued because continued manipulation may lead to urethral trauma. Urohydropulsion using an open-ended 4.5-in. polypropylene "tomcat" catheter (Monoject, St. Louis) or a silver abscess cannula (25-gauge) provides a nontraumatic means for relieving the urethral obstruction when massage of the cat's penis fails. Urohydropulsion involves the use of a 12-ml syringe filled with sterile saline to dislodge the obstruction by positive-pressure injection (backflushing) as the catheter/cannula is passed into the urethra. If the urethral plug is not immediately dislodged, several attempts should be made; continued flushing will loosen the plug in the majority of cases. It is important that the urethra be straightened as much as possible, this will aid in passing the catheter into the bladder and will decrease the chance of causing a urethral rupture.[24,56] In most cases, an indwelling urinary catheter (a 5.5-in. "tomcat" catheter with side holes, or a 3 to 5 French polyvinyl catheter) attached to a closed urine collection system should be left indwelling for 1 to 3 days. An indwelling urethral catheter ensures urethral patency. The closed collection system allows an accurate measurement of urine production (fluid requirements) and prevents saturation of the cat's fur with urine (prevents urine scalding).[48,56] The cat should be observed for 24 hours following removal of the catheter to ensure that obstruction does not recur and that temporary bladder atony due to overdistention is not present.

Occasionally, urohydropulsion does not relieve the obstruction; in these cases the bladder should be emptied via cystocentesis (22-gauge needle) and a repeated attempt made at urethral catheterization. In these cases, an emergency perineal urethrostomy should be performed following stabilization of the patient.

Fluid therapy. The fluid deficits, electrolyte and acid-base imbalances that may occur with obstructive uropathy in cats are similar to those discussed for urethral obstruction in the dog. The severity of the metabolic changes depends in large part on the duration of obstruction and the presence of any underlying disease.

Fluid therapy is very important in the treatment of cats with urinary tract obstructions. These cats are dehydrated and will experience a postobstructive diuresis that may last several hours to several days. Accurate measurement of urine production is essential to maintain adequate fluid therapy and adequate hydration for these cats during their polyuric state. Normal saline (0.9%) should be used for initial fluid resuscitation in these cats, and once electrolyte disturbances have been corrected, lactated Ringer's solution can be substituted for continued fluid administration. As postobstructive diuresis is almost inevitable, a 5% "push" (5% push = body weight [kg] × 0.05 × 1000 ml) is added to the fluid requirements calculated for rehydration and maintenance (Chapter 38). The calculated fluid requirements are divided into four treatments to be administered in 6-hour intervals. Urine production is measured to allow periodic calculations of urine output and appropriate changes in the fluid volume administered.[56]

Hyperkalemia. The most serious electrolyte abnormality encountered in the cat with urethral obstruction is hyperkalemia. Hyperkalemic cats often present as true life-threatening emergencies (laterally recumbent, hypothermic, dehydrated, and semicomatose). Electrocardiographic evaluation will usually confirm the suspicion of hyperkalemia. Electrocardiographic changes consistent with hyperkalemia include absence of P waves (atrial standstill), widened QRS complexes and large peaked T waves. In cats with life-threatening hyperkalemia, attempts are made to relieve the hyperkalemia before attempting to relieve the urethral obstruction.

An indwelling intravenous catheter for adminis-

MANAGEMENT OF URETHRAL OBSTRUCTION IN THE CAT

Relieve obstruction
  Gently massage penis between thumb and forefinger to remove plug
  Insert urethral catheter using hydropulsion*
    Relieve urethral spasm with topical anesthetic
    Sedate patient—inhalant anesthetic, short-acting thiobarbiturate intravenously; ketamine 5 to 10 mg intravenously
    Backflush 0.9% saline and pass the urethral catheter into the bladder
Secure and maintain indwelling urinary catheter
  Ensures patency of lower urinary tract
  Measure urine production
Diagnostic procedures/laboratory data
  Immediate electrocardiogram
  Complete blood count
  Serum biochemical profile
    Serum electrolytes
    Serum creatinine, blood urea nitrogen
    Determine anion gap
  Blood gas
  Urinalysis—culture and sensitivity
  Abdominal and pelvic radiography
    Survey films
    Contrast studies
Fluid therapy
  Intravenous fluids
    Initially 0.9% saline (ml fluid = replacement fluids + maintenance fluids + 5% push)
    Lactated Ringer's solution ± potassium chloride following correction of initial dehydration, electrolyte, and acid-base imbalances
Correct metabolic derangements
  Hyperkalemia
    Normal saline
    Sodium bicarbonate 1.0-2.0 mEq/kg intravenous slow bolus
    Regular insulin (1.0 unit/kg) and glucose (2 g/unit of insulin). Administer 25% of glucose dose over the initial 5 minutes, and place the remainder in intravenous fluids to be given over 12 hours
    10% calcium gluconate. 0.5-1.0 ml/kg intravenously slowly
  Metabolic acidosis
    Sodium bicarbonate (mEq) = 0.3 × body weight (kg) × base deficit (mEq/L)
Monitoring the patient post obstruction
  Urine production every 6 hours
  Packed cell volume and total serum solids every 12 hours
  Blood urea nitrogen, serum creatinine, serum electrolytes every 24 hours
  Electrocardiogram every 24 hours

---

*If unable to pass urethral catheter, cystocentesis and emergency surgical procedures (perineal urethrostomy) would be required.

tration of fluids and emergency drugs must be established. The treatment options for relieving hyperkalemia include intravenous administration of sodium bicarbonate, calcium gluconate and glucose/regular insulin (see box). Hyperkalemia is rapidly corrected following administration of these treatments, after relief of the urethral obstruction, and following intravenous administration of 0.9% saline. Hypokalemia may develop during the postobstructive diuresis, requiring potassium supplementation (Chapter 38).

Metabolic acidosis. Metabolic acidosis is invariably present in the hyperkalemic cat with urethral obstruction. This acidosis needs to be addressed specifically (administration of sodium bicarbonate) if the blood pH is <7.2 (Chapter 38). If the blood pH is above 7.2, then relief of the obstruction and intravenous fluid administration should allow the cat to correct its metabolic acidosis.

Surgical. Perineal urethrostomy, once a popular prophylactic treatment for urethral obstruction in cats, should only be considered for relief of urethral obstruction in cats that cannot be catheterized, the treatment of cats that have had multiple previous urethral obstructions, and the treatment of cats with poor urine streams secondary to urethral stricture formation following bouts of urethral obstruction.[48] Urethral obstruction from urolithiasis may be surgically corrected by removal of the calculi following stabilization of the patient.

Elimination of cause. Causes of urethral obstruction in cats such as urolithiasis and urethritis/cystitis are relatively easy to manage by surgical removal of the calculi or long-term treatment with administration of an appropriate antibiotic.

Unfortunately the cause(s) of idiopathic feline lower urinary tract disorders, including urethral obstruction from plug formation, remains unclear. These disorders often recur and some prophylactic measures that appear to be useful should be instituted. A low-magnesium or calculytic diet should be fed to cats with a history of lower urinary tract disease. These diets are designed to maintain urine pH between 5.5 and 6.0 to prevent struvite crystal precipitation. Water intake should be encouraged. The cats should be allowed to void frequently by allowing continued access to a clean litter box. Antispasmodic agents (flavoxate, oxybutynin, dicyclomine, propantheline bromide) can be used in cats with urge incontinence secondary to idiopathic urethritis/cystitis. Antiinflammatory drugs (corticosteroids) may be used with caution in cats with urethritis and persistent hematuria.

In most cases of idiopathic feline lower urinary tract disorder the urine is sterile. Bacterial infections will increase urine pH, so it is imperative to culture the urine of cats with lower urinary tract disease to make sure that infection is not present. Cats with an indwelling urinary catheter (open or closed collection system) are at increased risk for the development of urinary tract infections.[57-59]

ACUTE RENAL FAILURE

Acute renal failure (ARF) is a syndrome characterized by abrupt deterioration of renal function and inability to regulate solute and water balance adequately.[4,60-68] It is a tenuously reversible state, which must be quickly diagnosed and aggressively treated. Acute renal failure can be caused by acute prerenal failure, primary (intrinsic) failure, or postrenal failure. Differentiating intrarenal from prerenal ARF is the most important distinction to be made.[4] Acute renal failure occurs more frequently than is generally recognized and is often misdiagnosed as chronic renal failure. The importance of early recognition of ARF should be stressed, because it is a potentially reversible condition.

Pathophysiology

The primary cause of prerenal ARF is inadequate renal perfusion resulting from a variety of causes, including intravascular volume depletion (hemorrhage) or translocation of intravascular fluids (peritonitis, pancreatitis, burns); marked reductions in cardiac output (myocardial, valvular, or pericardial disease) or an abrupt decline in peripheral vascular resistance (vasodilation, sepsis).[63]

Interference with urine flow caused by a variety of traumatic, inflammatory or neoplastic processes in the upper or lower urinary tract may result in postrenal ARF. The cause, diagnosis, and management of postrenal ARF have been discussed elsewhere in this chapter.

Acute tubular necrosis is a syndrome of abrupt and sustained reduction in glomerular filtration rate (GFR) resulting from an ischemic or toxic renal insult and accounts for the majority of cases of primary (intrinsic) ARF.[67] Three mechanisms may contribute to decreased GFR or reduced renal tubular flow rate during ARF: tubular obstruction, tubular backleak, and primary filtration failure. Tubular obstruction may be intraluminal (casts, proteinaceous debris) or extraluminal (edema). The obstruction may elicit vasoconstriction at the level of the glomerulus and reduce filtration. Tubular backleak occurs when filtrate leaks back across or between damaged tubular cells and enters the renal venous circulation. Primary filtration failure results from inadequate glomerular capillary plasma flow, inadequate glomerular hydrostatic pressure, or altered glomerular permeability.[44,63,68]

Causes of acute intrinsic renal failure (see box)

Renal hypoperfusion/ischemia. The causes of hemodynamically mediated ARF are the same as those predisposing to prerenal ARF, except they are more profound and prolonged in intensity and duration with intrinsic ARF. Hypotension, hypovolemia, circulatory collapse, or other causes of insufficient renal perfusion (renal artery infarcts, disseminated intravascular coagulation, septic thrombi, vasculitis, peritonitis, and gastric torsion) can initiate ARF.[63] Animals that have experienced hemorrhage, trauma, extensive surgery, and prolonged anesthesia are at increased risk for the development of ARF.[62]

Intrarenal vasoconstriction is key to the development of ischemic ARF. In an attempt to maintain systemic arterial blood pressure during situations of hypoperfusion, increased vasopressor activity occurs as a result of increased activity of the sympathetic nervous system. The renal vasculature also experiences vasoconstriction from stimulation of renal catecholamine and angiotensin receptors. Under normal conditions, or during brief episodes of hypoperfusion, this effect is counterbalanced by the intrarenal production and action of prostaglandins.[68]

Renal vasoconstriction decreases renal blood flow in both the cortex and the medulla, with greater reduction in blood flow occurring in the cortex. Preservation of blood flow to the medulla may be a protective mechanism to supply oxygen to the metabolically active tubular cells in the outer medulla. The pars recta (straight portion of the proximal tubule) and the medullary thick as-

---

CAUSES OF ACUTE INTRINSIC RENAL FAILURE

Toxins
  Heavy metals
  Organic compounds, solvents
Drugs
  Antibiotics (aminoglycosides)
  Nonsteroidal antiinflammatory drugs
  Radiographic contrast agents
  Chemotherapeutic agents
Ethylene glycol
Ischemia
Infection
Acute hydronephrosis
Infarction
Hypercalcemia
Hemoglobinuria
Myoglobinuria
Biotoxins (snake venom)

cending limb of Henle's loop are cells with high metabolic activity, located in the outer medulla, and are at increased risk for ischemic injury. Swelling of proximal tubular cells located in the outer medulla further reduces renal blood flow, potentiating ischemic injury to the thick ascending limb of Henle. Renal tubular damage resulting from ischemia is characterized by a patchy distribution along nephrons, with a tendency toward disruption of the tubular basement membranes.[60,68]

Pigment nephropathy. Acute renal failure can be associated with endogenous toxins, usually breakdown products of muscle or blood. Pigment nephropathy is acute renal failure associated with the breakdown of muscle (myoglobin) or red blood cells (hemoglobin). Rhabdomyolysis should be considered in the differential diagnosis of ARF developing in patients with crush injuries or hyperthermia (Chapter 16). Rhabdomyolysis promotes a major shift of fluid from the intravascular space into injured tissue. The intravascular volume depletion reduces GFR and leads to slowing of tubular fluid flow rates, thereby predisposing to the intratubule precipitation of myoglobin. Ferrihemate, the nonglobin moiety derived from myoglobin degradation, may exert renal tubule toxicity by directly impairing cellular metabolism.[63,69]

Blood transfusion reactions are frequently complicated by acute tubular necrosis in people. Heme pigment nephropathy is an infrequent cause of ARF in dogs and cats in similar clinical situations.[62,63] The immune-mediated destruction of red blood cells and the release of free hemoglobin into the plasma may promote intravascular coagulation and the release of vasoactive substances that lead to increased vascular permeability, intravenous volume depletion, hypotension, and ARF.

Hypercalcemic nephropathy. Hypercalcemia from primary hyperparathyroidism, lymphoma, perianal adenocarcinoma, squamous-cell carcinoma, or excessive oral intake of calcium/vitamin D occasionally results in ARF.[62,70] The elevated plasma and ultrafiltrable calcium specifically damages tubular epithelium and glomeruli as well as inducing arteriolar constriction and ischemia.[62] Hypercalcemic nephropathy as a cause of ARF has been seen with increasing frequency with the advent of rodenticides (Quintox, Bell Laboratories; Rampage, Ceva Laboratories; Ortho Rat-B-Gone and Ortho Mouse-B-Gone, Chevron) that contain vitamin D_3 (cholecalciferol).

Infection. Sepsis or primary urinary tract infection is a common cause of ARF. A number of viral (infectious canine hepatitis, herpesvirus, canine distemper virus) and bacterial *(Escherichia coli, Streptococci, Staphylococci, Proteus, Klebsiella)* causes have been documented as the cause

of nephritis/pyelonephritis and of ARF. Pyelonephritis may be classified as acute or chronic. Patients with acute pyelonephritis have clinical signs that may vary from mild, nonspecific (pyrexia, lethargy, anorexia, vomiting) to profound (acute abdomen) consistent with septicemia (Chapter 13).[67] Clinical manifestations of chronic pyelonephritis are often subtle and nonspecific, commonly characterized by polyuria and polydipsia.[67] Leptospirosis is a recognized cause of ARF and should be entertained in the consideration of any differential diagnosis involving acute parenchymal failure.[62] Acute tubulointerstitial nephritis is associated with inflammatory-cell infiltrates and with tubular cell and glomerular necrosis of varying severity.[68]

Nephrotoxic chemicals and drugs. The administration of many chemicals and drugs has been associated with the development of ARF. The list of nephrotoxic agents is extensive and includes a variety of heavy metals, organic compounds, solvents, antimicrobials, and other miscellaneous drugs. Renal injury is attributed to attachment of the toxic agent to luminal, basolateral, or intracellular organelle membranes of renal tubular and glomerular cells. Increased membrane permeability and loss of cellular functions occur. The degradation of phospholipids in cell membranes appears to be central in initiating and perpetuating tubular-cell injury. The role of intracellular calcium in the development of nephrotoxic injury is unclear, but redistribution of calcium within the cell may be important in the early activation of phospholipase.[68]

Heavy metal (arsenic, lead, thallium, bismuth, mercury, and uranium) nephrotoxicity is rarely encountered in clinical practice, but was once a common cause of acute tubular necrosis. The heavy metals share a similar mode of action related to the interaction of the metal with membrane-bound sulfhydryl groups, thereby altering membrane permeability and a multitude of cellular enzymes, resulting in renal cell injury.[62,63] Excessive activation of the renin angiotensin system results in a decrease in GFR and renal blood flow (RBF), which leads to tubular necrosis; this effect has been observed with heavy metals.

Another heavy metal, platinum, in the form of cisplatin is an effective chemotherapeutic agent (Platinol, Bristol-Myers). Platinum clearance exceeds creatinine clearance, which indicates a predominant secretory process by the proximal renal tubular epithelium. Current evidence suggests that it shares the same affinity for membrane-bound sulfhydryl groups observed with other heavy metals. Platinum administration may be associated with oliguric or nonoliguric acute tubular necrosis. Augmentation of intravascular volumes by prehydration with saline and mannitol-induced diuresis has been known to decrease cisplatin toxicity.[63,71]

Methotrexate, cyclophosphamide, mithramycin, streptozocin, and doxorubicin are other cancer chemotherapy drugs whose administration has been associated with nephrotoxicity.[68,72]

Iodinated organic compounds (diatrizoate compounds: Hypaque, Cardiografin, Renografin) used as radiocontrast agents may cause ARF by direct toxicity to renal tubular cells and through hemodynamic mechanisms. In human medicine, ARF has been associated with the administration of these contrast agents to patients with diabetes mellitus, preexisting renal disease, or multiple myeloma.[69,73] Clinical cases have not been reported in veterinary medicine.

Administration of methoxyflurane and other fluorinated anesthetic agents has occasionally been associated with the development of ARF in human patients. Methoxyflurane is metabolized to several products including oxalate and inorganic fluoride. Nephrotoxicity is related to accumulation of both compounds. Dogs and cats may be as susceptible as humans to methoxyflurane-induced nephrotoxicity, but these animals may be at reduced risk in general because of the relatively shorter duration of anesthesia and surgery in veterinary medical patients.[63,74,75]

Nonsteroidal antiinflammatory drugs (NSAIDs) are widely used in veterinary medicine for the treatment of arthritis and other inflammatory conditions. There are a number of different categories of NSAIDs, including salicylates (aspirin), propionic acid derivatives (naproxen), pyrazolone derivatives (phenylbutazone), anthranilic acid derivatives (meclofenamic acid), and flunixin meglumine. All NSAIDs inactivate cyclooxygenase, a major enzyme in the biosynthetic pathway of eicosanoids. Acute renal failure results primarily from inhibition of local eicosanoid (prostaglandin) synthesis (local regulators of renal blood flow and renal tubular function).[74,76,77]

Ingestion of ethylene glycol (as antifreeze) is the most common cause of nephrotoxicity encountered in veterinary medical patients. Ethylene glycol is not toxic until metabolized to glycoaldehyde, glyoxylic acid, glycolate, and oxalic acid. Oxalic acid is the primary toxic intermediate, producing tubular epithelial-cell necrosis and intratubular obstruction secondary to calcium oxalate crystal deposition. Ethylene glycol and its metabolites also affect the central nervous system and heart of intoxicated animals.[62,78]

Aminoglycoside nephrotoxicity is the second most common cause of ARF in dogs and cats. Neomycin is the most nephrotoxic, streptomycin the least, and the toxicity of kanamycin, gentamicin, amikacin, tobramycin, and netilmicin is intermediate. Gentamicin is the aminoglycoside most commonly used in clinical veterinary practice.

Aminoglycosides are eliminated almost exclusively by glomerular filtration. Active uptake of aminoglycosides by the proximal tubules leads to accumulation of these drugs within the cells. The aminoglycosides then interfere with mitochondrial function and with normal lysosomal maturation and turnover. Lysosomal phospholipase is inhibited. The result is accumulation of lysosomes within the cells and a decrease in cellular respiration resulting in acute tubular necrosis.[68,74,79]

Cephaloridine, penicillins, tetracyclines, and sulfonamides are other antibiotics that have been associated either directly or indirectly with nephrotoxicity.[68,74] The polyene antifungal agent amphotericin B is reserved for the treatment of life-threatening fungal diseases because of its serious nephrotoxic side effects. Amphotericin B is the third most frequently reported cause of ARF in dogs and cats.[62,68] Amphotericin B causes disruption of the normal permeability of the distal tubules by altering the normal sterol-lipid interactions of the distal renal tubular epithelial membranes. Amphotericin B also causes intense vasoconstriction; renal blood flow decreases more than GFR, indicating disproportionate afferent arteriolar vasoconstriction.[74]

Phases of acute renal failure

Acute renal failure is typically divided into three phases; incipient, maintenance, and recovery. The incipient phase is the period from exposure to a nephrotoxin or ischemic event until detection of azotemia or change in volume of urine production is noted in the animal. Serum creatinine concentration and blood urea nitrogen levels increase progressively and urine specific gravity and osmolality decrease progressively as the renal injury is established. The incipient phase usually goes undetected, as clinical signs are minimal. Prompt treatment of the inciting cause of injury if detected during the incipient phase will result in rapid return to normal renal function. The maintenance phase is the period when established ARF is readily apparent. During this phase azotemia will be progressive or constant despite correction of prerenal factors. Treatment of the inciting cause will not result in an immediate return of normal renal function. This phase may last from 7 to 14 days or may be longer in duration. Serum creatinine and blood urea nitrogen levels reach plateau values; urine specific gravity remains isosthenuric, and oliguria may or may not be present.

Examination of urine sediment may reveal an increased number of renal tubular casts and renal epithelial cells. The recovery phase is characterized by return of normal renal function and resolution of the renal lesions. The time from the beginning of recovery to complete recovery is variable. Residual defects in renal concentrating and acidifying functions may persist but usually are not of clinical consequence. Functional hypertrophy of single nephrons restores GFR and renal blood flow to normal despite a smaller number of surviving nephrons.[44,60,64]

Diagnosis of acute renal failure

History. There is no age, breed, or sex predilection for ARF. A history of recent trauma, surgical intervention, or anesthetic procedure may suggest the possibility of ischemic nephropathy. Recent administration of known nephrotoxic drugs may offer further evidence suggestive of ARF. Access to ethylene glycol or actual observation of its ingestion is helpful in making that diagnosis, but often such information is not available. Owners may report the animal demonstrates a lack of urine production, hunching of the back, or a reluctance to move (renal pain).[44]

Clinical signs. Acute lethargy, anorexia, vomiting, diarrhea, and melena are common clinical signs in animals with ARF, yet these clinical signs are nonspecific for ARF. Animals with ARF do not produce a characteristic urine volume, although most of these animals are oliguric; anuria, polyuria, or normal urine volumes may be observed. Oliguria may be defined as a urine volume less than 1 ml/kg per hour.

Prerenal ARF is usually associated with a physiologic oliguria in response to dehydration or decreased renal perfusion. Because physiologic oliguria occurs in dehydrated patients, urine production rate is best determined after the dehydration has been corrected. Postrenal ARF is associated with a variable degree of urine production but is typically polyuric after the obstruction has been relieved. Nonoliguric ARF (polyuric or normal urine volumes) is being recognized with increased frequency. Nonoliguric ARF is thought to result from less severe renal injury than that which results in oliguric ARF.[44,62,63,67]

A number of complications may be encountered with ARF, depending on the duration and extent of renal injury and the nature of the underlying disorder. Loss of the ability to modify the character of the urine leads to disturbances in the volume and composition of body fluids. Abnormalities in sodium and water balance are the result of their continued ingestion in the presence of reduced excretory function and may lead to edema, hyperten-

sion, and congestive heart failure.[63] Cardiopulmonary problems usually occur secondary to fluid overload, but uremic pericardial effusions, pericarditis, and pleuritis may occur. Hyperkalemia is a frequent complication of ARF resulting from decreased excretion, metabolic acidosis, tissue injury, hemolysis, and increased tissue catabolism. Arrhythmias secondary to hyperkalemia represent a major cause of mortality in patients with ARF.[63] The development of metabolic acidosis occurs in nearly all patients with ARF. In rare instances, metabolic alkalosis may develop secondary to severe vomiting. Hypocalcemia and hyperphosphatemia are common in ARF, but the pathogenesis of these abnormalities is not completely understood. Ethylene glycol-induced ARF may result in severe (symptomatic) hypocalcemia as calcium is chelated from the plasma by oxalate metabolites of ethylene glycol.

Gastrointestinal abnormalities are among the most common complications of ARF. Diffuse erosive gastritis, septic ulcer disease, or uremic colitis may develop. Gastrointestinal hemorrhage remains a major cause of morbidity and mortality in patients with ARF.[63]

A number of hematologic disorders accompany ARF. Anemia may be seen secondary to hemodilution, hemorrhage, and hemolysis. Leukocytosis is often observed with septic (infectious) or inflammatory causes for ARF. Bleeding time and other tests of platelet function demonstrate abnormal results. A number of different factors may contribute to the bleeding diathesis seen with ARF; these include: a direct effect on platelet function by urea or guanidinosuccinic acid, reduced platelet factor III activity, abnormal capillary integrity, and increased prostacyclin (PGI_2) synthesis (an inhibitor of platelet aggregation).[63]

In people, secondary infections occur in 40% to 80% of patients with ARF, representing a second major cause of mortality. Data on the prevalence of infections associated with ARF in veterinary patients is not available.

Neurologic complications of ARF (stupor, coma, seizure) are usually observed as terminal events in veterinary medical patients.

Physical examination. Dogs and cats presenting with ARF are generally lethargic, hypovolemic, hyperpneic, bradycardic, and hypothermic. If fever is present this may be supportive evidence for inflammatory or infectious renal disease. Abdominal palpation may reveal a small, normal, or large urinary bladder. Renal pain may be elicited. The kidneys, if palpable, should be of normal size or slightly enlarged. Chronic renal disease is suggested by small and irregular kidneys.

Ancillary diagnostics. A combination of laboratory and diagnostic tests may be helpful in establishing a diagnosis of ARF and in determining its underlying cause. A complete blood count may reveal a leukocytosis (secondary to stress or infection). The red blood cell count is variable—either elevated secondary to dehydration, or decreased secondary to hemorrhage, hemolysis or hemodilution. The serum biochemical profile will reveal an elevated blood urea nitrogen, serum phosphorus, and serum creatinine level. Hyperkalemia will be evident in animals with oliguric ARF. Serum calcium concentration may be normal, low, or elevated depending on the cause of the ARF. Serum sodium concentrations can be normal, low, or elevated depending on the factors contributing to patient dehydration and the stage of the disease process. If diuresis occurs during the late incipient phase or early in the maintenance phase, free water loss may be greater and hypernatremia may result. Conversely, during the late maintenance phase when a marked diuresis occurs there may be a dramatic loss of sodium resulting from increased urine flow.[44,60] Abnormalities in acid-base balance should be evaluated by blood gas analysis. A moderate to severe metabolic acidosis is usually present. A concomitant partial compensatory respiratory alkalosis may be detected.

If urine is being produced, an urinalysis should be performed and urine should be submitted for bacteriologic culture and antibiotic sensitivity testing. Very often the urine specific gravity is in the isosthenuric range (1.007 to 1.015) and proteinuria, hematuria, and glucosuria are evident. Glucosuria despite normoglycemia and alkaline urine despite systemic metabolic acidosis are indicative of proximal tubular damage typical of acute tubular necrosis.[67] The urine sediment should be evaluated for evidence of bacteria, red blood cells, white blood cells, casts, and crystals. Acute tubular necrosis and nephritis may both result in the formation of significant numbers of renal tubular casts. The absence of casts, however, does not exclude the diagnosis of intrinsic ARF.[44] The presence of oxalate or hippurate crystals in urinary sediment of an animal with ARF supports a diagnosis of ethylene glycol poisoning.

Radiographic and ultrasonographic evaluation of the kidneys is not generally helpful in the diagnosis of ARF. The main indication is to aid in ruling out chronic renal disease. In ARF, radiographic or ultrasonographic examination of the kidneys should demonstrate normal or enlarged renal size and shape. Altered corticomedullary echogenicity and distinction between renal cortex and medulla can also be evident ultrasonographically. In dogs and cats with marked azotemia and oliguria, the excretory urogram rarely provides diagnostic information.

The value of renal biopsy in the diagnosis and evaluation of acute renal failure cannot be overemphasized. Information concerning the potential reversibility, chronicity, and specific pathologic basis of the disease can generally be obtained from examination of a renal biopsy. Histopathologic examination can demonstrate lesions compatible with ARF, including degenerative tubular changes, tubular necrosis, desquamation of tubular cells, denuding and disruption of tubular basement membranes, and intrarenal cast formation. Renal biopsy is helpful in evaluation for the presence of intact basement membranes, adequate tubular regeneration and repopulation of tubular cells, or significant fibrosis and nephron loss. The prognosis is particularly important when expense and effort must be justified in relation to the potential reversibility of the injury.[44,62] Bacteriologic cultures of renal tissue should be submitted to rule in or rule out an infectious cause of ARF. Silver stains may be useful in diagnosing the presence of spirochete organisms (leptospirosis). The diagnosis of glomerulonephritides may require electron microscopy.

There are a few special studies that may be helpful in the diagnosis of ARF. In any animal presenting with evidence of ARF, serology and darkfield microscopy for *Leptospira* should be performed, regardless of the animal's vaccination history. The finding of simultaneous large serum anion and osmolal gaps early in the course of the poisoning is helpful in supporting a diagnosis of ARF due to ethylene glycol intoxication.[44] Measurement of ethylene glycol concentration in whole blood, serum, or urine within 12 hours of poisoning using an Ethylene Glycol Test Kit (PRN Pharmacal) is helpful in confirming the diagnosis. Increases in urinary gamma-glutamyl transpeptidase (GGT) activity is a sensitive indicator of gentamicin-induced renal injury in dogs. One study revealed that the ratio of urinary GGT activity to urinary creatinine concentration correlated with 24-hour urine enzyme excretion; so a random urine sample may be used as a screening test.[80]

Fractional clearance studies may be useful in diagnosing ARF. In ARF, sodium is retained during the oliguric or anuric phase due to the reduction in GFR despite an increase in fractional sodium excretion (FE_{Na}). Normal FE_{Na} is <1%; in ARF it is usually >1.5%.[61] The values for the fractional excretion of sodium can be roughly calculated from random determinations of creatinine and sodium (Na) in plasma (P) and urine (U), according to the formula[62]:

$$FE_{Na} = \frac{(U/P)Na}{(U/P)\text{ creatinine} \times 100}$$

Fractional excretion of sodium has been used to differentiate ARF from other causes of azotemia such as decreased circulating volume from dehydration or congestive heart failure (FE_{Na}, <1%). The recovery phase of all forms of ARF, and all phases of nonoliguric ARF, are characterized by increased FE_{Na} (>1.5%) and sodium loss. As tubular function is reestablished, normal sodium excretion is restored.[61]

Treatment of acute renal failure

General management. Specific therapy directed at the inciting cause of ARF should be initiated whenever possible, for example, a postrenal obstruction should be relieved. Specific therapy for intrinsic ARF can be divided into conservative medical management and dialysis. The basic aims are to correct the renal hemodynamic disorders and alleviate the fluid and biochemical abnormalities until renal repair can take place.[62]

Fluid therapy. There are two main objectives of fluid therapy: (1) correction of fluid, acid-base, and electrolyte imbalances; and (2) initiation or augmentation of diuresis in order to improve renal function and enhance excretion of metabolic waste products and uremic toxins.[61]

It is extremely important to assess and continually reassess the animal's body weight, packed cell volume, total serum solids, skin turgor, central venous pressure, and urine production, as changes in these parameters form the basis for calculation of fluid, acid-base, and electrolyte requirements. All animals should be weighed twice daily using the same scale and with the bladder empty. Placing an indwelling urinary catheter attached to a closed collection system or the use of intermittent catheterization should be considered for precise monitoring of urine production.

Initial fluid therapy should consist of intravenous administration of a balanced electrolyte solution. The type of fluid administered should be dictated by serum sodium levels. Progressive hypernatremia may develop in hydrated patients receiving normal saline. Such patients should receive a balanced electrolyte solution (lactated Ringer's) or 5% dextrose in water (Chapters 18 and 38). Progressive hyponatremia may indicate excessive administration of electrolyte-free water or excessive sodium losses. In the overhydrated patient with hyponatremia fluid restriction is necessary. In the normally hydrated or dehydrated patient with hyponatremia sodium-containing fluids are indicated.[67]

Dehydration in animals with suspected ARF should be corrected more rapidly than in an animal with normal renal function in order to prevent further renal damage from ischemia and to differentiate physiologic oliguria from pathologic oliguria.[61] The initial estimated volume of fluid to be administered should be based on the animal's body weight, degree of dehydration, and ongoing losses (vomiting, diarrhea):

fluid replacement = BW × % dehydration × 1000 ml/kg + maintenance [66 ml/kg × BW] + ongoing losses,

where BW denotes body weight in kilograms. Measurement of central venous pressure and/or pulmonary capillary wedge pressure may be necessary for monitoring fluid administration in oliguric patients. In the case of physiologic oliguria, urine flow should increase to 2 to 5 ml/kg per hour depending on the rate of fluid administration, and once rehydration has been completed fluids should be administered at a rate of 1.5 to 3 times maintenance to achieve continued diuresis. If clinical signs of fluid overload (increased central venous pressure, dyspnea, edema) occur, fluid administration should be temporarily discontinued. If adequate urine production has not been established following rehydration, alternative therapy to restore urine production is indicated.[61]

Overly aggressive fluid therapy during the recovery phase of ARF may promote continued polyuria. As urine volume stabilizes, the volume of fluids should be reduced. It is imperative to carefully monitor body weight and assess clinically the status of hydration as rapid discontinuation of fluids may result in dehydration.[67]

Diuretics. When oliguria persists despite correction of all prerenal factors, additional therapeutic measures are indicated. Diuretic administration is commonly chosen by clinicians in the management of severe oliguria. Diuretic administration alone probably does not improve renal function despite increasing urine flow. Diuretics are beneficial in that they facilitate continued diuresis induced by intravenous fluid administration. Furosemide (2.2 mg/kg intravenously) is the diuretic of choice. Urine production should increase within 30 minutes following administration of furosemide or the dosage can be doubled or tripled at hourly intervals. However, dosages greater than 5 mg/kg seem to have no additional benefit.[44,61,62,67]

An osmotic diuretic may be tried if furosemide administration fails to increase urine production. Mannitol or dextrose 10% to 20% should be used (0.5 to 1.0 g/kg infused over 15 to 20 minutes). Urine production should begin within 15 to 30 minutes if the treatment is effective. Osmotic diuretics are contraindicated in the dehydrated patient. Mannitol administration is contraindicated in the overhydrated oliguric animal. Administration of an osmotic diuretic in that circumstance creates the danger of even greater plasma volume expansion, edema, and heart failure.[44,61,62,67]

Some animals will respond to administration of one diuretic but not the other. So, it is advisable to try both if administration of the initial choice fails to be effective in improving urine output. A combination administration of mannitol with furosemide may elicit a response when administration of either drug alone did not elicit a response. When diuretic therapy is unsuccessful in improving urine production the use of vasodilators may prove successful.

Vasoactive drugs. Dopamine is the vasodilator most often used to augment renal function and urine production in oliguric animals. Dopamine administration reduces renal vascular resistance and increases renal blood flow, particularly in the inner renal cortex. The effects are mediated through dopaminergic receptors in the renal vasculature. Dopamine is diluted in an isotonic fluid and administered intravenously at a rate of 2 to 5 μg/kg per minute. Infusion rates higher than 10 μg/kg per minute may cause renal vasoconstriction and should be avoided.[44,61] Dopamine is arrhythmogenic, and animals receiving an intravenous infusion of it should be monitored electrocardiographically.

If oliguria persists despite the use of aggressive treatment with intravenous fluid, diuretic, and vasodilator administration, peritoneal dialysis (or hemodialysis at institutions where it is available) will be necessary (Chapter 39).[44,61,62,64,67]

Management of acid-base and electrolyte abnormalities. A moderate to severe metabolic acidosis is the most common acid-base problem seen with ARF. Compensatory respiratory alkalosis is helpful in neutralizing pH changes in many animals so that alkali replacement is unnecessary unless the blood pH is <7.2. Blood gas analysis should be performed daily until the animal is stabilized. When the cause for the ARF is ethylene glycol intoxication, a severe metabolic acidosis (pH <7.0) is commonly encountered and usually requires very aggressive therapy (see box p. 309).

The most significant electrolyte abnormality associated with ARF is hyperkalemia. Hyperkalemia-induced myocardial conduction abnormalities are a prime cause of early mortality in patients with acute oliguric failure. The short-term management of severe hyperkalemia (potassium concentration >8 mEq/L) has been discussed (see box p. 309). Calcium gluconate administration acts as a specific antagonist to the cardiotoxic ef-

fects of hyperkalemia, but its effects are short-lived, and calcium administration has no influence on lowering serum potassium levels. Calcium administration should be used in conjunction with other therapies. A potential therapy for hyperkalemia involves administration of beta$_2$-agonists, which promote the intracellular uptake of potassium through a mechanism involving beta$_2$-adrenoreceptors. Intravenous administration of albuterol sulfate has been shown to reduce serum potassium levels rapidly in humans with ARF.[67] The intravenous form of this drug is not available in the United States. For prolonged control of hyperkalemia in patients with oliguric renal failure, a cationic exchange resin, sodium polystyrene sulfonate, can be administered orally at 2 g/kg per day in 3 divided doses. Effective long-term control of hyperkalemia is obtained with dialysis (peritoneal or hemodialysis)[62] (Chapter 39).

Hypokalemia (potassium level, <3.5 mEq/L) may occur with overcorrection of hyperkalemic states and in cases of decreased intake. It may also occur in nonoliguric ARF due to renal potassium losses. Hypokalemia is most prevalent with gentamicin-induced ARF and the recovery phase of acute tubular necrosis. Clinical signs associated with hypokalemia are extreme muscle weakness, vomiting, anorexia (associated with ileus and gastric stasis), and cardiac dysrhythmias. Symptomatic hypokalemia is a significant problem in cats.[67] Management of hypokalemia requires potassium supplementation, either intravenously or orally. Intravenous therapy consists of the addition of potassium chloride to the animal's fluids. The dose of potassium is based on the severity of the hypokalemia (Chapter 38). Potassium should not be administered at a rate greater than 0.5 mEq/kg per hour. Oral potassium chloride supplementation can be used if the animal is not vomiting (1 to 2 mEq/kg daily diluted 50% with water three times a day).[61,62,64,67]

Abnormalities in serum sodium levels may occur (hyponatremia or hypernatremia) with ARF. Serum sodium levels should be assessed daily and appropriate changes made in the type of fluid therapy administered. In general, animals with oliguric ARF retain sodium and often require administration of fluid solutions low in sodium (0.45% sodium chloride or 0.45% sodium chloride and 2.5% dextrose). Once the recovery phase of ARF has been reached urinary sodium loss increases and balanced (isosmotic) electrolyte solutions are indicated.[81]

Hypercalcemia is infrequently encountered with ARF, but has been associated with neoplasia and rodenticide intoxication. Treatment should consist of treating or removing the inciting cause. When serum calcium levels are greater than 14 mg/dl, specific treatment to decrease the hypercalcemia should be aggressively pursued. Fluid therapy should consist of the intravenous administration of normal saline. Furosemide is a calciuretic diuretic and should be administered parenterally. Glucocorticosteroid, calcitonin, diphosphonate, and anticancer chemotherapy administration may be required[44] (see Chapter 18).

Hypocalcemia may be observed with ARF but is usually mild to moderate and asymptomatic. Severe hypocalcemia resulting in tetany may be seen with ethylene glycol intoxication and severe crushing injuries. Intravenous calcium chloride or calcium gluconate should be given to effect to control tetany[44] (see Chapter 18).

Hyperphosphatemia occurs commonly with ARF because of the severe decrease in GFR. Treatment consists of fluid therapy and oral administration of intestinal phosphorus-binding agents (e.g., Amphojel, initial dose of 1 to 2 ml/kg/day with food) provided the animal is not vomiting.

Peritoneal dialysis. When intensive fluid therapy and diuretic administration does not reestablish urine flow or improve renal function, peritoneal dialysis is indicated. Dialysis is the recommended treatment for patients with acute reversible renal failure (aminoglycoside or ethylene glycol-induced ARF). Dialysis is a labor-intensive treatment and therefore is expensive. When ARF is due to a reversible toxic insult, is detected early, and/or when renal biopsy establishes a good prognosis then dialysis is a treatment technique worth considering. Peritoneal dialysis uses the peritoneum as a semipermeable membrane for the exchange of water and solute. Peritoneal dialysis can be used to correct acid-base and electrolyte imbalances, remove the toxic agent and other metabolic waste products, and maintain the animal until renal tissue has regenerated.[81-86] Peritoneal dialysis is discussed in detail in Chapter 39.

Additional treatments. In addition to the more life-threatening conditions that must be addressed and managed, other problems such as vomiting, hematemesis, melena, and anorexia should not be ignored. H_2-blockers have been recommended for control of uremic gastritis and ulcers. Cimetidine (3 to 6 mg/kg intravenously three or four times a day) is the agent most often used. Vomiting associated with ARF may be severe and persistent. The thorazine tranquilizers act as centrally acting antiemetics and seem to ameliorate nausea and vomiting in animals with ARF. Chlorpromazine (0.5 mg/kg every 8 hours), prochlorperazine (0.13 mg/kg every 6 hours), or trimethobenzamide (3 mg/kg every 8 hours) may be used by

parenteral administration for this purpose. It is important to monitor the animal for side effects (hypotension and sedation) that may occur with administration of these drugs.[67]

Animals in ARF are in a hypercatabolic state. These animals have vomiting, diarrhea, and anorexia; protein-calorie malnutrition rapidly results. Hyperalimentation, in the form of total parenteral nutrition, is indicated to establish a positive protein-calorie balance (Chapter 37). The supply of calories helps decrease the catabolic response, lessening the degree of protein breakdown products requiring renal excretion. Additionally, regeneration of renal tubular cells requires an extensive supply of energy and protein. By considering these demands early in the course of treatment of animals with ARF, complications may be avoided (weight loss, increased risk of infection, decubital ulcers).

Therapy for ethylene glycol toxicity (see also Chapter 27)

Ethylene glycol toxicity is the major cause of ARF in dogs and cats. The mortality rate is high. Successful treatment of the intoxicated patient hinges on a rapid diagnosis and early institution of therapy.

Ethylene glycol is rapidly absorbed from the gastrointestinal tract and distributed to all body tissues. Metabolism takes place primarily in the liver and secondarily in the kidney. The metabolites (glycoaldehyde, glycolate, glyoxalate, oxalate) of ethylene glycol are responsible for its toxicity. The conversion of glycolic acid to glyoxalate proceeds relatively slowly and is thought to be the rate-limiting step. It has been estimated that from 0.25% to 2.5% of ingested ethylene glycol is converted to oxalate.[79] Inhibition of alcohol dehydrogenase, the enzyme responsible for the first oxidative step in ethylene glycol metabolism, results in the excretion of unmetabolized ethylene glycol by the kidneys and forms the basis for treatment.[86] The minimum lethal dose of ethylene glycol is 4.2 to 6.6 ml/kg in dogs and 1.5 ml/kg in cats.[87] Cats produce relatively large amounts of oxalate during the metabolism of ethylene glycol, which may account for their increased sensitivity.[87]

Treatment. If an animal is seen within 2 hours of observed ingestion then vomiting should be induced and gastric lavage performed in an attempt to prevent absorption. The next step in treatment is to increase renal excretion of ethylene glycol, so intravenous fluid diuresis should be instituted (an isotonic fluid solution at 1.5 to 3 times maintenance). Metabolism of ethylene glycol to the toxic metabolites is prevented by administering

---

TREATMENT OF ETHYLENE GLYCOL INTOXICATION

Ethanol administration
Dogs
    5.5 ml of 20% ethanol/kg intravenously every 4
    hours for five treatments, then every 6 hours
    for four treatments
    0.6 gm/kg of 7% ethanol intravenously as a bolus
    followed by 100 mg/kg per hour as a
    continuous intravenous infusion continued until
    10 hours postdialysis*
Cats
    5 ml of 20% ethanol/kg intravenously every 6
    hours for five treatments, then every 8 hours
    for four treatments
4-Methylpyrazole—dog only
    20 mg/kg of a 5% solution intravenously initially,
    followed by 15 mg/kg intravenously at 12 hours
    and 24 hours, and 5 mg/kg intravenously at 36
    hours after the first dose
Peritoneal dialysis
    For acute removal of ethylene glycol (multiple
    exchanges [20 ml/kg per exchange, 1.5%
    dextrose concentration dialysate] continuing until
    8 hours after correction of metabolic acidosis)*

---

*Dr. Rebecca Kirby, personal communication.

agents that compete as substrates for the enzyme alcohol dehydrogenase. There are two protocols that have been established, one uses ethanol (dog and cat) and the other 4-methylpyrazole (dog only) (see box). Ethanol is an alternative substrate for alcohol dehydrogenase and it effectively interferes with ethylene glycol metabolism because alcohol dehydrogenase has a higher affinity for ethanol than for ethylene glycol. Unfortunately, ethanol enhances many of the metabolic effects of ethylene glycol. Both agents are central nervous system depressants and cause increased serum osmolality.

4-Methylpyrazole (Aldrich Chemical, Milwaukee) is an inhibitor of alcohol dehydrogenase and has been used with excellent results in dogs with experimentally induced and naturally acquired ethylene glycol toxicity. It does not appear to be effective in the treatment of ethylene glycol poisoning of cats. 4-Methylpyrazole does not contribute to central nervous system or to renal concentrating disorders (i.e., it does not induce diuresis as ethanol does). 4-Methylpyrazole forms an inactive complex with liver alcohol dehydrogenase. It must be given early in the course of intoxication (<8 hours after ethylene glycol ingestion) to be most effective as an antidote.[86,87] In dogs, the recommended dosage of 4-methylpyra-

zole (5% solution) is 20 mg/kg intravenously initially, followed by 15 mg/kg intravenously at 12 and 24 hours, and 5 mg/kg intravenously at 36 hours after the first dose.[87]

The use of peritoneal dialysis to remove ethylene glycol and its metabolites has been recently advocated in the acute treatment of animals with ethylene glycol intoxication (prior to the onset of ethylene glycol-induced ARF). In human medicine, peritoneal dialysis and hemodialysis have been highly effective methods for the removal of ethylene glycol from the body.

REFERENCES

1. Peterson NE. Emergency management of urologic trauma. Emerg Med Clin North Am 1988;6:579-599.
2. Morgan RV. Urogenital emergencies—Part 1. Compend Contin Educ Pract Vet 1982;4:908-918.
3. Zenoble RD. Trauma: disease of the kidney. In Morgan RV, ed. Handbook of Small Animal Practice. New York: Churchill Livingstone, 1988;591-593.
4. Christie BA. Kidneys. In Slatter DH, ed. Textbook of small animal surgery. Philadelphia: WB Saunders, 1985;1764-1777.
5. Christie BA: Ureters. In Slatter DH, ed. Textbook of small animal surgery. Philadelphia: WB Saunders, 1985;1777-1785.
6. Selcer BA. Urinary tract trauma associated with pelvic trauma. J Am Anim Hosp Assoc 1982;18:785-793.
7. Thornhill JA, Cechner PE. Traumatic injuries to the kidney, ureter, bladder and urethra. Vet Clin North Am 1981;11:157-169.
8. Crane SW. Evaluation and management of abdominal trauma in the dog and cat. Vet Clin North Am 1980;10:655-689.
9. Osborne CA, Finco DR. Urinary tract emergencies and renal care following trauma. Vet Clin North Am 1972;2:259-292.
10. Kirk RW, Bistner SI. Genitourinary emergencies. In Morgan RV, ed. Handbook of veterinary procedures and emergency treatment, ed. 4. Philadelphia: WB Saunders, 1985;130.
11. Guerriero WG, Devine CJ. Renal Trauma. In Guerriero WG, ed. Urologic injuries. Norwalk, CT: Appleton-Century-Crofts, 1984;9-44.
12. Kennedy TJ, McConnell JD, Thal ER. Urine dystick vs. microscopic urinalysis in the evaluation of abdominal trauma. J Trauma 1988;28:615-617.
13. Kerr DV, Koblick PD. Contrast radiography. In Morgan RV, ed. Handbook of small animal practice. New York: Churchill Livingstone, 1988;41-58.
14. Kealy JK. The urinary system. In Kealy KJ, ed. Diagnostic Radiology of the Dog and Cat, Philadelphia: WB Saunders, 1979;95-127.
15. Feeney DA, Barber DL, Johnston GR, Osborne CA. The excretory urogram: Part I. Techniques, normal radiographic appearance, and misinterpretation. Compend Cont Educ Pract Vet 1982;4:233-243.
16. Feeney DA, Barber DL, Johnston GR, Osborne CA. The excretory urogram: Part II. Interpretation of abnormal findings. Compend Contin Educ Pract Vet 1982;4:321-329.
17. Johnston GR, Feeney DA. Radiographic evaluation of the urinary tract in dogs and cats. In Bretschiverett EB, ed. Nephrology and urology. New York: Churchill Livingstone, 1986;203-275.

18. Bergren CT, Chan FN, Bodzin JH. Intravenous pyelogram results in association with renal pathology and therapy in trauma patients. J Trauma 1987;27:515-518.
19. Walter PA, Johnston GR, Feeney DA, O'Brien TD. Application of ultrasonography in the diagnosis of parenchymal kidney disease in cats: 24 cases (1981-1986). J Am Vet Med Assoc 1988;192:92-98.
20. Brasmer TH. Kidney and ureter. In Brasmer TH, ed. The Acutely traumatized small animal patient. Philadelphia: WB Saunders, 1984;158-159.
21. Zenoble RD. Trauma: Diseases of the ureter. In Morgan RV, ed. Handbook of small animal practice. New York: Churchill Livingstone, 1988;602-603.
22. Jones BR. Diseases of the ureters. In Ettinger SJ, ed. Textbook of veterinary internal medicine: Diseases of the dog and cat. ed. 2. Philadelphia: WB Saunders, 1983;1879-1890.
23. Guerriero WG, Devine CJ. Ureteral trauma. In Urologic injuries. Norwalk, CT: Appleton-Century-Crofts, 1984; 45-72.
24. Greene RW, Scott RC. Diseases of the bladder and urethra. In Ettinger SJ, ed. Textbook of veterinary internal medicine: Diseases of the dog and cat, ed. 2. Philadelphia: WB Saunders, 1983;1890-1936.
25. Zenoble RD. Trauma: Diseases of the bladder. In Morgan RV, ed. Handbook of small animal practice. New York: Churchill Livingstone, 1988;618-619.
26. Whitney WO, Mehlhaff CJ. High-rise syndrome in cats. J Am Vet Med Assoc 1987;191:1399-1403.
27. Hobson HP, Bushby P. Surgery of the bladder. In Slatter DH, ed. Textbook of small animal surgery. Philadelphia: WB Saunders, 1986;1786-1799.
28. Zenoble RD. Trauma: Disease of the urethra. In Morgan RV, ed. Handbook of small animal practice. New York: Churchill Livingstone, 1988;633-639.
29. Zenoble RD, Pechman RD. Urinary tract trauma. In Kirk RW, ed. Current veterinary therapy IX. Philadelphia: WB Saunders, 1986;1155-1159.
30. Anson LW. Urethral trauma and principles of urethral surgery. Compend Contin Educ Pract Vet 1987;9:981-988.
31. Bradley RL. Complete urethral obstruction secondary to fracture of the os penis. Compend Contin Educ Pract Vet 1985;7:759-763.
32. Smith CW. Surgical diseases of the urethra. In Slatter DH, ed. Textbook of small animal surgery. Philadelphia: WB Saunders, 1985;1799-1810.
33. Labato MA. Disorders of micturition. In Morgan RV, ed. Handbook of small animal practice. New York: Churchill Livingstone, 1988;621-628.
34. Brasmer TH. Urethra. In Brasmer TH, ed. The acutely traumatized small animal patient. Philadelphia: WB Saunders, 1984;159-160.
35. Barbagh G, Selli C, Stomaci N, et al. Urethral trauma: Radiological aspects and treatment options. J Trauma 1986;27:256-261.
36. Brown CC, Gibson KL, Kreegen JM. Obstructive urolithiasis in a six-week-old puppy. J Am Anim Hosp Assoc 1988;24:466-468.
37. Osborne CA, ed. Canine urolithiasisis I. Vet Clin North Am 1986;16(1).
38. Osborne CA, ed. Canine urolithiasisis II. Vet Clin North Am 1986;16(2).
39. Polzen DJ. Urocystolithiasis. In Morgan RV, ed. Handbook of small animal practice. New York: Churchill Livingstone, 1988;611-616.
40. Patnaik AK, Matthiesen DT, Zawie DA. Two cases of canine penile neoplasm: Squamous cell carcinoma and mesenchymal chondrosarcoma. J Am Anim Hosp Assoc 1988;24:403-406.
41. Bradley RL. Complete urethral obstruction secondary to fracture of the os penis. Compend Contin Educ Pract Vet 1985;7:759-763.
42. Morgan RV. Urogenital emergencies—Part II. Compend Contin Educ Pract Vet 1983;5:43-55.
43. Hall JA, Allen TA, Fettman MJ. Hyperammonemia associated with urethral obstruction in a dog. J Am Vet Med Assoc 1987;191:1116-1118.
44. Chew DJ, DiBartola SP. Acute renal failure. In van Marthens E, ed. Manual of Small Animal Nephrology and Urology, New York: Churchill Livingstone 1986;109-146.
45. Osborne LA, Johnston GR, Polzin DJ, et al.: Etiology of feline urologic syndrome: Hypothesis of heterogeneous causes. Proc Kal Kan Symp Treat Small Anim Dis 1983;7:107-124.
46. Barsanti JA, Finco DR, Shotts ED, et al. Feline urologic syndrome: Further investigation into therapy. J Am Anim Hosp Assoc 1982;18:387-390.
47. Barsanti JA, Finco DR, Shotts EB, et al. Feline urologic syndrome: Further investigation into etiology. J Am Anim Hosp Assoc 1982;18:391-396.
48. Lage AL. Feline urologic syndrome. In Morgan RV, ed. Handbook of Small Animal Practice. New York: Churchill Livingstone, 1988;608-611.
49. Finco DR. Feline urologic syndrome: Management of the critically ill patient. In Kirk RW, ed. Current veterinary in therapy VII. Philadelphia: WB Saunders, 1980;1188-1190.
50. Lees GE, Osborne CA. Feline urologic syndrome: Removal of urethral obstructions and use of indwelling urethral catheters. In Kirk RW, ed. Current Veterinary Therapy VII. Philadelphia: WB Saunders, 1980;1191-1196.
51. Osborne CA, Lees GE: Feline urologic syndrome: Medical aspects of prophylaxis. In Kirk RW, ed. Current veterinary therapy VII. Philadelphia: WB Saunders, 1980;1196-1201.
52. Tomchick TL, Greene RW: Feline urologic syndrome: Surgical aspects of prophylaxis. In Kirk RW, ed. Current veterinary therapy VII. Philadelphia: WB Saunders, 1980;1201-1203.
53. Osborne CA, Polzen DJ, Johnston GR, et al. Medical management of feline urologic syndromes. In Kirk RW, ed. Current veterinary therapy IX. Philadelphia: WB Saunders, 1986;1196-1206.
54. Sutor DJ, Wooley SE. Crystaline material from the feline bladder. Res Vet Sci 1970;11:298-299.
55. Finco DR, Barsanti JA. Obstructive uropathies. In Kirk RW, ed. Current veterinary therapy IX. Philadelphia: WB Saunders, 1986;1164-1167.
56. Garvey MS. Medical emergencies in cats. Ninth Annual Carnation Symposium on Feline Disease and Nutrition, Los Angeles: Friskie Pet Care Division, 1986.
57. Lees GE, Osborne CA, Stevens JB, et al. Adverse effects of open indwelling urethral catheterization in clinically normal male cats. Am J Vet Res 1981;42:825-833.
58. Smith CW, Schiller AG, Smith AR, et al. Effects of indwelling urinary catheters in male cats. J Am Anim Hosp Assoc 1981;17:427-433.
59. Barsanti JA, Blue J, Edmunds J. Urinary tract infection due to indwelling bladder catheters in dogs and cats. J Am Vet Med Assoc 1985;187:384-388.
60. Chew DJ. Acute renal failure. In Van Marthens E, ed. Proceedings of the Kal Kan Symposium for the Treatment of Small Animal Diseases. Vernon, CA: Kal Kan Foods Inc., 1983;9-17.
61. Ross LA. Fluid therapy for acute and chronic failure. Vet Clin North Am 1989;19:343-359.
62. Cowgill LD. Acute renal failure. In Bovee KC, ed. Canine nephrology. Philadelphia: Harwal, 1984;405-438.

63. Brenner BM, Coe FL, Rector FC. Causes of acute renal failure. In Brenner BM, ed. Clinical nephrology. Philadelphia: WB Saunders, 1987;36-72.
64. Breitschewerdt EB. Acute renal failure. In Morgan RV, ed. Handbook of small animal practice. New York: Churchill Livingstone, 1988;578-582.
65. Harrington JT, Cohen JJ. Acute oliguria. N Engl J Med 1975;292:89-91.
66. Myers BD, Moran SM. Hemodynamically mediated acute renal failure. N Engl J Med 1986;314:97-105.
67. Polzin D, Osborne C, O'Brien T. Diseases of the kidneys and ureters. In Ettinger SJ, ed. Textbook of veterinary internal medicine. Philadelphia: WB Saunders, 1989;1962-1981.
68. Chew DJ, Dibartola SP. Diagnosis and pathophysiology of renal disease. In Ettinger SJ, ed. Textbook of veterinary internal medicine. Philadelphia: WB Saunders, 1989;1926-1937.
69. Ellison DH, Bia MJ. Acute renal failure in critically ill patients. J Intern Care Med 1987;2:8-24.
70. Klausner JS, Bell FW, Hayden DW, et al. Hypercalcemia in two cats with squamous cell carcinomas. J Am Vet Med Assoc 1990;196:103-105.
71. Page R, Matus RE, Leifer CE, Loar A. Cisplatin, a new antineoplastic drug in veterinary medicine. J Am Vet Med Assoc 1985;186:288-290.
72. Cotter SM, Kanki PJ, Simon M. Renal disease in five tumor-bearing cats treated with Adriamycin. J Am Anim Hosp Assoc 1985;21:405-409.
73. Parfrey PS, Griffiths SM, Barrett BJ, et al. Contrast material-induced renal failure in patients with diabetes mellitus, renal insufficiency, or both. N Engl J Med 1989;320:143-148.
74. Englehardt JA, Brown SA. Drug-related nephropathies. Part II. Commonly used drugs. Compend Contin Educ Pract Vet 1987;9:281-288.
75. Ramazzotto LJ, Carlin RC, Barrett RJ, et al. Enflurane induced nephrotoxicity in renally compromised dogs. Can Assoc Lab Anim Sci Newslett 1985;17(2):33-37.
76. Rubin SI. Nonsteroidal anti-inflammatory drugs, prostaglandins, and the kidney. J Am Vet Med Assoc 1986;188:1065-1068.
77. Spyridakis LK, Bacia JJ, Barsanti JA, Brown SA. Ibuprofen toxicosis in a dog. J Am Vet Med Assoc 1986;188:918-919.
78. Grauer GF, Thrall MA. Ethylene glycol (antifreeze) poisoning in the dog and cat. J Am Anim Hosp Assoc 1982;18:492-497.
79. Brown SA, Barsanti JA, Crowell WA. Gentamicin-associated acute renal failure in the dog. J Am Vet Med Assoc 1985;186:686-690.
80. Gossett KA. Evaluation of gamma-glutamyl transpeptidase-to-creatinine ratio from spot samples of urine supernatant, as an indicator of urinary enzyme excretion in dogs. Am J Vet Res 1987;48:455.
81. Thornhill JA. Peritoneal dialysis in the dog and cat: An update. Compend Contin Educ Pract Vet 1981;3:160-172.
82. DiBartola SP, Chew DJ, Tarr MJ, et al. Hemodialysis of a dog with acute renal failure. J Am Vet Med Assoc 1985;186:1323-1326.
83. Shahar R, Holmbert DL. Pleural dialysis in the management of acute renal failure in two dogs. J Am Vet Med Assoc 1985;187:952-954.
84. Ross LA. Peritoneal dialysis. In Morgan RV, ed. Handbook of small animal practice. New York: Churchill Livingstone, 1988;585-588.
85. Vaamonde CA. Peritoneal dialysis—Current status. Postgrad Med 1977;62:148-156.
86. Dial SM, Thrall MA, Hamar DW. 4-Methylpyrazole as treatment for naturally acquired ethylene glycol intoxication in dogs. J Am Vet Med Assoc 1989;195:73-76.
87. Grauer GF, Thrall MA. Ethylene glycol (antifreeze) poisoning. In Kirk RW , ed. Current veterinary therapy IX. Philadelphia: WB Saunders, 1986;206-212.

22 Gastrointestinal Emergencies

Keith P. Richter

ALIMENTARY TRACT CONDITIONS
Esophageal foreign bodies

Esophageal foreign bodies frequently occur in the dog and cat, and can cause life-threatening problems, chronic dysphagia, regurgitation, or vomiting. Prompt management is necessary to prevent progression of the problem to sequelae such as esophageal perforation, mediastinitis, pleuritis, and aspiration pneumonia. The presence of a foreign body in the esophagus stimulates secondary peristaltic waves in an oral to aboral direction.[1] These waves result in pressure necrosis of the esophageal wall. The degree of damage to the esophagus depends on the size and shape of the foreign body, and the duration of its presence in the esophagus.[1] Once pressure necrosis is severe, transmural inflammation may occur, resulting in escape of bacteria and toxins into the mediastinal or pleural space. Eventually, perforation may occur, resulting in severe mediastinitis and pleuritis.

Clinical findings with esophageal foreign bodies. Clinical signs in animals with esophageal foreign bodies include dysphagia, excess salivation, regurgitation, and anorexia. The severity of clinical signs depends on the degree of esophageal obstruction, damage to the esophageal wall, and the presence of esophageal perforation. When transmural inflammation or perforation results in mediastinitis or pleuritis, animals will become febrile, depressed, and eventually dyspneic with signs of septic shock.

Physical examination may be normal, or some animals may have excess salivation, repeated swallowing attempts, and fever. If the foreign body is in the cervical esophagus, it may be palpable. If there is pleuritis, dyspnea or pleural friction rubs may be detected.

Survey radiography often reveals a radiopaque object in the esophagus (Fig. 22-1). In many cases, air can be seen in a dilated esophagus.[2] The most common place for a foreign body to lodge is just cranial to the diaphragm,[2] followed by directly over the heart base and at the thoracic inlet. Occasionally, contrast radiography is necessary to delineate an esophageal foreign body. In this setting, a water-soluble iodinated contrast medium (versus barium) should be used in the event a perforation is present or surgical esophagotomy is necessary. Radiography may also indicate the presence of mediastinitis and pleuritis.

The diagnosis of an esophageal foreign body can be confirmed by performing endoscopy. Flexible endoscopes are more versatile for this purpose, although rigid scopes are often adequate. Endoscopy also has the advantage of being the first line in the treatment of esophageal foreign bodies. The clinician can also endoscopically evaluate the esophageal mucosa before and after foreign body removal to determine whether surgical intervention is necessary.

Treatment of esophageal foreign bodies. The initial treatment of choice of esophageal foreign bodies is endoscopic removal. If possible, a large-bore, hollow, rigid endoscope is preferred to visualize the object, through which a long alligator-style forceps can be used to grasp the object. This method has the advantage of dilating the esophagus with the rim of the scope just cranial to the foreign object. Often this will dislodge sharp points of the object that were imbedded in the esophageal wall. Alternatively, a flexible endoscope can be used to retrieve the object. Various types of two-, three-, and four-pronged forceps are available that fit through the instrument channel of a flexible endoscope. Unfortunately, these instruments do not grasp objects as tightly as rigid forceps, and objects firmly imbedded in the esophageal wall are more difficult to remove.

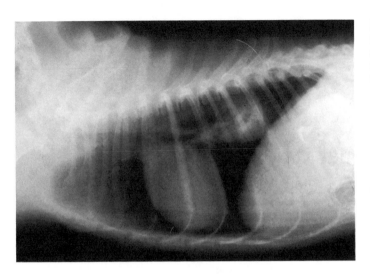

Fig. 22-1 Radiopaque foreign body (bone) is visible in the caudal esophagus of a dog. (Courtesy of David Hager, Radiology Consulting Service, Cardiff, CA.)

Sometimes the object can be freed from the wall by pushing it in an aboral direction, and subsequently retrieving it in the oral direction.

If an object has numerous sharp edges (Fig. 22-1) or cannot be easily freed from the esophageal wall, it is not recommended to remove it per os because of the risk of esophageal laceration or perforation. In this setting, propulsion into the stomach is recommended if possible. Objects that will not safely pass through the gastrointestinal tract can then be removed via gastrotomy, a much less invasive procedure than esophagotomy. If propulsion into the stomach with a forceps is not possible, a large-bore rigid endoscope or tube of any sort can be used for this purpose. In this manner, the tube acts to stretch the esophageal wall and frees it from sharp edges of the foreign object.

Once the foreign object is removed from the esophagus, the esophageal mucosa should be inspected for the presence of lacerations or perforations with the aid of the endoscope and the need for surgical intervention determined. Radiography can also be used to help determine the presence of an esophageal perforation. Since air is insufflated during the endoscopic procedure, perforation usually results in pneumomediastinum, which can be detected by thoracic radiography.

If endoscopic removal is unsuccessful, surgical intervention is indicated. The survival rate following thoracic esophagotomy is approximately 85%.[1] If the foreign object is in the caudal esophagus, it may be removed via a transdiaphragmatic approach through a gastrotomy incision.[3] Thoracotomy is also indicated if there is evidence of mediastinitis or pleuritis. Postoperative problems following esophageal surgery include leakage or dehiscence, infection, and stricture formation.[3]

Once the foreign body is removed (either endoscopically or surgically) esophagitis is often present. Esophagitis may also decrease lower esophageal sphincter pressure and allow gastroesophageal reflux to occur, further exacerbating esophagitis.[4] This is minimized by avoiding contact of esophageal mucosa with gastric acid by using drugs that inhibit gastric acid secretion and by increasing lower esophageal sphincter tone with metoclopramide. The drugs of choice for inhibiting gastric acid secretion are the histamine H_2-receptor blockers such as cimetidine (Tagamet) or ranitidine (Zantac). In addition, histamine H_2-receptor blocker administration results in increased lower esophageal sphincter pressure.[5] These drugs will be discussed in more detail in the section on "Treatment of Gastric Ulcers." Generally, these drugs are used for 2 to 3 weeks following foreign-body removal. A repeat endoscopic examination may be helpful in documenting resolution of esophagitis.

Antibiotics are indicated if there is esophageal mucosal damage. Since the bacteria that are likely to cause problems originate from the oral cavity, antibiotics effective against oral flora are used. Ampicillin and the cephalosporins are indicated for this purpose. More aggressive treatment is warranted if mediastinitis or pleuritis is present. In this setting, administration of an aminoglycoside antibiotic (either gentamicin or amikacin) parenterally is indicated, as well as irrigation through tube thoracostomy (see Chapter 25).

Restriction of oral alimentation is also important to allow proper healing of the esophageal mucosa following foreign-body removal. Esophageal healing may be impaired by the motion of swallowing as well as the presence of food.[3] Therefore, oral alimentation should be withheld for at least 5 days with severe esophageal injuries. An ideal way to provide nutritional support for this period or longer is through a percutaneous endoscopic gastrostomy (PEG) tube.[6] These are large-bore feeding tubes placed percutaneously into the stomach under endoscopic guidance (Chapter 37). Briefly, the stomach is inflated with air with the endoscope. Following surgical preparation of the abdomen, a 2-in. intravenous catheter is placed into the stomach through a percutaneous puncture. The catheter is easily visualized through the endoscope. The stylet of the catheter is removed and a guide wire is placed through the catheter into the stomach. The guide wire is grasped with retrieval forceps through the endoscope and brought out of the mouth. A tapered feeding tube is threaded over the guide wire and brought out through the stomach and body wall. A rubber retention disk at the end of the tube keeps it in the stomach. The tapered end is cut outside the body and a feeding adapter is placed. Thus, the tube enters the abdominal body wall and ends in the stomach. An alternative method involves placing a long length of suture material through the 2-in. catheter rather than a guide wire. This is then tied to a loop of suture material secured to the tapered end of the feeding tube, and the tube is pulled into the stomach and out the abdominal body wall using the long length of suture material.

Percutaneous endoscopic gastrostomy tubes have the advantage of not resting against the healing esophageal mucosa, whereas the use of pharyngostomy or nasogastric tubes is associated with delayed epithelial healing.[1] In addition, PEGs do not traverse the lower esophageal sphincter and subsequently do not predispose to gastroesophageal reflux. Most clients can easily manage PEGs at home, and they are well tolerated by dogs and cats. I have left them in place for up to 10 weeks without problems. If endoscopy is not available, a surgically placed gastrostomy tube to provide nutritional support is an acceptable alternative. Details of enteral nutrition are provided in Chapter 37.

Prognosis with esophageal foreign bodies. The prognosis for most animals with esophageal foreign bodies is good. Most foreign bodies can be removed endoscopically or pushed into the stomach. If surgical intervention is necessary to remove the foreign body, the recovery rate is still high. If there is severe esophagitis, mediastinitis, or pleuritis, the prognosis is guarded to poor. In these cases, aggressive medical management as described above is necessary. Stricture formation may result if there is severe necrosis extending beyond the mucosa.[3,4,7] Minimizing the degree of

esophagitis and withholding food initially will reduce the likelihood of this complication. If stricture formation occurs, I have had success in treating these with balloon dilation.[8] Surgical management of esophageal strictures is reserved for cases unresponsive to balloon dilation.

Penetrating wounds and laceration of the esophagus

Causes. Most esophageal wounds occur in the cervical esophagus, because the thoracic esophagus is protected by the chest wall. Causes of esophageal wounds or lacerations include bite wounds, external penetration by sharp objects, gunshot wounds, and ingested sharp foreign bodies (bones [see Fig. 22-1], fishhooks, sticks, needles). Complications of esophageal perforation include local infection or cellulitis, mediastinitis, pleuritis, pneumomediastinum, pneumothorax, shock, sepsis, and hemorrhage. When external trauma is the cause of esophageal rupture, there is often damage to other nearby structures, including the trachea, blood vessels, and nerves.

Clinical signs. Clinical signs of esophageal wounds include hemorrhage, excess salivation, dysphagia, regurgitation, and repeated swallowing attempts. In cases that involve the thoracic esophagus, respiratory distress may be seen. Many animals will be febrile and show signs of shock.

Diagnosis. The diagnosis of esophageal rupture is often suspected from a history of known trauma, animal fight, or penetrating wound. Physical examination may reveal external signs of trauma. In cases of rupture of the esophagus, there may be subcutaneous emphysema. This finding can also be caused by tracheal rupture.

Radiography may demonstrate a penetrating object if present (see Fig. 22-1). Additional radiographic findings in cases of esophageal rupture may include subcutaneous emphysema, pneumomediastinum, pneumothorax, and pleural effusion. If the diagnosis is in doubt, a contrast study can be performed by obtaining radiographs after oral administration of water-soluble iodinated contrast media. Barium sulfate should not be used for this purpose.

The diagnosis of esophageal rupture can also be made by endoscopic examination. Care should be taken not to cause further esophageal damage with the endoscope. The smallest diameter scope available should be used. Endoscopic signs of esophageal perforation include direct visualization of the tear or structures outside the esophagus, or inability to maintain air insufflation with worsening of subcutaneous emphysema or pneumomediastinum.

Treatment of esophageal rupture. All esophageal tears must be repaired surgically. Precise location of the site and number of tears must be made prior to surgery to aid in the surgical approach. In most cases, primary closure of the rupture can be accomplished. Since the esophagus does not have a serosal layer but only a thin outer fibrous covering, mucosal apposition is extremely important.[9-11] Therefore, devitalized tissue must be removed. In severe cases, esophageal resection and anastomosis may be necessary. The decision to excise a necrotic area followed by primary closure versus resection of a segment of the esophagus depends on the amount of tissue that is devitalized. Healing of esophageal wounds or anastomoses is more difficult than with intestinal anastomoses, as there is no omental structure in the thorax to provide a seal and vascular adhesions to the suture line, esophageal blood vessels are segmental in distribution and therefore easily disrupted, there is constant flow of saliva over the incision, and movement and tension on the incision site constantly occur from peristaltic waves associated with swallowing.[11] Following repair of cervical esophageal wounds, subcutaneous drain placement exiting the skin may be necessary to control infection. Following repair of thoracic esophageal wounds, drainage and lavage through tube thoracostomy may be necessary. Postoperative problems following esophageal surgery may occur, and include leakage or dehiscence, infection, and stricture formation.[3]

Broad-spectrum parenteral antibiotics are administered perioperatively and postoperatively. Since the bacteria that are likely to cause problems originate from the oral cavity, antibiotics effective against oral flora are used. Ampicillin and the cephalosporins are indicated for this purpose. Because subcutaneous infection, mediastinitis, or pleuritis is usually present, additional administration of an aminoglycoside antibiotic (either gentamicin or amikacin) parenterally is indicated. Aggressive intravenous fluid support is necessary since many animals will be in shock.

Postoperative care also includes food restriction and nutritional support through a PEG or nasogastric tube.

Megaesophagus

In most cases, animals with megaesophagus present with histories of chronic regurgitation, coughing, and weight loss. However, some animals have acute aspiration pneumonia secondary to inhalation of food present in the dilated esophagus. These animals often have life-threatening signs and present in an emergency situation. This discussion will be restricted to these cases.

CAUSES OF MEGAESOPHAGUS IN SMALL ANIMALS

Idiopathic esophageal motility disorder (acquired or congenital)
Myasthenia gravis
Hypothyroidism
Hypoadrenocorticism
Polyneuropathy
Polymyositis
Organophosphate intoxication
Lead or thallium intoxication
Brainstem lesion
Vascular ring anomaly
Esophageal stricture or mass
Feline dysautonomia (Key-Gaskell syndrome)

Causes of megaesophagus are listed above (see box).[10,12]

Clinical signs of megaesophagus. Animals with acute signs of megaesophagus usually are presented for severe dyspnea secondary to aspiration pneumonia. Approximately 15% of animals with megaesophagus have only respiratory signs[10] and present in acute respiratory distress. Eventually, pneumonia develops in 75% of dogs with megaesophagus, and 50% die from it.[12] These animals often have additional signs, including regurgitation, coughing, and weight loss.

Diagnosis. The diagnosis of megaesophagus is usually easily made by thoracic radiography. Survey radiographs usually demonstrate an air-filled, dilated esophagus. Poor esophageal motility can also be documented with contrast radiography. However, this is rarely necessary to establish a diagnosis and carries the risk of the patient aspirating the radiographic contrast media. Thoracic radiography also demonstrates features of aspiration pneumonia. These include an alveolar and peribronchial infiltrate with a ventral distribution, with the right middle lung lobe often most severely affected (this lobe has the most dependent bronchus in the dog).

Emergency treatment of megaesophagus. The emergency treatment of animals with megaesophagus deals with controlling aspiration pneumonia, preventing further regurgitation and aspiration, and providing nutritional support. Because many animals are in acute respiratory distress, oxygen administration is often necessary. This can be accomplished with the use of an oxygen cage, face mask, or nasal oxygen tube (see Chapters 25 and 36).

Parenteral administration of broad-spectrum antibiotics is essential. Oral administration is unreliable because the drug may not reach the stomach where it can be absorbed. The choice of antibiotics should ideally be based on microbiological culture and antibiotic sensitivity testing of the offending organisms. If the patient is stable, a transtracheal aspirate should be performed for this purpose. If the animal is showing signs suggestive of septicemia, multiple blood cultures are indicated. If these tests cannot be performed, empirical administration of a combination of a cephalosporin and aminoglycoside is indicated. Additional therapy for aspiration pneumonia includes ultrasonic nebulization with saline solution (30 minutes, every 4 to 6 hours) followed by coupage of the chest for 5 minutes.

While the aspiration pneumonia is being treated, it is imperative to minimize the amount of regurgitation. In some animals this can be accomplished by elevation while feeding. In other animals, however, complete cessation of oral intake is necessary to allow aspiration pneumonia to resolve. In these cases, it is helpful to provide nutritional support through a nasogastric or PEG tube. In many animals the placement of a nasogastric tube is impossible because the tip of the tube gets caught in redundant folds of the esophagus and the tube coils on itself. The use of a stylet (using a stiff wire or guitar string) often makes placement easier. If the placement of a nasogastric tube is attempted, its location must be confirmed radiographically.

Esophageal neoplasia

Occasionally, animals with esophageal neoplasia will be presented for signs of acute esophageal obstruction. Squamous-cell carcinomas, leiomyomas, carcinomas, and sarcomas occur in the esophagus.[13] The diagnosis may be suspected from contrast radiography and confirmed by endoscopy and biopsy. Treatment involves surgical resection. The prognosis is poor because a large segment of the esophagus is usually involved, making surgical intervention difficult. Metastasis and local recurrence is common.

Acute gastritis and vomiting

Acute vomiting can be caused by many problems, including primary gastrointestinal disease or extragastrointestinal metabolic problems. Causes of vomiting are listed in the box.[13] It is often difficult to determine the exact cause of vomiting. Often treatment is directed at symptomatic management until the problem resolves or until laboratory and ancillary testing determine a definitive diagnosis so that specific appropriate therapy can be instituted. This discussion will review the pathophysiologic mechanisms of vomiting and management of acute gastritis.

CAUSES OF VOMITING

Primary gastrointestinal disorders
  Acute gastritis
  Gastric or intestinal neoplasia
  Gastric or duodenal ulceration
  Chronic idiopathic inflammatory bowel disease
  Eosinophilic gastroenteritis
  Gastrointestinal parasitism
  Infectious enteritis
    Viral
    Bacterial
    Fungal
    Miscellaneous (e.g., prototheca)
  Gastric-outlet obstruction (functional or structural)
  Gastric or intestinal foreign body
  Intussusception
  Gastric or intestinal neoplasm
  Intestinal obstruction
Extragastrointestinal disorders
  Hepatic disease
  Renal disease
  Pancreatitis
  Endocrine disorders
    Hypoadrenocorticism
    Diabetes mellitus
    Hyperthyroidism
  Pyometritis
  Congestive heart failure
  Electrolyte abnormalities
  Drugs or toxins
  Central nervous system disorders

Pathophysiology of vomiting.[13] Vomiting is a reflex act with neural pathways that synapse in the medulla at the vomiting center. The vomiting reflex can be divided into afferent and efferent limbs. Many types of problems can initiate vomiting through input into various afferent limbs to the vomiting center. There are four principal pathways that provide afferent input to the vomiting center: peripheral sensory input, chemoreceptor trigger zone, higher brain center (psychic influences, pain), and the vestibular system. Most peripheral sensory receptors initiating vomiting are found in the abdominal cavity, including the stomach, duodenum, jejunum, mesentery, peritoneum, and pancreas. The highest concentration of receptors are found in the bowel, especially in the duodenum. Factors that stimulate these receptors include distention, acute erosions, chronic ulceration, inflammation, and chemical irritation. Distention of the small intestine produces vomiting more readily than distention of the stomach. The more proximal the small intestinal obstruction, the more likely it is to induce vomiting. When these receptors are stimulated, input to the vomiting center is carried by the vagus and sympathetic nerve supply.

The chemoreceptor trigger zone (CTZ) also provides input to the vomiting center. The CTZ lies on the floor of the fourth ventricle, and it is activated primarily by blood-borne substances. There is a minimal blood-brain barrier in this area, allowing circulating toxins and substances to cause stimulation. Afferent impulses from the CTZ stimulate neurons in the vomiting center to initiate vomiting. Substances causing vomiting through their stimulation of the CTZ include apomorphine, digitalis glycosides, chemotherapeutic agents, and uremic toxins. In addition, other metabolic disorders, motion sickness, and radiation sickness induce vomiting through stimulation of the CTZ.

Higher central nervous system centers in the cerebrum have input to the vomiting center. Psychogenic factors, fear, excitement, pain, and stress cause vomiting mediated through this pathway.

The vestibular system has input to the vomiting center directly or via the CTZ.[13,14] Vomiting arising from stimulation of the vestibular system can occur as a result of motion sickness or labyrinthitis.

All afferent impulses stimulate nerves in the vomiting center, and efferent impulses are initiated. The motor events of vomiting result in contraction of abdominal muscles and the diaphragm mediated by phrenic and spinal nerves. Preceding these events are hypersalivation, nausea, and retching. The gastric antrum and duodenum contract, whereas the body of the stomach, lower esophageal sphincter, and esophagus relax. The driving force to propel the vomitus out of the stomach is contraction of the diaphragm and abdominal muscles, rather than reverse peristalsis. Vomiting is still possible when there is loss of innervation to abdominal viscera, whereas vomiting is impossible with denervation of the diaphragm and abdominal muscles.

Evaluation and management of acute gastritis and vomiting

History. The history often gives the clinician important clues as to the cause of acute vomiting. It is important to review all body systems and obtain information regarding dietary changes, parasite control, travel history, environment, exposure to garbage or foreign bodies, illness of other pets, vaccination status, and current medication. It is also essential to distinguish regurgitation from true vomiting. Regurgitation is the passive ejection of food or saliva from the esophagus, usually as a result of gravity, changes in body position,

or increased intrathoracic or intraabdominal pressure. A neural reflex is not necessary to produce regurgitation as opposed to vomiting. Regurgitation is associated with abnormal esophageal motility or obstruction. Regurgitation has the following features: the regurgitated material is undigested, although only saliva may also be regurgitated; undigested food may be cylindrically shaped; the act of regurgitation is passive and unrelated to coordinated abdominal contractions; there is no hypersalivation or repeated swallowing motions preceding the event; the act of regurgitation is often preceded by changes in body position; and regurgitated material is not bile stained.[10] There is often no relation between feeding and the act of regurgitation, which can occur minutes or hours after eating. Vomiting, on the other hand, is associated with forceful ejection of food associated with repeated abdominal muscle contractions. If the distinction between regurgitation and vomiting cannot be made from the history, other studies are necessary, such as testing the pH of the fluid (which will be high with regurgitation, below 5 with vomiting of gastric contents, and possibly high with vomiting of intestinal contents), radiography, or endoscopy.

Physical examination. Physical examination should determine the overall health status of the animal, including hydration status, and the presence of possible septicemia, endotoxemia, and electrolyte imbalances. Abdominal palpation is important to detect foreign bodies, changes in other abdominal organs, and the presence of pain. Rectal palpation should be performed and the feces inspected for the presence of blood, melena (suggestive of esophageal, gastric, or upper intestinal hemorrhage), and parasites.

Laboratory evaluation. If the history and physical examination do not result in the diagnosis, further testing may be necessary. A diagnostic approach to the patient with acute vomiting is illustrated in Fig. 22-2.

The initial minimal laboratory testing should include a measurement of packed cell volume, total solids, and blood reagent strips to estimate blood urea nitrogen (Azostix) and blood glucose concentrations (Chemstrip bG). This will determine hydration status, estimate renal function, and help rule out diabetes mellitus. A urinalysis should also be obtained prior to fluid therapy, especially if the Azostix reading is high. This will allow the clinician to distinguish prerenal from renal elevations in blood urea nitrogen concentrations. A fecal flotation and direct fecal smear should also be obtained on any animal with gastrointestinal signs.

A more complete data base should be obtained

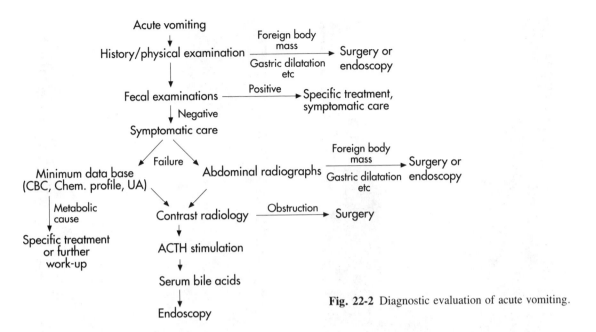

Fig. 22-2 Diagnostic evaluation of acute vomiting.

on severely ill animals, including a serum biochemistry profile and complete blood count. Abnormalities in the complete blood count may be nonspecific, but may also give clues as to the cause. Leukocytosis may be seen with bacterial infections, stress (neutrophilia, lymphopenia, and eosinopenia), septicemia, or as a nonspecific finding suggesting inflammatory disease. Leukopenia is seen with viral enteritides (canine parvovirus or feline panleukopenia virus) or septicemia. Eosinophilia is seen with eosinophilic gastroenteritis, parasitism, or hypoadrenocorticism. The finding of lymphocytosis in a stressed animal should also increase the index of suspicion of hypoadrenocorticism. Anemia may be seen with acute or chronic blood loss. When chronic iron deficiency occurs, there will be microcytic and hypochromic red blood cell indices. Serum biochemistry profiles may reveal evidence of metabolic diseases that cause vomiting, such as renal disease, hepatic disease, hypoadrenocorticism, diabetes mellitus, and pancreatitis (see box on p. 325). Many automated serum biochemical profiles include measurement of serum total carbon dioxide concentration, an estimate of bicarbonate concentration, which in conjunction with serum electrolyte concentrations allows the clinician to plan appropriate fluid therapy.

Radiography. Survey abdominal radiography is useful to evaluate a vomiting patient. A definitive diagnosis can be reached in certain conditions, such as radiopaque foreign bodies and small intestinal obstruction. Radiography is also useful to rule out abnormalities of other organs, such as hepatomegaly, uterine enlargement, and abdominal masses. However, it is often necessary to perform a radiographic contrast study to evaluate the stomach and small intestine.

The simplest radiographic contrast study to evaluate the stomach is a pneumogastrogram. This procedure is a quick, inexpensive technique to screen for radiolucent foreign bodies, and to evaluate the shape, size, and position of the stomach. The technique is performed by injecting air into the stomach via orogastric tube until there is slight abdominal tympany.[15] Sedation is usually not required. The main limitation of this technique is that it does not allow for good evaluation of mucosal detail.

A positive contrast upper gastrointestinal barium study is useful in evaluating for the presence of gastrointestinal obstruction (Fig. 22-3), foreign bodies, abnormal position of the bowel (as would occur with an abdominal mass), gastrointestinal ulceration (Fig. 22-4), abnormal motility, and changes consistent with inflammatory or neoplastic involvement of the bowel. Barium is the contrast agent of choice. The use of water-soluble iodinated contrast media results in poor mucosal coating, rapid transit, and because of its high osmolality, fluid entering the bowel, thus exacerbating systemic volume depletion. If the history does not adequately distinguish regurgitation from vomiting, survey thoracic radiography or a radiographic contrast evaluation of the esophagus should be performed prior to introducing barium

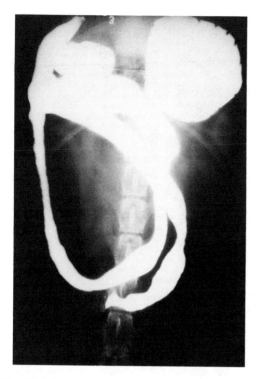

Fig. 22-3 Upper gastrointestinal barium series demonstrating complete small-intestinal obstruction in a dog. A corn cob was found at surgery.

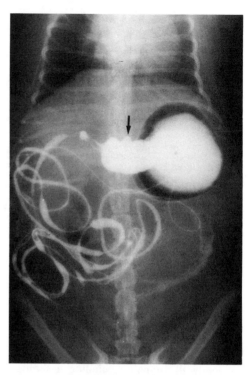

Fig. 22-4 Upper gastrointestinal barium series performed on a dog receiving aspirin. An ulcer is demonstrated by a smooth protrusion of barium beyond the normal contour of the stomach along the lesser curvature *(arrow)*. (Courtesy of David Hager, Radiology Consulting Service, Cardiff, CA.)

into the stomach. Blood tests to rule out metabolic causes of vomiting should be performed prior to radiographic contrast procedures.

Endoscopy. Endoscopic examination of the stomach and duodenum is now commonly performed in veterinary medicine. Either a flexible fiberoptic or electronic video endoscope can be used. The technique is a rapid, noninvasive method of evaluating the mucosa of the gastrointestinal tract. Endoscopy is useful for the detection of gastroduodenal foreign bodies, ulceration, neoplasia, or inflammatory changes. If a foreign body is not found, gastric or duodenal mucosal samples can be obtained for cytologic or histologic examination. The main disadvantage of endoscopy is the need for general anesthesia and the cost of the equipment. The techniques of gastrointestinal endoscopy have recently been reviewed.[16]

Surgery. Exploratory surgery of the abdominal cavity is often a valuable diagnostic and therapeutic procedure. It allows evaluation of all the abdominal organs, including the entire gastrointestinal tract, and allows for treatment of foreign bodies, obstructing neoplasms, and other surgically correctable problems. If no gross abnormalities are found during exploratory celiotomy, it is mandatory to obtain multiple gastrointestinal and hepatic biopsies.

Treatment of acute gastritis and vomiting. The therapy of acute vomiting should be directed toward correcting the primary problem and supportive care. Unfortunately, a definitive diagnosis is often not established, and treatment is symptomatic and supportive (see Fig. 22-2). This discussion will be directed toward the latter two efforts.

Fluid therapy. Vomiting may result in dehydration, electrolyte depletion, and acid-base abnormalities. Fluid lost by vomiting gastric contents is different from extracellular fluid in that it contains less sodium, more potassium, more hydrogen ions, and less bicarbonate.[13] Vomiting gastric contents can cause hypernatremia, hypokalemia, and alkalosis.[13] However, the changes in serum electrolytes and acid-base status are usually not predictable. In one series of cases, metabolic acidosis was the most common acid-base disturbance.[14] This was thought to occur from extracellular fluid loss and volume contraction, with minimal loss of gastric acid, possibly due to simultaneous loss of bicarbonate-rich duodenal fluid, and renal compensation.[14]

Gastric or proximal duodenal obstruction commonly results in hyponatremia, hypochloremia, hypokalemia, and metabolic alkalosis.[17] Hyponatremia and hypokalemia can result from sodium and potassium loss in the vomitus, followed by ingestion of water and subsequent volume expansion with sodium-free fluid. Hypochloremia and metabolic alkalosis can result from loss of hydrochloric acid in the vomitus. When this occurs, alkalosis is perpetuated by dehydration and chloride and potassium depletion.[14] The kidney attempts to maintain extracellular volume by reabsorbing sodium. Normally, sodium is absorbed with the anion chloride. With chloride depletion associated with severe vomiting, sodium is reabsorbed in the proximal tubule with the anion bicarbonate, thus exacerbating metabolic alkalosis. In addition, the distal tubule also reabsorbs sodium in an effort to expand extracellular fluid volume. Usually sodium is exchanged for potassium at this site, but when severe hypokalemia is present, sodium is exchanged for hydrogen ions. In this setting, proximal tubular bicarbonate reabsorption and distal tubular sodium-hydrogen ion exchange results in paradoxic aciduria in the face of metabolic alkalosis.[14] This condition will persist until chloride is replaced through fluid therapy.

Parenteral fluid therapy is indicated whenever there is dehydration, there are imbalances in electrolytes or acid-base status, or continued vomiting makes oral alimentation impossible. The intravenous route is preferred in most cases, especially in severely injured or critically ill patients. Subcutaneous fluid therapy may be useful with mild dehydration or with resolving problems. The volume of fluid to be administered is based on volume deficit, maintenance requirement, and ongoing fluid losses (Chapter 38).

The choice of fluids depends on the electrolyte and acid-base status of the patient. The acid-base status can be determined from arterial blood gas measurements or estimated from the serum total carbon dioxide concentration (an estimation of serum bicarbonate concentration). Serum biochemistry values may not be available or may be impossible to obtain in the acute situation. Therefore, the choice of fluids depends on expected changes in these parameters and on clinical judgment. In hypernatremic patients, half-strength (0.45%) saline plus 2.5% dextrose is the fluid of choice since it contains less sodium than plasma. With metabolic alkalosis, normal saline (0.9%) solution is preferred because of its acidifying

properties. This solution also contains high concentrations of sodium and chloride, which is appropriate since many patients have hyponatremia and hypochloremia. With metabolic acidosis, an alkaline buffering solution such as lactated Ringer's solution is preferred. This solution also replaces sodium, chloride, and potassium. Potassium depletion is common in most vomiting animals, so additional potassium should be added to the fluids. As a general rule, 20 to 25 mEq of potassium chloride should be added to each liter of the parenteral fluids initially if normal renal function is present. Once the serum potassium concentration is known, this amount can be adjusted (see Chapter 38).

Antiemetics. The antiemetic used depends on the cause of vomiting (see section on "Pathophysiology of Vomiting," above, and box on p. 325). Commonly used antiemetics with their mechanisms of action and dosages are listed in Table 22-1.

Antiemetics can be classified on the basis of broad spectrum (those inhibiting neural transmission through the vomiting center) or narrow spectrum (those inhibiting only one portion of an afferent limb to the vomiting center, such as antihistamines inhibiting vestibular input). In general, broad-spectrum antiemetics are more effective, whereas narrow-spectrum antiemetics may be completely ineffective unless used when the mechanism of vomiting will be affected by the specific action of the drug.

Phenothiazines are among the most effective antiemetics. They act by directly inhibiting the vomiting center, and their antiemetic effect is seen at dosages lower than those used for tranquilization. These drugs also inhibit neural activity through the chemoreceptor trigger zone and have weak anticholinergic activity.[13,18] The most common side effect of these drugs is hypotension, because they are alpha-adrenergic blockers. These drugs should not be used in dehydrated animals without intravenous fluid support. Many of these drugs can be administered via several routes, including orally, subcutaneously, intravenously, intramuscularly, and by rectal suppository.

Drugs that act on the CTZ are useful for vomiting caused by blood-borne irritants (drugs, chemotherapeutic agents, and uremia). Currently, the most useful drug in this category is metoclopramide (Reglan). In addition to its potent inhibition of the CTZ, metoclopramide is a prokinetic drug that has peripheral effects on the stomach and upper small intestine and also raises the threshold of activity in the vomiting center.[19-22] Unlike other nonspecific cholinergic drugs such as bethanechol, metoclopramide results in augmented motil-

TABLE 22-1 Antiemetic drugs used in small animals

Generic Drug	Trade Name	Site of Action	Dosage	Cautions/Side Effects
Metoclopramide	Reglan	CTZ, peripheral	0.2-0.4 mg/kg PO, SC, IM every 6 hours; or 1-4 mg/kg/24-hour IV infusion	Restlessness, behavior changes
Chlorpromazine	Thorazine	Vomiting center	0.2-0.4 mg/kg SC every 8 hours	Hypotension, sedation
Prochlorperazine	Darbazine, Compazine	Vomiting center	0.5 mg/kg SC, IM, rectal suppository, every 8 hours	Hypotension, sedation
Diphenhydramine	Benadryl	Vestibular system	2-4 mg/kg, PO, IM	Sedation
Dimenhydrinate	Dramamine	Vestibular system	8 mg/kg PO every 8 hours	Sedation
Trimethobenzamide	Tigan	CTZ	3 mg/kg IM every 8-12 hours	Allergic reaction
Atropine		Anticholinergic	0.04 mg/kg SC, every 8 hours	Gastric retention, intestinal ileus, tachycardia
Propantheline	Pro-Banthine	Anticholinergic	0.5-1.0 mg/kg PO, every 8 hours	Gastric retention, intestinal ileus, tachycardia
Isopropamide	Darbazine, Darbid	Anticholinergic	0.2-0.4 mg/kg PO, every 8-12 hours	Gastric retention, intestinal ileus, tachycardia
Aminopentamide	Centrine	Anticholinergic	0.1-0.5mg PO,IM,SC	Gastric retention, intestinal ileus, tachycardia

CTZ = chemoreceptor trigger zone; peripheral = prokinetic gastrointestinal motility modification; PO = orally; SC = subcutaneously; IM = intramuscularly; IV = intravenously.

ity in a coordinated manner and thus enhances gastric emptying and upper-small-intestine transit. Metoclopramide increases tone of the lower esophageal sphincter, increases frequency and amplitude of gastric fundic and antral contractions in coordination with pyloric relaxation, and increases duodenal contractions in a synchronized manner.[20-22] Metoclopramide has a rapid onset (30 to 60 minutes) and short duration (60-to-90-minute half-life) after oral administration. If administered by this route, metoclopramide should be given 30 minutes prior to feeding.[19,21,22] In animals receiving nothing orally, metoclopramide is best given mixed with the intravenous fluids and administered by constant infusion because of its short duration of effect when given by intravenous bolus (see Table 22-1). It is especially useful in this manner in patients with viral enteritis (gastric stasis and intestinal ileus). If intravenous administration is not possible and oral therapy is contraindicated, subcutaneous administration is preferred over intramuscular administration because the half-life is too short when metoclopramide is administered intramuscularly.[21] Side effects of metoclopramide are unusual, but include restlessness and behavior changes (especially in cats). The drug is contraindicated with gastrointestinal obstruction.

Trimethobenzamide (Tigan) is a drug that is a potent inhibitor of the CTZ without affecting the vomiting center and has virtually no other pharmacologic effects in the body.[18] Although this drug would seem to have promise in veterinary medicine, my limited experience with this drug has been disappointing.

Vomiting caused by vestibular stimulation (such as motion sickness) can be prevented by using various antihistamine drugs such as dimenhydrinate (Dramamine) and diphenhydramine (Benadryl). Their antiemetic effects are independent of their antihistaminic or sedative effects.[18] It should be emphasized that these drugs are ineffective for vomiting caused by any other mechanism. The main side effect of these drugs is sedation, which may be an advantage in an animal that is traveling.

Anticholinergic drugs such as atropine and propantheline inhibit contraction and spasm of smooth muscle in the gastrointestinal tract. Unless these specific processes are the cause of vomiting, these drugs will be ineffective. Anticholinergic drugs are rarely effective in controlling vomiting in small animals, because intestinal spasm rarely occurs in them. Because motility changes in the esophagus, stomach, and duodenum are not necessary for the vomiting to occur, anticholinergic drugs do not affect the efferent limb of the vomiting reflex.[13] In addition to their lack of effectiveness, these drugs can exacerbate vomiting because they decrease gastric emptying and can lead to gastric distention. Gastric distention can stimulate the vomiting reflex and gastrin release, resulting in increased gastric acid production.

Dietary considerations. One of the most important aspects of treating animals with acute vomiting or acute gastritis is proper dietary management. While an animal is vomiting, it is important to restrict all oral intake (including water) since gastric distention will elicit the vomiting reflex and increase gastric acid secretion. Twelve to 24 hours after the last episode of vomiting, the animal is offered water in small frequent increments. If no further vomiting occurs in the next 24 hours, the animal is offered food. Proper selection of food is important to minimize the probability for relapse. Nutrients should be selected that have minimal abrasiveness to the gastric mucosa (and are therefore low in fiber), minimal ability to stimulate gastric secretions, and do not delay gastric emptying.[13] Carbohydrates have the least propensity to stimulate gastric secretions.[13] The most easily digested starch is rice, and therefore this is the food of choice. Protein intake should be resumed gradually since amino acids are the most potent stimulators of gastric acid secretion.[13] Since fats delay gastric emptying, they should be avoided. Therefore, a diet of rice and a small amount of low fat cottage cheese is appropriate. This should be fed in small, frequent meals. If the animal does well after several days, the regular diet can be gradually reintroduced.

Antibiotics. In general, antibiotics are not indicated in cases of acute vomiting. Exceptions include animals at high risk for sepsis, such as patients with parvovirus enteritis, leukopenia, or gastrointestinal ulceration. In these cases, broad-spectrum antibiotic coverage is indicated. This will be discussed in more detail in the section on "Viral Enteritis." It is rare for a primary bacterial infection to cause vomiting. Adverse effects of antibiotics include alteration of the normal bacterial flora, and some antibiotics can induce vomiting.

Protectants and absorbants. Orally administered protectants such as preparations containing kaolin, pectolin, and bismuth are generally ineffective in controlling vomiting. Protectants may bind certain bacteria and toxins, but they do not coat the surface of the stomach or intestine and protect the mucosa. Since these drugs need to be administered orally, they may induce vomiting and therefore worsen the condition of the animal.

Antacid and antisecretory therapy. Antacids and drugs inhibiting gastric acid secretion will be discussed in the section on "Gastrointestinal Ulceration."

Gastrointestinal ulceration

Causes. Gastrointestinal ulceration or erosion can be defined as any disruption in the mucosal lining of the bowel. An ulcer is a mucosal defect extending through the lamina muscularis mucosae or deeper, whereas an erosion does not penetrate the lamina muscularis mucosae.[23] Ulcers can occur in any region of the bowel, but are most common in the stomach. Causes of gastrointestinal ulcers are listed below (see box).

The normal stomach has the ability to resist the harmful effects of hydrochloric acid, pepsin, and intraluminal abrasive products through several mechanisms, collectively termed the gastric mucosal barrier. The most important defense mechanisms include: (1) gastric mucus coating the surface of the stomach. Mucus is a viscous gel consisting of glycoprotein (5%) and water (95%) that adheres to the surface of the mucosa and protects it against mechanical abrasion and provides an undisturbed layer that maintains bicarbonate at the surface;[23] (2) production of bicarbonate, which neutralizes acid in the lumen; (3) barrier to "back-diffusion" of hydrogen ions into the mucosa, comprised of electrical interactions, phospholipids, epithelial cells, and mucus; (4) mucosal microcirculation, allowing rapid clearing of hydrogen ions that have "back-diffused" into the mucosa, and supplying nutrients and other factors to gastric mucosal cells; (5) rapid epithelial cell turnover; and (6) protective prostaglandins (especially of the E type), which inhibit acid secretion, in-

---

CAUSES OF GASTROINTESTINAL ULCERATION

Gastrointestinal neoplasia
Drugs (aspirin, glucocorticoids, nonsteroidal antiinflammatory drugs, others)
Hepatic disease
Renal failure
Acute pancreatitis
Chronic gastric retention
Nongastric mast cell tumor
Gastrin-secreting tumor (Zollinger-Ellison syndrome)
Intervertebral disk disease or other neurologic disease
Shock
Trauma
Bile reflux into stomach
Disseminated intravascular coagulation
Hypoadrenocorticism
Parasitism

---

crease bicarbonate secretion, maintain mucosal blood flow, and contribute to gastric mucus production.[23,24] Conditions or agents (see box on p. 331) that adversely affect these factors or cause increased gastric acid production can lead to gastric ulceration.

Drugs. The most common ulcerogenic drugs used in small animal patients are nonsteroidal antiinflammatory drugs (NSAIDs), including aspirin, flunixin (Banamine), meclofenamic acid (Arquel, Meclomen), phenylbutazone, piroxicam (Feldene), and ibuprofen (Motrin). In addition, glucocorticoids, especially dexamethasone, are potent ulcerogenic drugs in certain settings. The mechanisms of aspirin-induced injury include local cytotoxic effects on gastric mucosal epithelial cells and detrimental effects through cyclooxygenase inhibition, including decreasing prostaglandin activity.[24] As discussed above, prostaglandins are an important defense mechanism of the gastric mucosal barrier. Harmful effects of aspirin and other NSAIDs include local changes to mucosal epithelial cells unrelated to prostaglandin inhibition, and effects related to prostaglandin inhibition.[24,25] Local toxic changes include increased permeability, increased back-diffusion of hydrogen ions into mucosal epithelial cells, abnormal ion transport, and changes in the electrical potential difference.[25] Effects on mucosal defense related to cyclooxygenase inhibition include decreased endogenous prostaglandin production, decreased mucosal blood flow, decreased bicarbonate and mucus secretion, and decreased epithelial surface hydrophobicity.[25] Enteric-coated and buffered aspirin products are still ulcerogenic, primarily through their antiprostaglandin effects.[25] The most common location for ulcers induced by NSAIDs are along the lesser curvature near the pyloric antrum (Figs. 22-4 and 22-5). These ulcers are usually well demarcated, with smooth margins, and often very deep (Fig. 22-5).

Metabolic disease. The most common metabolic abnormalities leading to gastric ulceration are renal failure, hepatic failure, and hypoadrenocorticism. Gastric and duodenal ulcers commonly occur in renal failure because uremic toxins directly damage the mucosa, and because renal failure results in increased gastrin concentration, thus leading to hyperacidity.[26] Gastrointestinal ulceration occurs with hepatic failure because there are increased concentrations of histamine and gastrin (due to decreased gastrin clearance and due to bile acid-induced gastrin release), both leading to increased gastric acid production.[26] In addition, there is decreased mucosal blood flow (due to portal hypertension and microthrombi) and alteration in gastric mucus with hepatic failure, both

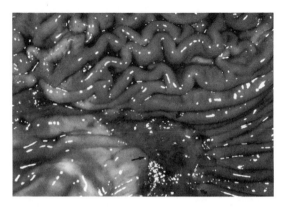

Fig. 22-5 Autopsy specimen of a dog with a deep ulcer *(arrows)* along the lesser curvature of the stomach caused by administration of a nonsteroidal antiinflammatory drug. Note the smooth contour and well demarcated margins. (Courtesy of Angell Memorial Animal Hospital, Boston.)

important components of the gastric mucosal barrier.[23,26] The mechanism of gastrointestinal ulceration in animals with hypoadrenocorticism is unclear.

Stress. Stress-induced gastrointestinal ulceration is uncommon in small animals as compared with human beings. Factors such as trauma, shock, and hypotension may decrease gastric mucosal blood flow and potentiate other ulcerogenic factors. Endogenous release of glucocorticoids and catecholamines may also contribute to gastrointestinal ulcers. In addition, gastric mucosal ischemia can occur as a result of sympathetically mediated vasoconstriction.[26]

Neurologic disease can also potentiate gastrointestinal ulceration, possibly due to the stress-related factors mentioned above and through an imbalance of the neural supply of the stomach resulting in decreased sympathetic tone and increased parasympathetic tone.[23,26] Administration of corticosteroids will further increase the likelihood of ulcers in these patients through their ability to decrease and alter gastric mucus, affect epithelial cell renewal, and decrease protective prostaglandins.[23] The administration of corticosteroids to dogs with neurologic injury has also been associated with colonic ulceration and rupture.[27] This will be discussed in detail in the section on "Nontraumatic Perforation of the Large Intestine."

Gastric hyperacidity. Gastric hyperacidity can lead to gastroduodenal ulceration. The mechanism of gastric acid production involves stimulation of the gastric parietal cell with gastrin, histamine, and acetylcholine. Conditions increasing these secretagogues can result in gastric hyperacidity.

This has been documented to occur in gastrin-producing tumors (Zollinger-Ellison syndrome) and in canine and feline systemic mast-cell tumors. In the latter syndrome, histamine is released by malignant mast cells, causing hyperacidity. The most common location for mast-cell-tumor-induced ulcers is at the proximal aspect of the duodenum. Disorders resulting in chronic gastric distention, such as the antral pyloric hypertrophy syndrome, can be associated with increased gastrin release and therefore gastric hyperacidity.[28]

Neoplasia. Gastrointestinal neoplasia frequently results in ulceration. The most common gastrointestinal tumors in the dog are lymphosarcoma and adenocarcinoma.[23,29] Lymphoma is by far the most common gastrointestinal neoplasm in the cat. Other gastrointestinal tumors that may result in ulceration include leiomyosarcoma, carcinoid, anaplastic sarcoma, mast-cell tumor, extramedullary plasmacytoma, adenomatous polyp, and leiomyoma.

Clinical findings. Animals with gastric ulcers may be asymptomatic, but a common clinical sign with gastric ulceration is vomiting. The vomitus may contain frank blood if hemorrhage is fresh, or material resembling coffee grounds if the blood was present in the stomach for a time. If the degree of bleeding is excessive, anemia will be present. With acute ulcers, the anemia will be regenerative. With chronic gastrointestinal blood loss, the anemia will be characterized as microcytic and hypochromic. Other signs include melena, abdominal pain, and anorexia. If the ulcer erodes through the serosa, signs of septic peritonitis will rapidly develop, including collapse, shock, and fever, leading to death. In animals receiving corticosteroids or NSAIDs, these signs are often delayed until therapeutic intervention is too late.

Diagnosis of gastric ulcers. An index of suspicion of gastric ulceration should be present when there are compatible clinical signs and associated ulcerogenic factors or conditions that lead to ulceration (see box on p. 331). Physical examination findings may reveal evidence of anemia or abdominal pain. In patients with systemic mast-cell tumor, cutaneous masses may be seen. A complete data base, including a complete blood count, serum biochemistry profile, and urinalysis should be obtained to exclude metabolic causes of ulceration (renal failure, hepatic failure, and hypoadrenocorticism).

Survey abdominal radiography is seldom helpful in the diagnosis of gastric ulceration, and the use of contrast radiography is necessary. If a perforation is suspected from physical examination or abdominal paracentesis findings, a water-soluble organic iodide contrast agent (such as Gastrografin) is preferred. Unfortunately, these contrast agents result in poor mucosal coating and have a lower diagnostic yield. Therefore, the use of barium sulfate is preferred in most cases. The appearance of an ulcer is characterized by protrusion of contrast material beyond the normal contour of the mucosa, or by retention of contrast material on a focal area of mucosa in multiple films (Fig. 22-4). The mucosal detail of the stomach can be improved with a double-contrast gastrogram using air and barium.[30] Several radiographic views may be necessary.

Endoscopy allows the most direct way to obtain a definitive diagnosis, allowing direct visualization of the ulcer. It is important to examine the entire circumference of the stomach and duodenum to avoid missing small ulcers or those along the lesser curvature. The scope should not be inserted into the duodenum too rapidly in order to avoid missing proximal duodenal ulcers, the most common location associated with systemic mast-cell tumor. Care should be taken to avoid perforation, which can occur with gastric overdistention with air insufflation, with introduction of the scope, or during biopsy.

The gross endoscopic appearance of gastric ulceration is quite variable. Superficial erosion appears as diffuse hyperemic mucosa with shallow disruptions of the surface. Ulcers induced by NSAIDs are usually found along the lesser curvature between the fundus and pyloric antrum. They are often deep, well demarcated from surrounding tissue, round, and regular (Fig. 22-5). Neoplastic ulcers, on the other hand, are often irregular, contain friable tissue, and are surrounded by hyperemic thickened tissue.

Since neoplasia is often associated with gastric ulceration, biopsy of all ulcers is mandatory. The rim of the ulcer should be sampled in addition to the center, since the center often contains only debris and inflammatory cells. I routinely obtain 10 to 20 endoscopic biopsies from each ulcer to minimize the likelihood of missing a neoplastic ulcer. It is often helpful to take multiple samples from the same site to obtain deeper tissue. If this is done, care and judgment must be used to avoid perforation.

Treatment of gastric ulcers. Several drugs can be used to treat gastric ulcers and erosions. Though this discussion will be primarily concerned with treatment of gastric ulcers, these drugs are often of benefit in other conditions, including acute or chronic gastritis, reflux esophagitis, chronic hypertrophic gastritis, gastritis associated with neurologic disease, gastritis associated with hepatic disease, and uremic gastritis.[24] The rationale for treatment of gastric ulceration relies on the old concept of "no acid, no ulcer." Though many causes of gastric ulceration do not involve increased gastric acid production, most drugs work by either neutralizing luminal gastric acid or suppressing gastric acid production. However, newer drugs protect against the deleterious effects of gastric acid or enhance the mucosal defense mechanism. Unfortunately there are no controlled clinical trials to substantiate the efficacy of these drugs in small animals, although clinical experience has shown them to be effective in many settings. Table 22-2 summarizes the use of these drugs.

Antacids. Antacids work by neutralizing gastric acid after it has been secreted into the gastric lumen.[31] Additional effects of antacids include reducing pepsin activity, stimulation of protective endogenous prostaglandins, and binding to bile salts.[23,24,31] Antacids have their buffering effect by combining with hydrochloric acid to form a neutral salt and water. The most commonly used antacids are magnesium hydroxide, aluminum hydroxide, calcium carbonate, or combinations of these compounds. Liquid antacids are preferred because in general they have more acid-neutralizing capacity.[24]

The main advantage of antacids are their relative safety and low expense. The therapeutic dosage is empirical and depends on the relative acid-neutralizing capacity of the product. A suggested starting dose is 0.5 to 1.0 ml/kg every 4 hours. It has been suggested that if antacids are not given frequently, there can be a rebound hypersecretion of acid.[13,23] One proposed explanation of this phenomenon is that since antacids are just intraluminal buffering agents and not antisecretory agents, gastric acid production continues.[13] When antacids are administered, gastric pH rises and feedback mechanisms result in increased gastrin production. When the buffering capacity of the antacid is exceeded, as would occur with infrequent administration, the increased gastrin release causes a rebound hypersecretion of acid.[13] More recent evidence suggests that acid rebound occurs from parietal-cell stimulation from divalent cat-

TABLE 22-2 Drugs used in the treatment of gastric ulcers

Drug	Mechanism of Action	Suggested Dosage	Side Effects
Magnesium hydroxide	Neutralizes gastric acid	0.5-1.0 ml/kg every 4 hours PO	Diarrhea, acid rebound, alkalosis, magnesium toxicity
Aluminum hydroxide	Neutralizes gastric acid	0.5-1.0 ml/kg every 4 hours PO	Constipation, acid rebound, alkalosis
Cimetidine (Tagamet)	H_2-receptor antagonist	5 mg/kg every 6 hours PO,SC,IM,IV	In human beings, may cause gynecomastia, decreased cell-mediated immunity, altered drug metabolism, headache, malaise, dizziness, nausea, constipation, skin rash, bradycardia
Ranitidine (Zantac)	H_2-receptor antagonist	2 mg/kg every 8 hours PO,SC,IM,IV	In human beings, may cause headache, malaise, dizziness, nausea, constipation, skin rash, bradycardia
Famotidine (Pepsid)	H_2-receptor antagonist	None available	Probably similar to ranitidine
Nizatidine (Axid)	H_2-receptor antagonist	None available	Probably similar to ranitidine
Sucralfate (Carafate)	Coats surface of ulcer	0.5-1 g every 6 hours PO	Constipation
Misoprostol (Cytotec)	Prostaglandin E_1 analog	3 μg/kg every 6-8 hour PO	Vomiting, diarrhea, abdominal cramps, abortions
Omeprazole (Losec)	Proton pump inhibitor	None available	Hypergastrinemia

PO = orally; SC = subcutaneously; IM = intramuscularly; IV = intravenously.

ions, as would be contained in calcium-containing antacids, and to a lesser extent from magnesium-containing antacids.[31] The calcium-induced acid rebound is due to a local effect of calcium acting on gastric and duodenal mucosa, and to a lesser extent mediated by gastrin and possibly by other neurohormonal factors.[31] This effect does not seem to depend on intraluminal pH or the buffering capacity of the antacid.[31] It is unclear whether acid rebound affects the efficacy of these products. In any case, frequent administration of a calcium-free product provides more continuous buffering action and minimizes the potential deleterious effects of rebound hypersecretion of gastric acid. Aluminum hydroxide has a longer duration of acid neutralization than magnesium salts.[24]

The most common side effects of antacids are diarrhea (most common with magnesium salts) and constipation (most common with aluminum salts). Antacids may also be associated with poor palatability, alkalosis, magnesium toxicity and interference with the absorption of cimetidine and other drugs.[23,24]

H₂-receptor antagonists. H₂-receptor antagonists are the drugs most commonly used to treat gastric ulceration. Since histamine stimulation of the parietal cell is necessary for gastric acid production, competitive blockage of the H₂-receptor with antagonist drugs effectively reduces gastric acid secretion. The H₂-receptor antagonists currently available include cimetidine (Tagamet), ranitidine (Zantac), famotidine (Pepsid), and nizatidine (Axid). The latter two drugs have not been used extensively in veterinary medicine.

Cimetidine in dogs will cause a 50% reduction of gastric acid lasting for 3 to 5 hours at a dosage of 5 mg/kg.[24] Therefore, it should be given every 4 to 6 hours to maintain constant acid suppression. Though similar information is not available in the cat, I have had good clinical success with this regimen in this species. Cimetidine can be given by the oral, subcutaneous, intramuscular, or intravenous route with similar effects (systemic availability following an oral dose is 95%).[24] In a vomiting patient, a parenteral route is preferred. Cimetidine is available in an oral liquid to allow more precise dosing in smaller patients. Ranitidine is approximately 5 to 12 times as potent as cimetidine in inhibiting gastric acid secretion in human beings.[32] Ranitidine dosed at a rate of 2 mg/kg (orally or systemically) three times a day will provide continuous acid suppression in dogs.[24] Its systemic availability following an oral dose is 81%.[24] Ranitidine can also be administered by the oral, intramuscular, and intravenous routes. Ranitidine undergoes he-

patic metabolism and renal clearance.[32] Neither cimetidine nor ranitidine affects pancreatic secretion or gastric motility.[23]

Famotidine and nizatidine are newer H₂-receptor antagonists that have not been thoroughly evaluated in veterinary medicine. However, these drugs may have theoretical advantages based on their effects in human beings. Famotidine is more potent than cimetidine or ranitidine (approximately eight to nine times) and has a longer duration of action, especially in hypersecretory states.[33,34] Therefore, it is possible that less frequent dosing may be efficacious in small animal patients, allowing once or twice a day administration. Clinical studies need to be performed to verify this. It is also unclear whether the increased potency of famotidine results in increased efficacy as compared with ranitidine in human patients with duodenal or gastric ulcers.[33,35]

Side effects of H₂-receptor antagonists in small animal patients are rare. In human beings several uncommon side effects are seen from use of these drugs. Side effects include headache, malaise, dizziness, constipation, nausea, bradycardia, and skin rash.[32] Specific side effects of cimetidine are related to specific binding sites. Cimetidine binds to androgen receptors and can result in gynecomastia and impotence.[32] In addition, cimetidine binds to the hepatic mixed-function oxidase system and peripheral lymphocytes.[32] This can result in altered metabolism of other drugs and decreased cell-mediated immunity, respectively. Studies to determine whether these side effects are important in small animals are needed.

It is not known whether there are long-term consequences of prolonged gastric acid suppression associated with the use of H₂-receptor blockers. Since gastric acid is a necessary component of the gastric barrier to systemic infection, reduced gastric acid secretion can result in gastric and intestinal bacterial and fungal overgrowth of normal flora and pathogens.[13,32]

Sucralfate. Sucralfate (Carafate) is a basic aluminum salt of a sulfated disaccharide that has selective binding to proteins at the ulcer site by way of strong electrostatic interactions.[35] At low pH, sucralfate dissociates into aluminum and sucrose sulfate.[35] The sucrose sulfate moiety remains fixed at the ulcer site at a concentration of six to seven times that of nonulcerated mucosa.[35]

Sucralfate has sustained local protective effects against acid, pepsin, and bile at the ulcer site, forming a protective barrier. Studies in human beings have shown sucralfate to be more effective than placebo or low-dose antacid in healing gastric and duodenal ulcers and that it is as effective as the H₂-receptor antagonist cimetidine.[35] Although it is thought that the main mechanism by which sucralfate protects against the effects of gastric acid and pepsin is by the formation of a local protective barrier at the ulcer site through selective binding, more recent evidence suggests that sucralfate may have beneficial effects on normal gastric mucosa.[36] The latter mechanism may explain sucralfate's effectiveness in preventing ulcer recurrence in human beings and in protecting the mucosa against several types of experimental injury. Changes in normal gastric mucosa following sucralfate administration include disruption and exfoliation of surface epithelial cells, mucus release, mucosal hyperemia, and edema of the lamina propria.[36] These changes are often seen after a normal meal; and they represent a stimulus for epithelial cell renewal.[36] In addition, sucralfate causes a reduction of the gastric mucosal potential difference and an increase in luminal concentration of prostaglandin E_2, both of which are protective against ulcerogenic factors.[36]

Because sucralfate is not absorbed from the gastrointestinal tract, it has virtually no systemic toxicity. Because of this wide safety margin, dosage is imprecise. I recommend 1 g four times a day for medium and large dogs, and 0.5 g four times a day for small dogs and cats. The only side effect that may be seen in rare instances is constipation (due to the aluminum moiety). Sucralfate may also inhibit the absorption of other drugs, including tetracyclines, phenytoin, cimetidine, and digoxin. Ideally, other drugs should be administered 30 to 60 minutes prior to sucralfate administration and sucralfate should be administered 30 to 60 minutes prior to feeding. Alternatively, other drugs could be administered with feeding.

Anticholinergic drugs. Because acetylcholine stimulates the parietal cell to produce gastric acid, anticholinergic drugs may decrease gastric acid secretion. However, these drugs also decrease gastric and intestinal motility. This can lead to gastric distention, a potent stimulus for gastrin release that increases acid secretion.[13] The net result may be increased gastric acid secretion.[13] Because of their questionable efficacy and undesirable side effects, these drugs have no place in the routine treatment of gastric ulcers or as antiemetics.

Prostaglandin analogs: misoprostol. As mentioned above, prostaglandins have important cytoprotective effects in the stomach and are an important part of the mucosal defense mechanism. Misoprostol (Cytotec) is a synthetic prostaglandin E_1 analog with activity when given orally. Misoprostol has many effects that are important in protecting against the development of gastroduodenal ulcers, including decreasing gastric acid secre-

tion, increasing bicarbonate secretion, increasing mucosal blood flow, increasing epithelial cell turnover, and increasing mucus secretion.[24,37,38] Therefore, misoprostol is both antisecretory and cytoprotective.

In human beings, misoprostol is especially useful to prevent and treat ulcers induced by NSAIDs.[37,38] The mechanism by which NSAIDs induce ulceration is multifactorial. Aspirin will cause gastric ulceration both by a systemic effect related to prostaglandin inhibition and by a local effect following accumulation in gastric epithelial cells.[25,39] These effects can be prevented and treated by using misoprostol.[37-39]

Although ranitidine may be efficacious in preventing duodenal ulceration following NSAID administration, H_2-receptor antagonists and sucralfate do not prevent NSAID-induced gastric ulcers in human beings.[38-40] In addition, it has been shown that cimetidine is not effective in preventing aspirin-induced gastric hemorrhage in dogs.[41] Misoprostol has been shown to have superior efficacy as compared with H_2-receptor antagonists and sucralfate in preventing NSAID-induced gastroduodenal ulcers in human beings.[37,38] Misoprostol has promise for this purpose in dogs, and I have had success for this purpose in a limited number of cases. Controlled clinical studies need to be performed to verify this finding.

I have had success using misoprostol at a dosage of 3 μg/kg three or four times a day in the dog. There is little information about its use in the cat. Common side effects are diarrhea, vomiting, and abdominal pain. These side effects are dose dependent and can be alleviated by lowering the dosage. Abortions may occur in pregnant animals because of prostaglandins' effects on the reproductive tract.

Proton pump inhibitors: omeprazole. Once the parietal cell is stimulated by histamine, acetylcholine, and gastrin, there is an increased cellular content of cyclic adenosine monophosphate and calcium.[13,24,42] This results in activation of hydrogen-potassium adenosine triphosphatase (the gastric proton pump), the pump that exchanges hydrogen for potassium ions across the apical membrane.[42] Omeprazole (Losec) is a substituted benzimidazole that effectively blocks the proton pump and results in inhibition of gastric acid secretion.[43] In human beings, omeprazole is a very potent and long-acting inhibitor of gastric acid secretion, even in hypersecretory states such as the Zollinger-Ellison syndrome.[43] It has been shown to promote rapid healing of duodenal ulcers and reflux esophagitis and to be superior to ranitidine in healing and preventing relapse of gastric ulcers.[44,45] In addition, omeprazole may be effective in healing NSAID-induced gastric ulcers.[44]

In dogs, omeprazole is 10 times as potent as cimetidine and has a long duration of action.[24] Although the plasma half-life is approximately 1 hour in dogs, it has a duration of effect lasting more than 24 hours.[24] Its long duration of effect is because it selectively accumulates in the parietal cell, chiefly because omeprazole is a weak base with an appropriate dissociation constant.[46] The main concern about the use of omeprazole is that it can result in hypergastrinemia secondary to prolonged gastric acid suppression.[24] Gastrin has a trophic effect on the gastric mucosa, and chronic elevations in gastrin concentration can lead to mucosal and muscular hypertrophy.[13,24] Omeprazole is now available in the United States, and it is a promising drug.

Prognosis of gastrointestinal ulcers. The prognosis of gastrointestinal ulceration depends on the underlying cause and severity of the ulcer. If predisposing causes can be eliminated (such as being drug induced) and the ulcer is aggressively treated pharmacologically, the outcome is often favorable. The use of endoscopy has made earlier and more accurate recognition possible, and recent advances in gastrointestinal pharmacology have provided newer and more effective drugs to treat this disorder.

Gastric foreign bodies

Clinical findings with gastric foreign bodies. Gastric foreign bodies frequently occur in dogs and cats. As opposed to esophageal foreign bodies, life-threatening signs seldom occur with gastric foreign bodies unless there is complete pyloric obstruction. Many animals will be asymptomatic or have occasional vomiting episodes. In cases in which the foreign body is large or sharp or when pyloric obstruction occurs, more severe vomiting will occur. When the foreign body is sharp or in longstanding cases, blood may be seen in the vomitus, reflecting gastric ulceration. Gastric perforation due to a foreign body is rare.

In most cases the foreign body will not be palpable, because the location of the stomach is under the rib cage in most animals. If there is gastric ulceration, there may be abdominal pain. Laboratory findings are usually normal. However, in cases of pyloric obstruction, there is often a metabolic alkalosis, hypochloremia, hypokalemia, and hyponatremia. These changes were discussed in detail in the section on "Fluid Therapy of Acute Gastritis and Vomiting."

Diagnostic evaluation of gastric foreign body. Survey abdominal radiography often reveals a radiopaque object in the stomach. Food must be distinguished from a foreign body. The appearance of the normal pylorus in the right lateral view can mimic a mass or foreign body, as gastric fluid pools in this area and gives a dense round appearance. Contrast radiology is often helpful in delineating a gastric foreign body. The simplest radiographic contrast study to evaluate for the presence of a gastric foreign body is a pneumogastrogram. This procedure is a quick, inexpensive technique to screen for radiolucent foreign bodies, and to evaluate the shape, size, and position of the stomach. The technique is performed by injecting air into the stomach via orogastric tube until there is slight abdominal tympany.[15] Sedation is usually not required. In cases of foreign body, the object is outlined by the negative contrast.

Barium radiography can also be used to help define the presence of a gastric foreign body. If a gastric foreign body is suspected, an initial dose of only 10 to 20 ml of barium should be administered in an attempt to coat the object and avoid obscuring it in a dense pool of barium.[15] If no foreign body is seen, the study can be completed by administering barium at the full dosage of 13 ml/kg.[15] Findings suggesting a foreign body include a filling defect, delayed gastric emptying, and coating of the object, with persistence of barium in the stomach.

The diagnosis of a gastric foreign body can be confirmed with endoscopy. Flexible endoscopes can completely evaluate the mucosal surface of the stomach. Endoscopy also has the advantage of allowing the removal of most gastric foreign bodies. The techniques of gastrointestinal endoscopy have been reviewed by Tams.[16]

Treatment of gastric foreign bodies. When a gastric foreign body is recognized, the clinician must decide whether it is likely to pass through the intestinal tract without causing obstruction. There are no firm guidelines to make this determination, although in general, objects larger than the resting diameter of the colon are less likely to pass. In addition, it is usually advisable to remove sharp objects, although these may occasionally pass safely through the intestinal tract. Bones often dissolve in the stomach, and therefore conservative management with radiographic monitoring is recommended. All longstanding gastric foreign bodies should be removed. If there is doubt whether to remove an object, it is usually safer to remove it while it is still in the stomach if the animal is a good surgical risk. Endoscopic or surgical removal from the stomach is less invasive and has less potential for complications than removal from the intestine via enterotomy.

Certain objects can be recovered by inducing emesis. This is recommended if the object is small and smooth, and if the animal is not dehydrated or clinically obstructed. Emesis can be induced by subcutaneous administration of apomorphine in dogs (a tablet is placed in a wet 3-ml syringe and made into a paste; this is then dissolved in 2 to 3 ml saline and given subcutaneously at a dosage of 0.1 mg/kg) and xylazine in cats (0.5 to 1.0 mg/kg intramuscularly).

Endoscopic removal is usually the treatment of choice if the equipment is available. Various types of two-, three-, and four-pronged forceps are available that fit through the instrument channel of the endoscope. Once the object is grasped, the endoscope is removed from the stomach with the forceps protruding and grasping the object. If the object is sharp, a large tube can be inserted into the stomach (an overtube) through which the endoscope can be introduced. Once the object is grasped, the scope is pulled through the tube, which protects the esophagus from laceration. Once the object is removed the stomach and esophagus should be inspected for damage. If endoscopic removal is unsuccessful, surgical intervention is indicated. If there is significant gastrointestinal ulceration, the animal should be treated with a 3-week course of an H_2-receptor blocker and/or sucralfate. These drugs were discussed in detail in the section on "Treatment of Gastric Ulcers."

The prognosis for animals with gastric foreign bodies is good, except in rare cases that result in gastric perforation. Prompt endoscopic or surgical management will minimize the likelihood of this occurring.

Acute diarrhea

Acute diarrhea, defined as in increase in frequency, volume, and/or fluidity of bowel movements, represents one of the most frequent gastrointestinal emergencies (see box). The severity of acute diarrhea can vary from severe and life threatening (as occurs with viral enteritides) to mild and self-limiting (as occurs with garbage ingestion). This discussion will be concerned with general principles of the pathophysiology, diagnostic evaluation, and management of acute diarrhea.

Pathophysiologic changes with acute diarrhea. There are four general mechanisms of diarrhea: osmotic diarrhea (decreased absorption), secretory diarrhea (hypersecretion), exudative diarrhea (increased permeability), and abnormal motility.[47] Though some disorders fall into one of these classifications, most disorders have more than one of these mechanisms involved in the pathogenesis of diarrhea.

CAUSES OF ACUTE DIARRHEA

Primary gastrointestinal disorders
  Infectious diseases
    Canine parvovirus
    Canine coronavirus
    Feline parvovirus (panleukopenia)
    Feline coronavirus
    Salmonella
    Campylobacter
    Yersinia
    Escherichia coli
    Clostridium spp.
    Salmon poisoning *(Neorickettsia helminthoeca)*
    Other infections
  Parasitic diseases
    Trichuris (whipworms)
    Ascarids (roundworms)
    Hookworms
    Giardia
    Coccidia
    Others
  Miscellaneous causes
    Hemorrhagic gastroenteritis
    Partial intestinal obstruction
    Intestinal lymphosarcoma
    Idiopathic inflammatory bowel disease
    Dietary indiscretion or intolerance
Extragastrointestinal disorders
  Renal disease
  Hepatic disease
  Pancreatitis
  Endocrine disorders
    Hypoadrenocorticism
    Diabetes mellitus
    Hyperthyroidism
  Drug- or toxin-induced
  Central nervous system disorders

Osmotic diarrhea. Osmotic diarrhea results when nonabsorbed particles pull fluid into the intestinal lumen. In most cases, the nonabsorbed solutes are dietary carbohydrates. Common causes of osmotic diarrhea with malabsorption include viral enteritides, dietary indiscretion, and small intestinal infiltrative diseases. Osmotic diarrhea from malabsorption usually improves or ceases during fasting.

Secretory diarrhea. Secretory diarrhea occurs when the mucosa is stimulated to secrete fluid into the lumen independent of the absorptive capacity of the mucosa.[47] Secretory diarrhea usually occurs in conjunction with other types of diarrhea in small animals. Agents that stimulate intestinal secretion include bacterial toxins, fatty acids, gastrointestinal hormones, prostaglandins, and non-absorbed bile acids.

Exudative diarrhea. Exudative diarrhea occurs when there is increased mucosal permeability, with leakage of protein-rich fluid, blood, or mucus into the intestinal lumen. Disorders that in part result in diarrhea by this mechanism include viral enteritides (with villous destruction), inflammatory diseases, bacterial infections, and hemorrhagic gastroenteritis.

Diarrhea caused by abnormal motility. Hypermotility as a primary cause of diarrhea has been poorly documented in dogs and cats,[13,47] whereas the most common motility derangement with diarrhea is hypomotility, which usually occurs as a result of diarrhea rather than as a cause.[13] Two types of normal intestinal motility occur—peristalsis and rhythmic segmentation.[13] Peristalsis represents the movements that propel ingesta in an aboral direction (the "accelerator"), whereas rhythmic segmentation represents random contraction of the circular smooth muscle that limits transport of ingesta in the aboral direction and promotes mixing and prolonged contact of ingesta with the mucosa (the "brake").[13] In most cases of diarrhea, the primary motility derangement is hypomotility associated with decreased rhythmic segmentation. This results in a flaccid tube with increased functional lumen diameter. In this setting, little peristaltic activity is required to propel ingesta in an aboral direction. Thus, therapeutic efforts should include drugs whose actions are directed at increasing rhythmic segmentation (including narcotic analgesics such as loperamide, diphenoxylate, and paregoric) rather than decreasing peristalsis.

Diagnostic evaluation of acute diarrhea. The diagnostic evaluation of animals with acute diarrhea should follow an orderly systematic approach. A suggested approach to the diagnostic evaluation of patients with acute diarrhea is depicted in Fig. 22-6. Many animals with acute diarrhea do not require an in-depth diagnostic approach, and signs will resolve with symptomatic management, whereas other animals require intensive care and specific treatment.

History and physical examination. The history and physical examination often gives important clues as to potential causes. Dietary changes, parasite control, environmental description, toxin ingestion, and aggravating factors should be part of the history. Answers to questions about these factors will give clues as to potential cause and will aid the clinician in determining how aggressive to be with the diagnostic and therapeutic plan. The history should also include a review of other systems that might suggest the possibility of extragastrointestinal causes of diarrhea (see box p. 338). An accurate description of the feces and the pattern of defecation should also be obtained in order to distinguish large- and small-bowel diarrhea.

The physical examination may reveal specific causes of acute diarrhea. Abdominal palpation may detect an intestinal foreign body causing a partial obstruction or intestinal thickening as is seen with infiltrative bowel diseases. Rectal palpation should always be performed and feces examined. This affords a good opportunity to obtain a fresh fecal sample to perform a direct saline fecal smear. The physical examination is also important to determine the degree of dehydration, shock, and debilitation, factors that determine whether outpatient treatment versus hospitalization will be most appropriate.

Initial data base. The extent of the initial data base depends on the clinical condition of the animal. If there is no evidence of shock, dehydration, abdominal pain, or systemic involvement, the initial data base can be restricted to fecal ex-

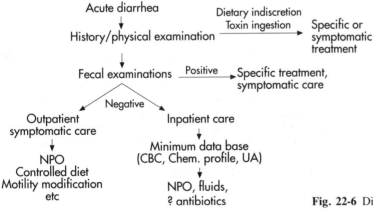

Fig. 22-6 Diagnostic evaluation of acute diarrhea.

amination. At least three fecal flotations should be obtained to rule out metazoan parasites. The zinc sulfate flotation method is the method of choice to detect *Giardia* cysts,[48] although trichrome staining of preserved feces is also a sensitive method in detecting this parasite.[49] Examination of direct fecal smears is used to detect motile trophozoites of *Giardia, Trichomonas, Balantidium,* and *Entamoeba.*[50] It is important to obtain the direct smear from a fresh fecal specimen or directly from a rectal glove or swab in order to detect motile trophozoites of protozoa.

Bacterial culture of feces may be indicated if an infectious cause is suspected. In general, bacterial cultures are only useful for detecting enteric pathogens, mainly *Salmonella* and *Campylobacter.* Invasive and enterotoxin-producing strains of *Escherichia coli* cannot be distinguished from nonpathogenic strains by standard microbiological culture techniques.[50] Since there are numerous bacteria normally present in feces, their identification and quantitation does not allow the clinician to speculate on their relative pathogenicity. A fecal hemagglutination or ELISA test may be used to detect canine parvovirus.

The hemogram, serum biochemistry profile, and urinalysis are usually indicated when there are signs of systemic illness. These tests evaluate other organ systems and may give specific clues as to cause (e.g., eosinophilia may suggest parasitism, leukopenia may suggest viral enteritis, electrolyte imbalance may suggest hypoadrenocorticism). Electrolyte concentrations, hematocrit, and measurements of total serum solids are also important to assess the degree of hemoconcentration and guide parenteral fluid administration.

Radiographic evaluation. Survey abdominal radiography is occasionally useful in the diagnostic approach to animals with acute diarrhea. Radiography is useful to detect the presence of gastrointestinal foreign body, peritonitis, ileus, and free abdominal fluid. Contrast radiography may be useful to detect complete (see Fig. 22-3) or partial obstructions (stagnant loop syndrome) and evaluate gastric and intestinal motility. Occasionally, ascarids may appear as intraluminal linear filling defects.

Endoscopic evaluation is rarely helpful in the diagnostic evaluation of patients with acute diarrhea. However, it may be a useful tool to obtain duodenal or colonic biopsies in animals with acute exacerbations of chronic diarrhea or in unresponsive cases of acute diarrhea.

Symptomatic treatment of acute diarrhea. Most cases of acute diarrhea are self-limiting and resolve without treatment or with symptomatic care only. If a specific cause is identified, specific treatment can be instituted.

Dietary management. Dietary restriction is an important part of treatment of acute diarrhea. Since the cause of diarrhea often has an osmotic component, withholding food will minimize the number of osmotically active particles in the lumen of the intestine. Resting the bowel also allows more rapid recovery of intestinal function.

When feeding is resumed, a bland, low-fat, highly digestible, controlled diet should be fed. A diet containing a limited number of nutrient sources should be used. Rice is the preferred carbohydrate source because its starch is more completely assimilated than starches in the flours from other cereal sources.[51] Suitable protein sources include low-fat cottage cheese or lean meat or poultry. Once the feces return to normal, the diet is gradually converted to the animal's regular food.

Motility modification. As mentioned previously, motility derangements include primarily a decrease in rhythmic segmental contractions, which normally provide resistance to flow of feces. Since the bowel is already hypomotile, there is no indication for the routine use of anticholinergic drugs that further depress rhythmic segmentation, and their use can exacerbate or prolong diarrhea.[13,47,50] Narcotic analgesics, on the other hand, act to increase rhythmic segmentation and thus help slow passage of feces and restore normal motility. These drugs may also favorably affect water and electrolyte transport.[47] Examples of narcotic analgesics with primarily gastrointestinal effects are loperamide (Imodium; 0.1 mg/kg, or about one 2-mg capsule per 15 kg body weight two or three times a day), diphenoxylate (Lomotil; 0.1 to 0.2 mg/kg or about one 2.5-mg tablet per 10 to 15 kg body weight three times a day), and paregoric (usually supplied with intestinal protectants and absorbants, given at 0.06 mg/kg two or three times a day).[50] On the rare occasion when intestinal spasm is contributing to clinical signs, anticholinergic drugs might be helpful, although long-term use is not justified.

Protectants and absorbants. Intestinal protectants such as kaolin-pectin, bismuth subsalicylate, activated charcoal, and barium sulfate are used with the intention of absorbing bacteria and toxins, and to provide a protective coating of the intestinal mucosa.[52] However, the efficacy of these agents is highly questionable, and there have been no controlled studies in animals to substantiate their effectiveness. Of these agents, bismuth subsalicylate (Pepto-Bismol, Corrective Mixture; 0.5 to 1.0 ml/kg three or four times a day) is most effective. This drug has many properties (including antienterotoxin, antibacterial, antisecretory, and antiinflammatory) attributed to the antiprostaglandin effects of the salicylate moiety.[52] Barium sulfate may also be effective by altering intestinal motility in a manner similar to that of narcotic analgesics (increasing rhythmic segmentation).[13] This may explain the improvement seen in some animals after barium administration for radiographic contrast studies.

Antibiotics. Antibiotics are rarely indicated to treat acute diarrhea since a primary bacterial cause is rare for diarrhea in dogs and cats. Occasionally, bacterial pathogens such as *Salmonella* and *Campylobacter* are the causative agents in diarrhea with accompanying systemic involvement. Intestinal bacterial overgrowth may also accompany other disorders, or a damaged intestinal mucosa might be further damaged by the effects of normal bacterial flora. In these settings, antibiotic therapy may result in improvement. Antibiotics are usually indicated in conditions in which there is severe mucosal damage, as occurs in viral enteritis or hemorrhagic gastroenteritis. In these conditions there is risk of secondary sepsis from absorption of bacteria or their products through a damaged mucosa. In these cases broad-spectrum parenteral antibiotics should be used, such as the combination of an aminoglycoside (such as gentamicin) and ampicillin or a cephalosporin. Alternatively, in less severe cases trimethoprim-sulfamethoxazole can be used because of its activity against gram-negative and anaerobic bacteria. Thus, the main indications for antibiotics are fever, leukocytosis, leukopenia, melena, hematochezia, and shock.[52] The routine use of antibiotics is not justified, and in some cases the condition will be worsened due to their disruptive effect on normal intestinal flora and the potential to promote resistant strains of bacteria.[50]

Fluid and electrolyte therapy. In most cases, there is not a serious derangement of fluid and electrolyte balance. However, in certain conditions, such as viral enteritis, hemorrhagic gastroenteritis, and bacterial enteritis, there may be life-threatening dehydration and electrolyte derangements. In these cases, parenteral fluids should be administered, with care taken to correct acid-base and electrolyte abnormalities. Details of fluid therapy will be discussed in the section on "Viral Enteritis" and in Chapter 38.

Intestinal obstruction

Causes. The most common cause of intestinal obstruction in dogs and cats is an intraluminal foreign body (Fig. 22-3). However, other causes of obstruction include stenosis induced by neoplasia, intussusception (Fig. 22-7), volvulus, stricture after trauma, intramural hematoma,[53] intesti-

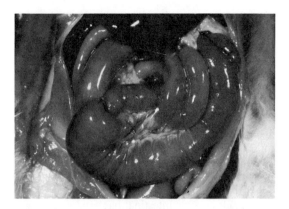

Fig. 22-7 Autopsy specimen of a cat with a jejunal intussusception causing complete small-intestinal obstruction. (Courtesy of Angell Memorial Animal Hospital, Boston.)

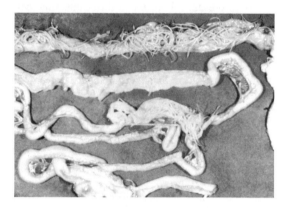

Fig. 22-8 Autopsy specimen of a dog with a severe burden of ascarids causing complete small-intestinal obstruction. (Courtesy of Angell Memorial Animal Hospital, Boston.)

nal incarceration in a hernia, intestinal pseudoobstruction associated with intestinal sclerosis,[54] a high burden of ascarids (Fig. 22-8), and extrinsic compression.[52-56]

Pathophysiology. When there is obstruction of the intestine caused by luminal blockage, intestinal distention occurs immediately proximal to the obstruction. This distention is caused by fluid (comprised mainly of intestinal and digestive secretions) and gas (about three fourths of which comes from swallowed air).[55,56] The results of this distention include increased intraluminal pressure. This can cause venous congestion and additional fluid loss into the bowel or peritoneal cavity.[55,56] Eventually distention can cause vascular compromise and anoxia of the bowel.[55,56] Fluid and electrolyte losses can result in dehydration and electrolyte derangements. This is exacerbated by vomiting, which is initiated by the obstruction and intestinal distention. The amount of vomiting, fluid, and electrolyte loss depends on the site of the obstruction. In general, the more proximal and complete the obstruction, the more severe the clinical signs, fluid, electrolyte, and acid-base derangements. With proximal intestinal obstructions (as with gastric-outlet obstructions) there is often a metabolic alkalosis, hypochloremia, hypokalemia, and hyponatremia. These changes were discussed in detail in the section on "Fluid Therapy of Acute Gastritis and Vomiting." With distal-small-intestine obstruction, there is usually metabolic acidosis.[52,55] Intestinal bacterial overgrowth occurs with chronic obstruction.[55,56]

With strangulation obstruction, there may be compromise of the intestinal blood supply, which can result in devitalization of the involved segment of bowel. When a foreign body is sharp or has been present for sufficient time, intestinal perforation may occur. This rapidly leads to septic peritonitis and death if immediate surgical intervention is not employed (Chapters 10, 13, and 15). Bacterial peritonitis and sepsis can also occur without perforation and is associated with anoxia of the intestinal wall, which allows breakdown of the mucosal barrier and therefore translocation of bacteria and toxins.[55,56]

Clinical signs. The severity of clinical signs depends on the site, cause, and completeness of the obstruction. With proximal obstructions, the signs are most severe, including persistent vomiting and anorexia. This will eventually progress to severe dehydration and eventual endotoxic and septic shock (Chapter 15). With more distal obstructions, the signs may be relatively mild, especially if the blockage is incomplete. Vomiting is often intermittent and may occur less than once daily. Anorexia may be partial or complete, and weight loss may be prominent in chronic cases.

Diagnosis. The diagnosis of intestinal obstruction can often be made by abdominal palpation. Foreign bodies, intussusception (see Fig. 22-7), and neoplasia are examples of conditions that are often readily palpable. In cases of bacterial peritonitis associated with intestinal perforation, there is often abdominal pain. In cats and puppies, particularly, the tongue should be lifted and the base of the tongue examined for the presence of a string.

Survey abdominal radiography may reveal the presence of intestinal obstruction. Radiopaque foreign bodies or calcified tumors are readily visible. In situations in which the cause of the obstruction is not readily visible on abdominal radiography, the presence of an obstruction is often suggested by the presence of multiple gas-distended loops of small intestine, often with hairpin turns.[30] In general, middle and distal obstructions are associated with more dramatic gas-distended loops of bowel than proximal obstructions. Care must be taken to distinguish a mechanical ileus from a functional ileus (as would be caused by viral enteritis), to avoid unnecessary surgical intervention. The presence of free peritoneal air (seen best caudal to the crura of the diaphragm) usually indicates a perforation. Occasionally, a radiographic contrast study is necessary to diagnose an intestinal obstruction (see Fig. 22-3). This is best accomplished with barium sulfate. If the animal is persistently vomiting, care must be taken to avoid aspiration of barium by the patient. Radiographic signs of intestinal obstruction include delayed transit time, intraluminal filling defects, and loops of bowel distended with contrast medium.

Treatment. The treatment for intestinal obstruction is surgery (with the exception of certain duodenal foreign bodies, which may be removed via endoscopy). Prior to surgical treatment, intravenous fluids should be administered to stabilize the patient. Electrolyte and acid-base derangements should be corrected, and these parameters should be closely monitored following surgery. In general, surgery should not be delayed for more than 3 to 6 hours while these parameters are being treated. Broad-spectrum antibiotic prophylaxis is indicated, especially in longstanding cases or those with suspected impending or confirmed perforation. The reader is referred to veterinary surgical textbooks for details about intestinal surgery.

Abdominal Trauma

Blunt abdominal trauma is usually caused by automobile accidents, kicks, or falls. Penetrating abdominal wounds are most commonly caused by bite wounds, gunshot wounds, and impalement or stab wounds. Virtually any abdominal organ can be traumatized (Chapters 10 and 13). However, this discussion will be primarily concerned with gastrointestinal trauma.

Clinical signs. Problems associated with abdominal trauma are due to hemorrhage, organ dysfunction, or peritonitis. Often shock can mask the nature of the abdominal injury. With massive hemorrhage, signs of anemia predominate. With peritonitis, clinical signs may be delayed or the manifestations of endotoxic shock may be obvious. Peritonitis can be due to bacterial contamination (as would occur with a bowel rupture) or due to chemical injury (as would occur with rupture of the biliary tree or pancreatic or urinary trauma). Bacterial peritonitis causes more severe fulminating signs.

Diagnosis. Physical examination findings may be nonspecific and often are compromised by the altered sensation associated with shock. In cases of penetrating abdominal wounds, physical examination predicts the presence or absence of visceral injury in only half the cases.[57] Serial evaluations are often helpful in detecting injury.

Abdominocentesis and peritoneal lavage are sensitive techniques to determine the presence of visceral injury. If no fluid is obtained on aspiration of multiple quadrants, peritoneal lavage can be performed by instilling saline at a volume of 20 ml/kg into the abdominal cavity. A sample is withdrawn 15 minutes later for analysis. Findings suggestive of visceral injury include grossly bloody or opaque fluid, more than 500 white blood cells per microliter, fluid amylase activity exceeding that of serum, presence of bilirubin, fluid creatinine concentration exceeding that of serum, presence of bacteria, presence of vegetable fibers, fluid packed cell volume greater than 5%, and presence of toxic neutrophils.[57] In cases of penetrating abdominal wounds, peritoneal lavage is approximately 90% accurate in identifying visceral injury.[57]

Abdominal radiography may be helpful in identifying abdominal injuries. The presence of free abdominal fluid or gas suggests the presence of visceral injury.

Laboratory tests are rarely helpful in the immediate posttraumatic period. In cases of hemorrhage, it takes up to 12 hours for the packed cell volume to drop to its lowest point. In cases of septic peritonitis, the white blood cell count can be low (reflecting sequestration of neutrophils) or high (reflecting a systemic inflammatory response). Serum activities of hepatic enzymes are often markedly elevated following blunt abdominal trauma. In most cases, however, there are no clinical manifestations of hepatic disease (unless there is biliary tract rupture).

Treatment. Initial treatment is directed at managing shock and treating life-threatening hemorrhage. Aggressive intravenous fluid administration is necessary. The administration of a blood transfusion and rapid-acting glucocorticoids (such as dexamethasone sodium phosphate or prednisone sodium succinate) may also be warranted. Broad-spectrum antibiotics (cephalosporin) should be administered to all patients with penetrating abdominal wounds and in any patient with evidence of peritonitis (cephalosporin, aminoglycoside, metronidazole).

If the patient cannot be stabilized or if there is evidence of visceral injury, immediate surgical intervention is warranted (Chapter 10). It must be emphasized that continual reevaluation of the patient (including physical examination, abdominocentesis, peritoneal lavage, and abdominal radiography) may be necessary to determine the need for surgical exploration (Chapter 13).

In cases of penetrating abdominal trauma, the high prevalence of visceral injury justifies immediate surgical exploration.[57] The low risk of a negative exploratory procedure is outweighed by the possibility of undiagnosed visceral injury by other means. If the animal is not stable for surgery and it is unclear whether there is visceral injury, it may be safer to pursue nonsurgical diagnostic means (lavage, contrast radiography, ultrasound, computed tomography) to establish the presence or absence of visceral injury.[57]

Nontraumatic perforation of the large intestine

Pathophysiology. The administration of corticosteroids to dogs with neurologic injury has been associated with colonic rupture in several cases.[27,58] Most of these animals have undergone a major surgical procedure, and most have received dexamethasone as the corticosteroid. The dosage and duration of dexamethasone given to these dogs varies, with cumulative doses ranging from 2.7 to 15.5 mg/kg (mean 6.4 mg/kg).[27] Causes of corticosteroid-induced colonic perforation are unknown, but may include the deleterious effect of corticosteroids on normal cytoprotective mechanisms and thus a predisposition to mucosal injury.[59] There might also be an autonomic nervous imbalance associated with neurologic injury and stress.[27] It has been suggested that the most common site of perforation, the proximal portion of the descending colon, is the location of a changeover between vagal and sacral sources of parasympathetic innervation and between celiomesenteric and caudal mesenteric sources of sympathetic innervation. An imbalance of innervation in the transition zone could affect motility and microvascular blood supply, thus increasing the likelihood of ulceration.[27]

Clinical findings. Perforation of the colon causes rapidly progressive septic peritonitis. Initial signs include abdominal pain, vomiting, and fever. Pale mucous membranes, slow capillary refill, and rapid pulse are seen as septic shock develops. Deterioration in animals is fulminant, making rapid diagnosis important.[60] Prior glucocorticoid administration may mask early signs of peritonitis; early detection may be difficult.[59]

Radiographic findings may include free air or lack of detail in the peritoneal cavity. Barium enema should not be used in cases of suspected colon rupture, as leakage of barium through the colon is almost always fatal.[60] The diagnosis can be confirmed by evaluating a peritoneal aspirate or diagnostic peritoneal lavage. Degenerate neutrophils and bacteria are seen microscopically, although these can also be seen in animals with localized intestinal devitalization without actual rupture.

Treatment and prognosis. Treatment consists of immediate surgical repair of the perforation. Broad-spectrum antibiotics are indicated before and after surgery. If the diagnosis is uncertain, continual reevaluation of physical parameters, radiography, and peritoneal lavage are used to determine if surgical exploration is indicated.

The prognosis for recovery is grave, as almost all cases are fatal despite surgical intervention. Therefore, careful monitoring of animals with neurologic conditions receiving corticosteroids is mandatory. Preventive measures include use of corticosteroids other than dexamethasone, limitation of dosage and duration of usage, avoidance of concurrent drugs with ulcerogenic potential, and avoidance of large-volume enemas, if possible.[58]

Acute bacterial enteritis

Primary bacterial infections are a relatively uncommon cause of diarrhea and vomiting in dogs and cats. There are several defense mechanisms to prevent bacterial overgrowth or colonization by pathogens, including normal motility, gastric acid secretion, the protective mucus layer, the local immune system, and microbial interactions.[13,50] Microbial interaction is especially important in the colon, and disruption of normal populations, as would occur with antibiotic therapy, can lead to certain bacteria causing disease.[61] This discussion will concern the effects of known pathogens not part of the normal flora.

Campylobacter. *Campylobacter jejuni* is now a recognized pathogen in human beings, although its pathogenicity in dogs and cats is less clear, mainly because of similar isolation rates in normal and diarrheic animals.[61,62] Attempts to induce diarrhea in puppies and kittens experimentally have been equivocal.[63,64] However, chronic diarrhea has resolved in clinical cases when specific antibiotic therapy has been used.[65] Failure to consider *C. jejuni* as a pathogen until recently may also stem from the special environmental and microbiological cultural requirements of the organism.[63,66,67] Different isolation rates may also reflect the environment and age of the animals. There seems to be a higher prevalence of infection in animals that are young, stray, kenneled, stressed, or have concurrent disease.[64,68] The organism survives poorly in the environment. Food or water contamination and fecal-oral spread are

the most likely routes of infection.[63] The organism can survive in feces for up to 4 weeks, and the duration of excretion in infected animals can vary from 1 to 4 months.[64]

Clinical findings. The incubation period following ingestion ranges from 1 to 7 days. The organism colonizes the mucosal surface of the terminal small intestine and colon, usually without epithelial invasion.[64] Clinical signs are most common in young pups and kittens, especially in those with concurrent diseases. Depression, mucoid or bloody diarrhea, and vomiting are the most common signs, usually lasting from 3 to 15 days.[63,68] Most animals are afebrile, and bacteremia and fatal cases are rare.[64] Infections in human beings are usually self-limiting.

Diagnosis. The diagnosis is based on a positive fecal culture. Fresh rectal swabs should be placed immediately into appropriate transport media. Selective enrichment and isolation media for *Campylobacter* have been described and are commercially available.[66] Cultures are incubated at 42 to 43°C in a microaerophilic, high-nitrogen environment.[64,66-68] Direct microscopic fecal smears can also be used to identify the curved, motile rods, but this method is unreliable.

Treatment. Treatment with antibiotics may not be necessary because some cases are self-limiting. However, if clinical signs are prolonged or the animal is debilitated, treatment is indicated. Animals that persistently shed the organism should be treated due to the zoonotic potential of the disease. The drug of choice for human *Campylobacter* infections is erythromycin, and it has been suggested that this is the drug of choice in animals.[62,64,65,68] A dose of 30 to 40 mg/kg per day for 5 days eliminates infection in dogs and cats.[62,65] An alternative antibiotic is oral tylosin at a dose of 45 mg/kg per day for 5 days.[62,64] The efficacy of treatment should be confirmed by fecal cultures 1 and 4 weeks after treatment. Negative cultures are usually obtained within 48 hours after treatment.[64,68] Other antibiotics that show in vitro effectiveness include tetracycline, aminoglycosides, clindamycin, chloramphenicol, and furazolidone. Variable susceptibility is seen with metronidazole, ampicillin, and trimethoprim-sulfamethoxazole. There is usually resistance to penicillin, cephalosporins, rifampin, vancomycin, and polymyxin B.[64] Antibiotic administration does not appear to prolong the carrier state, as is thought to occur with *Salmonella* infections.

Campylobacter infection should be considered zoonotic. It is estimated that only 5% of human infections are associated with a canine or feline source.[62,69] When pets are a source of human infections, the animals usually have diarrhea and are often kept in conditions of poor hygiene.[62] Appropriate hygiene should be stressed to clients as an important consideration in treatment of the animal(s) and in limiting the zoonotic potential of the disease.

Salmonella. Salmonella infections can be limited to the gastrointestinal tract (acute or chronic enterocolitis) or the animal can undergo systemic invasion by the bacteria, producing signs referable to other organ systems. The organisms are ubiquitous and are transmitted by the fecal-oral route, with contaminated food, water, or fomites the most likely source of infection.[52,64] The organisms can also survive long periods outside the host, making fomite transmission possible.[64]

Young animals and those with concurrent disease, immunodeficiency, and stress are more susceptible to infection and clinical illness. Animals housed in crowded, unsanitary, or hospitalized conditions are at higher risk.[52] Administration of immunosuppressive drugs, glucocorticoids, and antibiotics also predispose animals to infection. Normal bacterial flora is especially important in minimizing the likelihood of *Salmonella* colonization.[70] *Salmonella* requires a relatively large inoculum to produce colonization as compared with *Campylobacter.*[64] Once ingested, *Salmonella* colonizes the ileum and to a lesser extent the colon.[61] The organism is capable of mucosal invasion, although some strains cause intestinal secretion by stimulating cyclic adenosine monophosphate.[61] Bacteremia can occur with severe mucosal invasion, allowing the organism to disseminate throughout the body. When localized to the intestine, the infection is usually self-limiting. However, intermittent shedding of the organism can occur for 3 to 6 weeks.

Clinical findings. Clinical signs depend on the number of organisms, host status, and the presence or absence of concomitant disease. Gastrointestinal signs are usually acute and are typical of both small- and large-bowel diarrhea. When systemic invasion occurs, signs are referable to the organs involved.

Diagnosis. The diagnosis is based on a positive fecal culture. Because of subclinical carriers, positive cultures are not diagnostic of illness. Concurrent disease or stress can reactivate shedding in carrier animals.[64] Special enrichment broths (selenite or tetrathionate) and culture media (deoxycholate) are used to inhibit the growth of other organisms and favor the growth of *Salmonella.* A negative culture does not rule out *Salmonella.* Culture of other organs and body fluids can be used to detect systemic disease.

Treatment. The use of antibiotics in salmonellosis remains controversial. In cases in which clinical infection is confined to the intestine, it is doubtful that antibiotic therapy alters the course of illness, but the likelihood of increased shedding, the development of resistant strains, and the prolongation of the carrier state become much greater.[61,64] Therefore, in the absence of systemic involvement, only supportive care is indicated. In asymptomatic carriers, antibiotic therapy may reactivate clinical illness.

With systemic involvement, parenteral antibiotics are indicated, based on results of microbiological culture and antibiotic sensitivity testing. Indications for this include severe bloody diarrhea, dehydration, shock, leukopenia, leukocytosis, fever, and laboratory test results suggestive of disseminated intravascular coagulation. In these cases, chloramphenicol, trimethoprim-sulfamethoxazole, cephalothin, or gentamicin administration is usually effective, although resistance to these antibiotics may occur.[52,70] Intravenous fluid administration and other supportive measures are also indicated. *Salmonella* does have zoonotic potential, so clients must be made aware of the importance of proper hygiene.

Yersinia. Yersinia enterocolitica is a motile gram-negative coccobacillus capable of causing enterocolitis in humans and animals; however, there are few reports of documented clinical cases in animals.[71,72] The organism has been cultured in normal dogs and cats with a low prevalence. The pathogenesis of infection is unknown, although an enterotoxin is suspected,[73,74] and mucosal invasion may occur.[61,73]

Clinical findings. Clinical signs are typical of acute large intestinal involvement, including increased frequency of defecation, blood and mucus in the feces, and tenesmus.[71] Systemic involvement or fever has not been seen in dogs.

Diagnosis. The diagnosis is based on culture of the organism and subsequent response to an appropriate antibiotic. *Yersinia* selectively replicates in refrigerated temperatures, and cold enrichment with subculture is recommended.[61]

Treatment. Treatment is indicated in animals with persistent diarrhea from whom the organism is isolated. The organism is usually sensitive to chloramphenicol, trimethoprim-sulfamethoxazole, tetracycline, cephalosporins, and gentamicin.[64] In clinical cases reported to respond to treatment, one dog recovered following cephadrine therapy, and another dog recovered following trimethoprim-sulfamethoxazole therapy.[71] Because humans are susceptible to *Yersinia,* public health concerns should exist for this organism.

Other bacterial and rickettsial infections

Escherichia coli. Escherichia coli is part of the normal gastrointestinal flora. Although certain strains of *E. coli* are invasive or can produce an enterotoxin resulting in diarrhea in some species, their role in producing illness in dogs and cats is unknown. Since *E. coli* is part of the normal fecal flora, microbiological culture of feces would be expected to grow the organism. Documenting the presence of enterotoxin-producing strains requires specific in vivo and in vitro tests.[75] Demonstration of invasive strains requires laboratory animals inoculation.[61] When mucosal invasion occurs, it is difficult to say whether it results from decreased host resistance or from bacterial pathogenicity.[61] Antibiotics should be used with caution to prevent the development of multiply antibiotic resistant strains, which readily occurs with *E. coli.*[76] Since most pathogenic strains of *E. coli* are host-specific, the zoonotic potential is low.[61]

Clostridium. Clostridium difficile produces a toxin that results in pseudomembranous colitis in humans. The condition usually occurs with overgrowth of the organism following antibiotic suppression of normal flora. Many antibiotics have been associated with the disease, but lincomycin, clindamycin, ampicillin, and cephalosporins are most commonly involved. Gross findings in humans include an erythematous mucosa covered with small, raised plaques composed of mucin, fibrin, neutrophils, sloughed epithelial cells, and a variety of bacteria.[77] The disease is usually successfully treated with either vancomycin or metronidazole.[78]

There have been very few reports of pseudomembranous colitis in animals.[79,80] Diarrhea in dogs has also been associated with *Clostridium welchii* and *Clostridium perfringens* type A.[81,82] Despite these observations, the evidence linking *Clostridium* species as a causative agent of diarrhea in dogs is only circumstantial.

Salmon poisoning. Salmon poisoning is a highly fatal rickettsial disease of dogs caused by the helminth-transmitted *Neorickettsia helminthoeca.* The organism is primarily found in the Pacific Northwest, where the trematode vector *Nanophyetes salmincola* is found. The trematode is harbored by the intermediate host, the snail *Oxytrema silicula.*[83] Cercariae of *N. helminthoeca* leave the snail and penetrate a second intermediate host, usually a salmonoid fish.[83] Following ingestion of the fish by a dog, adult trematodes attach to the intestinal mucosa of the dog and inject the rickettsiae they harbor.[83]

Neorickettsiae cause severe bloody diarrhea and enter the blood and disseminate to the lymph nodes, spleen, and other organs. Signs generally occur 5 to 7 days after infection, and include fever, vomiting, bloody diarrhea, anorexia, depression, and peripheral lymphadenopathy.[52,83] I have seen one dog in which an intussusception developed during illness from the rickettsial infection. The mortality rate in untreated dogs is 50% to 90%, and death occurs 7 to 10 days after clinical signs appear.[52,83]

The diagnosis is suspected from the dog's travel history, and supported by the finding of operculated fluke eggs in a microscopic examination of feces. Diagnosis of the disease cannot be made on the basis of finding the fluke eggs alone, since the trematode does not necessarily carry the rickettsia. The rickettsia can be demonstrated by finding purple-staining bodies in macrophages from Giemsa-stained lymph node aspirates.[52]

Tetracycline is the treatment of choice (22 mg/kg orally three times a day for 2 to 3 weeks). If vomiting precludes oral treatment, intravenous oxytetracycline can be given (7 mg/kg twice a day for at least 3 days or until oral therapy is possible).[83] Chloramphenicol, sulfonamides, and penicillin may also be effective.[83] Supportive care with intravenous fluid administration may also be necessary. The trematode vector can be eliminated with oral fenbendazole (55 mg/kg per day for 10 to 14 days).[52]

Acute parasitic enteritis

The most common parasites to cause severe clinical signs in dogs and cats are ascarids, hookworms, whipworms, and *Giardia.* The diagnosis of intestinal parasites depends on finding ova, cysts, larvae, or trophozoites in the feces of affected animals. This can be accomplished by examining fresh fecal smears in saline, standard flotation methods, zinc sulfate flotation, or special stains of the feces. Certain parasites, such as whipworms and *Giardia,* are difficult to detect. If clinical signs are compatible with these organisms in an endemic area, treatment may be indicated, and positive response to therapy is suggestive of infection. Clinical signs in general are most severe in young animals (Chapter 29), those with concurrent illness, and in those receiving immunosuppressive drugs or corticosteroids.

Ascarids. Ascarids (roundworms) are the most common intestinal parasites of dogs and cats.[52] The ascarids of the dog are *Toxacara canis* and *Toxascaris leonina;* those of the cat are *Toxacara cati* and *Toxascaris leonina.*[84] Clinical signs include vomiting, diarrhea, abdominal pain, chronic weight loss, pot belly, and general malaise. If the worm burden is high, intestinal obstruction can occur (see Fig. 22-8). Intussusception and intestinal perforation have also been associated with a high ascarid burden.[52] The life cycle of ascarids has been described in detail elsewhere.[84] Several drugs are effective against roundworms. I prefer pyrantel pamoate in young animals and neonates (Nemex, Strongid; 15 mg/kg orally once, repeated at 2-week intervals), fenbendazole (Panacur; 50 mg/kg per day orally for 3 consecutive days), or febantel (Vercom; 10 mg/kg orally for 3 consecutive days).[85]

Hookworms. The most common hookworm of the dog is *Ancylostoma caninum*. The most common hookworm of the cat is *Ancylostoma tubaeforme*.[84] In addition, *Ancylostoma braziliense* and *Uncinaria stenocephala* occur in both species.[84] Only *Ancylostoma caninum* causes severe clinical signs, mainly because it is such a voracious blood sucker, and the worm burden of this species is often very high.[52,85]

Clinical signs include melena, frank bloody diarrhea, or diarrhea without overt signs of hemorrhage. In animals with a high worm burden, and especially in puppies, hookworms can cause life-threatening anemia. In longstanding cases, chronic blood loss can cause an iron-deficiency anemia, characterized by microcytic hypochromic indices with a poor reticulocyte response. The life cycle of hookworms has been described in detail elsewhere.[84] Several drugs are effective against hookworms. I prefer pyrantel pamoate in young animals and neonates (Nemex, Strongid; 15 mg/kg orally once, repeated at 2-week intervals), fenbendazole (Panacur; 50 mg/kg per day orally for 3 consecutive days), or febantel (Vercom; 10 mg/kg orally for 3 consecutive days.).[85]

Whipworms. Whipworm *(Trichuris vulpis)* infection is a very common cause of acute, chronic, or intermittent large-intestine diarrhea in the dog. Although *Trichuris* spp. have been reported in cats, it is extremely rare and not a significant pathogen in this species.[84,86,87] The parasite generally lives in the cecum and proximal colon of the dog, where the long threadlike esophageal region of the worm is imbedded in the mucosa and the stout "handle" portion of the worm is free in the lumen (Fig. 22-9).[84]

Clinical signs include diarrhea, with or without blood and/or mucus, vomiting, and anorexia. The severity of the signs depends on the number of parasites and the individual response of the host. Often, stress, concurrent disease, or the administration of corticosteroids will cause a previously asymptomatic dog to show clinical signs. The diagnosis of whipworms can be more difficult than diagnosis of previously mentioned intestinal parasites because dogs will shed the eggs in the feces intermittently, requiring at least three to four negative samples over a 3 to 4-day period before the presence of whipworms can be ruled out. Often I use an empirical trial of an appropriate anthelmin-

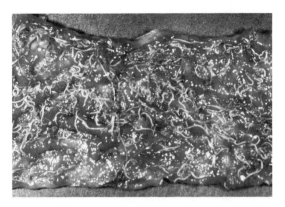

Fig. 22-9 Autopsy specimen of a dog with a large burden of whipworms causing severe diarrhea. (Courtesy of Angell Memorial Animal Hospital, Boston.)

tic against whipworms in an animal displaying clinical signs compatible with whipworm infection. The life cycle of whipworms has been described in detail elsewhere.[84] Several drugs are effective against whipworms. I prefer fenbendazole (Panacur; 50 mg/kg per day orally for 3 consecutive days) or febantel (Vercom; 10 mg/kg orally for 3 consecutive days) since these drugs are virtually 100% effective, with minimal side effects.[85] Animals should be re-treated or have repeated fecal examinations at 3-month intervals to check for reestablishment of patent infections. Supportive care is generally not necessary, and the prognosis for recovery is good.

Giardiasis. *Giardia* is a flagellate protozoan parasite thought to be primarily a small-intestine parasite, although some dogs will show signs typical of large intestine involvement.[50,52] Outside the host, *Giardia* exists as a resistant cyst.[88] The life cycle is simple and direct, with trophozoites becoming infective cysts in the large intestine and subsequently being passed in feces. When ingested, they excyst in the duodenum to the trophozoite stage.[88] The pathogenic mechanisms by which *Giardia* causes diarrhea remain unclear.

Clinical signs are most severe in young animals and most commonly include large volumes of loose, tan feces. This pattern of diarrhea may be acute or chronic. Some animals will have diarrhea more typical of large intestinal origin.[50] Dehydration may be a prominent feature in young animals.

The diagnosis of *Giardia* is made by identification of the parasite or by response to specific treatment. There are several methods by which *Giardia* can be detected. Motile trophozoites can be found in fresh saline smears of feces. However, a modified zinc sulfate concentration technique was found to be the most sensitive method of diagnosis, detecting the cyst stage of the parasite.[48] In another study, a trichrome stain of preserved feces was found to be the most sensitive method of detection.[49] Since shedding of the organism is often intermittent, repeated examinations may be necessary to identify the parasite. Identification of *Giardia* can also be made from duodenal aspirates obtained during endoscopy or surgery. However, response to treatment may be a less invasive diagnostic alternative.

Treatment of *Giardia* is usually successful with either metronidazole (Flagyl; 25 mg/kg orally twice a day for 5 days), or with quinacrine (Atabrine; 6.6 mg/kg orally twice a day for 5 days). Furazolidone (Furoxone; 4 mg/kg orally twice a day for 5 days) is also effective, especially in cats.[52] Ipronidazole hydrochloride is also effective and is added to the dog's drinking water at a concentration of 126 mg/L of water for 7 days.[89] Some animals require higher doses and longer duration of these drugs to clear the infection.

Viral enteritis (see also Chapter 29)

Several viral infections have been shown to cause acute diarrhea in dogs and cats. The most common viruses in the dog include canine parvovirus, canine coronavirus, and canine rotavirus. Feline panleukopenia virus is the most common cause of viral enteritis in the cat. Although the severity of clinical signs vary with the virus, host status, and concurrent disease, the pathophysiologic changes, diagnosis, and treatment are similar. This discussion will apply to enteric viruses in general, with specific differences pointed out where appropriate.

Pathophysiologic changes. Enteric viruses have a predilection for rapidly dividing cells, including those of the intestine. Certain viruses (rotavirus and coronavirus) will attack the villi, resulting in villous atrophy, malabsorption, crypt hyperplasia, and increased intestinal secretion.[52] Parvoviruses (canine parvovirus and feline panleukopenia virus) destroy the intestinal crypts, resulting in complete mucosal loss and a severe diarrhea.[52] Since parvoviruses have an affinity for rapidly dividing cells, they also affect the bone marrow (resulting in leukopenia), lymphoid tissue, and, in young puppies, the myocardium (resulting in myocarditis). The latter syndrome can result in sudden death or cardiopulmonary failure due to myocarditis following canine parvovirus infection in young puppies.[90-93]

Most animals with viral enteritis suffer severe dehydration. Since the intestinal mucosa is severely disrupted, malabsorption and intestinal secretion greatly exceed fluid absorption. In addition, most animals have anorexia and vomiting and are unable to utilize orally ingested water. Fluid shifts can result in severe hemoconcentration, reflected by marked increases in hematrocrit and measurements of total serum solids.

Electrolyte and acid-base disturbances are common in viral enteritis.[94] Since many animals have severe diarrhea and vomiting, electrolytes are lost in high concentrations in the feces and vomitus. Total body sodium, chloride, and potassium are usually depleted, although serum concentrations are variable. Metabolic acidosis is usually present, primarily because of intestinal bicarbonate loss and due to lactic acidosis associated with poor peripheral vascular perfusion. If vomiting is excessive, loss of hydrochloric acid can result in concurrent metabolic alkalosis. Therefore measurements of acid-base status and electrolyte concentrations are critical for appropriate fluid therapy.

Since animals with parvovirus enteritis are leukopenic, they are at risk for bacteremia, sepsis, and endotoxic shock.[95] The severe intestinal mucosal disruption also predisposes to bacterial entry into the circulation. Infection is usually with gram-negative, anaerobic organisms.

Clinical signs. Clinical signs of viral enteritis are variable, and depend on the virus, host status, and other factors. Since the signs observed with canine parvovirus infection are usually most severe, this discussion will apply primarily to this virus. Clinical signs are first observed 4 to 7 days after oral exposure.[96] Anorexia and depression occur initially, followed rapidly by vomiting, diarrhea, or both. The volume of diarrhea is usually profound, and it is often extremely foul-smelling. Both the vomitus and feces often contain frank blood. Fever, hypoglycemia, and signs of endotoxic shock often occur, especially in severe cases in all ages and in young puppies. Death can occur from a combination of these factors.

Diagnosis. The diagnosis of viral enteritis is often made by compatible clinical signs without confirmatory tests. Viral enteritis should be suspected in young animals with fulminant vomiting and/or diarrhea. A hemogram may be helpful in the diagnosis of parvovirus, since leukopenia is a common finding, present in approximately 85% of cases.[52] Hematocrit and measurements of total serum solids are variably increased or decreased. This is often helpful in distinguishing parvovirus enteritis from hemorrhagic gastroenteritis. In the latter syndrome, there is usually profound increases in both hematocrit and measurements of total serum solids resulting from hemoconcentration. Radiographic findings are nonspecific, but can include a generalized ileus mimicking intestinal obstruction.

A definitive diagnosis of viral enteritis requires demonstration of the virus in feces or specific IgM antibodies in the serum. Demonstration of canine parvovirus in feces can be accomplished by a hemagglutination test or the enzyme-linked immunosorbent assay.[52] Canine parvovirus and other enteric viruses can also be demonstrated by electron microscopy and virus isolation.[52] Since the treatment of viral enteritis is supportive, specific diagnosis is often not necessary for treatment. It is important, however, to distinguish viral enteritis from other diseases with specific treatment and/or management considerations (e.g., intestinal obstruction, *Salmonella* infection, salmon poisoning, and acute parasitic enteritis).

Treatment. The treatment of viral enteritis is supportive and is based on the pathophysiologic derangements that occur. Since diarrhea and vomiting predominate and result from intestinal mucosal destruction, resting the bowel is important to minimize these signs, prevent further fluid losses, and promote recovery. Therefore, animals should receive no oral fluids or food until there are minimal gastrointestinal signs remaining.

Fluid therapy is critical to correct dehydration, electrolyte imbalances, acid-base disturbances, hypovolemia, and shock. Since electrolyte changes and acid-base status are variable, these parameters should be measured in critically ill animals to determine the most appropriate therapy. If this information is unavailable, a balanced electrolyte solution such as lactated Ringer's solution is indicated. Since many animals are hypoglycemic, the use of 2.5% or 5% dextrose solution (in combination with an electrolyte solution) may be necessary. Since there is usually total body potassium depletion, potassium should be added to the fluids. Fluids should be administered in amounts to correct dehydration, meet maintenance requirements, and compensate for ongoing fluid losses (Chapter 38). In animals that are severely hypoproteinemic, the administration of plasma or dextrans may be necessary to maintain plasma oncotic pressure.

Broad-spectrum parenteral antibiotics are necessary because of systemic invasion of enteric organisms secondary to mucosal disruption and immunosuppression associated with leukopenia. An appropriate regimen includes a combination of an aminoglycoside (such as gentamicin or amikacin) and ampicillin or a cephalosporin. This combination is effective against most of the intestinal flora. An alternative in less severe cases is trimethoprim-sulfamethoxazole as a single-agent drug, since this has good activity against gram-negative aerobes and anaerobic organisms. Antibiotics can be discontinued when diarrhea and leukopenia resolve.

Antiemetics are usually necessary to control vomiting and prevent further fluid and electrolyte losses. I prefer metoclopramide as the initial drug, given as a constant intravenous infusion with parenteral fluids. This drug has central and peripheral effects and is helpful to control the ileus that is present with viral enteritis.[21] An alternative is to use a phenothiazine such as chlorpromazine or prochlorperazine. Since these drugs can cause hypotension, aggressive fluid support is necessary. Anticholinergic drugs are contraindicated since there is already a hypomotile gut predisposing to increased bacterial numbers and toxin formation. Antiemetic drugs were discussed in detail in the section on "Treatment of Acute Gastritis and Vomiting."

When feeding is resumed, the animal should be given small amounts of a bland diet. Ideally, cottage cheese and rice or chicken and rice should be fed. If clinical signs resolve, the animal can be weaned back onto a normal diet over a 1-week period. Prevention of infection by the use of vaccines has been reviewed elsewhere.[52,96]

ACUTE PANCREATITIS

Acute pancreatitis is a common clinical diagnosis in dogs, and on rare occasions in cats. The true incidence of pancreatitis is unknown because of the difficulty in obtaining a definitive diagnosis. The severity of the disease ranges from mild abdominal pain with occasional vomiting to a fatal syndrome accompanied by severe gastrointestinal signs. The disease is seen most frequently in middle-aged female dogs who are often overweight, although affected dogs can be of any age and sex.

Pathophysiology

There are many factors and pathophysiologic changes that are implicated in the development of acute pancreatitis. There are two stages in the development of acute pancreatitis. The first step involves pancreatic acinar damage, and the second step involves activation of digestive enzymes within the gland, with resultant pancreatic autodigestion.[97-99] In this setting, protective mechanisms against self-destruction, including storage of enzymes as inactive zymogens and the presence of inhibitors of enzyme activation, are lost.[97-99] Once there is enzyme activation, there is progressive damage to the gland, possibly mediated by oxygen-derived free radicals.[98,99] Associated with this is increased capillary permeability and pancreatic edema. There is also progressive activation of all pancreatic enzymes, which results in autodigestion and progression to hemorrhagic, necrotic pancreatitis with activation of kallikrein and bradykinin.[97-99] This process can be prevented by plasma and tissue protease inhibitors such as alpha-macroglubin, but once these are depleted, the progressive changes described above occur.[98,99]

Hypotension is an important feature of acute pancreatitis; it can result from several causes: bradykinin formation (resulting in systemic vasodilation and fluid loss from pancreatic edema), myocardial depressant factor released from ischemic pancreatic tissue, vomiting and diarrhea causing fluid loss, and disseminated intravascular coagulation.[97,100] Often there is prerenal azotemia, which can progress to overt renal damage and failure. Hepatic damage, biliary obstruction, and pulmonary edema can also occur.[100]

Peripancreatic inflammation results in leakage of pancreatic enzymes into the peritoneal cavity and a resultant chemical peritonitis.[97,100] This can progress to a septic peritonitis when pancreatic necrosis allows leakage of *Clostridium perfringens,* a normal inhabitant of the canine pancreas, into the abdomen.[97] In addition, transmural migration of bacteria through the intestine can occur due to severe enterocolitis occurring as a result of peritonitis.

The inciting cause of acute pancreatitis is often unknown, although several factors have been implicated in initiating pancreatic acinar damage (see box at right).[97,98,100] Of these factors, obesity, hyperlipidemia, and drugs are the most common causes of acute pancreatitis.

Clinical findings

Clinical signs are variable in acute pancreatitis. The most consistent clinical signs are vomiting, anorexia, and abdominal pain. Often animals will assume a "praying" position, indicative of peritonitis and pain. Diarrhea and fever may also be present. In severe cases, signs of shock and sepsis may be present. Other potential clinical signs include jaundice, respiratory distress, ascites, and cardiac arrhythmias. Often the diagnosis is based on these collection of signs, especially if associated with a typical signalment (middle-aged obese female) and the presence of any causative factors (see box).

Laboratory findings in pancreatitis are often nonspecific. The most specific findings include elevation in serum amylase and lipase activities. Unfortunately, these enzymes can be elevated with nonpancreatic disease, and confirmed cases of pancreatitis sometimes have normal serum activity of these enzymes. Amylase and lipase can also originate from the gastric and intestinal mucosa, and therefore serum activities increase with

CAUSES OF PANCREATITIS IN DOGS AND CATS

Nutritional
  Obesity
  High fat diet or fatty meal
Hyperlipidemia
  Familial hyperlipoproteinemia
  Hypothyroidism
  Hyperadrenocorticism
  Diabetes mellitus
Drugs
  Corticosteroids
  Azathioprine
  L-asparaginase
  Sulfonamides
  Thiazide diuretics
  Furosemide
  Tetracyline
Infection
  Toxoplasmosis (cats)
Duct obstruction
  Biliary calculi
  Parasite migration
  Tumor
  Surgery
Duodenal reflux
Trauma
  Surgery
  External blunt trauma
Pancreatic ischemia
Metabolic abnormalities
  Hypercalcemia
  Uremia

other causes of gastroenteritis.[97,98,100] In addition, since these enzymes may be cleared from the serum by the kidneys, azotemia can result in increased serum activity. Dexamethasone administration can induce up to a fourfold to fivefold increase in serum lipase activity without histologic damage to the pancreas.[101] Thus, there is no ideal laboratory test to document the presence of pancreatitis. Therefore, the diagnosis is based on clinical judgment, incorporating results of historical, physical examination, and laboratory findings. Promising tests in the future include the measurement of pancreatic isoamylases and trypsin complexed to alpha₁-antiprotease, although these are not yet commercially available.[98]

Laboratory findings in animals with pancreatitis may include leukocytosis, increased hematocrit (suggesting hemoconcentration), increased serum hepatic enzyme activities, increased concentration of serum bilirubin, hyperglycemia, hypocalcemia, hypoproteinemia, and lipemia. Fluid obtained by paracentesis or peritoneal lavage demonstrates a neutrophilic inflammatory response and a marked increase in amylase activity.

Radiographic findings are nonspecific but may include decreased abdominal detail (especially in the right cranial quadrant), displacement of the duodenum to the right and the stomach to the left, a static duodenal gas pattern, and increased density in the area of the pancreas.[98,100] Ultrasound findings are often diagnostic of pancreatitis. The normal pancreas is not visible ultrasonographically. In cases of pancreatitis there is often an enlarged pancreas viewed ultrasonographically, with peripancreatic fluid. This fluid can be aspirated under ultrasound guidance for analysis of amylase activity. In addition, there is often fluid seen within the wall of the duodenum along with static indentations of the duodenum. Ileus (bowel gas) may inhibit ultrasonographic evaluations.

Treatment

The goals of treatment of acute pancreatitis are to reduce pancreatic secretions, maintain hydration and tissue perfusion, and control sepsis. If underlying causes of pancreatitis can be identified (see box p. 350), these should be specifically treated, or if drug-induced, the offending drug should be discontinued.

Intravenous fluid administration is essential to maintain hydration and perfusion, especially in critical animals. Lactated Ringer's solution is appropriate and is usually supplemented with potassium. The administration rate varies with the condition of the patient (Chapter 38). In cases of severe pancreatitis, urine output must be closely monitored to guard against anuric renal failure. Often a urethral catheter with a closed collection system is required. Central venous pressure monitoring may also be helpful. In cases of septic shock, glucose supplementation may be necessary. Parameters that should be closely monitored are serum electrolytes, blood urea nitrogen, creatinine, and glucose concentrations. Acid-base status is variable and requires monitoring to choose appropriate fluids and assess the need for bicarbonate administration.

Despite aggressive treatment, some animals deteriorate. In these patients, fresh-plasma or whole-blood transfusions may be helpful (Chapter 34).[98,99] Consumption of plasma protease inhibitors such as alpha-macroglobulins, contribute to the progressive deterioration of these patients, eventually leading to disseminated intravascular coagulation. Transfusion replaces alpha-macroglobulin and other factors (such as albumin and antithrombin III).[98,99] The use of corticosteroids has not been shown to be helpful in acute pancreatitis, and should be given only in cases of shock.[97,98] Corticosteroid administration can cause pancreatitis.

The most important aspect of controlling pancreatic secretions is to withhold food. Drugs used to control pancreatic secretions have not been shown to be effective.[99] Anticholinergic drugs such as atropine have little effect on secretions in a fasting animal with pancreatitis, and they may worsen the condition by promoting gastric retention and subsequent gastrin release.[97] A new somatostatin analog, octreotide (Sandostatin), may have promise for reducing pancreatic secretions.

Antibiotics may be helpful in selected cases. In animals with risk or evidence of sepsis, when necrotic pancreatitis is suspected, or with severe abdominal pain suggesting peritonitis, broad-spectrum antibiotics are indicated. An appropriate regimen includes an aminoglycoside and ampicillin.

Peritoneal lavage may be effective in severe cases to remove toxins and help ameliorate a chemical peritonitis,[97,98,100] although studies in humans have shown no benefit of peritoneal lavage.[102]

When vomiting has not occurred for 24 to 48 hours, water can be given orally for 24 hours, followed by food. When feeding resumes, a low-fat, highly digestible diet should be fed. Cottage cheese and rice is the ideal diet for this purpose. Eventually the animal can be switched to a commercial low-fat diet such as R/D or W/D (Hills, Topeka, KS). There is evidence that oral pancreatic enzyme supplementation may be of value to decrease pancreatic secretions by a feedback mechanism, and may be useful in chronic or recurrent cases.[98,99]

HEPATIC FAILURE

Many types of hepatic diseases are managed with specific treatment methods. In addition to specific treatment, many patients with hepatic disease require general supportive care to manage the acute and chronic aspects of the derangements seen with hepatic failure. This discussion will concern therapeutic efforts common to the management of hepatic disease in general.

Causes

Severe hepatic failure can result as an end stage of any chronic hepatopathy or as a consequence of acute hepatic necrosis. Since the hepatocyte is exposed to an extensive portal and systemic venous circulation, it is susceptible to injury by a variety of agents. Hepatic necrosis can occur secondary to other hepatic processes

CAUSES OF HEPATIC NECROSIS

Chemicals
Drugs
Aflatoxins
Septicemia
Acute pancreatitis
Inflammatory bowel disease
Viral agents
Inflammatory hepatic disease
Systemic hypoxia
Anemia
Ischemic injury
Excessive copper storage
Heartworm-associated conditions (e.g., postcaval
    syndrome)
Trauma

DRUGS KNOWN TO CAUSE HEPATIC DISEASE

Acetaminophen
Anabolic steroids
Anticonvulsant drugs
Antineoplastic drugs (methotrexate, L-asparaginase,
    6-mercaptopurine)
Arsenicals (thiacetarsamide)
Diethylcarbamazine
Furosemide
Glucocorticoids
Inhalation anesthetics (halothane, methoxyflurane)
Ketoconazole
Mebendazole
Mitotane (o,p-DDD)
Sulfonamides
Tetracycline
Trimethoprim-sulfamethoxazole

such as infection inflammation, neoplasia, or hepatotoxins. Causes of hepatic necrosis are listed above. Hepatotoxic drugs are listed in the next column.

Clinical features

Clinical signs of hepatic disease depend on the severity of the hepatic insult. Many animals are asymptomatic, with disease detected only by biochemical screening, whereas other cases present with acute fulminant hepatic failure. In the latter instance, affected animals range from profoundly depressed to comatose, with the degree of hepatic encephalopathy depending on the cause and severity. Vomiting, anorexia, and fever are often seen. Icterus is often seen when there is periportal involvement. The presence of coagulopathies such as disseminated intravascular coagulation reflect the degree of severity and usually manifest with gastrointestinal bleeding, hematemesis, ecchymoses, and excessive bleeding at venipuncture sites.

Laboratory findings may include increases in serum alanine and aspartate aminotransferase activity. The concentrations of serum alkaline phosphatase, serum gamma-glutamyltransferase, serum bilirubin, serum glucose, and clotting factors are variable. Hepatic function tests such as serum bile acids and plasma ammonia concentration reflect the degree of hepatic failure.

Treatment of hepatic failure

The cornerstone of treating acute hepatic failure includes elimination of the inciting cause (such as drugs or toxins), providing optimal conditions for hepatic regeneration, preventing complications, and reversing derangements occurring with hepatic failure. The multitude of derangements occurring with acute hepatic failure relate to the many functions of the liver to maintain homeostasis. The important derangements seen include dehydration and hypovolemia, hepatic encephalopathy, hypoglycemia, acid-base and electrolyte abnormalities, coagulopathies, gastric ulceration, sepsis, and endotoxemia.

Management of dehydration, hypovolemia, and electrolyte disturbances. Many animals with severe hepatic disease have vomiting, diarrhea, and anorexia. Therefore dehydration can readily occur. Patients with ascites already are using all of their circulatory reserve function to maintain intravascular volume and tissue perfusion. When additional fluid losses (such as vomiting or diarrhea) occur, hypovolemic shock can result. In addition to volume depletion, these patients frequently have electrolyte and acid-base disturbances. Patients with hepatic disease frequently have hypokalemia in addition to total body potassium depletion. In addition to other deleterious effects, hypokalemia contributes greatly to the severity of hepatic encephalopathy. Potassium supplementation makes an enormous difference in the treatment of these patients. The most common acid-base disturbance with hepatic disease is alkalosis, although other disturbances can be seen.[13] If prerenal azotemia occurs, excess urea will diffuse into the colon, where it becomes a substrate for ammonia production and thus worsens encephalopathy. Appropriate fluid therapy will minimize this deleterious effect.

To manage these derangements, aggressive intravenous fluid therapy is often needed. The fluid of choice may be determined by measurement of serum electrolytes and arterial blood gases. If arterial blood gases are unavailable, the serum bicarbonate concentration can be estimated from the serum total carbon dioxide concentration. However, these values are usually not available immediately. In general, the fluid of choice is half-strength saline (0.45%) with 2.5% dextrose, supplemented with potassium chloride. Potassium chloride should be added at the rate of 30 mEq/L of fluids until serum potassium concentration is known, at which time the concentration can be adjusted. Ringer's solution or 0.9% saline are acceptable alternatives, but their higher sodium content makes them less desirable, because many patients with hepatic disease have excessive sodium retention and their administration can exacerbate ascites. Lactated Ringer's solution should be avoided because lactate is converted to bicarbonate in the liver and the alkalinization may exacerbate hepatoencephalopathy.[103] Care must also be taken not to administer fluids too aggressively, because patients with hepatic disease cannot efficiently excrete a salt and water load in response to volume expansion, thus exacerbating ascites and portal hypertension. Diuretics such as furosemide should be given with caution since these can exacerbate hypovolemia, prerenal azotemia, hypokalemia, and metabolic alkalosis.

Short-term management of hepatic encephalopathy. The approach to managing acute hepatic encephalopathy involves reducing the formation and absorption of encephalopathic toxins from the intestinal tract, avoiding drugs that exacerbate encephalopathy (e.g., tranquilizers, anticonvulsants, anesthetics), controlling gastrointestinal hemorrhage, and following an appropriate diet. Factors that precipitate metabolic changes that can lead to

encephalopathy are listed below (see box). These factors must be avoided or treated if possible.

Decreasing encephalopathic toxins. The therapeutic efforts designed to reduce formation and absorption of encephalopathic toxins are primarily directed toward reducing ammonia absorption, although other encephalopathic toxins are also important, including mercaptans, short-chained fatty acids, and aromatic amino acids. Since ammonia is produced primarily in the colon from bacterial action on dietary amines (proteins) and urea (which diffuses from the systemic circulation into the colon), efforts at lowering blood ammonia concentration are aimed at interrupting this process. This can be done in several ways. Initially, food is withheld to prevent dietary proteins from reaching the colon. In addition, large-volume (50 ml/kg body weight) cleansing enemas are used to decrease bacterial numbers. The enema solution should be composed of normal saline solution with betadine solution added to make a 1:10 to 1:100 solution to further decrease colonic bacterial numbers. Alternatively, gentamicin can be added (1 mg/kg body weight) to the saline solution to kill urease-producing bacteria. Saline also has the advantage of lowering colonic pH. This has the effect of converting freely absorbable ammonia (NH_3) to the nonabsorbable ammonium (NH_4^+) ion. Enemas should be retained as long as possible and repeated often (up to every 2 hours) as necessary to manage neurologic manifestations of encephalopathy and hepatic coma.

Lactulose (Cephulac) administration is another useful adjunct to decrease ammonia absorption. Lactulose is a disaccharide that undergoes minimal absorption in the stomach and small intestine, reaching the colon unchanged. In the colon it is metabolized by bacteria, resulting in the formation of low-molecular-weight acids that acidify the colonic contents. This has the effect of converting ammonia (NH_3) to the ammonium ion (NH_4^+), thus trapping it in the colon and preventing its absorption. In addition, the metabolic byproducts of lactulose induce an osmotic catharsis and therefore lower colonic bacterial numbers. The initial, empirical dosage of lactulose is 1.0 ml/kg. It can be given by several routes. The oral route is preferred if possible. In stuporous patients it can be administered via orogastric tube. Alternatively, it can be given mixed with a saline enema. In conscious patients, the liquid is given orally by syringe. In the acute situation, it can be given every 2 to 4 hours. In the long-term management of chronic hepatic encephalopathy, it is given at the above dosage orally three times a day. The dosage can be titrated by noting the consistency of the feces, since excessive amounts of

---

FACTORS THAT PRECIPITATE METABOLIC CHANGES LEADING TO HEPATIC ENCEPHALOPATHY

Increased dietary protein intake
Gastrointestinal hemorrhage
Diuretic administration
Sedative or barbiturate administration
Uremia
Infection or endotoxemia
Constipation
Large intestinal bacterial overgrowth
Methionine administration

lactulose will cause diarrhea. Ideally, the feces should be loose to slightly liquid.

Orally administered antibiotics can also be helpful to decrease colonic bacterial numbers. Since ammonia-generating bacteria in the colon are primarily gram-negative anaerobes, appropriate antibiotics can include neomycin, aminoglycosides (which undergo minimal intestinal absorption) and/or metronidazole. I have had more success with orally administered gentamicin (using the injectable product given orally at a dosage of 2 mg/kg three times a day) than neomycin (20 mg/kg orally three times a day), although the latter is an acceptable alternative. Metronidazole is given at a dosage of 6 to 10 mg/kg orally two or three times a day. This drug is also systemically absorbed and may be useful for anaerobic sepsis. Sepsis can occur with hepatic failure due to abnormal hepatic reticuloendothelial cell function and resultant decreased clearance of bacteria absorbed into the portal circulation.

Drugs that exacerbate encephalopathy. Drugs that can depress the central nervous system should be avoided because of their potential to exacerbate hepatic encephalopathy. These patients have increased cerebral sensitivity to central nervous system depressants. In addition, drugs that are cleared by the liver have prolonged activity due to decreased hepatic clearance in animals with liver failure. Analgesics, tranquilizers, sedatives, anesthetics, and barbiturates should be avoided if possible. If sedation is necessary, these drugs should be used in decreased dosages. If a convulsive state is present, diazepam is the safest drug to use to control seizure activity. If analgesia is required, I have had the least problems with meperidine (Demerol). This drug is used at a lower dosage than in patients with normal hepatic function.

Controlling gastrointestinal hemorrhage. Gastrointestinal hemorrhage must also be controlled. Patients with hepatic disease are prone to gastrointestinal hemorrhage. Gastrin concentration is increased due to decreased hepatic clearance and increased secretion stimulated by excess bile acids, resulting in gastric hyperacidity. Microthrombi in the mucosal microcirculation (if disseminated intravascular coagulation is present), resulting in inability to handle back-diffused hydrogen ions also contributes. In addition, patients with hepatic disease often have coagulopathies that exacerbate any bleeding tendency. The result of gastrointestinal hemorrhage is increased ammonia production because blood is a substrate for bacterial conversion to ammonia (100 ml of blood yields 15 to 20 g of protein).[104] In addition, gastrointestinal hemorrhage leads to hypovolemia, shock, and hypoxia. These effects also exacerbate encephalopathy, as discussed above.

The treatment of gastrointestinal hemorrhage involves several aspects. A bland diet with minimal residue is helpful to minimize potential inflammation in the bowel. In addition, specific drug therapy is indicated, including drugs that inhibit gastric acid secretion. These drugs were discussed in detail in the section on "Treatment of Gastric Ulcers."

It is important to note that blood transfusion should be avoided unless absolutely necessary. Red blood cells have a high ammonia content, and once blood is stored, ammonia is released. Storage of blood for 1 day results in the elaboration of 170 μg of ammonia per 100 ml of blood, after 4 days 330 μg per 100 ml, and after 21 days 900 μg per 100 ml.[104] It is not uncommon to see clinical deterioration shortly after blood is administered to patients with hepatic failure. If blood administration is necessary, freshly collected blood should be used. Ideally, plastic blood collection bags should be used, since platelets stick to glass and glass activates factor XII, exacerbating disseminated intravascular coagulation.

Dietary management. Dietary management is important in the acute and chronic stages of hepatic failure (see Chapter 37). In the acute stages, food restriction is important to minimize dietary substrates for ammonia production in the colon. Most encephalopathic animals are anorectic so this is not a problem. Once acute encephalopathy is controlled, dietary management is important. This involves protein restriction, small frequent meals, and the careful selection of ingredients in the diet.

Management of hypoglycemia. Many patients with severe hepatic failure are hypoglycemic because of inadequate gluconeogenic enzymes and depletion of glycogen stores. Hypoglycemia can significantly worsen hepatic encephalopathy in addition to its other deleterious effects. It has been shown that hypoglycemia is an accurate predictor of early death in patients with hepatitis.[105] Glucose supplementation will correct hypoglycemia, prevent catabolic processes, and may lower central nervous system and blood ammonia concentrations.[103] It is usually easy to restore normal blood glucose concentration with intravenous glucose supplementation in patients with hepatic failure, whereas it is more difficult to maintain euglycemia with other causes of hypoglycemia such as insulin-producing tumors. Glucose can be supplied in the intravenous fluids up to a concentration of 5% to 10%. It is rare that higher glucose concentrations will be necessary to maintain euglycemia.

Management of coagulopathies. The causes of coagulopathies associated with severe hepatic disease are numerous, and appropriate management depends on identifying the cause. The most common coagulopathy seen is disseminated intravascular coagulation. Appropriate treatment includes aggressive intravenous fluid administration to maintain tissue perfusion and treatment of the underlying hepatopathy if possible. Additional treatment measures include inhibition of platelet function with aspirin, and clotting factor and antithrombin III replacement with a fresh-whole-blood transfusion (collected in a plastic collection bag to prevent activation of factor XII) along with heparin therapy (150 units/kg units subcutaneously three times a day). Heparin can also be added to the transfused blood at a concentration of 75 units/500 ml of blood to activate antithrombin III. If there is antithrombin III depletion, and it is not supplied in the form of a fresh blood transfusion, heparin therapy will be deleterious.

If the cause of the coagulopathy is from abnormal clotting factor production, a fresh-whole-blood or plasma transfusion is indicated. As mentioned above, stored blood should be avoided because of its high ammonia content. In rare instances, such as prolonged biliary obstruction, vitamin K deficiency causes abnormal clotting ability. This can be corrected by administering vitamin K_1 orally or subcutaneously. In my experience, this seldom corrects abnormal clotting times, although it is a therapeutic measure that does little harm.

Management of sepsis and endotoxemia. Patients with severe hepatic disease are prone to systemic and hepatic infection due to abnormal hepatic reticuloendothelial-cell function. Because the liver is responsible for clearing bacterial products from the portal blood, therapy is directed primarily against intestinal flora. The main concern is with gram-negative enterics and anaerobes, as well as endotoxins. If sepsis is strongly suspected, multiple blood cultures (both aerobic and anaerobic) are indicated. If hepatic biopsy is performed, a culture of the specimen should always be obtained. If an organism can be cultured, specific antibiotic therapy can be employed; otherwise, animals should be placed on broad-spectrum antibiotics empirically.

Appropriate choices for empirical antibiotic usage are based on activity against intestinal flora, degree of hepatic clearance, and toxicity. Drugs requiring hepatic inactivation should be avoided, whereas drugs excreted by the liver should be beneficial, although they must be used with caution. Drugs with good activity against anaerobes include metronidazole (6 to 10 mg/kg two to three times a day), penicillins, and cephalosporins. These drugs are combined with an aminoglycoside such as gentamicin to combat gram-negative organisms. Aminoglycosides can be given systemically for septicemia, or orally to kill intestinal bacteria (since they are not absorbed when given by this route).

Tetracycline is concentrated in the bile and may be useful for biliary tract infections. However, it should be used with caution to avoid excessive blood levels and toxicity. The new quinolone antibiotics (enrofloxacin, ciprofloxacin) also have promise for use with hepatic disease since they have excellent activity against intestinal flora and reach high concentrations in the liver.

Antibiotics that should be avoided include chloramphenicol, lincomycin, sulfonamides, erythromycin, clindamycin, chlortetracycline, and hetacillin.[103,106] These drugs are either inactivated by the liver, require hepatic metabolism, or can cause hepatotoxicity.[103,104,106]

Methods used to control endotoxin absorption include nonabsorbed orally administered antibiotics (aminoglycosides) and cholestyramine. The latter drug binds to bile acids and endotoxins and prevents their absorption into the portal circulation.[104]

Amino acids and neurotransmitters. Therapeutic measures to treat acute hepatic coma include the intravenous administration of branched-chain amino acids. Since amino acid derangements (mainly increased aromatic amino acids) contribute greatly to hepatic encephalopathy, normalization of amino acid ratios are helpful. By administering branched-chain amino acids, less aromatic amino acids enter the central nervous system, since they compete for a common carrier to get across the blood-brain barrier. However, there is conflicting evidence as to the effectiveness of branched-chain amino acids in managing hepatic coma.[103] The high cost of these solutions will also limit their use. The use of conventional amino acid solutions or protein hydrolysates should be avoided since use of these solutions leads to a high serum ammonia concentration.

The use of the dopamine agonist, L-dopa, has also been proposed to treat acute hepatic coma.[103] It is thought that this and similar drugs act to alter neurotransmitter concentrations in the brain favorably. Clinical trials in dogs with hepatic coma are needed before these drugs can be recommended for routine clinical use.

Nutritional management. Nutritional management of chronic hepatic failure should include the following considerations: (1) Calories from protein should be moderately restricted, and ingredients that are of high biologic value and highly digestible should be used. (2) Protein sources with high branched-chain: aromatic amino acid ratios are preferred. Cottage cheese is an ideal protein source. (3) A palatable energy-dense diet in amounts sufficient to meet energy needs is necessary to avoid negative energy balance. (4) Carbohydrates supply most nonprotein calories, but should be from highly digestible sources. (5) Sodium and copper should be restricted. (6) Supplementation with zinc, ascorbic acid, and a salt and copper-free vitamin-mineral supplement may be helpful. (7) These elements must be present in a highly digestible, low-residue diet and fed in small frequent meals.

Management of ascites

Ascites results primarily from a combination of portal hypertension, renal sodium and water retention, and hypoalbuminemia. Starling's forces are disrupted by these changes, resulting in abdominal fluid accumulation. Therefore, therapy will be directed toward reversing these processes.

Emergency treatment of ascites is rarely necessary. Occasionally, however, the volume of ascitic fluid is large enough to result in respiratory distress due to compression of the diaphragm, limiting inspiratory efforts. In this setting, paracentesis may be helpful. The only other reasons to withdraw fluid from the abdominal cavity are for diagnostic fluid analysis and cytology and to make it easier to perform percutaneous hepatic biopsy, laparoscopy, or abdominal radiography. The risks of paracentesis are hypovolemic shock, iatrogenic infection, protein depletion, and perforation of abdominal viscera. Animals with ascites are already using their maximum cardiac and circulatory reserve to maintain tissue perfusion. When a large volume of fluid is rapidly removed, fluid shifts from the intravascular to extravascular compartment and can precipitate hypovolemic shock. Although this is rare in my experience, I recommend that if paracentesis is necessary, fluid should be withdrawn slowly and intravenous fluid support should be provided.

Dietary salt restriction, diuretics, and aldosterone-inhibiting drugs are used in the long-term control of ascites. Renal retention of salt and water (and thus the failure to excrete a salt and water load in response to volume expansion) is one of the initiating events in the development of ascites. Increased sensitivity to aldosterone, increased aldosterone secretion, and failure of the normal negative feedback system that governs the renin-angiotensin-aldosterone axis occur.

Dietary salt restriction is of prime importance to minimize sodium retention. Diuretics may be necessary to control ascites in some patients.

They should be administered with caution to avoid dehydration, as animals with hepatic failure and ascites are using their maximum circulatory and cardiac reserve to maintain perfusion. Aldosterone-inhibiting drugs are used initially. I recommend spironolactone at a dosage of 1 mg/kg orally twice a day. If this dose is ineffective, it should be doubled to 2 mg/kg orally twice a day. Spironolactone will not exacerbate hypokalemia. Loop diuretics such as furosemide (Lasix) can cause excessive urinary fluid loss, which will result in hypovolemia, hypokalemia, and alkalosis.

If ascites persists, captopril is added at a dosage of 0.5 to 2 mg/kg orally two or three times a day. Captopril is an angiotensin-converting enzyme inhibitor that decreases activity of the renin-angiotensin-aldosterone system. If ascites still remains a clinical problem, furosemide is added at a dosage of 1 to 2 mg/kg orally two or three times a day. Caution must be used to avoid hypovolemia and electrolyte imbalances. Therefore, serum electrolytes must be measured periodically in addition to continued clinical assessment.

REFERENCES

1. Zimmer JF. Canine esophageal foreign bodies: endoscopic, surgical, and medical management. J Am Anim Hosp Assoc 1984;20:669-677.
2. Houlton JEF, Herrtage ME, Taylor PM, Watkine SB. Thoracic esophageal foreign bodies in the dog: a review of ninety cases. J Small Anim Pract 1985;26:521-536.
3. Taylor RA. Transdiaphragmatic approach to distal esophageal foreign bodies. J Am Anim Hosp Assoc 1982;18:749-752.
4. Eastwood GL, Castell DO, Higgs RH. Experimental esophagitis in cats impairs lower esophageal sphincter pressure. Gastroenterology 1975;69:146-153.
5. Goodall RJR, Temple JG. Effect of cimetidine on lower oesophageal sphincter pressure in oesophagitis. BMJ 1980;280:611-612.
6. Bright RM, Burrows CF. Percutaneous endoscopic tube gastrostomy in dogs. Am J Vet Res 1988;49:629-633.
7. Knox WG, Scott JR, Zintel HA, Guthrie R, McCabe RE. Bouginage and steroids used singly or in combination in experimental corrosive esophagitis. Ann Surg 1967;166:930-941.
8. Sooy TE, Adams WM, Pitts RP, Beck KA. Balloon catheter dilatation of alimentary tract strictures in the dog and cat. Vet Radiol 1987;28:131-137.
9. Hoffer RE. Atlas of small animal surgery. St Louis: Mosby–Year Book, 1977.
10. Leib MS. Megaesophagus in the dog. Part II. Clinical aspects. Compend Contin Educ Pract Vet 1984;6:11-17.
11. Henderson RA, Pope ER. Principles of gastrointestinal surgery. Vet Clin North Am 1983;13:485-502.
12. Boudrieau RJ, Rogers WA. Megaesophagus in the dog: a review of 50 cases. J Am Anim Hosp Assoc 1985;21:33-40.
13. Strombeck DR. Small animal gastroenterology. Davis, CA: Stonegate Publishing, 1979.
14. Twedt DC. Differential diagnosis and therapy of vomiting. Vet Clin North Am 1983;13:503-520.

15. Brawner Jr WR, Bartels JE. Contrast radiography of the digestive tract. Indications, techniques, and complications. Vet Clin North Am 1983;13:599-626.
16. Tams TR. Endoscopy. In Kirk RW, ed. Current veterinary therapy X. Philadelphia: WB Saunders, 1989;864-868.
17. Moore FM. Personal communication. Boston.
18. Davis LE. Clinical pharmacology of the gastrointestinal tract. In Anderson NV, ed. Veterinary gastroenterology. Philadelphia: Lea & Febiger, 1980;277-310.
19. Tams TR. Newer concepts in gastrointestinal therapeutics. Proc Am Coll Vet Intern Med Forum 1987;5:126-129.
20. Mann NS. Metoclopramide and gut. Am J Proct Gastroenterol Colon Rect Surg 1982;33(9):9-11.
21. Burrows CF. Metoclopramide. J Am Vet Med Assoc 1983;183:1341-1343.
22. Albibi R, McCallum RW. Metoclopramide: pharmacology and clinical application. Ann Intern Med 1983;98:86-95.
23. Moreland KJ. Ulcer disease of the upper gastrointestinal tract in small animals: pathophysiology, diagnosis, and management. Compend Contin Educ Pract Vet 1988;10:1265-1279.
24. Papich MG. Medical therapy for gastrointestinal ulcers. In Kirk RW, ed. Current veterinary therapy X. Philadelphia: WB Saunders, 1989;911-918.
25. Kauffman G. Aspirin-induced gastric mucosal injury: lessons learned from animal models. Gastroenterology 1989;96:606-614.
26. Twedt DC. Gastric ulcers. In Kirk RW, ed. Current veterinary therapy VIII. Philadelphia: WB Saunders, 1989;767-770.
27. Toombs JP, Collins LG, Graves GM, Crowe DT, Caywood DD. Colonic perforation in corticosteroid-treated dogs. J Am Vet Med Assoc 1986;188:145-150.
28. DeNovo RC. Antral pyloric hypertrophy syndrome. In Kirk RW, ed. Current veterinary therapy X. Philadelphia: WB Saunders, 1989;918-921.
29. Crow SE. Tumors of the alimentary tract. Vet Clin North Am 1985;15:577-596.
30. Kleine LJ, Lamb CR. Comparative organ imaging: the gastrointestinal tract. Vet Radiol 1989;30:133-141.
31. Holtermuller K-H. Acid rebound: fact or fiction. Hepatogastroenterology 1982;29:135-137.
32. Zeldis JB, Friedman LS, Isselbacher KJ. Ranitidine: a new H_2-receptor antagonist. N Engl J Med 1983;309:1368-1373.
33. Friedman G. Famotidine. Am J Gastroenterol 1987;82:504-506.
34. Schunack W. What are the differences between the H_2-receptor antagonists? Aliment Pharmacol Therap 1987;1:493S-503S.
35. Dobrilla G, De Pretis G, Piazzi L, et al. Comparison of once-daily bedtime administration of famotidine and ranitidine in the short-term treatment of duodenal ulcer. Scand J Gastroenterol 1987;22(Suppl 134):21-28.
36. Tarnawski A, Hollander D, Krause WJ, Zipser RD, Stachura J, Gergely H. Does sucralfate affect the normal gastric mucosa? Gastroenterology 1986;90:893-905.
37. Jiranek GC, Kimmey MB, Saunders DR, Willson RA, Shanahan W, Silverstein FE. Misoprostol reduces gastroduodenal injury from one week of aspirin: an endoscopic study. Gastroenterology 1989;96:656-661.
38. Graham DY. Prevention of gastroduodenal injury induced by chronic nonsteroidal antiinflammatory drug therapy. Gastroenterology 1989;96:675-681.
39. Soll AH, Kurata J, McGuigan JE. Ulcers, nonsteroidal antiinflammatory drugs, and related matters. Gastroenterology 1989;96:561-568.
40. McCarthy DM. Nonsteroidal antiinflammatory drug-induced ulcers: management by traditional therapies. Gastroenterology 1989;96:662-674.
41. Boulay JP, Lipowitz AJ, Klausner JS. Effect of cimetidine on aspirin-induced gastric hemorrhage in dogs. Am J Vet Res 1986;47:1744-1746.
42. Wolfe JJ, Soll AH. The physiology of gastric acid secretion. N Engl J Med 1988;319:1707-1715.
43. Lamers CBHW, Lind T, Moberg S, Jansen JBMJ, Olbe L. Omeprazole in Zollinger-Ellison syndrome. N Engl J Med 1984;310:758-761.
44. Walan A, Bader J-P, Classen M, et al. Effect of omeprazole and ranitidine on ulcer healing and relapse rates in patients with benign gastric ulcer. N Engl J Med 1989;320:69-75.
45. Blum AL, Riecken EO, Dammann JG, et al. Comparison of omeprazole and ranitidine in the treatment of reflux esophagitis. N Engl J Med 1986;314:716.
46. Sachs G. Pump blockers and ulcer disease. N Engl J Med 1984;310:785-786.
47. Sherding RG. Diseases of the small bowel. In Ettinger SJ, ed. Textbook of veterinary internal medicine. Diseases of the dog and cat, ed. 2. Philadelphia: WB Saunders, 1983;1278-1346.
48. Zimmer JF, Burrington DB. Comparison of four techniques of fecal examination for detecting canine giardiasis. J Am Anim Hosp Assoc 1986;22:161-167.
49. Baker DG, Strombeck DR, Gershwin LJ. Laboratory diagnosis of *Giardia duodenalis* infection in dogs. J Am Vet Med Assoc 1987;190:53-56.
50. Richter KP. Diseases of the large bowel. In Ettinger SJ, ed. Textbook of veterinary internal medicine. Diseases of the dog and cat, ed. 3. Philadelphia: WB Saunders, 1989;1397-1420.
51. Washabau RJ, Buffington CA, Strombeck DR. Evaluation and management of carbohydrate malassimilation. In Kirk RW, ed. Current veterinary therapy IX. Philadelphia: WB Saunders, 1986;889-892.
52. Sherding RG. Diseases of the small bowel. In Ettinger SJ, ed. Textbook of veterinary internal medicine. Diseases of the dog and cat, ed. 3. Philadelphia: WB Saunders, 1989;1323-1396.
53. Moore R, Carpenter J. Intramural intestinal hematoma causing obstruction in three dogs. J Am Vet Med Assoc 1984;184:186-188.
54. Arrick RH, Kleine LJ. Intestinal pseudoobstruction in a dog. J Am Vet Med Assoc 1978;172:1201-1205.
55. Lantz GC. The pathophysiology of acute mechanical small bowel obstruction. Compend Contin Educ Pract Vet 1981;3:910-916.
56. Holder WD. Intestinal obstruction. Gastroenterol Clin North Am 1988;17:317-340.
57. Bjorling DE, Crowe DT, Kolata RJ, Rawlings CA. Penetrating abdominal wounds in dogs and cats. J Am Anim Hosp Assoc 1982;18:742-748.
58. Bellah JR. Colonic perforation after corticosteroid and surgical treatment of intervertebral disk disease in a dog. J Am Vet Med Assoc 1983;183:1002-1003.
59. Scott J. Physiological, pharmacological and pathological actions of glucocorticoids on the digestive system. Clin Gastroenterol 1981;10:627-652.
60. Abcarian H, Lowe R. Colon and rectal trauma. Surg Clin North Am 1978;58:519-537.
61. Dillon R. Bacterial enteritis. In Kirk RW, ed. Current veterinary therapy IX. Philadelphia: WB Saunders, 1986;872-880.
62. Holt PE. The role of dogs and cats in the epidemiology of human campylobacter enterocolitis. J Small Anim Pract 1981;22:681-685.

63. Fox JG, Moore R, Ackerman JI. Canine and feline campylobacteriosis: epizootiology and clinical and public health features. J Am Vet Med Assoc 1983; 183:1420-1424.

64. Greene CE. Enteric bacterial infections. In Greene CE, ed. Clinical microbiology and infectious diseases of the dog and cat. Philadelphia: WB Saunders, 1984;617-632.

65. Fleming MP. Association of *Campylobacter jejuni* with enteritis in dogs and cats. Vet Rec 1983;113:372-374.

66. Patton CM, Mitchell SW, Potter ME, Kaufmann AF. Comparison of selective media for primary isolation of *Campylobacter fetus* subsp. *jejuni*. J Linc Microbiol 1981;13:326-330.

67. Fox JG. Campylobacteriosis-a "new" disease in laboratory animals. Lab Anim Sci 1982;32:625-637.

68. Fox JG, Moore R, Ackerman JI. *Campylobacter jeuni* - associated diarrhea in dogs. J Am Vet Med Assoc 1983;183:1430-1433.

69. Skirrow MB. Campylobacter enteritis in dogs and cats: a 'new' zoonosis. Vet Res Commun 1981;5:13-19.

70. Dillon R. Therapeutic strategies involving antimicrobial treatment of the gastrointestinal tract. J Am Vet Med Assoc 1984;185:1169-1171.

71. Papageorges M, Higgins R, Gosselin Y. *Yersinia enterocolitica* enteritis in two dogs. J Am Vet Med Assoc 1983;182:618-619.

72. Farstad L, Landsverk T, Lassen J. Isolation of *Yersinia enterocolitica* from a dog with chronic enteritis. Acta Vet Scand 1976;17:261-263.

73. Mors V, Pai CH. Pathogenic properties of *Yersinia enterocolitica*. Infect Immun 1980;28:292-294.

74. Robins-Browne RM, Still CS, Miliotis MD, Koornhof HJ. Mechanism of action of *Yersinia enterocolitica* enterotoxin. Infect Immun 1979;25:680-684.

75. Olson P, Hedhammar A, Wadstrom T. Enterotoxigenic *Escherichia coli* infection in two dogs with acute diarrhea. J Am Vet Med Assoc 1984;184:982-983.

76. Moss S, Frost AJ. The resistance to chemotherapeutic agents of *Escherichia coli* from domestic dogs and cats. Aust Vet J 1984;61:82-84.

77. Onderdonk AB, Hermos JA, Bartlett JG. The role of the intestinal microflora in experimental colitis. Am J Clin Nutr 1977;30:1819-1825.

78. Cherry RD, Portnoy D, Jabbari M, Daly DS, Kinnear DG, Goreskyt CA. Metronidazole: an alternate therapy for antibiotic-associated colitis. Gastroenterology 1982;82:849-851.

79. Berry AP, Levett PN. Chronic diarrhoea in dogs associated with *Clostridium difficile* infection. Vet Rec 1986;118:102-103.

80. Burrows CF. Diseases of the colon, rectum, and anus in the dog and cat. In Anderson NV, ed. Veterinary gastroenterology. Philadelphia: Lea & Febiger, 1980;533-592.

81. Prescott JF, Johnson JA, Patterson JM. Haemorrhagic gstroenteritis in the dog associated with *Clostridium welchii*. Vet Rec 1978;103:116-117.

82. Carman RJ. Recurrent diarrhoea in a dog associated with *Clostridium perfringens* type A. Vet Rec 1983;112:342-343.

83. Gorham JR, Foreyt WJ. In Greene CE, ed. Clinical microbiology and infectious diseases of the dog and cat. Philadelphia: WB Saunders, 1984;538-544.

84. Georgi JR. Parasitology for veterinarians. Philadelphia: WB Saunders, 1974.

85. Cornelius LM, Roberson EL. Treatment of gastrointestinal parasitism. In Kirk RW, ed. Current veterinary therapy IX. Philadelphia: WB Saunders, 1986;921-924.

86. Kelly JD. Occurrence of *Trichuris serrata* von Linstow, 1879 (Nematoda: Trichuridae) in the domestic cat *(Felis catus)* in Australia. J Parasitol 1973;59:1145-1146.

87. Roberson EL, Cornelius LM. Gastrointestinal parasitism. In Kirk RW, ed. Current veterinary therapy VIII. Philadelphia: WB Saunders, 1983;797-810.

88. Kirkpatrick CE. Enteric protozoal infections. In Greene CE, ed. Clinical microbiology and infectious diseases of the dog and cat. Philadelphia: WB Saunders, 1984;806-823.

89. Abbitt B. Huey RL, Eugster AK, Syler J. Treatment of giardiasis in adult Greyhounds, using ipronidazole-medicated water. J Am Vet Med Assoc 1986;188:67-69.

90. Carpenter JL, Roberts RM, Harpster NK, King NW. Intestinal and cardiopulmonary forms of parvovirus infection in a litter of pups. J Am Vet Med Assoc 1980;176:1269-1273.

91. Hayes MA, Russell RG, Babiuk LA. Sudden death in young dogs with myocarditis caused by parvovirus. J Am Vet Med Assoc 1979;174:1197-1203.

92. Jezyk PF, Haskins ME, Jones CL. Myocarditis of probable viral origin in pups of weaning age. J Am Vet Med Assoc 1979;174:1204-1207.

93. Mulvey JJ, Bech-Nielsen S, Haskins ME, Jezyk PF, Taylor HW, Eugster AK. Myocarditis induced by parvoviral infection in weaning pups in the United States. J Am Vet Med Assoc 1980;177:695-698.

94. Heald RD, Jones BD, Schmidt DA. Blood gas and electrolyte concentrations in canine parvoviral enteritis. J Am Anim Hosp Assoc 1986;22:745-748.

95. Jeraj P, Manning PJ. Bacteremia concomitant with parvovirus infection in a pup. J Am Vet Med Assoc 1984;184:196-197.

96. Pollock RVH. The parvoviruses. Part II. Canine parvovirus. Compend Contin Educ Pract Vet 1984;6:653-661.

97. Mulvaney MH, Feinberg CK, Tilson DL. Clinical characterization of acute necrotizing pancreatitis. Compend Contin Educ Pract Vet 1982;4:394-404.

98. Williams DA. Exocrine pancreatic disease. In Ettinger SJ, ed. Textbook of veterinary internal medicine. Diseases of the dog and cat. ed. 3. Philadelphia: WB Saunders, 1989;1528-1554.

99. Williams DA. Pancreatitis-recent findings. Proc Am Coll Vet Intern Med Forum 1989;7:787-790.

100. Johnson S. Medical emergencies of the digestive tract and abdomen. In Sherding RG, ed. Medical emergencies. Contemporary issues in small animal practice, vol 1. New York: Churchill Livingstone, 1985;213-254.

101. Parent J. Effects of dexamethasone on pancreatic tissue and on serum amylase and lipase activities in dogs. J Am Vet Med Assoc 1982;180:743-746.

102. Mayer AD, McMahon MJ, Corfield AP, et al. Controlled clinical trial of peritoneal lavage for the treatment of severe acute pancreatitis. N Engl J Med 1985;312:399-404.

103. Tams TR. Hepatic encephalopathy. Vet Clin North Am 1985;15:177-195.

104. Hardy RM. Diseases of the liver. In Ettinger SJ, ed. Textbook of veterinary internal medicine. Diseases of the dog and cat, ed. 2. Philadelphia: WB Saunders, 1983;1372-1434.

105. Strombeck DR, Miller LM, Harrold D. Effects of corticosteroid treatment on survival time in dogs with chronic hepatitis: 151 cases (1977-1985). J Am Vet Med Assoc 1988;193:1109-1113.

106. Papich MG, Davis LE. Drugs and the liver. Vet Clin North Am 1985;15:77-95.

23 Hematologic and Oncologic Emergencies

C. Guillermo Couto and Alan S. Hammer

HEMATOLOGIC EMERGENCIES
Anemia

Clinical and laboratory evaluation. Anemia is defined as a decreased ability to transport oxygen; in practical terms it can be defined as a decrease in the packed cell volume or the red blood cell count below reference values for the species. When interpreting packed cell volume and red blood cell counts, the clinician should keep in mind that there are situations (e.g., puppyhood, pregnancy) when these parameters are below the reference value for the species (i.e., physiologic anemia).[1]

Owners' complaints in dogs and cats with anemia usually refer to the presence of pale mucous membranes and decreased overall activity. The owners may detect these changes "suddenly," after evaluating a pet that has actually been symptomatic for a considerable amount of time, thus leading to emergency presentation of a patient with chronic anemia.

When evaluating a patient with pallor, the clinician needs to determine if the change in the color of the mucous membranes is due to hypoperfusion or to anemia. The simplest approach to solve this problem is to evaluate the capillary refill time and the packed cell volume. Patients with cardiovascular disease and hypoperfusion usually have other clinical signs (see Chapter 17), including a prolonged capillary refill time. The capillary refill time may be difficult to evaluate in an anemic patient because of the lack of contrast due to pallor. In addition, patients should be evaluated for the presence of petechiae, ecchymoses, and deep bleeding, which may suggest the presence of an associated platelet or clotting factor deficiency. When evaluating a patient's packed cell volume, the plasma (or serum) protein content should also be determined with a refractometer and the plasma (or serum) evaluated for icterus or hemolysis. Also, the microhematocrit tube should be carefully inspected for evidence of autoagglutination (see below).

Once it is established that the patient is anemic, it should be determined whether the anemia is regenerative or nonregenerative. This is usually accomplished by obtaining a reticulocyte count during a routine complete blood count, and this reticulocyte index reflects the pathogenesis of the anemia (Table 23-1). This determination is important from the therapeutic standpoint, since the two groups of anemic patients are treated differently (see below). When the patient presents as an emergency, examination of the blood smear usually suffices to determine if the bone marrow is responding appropriately to the anemia (i.e., if the anemia is regenerative). Several pieces of information can be acquired from examining a good quality, properly stained blood smear, including red blood cell size and morphology, presence of autoagglutination, approximate numbers and morphology of white blood cells and platelets, presence of nucleated red blood cells, presence of

Table 23-1 Pathogenetic classification of anemias

Regenerative (RI ≥2.5)	Nonregenerative (RI ≤2.5)
Blood loss (after 48-96 hours)	Anemia of chronic disease
Hemolysis	Anemia of renal disease
	Hypoproliferative anemias (e.g., bone marrow disorder)
	Iron deficiency anemia
	Blood loss (first 48-96 hours)
	Endocrinopathy associated anemia

RI = reticulocyte index.

359

Table 23-2 Estimation of white blood cell and platelet counts from the blood smear

White blood cell count	Average number of white blood cells in 10 low power (10×) fields × 100 = white blood cells/μl
Platelet count	10 platelets/oil immersion field = 150,000 to 180,000 platelets per microliter (11 to 25 platelets per oil field is normal for dogs and 11 to 19 for cats)

Modified from Weiss DJ: Uniform evaluation and semiquantitative reporting of hematologic data. Vet Clin Pathol 1984; XIII:30. With permission.

polychromasia, presence of red blood cell parasites, and whether the red blood cell numbers are adequate (provided the clinician/technician is familiar with the way his/her blood smears should look). Table 23-2 summarizes some of the abnormalities detected by careful examination of the blood smear and their clinical implications. Tables 23-3 and 23-4 present guidelines to evaluate blood smears semiquantitatively. It is important to conduct this evaluation in a monolayer field (where the erythrocytes are in a monolayer and 50% of the cells are touching) under an oil immersion lens.

When a complete blood count and a reticulocyte count can be obtained in an anemic patient, they provide a more absolute parameter to evaluate the degree of regeneration:

1. If the red blood cell indices are macrocytic and hypochromic, that is most likely due to the presence of increased numbers of reticulocytes (which are larger and contain less hemoglobin than mature red blood cells), and therefore, the anemia is probably regenerative.
2. If the reticulocyte numbers are over 60,000 to 100,000/μl, and the degree of anemia is not severe (i.e., PCV in the range of 20 to 30), the anemia is probably regenerative.
3. If the reticulocyte index is over 2.5, the anemia is regenerative (see the box on the next page); this approach best applies to the dog, since cats have two types of reticulocytes (punctate and aggregate) with different circulation times, making calculations unreliable.

When evaluating a patient with regenerative anemia, it is beneficial to determine the serum or plasma protein concentration, since blood loss usually leads to hypoproteinemia, while hemolysis does not. Table 23-5 lists other physical examination and laboratory findings that allow clinicians to distinguish between blood loss and hemolytic anemias.

Table 23-3 Common abnormalities detected by examination of the blood smear and their clinical significance

Morphologic Abnormality	Commonly Associated Disorders
Macrocytosis	Breed characteristic (poodles), feline leukemia virus infection; regeneration; folate deficiency; dyserythropoiesis (bone marrow disease)
Microcytosis	Breed characteristic (Akitas): iron deficiency; portosystemic shunt; copper deficiency; polycythemia (erythrocytosis)
Hypochromia	Iron deficiency; copper deficiency
Polychromasia	Regeneration
Poikilocytosis	Regeneration; iron deficiency; hyposplenism
Schistocytosis (fragments)	Microangiopathy; hemangiosarcoma; disseminated intravascular coagulation
Spherocytosis	Immunohemolytic anemia; mononuclear phagocyte origin neoplasm; hypersplenism
Acanthocytosis (spur cells)	Hemangiosarcoma; liver disease; hyposplenism
Ecchinocytosis (burr cells)	Artifact; renal disease; pyruvate kinase deficiency anemia
Elliptocytosis	Congenital elliptocytosis (dogs)
Heinz bodies	Oxidative insult to red blood cells; normal in cats
Howell-Jolly bodies	Hyposplenism; regeneration
Autoagglutination	Immunohemolytic anemia
Leukopenia	See text
Thrombocytopenia	See text
Pancytopenia	Bone marrow disorder; hypersplenism

Table 23-4 Semiquantitative evaluation of red blood cell morphologic abnormalities based on average number of abnormal cells per 1000× microscopic field

Abnormality/Species	1+	2+	3+	4+
Anisocytosis				
Dog	7-15	16-20	21-29	>30
Cat	5-8	9-15	16-20	>20
Polychromasia				
Dog	2-7	8-14	15-29	>30
Cat	1-2	3-8	9-15	>15
Hypochromasia				
Dog and cat	1-10	11-50	51-200	>200
Poikilocytosis				
Dog and cat	3-10	11-50	51-200	>200
Spherocytosis				
Dog and cat	5-10	11-50	51-150	>150
Schistocytosis				
Dog and cat	1-2	3-8	9-20	>20
Acanthocytosis				
Dog and cat	1-2	3-8	9-20	>20

Modified from Weiss DJ: Uniform evaluation and semiquantitative reporting of hematologic data. Vet Clin Pathol 1984; XIII:30. With permission.

Table 23-5 Features that assist the clinician in differentiating blood loss from hemolytic anemias

	Blood loss	Hemolysis
Serum (plasma) protein	Normal to low	Normal to high
Evidence of bleeding	Common	Rare*
Icterus	No	Common
Hemoglobinemia	No	Common
Spherocytosis	No	Common
Red blood cell inclusions	No	Occasional
Hemosiderinuria	No	Yes
Autoagglutination	No	Occasional
Direct Coombs' test	Negative	Usually positive (in immune-mediated hemolytic anemia)
Splenomegaly	No	Common

*Unless the hemolysis is associated with thrombocytopenia (i.e., Evan's syndrome, canine ehrlichiosis, feline leukemia virus infection).

CALCULATION OF THE RETICULOCYTE INDEX IN DOGS

1. $\dfrac{\text{Patient's PCV}}{45} \times \text{Retic \%} = A$, where 45 is the average packed cell volume for dogs; this corrects for the artifact caused by the anemia (i.e., with a low packed cell volume the percent of reticulocytes exaggerates the absolute number of cells).
2. If there is polychromasia in the blood smear, divide A by 2, to correct for the maturation time in circulation.
3. If the results are >2.5, the anemia is regenerative.

Emergency treatment of the anemic patient. The first basic principle of treatment of anemic (or bleeding) patients, is to collect all blood samples prior to instituting any therapy. Since most of these patients present as true emergencies, often collecting samples is neglected until the patient has been completely stabilized, thus resulting in treatment-induced changes in the laboratory parameters.

As a general rule, due to the acute onset of these disorders, patients with regenerative anemias (i.e., blood loss or hemolysis) require more aggressive therapy than patients with nonregenerative forms. Once the clinician has determined that the patient is stable and that the anemia is regenerative, specific therapy should be initiated.

Regenerative anemias

Blood loss anemia. The source of bleeding should be identified, and the bleeding arrested. If the patient is bleeding from a systemic hemostatic defect, specific treatment should be initiated. Transfusion of blood or blood products is often required in patients with anemia due to acute blood loss. For a detailed discussion of this topic please refer to Chapter 34.

Hemolytic anemia. In humans, under maximal stimulation, the bone marrow is capable of undergoing hyperplasia until its production rate is increased approximately sixfold to eightfold.[2] As a consequence of this, significant destruction of red blood cells has to occur before anemia develops. It should also be remembered that patients with peracute hemolysis can present with nonregenerative anemia, since the bone marrow has not yet been able to mount a regenerative response (see below).

Anemia due to extravascular or, less commonly, to intravascular destruction of red blood cells is common in dogs, and relatively common in cats. Because of the acute nature of the hemolytic process, most patients present for emergency care.

In extravascular hemolysis, red blood cells are phagocytosed by the mononuclear phagocytic system in the spleen, liver, and bone marrow. Stimuli that result in red blood cell phagocytosis include mainly presence of intracellular inclusions (e.g., red blood cell parasites; Heinz bodies) and membrane coating with immunoglobulin (Ig) G or M. Once abnormal red blood cells are recognized, the mononuclear phagocytic system rapidly phagocytoses them, resulting in both a decrease in the number of circulating red blood cells and the generation of cells with specific morphologic changes (i.e., spherocytes). If the destruction of red blood cells continues, anemia develops. Spherocytes are red blood cell "leftovers" after a mononuclear phagocytic cell took a "bite" of cytoplasm and membrane, and are characteristic of immunohemolytic anemia and neoplasms of the mononuclear phagocytic system. Occasionally, spherocytes are seen in cases of hypersplenism, in which the spleen acquires significant phagocytic activity resulting in peripheral blood cytopenias. Immunohemolytic anemia is the most common cause of hemolytic anemia in dogs in our hospital; in cats, drug-induced hemolysis and hemobartonellosis are the two most common causes. Table 23-6 lists other causes of hemolytic anemia in dogs and cats.

Intravascular hemolysis can occur as a consequence of direct red blood cell lysis, usually by drugs or toxins, or by increased shearing of red blood cells (e.g., microangiopathy, disseminated intravascular coagulation). It is considerably less common than extravascular hemolysis in small animals.

Clinically, patients with congenital (familial) hemolytic anemias may present with relatively prolonged clinical courses, with the notable exception of phosphofructokinase deficiency-induced hemolysis in English springer spaniels, in which acute hemolytic episodes occur after hyperventilation during exercise (e.g., alkaline hemolysis).[3] Patients with acquired hemolytic anemias usually present with acute clinical signs, characterized by pallor, with or without icterus (in our experience only approximately half the dogs and cats with hemolytic anemia are icteric); splenomegaly may be a prominent finding. If there is associated thrombocytopenia (e.g., Evan's syndrome, hemoparasites), petechiae and ecchymoses may be present. Clinical signs and physical examination findings associated with the primary disease can also be present in cases of secondary hemolytic anemias.

When evaluating patients with hemolytic anemia, a careful examination of the blood smear is mandatory. Morphologic abnormalities pathognomonic for or highly suggestive of a particular cause are often detected (see Table 23-2). The sample should be evaluated for autoagglutination by placing a large drop of blood on a glass slide at both room temperature and at 4°C; agglutination can be distinguished from rouleau formation by diluting the blood 1:1 in saline solution (this procedure disaggregates rouleaux). A direct Coombs' test to detect red blood cell-bound immunoglobulins should always be performed in dogs and cats with suspected hemolysis. The presence of immunoglobulin coating the red blood cells is a good indication that there is immune-mediated hemolysis. A positive Coombs' test should be interpreted with caution, as certain drugs and hemoparasites can result in the formation of antibodies that bind to the red blood cells (see Table 23-6), thus causing secondary immune-mediated hemolysis. The clinician should be familiar with the dilutions (i.e., titers) of the Coombs' test used by referral laboratories, since minimally positive titers may range from 1:16 to 1:64.

If a causative agent cannot be identified (e.g., red blood cell parasite, drug), the patient should be treated for primary or idiopathic IHA, pending further test results (e.g; titers for hemoparasites). As mentioned above, primary immunohemolytic

Table 23-6 Causes of hemolytic anemia in dogs and cats

Disorder	Species	Breed
Congenital (inherited?)		
Pyruvate kinase deficiency	Dog	Basenji, beagle
Phosphofructokinase deficiency	Dog	English springer spaniel
Anemia/chondrodysplasia	Dog	Alaskan Malamute
Nonspherocytic hemolytic anemia	Dog	Poodles, beagles
Acquired		
Immunohemolytic anemia	Dog more than cat	All
Microangiopathic hemolytic anemia	Dog more than cat	All
Infectious	Cat more than dog	All
Hemobartonellosis		
Babesiosis	Dog more than cat	All
Cytauxzoonosis	Cat	All
Ehrlichiosis	Dog	All
Hypophosphatemia	Dog, cat	All
Oxidants		
Acetaminophen	Cat	All
Phenothiazines	Dog, cat	All
Benzocaine	Cat	All
Vitamin K	Dog, Cat	All
Methylene blue	Cat more than dog	All
Methionine	Cat	All
Zinc	Dog	All
Drugs that can cause immune-mediated hemolysis		
Sulfas	Dog more than cat	Doberman, labrador retriever
Anticonvulsants	Dog	All
Penicillins and cephalosporins	Dog more than cat	All
Propylthiouracil	Cat	
Methimazole	Cat	
Antiarrhythmics?	Dog	

anemia is considerably more common in dogs than in cats, so every effort should be made to identify a cause such as drugs or hemoparasites in the feline.

The treatment of choice for primary immune-mediated hemolytic anemia is based on the use of immunosuppressive dosages of corticosteroids (equivalent to 2 to 4 mg/kg of prednisone once to twice a day in a dog, and up to 8 mg/kg once to twice a day in the cat).[3a] Although dexamethasone can be used initially to induce remission, it should not be used for prolonged periods as maintenance therapy, due to its potential to cause gastrointestinal ulceration and pancreatitis, and because it cannot be used for alternate-day therapy (i.e., it still results in interference with the hypothalamic-pituitary-adrenal axis). A high percentage of cases thus treated improve dramatically within 24 to 96 hours (Fig. 23-1). Corticosteroids act by three different mechanisms: suppression of

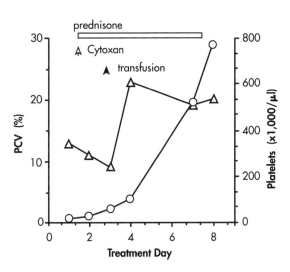

Fig. 23-1 Hematologic response in a 7-year-old, female, spayed dog with Evan's syndrome (immunohemolytic anemia and thrombocytopenia) treated with corticosteroids and cyclophosphamide.

the mononuclear phagocytic system, decrease of complement and antibody binding to the cells, and suppression of immunoglobulin production.[3b] The first two are rapid in onset (hours), while the latter is delayed (1 to 3 weeks).[3b]

We have observed an increasing number of dogs with acute Coombs' positive immunohemolytic anemia associated with icterus, that deteriorate rapidly (e.g., thromboembolism of the liver, lungs, and kidneys) despite the aggressive use of corticosteroids. In these cases, we recommend using cyclophosphamide (Cytoxan, Mead Johnson), at a dose of 200 to 300 mg/m^2 intravenously as a single dose administered over 5 to 10 minutes. We also advocate the use of heparin as a prophylactic measure (dogs with hemolysis are at high risk for disseminated intravascular coagulation). We routinely use mini-dose (5 to 10 IU/kg subcutaneously three times a day) or low-dose heparin (100 to 200 IU/kg subcutaneously three times a day). These dosages of heparin usually do not result in therapy-related prolongations of the activated clotting time or activated partial thromboplastin time, tests used routinely to monitor heparinization.[4] If there is evidence of thromboembolism, we recommend using high-dose heparin (700 to 1,000 IU/kg subcutaneously three times a day), or a dosage that will result in prolongation of the activated clotting time to 2.5 times normal. If excessive bleeding from overzealous heparinization occurs, intravenous protamine sulfate can be administered by slow intravenous infusion (1 mg for each 100 IU of the last dose of heparin; 50% of the calculated dose is given 1 hour after the heparin, and 25% 2 hours after the heparin). The remainder of the protamine sulfate dose can be administered if clinically indicated. Protamine sulfate should be administered with caution, since it can be associated with acute anaphylaxis in dogs. Aggressive fluid therapy should be used in conjunction with these treatments, realizing that, depending on the degree of anemia, hemodilution may be detrimental to the patient.

Drugs used for maintenance treatment of dogs with immunohemolytic anemia include prednisone (1 mg/kg orally every other day) and azathioprine (Imuran, Burroughs Welcome) (50 mg/m^2 orally once daily to once every other day), used either singly or in combination. Azathioprine is associated with few side effects, although close hematologic monitoring is necessary because of its potential to cause bone marrow suppression. Should myelosuppression occur, dosage reduction is necessary.

Alternative approaches used in the treatment of patients with refractory immunohemolytic anemia include the use of therapeutic plasmapheresis, danazol (Danacrine, Winthrop) (5 mg/kg to 10 mg/kg, twice to three times a day), and possibly splenectomy.[5-7] Splenectomy has never been of benefit in dogs with immunohemolytic anemia treated by us.

The biggest dilemma the clinician faces when treating a patient with immunohemolytic anemia is whether to administer a transfusion of blood or blood products. As a general rule, a transfusion should not be withheld if it represents a life-saving procedure. Patients with immunohemolytic anemia are already destroying their own antibody-coated red blood cells; therefore, they are also prone to destroying transfused red blood cells. Our recommendation is to administer a transfusion in any patient with immunohemolytic anemia that is "in dire need of red blood cells" (i.e., withholding a transfusion would result in the patient's death). We usually use pretreatment with dexamethasone sodium phosphate (0.5 to 1 mg/kg intravenously), administer fluids through an additional intravenous catheter, and continue the heparin therapy. Oxygen therapy can also be used if deemed necessary. Although cross matching is indicated (see Chapter 34), time is usually of the essence, so type A negative blood that is not cross matched is generally administered in animals not previously transfused. There is no rule-of-thumb (e.g., packed cell volume, lack of response to oxygen therapy) about when to transfuse a patient. The clinician should use his/her best clinical judgment to determine when a transfusion of blood or blood products is necessary. For further information, refer to Chapter 34.

Hemolytic anemias not associated with immune destruction of the red blood cells are treated by removal of the cause (i.e., drug, infectious agent) and supportive therapy. Corticosteroids can be administered to suppress mononuclear phagocytic system activity while the causative agent is removed. Tetracycline is used in dogs and cats with hemobartonellosis and in dogs with ehrlichiosis, at a dose of 20 to 25 mg/kg orally three times a day for 14 to 21 days.

Nonregenerative anemias. Patients with nonregenerative anemias rarely present as emergencies, given the chronic course of these disorders. However, the emergency clinician is occasionally faced with dogs and cats with chronic anemia in which the owners have just noticed the pallor after their pets were symptomatic for days or weeks. Moreover, two other forms of acute nonregenerative anemia may present as emergencies: acute blood loss (first 24 to 96 hours) and immunohemolytic anemia with delayed regeneration.[8]

When evaluating dogs and cats with nonregenerative anemias of acute onset, the clinician should try to answer the following questions:

- Does this patient have acute blood loss or hemolytic anemia and has not yet been able to mount a regenerative response (i.e., less than 48 to 96 hours from the event)?
- Does this patient have acute leukemia causing myelophthisis and cytopenias?
- Does this patient have pure red blood cell aplasia?
- Does this patient have chronic anemia, but is now symptomatic due to intercurrent disease (e.g., heart failure, sepsis)?

If the answer to the questions listed above is no, then the patient should be treated symptomatically and should probably receive packed red blood cell transfusion(s). Remember that one of the mechanisms of adaptation to chronic hypoxia (e.g., anemia) is the increase in the intraerythrocytic 2,3-diphosphoglycerate (2,3-DPG) concentration, resulting in lower oxygen affinity for hemoglobin (i.e., the delivery of oxygen to the tissues is facilitated). Since stored red blood cells have lower levels of 2,3-DPG, the transfused cells have a higher affinity for oxygen. As a consequence of this, transfusion of stored blood to a patient with chronic anemia may result in transient decompensation, since transfused stored red blood cells can regain 50% of the normal 2,3-DPG concentrations within 24 hours.[9] A detailed discussion of transfusion therapy can be found in Chapter 34.

Bleeding disorders

Bleeding disorders may be the primary reason for a client to seek emergency care for an animal, or bleeding disorders may occur as complicating factors of already existing systemic illnesses. Bleeding disorders can be classified as primary, secondary, or mixed (i.e., combination of primary and secondary). As our knowledge of primary diseases and our ability for therapeutic intervention increases, patient treatment is often limited by secondary disorders such as hemostatic abnormalities. Awareness of disease conditions associated with hemostatic abnormalities and rapid recognition and intervention in cases in which imbalance of the hemostatic system has occurred is necessary by all primary care clinicians.

Primary hemostasis

Pathophysiology. Primary hemostasis involves the initial interactions between the vessel wall and the platelets, culminating in a short-lived, unstable primary hemostatic plug. Following injury, sympathetic-mediated vasoconstriction occurs to slow blood flow. Exposure of the subendothelial components results in platelet adherence with the von Willebrand's factor (factor VIII-R:Ag) acting as a bridging molecule between the

endothelium and the platelet to enhance adherence. Following adherence, platelets release bioactive factors (for example, adenosine diphosphate, serotonin, epinephrine) that recruit more platelets for aggregation.[10-12] The aggregated platelet plug serves as a surface on which secondary hemostasis occurs. The aggregated platelets expose various phospholipids (for example, platelet factor-3) important in the common coagulation pathway) and synthesize thromboxane A_2 (a potent mediator of further vasoconstriction and platelet aggregation).[10,11,13]

Clinical and laboratory evaluation. There are tests to evaluate primary hemostatic disorders. However, only a few are applicable in an emergency care facility. Platelets are the component most often affected in primary hemostatic disorders. Quantitative platelet disorders can be detected by performing platelet counts. In an emergency facility, examination of a blood smear can rapidly determine if significant thrombocytopenia is present.[14] One should first examine the feathered edge for the presence of platelet clumps to detect artifactually decreased platelet numbers. Under an oil immersion lens, a monolayer field (where the erythrocytes are in a monolayer and 50% are touching) should be evaluated to make an estimate of platelet numbers. Each platelet in the field represents approximately 15,000 platelets/μl. Normal numbers are approximately 11 to 25 platelets per field.[14] The clinician should also evaluate platelet size, looking for macroplatelets, which may indicate a regenerative platelet response or a bone marrow disturbance.[14,15] Actual platelet counts can be obtained using automated or manual methods. Feline platelet numbers are best determined by manual means.

The bleeding time evaluates the entire primary hemostatic system (i.e., vessel wall and platelets) and is the most readily available test of vascular and platelet function. Platelet aggregation in response to low concentrations of aggregating agents is a much more sophisticated test of platelet function but is usually available only at referral and specialty hospitals. The bleeding time is subject to wide variations in technique. In an attempt to standardize this useful procedure, we use a commercial bleeding time template (Surgicutt; International Technidyne Corp.; Edison, NJ) to create a wound of standard size and depth on the buccal mucosa (Fig. 23-2).[16] The blood welling up from the incision is blotted away with a tissue (being careful not to touch the wound) and the time to cessation of bleeding is noted. For dogs, the normal bleeding time is 2.6 ± 0.5 minutes. Cats are lightly sedated with ketamine, and the bleeding time test is performed as in the dog; normal bleeding times in cats are 1.9 ± 0.5 min-

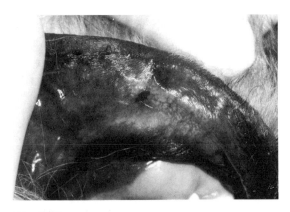

Fig. 23-2 Demonstration of mucosal bleeding time in a dog.

Table 23-7 Clinical features that characterize primary and secondary hemostatic disorders

Platelet Abnormalities	Coagulation Abnormalities
Petechiae/ecchymoses common	Petechiae/ecchymoses rare
Hematomas rare	Hematomas common
Bleeding at mucosal membranes	Bleeding into muscles, joints, and body cavities
Bleeding from multiple sites	

utes.[17] An alternative test is the nailbed bleeding time. Using a Resco nail trimmer, the nail is trimmed back to the quick so that blood wells from the wound. The time to cessation of bleeding is noted.[18,19] This technique is subject to marked variation. Normal bleeding times are 2 to 8 minutes.[18,19] Another crude test of platelet function is observation of clot retraction due to contraction of platelet thrombosthenin. This test is also partly dependent on fibrinogen concentration and may be affected by hypofibrinogenemia.

Clinical signs of primary hemostatic disorders include petechiae, ecchymoses, and mucosal bleeding at multiple sites (e.g., gastrointestinal bleeding such as hematochezia, melena, and hematemesis; epistaxis; and hematuria). Primary and secondary bleeding disorders can usually be distinguished on physical examination, since patients with primary hemostatic defects have primarily petechiae and ecchymoses, while patients with secondary defects have deep bleeding (e.g., hematomas) (Table 23-7).[11]

A classification of primary hemostatic disorders is presented in the box on p. 367. Because vascular disorders are extremely uncommon, they will not be discussed here. Quantitative platelet disorders (i.e., thrombocytopenia) are the most common cause of spontaneous bleeding in the dog.[11,20] Thrombocytopenia may result from decreased production or increased destruction or sequestration of platelets. The diagnostic approach to the patient with thrombocytopenia can be difficult due to the numerous disorders that result in low platelet counts.[11] Qualitative platelet disorders can be either hereditary or acquired, and are rare (see box on p. 367).

Clinical signs of bleeding (e.g., petechiae, ecchymoses, hematuria, epistaxis) do not occur until the platelet count is under 35,000/µl, though bleeding may occur at higher platelet counts if concomitant thrombocytopathia or a coagulopathy is present.[21,22] The secondary hemostatic mechanisms should be evaluated in patients with thrombocytopenia and spontaneous bleeding to exclude disseminated intravascular coagulation or concurrent vitamin K antagonist rodenticide poisoning (see Chapter 27).

If the secondary hemostatic mechanisms are normal, a bone marrow aspiration or biopsy is next indicated to evaluate megakaryocyte numbers (although published values are variable, we consider three to five megakaryocytes per smear to be normal). Megakaryocytic hypoplasia may be secondary to myeloproliferative or lymphoproliferative disease (i.e., myelophthisis), immune mechanisms, estrogen-secreting tumors, drug therapy, or chronic rickettsial disease; it can also be idiopathic. Normal to increased numbers of megakaryocytes in thrombocytopenic patients are suggestive of platelet sequestration, or increased utilization and destruction of platelets. Sequestration may be secondary to hepatomegaly or splenomegaly, or to "sticky" endothelial cells and platelets, as is seen in endotoxemia.[3b] Causes of increased utilization and destruction include disseminated intravascular coagulation and microangiopathy, immune-mediated, infectious (e.g., rickettsial), and drug-mediated thrombocytopenia.

When evaluating a patient with a presumed platelet function defect (i.e., normal platelet numbers but prolonged bleeding times), several factors need to be investigated. The drug history should be carefully appraised. In an emergency situation, the owner often neglects to mention the aspirin given several days ago, the vaccines or antibiotics given by another veterinarian, or other drugs the pet may have received.[10,11] A variety of disease states may cause platelet dysfunction and may be recognized from the physical examination or clinical tests. These include myeloproliferative or lymphoproliferative disorders, renal failure, se-

CAUSES OF PRIMARY BLEEDING DISORDERS IN SMALL ANIMALS

Vasculopathies
  Vasculitis
  Hyperadrenocorticism
  Ehlers-Danlos syndrome
Quantitative platelet disorders
  Decreased platelet production
    Immune-mediated megakaryocytic hypoplasia
    Idiopathic bone marrow aplasia
    Drug-induced megakaryocytic hypoplasia (e.g., estrogens)
    Myeloproliferative disorder
    Cyclic thrombocytopenia
    Myelofibrosis
  Increased platelet destruction and sequestration
    Immune-mediated thrombocytopenia (immune thrombocytopenic purpura, systemic lupus erythematosus, autoimmune hemolytic anemia)
    Live-virus-vaccine-induced thrombocytopenia
    Drug-induced thrombocytopenia
    Microangiopathy
    Disseminated intravascular coagulation
    Hemolytic uremic syndrome
    Vasculitis
    Splenomegaly
    Splenic torsion
    Endotoxemia
    Heparin-induced thrombocytopenia
    Acute hepatic necrosis
    Neoplasia (immune-mediated, microangiopathy)
Qualitative platelet disorders
  Hereditary
    von Willebrand's disease (many breeds)
    Canine thrombasthenic thrombopathia (otterhounds)
    Canine thrombopathia (basset hounds)
    Collagen deficiency diseases (Ehlers-Danlos syndrome)
  Acquired
    Drugs (prostaglandin inhibitors, antibiotics, heparin, phenothiazines, membrane active drugs)
    Secondary to disease states (myeloproliferative disorders, SLE, renal disease, liver disease, dysproteinemias)

vere liver disease, and multiple myeloma. If no cause for platelet dysfunction can be found, a hereditary disorder such as von Willebrand's disease (wide variety of breeds),[23] canine thrombasthenic thrombopathia (otterhounds),[24] canine thrombopathia (basset hounds),[25] or a collagen deficiency disorder such as Ehlers-Danlos syndrome should be considered.[10,11] The reader should be aware

that there is some evidence that the drug desmopressin acetate (DDAVP, USV Pharmaceutical), may have some beneficial clinical effect in Doberman pinschers with von Willebrand's disease who are actively bleeding.[26,27] Administration of 1 μg/kg subcutaneously has been reported to control postoperative bleeding in these patients.

Secondary hemostasis

Pathophysiology. Secondary hemostasis involves the circulating coagulation factors and results in the formation of a stable fibrin clot. The synthesis of fibrin is the result of a cascade of enzymatic reactions, many of which occur on the "activated" platelet surface and are capable of amplifying the initial event. The liver is responsible for synthesis of most of the clotting factors and anticoagulant proteins (including antithrombin III and proteins C and S) except calcium, factor VIII, and von Willebrand factor (the latter is apparently synthesized by the endothelial cells; the site of synthesis of factor VIII remains unknown).[27a] Vitamin K is necessary for the synthesis of factors II, VII, IX, and X and proteins C and S. Secondary hemostatic disorders can be classified as either congenital or acquired (see the box on p. 368).

There are two traditional pathways for activation of the coagulation cascade: intrinsic and extrinsic. Activation of the extrinsic pathway begins with release of tissue thromboplastin from damaged endothelium, damaged tissues, or hemolyzed red blood cells activating factor VII, which in turn activates factor X (common pathway). The tissue thromboplastin-factor VII complex is also capable of activating factor IX of the intrinsic system.

The contact phase of the intrinsic pathway involves factors XII and XI and activates the intrinsic pathway through factors IX and VIII, and then the common pathway (factor X); the fibrinolytic, kinin, and complement systems are also activated by the contact phase.

Activation of the common pathway results in the formation of thrombin, which acts on fibrinogen to form fibrin monomers that polymerize to form a delicate gel. Factor XIII crosslinks and stabilizes the gel.

Just as there are complex mechanisms to control hemorrhage, there are mechanisms to prevent inappropriate activation of the hemostatic system. At the vessel surface, heparan sulfate and glycocalyx repel platelets. Endothelial cells synthesize prostacyclin (PGI_2), which inhibits platelet aggregation. Thrombomodulin is also present at the endothelial surface and inhibits thrombin action, by reversibly binding to it.[27b] The thrombomodulin-thrombin complex activates protein C to a protease, which in conjunction with protein S specif-

CAUSES OF SECONDARY BLEEDING DISORDERS IN SMALL ANIMALS

Congenital coagulation defects
   Factor I hypofibrinogenemia & dysfibrinogenemia
      (St. Bernards and borzois)
   Factor II hypoprothrombinemia (boxers)
   Factor VII hypoproconvertinemia (beagles and
      malamutes)
   Factor VIII hemophilia A (many breeds)
   Factor IX hemophilia B (many breeds)
   Factor X Stuart-Prower trait (cocker spaniels)
   Factor XI Hemophilia C (English springer spaniels,
      Great Pyrenees, Kerry blue terrier)
   Factor XII Hageman factor (many breeds)
Acquired coagulation defects
   Liver disease
      Decreased production of factors
      Qualitative disorders
   Antithrombin III deficiency
      Nephrotic syndrome
      Disseminated intravascular coagulation
      Liver disease
      Heparin-induced
   Vitamin K antagonists
   Disseminated intravascular coagulation (neoplasia,
      sepsis, feline infectious peritonitis, leptospirosis,
      dirofilariasis, babesiosis, pancreatitis, shock, heat
      stroke, autoimmune hemolytic anemia, acute
      hepatic necrosis, gastric dilatation-volvulus,
      trauma)

ically inactivates the accelerating factors of coagulation—factors V and VIII.[28] Another element that regulates the extent of a local hemostatic response is blood flow. Adequate blood flow carries the activated components away to the liver, where they are metabolized.

Specific inhibitors of coagulation factors represent one of the main control mechanisms of hemostasis. Antithrombin III (ATIII) is the main "monkey wrench" capable of shutting down the fibrin synthesis factory complex on the platelet surface.[29] The liver is the primary site of synthesis of ATIII. ATIII can inhibit factors IX, X, XI, XII, and thrombin. ATIII's action is markedly potentiated by binding to heparin of either endogenous or exogenous origin.[29,30] Other inhibitory proteins include alpha$_2$-macroglobulin, alpha$_1$-antitrypsin, and C1-esterase inhibitor.

The final phase of hemostasis is fibrinolysis. During this phase, plasminogen is converted by tissue plasminogen activator and activation of the intrinsic pathway to plasmin. Plasmin cleaves fibrin and fibrinogen and inactivates factors V and

VIII. Usually plasminogen is incorporated within the clot so dissolution occurs from within as well as from the surface of the clot. Alpha$_2$-antiplasmin circulates to inhibit free plasmin and to prevent systemic fibrinolytic activity. The fibrinogen/fibrin fragments released during the fibrinolytic process are termed fibrinogen/fibrin degradation products. They are capable of decreasing platelet plug formation, fibrin polymerization, and thrombin activity, and as such are potent anticoagulants.

Clinical and laboratory evaluation. In emergencies, the following laboratory tests to evaluate hemostatic function should be accessible: activated clotting time, Thrombo-Wellcotest for FDPs (Wellcome Research Laboratory; Beckenham, England), and evaluation of the blood smear for fragmented erythrocytes (schistocytes). Additional tests include the activated partial thromboplastin time, the one-stage prothrombin time, and the plasma fibrinogen concentration. Fig. 23-3 illustrates the portions of the coagulation cascade each test evaluates.

Proper collection of blood samples for evaluation of hemostasis is vital to prevent misleading results. This includes an atraumatic venipuncture to prevent tissue factors from contaminating the sample (the APTT is particularly sensitive); sample collection into citrated siliconized glass or plastic tubes (except for FDP determinations and platelet counts); and using the proper blood-to-anticoagulant ratio (i.e., one part 3.8% citrate to nine parts blood). With proper handling, samples can be frozen for shipment or delayed analysis.

The presence of schistocytes (fragmented red blood cells) in blood smears is highly suggestive of microangiopathic hemolysis. Abnormalities in the microvasculature may result from disseminated intravascular coagulation or microvascular anomalies in neoplastic tissues (e.g., hemangiosarcoma). Red blood cells are sliced by the fibrin strands or endothelial abnormalities and the fragments reseal. Schistocytes are not exclusively seen in microangiopathic hemolysis and can be seen in Heinz body anemia, iron deficiency anemia, heartworm disease, structural defects of the heart and great vessels, and hyposplenism or asplenia. A quantitative technique for evaluating red blood cell morphology has been previously described in this chapter (see Table 23-4).

The activated partial thromboplastin time (APTT) evaluates the intrinsic and common pathways. Prolongation of the APTT is caused by contact phase defects (factors XI or XII, in which clinical bleeding is unlikely), factor VIII or IX deficiencies, common pathway defects, and hepa-

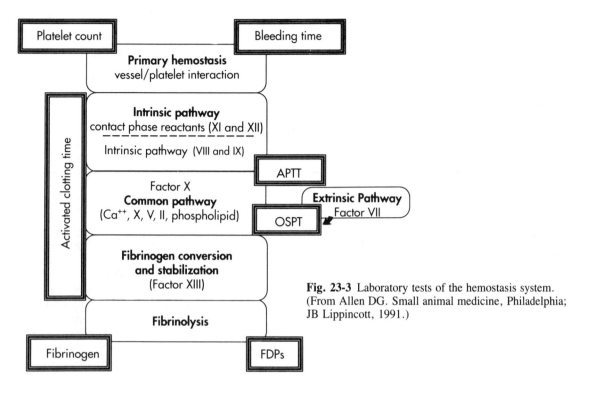

Fig. 23-3 Laboratory tests of the hemostasis system. (From Allen DG. Small animal medicine, Philadelphia; JB Lippincott, 1991.)

rin therapy. Factor concentration must be decreased to at least 30% of normal before prolongation of tests occurs.

The one-stage prothrombin time (OSPT) evaluates the extrinsic system and is prolonged in congenital or acquired factor VII deficiencies (e.g., liver disease, vitamin K deficiency). Common pathway defects also result in prolongation of the OSPT, but heparin administration usually does not. Prolongations of 25% over the control should be considered to be abnormal for both APTT and OSPT.[31]

Plasmin's action on fibrinogen/fibrin results in the release of various cleavage fragments termed fibrinogen/fibrin degradation products (FDPs). These can be measured using commercial kits with latex particles coated with anti-FDP antibody (Thrombo-Wellcotest, Burroughs Wellcome). Minor elevations of FDP concentrations may occur in many disease states and are not always diagnostic of disseminated intravascular coagulation. In general, FDP concentrations greater than 10 μg/dl are indicative of pathologic fibrinolysis.[32]

The activated clotting time provides a rapid evaluation of the intrinsic and common pathways. Two milliliters of blood are added to a tube containing diatomaceous earth (Becton Dickinson Tube no. 6522) to activate the clotting cascade. The sample is incubated at 37°C for 60 seconds and then evaluated every 5 seconds until clotting occurs. Normal clotting times are 60 to 125 seconds in the dog and cat.[33] Prolongation may occur from intrinsic or common pathway defects and severe hypofibrogenemia. It should be noted that mini-dose heparin (10 IU/kg) does not prolong the activated clotting time. The activated clotting time is a more sensitive test than the older Lee-White clotting time, which evaluates the time needed for clot formation to occur, when blood is placed in a plain glass tube (reference range; 6 to 7.5 minutes in the dog, and 8 minutes in the cat).[33] Observation of blood left in plastic syringes may lead to falsely prolonged clotting time due to the lack of activation of the contact phase reactants by the plastic.

Approach to the bleeding patient. The emergency treatment of a patient with a bleeding disorder is directed at halting or slowing the flow of blood, and at collecting appropriate blood samples for diagnostic purposes prior to instituting any therapy. The use of blood component therapy in patients with spontaneous bleeding disorders is discussed in Chapter 34. Supportive measures such as oxygen, pericardiocentesis, and removing blood (with or without autotransfusion) from the pleural or abdominal cavities may also be necessary.

The clinical signs of primary and secondary hemostatic disorders are listed in Table 23-7. The physical examination can be extremely helpful in

Table 23-8 Rapid classification of bleeding disorders

	Bleeding Time	Activated Clotting Time	Platelet Count	FDPs or Fragmented RBC
Warfarin toxicity	N	↑	N to ↓	Negative to positive
Thrombocytopenia	↑	N to slight ↑	↓	Negative to positive
Disseminated intravascular coagulation	↑	↑	↓	Positive
von Willebrand's disease	↑	N	N	Negative
Hemophilia	N	↑	N	Negative
Platelet dysfunction	↑	N	N	Negative

N = normal; ↑ = prolonged or increased; ↓ = shortened or decreased.

rapidly determining whether the bleeding disorder is of primary, secondary, or combined origin. Combined primary and secondary bleeding disorders (e.g., disseminated intravascular coagulation) are relatively common in the dog and can be life threatening. Two concurrent primary and secondary hemostatic disorders could also result in a similar situation (e.g., immune-mediated thrombocytopenia and warfarin toxicity).

Five simple "cageside" tests that can rapidly assess which aspect(s) of the hemostatic system are disrupted and what further tests/therapy are needed include: the bleeding time, activated clotting time, platelet count (or estimation from blood smear), FDPs, and examination of the blood smear for fragmented red blood cells (Table 23-8).

Immune-mediated thrombocytopenia. Idiopathic immune-mediated thrombocytopenia is probably the most common cause of spontaneous bleeding in dogs.[10,11,20,32,34] It affects primarily middle-aged female dogs, with toy breeds and Old English Sheepdogs being overrepresented.[34] Clinical signs include petechiae, ecchymoses, and superficial bleeding; if bleeding is pronounced, acute collapse may occur. The complete blood count in patients with immune-mediated thrombocytopenia is characterized by thrombocytopenia with or without anemia (depending on the degree of spontaneous bleeding); leukocytosis with a left shift may be present. Bone marrow cytology is usually characterized by megakaryocytic hyperplasia, although in rare instances, megakaryocytic hypoplasia may be present.[35] When immunohemolytic anemia is associated with immune-mediated thrombocytopenia (i.e., Evan's syndrome), a Coombs'-positive, extremely regenerative anemia with spherocytosis is present. In addition to the thrombocytopenia, the bleeding time is the only other laboratory test that commonly provides abnormal results (i.e., activated clotting time, APTT, OSPT, FDPs, and fibrinogen concentration are generally normal).

Canine ehrlichiosis, drug-induced thrombocyto-penia, disseminated intravascular coagulation and infectious thrombocytopenia *(Ehrlichia platys)* should be ruled out before establishing a diagnosis of immune-mediated thrombocytopenia. When the index of suspicion for immune-mediated thrombocytopenia is high, a therapeutic trial with immunosuppressive dosages of corticosteroids (equivalent to 2 to 8 mg/kg per day of prednisone) should be instituted. Responses are usually seen within 48 to 96 hours. Fresh whole blood is administered as needed to maintain oxygen-carrying capacity. In addition to immunosuppressive doses of corticosteroids, cyclophosphamide (as a single dose of 200 to 300 mg/m^2 intravenously) can be used for induction of remission. Azathioprine (Imuran, Wellcome) (50 mg/m^2 orally once a day to once every other day) is also indicated to maintain remission; in some dogs, azathioprine is better tolerated than long-term administration of corticosteroids. The androgenic steroid danazol (5 mg/kg to 10 mg/kg orally twice to three a day) has received recent attention as a potential therapy in immune-mediated thrombocytopenia.[36]

Vitamin K deficiency. Vitamin K deficiency in small animals is usually the result of ingestion of vitamin K antagonists (warfarin, diphacinone, or their derivatives, brodifacoum and bromadoline). If ingestion has occurred minutes to a few hours prior to presentation, inducing vomiting may remove most of the toxin. Due to the increased potency and slower metabolism of the newer vitamin K antagonists, it is often necessary to administer vitamin K for several weeks to control spontaneous bleeding.[37] If the ingestion of anticoagulant rodenticides is questionable and there are no clinical signs suggestive of coagulopathy (e.g., hemothorax, hemoabdomen), evaluation of the OSPT is recommended. Factor VII is the shortest-lived vitamin K-dependent protein (circulating half-life of 4 to 6 hours) and prolongation of the OSPT usually occurs before spontaneous bleeding becomes evident. Newer tests for proteins induced by vitamin K absence (PIVKA) may soon be commercially available and may aid in the early diagnosis of rodenticide toxicity.[38]

Most patients present with acute collapse and no history of rodenticide ingestion. These patients usually have clinical signs compatible with secondary bleeding, such as hematomas and bleeding into body cavities; other abnormalities include pale mucous membranes, anemia (usually regenerative if sufficient time has elapsed since the acute bleeding episode), and hypoproteinemia (which returns to normal values shortly after internal hemorrhage). Sudden death may occur due to central nervous system or pericardial hemorrhage.

Treatment of these patients may require immediate fresh whole blood or fresh frozen plasma transfusions for repletion of coagulation factors, as parenteral vitamin K may take 12 hours before an appreciable decrease in the OSPT and subsequent increased coagulability are seen. When animals severely depleted of coagulation factors are treated with vitamin K alone, it may take up to 48 hours for the OSPT to return to reference ranges.[37]

Vitamin K is available in several forms, with vitamin K_1 being the most effective. Vitamin K_3 (menadione) is less expensive but also appears to be a less effective antidote. Vitamin K_3 should not be used as the sole antidote in a rodenticide intoxicated animal. Vitamin K_1 is available for oral or parenteral use. Intravenous administration of vitamin K is not recommended due to the risk of anaphylactic reactions. Intramuscular injections in a dog with a coagulopathy usually result in hematoma formation. Subcutaneous administration of vitamin K_1 using a 25-gauge needle (loading dose of 5 mg/kg followed in 8 hours by 2.5 mg/kg subcutaneously divided three times a day) is preferred if the patient is properly hydrated. If the patient is stable and not vomiting after the first injection, vitamin K_1 may be given orally (2.5 mg/kg divided three times a day). Being liposoluble, vitamin K absorption is enhanced when given with fatty meals; animals with cholestatic or malabsorptive syndromes may require continued subcutaneous injections. In critical cases, the OSPT should be monitored every 8 hours until it normalizes.

If the anticoagulant is known to be warfarin or another first-generation hydroxycoumarin, 1 week of oral vitamin K_1 is sufficient. However, if the poison is not known, or if it is indandione or any of the second-generation anticoagulants, oral vitamin K_1 must be given for at least 3 weeks. The animals must be examined and an OSPT evaluated within 48 to 72 hours of cessation of vitamin K_1 therapy. If the OSPT is prolonged at that time, therapy should be reinstituted for another 2 weeks and the OSPT reevaluated.

Disseminated intravascular coagulation. Disseminated intravascular coagulation (DIC) (consumptive coagulopathy, defibrination syndrome) refers to the intravascular activation of the coagulation factors with resultant microcirculatory thromboembolism and attendant organ failure.[39] Depletion of clotting factors and platelets also leads to spontaneous bleeding episodes; the bleeding is due to abnormalities in both the primary (i.e., vessels and platelets) and secondary (i.e., coagulation factors) hemostatic systems. Organs affected by the thromboembolic process include brain, lungs, liver, kidneys, and intestines, among others. As fibrinolysis occurs, FDPs are produced, further adding to the coagulopathy by inhibiting platelet function and coagulation.[39] A paradoxical situation arises whereby what started out as excessive coagulation in the microcirculation, rapidly becomes a bleeding disorder due to the intravascular enzymatic degradation of the clotting precursors by active plasmin and the negative influence of the circulating FDPs.[39]

There are numerous causes of disseminated intravascular coagulation in animals (discussed below); however, most cases of spontaneous disseminated intravascular coagulation are multifactorial in nature. Activation of the contact phase of the intrinsic pathway by particulate or colloidal materials, endothelial damage, or antibody-antigen complexes constitutes one mechanism. Vasculitis, hemangiosarcoma, immune-mediated hemolytic anemia, sepsis, and feline infectious peritonitis are thought to initiate disseminated intravascular coagulation by this mechanism. The extrinsic pathway can be activated by massive release of thromboplastin, as often occurs in widespread neoplasia, hemolysis, tissue damage, necrosis, surgery, and endotoxemia. Finally, prothrombin may be directly activated by enzymes such as trypsin; this mechanism is believed to play a role in disseminated intravascular coagulation associated with pancreatitis.

The secondary "enhancers" of disseminated intravascular coagulation are no less important in the propagation of the disorder.[40] Decreased ATIII levels associated with liver disease, nephrotic syndrome, hereditary ATIII deficiencies, disseminated intravascular coagulation itself, and L-asparaginase therapy may potentiate (and self-perpetuate) disseminated intravascular coagulation. Acidosis and hypoxia inhibit ATIII and increase endothelial damage. Decreased blood flow, as occurs in shock, decreases removal of activated factors and exacerbates local acidosis and hypoxia. The mononuclear phagocytic system can be overwhelmed by soluble complexes and particulate matter resulting in inadequate removal of enzymes, FDPs, antigen-antibody complexes, cell fragments, and endotoxins. Severe liver disease may result in decreased removal of these complexes, also potentiating disseminated intravascular coagulation.

The clinical signs of disseminated intravascular coagulation can vary from thromboembolic events (e.g., renal and liver failure, neurologic signs, pulmonary thromboembolism, and intestinal infarcts) to hemorrhages (e.g., petechiae, ecchymosis, immediate or delayed bleeding from venipuncture sites, epistaxis, gastrointestinal hemorrhages, and hematoma formation). The diagnosis of acute (or fulminant) disseminated intravascular coagulation is usually easily made, but the diagnosis of chronic (or subclinical) disseminated intravascular coagulation may be more difficult. All the clinical and laboratory findings must be evaluated to make the diagnosis. Platelet consumption appears to be a constant feature in disseminated intravascular coagulation, and thrombocytopenia is almost invariably present. Fibrinogen levels are greatly decreased in acute DIC but can be elevated in chronic DIC due to compensatory overproduction. The APTT and OSPT may or may not be prolonged; however, the APTT is the more likely to be prolonged. Finding significant elevation of FDP concentrations is probably the most specific test for diagnosing DIC. However, significant liver disease may falsely elevate the FDPs due to poor clearance. Finally, a negative FDP test does not necessarily eliminate DIC from consideration. Schistocytes in the blood smear constitute a significant finding, although they are not specific for DIC. The ATIII levels are usually low in DIC, although they are also low in other disease states previously mentioned.

The most vital step in treating DIC is to identify and remove (if possible) the underlying cause (e.g., by surgically removing a neoplasm). Correction (or modification) of the secondary enhancers of DIC is also important. The major complication in most patients with DIC is hemorrhage; in these cases, transfusion may be necessary to replenish red blood cells, platelets, coagulation factors, and ATIII (see Chapter 34). In our experience, the adage of adding fuel to the fire has not proven true. The use of mini-dose heparin (5 to 10 IU/kg three times a day subcutaneously) appears to offer a possible mode of therapy in DIC by enhancing ATIII activity, therefore inhibiting further activation of coagulation.[40-40a]

Mini-dose heparin does not cause prolongation of the activated clotting time or APTT; therefore, if the activated clotting time or APTT increases during therapy, the clinician should consider worsening of the intravascular coagulation as the most likely cause. If plasma is to be administered, one dose of heparin can be added to the plasma and incubated at 37°C for 30 minutes prior to administration; this allows for interaction between the ATIII and heparin, thus resulting in prompt activation.[40a] Adequate administration of intravenous fluids, adjustments of blood pH, and correction of hypoxia are additional measures required when attempting to control DIC. The use of aspirin in acute DIC remains controversial and is currently not in wide use.

Leukemias

Leukemia is defined as a malignant proliferation of bone marrow hematopoietic precursors. These precursors can be affected at various levels, thus resulting in variable cytomorphologic features of the predominating leukemic cell. According to their origin, leukemias are classified as lymphoid or myeloid; according to their clinical course and cytomorphology, they are classified as acute or chronic. Acute leukemias are characterized by the acute onset of signs resulting from a proliferation of undifferentiated (blast) cells in the blood or bone marrow; if untreated, they result in death of the patient in a short time (days to weeks). Conversely, chronic leukemias are usually insidious disorders in which the predominant blood and bone marrow cell is well differentiated (i.e., neutrophil, mature lymphocyte). Dogs and cats with acute leukemias are more likely to present to the emergency room than patients with chronic forms, given the aggressive nature of the disease or its treatment (see Complications of Anticancer Chemotherapy below). Clinical signs in dogs and cat with acute leukemia are sudden in onset (days to weeks) and may include anorexia, depression, vomiting, diarrhea, bleeding, shifting leg lameness, abdominal distention, and central nervous system signs, among others. Physical examination findings include pallor, fever, hepatosplenomegaly, mild lymphadenopathy, petechiae, and ecchymoses. Most of these signs and findings are secondary to multiple organ infiltration by the leukemic cells.[41] Occasionally, if the white blood cell count is extremely high (i.e., over 1 million cells/μl), signs of hyperviscosity may occur (hyperleukocytic syndrome).

Hematologic changes in patients with acute leukemia include anemia, neutropenia, thrombocytopenia (either singly or in combination); leukoerythroblastic reactions; and presence of blasts in circulation (usually diagnostic). When confronted with these abnormalities, a bone marrow aspirate for cytologic and cytochemical evaluations should

Table 23-9 Cytochemical characteristics of leukemic cells in the dog and cat

Cytochemical stain	ALL	AML	AMoL	AMML
Peroxidase	−	+	−	+/−
Chloroacetate esterase (CAE)	−	+/−	−	+/−
Alpha-naphthyl butyrate esterase (ANBE)	−*	−	+	+/−
Alkaline phosphatase	−/+	+/−	−	+/−
Sudan black B	−	+	−	+/−

ALL = acute lymphoblastic leukemia; AML = acute myeloblastic leukemia; AMoL = acute monocytic/monoblastic leukemia; AMML = acute myelomonocytic leukemia.
*Can stain focally positive.

be performed. Blast cells are usually quite undifferentiated, and they may be difficult to classify morphologically on a smear stained with Wright-Giemsa stain. In these cases, cytochemical stains are usually beneficial in identifying the origin of the leukemic cells (Table 23-9). It is important to identify the leukemic cells if the owners are contemplating therapy, since the treatment used for acute myeloid leukemias (AML) is different than that used for acute lymphoid leukemias (ALL). The prognosis for the former is significantly worse than for the latter.[41]

Emergency treatment of the leukemic patient consists of preventing or controlling existing bleeding, preventing or controlling existing sepsis, decreasing the leukemic cell count, and correcting organ failure induced by neoplastic cells. The first two are discussed elsewhere in this chapter. The latter two are usually achieved by using intensive chemotherapy. The drug of choice to decrease leukemic cell counts rapidly in dogs and cats with acute leukemia is cytarabine (Cytosar-U, Upjohn) (100 to 200 mg/m^2 per day for 1 to 4 days). This drug is an S-phase-specific antimetabolite that kills only cycling leukemic cells. Due to its relatively short circulating half-life, it is better administered by continuous intravenous infusion. Cytarabine appears to be effective in decreasing cell counts in dogs and cats with both ALL and AML. In patients with ALL, vincristine (Oncovin, Eli Lilly) (0.5 to 0.75 mg/m^2 intravenously once a week), prednisone (40 to 60 mg/m^2 orally once a day); and cyclophosphamide (Cytoxan, Mead) (50 mg/m^2 orally every other day or 100 to 200 mg/m^2 intravenously once a week), can be added to the Cytosar-U. The addition of these drugs does not appear to be of benefit in the treatment of dogs with AML.

Erythrocytosis

Erythrocytosis refers to an increase in the circulating number of red blood cells, and is manifested hematologically as an increase in the PCV above reference values. Increased red blood cell numbers may lead to severe hemorrheologic alterations resulting in clinical signs secondary to hyperviscosity. These signs may occur acutely and manifest primarily as functional abnormalities of the central nervous system (i.e., behavioral, motor, or sensory changes). Cardiopulmonary signs may occasionally be present. Although the development of erythrocytosis is usually gradual, most patients do not exhibit clinical signs until the red blood cells have reached a critical mass (or the PCV a certain number). It is not unusual to find PCVs of 70% to 90% in dogs and cats with absolute erythrocytosis.

According to its pathogenesis, erythrocytosis can be classified as either relative or absolute.[42,43] Absolute erythrocytosis can be classified as primary or secondary, depending on the causes and the serum erythropoietin concentrations. Primary erythrocytosis (polycythemia rubra vera) results from an autonomous, erythropoietin-independent proliferation of red blood cell precursors in the bone marrow; as a consequence of this, most patients with primary erythrocytosis have low to nondetectable serum erythropoietin concentrations. Secondary erythrocytosis results from increased orthotopic or heterotopic erythropoietin production. Orthotopic erythropoietin production (i.e., physiologically appropriate) occurs in response to tissue hypoxia. Secondary erythrocytosis is encountered in adaptation to high altitude, chronic cardiopulmonary disease, cardiovascular right-to-left shunts, and in carboxyhemoglobinemia, among other causes. Tumor-associated erythrocytosis (i.e., heterotopic or orthotopic erythropoietin production) has been described in a wide variety of human neoplasms, in dogs with renal masses, and in a dog with a nasal fibrosarcoma.[44]

The initial therapeutic approach to the patient with absolute erythrocytosis involves decreasing the blood viscosity by reducing the number of circulating red blood cells. This can be accomplished by performing therapeutic phlebotomies, in which a certain volume of blood (20 ml/kg) is collected from a central vein through a blood collection set. In cats, a 19-gauge butterfly catheter coupled to a 60-ml syringe containing 500 to 600 units of heparin diluted in 3 to 5 ml of saline is usually used to collect blood from the jugular vein. Gradual phlebotomy (5 ml/kg, repeated as needed over several days) is recommended for patients with right-to-left shunts and erythrocytosis, because due to chronic hypoxemia, an increased red blood count cell mass appears to represent a compensatory mechanism to enhance oxygen delivery to the tissues. Additionally, in all patients, since sudden decreases in blood volume can result in significant hypotension, a peripheral vein catheter is used to administer an equivalent volume of saline solution simultaneously to blood collection.

Once the patient has been stabilized, the cause of the erythrocytosis should be investigated. If it is established that the patient has polycythemia rubra vera, hydroxyurea (Hydrea, Squibb) (30 mg/kg orally once a day) is administered for 7 to 10 days; subsequently, the dose and the interval of administration can be gradually decreased to fulfill the patient's needs.[43] The treatment of patients with relative erythrocytosis (i.e., dehydration) is discussed in Chapter 38.

Hyperviscosity syndromes

Normal blood viscosity is necessary to ensure proper blood flow to most tissues and organs. Different pathologic processes can increase blood viscosity by increasing the red blood cell mass (i.e., erythrocytosis), the plasma viscosity (i.e., gammopathies), or the white blood cell count (i.e., hyperleukocytic syndrome). The first two are occasionally seen in small animals, while the latter is extremely rare. Elevated whole-blood viscosity as a consequence of increased red blood cell mass is discussed in the section on "Erythrocytosis."

A marked increase in plasma viscosity usually results in hemorrheologic abnormalities (hyperviscosity syndromes).[2] This commonly occurs when there is an increased plasma concentration of molecules with high molecular weight and irregular shape, such as immunoglobulins. This situation is usually encountered in monoclonal gammopathies secondary to neoplastic disorders of the B lymphocytes, such as multiple myeloma, B-cell chronic lymphocytic leukemia, and B-cell lymphoma. It can rarely be seen in association with monoclonal gammopathies secondary to chronic infectious diseases such as canine ehrlichiosis and canine leishmaniasis.

As a general rule, the larger and more irregular the circulating molecule the higher the serum viscosity.[2] Hyperviscosity syndromes appear to be more common in IgM and IgA monoclonal gammopathies; IgG gammopathies are rarely associated with hyperviscosity syndromes. The serum or whole-blood relative viscosities can be roughly evaluated in practice by timing the flow of the fluid investigated through a small pipette (i.e., 0.5 to 1 ml) and dividing it by the time it takes

for an equal volume of water to flow through the same pipette (normal viscosity of plasma is similar to that of water). The value obtained represents the viscosity of the fluid in relation to that of water. Complex viscometers are also available in diagnostic laboratories to obtain absolute viscosity of a fluid.[2]

The clinical signs associated with hyperviscosity syndromes include functional abnormalities of the central nervous system, such as dementia, personality changes, and disorientation; ocular signs such as enlarged, tortuous retinal vessels, retinal hemorrhages and retinal detachment, which can result in acute onset of blindness; cardiopulmonary signs (i.e., exercise intolerance, syncope, cyanosis); and spontaneous bleeding due to coating of the platelets by the M component.[2,45] Abnormalities detected during physical examination are usually limited to the three organ systems discussed above, and include ocular changes, changes in the mucous membranes consistent with abnormal perfusion (i.e., brick-red color in erythrocytosis, delayed capillary refill time in other hyperviscosity syndromes), neurologic abnormalities, and evidence of primary hemostatic failure (i.e., petechiae and ecchymoses).[45]

It is extremely difficult to obtain a sample from a venipuncture site with a small-gauge needle (21 gauge or smaller) when the blood viscosity is markedly elevated. In these instances, an 18-gauge needle or larger is recommended. In cases of erythrocytosis or monoclonal gammopathies, it may be difficult to separate serum during routine centrifugation. In the former, this is due to the increased red blood cell mass, while in the latter, it results from the high-viscosity serum being entrapped among the red blood cells.

Emergency treatment of patients with hyperviscosity syndromes consists primarily of decreasing blood viscosity by removing red blood cells (in case of erythrocytosis), plasma (in case of gammopathies), or whole blood (in both). Plasmapheresis can be performed manually or with automated blood-cell separators.[46] Manual plasmapheresis is performed by collecting blood from the patient as described in the section on "Erythrocytosis"; the blood is then centrifuged at 1700 g for 30 minutes at 4° to 5°C and the plasma discarded. The packed red blood cells are resuspended in an appropriate amount of saline (or donor plasma, if available), and administered to the patient. In an emergency situation, blood collected from the patient can be discarded and replaced with packed red blood cells from a donor (suspended in saline solution).

ONCOLOGIC EMERGENCIES
Metabolic

Metabolic complications associated with neoplasia may be the underlying reason for patients to be presented to an emergency service. Often the tumor burden is low, but the patient's status is critical due to the severity of the paraneoplastic disease and the degree of metabolic derangement. Prompt recognition and correction of the metabolic abnormality usually leads to a dramatic improvement in the patient's condition.

Hypercalcemia. Hypercalcemia associated with malignancy is one of the most common paraneoplastic syndromes in small animals[47,48]; it is common in dogs and rare in cats. The increased use of automated blood chemistry analyzers has led to more frequent diagnoses of hypercalcemia and recognition of the underlying disorders. As a consequence of this, hypercalcemia has been identified as an important cause of morbidity in cancer-bearing animals. While malignancy represents the most common underlying disorder in older dogs with hypercalcemia, nonneoplastic conditions associated with this metabolic abnormality should not be ruled out until a complete evaluation has been performed.[48] For further discussion of the pathophysiology of hypercalcemia, see Chapter 18.

The clinical signs associated with hypercalcemia are nonspecific and include anorexia, vomiting, dysphagia, constipation, weight loss, muscular weakness, lethargy, polyuria/polydipsia, and depression.

Hypercalcemia has been reported in association with various neoplasms in animals, including lymphomas, anal sac adenocarcinomas, fibrosarcomas, and a variety of sarcomas and carcinomas.[49] The most common tumor types associated with hypercalcemia in dogs are lymphomas and apocrine gland adenocarcinoma of the anal sac.[48-50] Approximately 10% to 40% of dogs with lymphoma have paraneoplastic hypercalcemia.[51-53] The prevalence of hypercalcemia appears to be higher in dogs with mediastinal lymphoma than in dogs with the multicentric, alimentary, or extranodal forms. Apocrine gland adenocarcinomas of the anal sacs occur predominantly in females, in which they present as a nonulcerated perianal mass; iliac lymph node metastases are common early in the course of the disease. In cats, hypercalcemia has been associated almost exclusively with lymphoma.[54,55] We have recently evaluated two cats with hypercalcemia associated with a soft-tissue fibrosarcoma and a malignant fibrous histiocytoma, respectively.

The molecular mechanism underlying hypercalcemia of malignancy constitutes a subject of intense interest. Several mechanisms have been recognized, although not all appear to play a role in small animals. The first recognized mechanism was excessive parathormone from parathyroid hyperplasia or adenomas. A second mechanism is that of direct tumor lytic action on bone by a primary or a metastatic neoplasm. Most primary bone cancers in dogs (e.g., fibrosarcomas, osteosarcomas, chondrosarcomas) cause little or no change in serum calcium concentrations.[50] Tumors metastatic to bone in small animals are rarely associated with hypercalcemia. Markedly elevated serum levels of 1,25-dihydroxyvitamin D have been documented in human patients with lymphoma and hypercalcemia.[56-59] We have recently recognized a similar condition in two boxer dogs with mediastinal lymphomas and hypercalcemia. Transforming growth factors alpha and beta, parathyroid hormone-related protein, prostaglandins, and colony-stimulating factors are known to mediate hypercalcemia in humans and some animal models; however, their role in clinical cases is currently unknown.[60,61] Various cytokines have also been incriminated in the pathogenesis of hypercalcemia. These include osteoclast activating factor, interleukin-1, tumor necrosis factor, and lymphotoxin.[60] More than one mechanism may contribute to the development of hypercalcemia in any given case.

The pathogenesis of hypercalcemia in 34 dogs with lymphoma was investigated in two studies.[62,63] One report described subnormal immunoreactive parathyroid hormone and 1,25-dihydroxy vitamin D concentrations.[62] The other study evaluated only vitamin D concentrations, which were similar to those of normocalcemic dogs with lymphoma.[63] The mediator of hypercalcemia in these 34 dogs was not 1,25-dihydroxyvitamin D but, rather, appeared to be parathyroid hormone-related protein.

The diagnostic approach to the dog with hypercalcemia must not only be accurate, but must also be reasonably rapid in order to preserve renal function. Fortunately, the physical examination and laboratory abnormalities often lead to a presumptive diagnosis leaving only confirmatory tests to be performed. An algorithm describing the clinical approach to the hypercalcemic patient is depicted in Fig. 23-4.

Having determined the cause of the hypercalcemia, the clinician faces the question of whether to treat the patient. Parathyroid adenomas usually cause gradual serum calcium elevations and the renal function remains normal. In these cases, no medical therapy for the hypercalcemia may be needed if parathyroidectomy is performed within days. In other forms of hypercalcemia, serum cal-

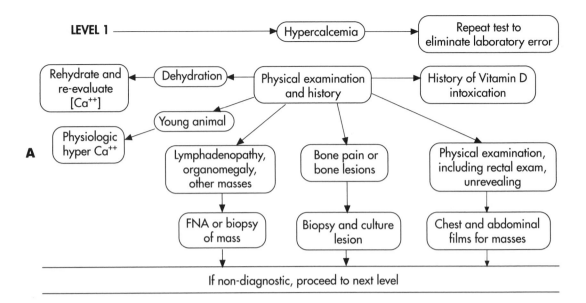

A

LEVEL 1 ——————————→ Hypercalcemia → Repeat test to eliminate laboratory error

Rehydrate and re-evaluate [Ca⁺⁺] ← Dehydration ← Physical examination and history → History of Vitamin D intoxication

Young animal

Physiologic hyper Ca⁺⁺

Lymphadenopathy, organomegaly, other masses

Bone pain or bone lesions

Physical examination, including rectal exam, unrevealing

FNA or biopsy of mass

Biopsy and culture lesion

Chest and abdominal films for masses

If non-diagnostic, proceed to next level

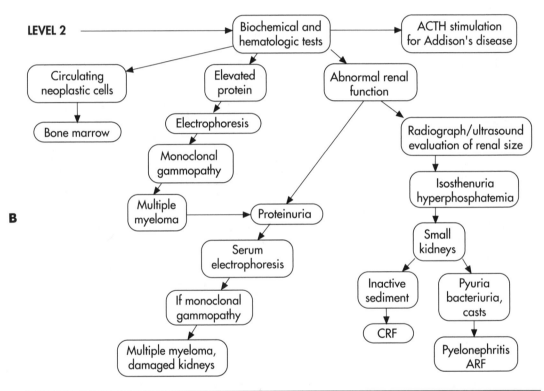

B

LEVEL 2 ——————————→ Biochemical and hematologic tests → ACTH stimulation for Addison's disease

Circulating neoplastic cells

Elevated protein

Abnormal renal function

Bone marrow

Electrophoresis

Monoclonal gammopathy

Multiple myeloma → Proteinuria

Serum electrophoresis

If monoclonal gammopathy

Multiple myeloma, damaged kidneys

Radiograph/ultrasound evaluation of renal size

Isosthenuria hyperphosphatemia

Small kidneys

Inactive sediment

Pyuria bacteriuria, casts

CRF

Pyelonephritis ARF

If non-diagnostic, proceed to next level

C

LEVEL 3

PTH levels

Ventral cervical exploratory

Steroid trial

Institute therapy pending diagnosis

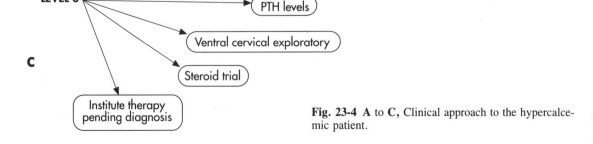

Fig. 23-4 A to **C,** Clinical approach to the hypercalcemic patient.

cium concentrations can rise rapidly and may require therapy even before a definitive cause is identified. It is important to avoid the use of corticosteroids, if possible, prior to establishing a definitive diagnosis, since their administration may make cytologic or histopathologic identification of lymphoid neoplasms difficult. Corticosteroids are cytotoxic to lymphocytes and usually decrease serum calcium concentrations in dogs with lymphoma by this mechanism. Lastly, glucocorticoids antagonize vitamin D metabolites, block absorption of calcium from the gut, and increase renal excretion of calcium. A resolution of hypercalcemia with glucocorticoid administration does not confirm a diagnosis of lymphoid neoplasia.

Therapy of malignancy-associated hypercalcemia can be directed at lowering the serum calcium concentrations or controlling the primary and metastatic neoplasm, thus indirectly lowering the serum calcium concentrations; often both approaches are combined in critical patients. The neoplasms can be treated with surgery, radiation, and/or chemotherapy. Surgical intervention and radiation are effective against local tumors producing humoral factors (e.g., anal sac adenocarcinomas). Institution of chemotherapy for metastatic or systemic neoplasms (e.g., lymphoma, myeloma) usually results in normocalcemia within 24 to 48 hours (Fig. 23-5).

Several methods to lower the serum calcium concentration without directly affecting the tumor (or while waiting to establish a definitive diagnosis) exist. The first line of therapy is saline diuresis. Intravenous 0.9% sodium chloride should be given at a rate of 120 to 200 ml/kg per day, provided cardiopulmonary function is adequate. The second line of therapy is furosemide diuresis,

which promotes calciuresis. It is important not to initiate furosemide therapy until the patient is well hydrated, as dehydration in the face of hypercalcemia potentiates renal toxicity. Drugs used in humans to reduce serum calcium concentrations in hypercalcemia of malignancy include nonsteroidal antiinflammatory agents, calcitonin, and mithramycin. These drugs have not been very effective in dogs with hypercalcemia of malignancy; moreover, they are usually associated with severe side effects. A new group of drugs that can be used to lower serum calcium concentrations directly are the diphosphonates.[64,65] These compounds inhibit osteoclast resorption of bone and are available for oral and intravenous use. The effect is not immediate; however, there are fewer side effects associated with diphosphonates than with the drugs previously discussed. One of the compounds used is ethane-1-hydroxy-1,1-diphosphonate (Didronel; Norwich Eaton) (10 to 40 mg/kg/day orally divided twice to three times a day).

Fig. 23-6 illustrates the serum calcium concentrations in a dog with a thyroid adenocarcinoma and hypercalcemia treated with diphosphonates. While this dog was not azotemic, there was evidence of mitral and tricuspid insufficiency and decreased myocardial contractility. Attempts at fluid diuresis resulted in pulmonary edema. Diphosphonates lowered the serum calcium concentration before appreciable chemotherapy-induced cytoreduction occurred.

Hypoglycemia. Hypoglycemia is another metabolic disease whose signs may prompt pet owners to seek emergency veterinary care. Islet-cell tumors (insulinomas, islet-cell carcinomas, beta-cell tumors) are the most common cause of tumor-associated hypoglycemia in dogs[47,66,67]; large intraabdominal or intrathoracic tumors have also

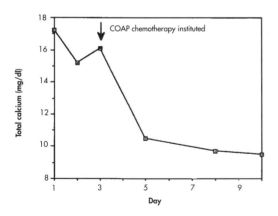

Fig. 23-5 Serum calcium concentrations in a dog with multicentric lymphoma and hypercalcemia treated with multiple agent chemotherapy.

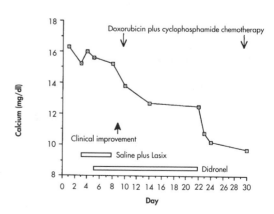

Fig. 23-6 Serum calcium concentrations in a dog with thyroid adenocarcinoma and hypercalcemia treated with oral diphosphonates.

been associated with hypoglycemia in this species.[66,68] The prevalence of tumor-associated hypoglycemia appears to be considerably higher in dogs than in cats.[69] The proposed mechanisms underlying hypoglycemia are numerous but some of the best substantiated are: (1) ectopic insulin production such as that seen with islet-cell tumors[67,68,70]; (2) nonsuppressible insulin-like activity such as that seen with mesenchymal tumors like leiomyosarcoma, fibrosarcoma, and hemangiosarcoma[66-68,70]; (3) overutilization of glucose by the tumor (a poorly documented phenomenon)[67,71,72]; and (4) severe hepatic infiltration with disruption of normal glucose metabolism.[67,71,73] Three other mechanisms resulting in hypoglycemia that are indirectly related to neoplasia are: (1) hypoglycemia induced by sepsis[73,74]; (2) severe cancer cachexia resulting in mild hypoglycemia[67]; and (3) hypoglycemia that is artifactually created by leukemic cell consumption of glucose if the serum is not separated soon after collection.[66] These last three mechanisms are usually not associated with clinical signs of neuroglycopenia.

The typical signs of hypoglycemia are mainly neurologic in nature (i.e., neuroglycopenic) due to the small carbohydrate reserve in neural tissue.[66,67] Disorientation, weakness and ataxia are typically followed by convulsions and coma. The cerebrum (with greater metabolic activity) is usually affected first. The onset and severity of signs are more often dependent on the rate of decrease in serum glucose concentration, rather than being dependent on the degree of hypoglycemia.[67] If the hypoglycemic event is prolonged, hypoxia may occur with attendant permanent neurologic damage. If untreated, death eventually ensues due to depression of the respiratory centers.

Documentation of a serum glucose of 40 mg/dl or less with attendant neurologic signs, and relief of neurologic signs by administration of glucose constitutes the Whipple's triad. Whipple's triad is not diagnostic for an insulinoma, only for hypoglycemia. Nonneoplastic diseases that should be considered in the differential diagnosis of hypoglycemia in an adult animal include hypoadrenocorticism, severe hepatic dysfunction, sepsis, hunting dog hypoglycemia, and severe malnutrition. Having drawn the appropriate blood samples, emergency treatment for hypoglycemia should be instituted by intravenous administration of 50% dextrose (0.5 ml/kg) followed by an intravenous drip of 5% or 10% dextrose in water. Feeding small meals frequently will usually alleviate clinical signs while test results are pending (insulin radioimmunoassay may take several days). A preliminary diagnosis of insulinoma can be made if the glucose and insulin concentrations are markedly disparate (i.e., marked hypoglycemia and normoinsulinemia or hyperinsulinemia) (see Chapter 18).

Surgery is the mainstay of treatment for dogs with insulinomas; it may result in palliation of the clinical signs (i.e., by tumor cytoreduction) and it permits tumor staging. In a study of 73 dogs with insulinomas, over 80% had evidence of metastatic disease at the time of surgery.[75] Survival in that study correlated well with the clinical stages. Dogs classified as Stage I (no gross invasion or metastatic disease) had a median survival of 11 months, while dogs classified as Stage III (gross metastases, usually in the liver) survived only 5 months. Another study had an overall mean survival of 14 months with gross metastases present in 46% of the dogs at the time of initial surgical treatment.[76]

Medical treatment of patients with insulinomas includes frequent feedings, glucocorticoids (0.25 to 0.5 mg/kg per day) for their gluconeogenic activity, and diazoxide at 10 mg/kg per day. Diazoxide inhibits insulin release and at high doses causes release of epinephrine. Side effects of diazoxide include nausea and vomiting. Chemotherapy using streptozocin has been disappointing in animals because of drug-associated nephrotoxicity.[77,78] Refer to Chapter 18 for further information on the acute and long-term management of hypoglycemia.

Other mechanisms for hypoglycemia include nonsuppressible insulin-like activity, glucose utilization by the tumor, and disruption of glucose metabolism in the liver. In a series of 13 extrapancreatic neoplasms with hypoglycemia, 10 were associated with the liver.[68] All 10 animals had large palpable abdominal masses. This is analogous to the situation in humans in which extrapancreatic tumors associated with hypoglycemia have an average weight of 2.6 kg and are readily detectable.[79] Of these 10 tumors, 8 were hepatocellular carcinomas, and the other 2 were a hemangiosarcoma and a leiomyosarcoma. Insulin concentrations were found to be in the low normal range (4.5 to 8.6 μU/ml) in five of these dogs. The extrapancreatic, extrahepatic tumors included a metastatic melanoma, a splenic hemangiosarcoma, and a salivary gland adenocarcinoma. The insulin levels in the dog with the hemangiosarcoma and the adenocarcinoma were 9.9 and 4.2 μU/ml, respectively. As each of the liver tumors involved only one lobe of the liver, it seems unlikely that severe liver dysfunction was the cause of the hypoglycemia in these cases.

Acute tumor lysis syndrome. Occasionally, animals with marginal renal function, chemosensitive neoplasms, and large tumor burdens, may develop a syndrome referred to as acute tumor lysis syndrome (ATLS).[80-82] This is not an uncommon side effect of chemotherapy in humans, in whom it occurs in approximately 10% of patients with lymphoma and leukemia.[83] In humans, this syndrome is characterized by hyperuricemia, hyperkalemia, and hyperphosphatemia, with attendant hypocalcemia. These metabolic derangements can result in renal failure due to mineral and uric acid precipitation within the renal tubules, and cardiac disease related to the hyperkalemia. Intensive diuresis and occasionally dialysis may be necessary to correct these derangements.

Acute tumor lysis syndrome is extremely rare in dogs, and to our knowledge, it has not been documented in cats. Typical clinical signs include acute onset of weakness, lethargy, and anorexia within 48 to 72 hours of instituting anticancer chemotherapy; vomiting and diarrhea may also occur. The prevalence of this syndrome is low. In the past 6 years, we have documented ATLS in three dogs with lymphoma treated with a combination of cyclophosphamide, vincristine, cytarabine, and prednisone (COAP protocol) (Fig. 23-7). Approximately 300 dogs were treated with COAP chemotherapy for lymphomas during the same period. All dogs that developed ATLS had high tumor burden and borderline renal disease.

It is important to recognize this syndrome as being an overload of tumor solute on the kidneys. The initial reaction to a vomiting, lethargic dog on chemotherapy is that the signs are due to drug toxicity. However, therapy should be continued while other supportive measures, such as fluid therapy, are instituted. Knowledge of renal function prior to therapy can aid in the early recognition of ATLS or prevention of it by judicious use of parenteral fluids.

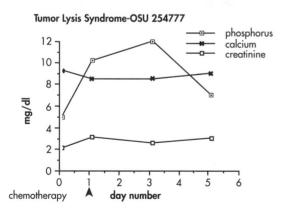

Fig. 23-7 Tumor lysis syndrome in a dog with pulmonary lymphoma treated with doxorubicin, prednisone, vincristine, and cyclophosphamide.

Tumor rupture

Pets may present to the emergency room in a state of acute collapse due to tumor rupture. The majority of these patients are in shock and are severely anemic due to blood loss. The most common neoplasm associated with acute rupture in the dog is hemangiosarcoma, although any large tumor can rupture or erode a major vessel, causing severe acute bleeding.

Approximately 50% to 60% of dogs with hemangiosarcoma present because of acute collapse due to tumor rupture and subsequent intracavitary bleeding.[84] Signs of intraabdominal tumor rupture are usually acute and include lethargy, anorexia, vomiting, dyspnea, distended abdomen, and pale mucous membranes. A presumptive diagnosis of tumor rupture can be established by finding blood during cavity centesis in a patient with the clinical signs discussed above. Cytologic evaluation of the fluid usually reveals hemorrhage or hemorrhage with increased numbers of neutrophils and macrophages (if the blood has been present for several days). A coagulation panel is indicated in these patients to differentiate tumor rupture from a coagulopathy; the presence of blood in only one cavity and the lack of other signs of systemic bleeding are suggestive of tumor (or organ) rupture. If a necrotic tumor has ruptured, the fluid cytology may be inflammatory in nature. Since it is usually difficult to remove sufficient abdominal fluid to obtain diagnostic radiographs of the abdomen, abdominal ultrasound is indicated to aid in detection of mass lesions under these circumstances (Fig. 23-8).

A special situation of tumor rupture is seen in dogs with atrial hemangiosarcoma resulting in pericardial tamponade. This acute emergency situation requires immediate attention to relieve the life-threatening cardiovascular changes. On physical examination, signs of right-sided failure (e.g., ascites, jugular pulsation) may be present; they may also be accompanied by other signs of pericardial effusion (e.g., pulsus paradoxus, electrical alternans, weak pulses, muffled heart sounds, globoid cardiac shadow on thoracic radiographs). It is desirable to establish a definitive diagnosis of pericardial effusion by echocardiography prior to pericardiocentesis in these patients; often, echocardiography allows for visualization of right atrial masses (Fig. 23-9). Refer to Chapter 17 for further discussion of treatment for pericardial tamponade.

Therapy for dogs with ruptured hemangiosarcomas and acute bleeding involves supportive measures until the bleeding tumor can be dealt with surgically. These measures include shock therapy, transfusion, and abdominal bandaging. Often,

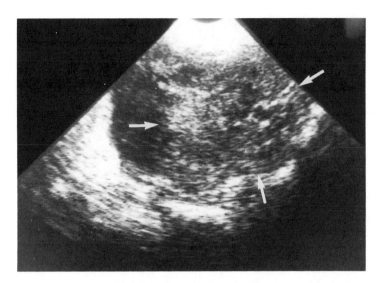

Fig. 23-8 Ultrasonographic characteristics of a splenic hemangiosarcoma.

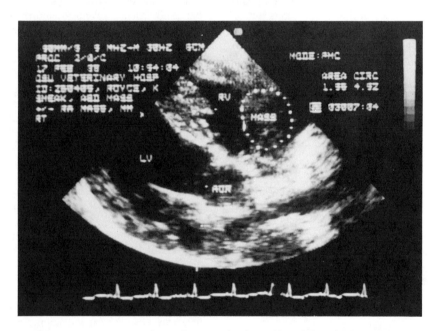

Fig. 23-9. Two-dimensional echocardiogram of a dog with a right atrial hemangiosarcoma.

surgical intervention cannot be delayed and must be performed before the patient is stable (see Chapter 10). Preoperatively and postoperatively, the patient must be observed carefully for the development of arrhythmias and hemostatic abnormalities such as disseminated intravascular coagulation. Occasionally, bleeding from a ruptured tumor is arrested by normal hemostatic mechanisms, and the blood collected in the affected body cavity is subsequently autotransfused. In these cases, the owners usually report recurrent collapsing episodes that last from minutes to hours.

Dogs with ruptured splenic hemangiosarcomas and no gross evidence of metastases at the time of surgery have a poor prognosis (median survival of 65 days in one report and 19 days in another).[84,85] The use of a combination of vincristine, doxorubicin, and cyclophosphamide postoperatively in these patients resulted in a median survival of 192 days.[86]

Respiratory complications

Many patients with cancer initially present with acute dyspnea directly related or secondary to the tumor. The dyspnea is usually related to the anatomic location of the tumor or its metastases, which can affect the upper airways (i.e., nasal

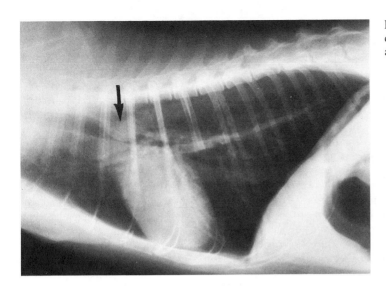

Fig. 23-10 Thoracic radiographs of a cat with acute onset of dyspnea due to an intratracheal lymphoma.

cavity, pharynx, larynx, trachea), mediastinum, pleural space, and lower airway or lung parenchyma.

Tumors commonly associated with upper airway obstruction include tonsillar, submandibular, intranasal, mediastinal, and tracheal lymphomas (Fig. 23-10); thymomas; tonsillar squamous-cell carcinomas; thyroid adenocarcinomas; and primary laryngeal neoplasms. The initial diagnosis is often made by physical examination, radiologic evaluation, or laryngoscopy. Ultimately, cytologic or histopathologic evaluation is required for a definitive diagnosis. Therapy for upper airway masses usually includes oxygen, acepromazine or morphine to relieve anxiety, an emergency tracheostomy, glucocorticoids to decrease inflammation, and cytotoxic chemotherapy or radiotherapy. The following chemotherapy protocol is recommended for dogs and cats with lymphoma: vincristine (0.5 mg/m^2 intravenously weekly), cytosine arabinoside (100 mg/m^2 subcutaneously divided twice a day for 4 days in dogs and 2 days in cats), cyclophosphamide (50 mg/m^2 orally every other day), and prednisone (50 mg/m^2 orally or subcutaneously daily for 1 week, then 25 mg/m^2 every other day).[87] This protocol usually results in remission in more than 85% of the patients. Tumor shrinkage usually occurs within hours of instituting chemotherapy or radiotherapy in dogs and cats with lymphomas. Surgical removal of nonlymphoid neoplasms is usually indicated for rapid resolution of the dyspnea.

Mediastinal masses such as lymphomas and thymomas can cause a rapid onset of cervicofacial edema by compression of the anterior vena cava (Fig. 23-11). The presenting signs are usually such that only thoracic radiography is needed to

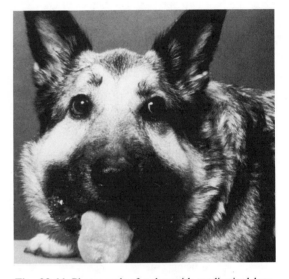

Fig. 23-11 Photograph of a dog with mediastinal lymphoma and anterior vena cava syndrome.

confirm the presence of a large thoracic mass. Cytologic specimens of the mass can be obtained by percutaneous fine needle aspiration through the thoracic inlet or through a right intercostal approach (at the second or third costochondral junction); ultrasound- or fluoroscopy-guided aspirates can also be obtained. If that does not yield diagnostic material, it may be necessary to perform a minithoracotomy to obtain a biopsy specimen. If cytologic evaluation yields a definitive diagnosis of lymphoma, multiple-agent chemotherapy should be instituted immediately.

Malignant pleural effusion may occur with mediastinal lymphomas, thymomas, mesotheliomas, and primary and secondary lung neoplasms (especially carcinomas). Dyspnea can be so severe that immediate removal of the pleural fluid is necessary for survival and may even precede radiography. These patients should be handled with extreme care, as undue stress may be fatal. If a high index of suspicion for pleural effusion exists from the physical examination (e.g., muffled heart and lung sounds, dyspnea, noncompressible cranial thorax), pleurocentesis is indicated. The fluid thus obtained can be analyzed cytologically, biochemically, and microbiologically to differentiate malignant effusions from the other causes. Attempts can be made to manage malignant pleural effusions in the dog by weekly intrapleural injections of 5-flourouracil (150 mg/m^2) diluted in 150 to 200 ml of saline per square meter of body-surface area. 5-fluorouracil cannot be used in cats because of its neurotoxicity in this species.

Complications of anticancer chemotherapy

Over the past two decades, anticancer drugs have become widely available for the management of small animal patients with systemic neoplasms (e.g., lymphoma), metastatic neoplasia (e.g., hemangiosarcoma), and nonresectable malignancies resistant to radiotherapy and hyperthermia (e.g., some adenocarcinomas and sarcomas).[88,89] Drug dosing, monitoring, and supportive care of small animals with cancer who are undergoing chemotherapy has greatly improved over the past decade, but significant toxicities and side effects still constitute a potential life-threatening complication associated with this treatment modality.[90-92] Antineoplastic agents have an extremely low therapeutic index (i.e., narrow therapeutic-to-toxic ratio).

Because most of the complications of anticancer chemotherapy have been recently reviewed,[92] only those requiring emergency care will be discussed herein.

Hematologic toxicity. The high mitotic rate and growth fraction (i.e., 40% to 60%) of the bone marrow cells predispose this organ to significant toxicity from anticancer drugs. Hematologic toxicity represents the most common toxicity of

chemotherapy, and often results in temporary or permanent discontinuation of the offending agent(s) due to severe (and often life-threatening) cytopenias.[91-93] Agents commonly implicated in this type of toxicity are listed in Table 23-10.

When one considers the bone marrow transit times and circulating half-life of formed elements in blood, it is easy to anticipate which cell line will be affected. The bone marrow transit time and circulating half life of red blood cells in the dog are approximately 7 days and 120 days, those of the platelets are 3 days and 4 to 6 days, and those of granulocytes are 6 days and 4 to 8 hours, respectively.[94] Therefore, it is anticipated that neutropenia will occur first, and it will be followed by thrombocytopenia. Anemia induced by chemotherapeutic agents is extremely rare in dogs and cats. If it occurs, it has a late onset (3 to 4 months following initiation of therapy). The degree of cytopenia is affected by several factors (see box).

Although thrombocytopenia is probably as common as neutropenia, it is rarely severe enough to cause spontaneous bleeding, and it will therefore not be discussed at length. In most dogs and cats with chemotherapy-induced thrombocytopenia the platelet counts remain above 50,000 cells/μl (with the exception of dacarbazine-induced

---

FACTORS THAT AFFECT THE DEGREE OF MYELOSUPPRESSION INDUCED BY CHEMOTHERAPY

Mechanism of action of the drug
Dosage of the drug
Patient's age (i.e., younger dogs and cats have higher numbers of marrow cells)
Neoplastic bone marrow involvement (i.e., hemolymphatic neoplasia, metastatic malignancy)
Prior use of chemotherapy or radiotherapy
Patient's nutritional status
Additive myelosuppressive effects in multiple-agent chemotherapy

---

Table 23-10 Myelosuppressive potential of anticancer drugs commonly used in small animal patients

Severe	Moderate	Mild to None
Doxorubicin	Chlorambucil	Corticosteroids
Cyclophosphamide	Methotrexate (low dose)	Bleomycin
Cytarabine	Cisplatin	L-asparaginase
Vinblastine	Vincristine (>0.5 mg/m^2)	Vincristine (0.5 mg/m^2)
Hydroxyurea	Melphalan	
Actinomycin D	5-Fluorouracil	

thrombocytopenia); spontaneous bleeding usually does not occur until platelet counts fall below 30,000 to 40,000/μl.[95] If spontaneous bleeding occurs in a patient with platelet counts >50,000/μl, an underlying coagulopathy should be suspected.

Granulocytopenia (neutropenia) usually constitutes the dose-limiting cytopenia and frequently leads to life-threatening sepsis.[91-93,96] The nadir (the lowest point in the curve) usually occurs 5 to 7 days following treatment, and the neutrophil counts usually return to normal values within 36 to 72 hours. Patients with neutrophil counts lower than 2,000 cells/μl should be closely monitored for the development of sepsis. Neutrophil counts under 100 cells/μl are almost invariably associated with sepsis. The pathogenesis of sepsis in neutropenic patients is as follows: chemotherapy-induced death and desquamation of gastrointestinal crypt epithelial cells occurs simultaneously with myelosuppression; enteric bacteria are absorbed through the damaged mucosal barrier into systemic circulation; the numbers of neutrophils in circulation are not sufficient to phagocytose and kill the invading organisms; and, as a consequence, microbial colonization of multiple organs occurs, and death ensues unless the patient is treated appropriately.[92]

From the clinical standpoint, it is important to identify the septic neutropenic patient, since the cardinal signs of inflammation (i.e., redness, swelling, increased temperature, pain, and abnormal function) may be absent due to insufficient numbers of neutrophils available to participate in the inflammatory process.[97] The same holds true for radiographic changes compatible with inflammation; for example, dogs with neutropenia and bacterial pneumonia diagnosed on the basis of cytologic and microbiologic findings in transtracheal washes, often have normal thoracic radiographs. As a general rule, when a severely neutropenic patient (neutrophil count <500/μl) presents with significant pyrexia (temperature >104°F), the fever should be attributed to bacterial pyrogens until proven otherwise, and the patient should be treated aggressively with antimicrobial therapy (see below).

Monitoring the patient on chemotherapy constitutes the most effective way to prevent severe, life-threatening myelosuppression. Complete blood counts should be obtained weekly or biweekly, and all patients undergoing chemotherapy should be current on their immunizations. Myelosuppressive agents should be temporarily discontinued (or their doses decreased) if the neutrophil count falls below 2000 cells/μl or if the platelet count is below 50,000 cells/μl. Discontinuing the offending agent(s) for two or three administrations is usually sufficient for the cell counts to return to normal range. When therapy is reinstituted, it is recommended that only 75% of the initial dose be used, escalating dosages over 2 to 3 weeks until the initially recommended dose is reached.

Treatment of neutropenic patients. From the clinical standpoint, neutropenic patients can be classified into two broad categories: those that are febrile, and those that are afebrile. Neutropenic febrile patients should be treated aggressively, since they are usually septic. Fever in a neutropenic patient constitutes a medical emergency.[92,97,98] The following protocol is recommended for neutropenic febrile patients: the patient undergoes a thorough physical examination in search of a septic focus, an indwelling intravenous catheter is placed aseptically, and intravenous fluids are administered as required. All anticancer agents with the exception of corticosteroids are discontinued at once. Corticosteroids should be discontinued gradually, since patients on long-term steroid therapy can have episodes of acute hypoadrenocorticism when the drug is abruptly discontinued. Blood samples for complete blood count and serum electrolyte, blood glucose, and blood urea nitrogen concentrations are obtained immediately; a urine sample for urinalysis and bacterial culture is also obtained. Two to three sets of aseptically collected blood samples are obtained for aerobic and anaerobic bacterial cultures and antibiotic susceptibility tests at 30-minute intervals. After collecting the second set of samples for blood cultures, therapy with an empirical bacteriocidal antibiotic combination is instituted. We prefer a combination of gentamicin (2 mg/kg intravenously three times a day), and cephalothin (40 mg/kg intravenously three times a day), because most bacterial isolates in these patients are *Enterobacteriaciae* and staphylococci, organisms commonly susceptible to these agents. Once the neutrophil count returns to normal and the patient is clinically normal (usually within 72 to 96 hours), the antibiotic combination is discontinued and the patient is released with instructions to administer sulfadiazine-trimethoprim (13 mg/kg orally twice a day for 5 to 7 days).

Neutropenic afebrile patients can be treated as outpatients with discontinuation of the drug(s) as above plus sulfadiazine-trimethoprim. Owners should be instructed to monitor their pet's rectal temperature twice daily, and call the veterinarian if pyrexia develops, in which case the patients are treated as neutropenic and febrile. Sulfa-trimethoprim combinations eliminate the aerobic intestinal flora but preserve the anaerobic bacteria, which are an important component of the local defense system because of their ability to produce local antibiotics. These drugs are active against a large number of pathogens isolated from patients with cancer, provide therapeutic blood and tissue concentrations, and also provide high intragranulocytic concentrations.

Gastrointestinal toxicity. Although less common than myelosuppression, gastrointestinal toxicity is a relatively common complication of cancer chemotherapy in pets. From the clinical standpoint, two major types of gastrointestinal complications can result in acute signs requiring emergency care: nausea/vomiting and gastroenterocolitis.[99]

Although controlled studies are not available, nausea and vomiting apparently are not as common in pets as in humans when using similar drugs and dosages. Drugs potentially associated with nausea and vomiting in the dog and cat include dacarbazine (DTIC), cisplatin, doxorubicin (primarily in cats), methotrexate, cyclophosphamide, and 5-fluorouracil.

Acute nausea and vomiting caused by injectable drugs can usually be alleviated by administering the offending agents by slow intravenous infusion. If these signs persist despite slow administration, the use of antiemetics such as metoclopramide (Reglan; 0.1 to 0.3 mg/kg intravenously, subcutaneously, or orally three times a day), or prochlorperazine (Compazine; 0.5 mg/kg intramuscularly two to three times a day) is indicated. In humans, high-dose intravenous dexamethasone (10-mg total dose) has proven effective in preventing or alleviating the nausea and vomiting associated with cisplatin and DTIC therapy.[99] Corticosteroids are thought to inhibit vomiting by blocking the synthesis of prostaglandins in the medulla.[100] The antiemetic properties of corticosteroids are poorly documented in small animals.

Gastroenterocolitis associated with the use of anticancer agents is rare in dogs and cats. Drugs that occasionally cause mucositis include methotrexate, 5-fluorouracil, and doxorubicin; it rarely occurs with other alkylating agents, such as cyclophosphamide. Of the drugs listed above, only doxorubicin (Adriamycin) and methotrexate (Mexate) appear to be of any clinical consequence for the patients. In this regard, dogs appear to be more susceptible than cats to the toxic effects of these drugs on the gastrointestinal system. In our experience, collies and collie crosses appear to be extremely susceptible to doxorubicin-induced enterocolitis. This syndrome is characterized by the development of hemorrhagic diarrhea, primarily the large-bowel type, 3 to 7 days following administration of the drug. Supportive fluid therapy (if deemed necessary) and treatment with thera-

peutic doses of bismuth subsalicylate-containing products (Pepto-Bismol) are usually effective in controlling the clinical signs, which usually resolve in 3 to 5 days.

Pancreatitis is a well-recognized entity in human patients undergoing chemotherapy.[100a] Drugs associated with pancreatitis in man include corticosteroids, azathioprine, 6-mercaptopurine, L-asparaginase, cytosine arabinoside, and combination chemotherapy.[100a] Sporadic reports of pancreatitis in dogs receiving chemotherapeutic and immunosuppressive agents have also appeared in the literature.[100b,c,d]

We have documented acute pancreatitis in at least five dogs receiving L-asparaginase and in 6 dogs receiving combination chemotherapy. Two dogs in the latter group were receiving COAP chemotherapy (cyclophosphamide, vincristine, cytosine arabinoside, and prednisone), two dogs were receiving ADIC (doxorubicin and DTIC), and two dogs were receiving VAC chemotherapy (vincristine, doxorubicin, and cyclophosphamide). Clinical signs developed 1 to 5 days after initiating chemotherapy and were characterized by anorexia, vomiting, and depression. Supportive therapy resulted in resolution of the clinical signs within days of diagnosis.

Hypersensitivity reactions. Acute Type I hypersensitivity reactions occasionally occur in dogs receiving L-asparaginase (Elspar), etoposide (VePesid), or doxorubicin (Adriamycin).[101-103] The latter does not appear to be a true hypersensitivity reaction, since doxorubicin apparently can induce direct mast-cell degranulation independently of IgE mediation.[101] Acute Type I hypersensitivity reactions were observed in 2 of 2 dogs treated by us with intravenous etoposide and also documented by Ogilvie et al.[104] Hypersensitivity reactions to this drug are extremely rare in humans. The vehicle of the etoposide contains polysorbate 80 (Tween 80), and it is suspected that the reaction is caused by this substance rather than by the drug itself. Polysorbate 80 has previously been implicated in acute reactions in dogs.[104] Etoposide can be safely administered orally to dogs; hypersensitivity reactions were not observed in 15 dogs treated by us with oral etoposide.

Clinical signs in dogs and cats with hypersensitivity reactions to anticancer agents are similar to other types of hypersensitivity reactions. In dogs the manifestations are primarily cutaneous and gastrointestinal, while in cats they are predominantly respiratory. These reactions are more common in dogs than in cats; therefore, the following discussion will refer only to the former species. Typical signs begin during or shortly after administration of the agent, and include head shaking (due to ear pruritus), generalized urticaria and erythema, restlessness, occasional vomiting, and (rarely) collapse due to hypotension.

Most systemic anaphylactic reactions can be prevented by pretreating the patient with H_1 antihistamines (e.g., diphenhydramine, 1 to 2 mg/kg intramuscularly 20 to 30 minutes prior to administration of the chemotherapeutic agent) and by administering certain drugs (such as L-asparaginase) by the subcutaneous, intramuscular, or intraperitoneal route, rather than intravenously. If the agent cannot be given by any other routes (i.e., doxorubicin), slow intravenous infusions should be used. Therapy of acute hypersensitivity reactions includes immediate discontinuation of the agent and administration of H_1 antihistimines (i.e., diphenhydramine, 0.2 to 0.5 mg/kg, slow intravenous infusion), intravenous dexamethasone sodium phosphate (1 to 2 mg/kg), and intravenous fluids. If the systemic reaction is severe, the administration of epinephrine (0.1 to 0.3 ml of a 1:1000 solution intramuscularly or intravenously) is indicated. Once the reaction subsides, the administration of certain drugs such as doxorubicin can be continued. Intravenous H_1 antihistamines should be used with caution in cats, since they can cause acute central nervous system depression leading to apnea.

Cardiotoxicity. Cardiotoxicity is a relatively common complication of doxorubicin therapy in the dog, but it appears to be rare in the cat. Two types of doxorubicin-induced cardiac toxicity are observed in animals: an acute reaction during or shortly after administration, and a chronic cumulative toxicity.[101,105] Both forms of cardiotoxicity can lead to acute clinical signs and therefore to presentation to the emergency room. Acute doxorubicin toxicity is characterized by the development of cardiac arrhythmias during or shortly after administration of the drug. Two to 20 weeks following repeated doxorubicin injections, persistent arrhythmias, including ventricular premature contractions, atrial premature contractions, paroxysmal ventricular tachycardia, second-degree atrioventricular blocks, and intraventricular conduction defects develop. These rhythm disturbances are usually associated with the development of cardiomyopathy.[105]

The hallmark of chronic doxorubicin toxicity is the development of dilated cardiomyopathy after surpassing a total cumulative dose of approximately 240 mg/m^2 in dogs. The cumulative cardiotoxic dose in cats is unknown, but one report describes histologic findings compatible with doxorubicin-induced cardiomyopathy in cats receiving between 130 and 320 mg/m^2 total dose.[106] Clinical signs of toxicity in dogs and cats are those of congestive heart failure. Although slow in onset, the acute signs associated with doxorubicin-induced cardiomyopathy usually require emergency care. Therapy consists of discontinuation of the drug and use of cardiac drugs such as digitalis glycosides or nonglycoside inotropic agents (see Chapter 17). Once cardiomyopathy develops prognosis is poor, since the myocardial lesions are irreversible.[101]

Monitoring patients receiving doxorubicin is critical in order to prevent the development of fatal cardiomyopathy. Dogs and cats that have underlying rhythm disturbances or impaired myocardial contractility, as determined by decreased fractional shortening on M-mode echocardiography should not be treated with doxorubicin. It is recommended that patients receiving doxorubicin undergo M-mode echocardiographic evaluation every three doxorubicin cycles (every 9 weeks) to assess myocardial contractility. The drug should be discontinued if appreciable decreases in fractional shortening or arrhythmias develop. Doxorubicin-induced cardiomyopathy can also be monitored by means of serial endomyocardial biopsies and radionuclide angiocardiography.

Urinary tract toxicity. The urinary tract is rarely affected by anticancer agents in small animal patients. Two specific complications may require emergency care: nephrotoxicity and sterile hemorrhagic cystitis.

Nephrotoxicity is rarely observed in dogs and cats undergoing chemotherapy. Although several potentially nephrotoxic drugs are commonly used in these species, only doxorubicin (primarily in the cat), cisplatin (in the dog), and intermediate-to high-dose methotrexate (in the dog) are of concern to the clinician. One report indicates that doxorubicin can be a potent nephrotoxin in cats and suggests that the limiting cumulative toxicity in this species is renal rather than cardiac.[106] In five cats treated with doxorubicin for different malignancies, renal lesions developed characterized by cytomegaly of tubular epithelial cells and stromal fibrosis after receiving a total cumulative dose of 130 to 320 mg/m^2. All three cats in which the hearts were examined by light microscopy had multifocal myocyte vacuolation compatible with doxorubicin-induced cardiomyopathy; however, none of these cats showed signs of congestive heart failure. In dogs, doxorubicin appears to cause nephrotoxicosis in animals with preexisting renal disease and in those concomitantly receiving other nephrotoxins such as aminoglycoside antibiotics (Couto, 1986, unpublished observations).

Cisplatin, a platinum-derived anticancer agent, commonly causes renal toxicity in humans.[93] Progressive azotemia developed in six of 65 dogs with malignancy treated with cisplatin and monitored by serum biochemical determinations and urinalyses, suggesting nephrotoxicosis.[107,108] Nephrotoxicity associated with methotrexate administration is extremely rare in dogs and cats. Management of chemotherapy-induced nephrotoxicity is similar to that of other acute or chronic nephropathies (see Chapter 21).

Sterile hemorrhagic cystitis is a relative common complication of cyclophosphamide therapy in dogs; this toxicity is uncommon in cats. Sterile cystitis apparently results from the irritating effects of one of cyclophosphamide's metabolites (acrolein). The prevalence of sterile hemorrhagic cystitis is approximately 5% to 30% in dogs and 1% to 3% in cats.[109,110] It appears from these two studies that female dogs are at a higher risk for the development of this complication and that cats are at an extremely low risk. Forced diuresis appears to prevent or minimize the frequency of this complication. We usually recommend administration of cyclophosphamide in the morning, allowing the pet to urinate frequently (if he/she is an indoor dog), salting the food, and administering prednisone on the same day that the patient receives the cyclophosphamide.

Clinical signs of sterile hemorrhagic cystitis are acute and similar to those of other lower urinary tract disorders, and include pollakiuria, hematuria, and dysuria. Urinalyses are characterized by the presence of blood, with mildly to moderately increased numbers of white blood cells and absence of bacteria. Therapy of this complication is aimed at discontinuing the offending drug, forcing diuresis, diminishing inflammation of the bladder wall, and preventing secondary bacterial infections. In one study, discontinuation of cyclophosphamide resulted in resolution of the cystitis in 77% of the affected dogs within 4 to 17 weeks.[109,110] In addition to discontinuing the cyclophosphamide, we use furosemide (Lasix; 2 mg/kg orally twice a day) for its diuretic effects; prednisone (0.5 to 1 mg/kg orally once a day) for its antiinflammatory and diuretic effects; and a sulfadiazine-trimethoprim combination (Tribrissen; 13 to 15 mg/kg orally twice a day) to prevent secondary bacterial contamination. If despite this approach the clinical signs worsen, instillation of 1% formalin solution in water into the bladder is recommended. In two dogs thus treated, gross hematuria resolved within 24 hours and did not recur.[111]

Neurotoxicity. Neurotoxicity from anticancer agents leading to emergency presentation is also extremely rare in dogs and cats. However, neurotoxicosis associated with the use of 5-fluorouracil

(5-FU) has been reported in dogs and cats.[112,113] Clinical signs occurred shortly (3 to 12 hours) after administration of the drug and consisted primarily of excitation and cerebellar ataxia, resulting in death in three of five dogs reported on by Ndiritu and Enos.[113] In another report, 5 of 13 dogs (38%) and the only cat treated with 5-fluorouracil developed similar signs, resulting in the death of 4 dogs and the cat.[112] One dog treated with cisplatin developed grand mal seizures that were attributed to the drug.[108] Due to its high neurotoxic potential, 5-fluorouracil should not be used in cats. Treatment of patients with chemotherapy-induced neurotoxicity involves supportive care.

Pulmonary toxicity. This complication of chemotherapy is extremely rare in pets. To our knowledge, only cisplatin has been documented as a cause of acute pulmonary toxicity in cats.[114] In that report, six cats with squamous-cell carcinomas and five normal cats treated with 20 to 60 mg/m^2 of cisplatin intravenously had acute signs of dyspnea and died 48 to 96 hours following administration of this agent. Autopsy findings consisted of pulmonary and mediastinal edema and microangiopathic changes in the pulmonary vasculature. Because of this significant toxicity, cisplatin is not recommended for use in cats.

REFERENCES

1. Tvedten HW. Hematology of the normal dog and cat. Vet Clin North Am Small Anim Pract, 1981;11:209-217.
2. Wintrobe MM, Lee GL, Boggs DR, et al. Clinical hematology, ed. 8. Philadelphia: Lea and Febiger, 1981:734-754,1726-1738.
3. Giger U, Harvey JW. Hemolysis caused by phosphofructokinase deficiency in English Springer Spaniels: Seven cases (1983-1986). J Am Vet Med Assoc 1987;191:453-459.
3a. Dodds WJ: Immune-mediated diseases of the blood. Adv Vet Sci Comp Med 1983;27:163-196.
3b. Hirsch J, Brain EA: Hemostasis and thrombosis: a conceptual approach, ed. 2, New York: Churchill Livingstone, 1983:54-65.
4. Hellebrekers LJ, Slappendel RJ, van den Brom WE. Effect of sodium heparin and antithrombin III concentration on activated partial thromboplastin time in the dog. Am J Vet Res 1985;46:1460-1462.
5. Ahn YS, Harrington WJ, Mylvaganam R, et al. Danazol therapy for autoimmune hemolytic anemia. Ann Intern Med 1985;102:298-301.
6. Feldman BF, Handagama P, Lubberink AAME. splenectomy as adjunctive therapy for immune-mediated thrombocytopenia and hemolytic anemia in the dog. J Am Vet Med Assoc 1985;187:617-619.
7. Matus RE, Schrader LA, Leifer CE, et al. Plasmapheresis as adjunctive therapy for autoimmune hemolytic anemia in two dogs. J Am Vet Med Assoc 1985;186:691-693.
8. Jonas LD, Thrall MA, Weiser MG. Nonregenerative form of immune-mediated hemolytic anemia. J Am Anim Hosp Assoc 1987;23:201-203.

9. Ou D, Mahaffey E, Smith JE. Effects of storage on oxygen dissociation of blood. J Am Vet Med Assoc 1975;167:56-58.

10. Davenport DJ, Breitschwerdt EB, Carakostas MC. Platelet disorders in the dog and cat. Part I: Physiology and pathogenesis. Compend Contin Educ Pract Vet 1982;4:762-772.

11. Davenport DJ, Breitschwerdt EB, Carakostas MC. Platelet disorders in the dog and cat. Part II: diagnosis and management. Compend Contin Educ Pract Vet 1982;4:788-796.

12. Troy GC. An overview of hemostasis. Vet Clin North Am 1988;18:5-20.

13. Demers LM. The prostaglandins and thromboxane in hemostasis. Lab Manage 1985;23:39-47.

14. Weiss DJ. Uniform evaluation and semiquantitative reporting of hematologic data in veterinary laboratories. Vet Clin Pathol 1988;13:27-31.

15. Feldman BF, Thomason KJ, Jain NC. Quantitative platelet disorders. Vet Clin North Am 1988;18:35-49.

16. Jergens AE, Turrentine MA, Kraus KH, Johnson GS. Buccal mucosa bleeding times of healthy dogs and of dogs in various pathologic states, including thrombocytopenia, uremia, and von Willebrand's disease. Am J Vet Res 1987;48:1337-1342.

17. Parker MT, Collier LL, Kier AB, Johnson GS. Oral mucosa bleeding times of normal cats and cats with Chediak-Higashi syndrome or Hagemann trait (factor XII deficiency). Vet Clin Pathol 1988;17:9-12.

18. Giles AR, Tinlin S, Greenwood R. A canine model of hemophilic (factor VIII:C deficiency) bleeding. Blood 1982;60:1135-1138.

19. Pynappels MIM, Briet E, Van der Zwet GT, et al. Evaluation of the cuticle bleeding time in canine hemophilia A. Thromb Haemost 1986;55:70-73.

20. Cockburn C, Troy GC. A retrospective study of sixty-two cases of thrombocytopenia in the dog. Southwest Vet 1986;37:133-142.

21. Feldman BF, Madewell BR, O'Neil S. Disseminated intravascular coagulation: Antithrombin, plasminogen, and coagulation abnormalities in 41 dogs. J Am Vet Med Assoc 1981;179:151-154.

22. Dodds WJ. Bleeding disorders. In Ettinger SJ, ed. Textbook of veterinary internal medicine. Philadelphia: WB Saunders, 1975;1679-1698.

23. Dodds WJ. Von Willebrand's disease in dogs. Mod Vet Pract 1984;65:681-686.

24. Dodds WJ. Familial canine thrombocytopathy. Thromb Diath Haemorrh 1967;26:241-247.

25. Johnstone IB, Lotz F. An inherited platelet function defect in Basset Hounds. Can Vet J 1978;20:211-215.

26. Kraus KH, Turrentine MA, Jergens AE, Johnson GS. Effect of desmopressin acetate on bleeding times and vWF in Doberman Pinscher dogs with von Wilebrand's disease. Vet Surg 1989;18:103-109.

27. Johnson GS, Turrentine MA, Kraus KH. Canine von Willebrand's disease. Vet Clin North Am 1988;18:195-229.

27a. Hoyer LW: Factor VIII. In Colman RW, Hirsch J, Marder VJ, Salzman EW: Hemostasis and thrombosis: basic principles and clinical practice, ed 2. Philadelphia: JB Lippincott, 1987;48-59.

27b. Owen WG: Protein C. In Colman RW, Hirsch J, Marder VJ, Salzman EW: Hemostasis and thrombosis: basic principles and clinical practice, ed 2. Philadelphia: JB Lippincott, 1987;235-241.

28. Esmon NL, Esmon CT. Protein C and the endothelium. Semin Thromb Hemost 1988;14:210-215.

29. Mammen EF, Miyakawa T, Phillips TF, et al. Human antithrombin concentrates and experimental disseminated intravascular coagulation. Semin Thromb Hemost 1985;11:373-383.

30. Ofosu FA, Gray E. Mechanisms of action of heparin: applications to the development of derivatives of heparin and heparinoids with antithrombotic properties. Semin Thromb Hemost 1988;14:9-17.

31. Johnstone IB. Clinical and laboratory diagnosis of bleeding disorders. Vet Clin North Am 1988;18:21-33.

32. Feldman BF. Coagulopathies in small animals. J Am Vet Med Assoc 1981;179:559-563.

33. Kirk RW, ed. Current veterinary therapy IX—Small animal practice. Philadelphia: WB Saunders, 1986;1270.

34. Williams DA, Maggio-Price L. Canine idiopathic thrombocytopenia: clinical observations and long-term follow-up in 54 cases. J Am Vet Med Assoc 1984;185:660-663.

35. Joshi BC, Jain NC. Detection of antiplatelet antibody in serum and on megakaryocytes of dogs with autoimmune thrombocytopenia. Am J Vet Res 1976;37:681-685.

36. Bloom JC, Meunier LD, Thiem PA, Sellers TS. Use of danazol for treatment of corticosteroid-resistant immune-mediated thrombocytopenia in a dog. J Am Vet Med Assoc 1989;194:76-78.

37. Mount ME, Woody BJ, Murphey MJ. The anticoagulant rodenticides. In Kirk RW, ed. Current veterinary therapy IX—Small animal practice. Philadelphia: WB Saunders, 1986;156-165.

38. Mount ME. Proteins induced by vitamin K absence or antagonists (PIVKA). In Kirk RW, ed. Current veterinary therapy IX—small animal practice. Philadelphia: WB Saunders, 1986;513-515.

39. Bick RL. Disseminated intravascular coagulation and related syndromes: a clinical review. Semin Thromb Hemost 1988;14:299-338.

40. Slappendel RJ. Disseminated intravascular coagulation. Vet Clin North Am 1988;18:169-184.

40a. Ruehl W, Mills C, Feldman BF: Rational therapy in disseminated intravascular coagulation. J Am Vet Med Assoc 1982;181:76-78.

41. Couto CG. Clinicopathologic aspects of acute leukemias in the dog. J Am Vet Med Assoc 1985;186:681-685.

42. Harrison BDW, Stokes TC. Secondary polycythemia: its causes, effects and treatment. Br J Dis Chest 1982;76:313-340.

43. Peterson ME, Randolph JF. Diagnosis and therapy of polycythemia. In Kirk RW, ed. Current veterinary therapy VIII—small animal practice. Philadelphia: WB Saunders, 1983;406-408.

44. Couto CG, Boudrieau RJ, Zanjani EZ. Tumor-associated erythrocytosis in a dog with nasal fibrosarcoma. J Vet Intern Med 1989;3:183-185.

45. MacEwen EG, Hurvitz AL. Diagnosis and management of monoclonal gammopathies. Vet Clin North Am 1977;7:119-132.

46. Matus RE, Leifer CE, Gordon BR, et al. Plasmapheresis and chemotherapy of hyperviscosity syndrome associated with monoclonal gammopathy in the dog. J Am Vet Med Assoc 1983;183:215-218.

47. Giger U, Gorman NT. Oncologic emergencies in small animals. Compend Contin Educ Pract Vet 1984;6:805-810.

48. Chew DJ, Carothers M. Hypercalcemia. Vet Clin North Am 1989;19:265-287.

49. Weller RE. Cancer associated hypercalcemia in companion animals Compend Contin Educ Pract Vet 1984;6:639-645.

50. Chew DJ, Meuten DJ. Disorders of calcium and phosphorus metabolism. Vet Clin North Am 1982;12:411-438.

51. Weller RE, Holmberg CA, Theilen GH, et al. Canine lymphosarcoma and hypercalcemia: clinical, laboratory and pathologic evaluation of twenty-four cases. J Small Anim Pract 1982;23:649-658.

52. Heath H, Weller RE, Mundy GR. Canine lymphosarcoma: a model for study of the hypercalcemia of cancer. Calcif Tissue Int 1980;30:127-130.

53. MacEwen EG, Siegel SD. Hypercalcemia: a paraneoplastic disease. Vet Clin North Am 1977;7:187-194.

54. Chew DJ, Schaer M, Liu SK. Pseudohyperparathyroidism in a cat. J Am Anim Hosp Assoc 1975;11:46-52.

55. McMillan F. Hypercalcemia associated with lymphoid neoplasia in two cats. Feline Pract 1985;15:31-35.

56. Zaloga GP, Eil C, Medbery CA. Humoral hypercalcemia in Hodgkin's disease. Arch Intern Med 1985;145:155-157.

57. Rosenthal N, Insogna KL, Godsall JW, et al. Elevations in circulating 1,25-dihydroxyvitamin D in three patients with lymphoma-associated hypercalcemia. J Clin Endocrinol Metab 1985;60:29-33.

58. Davies M, Mawer EB, Hayes ME, et al. Abnormal vitamin D metabolism in Hodgkin's lymphoma. Lancet 1985;1:1186-1188.

59. Breslau NA, McGuire JL, Zerwekh JE, et al. Hypercalcemia associated with increased serum calcitriol levels in three patients with lymphoma. Ann Intern Med 1984;100:1-7.

60. Mundy GR. The hypercalcemia of malignancy. Kidney Int 1987;31:142-155.

61. Burtis WJ, Wu TL, Insoga KL, et al. Humoral hypercalcemia of malignancy. Ann Intern Med 1988;108:454-457.

62. Meuten DJ, Kociba GJ, Capen CC, et al. Hypercalcemia in dogs with lymphosarcoma. Lab Invest 1983;49:553-562.

63. Weir EC, Norrdin RW, Matus RE, et al. Humoral hypercalcemia of malignancy in canine lymphosarcoma. Endocrinology 1988;122:602-608.

64. Mundy GR, Wilkinson R, Heath DA. Comparative study of available medical therapy for hypercalcemia of malignancy. Am J Med 1983;74:421-432.

65. Thiebaud D, Jacquet AF, Burckhardt P. Dose-response in the treatment of hypercalcemia of malignancy by a single infusion of the bisphosphonate AHPrBP. J Clin Oncol 1988;6:762-768.

66. Leifer CE, Peterson ME. Hypoglycemia. Vet Clin North Am 1984;14:873-889.

67. Weller RE. Cancer associated hypoglycemia in companion animals Compend Contin Educ Pract Vet 1980;7:437-444.

68. Leifer CE, Peterson ME, Matus RE, et al. Hypoglycemia associated with non-islet cell tumors in 13 dogs J Am Vet Med Assoc 1985;186:53-55.

69. McMillan FD, Barr B, Feldman EC. Functional pancreatic islet cell tumor in a cat. J Am Anim Hosp Assoc 1985;21:741-746.

70. Gordon P, Hendricks CM, Kahn CR, et al. Hypoglycemia associated with non-islet cell tumors and insulin-like growth factors N Engl J Med 1981;305:1452-1455.

71. Kahn CR. The riddle of tumor hypoglycemia revisited. Clin Endocrinol Metab 1980;9:335-360.

72. Brown NO. Paraneoplastic syndromes of humans, dogs, and cats. J Am Anim Hosp Assoc 1981;17:911-916.

73. Breitschwerdt EB, Loar AS, Hribernik TN, et al. Hypoglycemia in four dogs with sepsis. J Am Vet Med Assoc 1980;178:1072-1076.

74. Miller SI, Wallace RJ, Musher DM, et al. Hypoglycemia as a manifestation of sepsis Am J Med 1980;68:649-654.

75. Caywood DD, Klausner JS, O'Leary TP, et al. Pancreatic insulin secreting neoplasms: clinical diagnostic, and prognostic features in 73 dogs [abstract]. Proc Vet Can Soc 1987:16.

76. Melhaff CJ, Peterson ME, Patnaik AK, et al. Insulin-producing islet cell neoplasms: surgical considerations and general management in 35 dogs. J Am Anim Hosp Assoc 1985;21:607-612.

77. Meyer DJ. Pancreatic islet cell carcinoma in a dog treated with streptozotocin. Am J Vet Res 1976;37:1221-1223.

78. Meyer DJ. Temporary remission of hypoglycemia in a dog with an insulinoma after treatment with streptozotocin. Am J Vet Res 1977;38:1201-1204.

79. Odell WD, Wolfsen AR. Humeral syndromes associated with cancer. Annu Rev Med 1978;29:379-406.

80. Page RL, Leifer CE, Matus RE. Uric acid and phosphorous metabolism in canine lymphosarcoma. Am J Vet Res 1986;47:910-912.

81. Page RL. Acute tumor lysis syndrome. Semin Vet Med Surg 1986;1:58-60.

82. Laing EJ, Carter RF. Acute tumor lysis syndrome following treatment of canine lymphoma. J Am Anim Hosp Assoc 1988;24:691-696.

83. Allegretta GJ, Weisman SJ, Altman AJ. Oncologic emergencies. I: metabolic and space-occupying consequences of cancer and cancer treatment. Pediatr Clin North Am 1985;32:601-611.

84. Brown NO, Patnaik AK, MacEwen EG. Canine hemangiosarcoma: retrospective analysis of 104 cases. J Am Vet Med Assoc 1985;186:56-58.

85. Prymak C, McKee LJ, Goldschmidt MH, et al. Epidemiologic, clinical, pathologic, and prognostic characteristics of splenic hemangiosarcoma and splenic hematoma in dogs: 217 cases. J Am Vet Med Assoc 1988;193:706-712.

86. Hammer AS, Couto CG, Filppi J, et al. Efficacy and toxicity of VAC chemotherapy (vincristine, doxorubicin, and cyclophosphamide) in dogs with hemangiosarcoma. J Vet Intern Med 1991;5:160-166.

87. Couto CG. Canine extranodal lymphomos. In Kirk RW, ed. Current veterinary therapy IX—small animal practice. Philadelphia: WB Saunders, 1986;1473-1476.

88. Theilen GH, Madewell BR, Carter SK. Chemotherapy. In Theilen GH, Madewell BR, ed. Veterinary cancer medicine, ed. 2. Philadelphia: Lea & Febiger, 1987;157-166.

89. Norris AM, Withrow SJ. A review of cancer chemotherapy for pet animals. Can Vet J 1984;25:153-157.

90. Madewell BR. Adverse effects of chemotherapy. In Kirk RW, ed. Current veterinary therapy VIII. Philadelphia: WB Saunders, 1983;419-423.

91. Giger U, Gorman NT. Oncologic emergencies in small animals. Part I. Chemotherapy-related and hematologic emergencies. Compend Contin Educ Pract Vet 1984;6:689-698.

92. Couto CG. Toxicity of anticancer chemotherapy. In Couto CG, ed. Oncology: Kal Kan 10th Annual Symposium. Vernon, CA: Kal Kan Foods, 1987;37-46.

93. Dorr RT, Fritz WL. Cancer chemotherapy handbook. New York: Elsevier, 1980.

94. Jain NC. Schalm's veterinary hematology, ed. 4. Philadelphia: WB Saunders, 1986.

95. Hirsh J, Brain EA. Hemostasis and thrombosis, ed. 2. New York: Churchill Livingstone, 1983.

96. Barr RD, Perry S. Hematologic effects of antineoplastic therapy. In Holland JF, Frei E, eds. Cancer medicine. Philadelphia: Lea & Febiger, 1982;1288-1302.

97. Greene WH. Management of infection in myelosuppressed patients: clinical trails and common sense. Exp Hematol 1985;13(suppl 16):80-88.

98. Wiernik PH. The management of infection in the cancer patient. JAMA 1980;244:185-187.

99. Mitchell EP, Schein PS. Gastrointestinal toxicity of chemotherapeutic agents. Semin Oncol 1982;9:52-64.

100. Eyre HJ, Ward JH. Control of cancer chemotherapy-induced nausea and vomiting. Cancer 1984;54:2642.

100a. Woolley PW. Hepatic and pancreatic damage produced by cytotoxic drugs. Cancer Treat Rev 1983;10:117-137.

100b. Hahn KA, Richardson RC. Use of cisplatin for control of metastatic malignant mesenchymoma and hypertrophic osteopathy in a dog. J Am Vet Med Assoc 1989;195:351-353.

100c. Hansen JF, Carpenter RH. Fatal acute systemic anaphylaxis and hemorrhagic pancreatitis following asparaginase treatment in a dog. J Am Anim Hosp Assoc 1983;19:977-980.

100d. Moriello KA, Bowen D, Meyer DJ. Acute pancreatitis in two dogs given azathioprine and prednisone. J Am Vet Med Assoc 1987;191:695-696.

101. Bristow MR, Sageman WS, Scott RH et al. Acute and chronic cardiovascular effects of doxorubicin in the dog: The cardiovascular pharmacology of drug-induced histamine release. J Cardiovasc Pharmacol 1980;2:487-515.

102. Hansen JF, Carpenter RH. Fatal acute systemic anaphylaxis and hemorrhagic pancreatitis following asparaginase therapy in a dog. J Am Anim Hosp Assoc 1983;19:977-980.

103. Smith DM, Kirk GR. Some systemic effects of Adriamycin in the dog. J Am Anim Hosp Assoc 1976;12:92-97.

104. Ogilvie GK, Cockburn CA, Tranquilli WJ, Reschke RW, Weigel RM. Hypotension and cutaneous reactions associated with intravenous administration of etoposide in the dog. Am J Vet Res 1988;49:1367-1370.

105. Kehoe R, Singer DH, Trapani A, et al. Adriamycin-induced cardiac dysrhythmias in an experimental dog model. Cancer Treat Rep 1978;62:963-978.

106. Cotter SM, Kanki PJ, Simon M. Renal disease in five tumor-bearing cats treated with Adriamycin. J Am Anim Hosp Assoc 1985;21:405-409.

107. Shapiro W, Kitchell BE, Fossum TW, Couto CG, Theilen GH. Use of cisplatin for treatment of appendicular osteosarcoma in dogs. J Am Vet Med Assoc 1988;192:507-511.

108. Knapp DW, Richardson RC, Bonney PL, Hahn K. Cisplatin therapy in 41 dogs with malignant tumors. J Vet Intern Med 1988;2:41-46.

109. Crow SE, Theilen GH, Madewell BR, et al. Cyclophosphamide-induced cystitis in the dog and cat. J Am Vet Med Assoc 1977;171:259-262.

110. Henness AM. Treatment of cyclophosphamide-induced cystitis. J Am Vet Med Assoc 1985;187:984.

111. Weller RE. Intravesical instillation of dilute formalin for treatment of cyclophosphamide-induced cystitis in two dogs. J Am Vet Med Assoc 1978;172:1206-1209.

112. Harvey HJ, MacEwen EG, Hayes AA. Neurotoxicosis associated with use of 5-fluoruracil in five dogs and one cat. J Am Vet Med Assoc 1977;171:277-278.

113. Ndiritu CG, Enos LR. Adverse reactions to drugs in a veterinary hospital. J Am Vet Med Assoc 1977;171:335-339.

114. Knapp DW, Richardson RC, DeNicola DB, Long GG, Blevins WE. Cisplatin toxicity in cats. 1988;1:29-35.

24 Dermatologic Emergencies

Stephen D. White

Dermatology has an impact on the area of emergency medicine in three basic ways. First, there are a small number of dermatologic diseases that require immediate attention on the part of the emergency clinician. A large number of skin diseases exist that may develop life-threatening complications. Finally, life-threatening systemic disorders may present with cutaneous lesions concurrent with or prior to other clinical signs.

SKIN DISEASES REQUIRING IMMEDIATE THERAPY
Anaphylaxis

Anaphylaxis (an IgE-mediated hypersensitivity response) in small animals is most often the result of an arthropod bite or sting. Drug administration and hyposensitization injections have also been implicated as causes.[1] Localized wheals or a generalized urticarial reaction with facial and pedal edema are the most common clinical signs. Arthropod bites can cause a necrotizing vasculitis (skin erythema, ulceration, and sloughing). Vomiting, diarrhea, airway obstruction (laryngeal edema), and cardiovascular collapse may be seen with severe anaphylaxis.

Corticosteroids (prednisone, prednisolone, or methylprednisolone preparations; 2.2 mg/kg body weight as needed) should be administered intravenously to treat anaphylaxis. The animal should be hospitalized for 24 hours. A thorough search of the animal's coat should be made for arthropods (ticks). Epinephrine and antihistamines can be used in the treatment of anaphylaxis.[2] I have rarely used these drugs because of the consistent efficacy of the corticosteroids. Intravenous administration of antihistamines may initiate an anaphylactic reaction.

Pyotraumatic dermatitis

Pyotraumatic dermatitis ("hot spots" or acute moist dermatitis), is a frequent and poorly understood disease in dogs.[3] Pyotraumatic dermatitis may occur and worsen over the course of just a few hours, and owners commonly contact emergency clinics for assistance. The disease is typified by pruritic, erythematous, ulcerated, and exudative lesions. These lesions are most often found on the dorsal caudal trunk, but may occur on the lateral limbs, neck, and face. Long-haired breeds may be more commonly affected. Most cases are seen in the warm months. Bacteria isolated from the lesions are colonizers, therefore antibiotics are seldom effective in treating the condition.

Deep skin scrapings should be performed on lesions to rule out demodicosis. Characteristic lesions on the face or jowls may be pyoderma masquerading as "hot spots," particularly in breeds such as the golden retriever, Saint Bernard, and Rottweiler.[4] These particular cases should be treated with antibiotics for 2 to 4 weeks. Most cases of pyotraumatic dermatitis respond to treatment with corticosteroids. I prefer an initial dosage of 1 mg/kg of predisone or prednisolone administered orally every 24 hours for 1 week. The dosage is tapered and the drug is discontinued after 2 to 3 weeks. In my experience, flea allergy dermatitis is the most common cause for pyotraumatic dermatitis. Flea control should always be instituted if no other underlying cause is found.[3]

SKIN DISEASES WITH LIFE-THREATENING COMPLICATIONS
Generalized demodicosis

The mite *Demodex canis* is a normal inhabitant of most dogs' hair follicles.[5,6] Skin lesions (patchy alopecia, fistulous tracts) arise when the mite population increases as a result of an altered host immune response[6] and damages the hair follicles. Diagnosis is based on skin scrapings demonstrating *Demodex canis*. Bacterial folliculitis and furunculosis are common complications. When these lesions become body-wide (generalized demodicidosis) the secondary bacterial infection may become systemic. *Staphyloccocus intermedius* is the usual initial bacterial pathogen and, *Pseudomonas* species are often isolated in cases that progress to sepsis. Clinical signs in generalized demodicosis include depression, fever, draining cutaneous tracts, and friable skin. Blood samples should be taken for microbiological culture and antibiotic sensitivity testing.[5] Empirical antibiotic therapy pending culture results should involve administration of a penicillinase-resistant penicillin (oxacillin), or a cephalosporin, in combination with an aminoglycoside (gentamicin). Aminoglycoside administration in a debilitated dog necessitates careful monitoring of renal function and hydration status. Use of an acaricidal dip such as amitraz (Mitaban, Upjohn) should be delayed until the draining tracts and friability of the skin are improved, in order to prevent excessive systemic absorption of the amitraz that could cause adverse signs (hypothermia, depression, death).[6] Gentle washing or whirlpooling with a dilute bactericidal solution (1 cup concentrate to 20 gallons water) such as chlorhexidine (Nolvasan, Fort Dodge) may aid in treatment. Corticosteroids are strictly contraindicated except for treatment of septic shock, in which a short-acting intravenous corticosteroid may be used.

The occurrence of generalized demodicosis in an old dog should initiate a search for underlying immunosuppressive disease such as hyperadrenocorticism or neoplasia.[5,6] Generalized demodicosis is rare in cats. Diabetes mellitus, feline leukemia virus or feline T-cell lymphotrophic (immunodeficiency) virus should be suspected as underlying causes in a cat with generalized demodicosis.[7]

Autoimmune disorders

Pemphigus and pemphigoid. These diseases are caused by cytotoxic antibodies (usually IgG but occasionally IgM or IgA) directed against the intercellular cement substance (pemphigus) or the basement membrane zone (pemphigoid).[8] Pemphigus has been seen in both dogs and cats, whereas pemphigoid has only been reported in dogs.[8,9] Breed predilection has been reported in the Japanese Akita, dachshund, bearded collie, Newfoundland, and schipperke for pemphigus foliaceus[9,10] and in the collie for bullous pemphigoid.[9]

The cytotoxic antibodies attach to the skin antigens and trigger a series of reactions leading to a loss of intercellular cohesion causing epidermal acantholysis and blisters. The subsequent loss of the normal cutaneous barrier to the environment predisposes the animal to infection and sepsis.

Clinical signs include pustules, vesicles, crusts, and ulcerations around the mucocutaneous junctions (Fig. 24-1). In bullous pemphigoid, skin lesions may be especially evident in the inguinal or axillary regions.[9] These lesions are generalized throughout the skin in severe cases. Swelling of the extremities, fever, and depression are common signs in severe cases.

Diagnosis of pemphigus and pemphigoid is based on histologic findings and immunohistochemical evaluation (direct immunofluorescence or immunoperoxidase staining) of the skin biopsies to demonstrate evidence of the cytotoxic antibodies.[8] Intact pustules or vesicles offer the best biopsy sites, but histologic evaluation of crusted lesions or elliptical biopsies from ulcerated to normal skin frequently confirm the clinician's diagnosis of the disease. Cytologic examination of

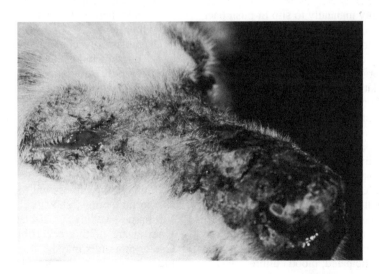

Fig. 24-1. Crusts on face of 10-year-old setter-cross with pemphigus foliaceus.

pustular contents may demonstrate acantholytic cells (rounded epidermal cells) in pemphigus (but not in pemphigoid).[8] Therapy of these conditions involves administration of immunosuppressive drugs (prednisone, azathioprine, or gold salts).[8,10] It is important to obtain biopsy samples before initiating immunosuppressive therapy. Blood cultures should be performed and broad-spectrum antibiotics (cephalosporins) administered if sepsis is suspected.

Immune-mediated disorders

Erythema multiforme/toxic epidermal necrolysis. Whether these rare diseases in dogs and cats are actually a continuum or two separate syndromes is controversial.[11,12] Erythema multiforme is the more benign of the two diseases; it has been associated with reactions to drugs and observed secondary to infections.[12,13] Typically, the disease presents as erythematous, circular, nonpruritic lesions on the trunk of the animal, often spreading peripherally and clearing centrally, producing "target" lesions.[1,13] Diagnosis is based on histologic examination of affected skin. Biopsies reveal individual cell death and intracellular edema (hydropic degeneration) in the epidermis, with or without a lichenoid reaction in the dermis. A search for and elimination of the cause (drugs, infection) is indicated. No specific treatment exists, and the role of corticosteroids is controversial.[1,12]

Toxic epidermal necrolysis is a more serious disease.[12] The loss of the epidermis may be precipitated by drugs, infection, or neoplasia.[1,14] In humans, 25% of the cases do not have a determined cause. Clinical signs include presence of cutaneous vesicles or the resultant ulceration (frequently widespread) as well as fever and depression.[8,14] The ability manually to slip or push back areas of epidermis, thus creating new ulcers (Nikolsky's sign) is frequently present.[8] Diagnosis is based on histologic examination of affected skin. Hydropic degeneration of the basal cells and full-thickness coagulation necrosis of the epidermis are noted.[8,14] There is minimal dermal inflammation unless the dermal-epidermal junction is disrupted. Therapy, as with erythema multiforme is controversial. Cessation of the offending cause represents the most important aspect.[1] High-dose corticosteroid administration (1 to 2 mg/kg prednisone or prednisolone) has been recommended.[1,12,14]

Erythema multiforme and toxic epidermal necrolysis are potentially life threatening because of their ability to deprive large areas of the body of the cutaneous barrier against the environment. Sepsis must be anticipated; blood cultures must be performed and the appropriate antibiotic regimen initiated when indicated. Fluid and electrolyte losses should be monitored and replaced.[8]

Parasitoses

Fleas. Severe anemia may also be associated with flea infestation. The animal is often a neonate in a poor husbandry situation. Therapy consists of blood transfusions followed by use of an insecticidal spray. Use of an insecticide on a debilitated animal should be done with caution. An aqueous spray licensed for use in cats and applied in small amounts every 48 hours is probably safe.

Myiasis. Myiasis is the invasion of tissue by the larvae (maggots) of various dipterous flies. These animals are often debilitated and need supportive care. Affected areas should be gently flushed with sterile saline solution to remove the maggots and any diseased tissue. Ivermectin administration (0.3 mg/kg orally) may also be effective in eliminating larvae. Ivermectin should be used with caution in collies and related breeds. Antibiotics are indicated to treat secondary bacterial infections.

Neoplasia

Two malignant neoplastic conditions of the skin are important, as the syndromes they cause may not present with typical nodules and tumors. The first is cutaneous lymphoma, specifically, epidermotropic lymphoma, or mycosis fungoides.[15] This disease occurs primarily in older dogs and may present as seborrhea (Fig. 24-2), erythema, or ulceration (especially of the oral cavity and other mucocutaneous junctions). Pruritus that is poorly responsive to corticosteroids may be associated with the skin lesions. Lymphadenopathy is often present, usually caused by the inflammatory skin component rather than by tumor invasion of the lymph nodes.

Diagnosis of epidermotropic lymphoma is based on skin biopsy, which reveals a lichenoid cellular infiltrate composed primarily of large atypical mononuclear cells with irregular folded and grooved nuclei. Pautrier's microabscesses (collections of these cells in the epidermis) are usually present.[15] Suggested therapies include topical nitrogen mustard, systemic chemotherapeutic agents or the retinoids (vitamin A derivatives).[15-17]

Primary lung tumors will occasionally metastasize to the dermis, subcutis, or skeleton, causing soft-tissue swelling, crusts, and draining tracts.[18] I am aware of this occurring in cats and dogs. One or more feet may be affected, and the animal may present as having a pododermatitis. Diagnosis is by demonstration of the neoplasm on biop-

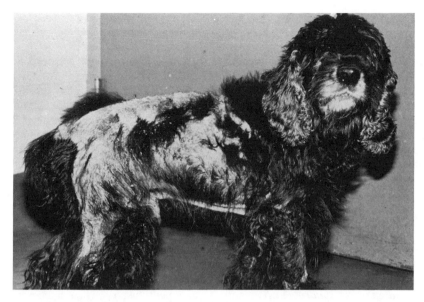

Fig. 24-2. Alopecia and seborrhea in association with pruritus in an 11-year-old cocker spaniel with canine epidermotropic lymphoma (mycosis fungoides).

sies of the subcutaneous and pulmonary tissues. Suspected neoplastic pulmonary lesions may be visualized on thoracic radiography. The tumor is frequently in its advanced metastatic stages, and there is no recommended therapy.

Juvenile cellulitis

Juvenile cellulitis (juvenile pyoderma, puppy strangles) is a disease of pups less than 4 months old. The cause is unknown.[8] Clinical signs observed are lymphadenopathy (especially the mandibular lymph nodes), anorexia, fever, and lethargy. Edema, pustules, papules, and crusts are observed at the mucocutaneous junctions of the face. Severely affected cases will present with high fevers, fistulous draining tracts (usually originating from lymph nodes), and purulent exudate from the ear canals and the face. Compromised respiration may occur due to the impingement of the mandibular and retropharyngeal lymph nodes on the larynx and trachea. A nonseptic purulent arthritis occurs in a small number of cases.[19]

Diagnosis is based on clinical signs. Skin scrapings should be done to eliminate demodicosis. Antibiotics (usually cephalosporins) and corticosteroids (prednisone or prednisolone 1 mg/kg twice a day for 1 week then slowly tapered down over the course of 30 days) is my preferred therapy. Care must be taken to avoid harsh or roughly applied topical therapy, as this disease may frequently result in scarring.[8] If corticosteroids are not used, a certain percentage of these dogs will die.

LIFE-THREATENING SYSTEMIC DISORDERS WITH CUTANEOUS MANIFESTATIONS
Congenital/hereditary disorders

Ehlers-Danlos syndrome. This congenital disease affects collagen fiber formation. A deficiency of the enzyme P-collagen peptidase has been documented in cats and a fibrillar packing defect identified in the dog.[8] A clinical consequence is hyperextensible, friable skin. Diagnosis is based on clinical signs.

The life-threatening aspect of this disease is directly related to the degree of cutaneous friability. Animals with only hyperextensible skin may be maintained as pets as long as trauma is avoided. Animals with friable skin develop continuous problems with ulcerations and lacerations either self-induced or environmentally caused. These wounds predispose the animal to recurrent sepsis and euthanasia. There is no cure for this condition. Affected animals should not be bred.[8]

Dermatomyositis. This disease affects collie dogs, Shetland sheepdogs, and their crosses.[20,21] It usually manifests itself prior to 6 months of age and is transmitted as an autosomal dominant gene with variable penetrance. Affected animals should not be bred. Cutaneous signs include erythema, alopecia, ulceration, and vesiculation of the mucocutaneous junctions, the pinna, and the trauma surfaces (especially of the front legs). Muscle atrophy, especially of the temporal, masseter, and limb girdle groups, and dysphagia may occur. Diagnosis is based on abnormal electromyography and histologic examinations of affected skin and muscle.[20,21]

Dermatomyositis varies in its clinical expression. Some pups show very minor signs that resolve. Sepsis, inhalation pneumonia, or euthanasia are the causes of death in severely affected dogs. Vitamin E and corticosteroids have been advocated and questioned as treatments. Vitamin E, as the more innocuous drug, is a candidate for empirical therapy (200 to 400 IU twice daily on an empty stomach).

Cyclic neutropenia. The cyclic neutropenia syndrome is found in all gray (not merle) collies.[22] Clinical signs (retarded growth, chronic diarrhea, arthralgia, lameness, gingivitis, anorexia, recurrent infection) begin at 6 to 8 weeks of life.[22] This is a progressive disease, usually terminating in death from sepsis of affected dogs. Therapy is limited to supportive care and antibiotics.

Nodular dermatofibrosis syndrome. A generalized nodular dermatofibrosis syndrome has been reported in mature (average age, 8 years) German shepherds.[1,23] (I have also seen this in a mixed breed dog.) These dogs have concurrent renal cystadenocarcinomas and may be presented in various stages of renal failure. The nodular growths affect the feet and the face and can be generalized along the trunk. Histopathology of the skin lesions reveals dense collagenous dermal fibrosis.[1,23] There is no known therapy for this disorder.

Endocrine diseases

Hyperadrenocorticism. Dogs with hyperadrenocorticism have an increased susceptibility to infections and are prone to bacterial urinary tract infection, pyoderma, and life-threatening bacterial pneumonia.[8,24] Sepsis can develop from any of the infections. Hypercortisolemia can also initiate pancreatitis, a common reason that dogs with hyperadrenocorticism are admitted to the intensive care unit. Dogs with hyperadrenocorticism may present in respiratory distress due to pulmonary thromboembolism. Diagnosis of pulmonary thromboembolism is confirmed by pulmonary radiography, nuclear scintigraphy, pulmonary arteriography, and blood gas evaluation. Appropriate anticoagulant therapy and supportive care should be initiated in these cases.[25] A clinical sign unique to cats with hyperadrenocorticism is the presence of friable, stretchable skin, similar to the congenital Ehlers-Danlos syndrome.[26]

The classic signs of hyperadrenocorticism in dogs are bilateral trunkal alopecia, hyperpigmentation, and calcinosis cutis.[8] Unilateral trunkal alopecia, alopecia of the extremities, deep or superficial pyoderma, demodicosis and seborrhea are less classic signs that can occur.[24] Dogs with seborrhea, demodicosis, pyoderma, or calcinosis cutis may be pruritic.[24]

Diagnosis of hyperadrenocorticism involves use of endocrine response tests (adrenocorticotropin [ACTH] stimulation, low-dose dexamethasone suppression test, high-dose dexamethasone suppression test) and measurement of endogenous ACTH levels.[8,24,25] Therapy involves aggressive treatment of complications (infections, pancreatitis) and adrenalectomy (in adrenal neoplasia in dogs[24] and perhaps for all forms of hyperadrenocorticism in cats[26]) or the adrenocorticolytic agent mitotane (in dogs with pituitary-dependent hyperadrenocorticism).[24] Diagnosis of iatrogenic hyperadrenocorticism is based on clinical signs of hyperadrenocorticism and on a *hypo*adrenocorticism-like response to an ACTH stimulation test.[8] Care should be taken to obtain a thorough drug treatment history when hyperadrenocorticism is suspected from clinical signs. Otic, ophthalmic, or topical corticosteroid-containing preparations may cause laboratory test results and clinical findings indicative of iatrogenic hyperadrenocorticism.[27-29]

Sertoli-cell tumor. This disease, thought to be caused by estrogen-like substances produced by the Sertoli cells, affects the behavior (loss of libido) and skin (bilateral alopecia, mammary gland hypertrophy) of dogs.[8] Pancytopenia, thought to be estrogen induced, occurs in approximately 13% of dogs with Sertoli-cell tumors.[30] The presence of normal testicles on palpation does not preclude the presence of Sertoli-cell tumors.[8] Diagnosis is based on histologic examination of the testicles following castration. The ability to detect abnormal serum estrogen levels is inconsistent.[30] Transfusions of fresh whole blood or platelet-rich plasma are indicated as a means to prepare a dog with thrombocytopenia for surgery and to maintain an animal with bone marrow suppression postoperatively. The presence of pancytopenia carries a poor prognosis.[8] In cases that respond to castration hematologic parameters can return to normal 20 to 30 days after castration.[30]

Hypothyroidism. Hypothyroidism is uncommon as an underlying life-threatening disease. Myxedema, stupor, coma, and eventual death have been reported in dogs[31] (see Chapter 18). Clinical signs in these severe cases include hypothermia, nonpitting edema, mental dullness, depression, nonresponsiveness to stimuli, inappetence, bradycardia, and hypoventilation. Hyponatremia and hypercholesterolemia are noted in biochemical serum analyses.[31] Diagnosis is based on results of a thyroid-stimulating hormone response test. Therapy in severe cases is reported as intravenous levothyroxine (300 μg given once)[31] followed by supplementation of the drug orally at 0.01 mg/kg body weight divided twice a day.

Diabetes Mellitus. Cutaneous signs related to diabetes mellitus are uncommon in small animals. Seborrhea, alopecia, xanthoma, and demodicosis (cats) have been reported.[7,8] Diabetic dermatopathy is an uncommon and poorly understood condition associated with diabetes mellitus (as well as pancreatic neoplasia or hepatic disease).[1,32,32a] Clinical signs are suppurative crusting of the muzzle and feet[1,32] Diagnosis is based on biopsy of affected skin (marked edema of the upper half of the epidermis and diffuse parakeratosis).[1,32] Cutaneous signs may precede the signs of metabolic derangements and internal organ dysfunction.

Infectious diseases

Sepsis. Sepsis may cause petechiae, papules, pustules, or ulcers.[33] The pathogenesis of these lesions is unknown. Factors thought to be responsible are septic embolization, bacterial invasion, deposition of antibody-antigen complexes, and circulating endotoxins.[33] In my experience, *Staphyloccocus intermedius* and *Pseudomonas* spp. are the organisms that will most commonly cause cutaneous signs of sepsis. Sepsis may also result from severe cases of deep pyoderma (common in German shepherds and in dogs with hyperadrenocorticism or generalized demodicosis).[38] Blood cultures should be obtained in all septic patients. I choose to treat such dogs with a cephalosporin and gentamicin pending culture results.

Plague. Bubonic plague is an acute febrile zoonotic disease with a high mortality rate caused by the gram-negative bacterium *Yersinia pestis*.[8] The disease is primarily found in the western United States (including Hawaii) as a disease of rodents. Plague is transmitted by fleas or by direct contact with infected animals or exudates.

Cats with plague usually present with severe fevers, subcutaneous abscesses, and lymphadenopathy. Septicemia without lymph node enlargement and primary pneumonic plague are uncommon forms of the disease in animals. Bubonic plague in cats cannot be differentiated clinically from fight wound abscesses caused by *Pasteurella multocida* or other pyogenic bacteria.[34] Plague should always be suspected in any cat from an enzootic area that presents with a high fever, lymphadenopathy and/or abscesses.[34] Dogs are highly resistant to plague and generally only mild fevers develop in them.

Diagnosis is confirmed by culturing the organism. *Yersinia pestis* is usually easily isolated from lymph node aspirates, abscess exudates, and peripheral blood. A fluorescent-antibody test (Plague Branch of the Centers for Disease Control, Fort Collins, CO) performed on two air-dried smears of exudate or lymph node aspirate is almost as reliable as culture, and the results are obtained much quicker. A passive hemagglutination test may also be performed on the serum. It is important to realize that *Pasteurella multocida* may also be cultured concurrently from abscesses or lymph nodes.

All animals suspected of plague should be treated for fleas to minimize exposure of people handling the animal. Systemic antibiotic therapy is indicated in all cases of plague except those in which there are signs of lung involvement. Animals with pneumonic plague are highly infectious and should be euthanized rather than treated. The antibiotics of choice for the treatment of plague are streptomycin (30 to 50 mg/kg divided twice a day given intramuscularly), tetracycline (75 mg/kg divided three times a day orally or 15 mg/kg divided twice a day given parenterally), and chloramphenicol (100 to 150 mg/kg divided three times a day orally).[34] Penicillin and ampicillin are not effective in the treatment of plague.

Sporotrichosis. This disease is caused by the organism *Sporothrix schenckii*.[8,35] The disease causes nodules, ulcers, corded lymphatics, and in generalized cases, pulmonary signs and death. Diagnosis is based on culture of the organism. In cats, microscopic examination of the exudate and/or biopsy of the affected skin (fungal stains) may show the organism.

This disease is a zoonosis and extreme care (gloves, hand washing) should be taken in handling suspected cases.[1,8,35] The organism can penetrate undamaged human skin. As a result of public health considerations, euthanasia of affected animals should be discussed with owners. Treatment involves administering sodium or potassium iodide, ketoconazole, or amphotericin B.[8]

Systemic mycoses. Systemic mycoses such as coccidioidomycosis, histoplasmosis, blastomycosis, and cryptococcosis can manifest cutaneous lesions.[8] Clinical signs are variable because of the multitude of organs that may be affected. Cutaneous lesions include nodules, draining tracts, ulcers, plaques, seborrhea, and alopecia. Cryptococcosis usually involves the nasal area. Diagnosis is based on demonstration of the organism on culture, histopathology, or aspirate cytology of affected organs. Effective therapy involves administration of ketaconazole with or without amphotericin B.[8,36] Blastomycosis has been reported to be directly transmissible from animals to humans.[37]

Leishmaniasis. Leishmaniasis is a protozoal disease of dogs that is rare in the United States. Leishmaniasis of dogs with no travel history outside the United States has been reported,[38] but most affected dogs have been imported from or vacationed with the owner in endemic areas, especially the Mediterranean basin. Leishmaniasis may present as purely cutaneous or as a visceral-cutaneous syndrome. Dogs from the Mediterranean area almost always have the latter form.[39] Clinical signs may include chronic debilitation, arthropathy, generalized lymphadenopathy, non-regenerative anemia, exfoliative dermatitis, periorbital and perioral alopecia and ulceration, keratoconjunctivitis, and diarrhea.[39] These clinical signs are nonspecific, and they mimic more common diseases (particularly the autoimmune skin diseases). Diagnosis is based on results of serologic tests, isolation of the organism from cultures of the skin or other organs, and demonstration of the organism on lymph node, joint fluid, or bone marrow aspirate cytology. [38-41] The pentavalent antimonials are the most effective drugs leading to remission or cure. In the United States these drugs are available only from the Centers for Disease Control in Atlanta.[8]

Direct transmission between dogs and humans is very unlikely (a sandfly vector is usually necessary), but not impossible.[39] Children under 5 years old are at greater risk of contracting the Mediterranean form. Euthanasia of dogs with leishmaniasis should be considered in cases in which there are children in the household.

Babesiosis. This protozoal disease usually presents with nondermatologic clinical signs (anorexia, lethargy, hematuria, fever, anemia, hemoglobinuria, icterus, generalized lymphadenopathy, splenomegaly, and emesis).[42] Occasionally, cases will present with dramatic petechiae due to thrombocytopenia[43] and/or bullous impetigo, urticaria, or edema of the distal extremities of the face. Diagnosis is by demonstration of the organism (*Brucella canis* or *B. gibsoni*) in red blood cells sampled from capillaries (ear pinna). Alternatively, serodiagnostic methods may be employed. These include complement fixation, indirect hemagglutination, indirect fluorescent antibody and, enzyme-linked immunosorbent assay.[44] Therapy has been reviewed elsewhere.[42]

Rocky Mountain spotted fever/ehrlichiosis. These tickborne rickettsial diseases usually present with nondermatologic clinical signs. However, about 20% to 30% of these dogs will present with edema of the extremities, petechiae of the skin, or scrotal dermatitis.[45] Diagnosis is confirmed by serology or demonstration of the organism on blood smears. Tetracycline (22 mg/kg

every 8 hours for 2 weeks) is the common treatment, but other therapies have been reported.[46]

Environmental diseases

Thallium toxicosis. Thallium is a rodenticide that often produces cutaneous and oral lesions when ingested over a long term. Lesions consist of nonpruritic alopecia, erythema, and crusts and ulceration of the perioral, interdigital, facial, and genital areas.[8] Histopathologic evaluation of these lesions reveals marked parakeratosis with intraepidermal microabscesses.[8] Antemortem diagnosis is made by determination of urine thallium concentration. Any thallium detected is diagnostic for thallium toxicosis (Gabriel's test with rhodamine B may give false positive results in cats).[8] Treatment involves the administration of Prussian blue (100 mg/kg orally three times a day). Thallium toxicosis has an extremely grave prognosis. The animal frequently dies of multiple-organ failure.[8]

Autoimmune diseases

Systemic lupus erythematosus. Cutaneous lesions (30% to 50% prevalence) in systemic lupus erythematosus in the dog are usually described as depigmentation, erythema, crusting, and ulceration of the mucocutaneous junctions, although stomatitis and panniculitis have also been reported.[47,48] Dogs with systemic lupus erythematosus will present on an emergency basis for development of immune-mediated hemolytic anemia (with or without thrombocytopenia) or for signs of renal failure. The presence of these signs carries a poorer prognosis than cutaneous signs alone.[8]

Diagnosis is based on the constellation of clinical signs, positive serum antinuclear antibody (ANA) test and/or lupus erythematosus-cell test, characteristic histopathology of the skin (interface, hydropic or lichenoid dermatitis, and thickening of the basement membrane zone), and demonstration of immunoglobulin deposition along the basement membrane zone.[8,47,49] Therapy most commonly includes high doses of corticosteroids and other immunosuppressive drugs (azathioprine, cyclophosphamide).[49]

Cold agglutinin disease. This is an uncommon disease of dogs and cats and is caused by the presence of cold-reacting (usually IgM) erythrocyte autoantibodies.[8] The autoantibody is most active at colder temperatures (0 to 4°C) but has a wide range of activity (0 to 30°C). Clinical signs of cold agglutinin disease relate to development of anemia, intracapillary hemagglutination, or both. Skin lesions include erythema, purpura, acrocyanosis, necrosis, and ulceration of the extremities (paws, ears, nose, tip of tail).[8] The lesions are precipitated or exacerbated in affected animals by exposure to cold that causes hemagglutination in capillary beds of extremities with resultant tissue ischemia.

Definitive diagnosis of cold agglutinin disease is made by in vitro autohemagglutination of blood at room temperature for the presence of cold-reacting autoantibodies.[8] This finding may be confirmed via a Coombs' test performed at 4°C with Coombs' reagent with activity against IgM. Normal dogs and cats may have titers up to 1:100.[8] Therapy for cold agglutinin disease includes correction of the underlying cause, avoidance of cold exposure and administration of immunosuppressive drugs.[8]

Drug eruption. In humans the most common drugs implicated as causing drug eruptions are sulfonamides (especially trimethoprim-sulfonamide combinations), penicillins (including semisynthetic penicillins and ampicillin), blood products, and nonsteroidal antiinflammatory drugs.[50,51] No data on the prevalence of drug eruptions is available in small animals, although a number of drugs have been implicated. Probably the best-documented reactions are those of Doberman pinschers (and other breeds) to trimethoprim-sulfadiazine preparations.[52]

Rashes (erythema with macules or papules) are probably the most common cutaneous response in people,[50] and this reaction has been noted in dogs and cats. Clinical signs can include pruritus unresponsive to corticosteroids.[8] Nondermatologic signs accompanying drug eruptions include anemia, leukopenia, thrombocytopenia, glomerulonephritis, and polymyositis.[52]

Diagnosis is made by observing improvement in clinical signs following identification and discontinuation of the administration of the offending drug. This process may be more difficult than it sounds, especially if multiple drugs are being administered. In such cases, the least essential and/or most likely drugs should be discontinued first. Most drugs initiate adverse eruptions soon after starting therapy (i.e., recently initiated drugs should elicit more suspicion than drugs administered over a long term). Ampicillin and the semisynthetic penicillins may cause eruptions that begin up to several weeks after the drug is discontinued.[50]

On cessation of clinical signs referable to a drug eruption, that drug and all related drugs should be avoided in the patient. Reinstitution of therapy with the offending drug as a diagnostic test is undesirable and potentially dangerous.

REFERENCES

1. Ihrke PJ. Life threatening dermatoses in small animal practice. Proc Eleventh Kal Kan Symp, 1987;11:103-107.
2. Wilcke JR. Allergic drug reactions. In Kirk RW, ed. Current veterinary therapy IX. Philadelphia: WB Saunders, 1986;444-448.
3. White SD, Ihrke PJ. Pyoderma. In Nesbitt GH, ed. Contemporary issues of small animal practice dermatology. New York: Churchill-Livingstone, 1987;95-121.
4. Reinke SI, Stannard AA, Ihrke PJ, Reinke JD. Histopathologic features of pyotraumatic dermatitis. J Am Vet Med Assoc 1987;190:57-60.
5. White SD, Stannard AA. Canine demodicosis. In Kirk RW, ed. Current veterinary therapy VIII. Philadelphia: WB Saunders, 1983;484-487.
6. Kwochka KW. Canine demodicosis. In Kirk RW, ed. Current veterinary therapy IX. Philadelphia: WB Saunders 1986;531-537.
7. White, SD, Carpenter JL, Moore FM, Ogilvie GL. Generalized demodicosis associated with diabetes mellitus in two cats. J Am Vet Med Assoc 1987;191:448-450.
8. Muller GH, Kirk RW, Scott DW. Small animal dermatology, ed 3. Philadelphia: WB Saunders, 1983.
9. Scott DW, Walton DK, Slatter M, Smith CA, Lewis RM. Immune-mediated dermatoses in domestic animals: ten years after. Part I. Compend Contin Educ Pract Vet 1987;9:424-437.
10. Ihrke PJ, Stannard AA, Ardans AA, Griffin CE. Pemphigus foliaceus in dogs: a review of 37 cases. J Am Vet Med Assoc 1985;186:59-66.
11. Goldstein SM, Wintroub BW, Elias PM, Wuepper KD. Toxic epidermal necrolysis: unmuddying the water. waters. Arch Dermatol 1987;123:1153-1156.
12. Berman RS, Silvestri DL. Dermatologic problems in the intensive care unit: Part I. J Intensive Care Med 1986;1:15-28.
13. Scott DW, Miller WH, Goldschmidt MH. Erythema multiforme in the dog. J Am Anim Hosp Assoc 1983;19:453-459.
14. Scott DW, Halliwell REW, Goldschmidt MH, DiBartola S. Toxic epidermal necrolysis in two dogs and a cat. J Am Anim Hosp Assoc 1979;15:271-279.
15. Walton DK. Canine epidermotropic lymphoma. In Kirk RW, ed. Current veterinary therapy IX. Philadelphia: WB Saunders 1986;609-614.
16. Couto GC. Cutaneous lymphomas. Proc Eleventh Kal Kan Symp 1987;11:71-78.
17. Kessler JF, Jones SE, Levine N, et al. Isotretinoin and cutaneous helper T-cell lymphoma (mycosis fungoides). Arch Dermatol 1987;123:201-204.
18. Pool RR, Bodle JE, Mantos JJ, et al. Primary lung carcinoma with skeletal metastases in the cat. Feline Pract 1974;4(4):36-41.
19. White SD, Rosychuk RAW, Stewart LJ, et al. Juvenile cellulitis in dogs: 15 cases (1979-1988). J Am Vet Med Assoc 1989;195:1609-1611.
20. Kunkle GA, Chrisman CL, Gross TL, Fadok V, Warner LL. Dermatomyositis in collie dogs. Compend Contin Educ Pract Vet 1985;7:185-192.
21. Hargis AM, Haupt KH, Prieur DJ, Moore MP. A skin disorder in three Shetland sheepdogs: comparison with familial canine dermatomyositis of collies. Compend Contin Educ Pract Vet 1985;7:306-315.
22. Campbell KL. Canine cyclic hematopoiesis. Compend Contin Educ Pract Vet 1985;7:57-62.
23. Lium B, Moe L. Hereditary multifocal renal cystadenocarcinomas and nodular dermatofibrosis in the German shepherd dog: macroscopic and histopathologic changes. Vet Pathol 1985;22:447-455.

24. White SD, Ceragiloli KL, Stewart LJ, Bullock LP, Mason GD. Cutaneous markers of canine hyperadrenocorticism. Compend Contin Educ Pract Vet 1989;11:446-465.
25. Burns MG, Kelly AB, Hornof WJ, et al. Pulmonary artery thrombosis in three dogs with hyperadrenocorticism. J Am Vet Med Assoc 1981;178:388-393.
26. Nelson RW, Feldman EC, Smith MC. Hyperadrenocorticism in cats: seven cases (1978-1987). J Am Vet Med Assoc 1988;193:245-250.
27. Zenoble RD, Kemppainen RJ. Adrenal cortical suppression by topically applied corticosteroids in healthy dogs. J Am Vet Med Assoc 1987;191:685-688.
28. Glaze MB, Crawford MA, Nachreinder RF, Casey HW, Nafe LA, Kearney MT. Ophthalmic corticosteroid therapy: systemic effects in the dog. J Am Vet Med Assoc 1988;192:73-75.
29. Moriello KA, Fehrer-Sawyer SL, Meyer DJ, Feder B. Adrenocortical suppression associated with topical otic administration of glucocorticoids in dogs. J Am Vet Med Assoc 1988;193:329-331.
30. Morgan RV. Blood dyscrasias associated with testicular tumors in the dog. J Am Anim Hosp Assoc 1982;18:970-975.
31. Kelly MJ, Hill JR. Canine myxedema and stupor. Compend Contin Educ Pract Vet 1984;6:1049-1057.
32. Walton DK, Center SA, Scott DW, Collins K. Ulcerative dermatitis associated with diabetes mellitus in the dog: A report of four cases. J Am Anim Hosp Assoc 1986;22:79-88.
32a. Miller WH, Scott DW, Buerger RG, et al. Necrolytic migratory erythemia in dogs: a hepatocutaneous syndrome. J Am Anim Hosp Assoc 1990;26:573-581.
33. Berman RS, Silvestri DL. Dermatologic problems in the intensive care unit: Part II. J Intensive Care Med 1986;1:111-118.
34. Thilsted JP. Plague. In Barlough JE, ed. Manual of small animal infectious disease. New York: Churchill Livingstone, 1988;169-176.
35. Dunstan RW, Reimann KA, Langham RF. Feline sporotrichosis. J Am Vet Med Assoc 1986;189:880-883.
36. Legendre AM, Selcer BA, Edwards DF, Stevens R. Treatment of canine blastomycosis with amphotericin B and ketoconazole. J Am Vet Med Assoc 1984;184:1249-1254.
37. Knoll JS, MacWilliams PS. Blastomycosis. In Barlough JE, ed. Manual of small animal infectious diseases. New York: Churchill Livingstone, 1988;299-308.
38. White SD. Diseases of the lips and oral cavity of domestic animals. Clin Dermatol 1987;5:190-201.
39. Anderson DC, Buckner RG, Glenn BL, MacVean DW. Endemic canine leishmaniasis. Vet Pathol 1980;17:94-96.
40. Longstaffe JA, Guy MW. Canine leishmaniasis—United Kingdom update. J Small Anim Pract 1986;27:663-671.
41. Macianti F, Meciani N. Specific serodiagnosis of canine leishmaniasis by indirect immunofluorescence, indirect hemagglutination, and counter immunoelectrophoresis. Am J Vet Res 1988;49:1409-1411.
42. Abdullahi SU, Sannusi A. Canine babesiosis. In Kirk RW, ed. Current veterinary therapy, IX. Philadelphia: WB Saunders, 1986;1096-1098.
43. Pages J-P, Trouillet J-L. Thrombocytopenie dans la babesiose du chien. Pract Med Chir Anim Compagnie 1984;19:222-227.
44. Huxsoll DL. Babesiosis. In Barlough JE, ed. Manual of small animal infectious disease. New York: Churchill Livingstone, 1988;383-389.
45. Greene CE, Burgdorfer W, Cavagnolo R, Philip RN, Peacock MG. Rocky Mountain spotted fever in dogs and its differentiation from canine ehrlichiosis. J Am Vet Med Assoc 1985;186:465-472.
46. Greene CE. Rocky Mountain spotted fever and ehrlichiosis. In Kirk RW, ed. Current veterinary therapy IX. Philadelphia: WB Saunders, 1986;1080-1084.
47. Scott DW, Walton DK, Manning TO, Smith CA, Lewis RM. Canine lupus erythematosus. I. Systemic lupus erythematosus. J Am Anim Hosp Assoc 1983;19:461-479.
48. Grindem CB, Johnson KH. Systemic lupus erythematosus: literature review and report of 42 new canine cases. J Am Anim Hosp Assoc 1983;19:489-503.
49. Scott DW, Walton DK, Slatter M, Smith CA, Lewis RM. Immune-mediated dermatosis in domestic animals: ten years after. Part II. Compend Contin Educ Pract Vet 1987;9:539-554.
50. Berman RS, Silvestri DL. Dermatologic problems in the intensive care unit: Part IV. J Intensive Care Med 1986;1:224-239.
51. Guillaume J-C, Roujeau J-C, Revuz J, Penso D, Touraine R. The culprit drugs in 87 cases of toxic epidermal necrolysis (Lyell's syndrome). Arch Dermatol 1987;123:1166-1170.
52. Giger U, Warner LL, Millichamp NJ, Gorman NT. Sulfadiazine induced allergy in six Doberman pinschers. J Am Vet Med Assoc 1985;186:479-484.

25 Respiratory Emergencies

Geoffrey Gibbons

The function of the emergency clinician is to stabilize and to maintain the patient as well as perform the tests and interventions necessary to achieve these goals. As an organism depends on its respiratory system every minute of its life, intervention in respiratory emergencies must be prompt and efficient to maintain life and to preserve the functional integrity of all organ systems.

EMERGENCIES OF THE UPPER AIRWAY
The nose

Nasal conditions rarely are of urgent concern to respiration, as the mouth serves as an alternative airway. However, severe, persistent epistaxis can result in significant blood loss and shock. Traumatic nosebleeds are usually self-limiting. Epistaxis can be treated by dripping epinephrine (adrenalin) 1:100,000 solution into the affected nasal cavity and, if necessary, packing the nares and nasopharynx under general anesthesia with epinephrine soaked gauze.[1] Acute onset of sneezing can be associated with nasal foreign bodies, hypocalcemia, or focal epilepsy. Foreign bodies can be removed from the nose with an alligator forceps, preferably with the help of an otoscope, arthroscope, or urethroscope under general anesthesia.[1]

Upper esophagus

Esophageal obstruction by foreign bodies often causes significant respiratory distress due to extraluminal compression of the trachea. In these cases, dyspnea and wheezing may be the presenting signs.[2] Common sites for esophageal obstruction include the thoracic inlet, the heart base, and the diaphragmatic hiatus.

Small rubber balls occasionally are swallowed by dogs; these tend to lodge in the cervical esophagus caudal to the larynx. External digital manipulations to the neck can often move the ball into the oropharynx and mouth. The obstruction of the pharynx that occurs as the ball exits the esophagus prevents respiration. The severe respiratory distress that results prevents adequate restraint of the patient and manipulation of the ball into the mouth. Sedation or anesthesia and the insertion of an endotracheal tube, prior to commencing manipulations, will maintain the airway during retrieval. Alternative methods that can be used include an endoscope with retrieval forceps, sponge forceps or Foley catheter(s). The Foley catheter is inserted past the obstruction, the cuff is blown up, then the catheter is retracted with the foreign object. A second Foley catheter inflated proximal (cranial) to the foreign body and retracted in concert with the caudal catheter may decrease esophageal damage.

Trachea and larynx

Obstructive lesions of this major airway include foreign bodies, tracheal stenosis, tracheal collapse, laryngeal paralysis, intratracheal neoplasms and parasitic granulomas, inflammatory edema (burns), and compression from extratracheal masses (neoplasia and lymphadenopathy). Neoplastic and infectious causes are least likely to present as emergencies.[3,4]

Upper airway obstructions usually produce inspiratory stridor and referred upper airway sounds heard on auscultation of the chest. Exercise intolerance, dyspnea, and cyanosis may also be noted to varying degrees and for varying durations depending on the cause of the obstruction. Heavy sedation or light general anesthesia will allow visualization of the larynx and observation of its function. Radiography is useful in diagnosis but should be performed after the animal is stable. Foreign bodies often stand out well against an inflated lung. If foreign bodies become lodged in a bronchus, the lung distal to the obstruction be-

399

comes atelectatic, diminishing contrast and making it harder to identify the foreign body on the radiograph.

Removal of a tracheal foreign body may be attempted by holding the animal's head down and rapidly compressing the chest. This is a noninvasive and simple maneuver that may be successful in a small percentage of cases. Obstructions proximal and immediately caudal to the larynx can be bypassed by a tracheostomy between the obstruction and the lung (see Chapter 10). This surgical incision may be extended to allow better access to the obstruction, facilitating its removal. A bronchoscope may be necessary to visualize and remove tracheal foreign bodies. If the foreign body is situated near the carina and cannot be removed with a bronchoscope and retrieval instruments, the object can be pushed into a bronchus, clearing ventilation to half the lung and allowing for routine surgical removal.

Laryngeal paralysis. The respiratory distress of laryngeal paralysis and collapsing trachea can usually be alleviated by sedation (acetylpromazine 0.05 mg/kg intravenously) and placing the animal in an oxygen-enriched atmosphere (40% to 100% oxygen). An alternative approach for oxygen administration is to use a long through-the-needle, 14- to 17-gauge intravenous catheter (Intracath, Becton Dickinson, Sandy, UT) inserted through the cricothyroid membrane and advanced down the trachea toward the carina. Oxygen, humidified by bubbling it through water, can be supplied directly to the lungs in this fashion. The catheter can also be used to suction out fluids but may become occluded during suction and have to be replaced.

Complications of acute upper airway obstruction that may have to be dealt with include pneumonia, management of a tracheostomy, and pulmonary edema. Pulmonary edema has been reported to occur in the dog and in 10% of humans suffering an acute upper airway obstruction.[5]

Acute laryngeal trauma. In the early stages, laryngeal injury may be deceptively silent, only to manifest hours later, as an acute, life-threatening problem. Clinical signs include hoarseness, dyspnea, dysphagia, subcutaneous emphysema, hemoptysis, and paralysis of the vocal chords. Mucosal tears, fractures of laryngeal cartilages, laryngotracheal avulsion, and damage to the nerve supply of the larynx can occur following laryngeal trauma. Diagnosis is made by direct visualization, palpation, laryngoscopy, and radiography. In human medicine, the CT scan has proved useful in the diagnosis of laryngeal cartilage fracture.[6] In cases with severe respiratory embarrassment, a tracheostomy should be performed in preference to endotracheal intubation, as endotracheal intubation may be difficult, may cause further trauma, and may increase the risk of infection. Corticosteroids may be administered to decrease concomitant laryngeal edema. Empirical broad-spectrum antibiotics may be used if observation and cytologic or bacteriologic examination indicates gross contamination. In these situations, microbiologic cultures should be obtained prior to the commencement of antimicrobial therapy. In humans, esophagoscopy and bronchoscopy are advised to define completely the extent of injuries. Definitive repair should not be delayed more than a few days, otherwise infectious complications are more likely to ensue.[6]

EMERGENCIES OF THE CHEST
Space-occupying lesions of the pleural space

Animals with compromise of their pleural space will generally present as emergencies due to respiratory embarrassment from marked lung collapse. These patients can demonstrate dyspnea, open-mouth breathing, and cyanosis. The animal's survival often depends on rapid diagnosis and removal of the space-occupying substance. Animals with uncomplicated diaphragmatic hernias are usually not severely compromised and can usually await routine surgical correction. Severe respiratory compromise due to space-occupying pleural masses or diffuse pulmonary metastases is often a terminal event, so a rapid, accurate diagnosis will allow confident termination of the animal's suffering.

Two useful manual diagnostic methods for detection of space-occupying pleural and pulmonary diseases are percussion and auscultation. The stethoscope bell is best for auscultation of low-pitched sounds and the diaphragm for high-pitched sounds. Holding the animal's mouth closed and occluding one nostril will cause it to breathe more deeply and quietly, aiding the auscultation of abnormal sounds. Harsh or dry lung sounds occur on inspiration and expiration and may be due to bronchial inflammation; moist crackles occur with fluid in the bronchi and are also heard on inspiration and expiration; crepitations are heard only on inspiration as fluid-filled alveoli are opened.[7] Percussion can be an inaccurate diagnostic technique when used alone, but it is useful in the emergency room, as it is a nonstressful and informative technique. Percussion involves using the middle finger of the left hand as the pleximeter—tapping it on the middle phalanx with the middle finger of the right hand. Wrist motion of the right hand should be loose and flexible. Keep the pleximeter finger parallel to the boundary being percussed and move it perpendicularly to the boundary.[7] A dull area on percussion with air-filled lung above it may suggest a space-occupying mass (fluid or tissue),[8] while the presence of hyperresonance may suggest pneumothorax. Auscultation for lung sounds, or their absence, when used with percussion aids diagnosis (Table 25-1).

Radiography is one of the most useful diagnostic techniques in the evaluation of pleural disease. However, restraint for radiography in the severely dyspneic animal can be fatal and radiography may be contraindicated during the initial evaluation.[9] With care, one radiograph with the animal in its most comfortable position may be obtained safely.[8] Full radiographic examination (lateral, ventrodorsal, dorsoventral, and other studies as indicated) should be performed after patient stabilization. To demonstrate air in the pleural space, the dorsoventral view is preferable, and to demonstrate pleural fluid, the ventrodorsal view is better.[10] Ultrasound is useful in noninvasively evaluating cardiac structure and function and in determining the presence and position of any pleural fluid or extracardiac mass lesions.

Thoracocentesis will alleviate signs of respiratory distress in cases of pleural effusion and pneu-

mothorax and should be performed without delay. Samples of fluid obtained by thoracocentesis should always be submitted for detailed clinicopathologic analysis (e.g., microbiologic culture, cytologic evaluation). Ultrasound guidance may aid in the detection and removal of pleural fluid.

Pleural effusion. The presence of free fluid in the pleural space can cause severe respiratory distress depending on the fluid involved and the rate of its accumulation. This compromise of pulmonary function causes hypoxia and hypercapnia.[8] Pleural fluid can be classified as a pure transudate (hydrothorax), modified transudate (chylothorax, neoplastic, cardiac) or exudate (pyothorax, hemothorax) according to its cellularity and protein content (Table 25-2). Physical characteristics such as color and odor, specific gravity, hematocrit, total solid content, and cellularity (from stained smears) can all be determined in the emergency room.

Hydrothorax. Hydrothorax refers to a clear fluid with a specific gravity less than 1.017 and little protein content. Hypoproteinemia and heart failure, particularly right-sided heart failure in cats, are common causes. Fluid present as a result

Table 25-1 Summary of the findings of auscultation and percussion in various pleural and pulmonary parenchymal diseases*

Disease Condition	Findings on Auscultation	Findings on Percussion
Pleural effusion (normally similar findings bilaterally)	"Fluid line" detectable where lung sounds are decreased or absent ventrally, and normal to increased bronchovesicular sounds dorsally; heart sounds may be muffled	"Fluid line" detectable where resonance is decreased below the line and normal to slightly increased above the line
Pneumothorax (normally similar findings bilaterally)	Line of demarcation noted with normal lung sounds ventrally, and decreased intensity (or absent) sounds dorsally; heart sounds normal	Line of demarcation noted with normal resonance ventrally, and a noticeably increased resonance dorsally
Diaphragmatic hernia (normally unilateral findings)	Increased bronchovesicular and heart sounds on the normal side, with absent or decreased heart and lung sounds on the hernia side	Decreased resonance on side of hernia (Exception: when stomach herniates it may fill with gas and an increased resonance may be detected)
Lung consolidation (normally unilateral findings)	Increased bronchovesicular sounds over affected area; absence of all sounds if bronchus is occluded	Localized area of decreased resonance over affected area
Parenchymal mass (normally unilateral findings)	Small size: no change; large size: shifting of the location of heart sounds (depending on mass location) with an absence of regional lung sounds	Small size: no change; large size: localized area of decreased resonance

*Animals should be in sternal recumbency or standing when examined. (From McKiernan BC. Lower respiratory tract diseases. In Ettinger SJ, ed. Textbook of veterinary internal medicine, ed. 2, Philadelphia: WB Saunders 1983.)

TABLE 25-2 Serous cavity effusions of the dog and cat

Type of Effusion	Color/Turbidity	Examples of Associated Diseases	Specific Gravity/Total Solids (g/dl)	Typical Nucleated Cell Count and Types
Pure transudate	Clear, colorless	Hypoalbuminemia	≤1.017/<2.0	<1000 to 1500/μl, polymorphonuclear leukocytes, macrophages, and mesothelial cells
Modified transudate				
Nonspecific	Yellow, pink, red, cloudy	Lung lobe torsion, cardiac disease, idiopathic, neoplasms	≥1.017/2.0-5.0	300 to 5000/μl, polymorphonuclear leukocytes, macrophages, mesothelial cells, ± neoplastic cells
Chylous	White/pink, milky	Ruptured or obstructed thoracic duct, cardiomyopathy, lymphoma	Invalid owing to turbidity	<10,000/μl, small lymphocytes usually predominate or a mixed population of polymorphonuclear leukocytes, lymphs and macrophages
Pseudochylous	White/pink, milky	Chronic inflammation, neoplasia, cardiomyopathy, lymphoma, idiopathic	Invalid owing to turbidity	<10,000/μl, mixed population of polymorphonuclear leukocytes, lymphs and macrophages, occasional plasma cells, mast cells, and eosinophils
Lymphoma	White/pink, cloudy	Thymic, mediastinal and/or abdominal neoplasms	Variable, usually <1.025	4500 to 45,000/μl immature lymphoid cells
Exudate				
Nonseptic	Pale yellow, cloudy	Sterile foreign body, ruptured urinary bladder, neoplasia	>1.025/73.0	3000 to >50,000/μl, nondegenerate PMN's, macrophages, ± elevated BUN/creatinine in fluid, ±neoplastic cells
	Green, yellow, cloudy	Ruptured bile duct or gallbladder	Variable owing to dilution, usually >1.025	Many polymorphonuclear leukocytes and macrophages, bilirubin crystals

TABLE 25-2 Serious cavity effusions of the dog and cat—cont'd

Type of Effusion	Color/Turbidity	Examples of Associated Diseases	Specific Gravity/Total Solids (g/dl)	Typical Nucleated Cell Count and Types
Septic	White, red, yellow, cloudy	Bacterial or fungal infections	>1.025	>3,000/μl, polymorphonuclear leukocytes usually showing at least minimal degenerate changes
	Green/brown, granular, hazy	Ruptured gastrointestinal tract	Variable owing to dilution	Variable, degenerate polymorphonuclear leukocytes, mixed bacterial population, perhaps yellow-staining fecal material
Hemorrhagic	Red	Trauma, coagulopathy, neoplasia	>1.017	>3,000/μl, packed cell volume >10, erythrophagocytosis, macrophages containing hemosiderin (unless acute)

From Freden G.: Clinical pathology course notes, Tufts University Veterinary School, MA, 1989

of heart failure is rapidly altered to a modified transudate. The mediastinum of dogs and cats is perforate, so fluid will generally be found bilaterally.[9] Echocardiography, electrocardiography, and radiography will assist in the diagnosis of heart failure. Determination of total serum solids will assist in the diagnosis of hypoproteinemia. Evaluation for renal, gastrointestinal, and hepatic disorders is required following identification of hypoproteinemia.

Hemothorax. Blood in the thoracic cavity nearly always occurs secondary to traumatic injury; however, spontaneous ruptures of major vessels have been reported[9] and I have seen two cases of lymphoma with hemorrhagic effusions. Clotting defects must also be considered. The presence of hemorrhage in multiple sites of the body, together with a suspicious history, suggests poisoning with an anticoagulant rodenticide. Petechiae of the gingiva or skin suggest a primary platelet disorder or consumptive coagulopathy. Blood samples should be obtained to determine the activated clotting time and for submission of a clotting profile and platelet count. A stained blood smear should be examined for platelet numbers (see Chapter 23). Platelet counts should be done within 6 hours of sample collection. Administration of a blood transfusion prior to sample collection may interfere with the diagnostic evaluation of the clotting profile and platelet count.

Collection and holding of the aspirated blood under sterile conditions may permit autotransfusion. Autotransfusion can be life saving when blood loss has been severe and a rapid transfusion is necessary. Blood may be aspirated from the chest cavity into a syringe containing anticoagulant (9 ml acid citrate dextrose in a 60-ml syringe).[11] Commercial units are also available to perform autotransfusions (Solcotrans, Solco Basle, Rockland, MA; Fig. 25-1). If blood has been present in the thoracic cavity longer than 45 minutes, it will not clot and anticoagulation is not required. Any hemorrhagic fluid from the chest should be analyzed carefully because the presence of neoplastic cells, bacteria, or other fluids (e.g., urine, bile) in the chest are contraindications for autotransfusion. The patient's own blood is reinfused intravenously through a 40-μm filter, though a standard 170-μm filter may suffice. Filtering through the 170-μm filter, then through the 40-μm filter will help prevent excessive clogging of the filters.

The packed cell volume should be determined

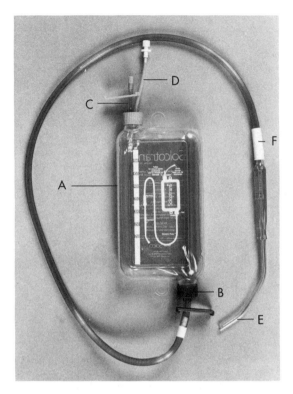

Fig. 25-1 Solcotrans Autologous Whole Blood Transfusion System (Solco Basle, Rockland, MA). The outer shell *A,* is semirigid and contains a 500-ml collapsible blood bag. The blood bag opens to the outside at the tubes marked *B* and *C.* The tube marked *D* connects into the space between the bag and the shell and is initially closed to preserve the negative pressure in the space and prevent collapse of the blood bag during aspiration. The tube marked *B* is connected to the aspiration tube *E,* through *F,* a 170-μg filter. The tube marked *C* is connected to the vacuum source for aspiration and to the patient for delivery of collected blood. The clamp on the tube marked *D* is released during blood reinfusion so that the inner blood bag can collapse to release its contents. Prior to harvesting exsanguinated blood from a body cavity, anticoagulant must be sucked into the blood bag.

frequently (every 1 to 4 hours), while shock fluids are being administered to animals with hemothorax, so that substantial blood loss can be determined and corrected quickly. An animal's packed cell volume often decreases about 10% with the administration of shock fluids. A greater decrease is generally only seen with severe or ongoing blood loss. Excessive, unceasing blood loss can be an indication for exploratory thoracotomy (Chapter 10).

Serous pleuritis.[9] This exudate occurs as a result of damage to the vascular endothelium of pleural vessels. Serous pleuritis can be caused by feline infectious peritonitis, feline respiratory viruses, leptospirosis, canine hepatitis, pulmonary parasitic infections, and mediastinitis. Treatment includes thoracocentesis and therapies specific to the cause, which is determined from results of cytologic and serologic tests.

Neoplastic effusion. Neoplasms within the chest cavity often produce a serosanguineous exudate.[9] Respiratory compromise can be extreme in cases of neoplastic effusions and must be relieved promptly by thoracocentesis. Microscopic examination of the aspirated fluid for neoplastic cells is essential. Round-cell tumors (lymphoma) shed cells readily, and a diagnosis of these neoplasms can usually be confirmed by cytologic examination of the pleural fluid. Adenocarcinomas may shed their cells in sheets, also occasionally permitting cytologic confirmation. Ultrasound-guided thoracocentesis is particularly useful, as fluid pockets can be identified readily and needle aspirates or biopsies of the tumors may also be obtained. Intrathoracic lymphoma and its associated effusion will respond dramatically to administration of glucocorticoids, often overnight, so immediate administration of prednisolone (1 mg/kg) is suggested following diagnosis. Once the animal is stabilized, continuation of chemotherapy with standard protocols is advised (see Chapter 23).

Pyothorax. This entity is an accumulation of purulent exudate and bacteria in the pleural space. Pyothorax can result from penetrating chest wounds, bite wounds, foreign bodies, rupture of the esophagus or respiratory passages, or from rupture of a lung abscess.[9] Numerous organisms have been isolated, including *Pasteurella, Bacteroides, Fusobacterium, Peptostreptococcus, Escherichia coli, Klebsiella, Actinomyces, Nocardia,* and *Coccidioides.* Affected animals may have septicemia due to the toxic nature of the exudate. Clinical signs include dehydration, anorexia, weight loss, fever, and dyspnea, often accompanying a history of other illness, surgery, or absence from home.[12]

A wide-bore needle (e.g., 19 gauge) or placement of a chest drain will assist initial aspiration of the thick, viscid pus. The exudate may have a putrid smell if anaerobic bacteria are present. Sulfur granules may be seen with *Actinomyces* and *Nocardia.* As the effusion is often loculated, aspiration at multiple sites may be necessary. The exudate from the chest should be submitted for fluid analysis, microbiologic culture (aerobic and anaerobic), and antibiotic sensitivity tests. In the emergency room, smears of the exudate should be stained with Gram stain and acid-fast stains in addition to routine cytologic stains. As anaerobes are slow growers in culture, the examination of stained smears is essential to guide empirical antimicrobial therapy.

A wide-bore, indwelling chest tube should be inserted (bilaterally if necessary) and connected to continuous suction with an underwater seal. This suction drainage is continued until less than 2 ml/kg per day of fluid is obtained, Gram stains are negative, and radiography shows no fluid accumulation in the chest over 48 hours.[12] Lavage of the chest cavity is often used; however, it has never been shown to improve resolution time, and it increases the risk of introducing external bacterial contamination and of causing iatrogenic pneumothorax.

Intravenous penicillin G or the synthetic penicillins are the drugs of choice for initial treatment when anaerobes are present or suspected. Aminoglycosides may also be used in initial treatment, as they have a relatively broad gram-negative (and gram-positive) spectrum, although they are ineffective against anaerobes. *Bacteroides* spp. have shown resistance to penicillins in humans, less so in animals; chloramphenicol is a broad-spectrum antibiotic that is well absorbed orally, penetrates tissues well, and is usually effective against *Bacteroides* spp.; clindamycin should also be effective. Metronidazole is a very useful drug against anaerobes, including *Bacteroides* spp. but may not be effective against *Actinomyces* and some *Streptococci*. Cefoxitin is a second-generation cephalosporin effective against obligate anaerobes and the Enterobacteriaceae.[12] Sulfa drugs are often used when *Nocardia* is present, and they have also a gram-positive and gram-negative spectrum (ineffective against *Pseudomonas*). The response to antibacterial therapy should be monitored daily by examining Gram-stained smears. The appearance of a new organism, the apparent failure of initial therapy, or culture results may suggest the need for a change in the antibiotic regimen.

Chylothorax. Chylothorax[8,12,13] is the accumulation of thoracic-duct lymph in the pleural space and may be caused by rupture of the thoracic duct but usually is caused by leakage from a dilated or obstructed lymph duct (lymphangiectasia).[14] The differential diagnoses for chylous-like effusions include neoplasia, infections, and pseudochylous effusions. Thoracic-duct lymph flow is estimated at 2 ml/kg per hour in the fasting animal and increases after intake of food or water. The accumulation of chyle in the thorax can be rapid. Thoracic-duct obstruction can occur with cranial mediastinal masses, fungal granulomas, vena caval thrombosis, dirofilariasis, lung-lobe torsion, or right-sided congestive heart failure. Trauma to a dilated thoracic duct, even mild trauma (cough), has been postulated as a cause of chylothorax.

Chylothorax is confirmed by fluid analysis and submission of serum and the chylous fluid for triglyceride and cholesterol estimations. Chyle is white to pink-white, does not clear on centrifugation, forms a cream layer on top when left standing (preferably refrigerated), demonstrates predominantly neutrophils (usually)[14] or lymphocytes on cytologic evaluation, and often clears when subjected to the ether test. To perform the ether clearance test, put equal volumes of the fluid in two tubes, add two drops of 10% potassium hydroxide to each, then add water to one to double its volume and add the same quantity of ether to the other. Chyle should clear in the ether tube. Sudan III or oil red O are lipophilic stains that can be used to identify the chylomicrons on smears of a chylous effusion. The cholesterol:triglyceride ratio is more useful than the ether or lipophilic stain tests, which can both be inconsistent. True chyle has more triglyceride than serum and the same or less cholesterol. Pseudochylous fluid has a high cholesterol content and a triglyceride content less than 110 mg/dl (1.25 mmol/L).[5] Chylous fluid can be submitted for bacterial cultures; however, infection in chylothorax is rare due to the bacteriostatic nature of chyle.

Lung-lobe torsion.[12] This condition is rare in dogs and rarer in cats. Clinical signs are nonspecific and may include tachypnea, dyspnea, fever, vomiting, and shock. The occurrence of lung-lobe torsion is predisposed by trauma, prior surgery, and pleural effusion, but may be spontaneous. The effusion is often hemorrhagic and is usually localized to the area of the torsion (most commonly the right middle lobe). The rapid development of hemorrhagic pleural effusion or a hemorrhagic appearance of a known chylous effusion is suspicious for development of a lung-lobe torsion. Diagnosis is by radiography, bronchography, ultrasonography, and bronchoscopy. Differential diagnosis includes atelectasis or consolidation of a lung lobe due to pleural effusion, pneumonia, pulmonary embolism, diaphragmatic hernia, hemorrhage, and neoplasia. Thoracocentesis and treatment for shock are instituted initially. Lung lobectomy can be performed when the patient is stabilized and able to tolerate surgery.

Pneumothorax. Pneumothorax[13,15]   occurs when air is admitted to the pleural space and is classified according to pathophysiology or type (see the box on p. 406). It is a potentially life-threatening condition that should be relieved immediately when it is the cause of dyspnea. Diagnosis is obtained in the compromised patient by auscultation, percussion, and bilateral thoracocentesis. All accumulated air should be removed at this time. After the patient has been stabilized by thoracocentesis, radiographs may be taken to

TYPES OF PNEUMOTHORAX

Open	Resulting from a tear in the chest wall
Closed	Resulting from a tear in the visceral pleura
Tension	Results when the leaking area acts like a valve, pumping air into the pleural space but not permitting it to exit; the chest cavity rapidly fills with air; also called valvular pneumothorax
Spontaneous	A closed pneumothorax that suddenly forms unexpectedly; usually due to rupture of a pulmonary bulla or bleb
Traumatic	Resulting from a traumatic incident; often due to laceration of the lung by a broken rib

CAUSES OF PNEUMOTHORAX

Perforation of the chest wall
Rupture of a pulmonary cyst, bulla, or bleb
Rupture of a bronchus
  Bronchiectasis
  Foreign body
  Tumor
  Trauma
Rupture of the trachea
  Parasite
  Trauma
  Foreign body
Rupture of the esophagus
  Trauma
  Foreign body
  Neoplasia
  Parasite
Rupture of the lung parenchyma
  Trauma
  Rib fracture
  Surgery
  Thoracocentesis
  Pneumonia
  Foreign body
  Positive-pressure ventilation
Rupture of a pneumomediastinum into the pleural space

assess the severity of the pneumothorax and its cause. Causes of pneumothorax are listed in the box, right.

A respiration rate of 45 to 60 breaths per minute or more indicates that thoracocentesis is required. Small air leaks from lung parenchyma may self-seal and require only limited thoracocenteses. If the pneumothorax is extensive, persistent and frequent thoracocenteses are required; a wide-bore chest tube should be inserted (bilaterally if necessary) and connected to continuous suction through an underwater seal (Fig. 25-2). If the pneumothorax is unresponsive to an effective chest drain with continuous suction, emergency thoracotomy may be required to close the leak or remove the affected lung lobe (Chapter 10).

A wound in the chest wall that causes pneumothorax should be packed with gauze or surgically closed to allow evacuation of the chest. When the animal is stable, a definitive surgical repair can be performed.

Tissue

Diaphragmatic hernia. This condition occurs when abdominal contents herniate into the thoracic cavity unilaterally or bilaterally through a rent in the diaphragm, usually as the result of trauma. Congenital hernias also occur, but are less often presented as emergencies.

Animals with diaphragmatic hernias present with varying degrees of dyspnea, polypnea, abdominal breathing, cyanosis, and shock. Concurrent injuries often include fractured ribs, flail chest, pulmonary contusions, pulmonary edema, traumatic myocarditis, and pleural effusion. Hypoxemia is due to restriction of respiration due to pain, low cardiac output (shock, hemorrhage, traumatic myocarditis, pericardial effusion), ventilation/perfusion mismatch (poor pulmonary compliance due to pulmonary edema and contusions, atelectasis) and restriction of pulmonary volume (effusion, abdominal organ herniation) (Fig. 25-3).[16,17] Auscultation may detect diminished heart and lung sounds on the affected side and accentuated sounds on the unaffected side of the chest. Percussion of the thorax may produce dullness over the affected areas. Borborygmus may be auscultated in the chest if intestine or stomach is herniated. These findings may not be evident in the first 24 to 36 hours after trauma. In a minority of cases, an empty feel to the abdomen may be noted. Auscultation and percussion findings can be confused with those obtained with pleural effusion or intrathoracic neoplasia.[18,19] In humans, only about 40% of diaphragmatic hernias are diagnosed preoperatively,[20-24] and similar diagnostic inaccuracies occur in small animals.

Radiography has been the most important, noninvasive method of diagnosis[25]; however, ultrasound is now being used as an adjunct.[26] Radiographic findings accompanying diaphragmatic hernias include disruption of the diaphragmatic outline, cranial displacement of the stomach or duodenum, or abdominal viscera in the thorax. Examination of radiographs obtained with the an-

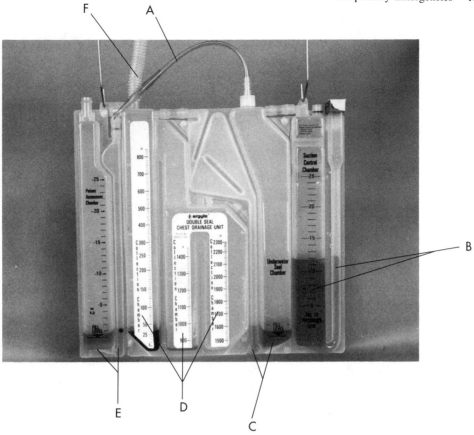

Fig. 25-2 Chest suction unit. A vacuum source A, is connected to a water manometer B, which regulates the negative pressure applied to the pleural cavity. An underwater seal C, prevents aspiration of air into the chest and allows observation of the amount of air (slow bubbling) harvested from the pleural space. This water seal also allows rapid detection (furious bubbling) of a leaking patient tube (e.g., from a hole bitten in the tube). D, Containers are provided for collection and measurement of aspirated fluid. Another water manometer E, measures the actual vacuum applied to the patient's chest tube F.

imal in ventrodorsal, dorsoventral, and right and left lateral positions is a useful diagnostic procedure. If the cardiophrenic angle is clearly outlined in the lateral view, and if the cupola is unobstructed in all projections, then a diagnosis of diaphragmatic hernia can be eliminated.[25] The presence of pleural effusion and pulmonary contusion may make the radiographic diagnosis of diaphragmatic hernia difficult.

Contrast radiography has been used to assist in the diagnosis of diaphragmatic hernia. An upper gastrointestinal series may demonstrate stomach or intestine in the thorax, though an entrapped loop may not fill for several hours after barium administration. Positive contrast peritoneography using 1 ml/kg sodium iothalamate (66.8%)[27] or 1 ml/kg of diatrizoate sodium with an equal volume of sterile saline[28] has been reported as useful in the diagnosis of diaphragmatic hernia. Abnormalities detected with peritoneography in patients

with diaphragmatic hernia include contrast medium in the pleural cavity, absence of normal liver outline, and inability to see the normal outline of the abdominal surface of the diaphragm. The last sign is the most consistent, as adhesions often prevent the passage of contrast medium into the chest.[25] Intraperitoneal diatrizoate administration can cause discomfort in some animals.[28] Alternatively, negative-contrast peritoneography with air or carbon dioxide may be performed.

Treatment is surgical in all cases, but carries a significant death risk (20%), which is higher for operations performed within the first 24 hours or more than 1 year after trauma. Immediate surgical intervention is contraindicated unless an entrapped stomach or strangulated loop of bowel is present.[16] Stabilization of the patient for shock, hypoxia, flail chest, cardiac arrhythmias, pulmonary contusions, and other abnormalities is essential prior to surgery. Respiratory compromise is

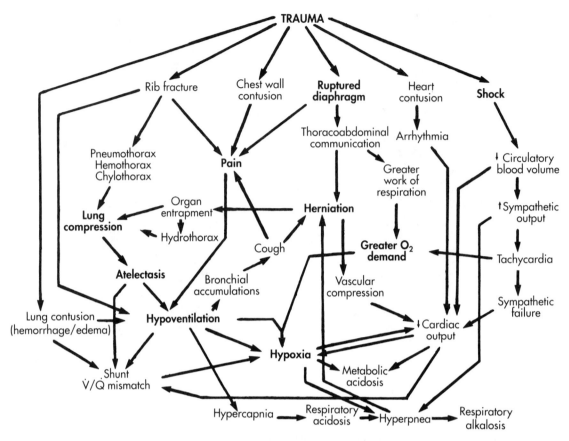

Fig. 25-3 Mechanisms in the pathogenesis of thoracic trauma. (From Boudrieau RJ, Muir WW. Pathophysiology of traumatic diaphragmatic hernia in dogs. Compend Contin Educ Pract Vet 1987;9:379.

more than likely due to these factors than to mechanical restriction of lung volume by herniated viscera.[1] The presence of severe respiratory compromise due to large-volume hernias with associated effusion may require surgical correction within 48 hours, but after hemodynamic stabilization has been achieved. Anesthetic considerations are discussed in Chapters 12 and 33.

Neoplasia. Solid neoplasms within the pleural space that are not associated with an effusion and are causing dyspnea are difficult for the emergency clinician to manage. Sedation, oxygen therapy, and ventilatory support may be the most suitable emergency treatment until a cytologic/histologic diagnosis can be made and a specific treatment regimen proposed. Euthanasia is often advised for terminal cases (confirmed malignancies) to avoid unnecessary patient suffering.

Lesions within the mediastinum

Pneumomediastinum.[9] Pneumomediastinum can result from disruption of mediastinal structures, including perforation of the trachea or bronchi, deep neck wounds, rupture of the esophagus, and leakage from the lung along its central surface. Pneumomediastinum has also been reported following coughing bouts and iatrogenically from transtracheal aspirates, mediastinoscopy, or large-bore central venous catheter insertion. Pneumomediastinum[29] may be asymptomatic, cause subcutaneous emphysema and, in some cases, very high intramediastinal pressure can cause acute hypotension and respiratory failure. Clinical signs are also referable to concurrent disorders (esophageal dysfunction, septic mediastinitis, pneumothorax).[29] Pneumomediastinum can be recognized radiographically by the abnormal lucency of the chest radiograph, which makes the structures of the mediastinum (azygos vein, tracheal walls, precava, brachiocephalic trunk, esophagus) more visible, silhouetted against a background of air. The air may migrate into the subcutis of the neck and spread from there along the trunk. Air may also leak past the diaphragm into the retroperitoneal space. It is prudent to watch for damage to other mediastinal structures following trauma—

Horner's syndrome from damage to the sympathetic trunk or hemorrhage from damage to mediastinal vessels are two examples. Pneumomediastinum may lead to pneumothorax but the reverse is not possible.[9]

Traumatic damage to the neck from gunshots, bites, or other penetrating injuries deserve surgical exploration but not necessarily as an emergency procedure. Clipping, culturing, cleansing, and covering the wound may be sufficient emergency treatment until surgical exploration can be performed. Esophageal rupture is best explored immediately because of the potential for septic mediastinitis and/or pleuritis. Tracheal perforations should be surgically repaired but spontaneous air leaks from the lung may self-seal.

Septic mediastinitis. Perforation of the esophagus and the development of septic mediastinitis in animals is most commonly due to foreign-body entrapment in the thoracic esophagus.[21] The presence of a foreign body causes esophagitis, predisposes to inhalation pneumonia,[22] and stimulates peristalsis, which eventually aids perforation. Esophagitis compromises the tone of the cardia and predisposes to gastric reflux, which aggravates the esophagitis, even after the foreign body is removed (see Chapter 22).

Diagnosis of esophageal perforation and mediastinitis is aided by white-cell count as well as radiographic, endoscopic, and contrast esophagographic evaluations. In one study, a rise in the number of band neutrophils on complete blood count was a significant indicator of perforation; mature neutrophil and toxic neutrophil numbers were elevated in cases of perforation, but not significantly more than in nonperforated cases. Radiographic evidence of mediastinitis around the foreign body is related to perforation; gas can be present around the foreign body whether the esophagus is perforated or not.[21] Iodine-based soluble contrast media are used in the definitive demonstration of perforation, but if the initial study fails to demonstrate leakage, a barium swallow is advised. Barium is more radiodense and coats mucosal surfaces better, and complications of leakage may not be clinically significant.[21] False negative results are not uncommon (14.5%) in contrast studies. If the esophagus is not perforated, an endoscope and retrieval instruments may be used to retrieve the foreign object, or it may be pushed into the stomach, from which it can be surgically removed if necessary. Certain circumstances may dictate an endoscopic approach prior to or followed by radiographic evaluations. If the esophagus is perforated or the foreign object cannot be safely moved with the endoscope, then an esophagotomy will be required.

Treatment of esophageal perforation is surgical (resection, anastomosis, stenting) in all cases except for very minor perforations that self-seal and minimally contaminate the mediastinum. Treatment of esophageal perforation and of septic mediastinitis includes the administration of broad-spectrum antibiotics to guard against aerobic and anaerobic infection. In humans, perforations of greater than 24 hours' duration prior to surgical intervention are associated with significantly higher mortality.[23] The mortality rate from esophageal perforation even with prompt diagnosis and treatment, is still high.

Abscesses in the mediastinal lymph nodes, formed as the result of a previous mediastinitis, can rupture and cause an acute problem. Adhesions and scarring from previous mediastinitis can constrict mediastinal structures such as the esophagus, trachea, or great vessels and cause acute, problems (regurgitation, dyspnea and edema). These conditions require surgical exploration.

Hemomediastinum. Blood accumulation in the mediastinum is rare but usually due to traumatic damage to the great vessels of the neck or mediastinum. Coagulopathies caused by problems such as sepsis, anticoagulant poisons, or disseminated intravascular coagulation should also be considered. Treatment is as for severe hemorrhage elsewhere in the body—maintain normovolemia with crystalloids and/or blood transfusions, ventilatory support, and exploratory surgery with vessel ligation in some cases. Many mediastinal bleeds are self-limiting but major vessel ruptures are likely to cause exsanguination before treatment can be provided.

Neoplasia. Animals with tumors in the mediastinum are presented to the emergency clinician when the mass or secondary effusions into the mediastinal and pleural spaces cause severe respiratory compromise. Conditions that may be observed with mediastinal neoplasia include edema of the head or forelimbs (venous or lymphatic obstruction), paraneoplastic syndromes (thymoma-associated polymyositis or myasthenia gravis), and ruptures of the trachea, esophagus, or blood vessels. These syndromes may all require appropriate emergency care.

Lesions within the lungs

Pulmonary edema. Pulmonary edema[15,30,31] is an accumulation of excessive fluid in the pulmonary interstitium or alveoli. The causes of pulmonary edema are listed in the box on p. 410. Pulmonary edema is usually caused by aberrations in more than one of these causative factors. Edema is initially interstitial, then progresses to involve the alveoli. Auscultation provides diagnostic in-

---

CAUSES OF PULMONARY EDEMA

Increased pulmonary capillary pressure
  Left ventricular failure
  Mitral-valve incompetence
    Endocardiosis
    Ruptured chordae tendineae
  Mitral stenosis
  Masses restricting left atrium, pulmonary veins
  Left-to-right shunts
  Iatrogenic fluid overload
Increased capillary permeability
  Pneumonia (septic and aspiration)
  Toxic fumes, smoke inhalation
  Electric shock
  Near drowning
  Anaphylaxis
  Disseminated intravascular coagulation
Hypoproteinemia
  Renal disease
  Liver disease
  Protein-losing enteropathy
  Starvation, malnutrition
Other causes
  High-altitude disease
  Pulmonary thromboembolism
  Neurogenic (increased intracranial pressure)
  Acute (adult) respiratory distress syndrome

---

formation in most instances. Pulmonary compliance, vital capacity, and pulmonary gas exchange are severely impaired in pulmonary edema (a life-threatening emergency).

Radiography aids in the diagnosis of pulmonary edema; however, the stress of restraint necessary to obtain diagnostic films may be fatal in unstable patients. Ultrasound and electrocardiographic examination of the heart are less stressful and results may be useful, in combination with auscultation findings, for guiding treatment during stabilization of the patient.

The presence of hypoproteinemia can easily be confirmed. Large volumes of plasma (2 to 6 units) may need to be administered to correct hypoproteinemia, which makes this treatment impractical in many cases. However, plasma oncotic pressure in cases of pulmonary edema and hypoproteinemia may be raised with administration of other colloidal fluids (dextran 70 or hydroxyethyl starch).

Cardiogenic pulmonary edema. Emergency treatment involves rest and sedation to lower oxygen demand, an increase in the fractional inspired oxygen, bronchodilation, lessening of venous return and reduction of excess body fluid. Use of an oxygen cage set at between 40% and 100% oxygen concentration (50% is the maximum for the long term) or humidified oxygen administered via nasal catheter or tracheal catheter are indicated. A potent diuretic (furosemide: dogs, 2 to 8 mg/kg intravenously; cats, 2 mg/kg intravenously) is administered hourly until diuresis is achieved. Morphine sulfate (0.2 to 0.5 mg/kg intramuscularly or subcutaneously to a dog) will help to sedate the patient, relieve anxiety, and shift blood out of the pulmonary vascular compartment. Bronchodilators such as aminophylline (10 mg/kg three times a day orally, intramuscularly, or intravenously in dogs; 6.5 mg/kg twice a day orally in cats) or terbutaline (0.05 to 0.1 mg/kg two or three times a day intravenously; 1.25 to 5.0 mg two or three times a day orally) are also used as adjunct therapy. Terbutaline is a semiselective β_2-agonist and primarily a bronchodilator, but its other systemic, adrenergic effects can be observed with systemic administration. Terbutaline should not be used in conjunction with other adrenergic drugs. Nitroglycerin ointment reduces preload by venodilation and reduces pulmonary vascular resistance by shifting blood from the pulmonary to the systemic circulation. Effects are apparent in 60 minutes and last 4 to 8 hours in humans.[32] The ointment is applied to the inner surface of the pinna (3 to 6 mm on cats; 5 to 50 mm on dogs) and a piece of white tape is placed on the outer surface of the pinna to warn personnel to avoid skin contact. Dobutamine and nitroprusside can be used as continuous infusions to assist cardiac output. Each drug is infused concurrently at a rate of 2.5 μg/kg per minute for 2 hours, then 5.0 μg/kg per minute for 24 hours. The actual infusion rate of nitroprusside must be titrated against systemic arterial blood pressure. In refractory cases of pulmonary edema, it may be necessary to insert an endotracheal or tracheostomy tube and use continuous positive airway pressure or to paralyze the animal and use positive end-expiratory pressure in order to force fluid out of the alveoli and to reexpand the air spaces (Chapter 36).

Smoke inhalation. The respiratory system of smoke inhalation victims is threatened by thermal burns, carbon monoxide, secondary bacterial pneumonia and pulmonary edema. Burns of the larynx and upper airway can cause airway obstruction due to severe edema of these structures. The efficient heat-dissipating system of the upper airway is protective of the more sensitive structures beyond it, so thermal injury to the lower airways is less common. Upper-airway compromise may necessitate an endotracheal or tracheostomy tube (see Chapter 10) with or without forced ventilation. Strict asepsis is essential in the placement and management of these tubes due to the high risk of bacterial bronchopneumonia following smoke-inhalation injury. Carbon monoxide has 240 times the affinity for hemoglobin that oxygen has. Carboxyhemoglobin concentrations of 10% to 20% will cause confusion and dyspnea; higher levels cause nausea, vomiting, incoordination and convulsions; 50% to 60% carboxyhemoglobin concentration is fatal.[33] Measurements of arterial partial pressure of oxygen (Pa_{O_2}) can be normal in the presence of severe carbon monoxide poisoning. The half-life of carboxyhemoglobin with the patient breathing 100% oxygen is about half an hour; it is 4 hours when breathing room air.

Smoke inhalation produces toxic chemicals when fumes combine with respiratory secretions. These chemicals poison alveolar macrophages and predispose to bacterial pneumonia.[33] It is preferable not to administer corticosteroids to smoke inhalation victims, as this treatment has been associated with higher mortality.[33] Immediate administration of antibiotics is not advised, as this practice will encourage growth of resistant bacterial organisms. If bacterial pneumonia develops, appropriate antibacterial therapy should be instituted based on the result of culture, Gram stain, and cytologic evaluation of a transtracheal aspirate. Aminophylline (10 mg/kg three times a day in dogs or 5 mg/kg three times a day in cats) can help to alleviate bronchospasm.[4,34] Careful monitoring during the administration of intravenous fluids to patients suffering from smoke inhalation is essential, as damage to alveolar membranes predisposes a patient to the development of pulmonary edema. Pulmonary edema will usually be radiographically evident 16 to 24 hours after injury.

Drowning. Four stages of drowning in the dog have been described: breath-holding and swimming movements initially; aspiration of water, choking, and struggling; vomiting; and finally relaxation and death.[35] The principle causes of death in any type of drowning are hypoxia and acidosis. About 10% of humans die from laryngospasm without aspiration of water; most nearly drowned humans aspirate less than 20 ml/kg body weight of water. Aspiration of greater amounts of water is often associated with serum electrolyte changes in resuscitated individuals.[36] If the water temperature is less than 15°C, hypothermia occurs and partially protects against hypoxic damage by lowering oxygen demand. Hypothermia also reduces the ability to swim, increases fatigue, interferes with the immune response, and can precipitate fatal cardiac arrhythmias. Sudden immersion in very cold water can cause immediate reflex hyperventilation or can activate the diving reflex. The diving reflex imposes severe bradycardia and

shunts blood to the brain and heart, helping to delay cerebral damage.

Aspiration of water decreases pulmonary compliance and causes pulmonary edema, which can be aggravated by neurogenic pulmonary edema if cerebral anoxia has occurred. Salt water is hypertonic and draws fluid into the alveoli, causing a severe intrapulmonary shunt. Fresh water aspiration dilutes surfactant, causing alveoli to become unstable, collapse, and be poorly ventilated, creating an intrapulmonary shunt. This problem will recur until the surfactant is replaced. A large volume of aspirated fresh water will cause transient hypervolemia, but the central venous pressure will return to normal in about an hour. At this stage, fluid may leak back into the alveoli, creating hypovolemia. Victims of near-drowning can present with severe bradycardia and/or peripheral vasoconstriction.[36] Bradycardia can be initiated by the diving reflex or by hypoxia; peripheral vasoconstriction can follow hypothermia or catecholamine release.

Immediate application of cardiopulmonary resuscitation (at the scene of the accident) to the patient is essential in order to reduce hypoxia and metabolic acidosis, both of which occur rapidly in the compromised individual. A very brief attempt to clear the airway and respiratory passages is in order, by inspection and manual removal of debris and by turning the patient head down and compressing the chest. It should be remembered that many nearly drowned patients have swallowed large volumes of water and are at risk for aspiration, particularly if pressure is applied to the abdomen. Cardiopulmonary resuscitation techniques including mouth-to-snout resuscitation and closed-chest massage (if cardiopulmonary arrest is present) should be commenced immediately. Supplemental oxygen should be given even if the patient is breathing spontaneously and is coherent, because marked acidosis and hypoxemia can still be present. The only indication for cessation of oxygen therapy is a normal partial pressure of arterial oxygen (Pa_{O_2}). Application of positive end-expiratory pressure (PEEP) will help clear alveoli, particularly in seawater drowning. If the patient can maintain a normal partial pressure of arterial carbon dioxide unassisted, continuous positive airway pressure (CPAP) may be sufficient. The amount of PEEP or CPAP used must be tailored to the individual's needs by observing oxygen tensions and cardiac output. Maintaining a normal circulating fluid volume will help reduce the risk of poor cardiac output that can occur with PEEP or CPAP. Metabolic acidosis is certain to occur with hypoxia, so intravenous bicarbonate should be given if indicated by blood gas measurements.

If blood gas estimations are unavailable, the clinician may consider administering 1 to 2 mmol/kg of sodium bicarbonate. Cerebral edema should be treated nevertheless, and reducing arterial carbon dioxide (by hyperventilation if necessary) is the most effective way to do this.[36] High-dose barbiturate administration and induction of hypothermia may have a place in reducing cerebral oxygen demand. These treatments are not without risk and are probably unnecessary if the Pao_2 is normal. Antibiotic usage is ill advised unless bacterial pneumonia is present. Corticosteroid administration is probably of little value.

Radiography is a secondary consideration, as the history alone is usually adequate for a diagnosis; however, radiography is useful for prognostication. Pulmonary edema may not be detectable radiographically for up to 48 hours after near-drowning. The initial alveolar pattern dissipates in 7 to 10 days with recovery, but disseminates and increases in density if pneumonia or acute respiratory distress syndrome develops.[35] The presence of "sand bronchograms" is a very poor prognostic sign.

As the owner of a drowned animal usually blames himself or herself, his or her family, or even the attending veterinarian, care should be taken to counsel all parties involved so as to help them overcome their emotional distress (Chapter 7).

Neurogenic pulmonary edema. This is thought to be caused by massive sympathetic overactivity, often following an increase in intracranial pressure. The sympathetic discharge raises blood pressure and peripheral resistance, causing a blood-volume shift from the peripheral to the pulmonary circulation (see Chapters 20 and 29). Volume overload of the pulmonary capillaries causes damage that persists beyond the duration of the initiating cause. Sympatholytics,[37] diuretics, vasodilators, or general anesthetics can be considered in its treatment.[30]

Pneumonia. Clinical signs and laboratory abnormalities associated with pneumonia include fever, neutrophilia, dyspnea, pulmonary crackles heard on auscultation, areas of dullness on percussion and/or auscultation of the chest, cough, depression, and dehydration. Radiographic assessment and blood gas analysis will demonstrate the severity of disease and alterations in pulmonary function. Continuous oxygen administration is indicated if the Pao_2 is below 65 mm Hg. Cytologic examination, Gram stain, and microbiologic culture of a transtracheal aspirate will confirm pneumonia and guide antibiotic therapy. Ultrasonic nebulization of the inspired air and frequent coupage will help loosen thick secretions and aid expectoration of accumulated discharge from small airways (0.5 to 1.0 mm).[38] Steam should not be substituted, as its particles are not small enough to reach the terminal airways. Bronchodilators such as aminophylline or terbutaline can be useful in the treatment of patients with pneumonia. Ventilatory support with PEEP or CPAP may be necessary to expand collapsed or fluid-filled alveoli (Chapter 36).

Pulmonary contusion. Contusions are caused by traumatic injury and consist of hemorrhage and edema within the lung. Blood or serum within the alveoli can interfere with gas exchange, causing dyspnea and hypoxemia. Associated conditions such as pleural space-occupying substances (air, blood), rib fractures, diaphragmatic hernias, traumatic myocarditis (Chapter 17), and circulatory shock can aggravate the hypoxemia.

A history of trauma (motor vehicle, bite) should lead to investigation for pulmonary contusions. Diagnosis is made from auscultation (crackles from alveolar fluid, alteration of lung sounds from consolidation) and from radiography. Radiographic signs include increased focal to diffuse alveolar and interstitial patterns, but these radiographic signs may not appear for up to 12 hours posttrauma. Diagnostic evaluations should include blood gas analysis (Chapter 36) and the patient should be confined and carefully monitored especially during the first 24 to 36 hours following injury.

There is no specific treatment for pulmonary contusions. If the Pao_2 is less than 65 mm Hg, oxygen supplementation should be provided by nasal catheter or oxygen cage. If alveolar consolidation is severe, ventilatory support with intermittent positive-pressure ventilation (IPPV) and PEEP or continuous positive airway pressure CPAP may be required (Chapter 36). If the cause is a bite wound or secondary pneumonia is documented by subsequent radiographic evaluation and tracheal or bronchial aspiration, then a suitable antibiotic should be administered after appropriate cultures are submitted. Iatrogenic fluid overload must be avoided in animals with pulmonary contusions. Diuretics are not beneficial in the treatment of pulmonary contusions unless fluid overload occurs subsequent to treatment for shock. Complete resolution of the contusions can be expected in 3 to 10 days unless complications (pneumonia, lobar collapse or torsion, traumatic pulmonary cysts) occur.[37]

Pulmonary embolism. Pulmonary embolism has rarely been diagnosed antemortem in veterinary medicine because of its subclinical or nonspecific signs. Risk factors in humans include deep venous thrombosis, age (50 to 60 years), immobilization (postsurgical, posttrauma), heart disease, pulmonary hypertension, major trauma, malignancies, obesity, pregnancy, and diabetes mellitus.[39] In the dog, heartworm disease, nephrotic syndrome (due to loss of antithrombin III), disseminated intravascular coagulation, sepsis, severe polycythemia, intravenous catheterization, hypothyroidism, immune-mediated hemolytic anemia[40] and hypoadrenocorticism have been reported as predisposing causes.[41] In humans, abnormalities present in confirmed pulmonary embolism include a drop in the Pao_2 (15% to 20% of the pulmonary circulation obstructed), an increase in pulmonary arterial pressure (25% to 30% obstructed), an increase in the central venous pressure (35% obstructed), and a decrease in cardiac output (more than 40% obstructed).[42] Dyspnea, panting, trembling, cyanosis, and apprehension in the dog[41] and dyspnea, pleuritic pain, apprehension, cough, hemoptysis, and syncope in humans,[39] are frequent, nonspecific clinical signs. Radiographic signs that have been associated with pulmonary embolism are presented in the box. The radiographic, blood gas, electrocardiogram, or serum enzyme changes associated with pulmonary thromboembolism are nonspecific. Combined ventilation/perfusion scintigraphic scans and pulmonary angiography are the only reliable methods currently available for the diagnosis of pulmonary embolism.[39,42,43]

Treatment involves symptomatic therapy (oxygen), treatment of the underlying disease, and anticoagulation or thrombolytic therapy. Thrombolytic therapy, using urokinase or streptokinase, has been shown to be effective in humans,[42] but the cost is still prohibitive for its use in veterinary medicine. Anticoagulant therapy with heparin or warfarin sodium (coumadin) is used to prevent further thrombus formation but has no effect on

---

RADIOGRAPHIC SIGNS ASSOCIATED WITH PULMONARY EMBOLISM[38,41]

A normal radiograph is the most common sign
Lobar or sublobar hyperlucency with normal to reduced lung density
Small lung vessels in affected area(s), indicating reduced perfusion
Low-volume pleural effusion
Enlarged hilar pulmonary arteries
Right ventricular enlargement
Radiographic signs not commensurate with the severe respiratory distress
Atelectasis

---

existing thrombi. Heparin acts by binding with antithrombin III, and the complex created is a potent inhibitor of factors II, IX, XI, and XII. Intravenous administration of 50 U/kg is followed 15 minutes later by a measurement of the activated clotting time or the prothrombin time. Subsequent heparin doses can be given as an intravenous infusion or intravenous boluses every 1 to 4 hours (25-200 IU/kg per 4 hours) until the activated clotting time is prolonged by 2 to 3 times the reference value or the prothrombin time by 1.5 to 2.5 times reference value. As the patient's prothrombin time/activated clotting time may be normal or shortened, laboratory reference values should be used rather than the values with which the patient initially presented. Frequent monitoring of clotting times is essential because of the potential risk of bleeding and subsequent death[39,41] and the wide variability in heparin dosage required (possibly 100 to 1200 U/kg per day, usually given as four divided doses subcutaneously for maintenance). Intramuscular injections are best avoided because of the risk of hemorrhage in an anticoagulated patient. Once the animal is stabilized, as judged by clinical improvement and blood gas values, heparin can be gradually replaced by coumadin. Over 2 to 3 days, the heparin dose is gradually reduced while the coumadin dose is gradually increased up to 10 to 20 mg/kg two or three times a day orally. After 2 weeks, the coumadin dose can be reduced to 5 mg/kg per day, to keep the prothrombin time at 1.5 to 2.5 times normal. The longer half-life of coumadin (36 hours) means that dose changes will not be reflected in the prothrombin time for 3 to 4 days.[41] The reagent used in the United States (simplastin) is less sensitive than BCT (British Comparative Thromboplastin) used in the United Kingdom, so a prolongation of 1.5 times with simplastin is equivalent to 2.5 times with BCT. Aspirin is given to reduce prostaglandin production and platelet adhesion (15 to 25 mg/kg twice a day to dogs[15]; 80 mg every third day to cats). As intravascular stasis is believed to contribute to thrombosis, appropriate fluid therapy to maintain hydration and circulatory volume is advised. Thoracocentesis and other invasive procedures should be avoided both before and during anticoagulant therapy.[39]

End airway disease. The lower airways normally cause less than 30% of the frictional resistance to breathing due to laminar airflow. Obstructions can be caused by smooth-muscle contraction (asthma, irritating substances), mucus accumulation (bronchitis, asthma), anatomic defects (tumors), foreign bodies, or dynamic collapse (forced exhalation).[44]

Animals with lower airway disease can present with life-threatening dyspnea as a new problem or as an exacerbation of a chronic one. History, clinical signs, complete blood count, serum biochemistry profile, radiography, thoracocentesis, echocardiography, transtracheal aspiration (asthma, bronchitis, neoplasia), and bronchoscopy can all be used in the diagnosis and differentiation of lower airway disease.

Allergic bronchitis. Asthma is primarily a disease of cats, though dogs can be affected. In asthma, the tracheobronchial tree is overresponsive to allergens and irritants, such as household dust and cigarette smoke. Irritants cause reversible bronchoconstriction and airway inflammation; the latter is the cause of the increased ventilatory drive of the patient with asthma.[45] The emergency clinician should obtain a good history of substance contact, but the nature of the allergen bears no relationship to emergency management of the disease. Affected cats may be of any age and are predominantly female.[46]

Clinical signs may include paroxysmal, nonproductive coughing, wheezing, dyspnea, and cyanosis. Affected cats are often anxious and may have a distended stomach from aerophagia. Radiography of the thorax may reveal an increased peribronchial pattern ("donuts," "tram tracks"), hyperlucency of the lung fields from air trapping, flattening of the diaphragm, increased space between the diaphragm and the heart, collapse of the right middle lung lobe (the bronchus is dependent and therefore plugs easily), lung borders extending caudal to T-13, separation of lung borders by the sublumbar muscles, and right heart enlargement. Peribronchial patterns may also be seen with *Aelurostrongylus* and *Dirofilaria* infestations, with bacterial bronchitis, and with bronchoalveolar carcinoma. Bronchial or tracheal washings produce predominantly eosinophils in about 50% to 75% of cases, neutrophils in about 30%, and macrophages in about 20%.[46] Cultures should be obtained irrespective of the cell type found on tracheobronchial aspirates.

Treatment must produce rapid bronchodilation and includes administration of corticosteroids, sympathomimetics, bronchodilators (methylxanthines), and sometimes parasympatholytics. Corticosteroids are the mainstay of treatment in cats and are often used for short-term management even though they take about 3 hours to produce clinically noticeable improvement. Dexamethasone sodium phosphate (0.2 to 1.0 mg/kg intravenously) or prednisolone sodium succinate (1 to 4 mg/kg intravenously) can be used. Long-term corticosteroid therapy is often required and is given at tapering dosages following control of clinical

signs, until a suitable maintenance dosage is established for the patient.[47,48] The methylxanthines (theophylline, caffeine, aminophylline) are phosphodiesterase inhibitors and cause central nervous system stimulation, diuresis, stimulate cardiac muscle and the respiratory center, and cause bronchodilation.[49] Adrenergic agonists that can be administered include epinephrine (adrenalin) (1:10,000 solution, 0.5 to 0.75 ml subcutaneously) or isoproterenol (0.1 to 0.2 ml of 1:200 solution subcutaneously). These adrenergic drugs may be repeated hourly; cardiac monitoring is required. These parenteral treatments may be followed by terbutaline administration (0.6 to 2.5 mg per cat orally two or three times a day) for maintenance treatment. In asthmatic people, combination terbutaline and theophylline has been shown to improve pulmonary function without cardiotoxic effects[50]: however, a rising death rate since the advent of this combination therapy has caused some concern. Atropine is a bronchodilator, but it is not superior to the adrenergics and is not necessarily recommended, because it has a drying effect on respiratory secretions. Studies in humans demonstrate conflicting data concerning the efficacy of atropine administration on bronchodilation.[51] In acute asthma, combination sympathomimetic and anticholinergic administration has demonstrated increased efficacy to the effects of either agent alone.[52] Some investigators claim that the parasympathetic system is the dominant reversible component of airway obstruction in emphysema.[53]

Infectious bronchitis. Infectious bronchitis is usually associated with an initiating cause such as viral upper respiratory infection, allergic bronchitis, aspiration of foreign material, or aspiration of infected discharges from the upper airway. Clinical signs may include productive cough, expiratory dyspnea, purulent nasal discharge, fever, weight loss, and loud breath sounds with crackles and wheezes. Radiography may demonstrate an increased bronchial pattern and mild peribronchial thickening (donuts). The complete blood count may demonstrate neutrophilia. Bronchial mucus usually contains increased numbers of macrophages and/or neutrophils and should be cultured to identify the causative organisms and their antibiotic sensitivities. Gram staining the tracheal or bronchial washings in the emergency room can aid in the choice of empirical antibiotic therapy. Viruses or mycoplasma may also cause acute bronchitis. Their presence is difficult to diagnose definitively.

Treatment is with antibacterials appropriate to the organism involved, nebulization of the tracheobronchial tree and bronchodilators. Response to treatment is often favorable with clinical signs resolving over a period of days.[47,48]

Emergencies of the chest wall

Rib fractures. Simple rib fractures are rarely of major clinical significance unless they penetrate the chest, causing pneumothorax, lung contusions, pericardial tears,[15] myocardial damage, hypoxemia from hypoventilation (pain), or cardiac arrhythmias (from myocardial damage). Analgesia from selective local intercostal nerve block with 0.5% bupivicaine (0.5 ml per site) has been shown to be superior to that from systemic administration of opiates in preventing hypoventilation and maintaining Pao_2.[54] Bandaging of the chest is ill-advised due to the restriction of chest-wall movement.[15]

Flail chest. Flail chest occurs when a section of thoracic wall has ribs fractured dorsally and ventrally so that the isolated section moves paradoxically with respiration. Severe respiratory compromise ensues due to the difficulty in creating enough negative intrathoracic pressure to expand the lungs. A technique for stabilization of a flail segment is described under "Special Techniques" at the end of this chapter. Endotracheal intubation or tracheostomy-tube insertion and positive-pressure ventilation with PEEP requires sedation but is effective in maintaining adequate ventilation during stabilization of the patient (see Chapters 10 and 36). Pneumothorax can develop as a result of lung puncture by the rib fragments, in which case

chest-tube placement and continuous suction drainage should be applied.

Chest-wall perforation. The normal canine and feline mediastinum is usually perforate, so a large, open chest wound is likely to be rapidly fatal. Treatment in less severe cases is initially aimed at closing the chest wound, evacuating the pneumothorax, and attending to other urgent problems (cardiac arrhythmias). Cultures of the wound will guide subsequent antibiotic therapy, if wound infection or pyothorax occurs. Exploration of the thorax to retrieve foreign material, debride devitalized tissues, and lavage the pleural space is recommended after the animal is stabilized.

SPECIAL TECHNIQUES
Oxygen therapy (see also Chapter 36)

Insertion of an intranasal oxygen catheter. The technique of the tube insertion is the same as described for insertion of a nasogastric tube.[55,56] A red rubber urinary catheter is ideal for this purpose, but polyurethane and polyvinylchloride catheters have also been used.[55,56] The tube is passed through the ventral nasal meatus of the dog or cat after anesthetizing the nasal passages with two or more drops of local anesthetic solution. Premeasuring and marking the tube will facilitate its passage to the level of the medial canthus. It is important to secure the tube as close to its exit from the nose as possible. I use a "Chinese finger tie"[57] on the tube and fasten it to the caudolateral corner of the planum nasale. The

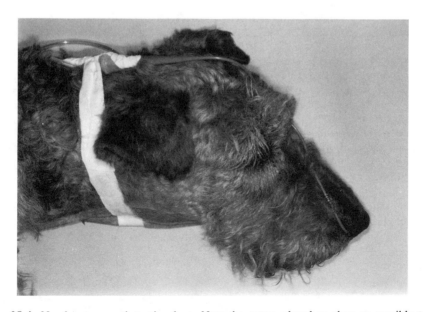

Fig. 25-4. Nasal oxygen catheter in place. Note the suture placed as close as possible to the tube's exit from the nose and the "Chinese finger tie." Cyanoacrylate glue was used as an additional fastening between tube, hair, and suture.

tube then passes over the midline of the head to the collar and is held in place by single interrupted sutures on the nasal midline and on the head. Cyanoacrylate glue is applied to the tube, the ligatures and the underlying hair (Fig. 25-4). The free end of the nasal catheter is connected to a source of humidified oxygen (50 to 100 ml/kg/min).[58] This method of oxygen delivery can potentially raise the Pao_2 to more than 100 mm Hg and is adequate for oxygen supplementation in most cases that do not require assisted ventilation.

Tracheostomy (see also Chapter 10)

Tracheostomy is indicated to bypass an upper-airway obstruction, to facilitate removal of lower-airway secretions (when the cough reflex is abolished), to enable assisted ventilation, to create a vent to reduce closed glottis pressure (which undesirably raises cerebrospinal fluid pressure in patients with cerebral edema), to decrease dead space, and to allow anesthesia for laryngeal or oral surgery.[59,60]

Technique. Under general anesthesia or heavy sedation, a midline skin incision about 3 cm long is made on the ventral neck equidistant from the larynx and the manubrium. The two sternohyoid muscles are parted on the midline and blunt dissection is continued down to the tracheal rings. A transverse incision between rings will give enough space for insertion of the tracheostomy tube. Placement too close to the first tracheal ring can potentially damage the cricoid cartilage and lead to subglottic laryngeal stenosis. The entry into the trachea can be enlarged with a longitudinal incision through the cartilage ring(s) immediately below the initial incision. Alternatively, a plate of tracheal tissue can be created with two longitudinal incisions about 1 to 2 cm apart through the two to three rings below. This plate is sutured to the skin to provide an entry guide should the tube need replacement. In both methods, stay sutures are placed through the skin and tracheal cartilage adjacent to the transverse incision on either side of the opening. These sutures will aid placement of the tube. The tube should ideally be two thirds to three quarters of the tracheal diameter and should have a high-volume, low-pressure cuff. The cuff is only inflated if positive-pressure ventilation is required or it is necessary to stop aspiration of oropharyngeal contents (comatose patient). If a seal cannot be obtained with an inflation pressure less than 25 mm Hg, then a larger-diameter tube should be used.[61] The tube is fastened in place by tying it around the patient's neck with umbilical tape or gauze. It can also be sutured to the skin, but care must be taken to avoid movement of the tube within the trachea

so that the mucosa is not abraded. To allow drainage, the caudal end of the skin incision is not completely closed around the tube. Tubes designed for human use may not center properly in the trachea of a dog or cat. The tip of the tracheostomy tube may abrade the ventral tracheal wall or damage the proximal border of the stoma. A method of manufacturing a tracheostomy tube recommended as being more suitable for the dog has been described.[62] It is molded from a semirigid siliconized vinyl tube 10 cm long with an internal diameter of 7 mm and an external diameter of 9 mm (the sizes of dogs used were not specified).

An alternative method of tracheostomy tube placement has been described.[63] A 13-gauge needle containing a 16-gauge inner needle is inserted between appropriate tracheal rings, and air is aspirated to confirm that the needle is in the trachea. The inner needle is removed and replaced with a dilator to which is attached the tracheostomy tube. The outer needle is removed, the dilator is pushed in with the accompanying tube, then the dilator removed, leaving the tube in place.

Postoperative care. Humidification is essential and can be provided by a commercial tap water humidifier[62] or by injecting 1 to 5 ml of normal saline into the tube every hour.[64] It is essential to monitor the tube frequently, as secretions can build up and block the tube. Suctioning has to be performed frequently (15 to 30 minutes initially) using a soft, sterile rubber or vinyl tube with a side port or T connecter to allow application of intermittent suction.[57] Many tubes are equipped with an internal cannula that can be removed, cleaned, and resterilized, making maintenance of the airway much easier in patients producing copious secretions. Tracheostomy is a major risk factor for nosocomial pneumonia. In humans, pneumonia develops in one half to two thirds of patients with tracheostomies, and in most of these patients *Pseudomonas* or other gram-negative enteric infections, which are often antibiotic resistant, develop. Poor nutritional status, severity of primary illness (debilitation) and infection of the tracheostomy stoma are risk factors for the development of pneumonia.[61]

When the tube is removed, the wound is allowed to heal by secondary intention to avoid subcutaneous emphysema.

Thoracocentesis

Indications. The indications for thoracocentesis include diagnostic and/or therapeutic removal of air or fluid from the chest cavity.

Diagnosis. Radiography can be used to determine the location of the fluid or air. Ventrodorsal and standing lateral views should be taken if possible, but in an animal with critical dyspnea it may be prudent to perform thoracocentesis prior to radiographic evaluation.[9,65] The use of ultrasound to identify fluid accumulations and to guide the needle is recommended. Ultrasound is of no use in pneumothorax.

Equipment. The size of needle or catheter recommended varies from 21-gauge to 15-gauge.[9,65,66] One author prefers a Duke's trochar in dogs over 9 kg, and for cats and small dogs he recommends a 21-gauge, 19-mm butterfly catheter.[8] The larger needle or catheter enables more rapid withdrawal of air or fluid, particularly thick, purulent exudates. Smaller needle holes may reduce the relatively high risk of iatrogenic pneumothorax. The use of flexible tubing and a three-way stopcock between the syringe and the puncturing needle makes it easier to apply pressure on the syringe and to empty it without moving the needle in the thorax and lacerating the lung.

Technique. An area from the sternum to the level of the transverse processes over the sixth to eighth intercostal spaces is clipped bilaterally and scrubbed as for surgery. With the animal in sternal recumbency or standing, the needle is inserted in the seventh intercostal space near the costochondral junction, taking care to avoid the vessels behind the seventh rib. Elevating the forequarters will assist aspiration of fluid, and inserting the needle more dorsally in the seventh space will aid the removal of air. Inserting the needle too far may cause it to "grate" against the lung, lacerating it; and inadequate depth of insertion will not "pop" the needle through the pleura. Fluid collected should be submitted in an ethylenediamine tetraacetic acid tube for fluid analysis. Aerobic and anaerobic microbiologic cultures should also be obtained. Cytologic evaluation, Gram stain, specific gravity, and total solids can be assessed on the fluid, along with color, consistency, and odor.

Insertion of a chest tube

Indications. The presence of unrelenting pneumothorax or pleural effusion that requires repeated thoracocenteses justifies the insertion of an indwelling chest tube.

Equipment. I prefer a trochar catheter (Argyle Trocar Catheter, Sherwood Medical, St. Louis, MO) and use a size and gauge appropriate to the patient (12 French/23 cm; 16 French/25 cm; 20 French/41 cm). This catheter has a sharp pointed trochar inside the tube, a hole at the end with two fenestrations on the side near the tip of the tube, measurements along its length and a radiopaque line running the length of the tube. Another three

to five holes should be made near the end of the tube; the one furthest from the tip should be through the radiopaque line. The break in the radiopaque line enables radiographic detection of the most external hole.

Technique. The chest tube is inserted on the side that has been the most productive during thoracocentesis or that has been identified radiographically (air) or ultrasonographically (fluid) as being the most severely affected. In severe cases, tubes may need to be inserted bilaterally. An area bound cranially by the shoulder, caudally by the 12th or 13th rib, ventrally by the sternum, and dorsally by the region of the lateral spinous processes is clipped and prepared as for sterile surgery. The insertion point through the skin is about midthorax over the 10th or 11th intercostal space and the insertion into the thorax is through the 7th intercostal space. Local anesthetic is infiltrated around both these points and along the line connecting them. It is useful to anesthetize the pleura at the thoracic entry point if this can be done without entering the chest. Cats may require sedation or general anesthesia.[28] A hemostat to clamp the tube should be available and a suction apparatus should be present and functional before the next stage is started. A small nick is made in the skin over the anesthetized area and a purse-string suture is preplaced. An estimate is made of the length of tube to be inserted, then the trochar with its tube is introduced through the hole and tunneled subcutaneously, parallel to the chest wall and cranially toward the anesthetized entry point. The tube is stood up perpendicular to the chest wall with the trochar point resting on the caudal part of the seventh intercostal space (to avoid the intercostal vessels behind the seventh rib) and a firm blow delivered with the heel of the hand to the top of the trochar to force the trochar into the chest. Too soft a blow will not deliver the unit into the chest and too hard a blow could damage intrathoracic structures. Pass the tube down the trochar a couple of centimeters to cover the sharp tip, then, pointing the end in the required direction (cranioventrally for fluid, craniodorsally for air), advance the tube and trochar as a unit into the desired position in the chest. Withdraw the trochar while holding the tube in place. Clamp the tube with a hemostat before the trochar is fully withdrawn from the tube so as not to permit an ingress of air to the chest cavity. Should this inadvertently happen, the suction is available to correct it. The chest is sealed by tying the purse-string suture around the tube as it exits the skin. The tube is anchored by placing a cruciate suture through the skin and around the tube at about the level of the eighth or ninth rib. A "Chinese finger tie" is placed around the tube to prevent it from slipping out of the chest. An encircling bandage is wrapped around the chest to cover the exit point. The tube can then be connected to a continuous suction apparatus or Heimlich valve as desired. Radiography of the chest will confirm correct placement of the chest tube. The use of prophylactic antibiotics in human tube thoracostomy patients is controversial; some studies are published showing significant reduction in infections when antibiotics are used, whereas others show no significant difference in infection rate.[67,68]

Stabilization of a flail chest

Emergency stabilization of the flail segment can be achieved with towel clamps, orthoplast,[15] or a splint manufactured from tongue depressors. The towel clamps are used to grip the center of the flailing segment and can be bandaged in place. Orthoplast is bridged over the flail segment and rests on the normal ribs to which it is fastened with sutures. Traction sutures through the orthoplast and around the flailing rib segment will hold the segment up so that it will move normally with the chest wall. The same effect can be achieved with tongue depressors in an H pattern. The upright parts rest on normal ribs and the traction sutures are placed around the crossbar. A rigid H is made to the appropriate size and shape with a suitable number of wooden tongue depressors held together with padding such as rolled cotton (cotton wool) or cast padding, bound by surgical tape. If necessary, the crossbar can be reinforced on its outer side with an aluminum rod. The traction sutures around the flail ribs are usually sufficient to hold the apparatus in place without placing sutures around the normal ribs.

REFERENCES

1. Murtaugh RJ, Spaulding GL. Initial management of respiratory emergencies. In Kirk RW, ed. Current veterinary therapy X—Small animal practice. Philadelphia: WB Saunders, 1989;195-201.
2. Jones BD, Jergens AE, Guilford WG. Diseases of the esophagus. In Ettinger SJ, ed. Textbook of veterinary internal medicine, ed. 3. Philadelphia: WB, Saunders, 1989;1269.
3. Ettinger SJ, Ticer JW. Diseases of the trachea. In Ettinger SJ, ed. Textbook of veterinary internal medicine, ed. 2. WB Saunders, 1983;723-746.
4. Kirk RW, Bistner SI. Handbook of veterinary procedures and emergency treatment, ed. 4. Philadelphia: WB Saunders, 1985;205-206.
5. Tami TA, Chu F, Wildes TO, Kaplan M. Pulmonary edema and acute upper airway obstruction. Laryngoscope 1986;96:506-509.
6. Myers EM, Iko BO. The management of acute laryngeal trauma. J Trauma 1987;27:448-452.
7. Kirk RW, Bistner SI. Special systems examination: respiratory system. Kirk RW, Bistner SI, eds. Handbook of veterinary procedures and emergency treatment, ed. 4. Philadelphia: WB Saunders, 1985;451-454.
8. Harpster NK. Chylothorax. In Kirk RW, ed. Current veterinary therapy IX. Philadelphia: WB Saunders, 1985;295-303.
9. Suter PF, Zinki JG. Mediastinal, pleural and extrapleural thoracic diseases. In Ettinger SJ, ed. Textbook of veterinary internal medicine, ed. 2. Philadelphia: WB Saunders, 1983;840-883.
10. Kneller SK. Thoracic radiography. In Kirk RW, ed. Current veterinary therapy IX—Small animal practice. Philadelphia: WB Saunders, 1986;250-261.
11. Weiser MG. Erythrocytes and associated disorders. In Ettinger SJ, ed. Textbook of veterinary internal medicine, ed. 3. Philadelphia: WB Saunders, 1989;2177.
12. Bauer T. Pyothorax. In Kirk RW, ed. Current veterinary therapy IX—Small animal practice. Philadelphia: WB Saunders, 1986;292-295.
13. Fossum TW, Birchard SJ. Chylothorax. In Kirk RW, ed. Current veterinary therapy X—small animal practice. Philadelphia: WB Saunders, 1989;393-399.
14. Fossum TW, Birchard SJ. Chylothorax. In Kirk RW, ed. Current veterinary therapy X—small animal practice. Philadelphia: WB Saunders, 1989;393-394.
15. Kirk RW, Bistner SI. Handbook of veterinary procedures and emergency treatment, ed. 4. Philadelphia: WB Saunders, 1985;208-210.
16. Boudrieau RJ, Muir WW. Pathophysiology of traumatic diaphragmatic hernia in dogs. Compend Contin Educ Pract Vet 1987;9:379.
17. Young PN, Gorgacz EJ, Barsanti JA. Respiratory failure associated with diaphragmatic paralysis in a cat. J Am Anim Hosp Assoc 1980;16:933-936.
18. Morgan RV. Respiratory emergencies Part II. Compend Contin Educ Pract Vet 1983;5:305-310.
19. Wilson GP, Newton CD, Burt JK. A review of 116 diaphragmatic hernias in dogs and cats. J Am Vet Med Assoc 1971;159:1142-1145.
20. Morgan AS, et al. Blunt injury to the diaphragm: an analysis of 44 patients. J Trauma 1986;26:565.
21. Parker NR, Walter PA, Gay J. Diagnosis and surgical treatment of esophageal perforation. J Am Anim Hosp Assoc 1989;25:587-594.
22. Zimmer JF. Canine esophageal foreign bodies: endoscopic, surgical, and medical management. J Am Anim Hosp Assoc 1984;20:669-677.
23. Azalat GM, Mulder DG. Esophageal perforations. Arch Surg 1984;119:1318-1320.
24. Rodriquez-Morales G, Rodriguez A, Shatney CH. Acute rupture of the diaphragm in blunt trauma: analysis of 60 patients. J Trauma 1986;26:438.
25. Farrow CS. Radiographic diagnosis of diaphragmatic hernia. Modern Vet Pract 1983;64:979-982.
26. Schulman AJ, et al. Congenital peritoneopericardial diaphragmatic hernia in a dog. J Am Anim Hosp Assoc 1985;21:655-662.
27. Stickle RL. Positive contrast celiography (peritoneography) for the diagnosis of diaphragmatic hernia in dogs and cats. J Am Vet Med Assoc 1984;185:295-298.
28. Roe SC, Smith CW, Stowater LJ. Diaphragmatic hernia producing gastric outflow obstruction, metabolic alkalosis and hypokalemia in the dog. Compend Contin Educ Pract Vet 1986;8:943-948.
29. Bauer T. Mediastinal, pleural and extrapleural diseases. In Ettinger SJ, ed. Textbook of veterinary internal medicine, ed. 3. Philadelphia: WB Saunders, 1989;890.
30. Suter PF, Ettinger SJ. Pulmonary edema. In Ettinger SJ, ed. Textbook of veterinary internal medicine, ed. 2. Philadelphia: WB Saunders, 1983;747-759.

31. Harpster NK. Pulmonary edema. In Kirk RW, ed. Current veterinary therapy X—Small animal practice. Philadelphia: WB Saunders, 1989;385-392.

32. Needleman P, Corr PB, Johnson EM. Drugs used for the treatment of angina. In Goodman LS, Gillman AG, Rall TW, Murad F, eds. The pharmacological basis of therapeutics, ed. 7. New York: Macmillan, 1985;806-816.

33. Hawkins EC, Ettinger SJ, Suter PF. Diseases of the lower respiratory tract (lung) and pulmonary edema. In Ettinger SJ, ed. Textbook of veterinary internal medicine, ed. 3. Philadelphia: WB Saunders, 1989;843-845.

34. Tams TR. Pneumonia. In Kirk RW, ed. Current veterinary therapy—small animal practice. Philadelphia: WB Saunders, 1989;382-384.

35. Farrow CS. Near-drowning (water inhalation). In Kirk RW, ed. Current veterinary therapy VII—small animal practice. Philadelphia: WB Saunders, 1980;182-186.

36. Modell JH, Boysen PG. Drowning and near-drowning. In Shoemaker WC, Ayres S, Grenvik A, Holbrook PR, Thompson WL, eds. Textbook of critical care medicine, ed. 2. Philadelphia: WB Saunders, 1989;64-69.

37. Hawkins EC, Ettinger SJ, Suter PF. Diseases of the lower respiratory tract (lung) and pulmonary edema. In Ettinger SJ, ed. Textbook of veterinary internal medicine, ed. 3. Philadelphia: WB Saunders, 1989;840-841.

38. Amis TC. Clinical respiratory physiology. In Kirk RW, ed. Current veterinary therapy VIII—small animal practice. Philadelphia: WB Saunders, 1983;192-199.

39. Rubin LJ. Southwestern internal medicine conference: pulmonary thromboembolic disease-diagnosis, management and prevention. Am J Med Sci 1985;290:167-177.

40. Klein MK, Dow SW, Rosychuk RAW. Pulmonary thromboembolism associated with immune-mediated hemolytic anemia in dogs: ten cases (1982-1987). J Am Vet Med Assoc 1989;195:246-250.

41. Suter PF. Miscellaneous diseases of the thorax. In Ettinger SJ, ed. Textbook of veterinary internal medicine, ed. 2. WB Saunders, 1983;887.

42. Sasahara AA, Sharma GVRK, McIntyre KM, Cella G. Does thrombolytic therapy alter the prognosis of pulmonary embolism? Haemostasis 1986;16(suppl 3):51-57.

43. McBride K, La Morte WW, Menzoian JD. Can ventilation-perfusion scans accurately diagnose acute pulmonary embolism? Arch Surg 1986;121:754-757.

44. Robinson NE. Pathogenesis of airway disease. In Proceedings of the 6th Annual Veterinary Medical Forum, American College of Veterinary Internal Medicine. Blacksburg VA: ACVIM, 1988;391.

45. Rebuck AS, Chapman KR. Asthma: 1. Pathophysiologic features and evaluation of severity. Can Med Assoc J 1987;136:351-354.

46. Moise NS, Spaulding GL. Feline bronchial asthma: pathogenesis, pathophysiology, diagnostic and therapeutic considerations. Compend Contin Educ Pract Vet 1981;3:1091-1101.

47. Bauer TG. Diseases of the lower airway. In Morgan RV, ed. Handbook of small animal practice. New York: Churchill Livingstone, 1988;185-193.

48. Moise NS, Dietze AE. Bronchopulmonary diseases. In Sherding RG, ed. The cat: diseases and clinical management. New York: Churchill Livingstone, 1989;798-810.

49. Rall TW. Central nervous system stimulants (continued). In Goodman LS, Gillman AG, Rall TW, Murad F, eds. The pharmacological basis of therapeutics, ed. 7. New York: Macmillan, 1985;589-601.

50. Vandewalker ML, et al. Addition of terbutaline to optimal theophylline therapy. Chest 1986;90:198-203.

51. Karpel JP, Appel D, Breidbart D, Fusco MJ. A comparison of atropine sulfate and metaproterenol sulfate in the emergency treatment of asthma. Am Rev Respir Dis 1986;133:727-729.

52. Rebuck AS, et al. Nebulized anticholinergic and sympathomimetic treatment of asthma and chronic obstructive airways disease in the emergency room. Am J Med 1987;82:59-64.

53. Gross NJ, Skorodin MS. Role of the parasympathetic system in airway obstruction due to emphysema. N Engl J Med 1984;311:421-425.

54. Berg RJ and Orton CE. Pulmonary function in dogs after intercostal thoracotomy: comparison of morphine, oxymorphone and selective intercostal nerve block. Am J Vet Res 1986;47:471-474.

55. Crowe DT. Clinical use of an indwelling nasogastric tube for enteral nutrition and fluid therapy in the dog and cat. J Am Anim Hosp Assoc 1986;22:675-682.

56. Crowe DT. Methods of enteral feeding in the seriously ill or injured patient: Part I. J Vet Emerg Crit Care 1986;3:1-3.

57. Crowe DT. Methods of enteral feeding in the seriously ill or injured patient: Part II. J Vet Emerg Crit Care 1986;3:7-17.

58. Fitzpatrick RK, Crowe DT. Nasal oxygen administration in dogs and cats: experimental and clinical investigations. J Am Anim Hosp Assoc. 1986;22:293-300.

59. Oliver JE. Tracheotomy in the dog. VM/SAC 1966;61:221-228.

60. Heffner JE, Scott-Miller K, Sahn SA. Tracheostomy in the intensive care unit, Part I: indications, technique, management. Chest 1986;90:269-274.

61. Heffner JE, Scott-Miller K, Sahn SA. Tracheostomy in the intensive care unit, Part II: complications. Chest 1986;90:430-436.

62. Leverment JN, Rae S. Cuffed tube tracheostomy in the dog. Lab Anim 1978;12:203-206.

63. Silverman BS, Robello G, Fowell E. Percutaneous tracheostomy in the dog. Modern Vet Pract 1982;63:62-63.

64. Eiseman B, Spencer FC. Tracheostomy: an underrated surgical procedure. JAMA 1963;184:684.

65. Todoroff RJ. Soft tissue surgery. In Holzworth J, ed. Diseases of the cat, vol. 1. Philadelphia: WB Saunders, 1987;279.

66. Kirk RW, Bistner SI, eds. Handbook of veterinary procedures and emergency treatment, ed. 4. Philadelphia: WB Saunders, 1985;524.

67. Lo Curto JJ, et al. Tube thoracostomy and trauma—Antibiotics or not? J Trauma 1986;26:1067.

68. Mandal AK, Montano J, Thadepalli H. Prophylactic antibiotics and no antibiotics compared in penetrating chest trauma. J Trauma 1985;25:639.

26 Reproductive Tract Emergencies

Frances O. Smith

FEMALE REPRODUCTIVE EMERGENCIES
Dystocia

Dystocia is defined as a difficult birth or as the inability to expel the fetus through the birth canal. Fetal position, shape, size, number, and viability contribute to fetal causes for dystocia. Single-puppy litters often result in dystocia for poorly defined reasons. Maternal dystocia is associated with maternal, anatomic, behavioral, endocrine, and fitness considerations.[1-5]

Stage II labor begins with fluid expulsion from the vulva or active straining on the part of the dam (see box). If the dam strains, without delivering offspring, for more than 1 hour after the onset of Stage II labor, she should be examined by a veterinarian. Likewise, if a gravid bitch rests for more than 3 hours between delivery of individual puppies she should be examined. Queens frequently have long delays between delivery of individual kittens, with no apparent ill effect on the queen or kittens. This makes the length of time between deliveries an inconsistent determinant for dystocia in queens.

The management options for cases of dystocia in animals depend on the condition of the dam, the value of the offspring and dam, the cause of dystocia, the availability of personnel and equipment, the owner's wishes, and the clinical judgment of the veterinarian. If the offspring are valuable, cesarean section may often be the most efficient and cost-effective method of treatment. The anesthetic and surgical risks to a dam in good condition are minimal.

When contemplating an initial medical approach to therapy of dystocia, it is important to assess fetal size relative to the maternal pelvic canal, the position and presentation of the caudal fetus, and the anatomic aspects of the vulva and vagina. Oxytocin should not be used in cases of obstructive dystocia (i.e., decreased pelvic canal size associated with healed pelvic fractures). Approximately 40% of canine and feline fetuses are presented posteriorly[6]; this presentation does not commonly result in dystocia. Forceps can be used to extract manually a fetus trapped in the birth canal, but their use requires careful manipulation due to the minimal space available in the birth canal.

Oxytocin (5 to 20 units intramuscularly) is the drug of choice for administration to dams with weak or ineffective labor. If there is no response within 20 minutes following initial oxytocin therapy, a second dose accompanied by 10% calcium gluconate (0.5 to 2 ml intravenously, given with caution) and glucose administration (equivalent of 2 ml/kg of 50% dextrose intravenously) can be used in an attempt to increase the strength of uterine contraction. Cesarean section should be undertaken in dams failing to whelp/queen following this attempt at medical treatment for dystocia.

STAGES OF LABOR

Stage I	Initiation of uterine contraction and dilation of the cervix; behavioral signs (nesting, restlessness), lasts 6-24 hours
Stage II	Stage of parturition; abdominal contractions visible; fetuses pass through cervix and vagina; lasts 3-24 hours (average 1 hour per fetus in bitch; unpredictable intervals in queens, but usually litters are delivered rapidly)
Stage III	Expulsion of the placentas, usually immediately with each fetus (may occur 5 minutes to hours later)

The uterus can become refractory to repeated administration of oxytocin. If there is a large litter, and the dam requires oxytocin to initiate labor with each offspring to be delivered, it is likely that the uterus will become refractory to the effects of oxytocin prior to delivery of the entire litter. Cesarean section should be considered when it appears that multiple doses of oxytocin are required.

Primary uterine inertia occurs when the uterus fails to respond to appropriate signals to begin labor. Primary uterine inertia may be seen with subsequent pregnancies in the same bitch. If a bitch experiences a temperature drop to 99°F or below and does not show signs of labor within 24 hours, she may have primary uterine inertia. Medical therapy may be attempted in these cases, but it often fails. Vaginoscopy should reveal an open cervix with fetal membranes visible. Cesarean section is indicated if there is no response to the oxytocin administration or if ultrasonography reveals signs of fetal distress (slowing of fetal heart rate).

Postpartum emergencies

Eclampsia. Puerperal tetany/hypocalcemia is an acute, potentially life-threatening syndrome occurring primarily in small to medium-sized bitches nursing large litters during the first 3 weeks of lactation.[2,7] This problem can also occur just prior to weaning in queens nursing large litters and occasionally manifests in bitches during late gestation. Eclampsia evolves when calcium loss in the milk occurs more rapidly than calcium absorption from the gut or mobilization from the bone. Ionized calcium levels in extracellular fluids are reduced. Hypocalcemia causes restlessness, nervousness or aggression, hypersalivation, pupillary dilatation, panting, vocalization, fever, muscle fasciculations, stiffness of gait, and tetany. The treatment of choice is slow intravenous administration of calcium gluconate (5 to 20 ml of a 10% to 20% solution) to effect. Auscultation and/or electrocardiography should be used to monitor the animal's heart during administration of therapy. Therapy should stop if bradycardia or other arrhythmias occur and may be reinstituted following resolution of the cardiac arrhythmias if therapeutic response has not occurred. Therapeutic response is often immediate and dramatic. The litter should be removed from the bitch/queen for 12 to 24 hours and bottle or tube fed. If signs of hypocalcemia recur when the litter is returned to the bitch/queen, hand raising of the litter will be necessary (see Chapter 29). Vomiting often occurs if intravenous administration of calcium is too rapid.

Calcium supplementation of the bitch/queen prior to whelping may predispose to eclampsia. Excess dietary calcium intake decreases the efficiency of intestinal calcium absorption, inhibits parathyroid hormone secretion, and stimulates thyrocalcitonin release. These factors limit the bitch's or queen's ability to mobilize calcium following parturition.[8-10]

During peak lactation, bitches with a history of eclampsia may benefit from calcium administration (calcium carbonate, 500 mg per 5 kg body weight per day). Some authors recommend the use of corticosteroids to reduce the risk of eclampsia.[11] This treatment may be contraindicated, as glucocorticoids decrease intestinal calcium absorption and enhance renal excretion of calcium. If used, corticosteroids should not be administered in the first 24 to 48 hours following an acute episode of eclampsia, as the immediate effect of administration is to lower serum calcium.

Metritis. Acute metritis is a disease of bacterial origin that occurs in the immediate postpartum period. Metritis may occur following an apparently uncomplicated parturition and following parturition complicated by retained placentas, retained puppies, fetal infection and death, obstetrical manipulations, whelping in a contaminated environment, or abortion.

Clinical signs in the dam usually begin 1 to 3 days after the delivery of the litter and include a foul-smelling vaginal discharge, depression, fever, anorexia, palpable uterine enlargement, decreased lactation, and maternal neglect of the litter. The bitch or queen should undergo radiography for the presence of retained fetuses. Ultrasonography can be used to assess the viability of any remaining fetuses.

Cytologic evaluation of the vaginal discharge demonstrates large numbers of neutrophils, red blood cells, debris, and bacteria. An increased white blood cell count with a neutrophilic left shift is observed on a complete blood count. Treatment involves the administration of local and systemic antibiotics, fluid therapy (Chapter 38), and the stimulation of uterine drainage. Pending microbiologic evaluation of the vaginal discharge, a broad-spectrum antibiotic such as amoxicillin or chloramphenicol is administered. Antibiotic therapy is continued for 21 days. Uterine evacuation may be accomplished with administration of oxytocin (5 to 20 units intramuscularly), ergonovine (0.2 mg per 13.6 kg intramuscularly) or prostaglandin $F_{2\alpha}$ (0.1 to 0.25 mg/kg subcutaneously once daily for 2 days). Some authors report success with uterine lavage using sterile saline or dilute povidone iodine solution. However, the cervix is difficult to cannulate and the uterus is friable in many cases, suggesting that this form of treatment may not be effective or ideal. The litter may be returned to the dam once treatment has been initiated unless severe systemic illness is present in the dam (toxic milk).

Mastitis. Acute septic mastitis during lactation may result when bacteria are introduced into the gland by nursing, trauma, or by the hematogenous route. One or more of the mammary glands will be firm, painful, warm, and discolored. Milk from the affected gland or glands may be blood-tinged or gray and purulent. The litter is usually ignored and the bitch or queen is usually febrile, anorectic, reluctant to move, and may vomit. Cytologic evaluation of the milk from the affected glands reveals variably increased numbers of white blood cells and bacteria. Because of the observed variability, milk cell counts may not be reliable criteria for the diagnosis of mastitis.[2,7,9,12,13]

Therapy involves administration of broad-spectrum antibiotics (amoxicillin) for 7 to 10 days, frequent stripping, hot packing, and hydrotherapy of the gland; and parenteral administration of fluid therapy (Chapter 38). Glands that are black or dark purple generally become gangrenous. Gangrenous tissue should be surgically debrided, with an attempt to preserve the nipple and associated ductular tissue, and allowed to heal as an open wound. Despite significant tissue losses most bitches or queens will lactate from previously affected glands during subsequent lactations. In most cases, offspring may nurse from all but abscessed or gangrenous glands following initiation of antibiotic therapy in the dam.

Uterine prolapse. Prolapse of the uterus is a rare but reported condition of the queen and bitch.[14] Complete or partial uterine prolapse occurs periparturiently when the cervix is open. Diagnosis is based on physical examination of the animal, visual examination of the prolapsed mass, and careful digital examination of the animal's vagina.[9] Goals of treatment are to replace the uterus and prevent infection. The prolapsed mass must be thoroughly and gently cleansed; minimal debridement is generally required with prolapses of recent onset. Application of hyperosmotic agents (50% dextrose) may be used to reduce swelling and ease reduction of the tissue. Episiotomy and laparotomy may be necessary to aid in reduction of the prolapse. If the prolapsed tissue is greatly devitalized or if severe external or intraabdominal hemorrhage occurs (torn broad ligament), ovariohysterectomy should be performed. Laparotomy, following or in conjunction with reduction of the prolapse, may be required to assess uterine viability. The prognosis is guarded for re-

productive function in animals undergoing corrective measures for uterine prolapse; there are no reports of reproductive outcome following correction of the prolapse.

Postpartum hemorrhage. The most common cause of postpartum hemorrhage (which is not a common problem) is an inherited coagulopathy, often von Willebrand's disease.[2,5,10.12,15] Causes of hemorrhage postpartum include rodenticide intoxication, immune-mediated disease (thrombocytopenia) and disseminated intravascular coagulation induced by parturition. The packed cell volume of the pregnant bitch at term is approximately 30% and a rapidly declining packed cell volume following parturition is cause for concern. If coagulopathy is suspected, citrated plasma samples should be sent to specific diagnostic centers for evaluation of coagulation tests and for coagulation factor analysis. Postpartum hemorrhage, without the appearance of blood clots, requires initial therapy with oxytocin (5 to 20 units intramuscularly) or ergonovine maleate (0.2 mg per 13.6 kg intramuscularly). Administration of these drugs indirectly constricts uterine wall vasculature and causes involution of placental sites, decreasing the bleeding surface. Persistent and severe hemorrhage may require transfusion therapy (Chapter 34) and/or ovariohysterectomy.

Cystic endometrial hyperplasia/pyometra

Cystic endometrial hyperplasia (CEH)/pyometra complex in the bitch is common.[2,16-19] This disease complex is likely to cause critical illness in the patient and difficulties in diagnosis. The disease complex occurs less commonly in the queen, as would be expected in an induced ovulator (progesterone levels not elevated in nonovulatory cycles). The pathophysiology of the CEH/pyometra complex has been investigated and classified (Table 26-1).[17]

Progesterone administration to ovariectomized bitches results in lesions and clinical signs typical of CEH/pyometra complex.[17] Similar changes have been described after administration of exogenous progestational analogues (megestrol acetate and medroxyprogesterone acetate). Exogenous estrogen administration potentiates the effects of progesterone on the uterus.[17] A significant risk for pyometra has been observed in bitches given estradiol cypionate for the treatment of mismating.[20]

Pyometra commonly develops 4 weeks to 4 months after ovulatory estrus or treatment with progestins. Clinical signs of disease in affected animals are highly variable and include polydipsia, polyuria, anorexia, depression, vomiting, and diarrhea. Some animals may be presented in a

TABLE 26-1 Classification of cystic endometrial hyperplasia (CEH)/pyometra in the bitch

Category	Clinical Signs	Complete Blood Count	Uterine Characteristics
Dow Type I—uncomplicated CEH	No clinical illness Mucoid vaginal discharge possible	No abnormal findings	Bacteria present; no inflammation Mucometra possible (uncommon)
Dow Type II—CEH plus plasma-cell infiltration	Vaginal discharge present consistently	Mild neutrophilia	Bacteria present; plasma-cell infiltration of uterine wall Uterine enlargement (<2-cm diameter)
Dow Type III—CEH plus acute endometritis and periendometrial gland abscessation	Clinical signs present Anorexia, fever, polyuria, depression, vomiting, abdominal distention Closed-cervix animals have more severe clinical signs	Neutrophilia or neutropenia with left shift	Neutrophilic infiltration of endometrium or myometrium
Dow Type IV—chronic endometritis	Clinical signs present Anorexia, fever, polyuria, depression, vomiting, abdominal distention Closed-cervix animals have more severe clinical signs	Neutrophilia or neutropenia with left shift	Fibrosis and myometrial hypertrophy causing uterine wall thickening (open cervix) Large accumulation of purulent exudate and endometrial atrophy with closed cervix

state of circulatory collapse. A septic, purulent, "tomato-soup-like" vaginal discharge may be present, and the animal's uterus may be palpably enlarged. Results of laboratory evaluations may include leukocytosis or leukopenia with a left shift, increased total serum protein concentrations (dehydration, hyperglobinemia, hyperfibrinogenemia), anemia, and azotemia accompanied by isosthenuria and proteinuria. The renal lesions are attributable to immune complexes causing glomerular and renal tubular dysfunction.[3,21,22] These changes are potentially reversible once the pyometra is resolved.

The diagnosis of pyometra is usually determined by careful history and physical examination. A complete blood count, urinalysis and serum biochemistry profile, abdominal radiography, and abdominal ultrasonography should be performed to confirm the diagnosis, determine the extent and severity of the disease process, and identify any concomitant diseases in the animal. A normal (nongravid) uterus may not be visible on radiographs or sonograms. The major differential diagnosis for pyometra in cases of uterine enlargement is pregnancy. The two conditions are generally readily differentiated by ultrasonographic examination of the animal. Fetal structures and heartbeats are usually detectable by day

17 to 19 of gestation. A leukocytosis and a purulent vaginal/uterine discharge may be observed late in gestation in pregnant bitches that subsequently whelp live litters. Uterine infection may occur during pregnancy, with only partial loss of the litter.

The treatment of choice for pyometra is ovariohysterectomy. Aggressive fluid therapy should be used to stabilize the patient, correct dehydration, and improve tissue perfusion during and prior to surgery (Chapter 38). Septicemia and endotoxemia are significant risks to the animal with pyometra (Chapter 15). Broad-spectrum antibiotics should be administered perioperatively and administration continued in animals with sepsis. Glucocorticoid administration may be beneficial for the treatment of endotoxic shock. Complications of ovariohysterectomy in cases of pyometra include peritonitis, hemorrhage, thromboembolic disease, and disseminated intravascular coagulation.

If the cervix is open in a young (less than 6 years old) bitch or queen with pyometra and the animal has potential reproductive value, medical therapy may be considered. Prostaglandin $F_{2\alpha}$ in combination with long-term antibiotic administration (3 to 4 weeks' duration) has been used for the treatment of pyometra in bitches, with varying degrees of success. Prior to the initiation of treatment, a culture of the purulent material is obtained from the anterior vagina. Dosages recommended for $PGF_{2\alpha}$ administration include 0.1 mg/kg, 0.25 mg/kg, and 0.5 mg/kg administered subcutaneously daily for 2 to 5 days. Prostaglandin $F_{2\alpha}$ at these dosages is not luteolytic in the bitch, and its efficacy is attributable to stimulation of myometrial contraction and uterine evacuation.[23,24] Uterine diameter should decrease with each dose of $PGF_{2\alpha}$ administered, and following administration of the initial dose, the uterus should decrease in diameter by 50%. Some bitches may require two courses of prostaglandin administration in order to achieve a good response.

The median lethal dose for $PGF_{2\alpha}$ in the bitch is 5.13 mg/kg.[23] This drug is not licensed for use in small animals. Clients should be well informed, and treatment consent forms should be signed when deemed appropriate. Side effects are very common with prostaglandin administration, but are seldom serious; they commonly include salivation, vomiting, defecation, panting, and restlessness. The prostaglandin analogs (fluprostenol, cloprostenol) should not be used in the bitch or queen, as serious side effects (including death) have been observed following their administration.

Reported success rates for treatment with $PGF_{2\alpha}$ of pyometra in bitches vary tremendously. Resolution of clinical signs occurs in 82% to 100% of the cases treated.[25] Pregnancy rates of 40% to 82% during the next reproductive cycle have been reported for treated bitches.[25] For best results in reestablishing fertility, the treated bitch should have a vaginal culture at her next estrus, be bred with a fertile male, and be treated with appropriate antibiotics for 3 to 4 weeks (during pregnancy). Antibiotic selection (e.g., amoxicillin, trimethoprim-sulfamethoxazole) should be based on considerations of safety (fetal development) and the antibiotic sensitivity of the organism involved. Many bitches that have resolution of pyometra following $PGF_{2\alpha}$ administration have recurrences of pyometra during subsequent estrous cycles. Prostaglandin therapy should be reserved for young healthy bitches with an open-cervix pyometra and owned by compliant individuals wishing to have the dogs bred in the near future.

Uterine torsion

Uterine torsion (180 to 1440 degrees) is an uncommon disorder of the bitch and queen. At least five cases of uterine torsion in the queen have been reported since 1984.[3,26-30] Clinical signs can include pain, collapse, abdominal distention, and dehydration. As most cases of uterine torsion occur in pregnant animals, dystocia can result from the torsion. Survey abdominal radiography reveals a large fluid-filled uterus, occasionally intrauterine gas, and commonly fetal skeletons. Appropriate supportive medical care and surgical management involving derotation and cesarean section, with or without ovariohysterectomy, is indicated. In contrast to large animals with uterine torsion, medical derotation, including rolling, is ineffective in the treatment of small animals with the condition. There has been a report of uterine torsion in a nongravid bitch.[30]

MALE REPRODUCTIVE REPRODUCTION EMERGENCIES
Acute bacterial prostatitis

Acute bacterial prostatitis is a disease of adult male dogs. Infection most commonly occurs following prostatic colonization with gram-positive or gram-negative bacteria ascending from the urethra or urinary bladder.[2,18,31,32] The bloodstream or the reproductive tract may also serve as routes for introduction of bacteria into the prostate. Common clinical signs include anorexia, depression, fever, vomiting, and pain on palpation of the caudal abdomen or the prostate per rectal examination.

The diagnosis is confirmed by evaluation of prostatic fluid (culture and cytology). In many dogs prostatic fluid can be obtained by ejaculation. If the dog is in extreme pain and will not ejaculate, prostatic washes or other techniques may be required to obtain prostatic fluid (Chapter 21). Urinalysis and urine culture with antibiotic sensitivity should be performed for comparison with the results of similar tests on prostatic fluid.

The treatment for bacterial prostatitis involves antibiotic therapy for several weeks. Fluid therapy and other treatment methods may be required for the severely ill (septic) dog (Chapters 15 and 38). Castration of the animal is recommended, although owners of breeding dogs may be resistant to this suggestion.

Prostatic abscess

Prostatic abscess formation can be a sequela to acute or chronic bacterial prostatitis. Prostatic abscess often becomes an emergency when the animal becomes septic (usually associated with rupture of the abscess and the development of peritonitis) or when the abscess(es) increase in size to the extent that they interfere with the animal's defecation and/or urination.[18,32,33]

The diagnosis of prostatic abscess is confirmed by the use of radiography, ultrasonography, and prostatic fluid analysis (culture, cytology).

Surgical drainage of the prostatic abscesses (in combination with supportive treatment, antibiotic administration, and castration) is the treatment of choice. The prognosis for animals with prostatic abscess is guarded.

Penile trauma

Penile trauma may occur in the tom or dog for a variety of reasons, including bite injury, automobile trauma, and jumping fences.[34,35] Maintenance of urethral integrity and hemorrhage control are important therapeutic considerations. Therapy of penile wounds requires thorough cleansing, flushing, and suturing with absorbable suture material. Fracture of the os penis can occur and may or may not require surgical repair (see Chapter 21). Rarely, prolapse of the urethra may occur and surgical resection of the affected area may be required (see Chapter 21).

Following repair of penile trauma, the animal's penis should be protruded and visually inspected twice daily for several weeks. Topical therapy involving application of an antibiotic and corticosteroid cream will aid in healing and decrease the risk of adhesion formation. The animal should be restricted from engaging in sexual activity during the healing period.

Paraphimosis

Paraphimosis is the failure of the glans penis to be fully retracted into the prepuce. It may occur with an erect or nonerect penis.[36] Paraphimosis is most commonly seen in long-haired dogs following copulation, when the penis becomes entrapped in preputial hair or the inverted prepuce. Paraphimosis is diagnosed on physical examination. Therapy involves cleaning, lubricating, and replacing the penis into the prepuce. Application of hyperosmotic agents (50% dextrose) may help to shrink the entrapped tissue. Debridement may be necessary; however, dramatic healing of damaged penile tissue can occur quickly following resolution of paraphimosis.

Orchitis

Orchitis may occur in a tom or dog following external trauma or as a secondary complication of inguinal hernias or urinary tract infection.[2,37-39] Following trauma to the testicle, pain, hematomas, and swelling result. The goal of therapy should be to reduce testicular swelling and inflammation. Glucocorticoid administration and cool compresses should be used in the treatment of testicular injuries in order to reduce inflammation. Penetrating testicular wounds usually require removal of the testicle.

Leakage of sperm from traumatized tissue into the interstitium of the testicle may cause sperm granulomas or disruption of the blood-testis barrier resulting in an antigenic response to the sperm and thus infertility. In addition, immune-mediated orchitis (nonpainful) has been recognized in dogs with immune-mediated thyroiditis.[39]

The prognosis for return of fertility following bilateral testicular or epididymal inflammation or infection is poor. With unilateral involvement, fertility is often regained. Fertility evaluations of male animals should be delayed for at least 12 weeks following resolution of orchitis.

Inguinal hernia

Whenever there are intermittent changes in scrotal size accompanied by pain, an inguinal hernia should be suspected.[39,40] The presence of material (fluid or tissue) in the scrotum that can be pushed back into the peritoneal cavity (reduced), suggests inguinal hernia. Breeds of dogs with increased risk of inguinal hernia include basenji, bassett hound, Pekingese, cairn terrier and West Highland white terrier.[39] Animals with inguinal hernias can be presented as emergencies when a loop of intestine becomes entrapped and strangulated in the scrotum.[40] Treatment is careful herniorrhaphy and castration, as the condition is probably heritable.

Testicular torsion

Testicular torsion is most common in dogs with intraabdominal testes. Dogs with intraabdominal testicular torsion present with signs of acute abdomen, including pain, anorexia, vomiting, and occasionally collapse. This condition may be associated with neoplastic enlargement of a retained testis, as cryptorchid dogs are at tremendously increased risk (7 to 21 times that of normal males) for the development of testicular neoplasia.[31,19] Occasionally, an animal with scrotal testes will develop a testicular torsion. The dog will usually walk stiffly, and swelling/edema of the testicle will be evident. The treatment for testicular torsion in any case is orchiectomy.

REFERENCES

1. Gaudet DA, Kitchell BE. Canine dystocia. Compend Contin Educ Pract Vet 1985;7:406-416.
2. Hall MA, Swenberg LM. Genital emergencies. In Kirk RW, ed. Current veterinary therapy VI. Philadelphia: WB Saunders, 1977;1221-1227.
3. Johnson CA. Uterine diseases. In Ettinger SJ, ed. Textbook of veterinary internal medicine, ed. 3, Philadelphia: WB Saunders, 1989.
4. Johnston SD. Management of pregnancy disorders in the bitch and queen. In Kirk RW, ed. Current veterinary therapy VIII. Philadelphia: WB Saunders, 1983;954-955.

5. Thornberg LP, Raisbeck MF. A study of hepatobiliary diseases. Part 9: hemolytic disease, mycotoxicosis and pregnancy toxemia in the bitch. Compend Anim Pract 1988;2(12):13-17.

6. Concannon PW. Canine pregnancy and parturition. Vet Clin North Am Small Anim Pract, May 1986;16:453-475.

7. Johnston SD. Management of the postpartum bitch and queen. In Kirk RW, ed. Current veterinary therapy VIII. Philadelphia: WB Saunders, 1983;959-961.

8. Lewis LO, Morris ML. Feeding dogs. In Lewis LA, Morris ML, Hand MS, ed. Small animal clinical nutrition, Topeka KS: Mark Morris Foundation, 1983;3-9.

9. Smith FO. Postpartum diseases. Vet Clin North Am Small Anim Pract 1986;16:521-524.

10. Wheeler SL, et al. Postpartum disorders in the bitch. Compend Contin Ed Pract Vet 1984;6:493-500.

11. Tiovola BE, Mather GU. Puerperal tetany of the bitch. Nordon News 1968;Winter:16.

12. Burke TJ. Post-parturient problems in the bitch. Vet Clin North Am 1977;7:693-698.

13. Olson PN, Olson AL. Cytologic evaluation of canine milk. Vet Med Small Anim Clin 1984;79:641-646.

14. Roberts DD. Uterine prolapse in a cat. Compend Contin Educ Pract Vet 1988;10:1294-1296.

15. Hamilton H, Olson PN, Jonas L. Von Willebrand's disease manifested by hemorrhage from the reproductive tract: two case reports, J Am Anim Hosp Assoc 1985;21:637-641.

16. Dorn AS, Craig JA, Van Ee RT. Sex hormone related diseases treated surgically in bitches. Mod Vet Pract 1985;6:621-625.

17. Dow C. The cystic hyperplasia-pyometra complex in the bitch. Vet Rec 1957;69:1409.

18. Dow SW, Jones RL, Adney WS. Anaerobic bacterial infections and response to treatment in dogs and cats: 35 cases (1983-1985). J Am Vet Med Assoc 1986;189:930-936.

19. Frank N, Thornton ST. Have you seen this complication of canine pyometra? Vet Med Small Anim Clin 1985;80(4):34.

20. Bowen RA, et al. Efficacy and toxicity of estrogens commonly used to terminate canine pregnancy. J Am Vet Med Assoc 1985;186:183.

21. Hardy RM, Osborne CA. Canine pyometra: pathophysiology, diagnosis and treatment of uterine and extrauterine lesions. J Am Anim Hosp Assoc 1974;10:245.

22. Kenney KJ, et al. Pyometra in cats: 183 cases (1979-1984). J Am Vet Med Assoc 1987;191:1130-1132.

23. Sokolowski JH, Geng S. Effect of prostaglandin $F_{2\alpha}$ THAM in the bitch. J Am Vet Med Assoc 1977;170:536.

24. Baker BA, et al. Luteal function in the hysterectomized bitch following treatment with prostaglandin $F_{2\alpha}$. Theriogenology 1980;14:195.

25. Nelson RW, et al. Treatment of canine pyometra and endometritis with prostaglandin $F_{2\alpha}$. J Am Vet Med Assoc 1982;181:899.

26. Biller DS, Habel GK. Torsion of the uterus in a cat. J Am Vet Med Assoc 1987;191:1128-1129.

27. Freeman LJ. Feline uterine torsion. Compend Contin Educ Pract Vet 1988;10:1078-1082.

28. Jolivet MR. Uterine torsion in a pregnant cat. Mod Vet Pract 1987;68:240.

29. Manda JA. Identifying uterine torsion in pregnant cats. Vet Med Small Anim Clin 1986;81:936-938.

30. Partington BP. What is your diagnosis. J Am Vet Med Assoc 1988;193:1451-1452.

31. MacIntire DK. The acute abdomen—differential diagnosis and management. Semin Vet Med Surg 1988;3:202-310.

32. Olson PN, Wrigley RH, Thrall MA, Husted PW. Disorders of the canine prostate gland: pathogenesis, diagnosis and medical therapy. Compend Contin Educ Pract Vet 1987;9:613-623.

33. Bauer MS. Prostatic abscess rupture in 3 dogs. J Am Vet Med Assoc 1986;188:735-737.

34. Bradley RL. Complete urethral obstruction secondary to fracture of the os penis. Compend Contin Educ Pract Vet 1985;7:759-763.

35. McDonald RK. Urethral prolapse in a Yorkshire Terrier. Compend Contin Educ Pract Vet 1989;6:682-683.

36. Elkins AD. Canine paraphimosis of unknown etiology: a case report. Vet Med Small Anim Clin 1984;79:638-639.

37. Allison N, et al. Eumycotic mycetoma caused by Pseudallescheria boydii in a dog. J Am Vet Med Assoc 1989;195:797-799.

38. Dunn JK, Gorman NT. Fever of unknown origin in dogs and cats. J Small Anim Pract 1987;28:167-181.

39. Larsen RE, Smith FO. Lesions of the scrotum and scrotal structures. In Burke TJ, ed. Small animal reproduction and infertility. Philadelphia: Lea & Febiger, 1986;240-242.

40. Manderino D, Bucklan L. Complete small bowel obstruction caused by scrotal hernia in a dog. Mod Vet Pract 1987;68:365-368.

27 Toxicologic Emergencies

E. Murl Bailey, Jr., and Tom Garland

Acutely ill animals are often diagnosed as "poisoned" when no other diagnosis is obvious. The clinician should direct efforts toward stabilizing the patient. Preexisting conditions and the diagnosis should be determined following initial control of the clinical signs.

The goals of therapy in cases of intoxication include emergency intervention and prevention of further exposure, preventing further absorption, application of specific antidotes, hastening elimination of the absorbed toxicant, supportive measures, and client education.

Veterinarians are frequently contacted by telephone concerning an intoxicated animal. Instructions provided at this time can assist subsequent therapeutic measures. In most cases, the owner should be urged to bring the animal to the clinic promptly.

When transportation is delayed, the client should be instructed to protect the affected animal, including keeping the animal warm and avoiding any other stress. Onlookers should be warned about the condition of the animal, and it may be desirable to muzzle the animal.

The animal owner should be instructed to cleanse the animal's skin or eye with copious amounts of water in cases of topical exposure. The client should be instructed to be careful to avoid exposure to the toxicant. Some type of protective clothing (e.g., rubber gloves, apron) should be used.

The client, in many instances, will be concerned about inducing emesis in the animal. The clinician should cite the contraindications to emesis (e.g., central nervous system depression; ingestion of petroleum distillates, acids, or alkalis). Emetic preparations and techniques easily available to the lay individuals (e.g., hydrogen peroxide, table salt, copper sulfate, and sticking the finger in the back of the animal's mouth) are generally ineffective and sometimes dangerous. One-half to 2 teaspoons of syrup of ipecac may be administered, if the animal is fully awake.

An insistent client may be advised to allow the animal to drink water, as this will act as a diluent. In most cases, the administration of milk, egg whites, and activated charcoal tablets may be advised. The client should be cautioned about oral administration if the animal is convulsing, depressed, or unconscious.

The client should not waste time. The animal must be taken to the veterinarian as soon as possible. The owner should be instructed to bring uncontaminated vomitus and suspected toxic materials and/or their containers with the animal. The client should be advised to bring the specimens in clean plastic or glass containers. In many instances, valuable time can be saved by applying the proper therapeutic measure when the suspected intoxicant is known. The clinician should not bias the diagnosis and treatment of an animal based on labels or material brought with the animal.

Suspected toxic materials and specimens may be valuable from a medicolegal aspect. A proper chain of physical evidence and good medical records should be maintained in cases of suspected intoxications.

Emergency intervention may include establishment of a patent airway, artificial respiration, cardiac massage (external or internal), and perhaps the application of defibrillation techniques. Following patient stabilization, the clinician should proceed with subsequent therapeutic measures.

Supported by Texas Agricultural Experiment Station (TAES) project no. H-6255. Published as TAES publication no. TA-25034.

427

Preventing absorption of additional toxicant(s) is a major factor in treating cases of intoxication. In many instances, intoxications may be prevented in this manner if undertaken shortly after an animal was observed coming in contact with or ingesting the suspected material. Removal of the animal from the affected environment is a necessary first step. If an external toxicant is involved, prevention of further absorption may entail washing the animal's skin to remove the noxious agent. Caution must be exercised to avoid contamination of persons handling the animal. The judicious use of emetics, gastric lavage techniques, adsorbents, and cathartics will aid in the prevention of further absorption of toxic materials that are ingested.

EMESIS

Emesis may be considered as a method of emptying the stomach of toxic materials. Some commonly available agents are not very reliable. Emesis may be of little value 4 hours after ingestion of a toxicant, as most materials will have passed to the duodenum, rendering emesis ineffective in its removal.

Apomorphine (Eli Lilly) is the most effective and most reliable emetic available for use in dogs and cats. The effective dose in small animals is 0.04 mg/kg intravenously or 0.08 mg/kg intramuscularly or subcutaneously. Apomorphine sometimes causes respiratory depression and protracted emesis in humans, but these adverse signs are not common in dogs. These signs may be effectively controlled with appropriate narcotic antagonists injected intravenously (naloxone [Narcan, Endo] 0.04 mg/kg; levallorphan [Lorfan, Roche] 0.02 mg/kg; or nalorphine [Nalline, Merck] 0.1 mg/kg).

Syrup of ipecac is an effective general emetic in 50% of the cases in which it is administered. Its mechanism of action involves gastric irritation and central stimulation. The dose is 1 to 2 ml/kg, with a maximum dosage of 15 ml (1 tablespoon) in small animals. The dosage may be repeated in 20 minutes if necessary. If the patient does not vomit, gastric lavage should be instituted to recover the ipecac to avoid any cardiotoxic effects. Ipecac should never be used when activated charcoal is part of the therapeutic regimen, since it markedly reduces the effectiveness of the charcoal. The drug should not be confused with ipecac fluid extract, which is 14 times stronger than the syrup. Outdated syrup of ipecac can be used since it is still effective.

Copper sulfate, table salt, or hydrogen peroxide have been advocated as locally acting emetics. The emetic effect of these agents is highly questionable. Intravenous xylazine has been used with some effect as an emetic in dogs and cats.

Emesis should not be induced in unconscious or severely depressed animals, or following ingestion of strong acids, alkalis, petroleum distillates, tranquilizers, and other antiemetics. Intoxication with acids or alkalis maybe diagnosed by the presence of burns on the mouth, forepaws, and other areas of the cranial portions of the body. Vomiting of caustic agents could cause additional damage to the esophagus and oral cavity. Caustic agents often weaken the gastric wall, predisposing it to rupture during forceful emesis.

Administration of activated charcoal in combination with emetics increases the efficacy of toxicant elimination by emesis. The clinician should induce emesis with apomorphine, administer the charcoal, and reinduce emesis with a subsequent dose of apomorphine (0.04 mg/kg intravenously).

GASTRIC LAVAGE

Gastric lavage, as an emergency procedure in treatment of intoxications, has at times been maligned as being inefficient. Use of a large-bore tube, large volumes of lavage fluids, and frequent lavages make this a very reliable procedure when undertaken within 2 to 4 hours of ingestion of a toxicant. The animal should be unconscious or under light anesthesia. A cuffed endotracheal tube should be positioned with the distal end of the tube extending 2 in. (5 cm) beyond the teeth. This will increase the animal's dead space but is required to prevent any inhalation of lavage fluid. The head and thorax should be lowered slightly but not enough to compromise respiration. The stomach tube should be premeasured from the tip of the animal's nose to the xiphoid cartilage and introduced into the stomach. A stomach tube as large as possible should be used. A good rule is to use the same size stomach tube as the cuffed endotracheal tube (1 mm = 3 French). The volume of water or lavage solution to be used for each washing is 5 to 10 ml/kg body weight. Following infusion of the solution, the fluid should be aspirated via the stomach tube with either a large aspirator bulb, 60-ml syringe, or stomach pump. The infusion and aspiration cycle of the lavage solution should be repeated 10 to 15 times. Activated charcoal in the solution will enhance the effectiveness of this procedure. Some precautions to be taken with this technique are (1) using low pressure to prevent forcing the toxicant into the duodenum, (2) reducing the infused volume in obviously weakened stomach walls, and (3) making sure not to force the stomach tube through either the esophagus or the stomach wall.

ACTIVATED CHARCOAL

Activated charcoal is probably the best adsorbing agent available. Although it does not detoxify toxicants, it will effectively prevent absorption of a toxicant if properly used. Activated charcoal is highly adsorptive for many toxicants, including organophosphate insecticides, other insecticides, rodenticides, mercuric chloride, strychnine, other alkaloids (morphine and atropine), barbiturates, and ethylene glycol. It is ineffective against cyanide.

The proper type of activated charcoal for treatment of intoxications is of petroleum or vegetable origin, not mineral or animal. A highly activated charcoal (SuperChar-Vet, Gulf Biosystems) made from petroleum is currently available and is two to three times more adsorptive than activated charcoal, USP. There are several commercial types of activated charcoal available including a mixture of activated charcoal and kaolin (Toxiban, Vet-A-Mix). Compressed activated charcoal tablets (5 g, B.C. Crowley and Requa Mfg.) are also available. These tablets may be easier to handle than the powdered charcoal and are as effective as activated charcoal, USP.

A bathtub or some other easily cleansed area is the best location to use when administering activated charcoal to small animals. Activated charcoal is used as follows: (1) Make a slurry of the charcoal with water. A proper dose is 1 to 5 g/kg body weight in a concentration of 1 g charcoal to 5 to 10 ml water. (2) Administer the charcoal by a stomach tube using either a funnel or a large syringe. (3) A cathartic of sodium sulfate should be administered 30 minutes after administration of the charcoal. This technique may be modified if the charcoal is used in conjunction with emetic or lavage techniques. When combined with these techniques, some charcoal should remain in the stomach and be followed by a cathartic to prevent desorption of the toxicant. The administration of activated charcoal three to four times a day for 2 to 3 days after occurrence of an intoxication may be beneficial in some cases. The "universal antidote," consisting of two parts activated charcoal, one part magnesium oxide and one part tannic acid, is very inefficient. The magnesium oxide and tannic acid decrease the adsorptive capability of the charcoal. Burned or charred toast is highly ineffective as an adsorbing agent. Mineral oil or vegetable oils are of value if lipid-soluble toxicants are involved. Mineral oil (liquid petrolatum) is inert and is less likely to be absorbed.

CATHARTICS

Sodium sulfate is a more efficient agent for evacuation of the bowel than is magnesium sulfate, and it is the preferable agent to use with activated charcoal and mineral oils. The oral dose of sodium sulfate is 1 g/kg.

A colonic lavage or high enema may be of value to hasten the elimination of toxicants from the gastrointestinal tract. Warm water with castile soap makes an excellent enema solution. Hexachlorophene soaps should be avoided in cats. There are several commercially available enema preparations that act as osmotic agents. Care should be taken to avoid the induction of dehydration and electrolyte imbalances with overzealous treatment.

There are some specific antidotal agents or procedures available for the more common animal toxicants. A list of these specific antidotal procedures is presented in the section on specific toxicants.

HASTENING ELIMINATION OF ABSORBED TOXICANTS

Absorbed toxicants are generally excreted via the kidneys. Some toxicants may be excreted by other routes (bile-feces, lung, other body secretions). Renal excretion can be manipulated in many instances. Urinary excretion of toxicants may be enhanced by the use of diuretics or altering the pH of the urine.

The use of diuretics to enhance urinary excretion of toxicants requires maintenance of adequate renal function (normal minimum urine output is 0.01 ml/kg per minute, i.e., 20 ml/kg per day[1]) and hydration of the affected animal. Once these requisites are established, diuretics are indicated. However, if a minimum urine flow cannot be established, peritoneal dialysis must be performed (Chapter 39). The diuretics of choice are mannitol and furosemide (Lasix, Hoechst-Roussel). Both of these agents are very potent diuretics. The dosage for mannitol is 1.0 to 2.0 g/kg every 6 hours intravenously and for furosemide 5 mg/kg every 6 to 8 hours intravenously. Careful serial monitoring of fluid and electrolyte balance in the animal is required with repeated administrations of these diuretics.

Alteration of urinary pH to expedite the excretion of toxicants and foreign chemicals is a classic pharmacologic technique. The technique relies on the physiochemical phenomenon that ionized compounds do not readily traverse cell membranes and hence are not reabsorbed by the renal tubules. Consequently, acid compounds such as acetylsalicylic acid (aspirin) and some barbiturates remain ionized in alkaline urine, while alkaline compounds such as amphetamines remain ionized in acidic urine. For long-term urinary acidification, oral ammonium chloride (200 mg/

kg per day in divided doses) or ethylenediamine dihydrochloride (Chlorethamine, Pitman-Moore, 1 to 2 tablets three times a day for the medium-sized dog) are available. Physiologic saline is a good, rapid, urine-acidifying agent. Sodium bicarbonate (5 mEq/kg per hour) may be used as an alkalinizing agent.

Peritoneal dialysis is indicated when an intoxicated animal exhibits oliguria or anuria. Dialysis is also indicated for simple removal of absorbed toxicants in animals with normal renal function. It is a rather time consuming, but effective, technique in many conditions. The process of peritoneal dialysis involves the infusion of 10 to 20 ml/kg of a dialyzing solution into the peritoneal cavity, waiting 30 to 45 minutes, withdrawing the dialyzing solution, and reinfusing a fresh solution. After the first two exchanges of dialyzing solutions, the interval between exchanges can be lengthened to 2 to 4 hours. The infusion and withdrawal cycles should be maintained for a minimum of 24 hours or until normal renal function is restored. The pH of the dialyzing solutions may be altered to maintain the ionized state of the offending compound.

SUPPORTIVE TREATMENTS

Supportive treatments are very important in cases of intoxications. These measures include control of body temperature, maintenance of respiratory and cardiovascular function, control of acid-base imbalances, alleviation of pain, and control of central nervous system disorders.

Hypothermia may be controlled with the use of blankets and by keeping the animal in a warm, draft-free cage. Infrared lamps or heating pads should be used with caution and under constant observation. A pad with circulating warm water may be of greater value and is less dangerous than lamps or conventional heating pads (Aquamatic K Pad, American Hospital Supply).

Hyperthermia is controlled through the use of ice bags, cold water baths, administration of cold intravenous fluids, and possibly cold-water enemas or cold peritoneal dialysis solution. It is vitally important that the animal's body temperature be constantly monitored to ensure that overcorrection does not occur.

Respiratory support requires the presence of an adequate, patent airway and may require the use of a cuffed endotracheal tube in an unconscious animal or a tracheostomy. Intermittent positive-pressure ventilation (Bird Respirator, Bird Corp., or Ohio Ventilator, Ohio Medical Products) is needed to treat cases of respiratory depression. An anesthetic machine with manual compression of the bag, may be used as a short-term alternative. A mixture of 50% oxygen and 50% room air is generally adequate unless there is a thickened respiratory membrane, in which case greater concentrations (up to 100% oxygen) and/or positive end-expiratory pressure/continuous positive airway pressure (Chapter 36) may be necessary. The use of analeptic drugs in cases of severe respiratory depression or apnea is questionable, due to the short duration of their effects and other undesirable side effects.

Cardiovascular support requires the presence of adequate circulating blood volume, cardiac performance, tissue perfusion, and acid-base balance. Hypovolemia due to fluid loss alone can be treated with the administration of lactated Ringer's solution or plasma expanders. Central venous pressure should be monitored in these cases to prevent cardiac overload. In the presence of hypovolemia due to loss of both cells and volume, administration of whole blood is necessary. A good rule is to give a sufficient quantity of whole blood (10 to 20 ml/kg) to raise the packed cell volume to 75% of the animal's estimated normal level. Tissue perfusion should also be monitored periodically to determine the adequacy of the replacement therapy. In some cases, it may be necessary to administer corticosteroids intravenously to restore appropriate tissue perfusion (dexamethasone [Azium, Schering], 2 to 10 mg/kg). Caution should be exercised in the use of these steroids since hypovolemia may ensue. Therefore, large intravenous doses of corticosteroids should never be administered unless volume-replacement therapy is ongoing. Cardiac activity can be aided by the application of closed-chest cardiac massage for immediate requirements, but the administration of pharmaceutical agents may be necessary to aid inotropic and chronotropic activity (Chapters 17 and 32). Care must be taken to avoid overdosage with cardioactive agents, since they are highly toxic to the myocardium. The electric activity of the heart should be closely monitored during administration of cardioactive agents.

The most common acid-base disturbance seen in intoxicated animals is metabolic acidosis. However, acidosis or alkalosis may occur in cases of intoxication.

The drug of choice for correcting metabolic acidosis is sodium bicarbonate, administered intravenously at a dosage rate of 5 mEq/kg per hour. Alternatively, if blood gas measurements are available, a method of calculating the replacement amount is 0.3 times the body weight in kilograms times the base deficit. With the use of blood gas monitoring, a quarter of this calculated deficit is given as an intravenous bolus and a quarter given in a drip over a 6-to-8-hour period. Then, blood gas measurements should be repeated. The empirical administration of 2 to 4 mEq/kg once or perhaps twice is another method of estimating the replacement amount. Other alkalinizing solutions include: 0.17 M sodium lactate, 16 to 32 ml/kg; lactated Ringer's solution, 120 ml/kg; or tromethamine (THAM) buffer, 300 mg/kg. Bicarbonate is generally the easiest to administer with respect to volume and requires no metabolic conversion. Caution must be exercised with all alkalinizing agents to avoid the induction of alkalosis.

Alkalosis, unless drug-induced, does not generally occur in animals suffering from intoxication. If alkalosis is present, the intravenous administration of 0.9% sodium chloride (physiologic saline), or Ringer's solution, 10 ml/kg, is usually sufficient for initial therapy. This should be followed by the oral administration of ammonium chloride, 200 mg/kg per day in divided doses. As in the case of acidosis, the clinician should be cautious about overtreatment of the alkalotic patient.

The control of pain is an important supportive measure in cases of intoxications. A minimal dose of morphine (dogs, 1 to 2 mg/kg; cats, 0.1 to 0.2 mg/kg) or meperidine (Demerol, Winthrop) (dogs, 5 to 10 mg/kg; cats, 1 to 2 mg/kg) is indicated in animals showing pain.

Management of central nervous system disorders in cases of intoxication is simple in appearance but complex in actuality. The type of therapy will depend on the presence of central nervous system depression or hyperactivity. Either disorder can easily be turned into the opposite problem by overzealous therapeutic measures. Respiratory depression can occur with central nervous system depression. The intravenous administration of analeptic agents such as doxapram (Dopram, Robins), 3 to 5 mg/kg; or pentylenetetrazol (Metrazol, Knoll), 6 to 10 mg/kg, is reported to be efficacious in these conditions, their actions are short-lived, and central nervous system/respiratory depression can return if the animals are not monitored continuously. Analeptics can induce convulsions. Ventilatory support is of greater value than analeptics in animals exhibiting central nervous system/respiratory depression and is the treatment of choice (Chapter 36).

Cases of central nervous system hyperactivity, including convulsions, can be managed by the administration of central nervous system depressants or tranquilizers. Pentobarbital sodium is generally the agent of choice for convulsions and hyperactivity. The dose required to alleviate the neurologic signs may cause respiratory depression, necessitating ventilatory support. Inhalant anesthetics have been reported as excellent for long-term management of central nervous system hyperactivity. Central-acting skeletal muscle relaxants and minor tranquilizers have been reported for use with convulsant intoxicants: methocarbamol (Robaxin, Robins), 110 mg/kg intravenously; glyceryl guaiacolate (Gecolate, Summit Hill Labs), 110 mg/kg intravenously; and diazepam (Valium, Roche), 0.5 to 1.5 mg/kg intravenously or intramuscularly. In cases of central nervous system stimulation due to amphetamines and hallucinogens such as lysergic acid diethylamide (LSD) or phencyclidine, phenothiazine tranquilizers are indicated. Animals with central nervous system hyperactivity should be placed in a quiet, dark room to prevent additional stimulation from auditory or visual stimuli.

POISON CONTROL CENTERS AND DIAGNOSTIC LABORATORIES

Poison control centers and animal diagnostic laboratories can be of great value to the clinician in cases of suspected intoxications, especially when labels or containers are presented with the acutely ill animal. *When the suspected compound and the signs exhibited by the animal do not concur, the signs should be treated and the label should be disregarded.*

The diagnosis should be confirmed by chemical analysis, even though this may occur after the fact. An accurate diagnosis, as well as detailed records, may help the veterinarian faced with subsequent cases from the same intoxicant. Detailed records will be invaluable considerations in any medicolegal proceedings.

The National Animal Poison Control Center (NAPCC) is an excellent resource for toxicologic emergencies (1-900-680-0000). Veterinarians, practice groups, or clinics may become members of the NAPCC support group and receive quarterly reports and the free use of a WATS telephone line for use in emergencies.

Listed in the box on pp. 432-435 are federal, state, and private diagnostic laboratories.

SPECIFIC TOXICANTS
Acetysalicylic acid intoxication (salicylism)

Aspirin is a weak organic acid (acetylsalicylic acid) (ASA) that is readily absorbed from the stomach in its non-ionized form; however, it is primarily absorbed from the duodenum. Since the cat, young animals, and children have reduced capability of glucuronide conjugation, this may account for the higher toxicity of aspirin in these groups. The effects of salicylates are attributed to the inhibition of the synthesis of prostaglandins (prostaglandin synthetase).

In animals, especially cats, aspirin can cause excitation and ataxia in early stages of acute toxicity. The animals subsequently become depressed and comatose. Hyperpnea results from di-

Text continued on p. 436.

DIAGNOSTIC LABORATORIES[5]

ALABAMA
State of Alabama Veterinary Diagnostic Laboratory
P.O. Box 2209
Auburn, AL 36830
205-887-8681   (FTS) 534-4551

Poultry Producers Diagnostic Laboratory
P.O. Box 1010
Cullman, AL 35055
205-739-1414

ALASKA
Alaska State Federal Laboratory
P.O. Box 720
Palmer, AK 99645
907-745-3236

ARIZONA
Arizona State Department of Health
1520 West Adams Street
Phoenix, AZ 85007
602-765-4551

Department of Veterinary Science
University of Arizona
Tucson, AZ 85721
602-621-2356

ARKANSAS
Arkansas Livestock and Poultry Commissions
Diagnostic Laboratory
Highway 71 N. Box 766
Springdale, AK 76764
501-751-4869

Fish Farming Experimental Station
Box 860
Stuttgart, AK 72160
501-673-8761

CALIFORNIA
County of Los Angeles
Department of Health Services Division
Comparative Medical and Veterinary Public Health
  Service
12824 Horton Avenue
Downey, CA 90242
213-923-0641

State of California Department of Food and
  Agriculture Laboratory Services
2789 South Orange Avenue
Fresno, CA 93725
209-266-9418

California Department of Agriculture
  Veterinary Laboratory Services
3290 Meadowview Road
Sacramento, CA 95823
916-428-3172

Wildlife Investigations Laboratory
987 Jedsmith Drive
Sacramento, CA 95819
916-465-0157

San Diego County Veterinary Laboratory
5555 Overland Avenue, Bldg. 4
San Diego, CA 92123
714-565-5395

California Department of Agriculture
  Veterinary Laboratory Services
P.O. Box 255
San Gabriel, CA 91778
213-282-6127

Intermountain Laboratories Incorporated
  Veterinary Reference Laboratory, Inc.
800 Charcot Avenue
San Jose, CA 95131
415-845-8844

Department of Clinical Pathology
School of Veterinary Medicine
University of California
Davis, CA 95616
916-752-6026

COLORADO
Veterinary Diagnostic Laboratory
Colorado State University
Fort Collins, CO 80523
303-491-6128

CONNECTICUT
Department of Pathology
Box U-89 University of Connecticut
Storrs, CT 06268
203-486-4000

DELAWARE
Division of Standards and Inspection
State Department of Agriculture Poultry and Animal
  Health Section
P.O. Drawer D
Dover, DE 19901
302-678-4821   302-678-4823   (FTS) 302-487-5122

FLORIDA
Kissimmee Animal Disease Diagnostic Laboratory
P.O. Box 460
Kissimmee, FL 32741
305-847-3185

Miami Springs Diagnostic Laboratory
8701 N.W. 58th Street
Miami, FL 33178
305-592-3059

GEORGIA
Department of Health, Education and Welfare
U.S. Public Health Service,
Centers for Disease Control
Atlanta, GA 30333
404-633-3311

Diagnostic Assistance Laboratory
College of Veterinary Medicine
University of Georgia
Athens, GA 30602
404-542-5568

Diagnostic and Investigational Laboratories
Route 2 Brighton Road
Tifton, GA 31794
912-386-3340

HAWAII
Hawaii Department of Agriculture
Veterinary Laboratory Branch
1428 South King Street
Honolulu, HI 96814
808-941-3071, ext. 158

IDAHO
Idaho Bureau of Animal Laboratories
P.O. Box 7249
Boise, ID 83707
208-384-3111

ILLINOIS
Laboratories of Veterinary Diagnostic
    Medicine
University of Illinois
Urbana, IL 61801
217-333-3611

INDIANA
Animal Disease Diagnostic Laboratory
School of Veterinary Medicine
Purdue University
West Lafayette, IN 47906
317-494-7448

IOWA
Veterinary Diagnostic Laboratory
Iowa State University
Ames, IA 50011
515-294-1950

Veterinary Services Laboratories
U.S. Department of Agriculture
Animal and Plant Health Inspection Service
Ames, IA 50010
515-232-0252

KANSAS
Veterinary Diagnostic Laboratory
College of Veterinary Medicine
Manhattan, KS 66506
913-532-5650

LOUISIANA
Central Louisiana Livestock Diagnostic
    Laboratory
Route 2, Box 51-F
Lecompte, LA 71346
318-443-6993

Northwest Louisiana Livestock Diagnostic
    and Research Laboratory
P.O. Box 2156
Natchitoches, LA 71457
318-352-6272

School of Veterinary Medicine
Louisiana State University
Baton Rouge, LA 70803
504-388-4141

MAINE
University of Maine Pathology Diagnostic
    and Research Laboratory
Hitchener Hall
Orono, ME 04473
207-581-7521

MARYLAND
Maryland Department of Agriculture
Animal Health Laboratory
4901 Calvert Road
College Park, MD 20740
301-454-3631

MASSACHUSETTS
Large Animal Diagnostic Laboratory
Paige Laboratory
University of Massachusetts
Amherst, MA 01002
413-545-2427

MICHIGAN
Wildlife Pathology Laboratory
Michigan Department of Natural Resources
8562 E. Stoll Road R1
East Lansing, MI 48823
517-339-8638

Michigan Department of Agriculture
Laboratory Division
1615 S. Harrison Road
East Lansing, MI 48823
517-373-6410

Animal Health Diagnostic Service
College of Veterinary Medicine
Michigan State University
East Lansing, MI 48913
517-353-5034

MINNESOTA
Veterinary Diagnostic Laboratories
E220 Diagnostic and Research Building
College of Veterinary Medicine
University of Minnesota
St. Paul, MN 55108
612-625-3179

Continued.

MISSISSIPPI
Mississippi Veterinary Diagnostic Laboratory
P.O. Box 4389
Jackson, MS 39216
601-354-6091

College of Veterinary Medicine
P.O. Drawer V
Mississippi State University, MS 39762
601-325-3432

MISSOURI
Veterinary Medical Diagnostic Laboratory
College of Veterinary Medicine
University of Missouri
Columbia, MO 65122
314-882-6811

Ralston Purina Veterinary Laboratory
Veterinary Service Department
Checkerboard Square
St. Louis, MO 63188
314-982-2611

MONTANA
State of Montana Animal Health Division
Diagnostic Laboratory
P.O. Box 997
Bozeman, MT 59715
406-586-5952   (FTS)555-4339

NEBRASKA
Diagnostic Laboratory
Department of Veterinary Science
University of Nebraska
Lincoln, NE 68583-0907
402-472-1434   (FTS) 472-3818

NEVADA
Animal Disease Laboratory
Nevada Department of Agriculture
P.O. Box 11100 350 Capital Hill Avenue
Reno, NV 89510
702-784-6229

NEW HAMPSHIRE
Veterinary Diagnostic Laboratory
University of New Hampshire
Durham, NH 03824
603-862-2726

NEW JERSEY
Rutgers Poultry Diagnostic Laboratory
Thompson Hall
New Brunswick, NJ 08903
201-932-9320

NEW YORK
Cornell University Duck Research Laboratory
Box 217 Old Country Road
Eastport, NY 11941
516-326-0600

Plum Island Animal Disease Center
United State Department of Agriculture
P.O. Box 848
Greenport, NY 11944
516-323-2508

Diagnostic Laboratory
New York State Veterinary College at Cornell
  University
Box 786
Ithaca, NY 14860
607-256-3117

NORTH CAROLINA
Rollins Animal Disease Diagnostic Laboratory
P.O. Box 12223
Cameron Village Station
Raleigh, NC 27605
919-733-3986

Laboratory of Toxicology
North Carolina State University
Raleigh, NC 27606
919-829-4200

NORTH DAKOTA
North Dakota State Veterinary Diagnostic Laboratory
North Dakota State University
Fargo, ND 58102
701-237-7511

OHIO
Ohio State University
Department of Veterinary Clinical Sciences
Clinical Pathology Laboratory
1935 Coffey Road
Columbus, OH 43210
614-292-1202

OKLAHOMA
Oklahoma Animal Disease Diagnostic Laboratory
College of Veterinary Medicine
Oklahoma State University
Stillwater, OK 74078
405-624-6623

OREGON
Oregon State Veterinary Diagnostic Laboratory
Oregon State University
Corvallis, OR 97331
503-424-3261

PENNSYLVANIA
Division of Clinical Laboratory Medicine
School of Veterinary Medicine
Department of Clinical Studies
University of Pennsylvania
3800 Spruce Street
Philadelphia, PA 19104
215-898-7891

Laboratory of Pathology
School of Veterinary Medicine
University of Pennsylvania
3800 Spruce Street
Philadelphia, PA 19104
215-898-8858

Pennsylvania Department of Agriculture
Bureau of Animal Industry Laboratory
Summerdale, PA 17093
717-637-8808

PUERTO RICO
Institute of Health Laboratory
Box 10427
Caparra Heights, PR 00922
809-764-8585

RHODE ISLAND
Diagnostic Laboratory
Department of Animal Pathology
University of Rhode Island
Kingston, RI 02881
401-792-2487

SOUTH CAROLINA
Clemson University
Livestock-Poultry Health Department
P.O. Box 218
Elgin, SC 29045
803-788-2260

SOUTH DAKOTA
Animal Disease Research and Diagnostic
    Laboratory
South Dakota State University
Brooking, SD 57006
605-688-5171

TENNESSEE
C.E. Kord Animal Disease Laboratory
P.O. Box 40627 Mel Station
Nashville, TN 37204
615-853-1559

College of Veterinary Medicine
University of Tennessee
Knoxville, TN 37901
615-546-9230

TEXAS
Texas Veterinary Medical Diagnostic
    Laboratory
P.O. Drawer 3040
College Station, TX 77841
409-845-3414

Texas Veterinary Medical Diagnostic
    Laboratory
P.O. Box 3200
Amarillo, TX 79116
806-353-7478

Southwest Foundation for Research and
    Education
P.O. Box 28147
San Antonio, TX 78228
512-674-1410

UTAH
Utah State University Veterinary Diagnostic
    Laboratory
Utah State University
Logan, UT 84312
801-752-4100, ext. 7584

Intermountain Laboratories Incorporated
Veterinary Reference Laboratory, Inc.
870 E. 7145 South
Midvale, UT 84047
801-561-2244

State Chemist Office and State Federal
    Cooperative Laboratory
412 Capitol Building
Salt Lake City, UT 84114
801-533-5421

VERMONT
Animal Pathology Laboratory
Hills Science Building
University of Vermont
Burlington, VT 05401
802-656-2650

VIRGINIA
Division of Animal Health and Dairies
Regulatory Laboratory
116 Reservoir Street
Harrisonburg, VA 22801
703-434-3897

Virginia Tech
Regional College of Veterinary Medicine
Blacksburg, VA 24061
703-961-7666

WASHINGTON
Department of Veterinary Pathology
Pullman, WA 99164
509-335-9696

Poultry Diagnostic Laboratory
Western Washington Research and Extension
    Center
Washington State University
Puyallup, WA 98371
206-843-6613

WEST VIRGINIA
State Federal Cooperative
Animal Health Laboratory
Rm. B86 Capital Bldg.
Charleston, WV 25305
304-885-2231   304-885-3418

WISCONSIN
National Fish and Wildlife Health Laboratory
University of Wisconsin
Department of Veterinary Science
1655 Linden Drive
Madison, WI 53706
608-252-5411   (FTS) 364-5411

WYOMING
Wyoming State Veterinary Laboratory
Box 950
Laramie, WY 82070
307-742-6638

rect and indirect stimulation of the medullary respiratory center. This may cause a transitory respiratory alkalosis; however, metabolic acidosis is a major problem in later stages of intoxication. Clinical signs resulting from gastrointestinal mucosal irritation and ulceration include vomiting, hematemesis, salivation, anorexia, and hemorrhagic diarrhea. A coagulopathy may occur in subacute or chronic intoxications.

The diagnosis of aspirin intoxication is made from the history, clinical signs, postmortem lesions, and possibly chemical identification. The treatment of animals with aspirin intoxication includes induced emesis or gastric lavage with activated charcoal, alkalinizing agents and diuresis, and fluid and electrolyte therapy. In severely intoxicated cats, the prognosis is marginal to poor.

Onion poisoning

In the past, onion (*Allium* spp.) poisoning was more of a problem in large animals. Onion soup has become problematical, especially in cats. The toxic principle in onions is *N*-propyl disulfide. The clinical signs of onion intoxication include Heinz-body anemia, hemoglobinuria, and sometimes icterus. The onset of clinical signs occurs 1 to 6 days after ingestion, and clinical signs often resolve with cessation of exposure.

Treatment of animals with onion intoxication includes removal of the animal from the source of toxin exposure, blood transfusions, and fluid therapy. Rapid recovery will occur unless animals are severely affected.

Acetaminophen intoxication

Acetaminophen (*N*-acetyl-*p*-aminophenol, Tylenol, Paracetamol) is a popular analgesic/antipyretic that has been promoted as a "safe" aspirin substitute, as it is equipotent to aspirin in these respects. Unlike aspirin, it has little antiinflammatory activity and is much less effective as an antirheumatic agent. The antipyretic activity of this compound appears to be due to its aminobenzene structure. It is a weak inhibitor of prostaglandin synthesis, but it may be more active against enzymes in the central nervous system than in the periphery.

Acetaminophen, a weak acid (pKa = 9.5), is rapidly and almost completely absorbed from the gastrointestinal tract. Peak plasma levels are reached in 0.5 to 1.0 hour after ingestion and the half-life ranges from 1 to 3 hours. It is relatively uniformly distributed throughout most body fluids and may be 20% to 50% protein bound. Acetaminophen is biotransformed in most species via Phase II reactions yielding glucuronides and sul-

fates. There is some conjugation with hepatic glutathione. A decrease in hepatic glutathione leads to covalent binding of the reactive intermediate (theorized to be *N*-acetyl-imidoquinone or *N*-acetyl-*p*-benzoquinone) to nucleophilic macromolecules in the cells, leading to necrosis in the liver and other tissues. During dehydration, acetaminophen may also accumulate in the renal papillae, leading to renal necrosis. Methemoglobin formation is also an important cause of disease and death, especially in cats. Dosage levels of 160 to 600 mg/kg are required to produce toxicosis in dogs, whereas a single 325-mg tablet of acetaminophen is sufficient to produce toxicosis in cats.

Clinical signs in dogs and cats are similar. Signs of toxicity may occur within 4 to 12 hours after ingestion. These include cyanosis due to methemoglobin formation and hemolysis, which may be the major findings in cats. Nausea, vomiting, abdominal pain, and anorexia are often present, followed by signs of dehydration. Hemoglobinuria and icterus (due to both hemolysis as well as hepatic necrosis) occur in dogs but are not common in cats. Facial and paw edema with lacrimation and pruritus are common observations in cats. Increased liver enzymes can be detected in the blood of dogs.

Postmortem findings include facial and paw edema in cats, icterus, and/or dark tissues due to methemoglobin formation. A mottled liver due to centrilobular necrosis is a frequent finding. Hemoglobinuria and swollen kidneys frequently occur in dogs.

The treatment for acetaminophen intoxication is acetylcysteine (Mucomyst), 140 mg/kg orally every 8 hours. Acetylcysteine is a glutathione stimulator that helps to protect the liver. In cats, ascorbic acid at a dosage rate of 200 mg orally three times a day is used for the methemoglobinemia. Additionally, blood transfusions should be used in the treatment of the methemoglobinemia in affected cats. The prognosis in these cases should be guarded to poor if significant hepatic necrosis has occurred or if more than 50% methemoglobin is present.

Plant-related insecticides

Rotenone. Rotenone is a botanical insecticide from the *Derris* spp. The fresh root is toxic to mammals; however, the insecticidal preparation is practically harmless, having toxicity at 1 to 3 g/kg. Rotenone is extremely safe and highly unlikely to be a cause of intoxications even in very young animals.

The clinical signs in intoxicated animals might include vomiting due to gastric irritation, incoordination, muscle tremors, clonic convulsions, and respiratory failure. Treatment of intoxicated animals is directed toward controlling the clinical signs. Sedative/hypnotics should be adequate to control the central nervous signs. Activated charcoal should be administered.

Limoline. Limoline is a monocyclic terpene, which is a major fraction from the oil of several citrus plants. It has been used in a commercially available flea and tick dip. Limoline has a low order of toxicity, i.e., the acute oral median lethal dose in rats is greater than 5 g/kg. Some cats are apparently extremely sensitive to this preparation and present with clinical signs including a mild hypersalivation of short duration, ataxia, and muscle tremors resembling shivering. Severe hypersalivation lasting up to 30 minutes, and moderate to severe ataxia and tremors lasting 4 to 5 hours may occur. In the rare deaths associated with limoline, there have been no gross lesions except for self-induced trauma and possibly acute dermal inflammation. The intoxication is apparently self-limiting and does not produce mortality at levels of 15 times the concentration for normal use. Treatment in cases of intoxications includes general therapy with internal and external decontamination.

Pyrethrum and synthetic pyrethroids. Pyrethrum is derived from the powdered flowering head of *Chrysanthemum* spp. It is the least toxic of all insecticides. The synthetic prethrins have been found to be somewhat toxic to fish, exotic fowl, and juvenile female cats. Some of the synthetic names include Allethrin, Cyfluthrin, Cypermethrin, Deltamethrin, Decamethrin, Fenpropathrin, Fenvalerate, Flumethrin, Kadethrin, Permethrin, Resmethrin, Terallethrin, Tetramethrin (*-rin* suffix). The mechanism of action in insects is to slow nerve conduction. Generally, pyrethrins have a very quick "knock down" but are rapidly metabolized by insects. Therefore, piperonyl butoxide is used as a synergist because it inhibits the insects from metabolizing the pyrethrins. Insecticidal mixtures generally have a ratio of pyrethrin to piperonyl butoxide of 1:10, i.e., 0.05% pyrethrin and 0.5% piperonyl butoxide.

The clinical signs of intoxication in some animals is an increased sensitivity to external stimuli, with the variation from fine tremors to gross tremors and finally prostration in extreme circumstances. In rodents, pawing, burrowing, salivation, writhing, and convulsions may be seen. The treatment for intoxicated animals is general in nature although diazepam may be used to control the central nervous system signs.

Deithyltoluamide (DEET). DEET is used as an insect repellent. It is effective against mosquitoes, biting flies, gnats, chiggers, ticks, and fleas. The DEET content in various products ranges from 5% to 100%. DEET has been used in dog and cat flea collars and in combination with synthetic pyrethrins in spray preparations for pets (Blockade, Hartz). There have been pet deaths reported from use of these mixtures. While many intoxications have occurred in juvenile, female cats, intoxications have occurred in mature cats of both sexes and in dogs.

DEET is absorbed through the skin. It will produce blisters, skin necrosis, erythema, central nervous system disturbances, and death. In humans it also produces blisters, skin necrosis, a burning sensation, erythema, ulcerations, slurred speech, confusion, convulsions, and without treatment, even death. It may be more toxic to human females than males. This may be an occupational phenomenon of females associated with dipping and spraying of animals. Although neurologic signs, in animals and people, may resolve, the parent compound and its metabolites are detectable for up to 2 weeks after the episode. Treatment of affected animals includes dermal cleansing, activated charcoal and cathartics, and control of central nervous system signs.

Organochlorine insecticides

Currently, the only chlorinated insecticides with uses approved by the Environmental Protection Agency are lindane and methoxychlor. While cases of organochlorine insecticide intoxications are rare, they occasionally occur. Organochlorine insecticides are extremely water insoluble and extremely lipid soluble and can easily penetrate the skin. Large amounts may be required to produce acute toxicity in animals, although cats are generally more sensitive than dogs. Dogs are, however, extremely sensitive to toxaphene.

The exact mechanism of action of organochlorine insecticides is unknown, with the possible exception of dichlorodiphenyltrichloroethane (DDT). DDT decreases the membrane potential of nerves, decreasing the threshold for activation. Insect sensory nerves are affected more than motor nerves, whereas the cerebellum and higher motor centers in the cortex are affected in mammals. Chlorinated insecticides act as diffuse stimulants or depressants of the central nervous system in animals.

In cases of acute oral intoxication, the presenting signs may include salivation, nausea, and vomiting. These are not generally seen after dermal exposures. Early neurologic signs include nervousness, restlessness, hyperexcitability, incoordination, and muscle spasms. Advanced neurologic signs may include tonic-clonic convulsions or generalized epileptiform convulsions. Elevated rectal temperatures are common in intoxicated animals. Ventricular fibrillation may occur as the myocardium becomes sensitized to endogenous epinephrine and certainly to administered epinephrine. The cause of death is respiratory failure.

Subacute exposures to organochlorine insecticides may cause anorexia and weight loss with subsequent emaciation. Additionally, hyperirritability, tremors, convulsions, and coma may be seen in these cases. Liver enlargement, hepatocellular degeneration, and cellular degeneration of kidneys and brain may occur. In cases of long-term exposures, clinical signs may be absent or follow those of subacute intoxication.

The treatment of intoxicated animals involves removal of the source of toxicity from the animal and symptomatic care. The acute clinical signs may be controlled with diazepam or pentobarbital.

Organophosphate and carbamate insecticide

Organophosphate (OP) and carbamate insecticides act by inactivating or inhibiting, noncompetitively, cholinesterases, specifically acetylcholinesterase, thereby preventing the biotransformation of acetylcholine (ACH) and prolonging its action. This leads to the buildup of ACH at the cholinergic sites of the autonomic and somatic nervous systems, leading to the typical clinical signs of cholinesterase inhibition. These compounds are lipid soluble and readily absorbed by all routes of exposure.

The clinical signs associated with these insecticides have been characterized as muscarinic, nicotinic, and central nervous system. The muscarinic signs may include dyspnea, bronchorrhea, bronchoconstriction, laryngeal spasms, sialorrhea, lacrimation, bradycardia, micturition, gastrointestinal hypermotility, colic, defecation to profuse diarrhea, and miosis. Nicotinic signs may include skeletal muscle stimulation leading to fasiculations, weakness, and generalized paralysis. Central nervous system signs include ataxia, anxiety, convulsions, and respiratory depression. The cause of death is respiratory failure.

Postmortem lesions in animals succumbing to cholinesterase inhibition may be nonspecific without circumstantial evidence. There may be pulmonary edema and emphysema and other signs of agonal struggling, such as petechial hemorrhages on the myocardium and serosal surfaces of the viscera. The diagnosis of organophosphate or carbamate insecticide intoxications is difficult. The diagnosis may be based on circumstantial exposure or potential for exposure, clinical signs, or chemical evidence of the offending chemical or demonstration of depressed cholinesterase activity of the red blood cells.

Some organophosphates, insecticides and noninsecticides, have been linked to a neurologic disorder termed "delayed neurotoxicity." Signs begin to occur several days after exposure to a single dose or multiple doses of the toxicant. Some organophosphates, in certain individual animals and humans, bind with a so-called neurotoxic esterase, which then causes degeneration of myelin in the spinal cord and peripheral nerves. Signs include sensory disturbances, weakness, ataxia, and eventual paralysis of the lower extremities. Insufficient transport of essential nutrients down the axons appears to play a role in the disorder. The "delayed neurotoxicity" syndrome is not common in small animals.

The aims of treatment in cases of cholinesterase depression due to organophosphate or carbamate insecticides include maintaining respiration, decreasing muscarinic effects, reactivating phosphorylated enzymes, and limiting further absorption. Animals should be ventilated if signs of hypoxia exist. Atropine should be administered at a dosage rate of 0.2 to 0.4 mg/kg, with half the dose given intravenously and the remainder subcutaneously or intramuscularly. If bradycardia or hypoxia exist, be sure to ventilate prior to administering intravenous atropine. Atropine should be repeated as necessary to control muscarinic signs. Atropine will not completely control all the clinical signs, and animals can become intoxicated through the overzealous use of atropine. The clinical signs of atropine intoxication include tachycardia and central nervous system disturbances (ataxia, staggering, and depression).

Pralidoxime chloride (2-PAM) can be administered intravenously at a slow rate at a dosage of 20 mg/kg, over a 2-hour period twice a day for several days to reactivate cholinesterase in cases of recent organophosphate intoxication. 2-PAM should not be used in most cases of carbamate intoxications. Carbamates are reversibly bound to cholinesterase, and 2-PAM administered in those situations can worsen or prolong clinical signs since it can also inhibit cholinesterases.

For dermal exposures, bathe the animal. Following organophosphate ingestions, activated charcoal and cathartics are indicated. Morphine, succinylcholine, and phenothiazine tranquilizers should not be administered to organophosphate or carbamate insecticide-intoxicated animals.

Strychnine intoxication

Strychnine is a spinal convulsant predacide primarily used for small mammals and coyotes. It is a restricted-use pesticide. Strychnine is still involved in malicious poisonings, primarily in the canine.

Strychnine is readily absorbed from the gastrointestinal tract, probably from the stomach as the sulfate form, which remains non-ionized at gastric pH. The rate of absorption depends on the quantity and characteristics of the gastrointestinal contents and the quantity and form of the alkaloid ingested. Absorption generally occurs within 30 minutes to 2 hours following ingestion. Strychnine is rapidly metabolized by liver microsomal enzymes. Sublethal dosages are eliminated within 10 hours. Eighty percent is biotransformed by the liver, and 20% is eliminated unchanged in the urine. In the dog, two lethal doses may be metabolized over a 24-hour period without producing clinical signs if administered in divided dosages.

Strychnine is a spinal convulsant that blocks glycine receptors in the spinal cord and medulla. It is not considered a central convulsant. The clinical signs are due to a blockade of postsynaptic inhibitory activity, possibly competing with glycine, allowing nerve transmissions to proceed unchecked. This causes an effect on the normal reflex relaxation of antagonistic muscle groups, mediated through the Renshaw cells. The action of the most powerful muscle groups predominate, therefore, extensor rigidity is most evident.

The clinical signs of strychnine intoxication may be separated into initial signs and classic signs. The initial signs include anxiety, restlessness, and increased respiration. These clinical signs progress to constant panting, muscle tremors, and contraction of antagonistic muscle groups. The lack of nausea and vomiting is characteristic of strychnine intoxication. Uneasy movements may develop in affected animals; these movements simulate walking on egg shells or ground glass. Tetanic seizures may occur spontaneously following exposure to touch, light, or noise stimuli. The limbs become extended, and the head curves upward and backward. The lips may be retracted into what has been characterized as a "sardonic grin." The severity and duration of convulsions are not prognostic. Death is from hypoxia due to prolonged paralysis of the respiratory muscles.

Postmortem lesions in animals dying from strychnine intoxication are nonspecific in nature. There is the rapid development of rigor mortis, and the stomach is generally filled with ingesta. Petechial hemorrhages and self-induced traumatic lesions may be present.

A presumptive diagnosis of strychnine intoxication can be made based on the characteristic clinical signs, lack of vomiting, and history of potential exposure. Exposure to other convulsant toxicants must be considered. Determination of strychnine or an alkaloid in urine is helpful in making a diagnosis. Strychnine remains in tissues for a considerable time following death. Tissue samples appropriate for submission to a laboratory for confirmatory diagnosis should include liver, kidney, urine, and stomach contents. Any baits or other materials suspected of containing strychnine should also be submitted.

Emesis should be induced in animals observed ingesting a bait, and not showing clinical signs. Strychnine convulsions should be controlled with the use of pentobarbital, to effect, with ventilatory support, if necessary. Activated charcoal should always be administered to these patients, followed by a saline cathartic, forced diuresis, and acidification of urine. Inhalant anesthetics, central-acting skeletal-muscle relaxants, and minor tranquilizers may be used in certain cases; however, there are many disadvantages to their routine use in strychnine intoxication. Treated animals should be turned periodically to prevent hypostatic congestion. Convulsions sometimes recur 1 to 3 days after apparent recovery. Animals should be given activated charcoal 2 to 3 times a day for 3 days after apparent recovery.

Anticoagulant rodenticides

Warfarin and/or dicoumarol are commonly used anticoagulants in human medicine for treatment of thrombophlebitis or undesirable clotting. These agents inhibit the production of biologically active clotting factors II, VII, IX, and X. Warfarin was once considered to be the most effective rat poison available; however, newer anticoagulant rodenticides (i.e., diphacinone, brodaficoum, etc.) have recently been introduced to control warfarin-resistant rats. These rodenticides have a much longer biologic half-life, and intoxications require much longer treatment regimens.

Clinical signs are manifested by internal and external hemorrhages resulting in anemia. These signs may include nonpainful swellings around pressure points (rump, thigh, pectoral, shoulder, and ventral thoracic regions); persistent bleeding from superficial lacerations and surgical procedures; extensive hemorrhage into subcutaneous tissues, intermuscular planes, and under serous surfaces and into serosal cavities; ataxia, depression, and hemorrhagic diarrhea; ecchymosis of skin and conjunctiva; epistaxis; pale mucous membranes; dyspnea; tachycardia; and in the terminal stages, asphyxial convulsions. Lameness can also occur due to hemorrhages over the bony prominences of the limbs or hemorrhages into joint capsules. Neurologic signs may occur if hemorrhage develops in the cranial vault or spinal column. Sudden death occurs in some animals. Postmortem lesions observed include multiple hemorrhages throughout the body musculature, masses of unclotted or poorly clotted blood, and diffuse hemorrhages that may involve any or all organs or tissues. The heart may be rounded and flaccid. Centrilobular hepatic necrosis sometimes occurs. In prolonged cases, icterus may be present due to absorption of blood pigments from areas of internal hemorrhage.

Anticoagulant toxicity may be suspected in cases having prolongation of any clotting test. The one-stage prothrombin test (OSPT) may be the most helpful, as it measures factors II, VII, and X. Differential diagnosis based on clinical signs may include hemophilia, autoimmune problems, disseminated intravascular coagulation, *Ehrlichia,* or blood loss anemia in dogs.

Detection of specific anticoagulants in patient tissue specimens and suspect baits by suitable chemical methods is possible. Liver, unclotted blood, stomach contents, feces, spleen, and kidney should be submitted for analysis. The tissues should be frozen.

Treatment of affected animals includes removal of animals from the source of the intoxication. Signs may persist for 4 to 10 days after removal if therapy is not initiated. In some cases fresh whole blood must be administered for clotting factors, whereas autotransfusions may be performed where only volume replacement is required. Ten to 20 ml of blood per kilogram should be used as required. Perivascular hematomas should be prevented. Vitamin K_1 should be administered orally at a dosage rate of 3 to 5 mg/kg per day with canned dog food. The fat in the diet will enhance absorption. The oral administration of vitamin K_1 has been found to be more efficacious than either intravenous or subcutaneous routes.[2] In the case of diphacinone or brodifacoum, the oral vitamin K_1 therapy should be continued for 21 days. Vitamin K_1 induces the production of clotting factors within 30 minutes of administration, and the clotting tests return to normal within 24 to 36 hours.

Metaldehyde

Metaldehyde is marketed as a liquid or meal preparation of 3.5% as a snail or slug killer. Some baits look and taste like cat or dog food. Metaldehyde is also available as a solid fuel.

Clinical signs of metaldehyde intoxication occur rapidly. There may be emesis with the odor of acetaldehyde. The typical signs include incoordination, hyperpnea, tachycardia, hypersalivation, hyperesthesia, convulsions, opisthotonos, and often continuous convulsions. An elevated rectal temperature is often present, and cats show nystagmus. There may be deep depression and cyanosis with death due to respiratory failure. There may be apparent recovery in some cases, followed by death from secondary liver damage several days after acute intoxications.

Postmortem lesions can include hyperemia of the liver, kidney, and lungs; hepatic degeneration; hemorrhages in the lungs; acetaldehyde odor in stomach and vomitus; and gastrointestinal inflammation. The diagnosis is confirmed by history and chemical evidence.

Treatment of metaldehyde-intoxicated animals includes control of central nervous system hyperactivity with the administration of pentobarbital or central-acting muscle relaxants. Ventilatory support may be required in some cases. The stomach should be evacuated by gastric lavage and the animal given activated charcoal followed by a laxative. Treatment should be directed at correcting the acidosis and preventing possible liver damage.

Herbicides and fungicides

Herbicides and fungicides have been used in American agriculture for over 20 years. Subsequently, their use in and around homes has increased the hazard for the intoxication of dogs and cats. Relatively little has been published on the toxicity of herbicides and fungicides in small animals. To date, intoxications in small animals caused by these agents have not been recognized as important.

The occurrence of intoxications caused by herbicides and fungicides is rare, following the application of the agents to plants, especially in animals that do not rely on plants as foodstuffs. With improper storage of these toxic agents, there is a poisoning hazard to cats and dogs because of the inquisitive nature of these animals. The reported distastefulness of most chemicals probably reduces the amount ingested. The clinical signs generally associated with experimental intoxications with these agents in dogs and cats are nonspecific gastroenteritis disturbances, listlessness, and depression. Staggering and other neuromuscular signs may be present.

The treatment of intoxicated animals is for the most part, symptomatic. Arsenicals, mercurials, and sodium chlorate have specific treatments if the condition is diagnosed in the early stages. Tables 27-1 and 27-2 are listings of some of the more commonly used herbicides and fungicides.

Clinical signs associated with herbicide intoxications in small animals are nonspecific. These signs include anorexia, muscular weakness, myotonia, vomiting, diarrhea, and death. There may be a contact dermatitis associated with agents such as trichloroacetic acid and paraquat. In addi-

TABLE 27-1 Some common herbicides

Chemical Groups	Common Names
Chlorophenoxy compounds	2,4-D, 2,4,5-T
Chlorinated aliphatic acids	Erbon, trichloroacetic acid
Amide compounds	Bensulide, Chlorthiamid
Carbamate	Chlorpropham
Thiocarbamate	Pebulate, Vernolate
Phenylurea	Norea, Chloroxuron, Linuron
Arsenicals, inorganic	$K_3As_3O_3$
Arsenicals, organic	Monosodium methanearsonate (MSMA)
Substituted dinitroaniline compounds	Trifluran, Benefin
Dipyridyl compounds	Paraquat, Diquat
Phthalmic acid compounds	Naptalam, Dinoseb
Sodium chlorate	Sodium chlorate
Triazines	Atrazine, Prometone
Dinitrophenols	Dinitro-o-cresol

TABLE 27-2 Some common fungicides

Chemical Group	Common Names
Chlorophenols	Pentachlorophenol
Organomercurials	Ceresan-M
Organotin	Triethyltin
Chloroneb	Demosan
Organozinc	Zineb
Organosulfur	Captan

tion, paraquat poisoning may induce cyanosis and convulsions. Sodium chlorate, a methemoglobin former, may produce cyanosis, respiratory distress, and chocolate-brown blood. Alkyl mercurials can induce mental disturbances, ataxia, gait disturbances, incoordination, paddling, posterior paralysis, blindness, and mental deficiencies. There may be a latent period for clinical signs to arise. Prenatal toxicity has been associated with ingestion of treated seeds by pregnant animals. Alkyl mercurials do not induce gross changes but cause neuronal degeneration in the cerebral cortex, cerebellum, spinal cord, and peripheral nerves.

Clinical signs observed with fungicide poisoning may be similar to those observed in herbicide intoxication. In addition, there may be greater involvement of the central nervous system, including ataxia, tremors, collapse, depression, and rapid respiration.

Lesions observed in animals poisoned by herbicides or fungicides are mainly located in the gastrointestinal tract. Severe gastroenteritis with ulcerations may be found. In addition, congestion of the cerebral vessels may occur.

Treatment of most poisonings caused by herbicides or fungicides is symptomatic and supportive in nature because of the lack of specific antidotes. The recommendations in the introduction on nonspecific treatment of poisonings should be followed in treating animals poisoned by these agents.

Proper storage of lawn, garden, and agricultural chemicals is the best preventive measure against herbicide or fungicide intoxication in pet animals. This precaution will help to keep poisonings caused by these agents to a minimum.

Arsenic

Arsenicals have been known for over 2000 years and they have been used as insecticides, medicinals, wood preservatives, and as "hematinics." There are two different and distinct syndromes associated with arsenicals, depending on the type of arsenic preparation involved. Inorganic arsenicals and trivalent organic arsenicals produce a disease syndrome characterized by an effect on the gastrointestinal tract and capillaries, whereas the pentavalent organic arsenicals may also produce a neurologic syndrome.

Inorganic pentavalent arsenic may uncouple oxidative phosphorylation, whereas arsenites react with sulfhydryl groups (-SH) of proteins and inhibit enzymes by blocking active groups (dimercaprol will reverse this action). Arsenic induces vasodilation and capillary damage. Organic pentavalent arsenicals have an unknown mechanism of action but may interfere with vitamins B_6 and B_1. Low doses over a long period may allow a "tolerance" to arsenicals to develop. In some circles, arsenicals are considered carcinogenic. However, long-term dosing trials in rats and dogs have not shown this to be the case. The toxicity of arsenicals is as follows. trivalent, As + 3 (Arsenite) > Pentavalent, As + 5 (Arsenate) > trivalent organics > pentavalent organics.

The typical clinical signs in animals include abdominal pain, staggering, collapse, and death in the peracute form. In the acute form, salivation, thirst, grinding of teeth, vomiting, moaning, weakness, muscular incoordination, trembling, abdominal pain, thready pulse, diarrhea (watery and sometimes hemorrhagic), rear-limb paralysis, hematuria, prostration, skin lesions, and death often occur. Animals with the subacute form of arsenic intoxication may live several days and demonstrate depression, anorexia, difficult movement, convulsions, and fluid feces containing mucosa and blood. Feces may be dark, and hematuria may be evident.

Chronically intoxicated animals are easily fatigued, and have violent breathing when excited. Affected animals may also demonstrate thirst, be unthrifty, have dry, rough hair coats, and a brick-red coloration to mucous membranes.

Treatment within 4 hours of ingestion or exposure to arsenicals is general and consists of emetics, activated charcoal, gastric lavage, milk, egg white, and sodium thiosulfate, orally, 0.5 to 1 g. If more than 4 hours after ingestion or exposure, the treatment consists of the above with the addition of dimercaprol, 2.5 to 5 mg/kg intramuscularly 2 to 4 times a day for 10 days or until recovery.

The diagnosis of arsenic intoxication is by history, clinical signs, and lesions. Liver and/or kidney arsenic levels greater than 8 to 10 ppm are diagnostic unless several days have elapsed since the last exposure, and then tissue levels may have declined to 2 to 4 ppm. Urine and fecal levels should be greater than 10 to 20 ppm to be diagnostic.

Lead

Lead is widely distributed in nature and readily forms organic compounds in many plants. Since lead is a cumulative poison, repeated small doses may prove toxic. Most animals are susceptible. Lead poisoning has been reported in dogs, cats, birds, cattle, horses, sheep, swine, primates, exotic birds, and humans.

Paints applied to buildings prior to World War II contained lead carbonate (white lead) and lead oxide (red lead). Lead in paints can constitute 5% to 50% of the dried solids. Children and pets are commonly poisoned by nibbling at lead-painted windowsills, frames, and toys. Lead-painted wood or cages are common sources of poisoning in exotic birds. Gasoline formulated with tetraethyl lead has also been a major source of environmental exposure. Dogs have become intoxicated drinking lead-based gasoline and by ingesting fishing weights. Ingested lead shot causes toxicosis in water fowl.

Lead is absorbed primarily via the gastrointestinal tract, distributed by erythrocytes, and initially deposited in soft tissues (liver and kidney). It is excreted very slowly via the bile (feces) and minimally via the urine. Lead concentrates in the renal cortex at high levels. Twenty-five percent of absorbed lead may be deposited in the liver, and the remaining 75% is eventually deposited in the bone. Inorganic lead is not biotransformed to any extent. Alkyl lead compounds (tetraethyl lead and tetramethyl lead) are dealkylated to trialkyl compounds. These are extremely toxic and are slowly biotransformed to inorganic lead.

Interference with -SH groups on enzymes may be the important mechanism of lead intoxication. Many of the manifestations of lead intoxication cannot be explained on the basis of enzyme inhibition. The major organ systems affected by lead are central nervous system, peripheral nervous system, kidney, and hematopoietic systems. Lead affects the gastrointestinal system causing vomiting, diarrhea, colic, abdominal pain, and dehydration. Acute, severe lead intoxication is manifested by gastrointestinal signs, hypovolemic shock, and death within 3 to 4 days.

The erythrocytic and renal signs require time to develop. The clinical signs may occur from several days to several weeks after exposure. Neurologic signs, often seen in dogs, include hyperirritability, viciousness, chomping of the jaws, hypersalivation, and paralysis of the masseter muscles.

In small animals, abdominal radiographic findings may be useful. Recently ingested lead-containing substances appear radiopaque on abdominal radiography. The findings must be differentiated from gravel, stones, and other foreign bodies. The metaphysis of long bones may develop lead lines in immature dogs poisoned 10 days or more before radiography. Radiopaque bands may be seen just above the open epiphyses of distal radius, ulna, and metacarpal bones. Shot and bullets are common incidental findings in the soft tissues of the trunk and limbs on radiographs of small animals. This is not generally a cause of lead intoxication in mammals but is a problem in game birds and other fowl.

Laboratory findings may include a neutrophilic leukocytosis with a left shift. The packed cell volume is usually normal, but a mild to moderate hypochromic anemia may be seen in chronic lead intoxication. Erythrocytes with basophilic stippling ($>0.1\%$) and large numbers of nucleated red blood cells are found in nearly all dogs with chronic lead poisoning (50 to 300 or more/100 white blood cells). Blood lead levels >0.4 ppm with associated clinical signs are considered diagnostic (normal, 0.05 to 0.25 ppm). Liver lead values >5 ppm are significant, even with low kidney cortex levels. Kidney cortex lead levels >10 ppm are significant, especially with clinical signs. Significant changes seen in chronic lead intoxication include chronic anemia, varying from mild to moderate hypochromia. Lead causes the red blood cell to be more fragile. The kidneys may be degenerated and fibrotic, with renal tubular damage and intranuclear inclusion bodies. Vascular endothelial swelling occurs in the brain with degenerative to necrotic vascular changes.

The primary aim of therapy in lead intoxication is immobilizing (chelating) the lead and removing it from the body (Table 27-3). Therapy should be

TABLE 27-3 Specific intoxicants and their systemic antidotes[3]

Toxic Agent	Systemic Antidote	Dosage and Method for Treatment
Acetaminophen	N-acetylcysteine (Mucomyst, Mead Johnson)	150 mg/kg loading dose, orally or IV, then 50 mg/kg every 4 hours for 17 to 20 additional doses
Amphetamines	Chlorpromazine	1 mg/kg IM or IV; administer only half dose if barbiturates have been given: blocks excitation
Arsenic, mercury and other heavy metals except cadmium, lead, silver, selenium, and thallium	Dimercaprol (BAL, Hynson, Wescott & Dunning)	10% solution in oil; give small animals 2.5 to 5.0 mg/kg IM qid for 2 days then bid for the next 10 days or until recovery (*Note:* In severe acute poisoning 5 mg/kg dosage should be given only on the first day)
	D-Penicillamine (Cuprimine, Merck)	Developed for chronic mercury poisoning, now seems most promising drug; no reports on dosage in animals; give 3 to 4 mg/kg q.i.d.
Atropine, belladonna alkaloids	Physostigmine salicylate	0.1 to 0.6 mg/kg (do not use neostigmine)
Barbiturates	Doxapram	2% solution: give small animals 3 to 5 mg/kg IV only (0.14 to 0.25 ml/kg); repeat as necessary (*Note:* The above is reliable only when depression is mild; in deeper levels of depression, ventilatory support [and oxygen] is preferable)
Bromides	Chlorides (sodium or ammonium salts)	Orally 0.5 to 1.0 g daily for several days; hasten excretion
Carbon monoxide	Oxygen	Pure oxygen at normal or high pressure; artificial respiration; blood transfusion
Cholecalciferol	Calcitonin (Calcimar, Rorer Pharm)	4 IU/kg every 8 to 12 hours SC or IM
Cholinergic agents	Atropine sulfate	0.02 to 0.04 mg/kg, as needed
Cholinesterase inhibitors	Atropine sulfate	Dosage is 0.2 mg/kg, repeated as needed for atropinization; treat cyanosis (if present) first; blocks only muscarinic effects; atropine in oil may be injected for prolonged effect. *Avoid atropine intoxication!*
Cholinergic agents and cholinesterase inhibitors (organophosphates, some carbamates; but not carbaryl, dimethan, or carbam piloxime)	Pralidoxime chloride (2-PAM)	5% solution; 20 to 50 mg/kg IM or by slow IV (0.2 to 1.0 mg/kg) injection (maximum dose is 500 mg per minute), repeat as needed; 2-PAM alleviates nicotinic effect and regenerates cholinesterase; morphine, succinylcholine, and phenothiazine tranquilizers are contraindicated
Copper	D-Penicillamine (Cuprimine)	See arsenic
Coumarin-derivative anticoagulants	Vitamin K₁ (Aqua-mephyton, 5-mg capsules or 1% emulsion, Merck) (Vita K₁, 25-mg capsules, Eschar)	Give 3 to 5 mg/kg SC or orally per day with canned food; treat 7 days for warfarin-type, treat 21 to 30 days for second-generation anticoagulant rodenticides; oral therapy more efficacious than parenteral
	Fresh whole blood, fresh plasma, or fresh frozen plasma	Blood transfusion, 10 to 25 ml/kg, as required

IV = intravenously; IM = intramuscularly; b.i.d. = twice a day; q.i.d. = four times a day; SC = subcutaneously; q.s. = in sufficient quantity; ECG = electrocardiographic; CNS = central nervous system; t.i.d. = three times a day. *Continued.*

TABLE 27-3 Specific intoxicants and their systemic antidotes—cont'd

Toxic Agent	Systemic Antidote	Dosage and Method for Treatment
Curare	Neostigmine methylsulfate	Solution: 1:5000 or 1:2000 (1 ml = 0.2 or 0.5 mg/ml); dose is 0.005 mg/5 kg SC; follow with IV injection of atropine (0.04 mg/kg)
	Edrophonium chloride (Tensilon, Roche) Ventilatory support	1% solution; give 0.05 to 1.0 mg/kg IV
Cyanide	Methemoglobin (sodium nitrite is used to form methemoglobin)	1% solution of sodium nitrite , dosage is 16 mg/kg IV (1.6 ml/kg)
	Sodium thiosulfate	Follow with 20% solution of sodium thiosulfate at dosage of 30 to 40 mg/kg (0.15 to 0.2 ml/kg) IV; If treatment is repeated, use only sodium thiosulfate.
		(NOTE; Both of the above may be given simultaneously as follows: 0.5 ml/kg of combination consisting of 10 g sodium nitrite, 15 g sodium thiosulfate distilled water q.s. to 250 ml; dosage may be repeated once; if further treatment is required, give only 20% solution of sodium thiosulfate at level of 0.2 ml/kg)
Digitalis glycosides, oleander, and *Bufo* toads	Potassium chloride	Dog: 0.5 to 2.0 g, orally in divided doses, or in serious cases, as diluted solution given IV by slow drip (ECG monitoring is essential)
	Diphenylhydantoin	25 mg/minute IV, until ventricular arrhythmias are controlled
	Propranolol (β-blocker)	0.5 to 1.0 mg/kg IV or IM as needed to control cardiac arrhythmias (ECG monitoring is essential)
	Atropine sulfate	0.02 to 0.04 mg/kg as needed for cholinergic and arrhythmia control
Fluoride	Calcium borogluconate	3 to 10 ml of 5% to 10% solution
Fluoracetate (Compound 1080)	Glyceryl monoacetin (Sigma)	0.1 to 0.5 mg/kg IM hourly for several hours (total 2 to 4 mg/kg), or diluted (0.5 to 1.0% solution IV, (danger of hemolysis); monoacetin is available only from chemical supply houses
	Acetamide	Animal may be protected if acetamide is given prior to or simultaneously with Compound 1080 (experimental)
	Pentobarbital	May protect against lethal dose (experimental) (NOTE: All treatments are generally unrewarding)
Hallucinogens (LSD, phencyclidine [PCP])	Diazepam (Valium, Roche)	As needed—avoid respiratory depression (2 to 5 mg/kg)
Heparin	Protamine sulfate	1% solution; give 1.0 to 1.5 mg to antagonize each 1 mg of heparin, slow IV injection; reduce dose as time increases between heparin injection and start of treatment (after 30 minutes give only 0.5 mg) (see Chapter 23)

TABLE 27-3 Specific intoxicants and their systemic antidotes—cont'd

Toxic Agent	Systemic Antidote	Dosage and Method for Treatment
Iron salts	Deferoxamine (Desferal, Ciba)	Dosage for animals not yet established; dosage for humans is 5g of 5% solution given orally, then 20 mg/kg IM every 4 to 6 hours; in case of shock, dosage is 40 mg/kg by IV drip over 4-hour period; may be repeated in 6 hours, then 15 mg/kg by drip every 8 hours
Lead	Calcium disodium edetate (CaEDTA)	Dosage: maximum safe dose is 75 mg/kg per 24 hours (only for severe case); EDTA is available in 20% solution; for IV drip, dilute in 5% glucose to 0.5%; for IM, add procaine to 20% solution to give 0.5% concentration of procaine
	EDTA and BAL	BAL is given as 10% solution in oil Treatment: (1) In severe cases (CNS involvement with >100 μg lead per 100 g whole blood) give 4 mg/kg BAL only as initial dose; follow after 4 hours, and every 4 hours for 3 to 4 days, with BAL and EDTA (12.5 mg/kg) at separate IM sites, skip 2 or 3 days and then treat again for 3 to 4 days; (2) In subacute case with <100 μg lead per 100 g whole blood, give only 50 mg EDTA/kg per 24 hours for 3 to 5 days;
	Penicillamine (Cuprimine, Merck)	(3) May use after either treatment (1) or (2) with 100 mg/kg per day orally for 1 to 4 weeks
	Thiamine hydrochloride	Experimental for CNS signs; 5 mg/kg IV b.i.d. for 1 to 2 weeks; give slowly and watch for untoward reactions
Metaldehyde	Diazepam (Valium, Roche) Triflupromaize Pentobarbital	2 to 5 mg/kg IV to control tremors 0.2 to 2.0 mg/kg IV To effect
Methanol	Ethanol	Give IV, 1.1 g/kg (4.4 ml/kg) of 25% solution; then give 0.5 g/kg (2.0 ml/kg) every 4 hours for 4 days; to prevent or correct acidosis, use sodium bicarbonate IV, 0.4 g/kg; activated charcoal, 5 g/kg orally if within 4 hours of ingestion
Methemoglobinemia-producing agents (nitrites, chlorates)	Methylene blue (not recommended for cats)	1% solution (maximum concentration), give by *slow* IV injection, 8.8 mg/kg (0.9 ml/kg) repeat if necessary; to prevent fall in blood pressure in case of nitrite poisoning, use a sympathomimetic drug (ephedrine or epinephrine)

Continued.

TABLE 27-3 Specific intoxicants and their systemic antidotes—cont'd.

Toxic Agent	Systemic Antidote	Dosage and Method for Treatment
Morphine and related drugs	Naloxone chloride (Narcan, Endo)	0.1 mg/kg IV; do not repeat if respiration is not satisfactory
	Levallorphan tartrate (Lorfan, Roche)	Give IV, 0.1 to 0.5 ml of solution containing 1 mg/ml
		(NOTE: Use either of the antidotes only in acute poisoning. Ventilatory support may be indicated. Activated charcoal is also indicated.)
Oxalates	Calcium	Treatment: 10% solution of calcium gluconate IV; give 3 to 20 ml (to control hypocalcemia)
Phenothiazine	Methylamphetamine (Desoxyn, Abbot)	0.1 to 0.2 mg/kg; treatment for hypovolemic shock may be required.
	Diphenhydramine hydrochloride	For CNS depression, 2 to 5 mg/kg IV for extrapyramidal signs
Phytotoxins and botulin	Antitoxins not available commercially (attempt to obtain through Centers for Disease Control)	As indicated for specific antitoxins, examples of phytotoxins: ricin, abrin, robin, crotin
Plants		Treat signs as necessary.
Red squill	Atropine sulfate, propranolol, potassium chloride	As for digitalis and oleander
Snake bite		
Rattlesnake Copperhead Water moccasin	Antivenin (Wyeth), Trivalent Crotalidae (Fort Dodge)	*Caution:* equine origin; administer 1-2 vials IV, slowly, diluted in 250-500 ml of saline or lactated Ringer's solution; also administer antihistamines. *Corticosteroids are contraindicated.*[4]
Coral snake	(Wyeth)	*Caution:* equine origin; may be used as with pit viper antivenin
Spider bite		
Black widow	Antivenin (Merck)	*Caution:* equine orgin; Administer IV undiluted
	Dantrolene sodium (Dantrium, Norwich-Eaton)	For neurologic signs, 1 mg/kg IV, followed by 1 mg/kg orally every 4 hours
Brown recluse	Dapsone	1 mg/kg b.i.d. for 10 days
Strontium	Calcium salts	Usual dose of calcium borogluconate
	Ammonium chloride	0.2 to 0.5 g orally 3 to 4 times daily
Strychnine and brucine	Pentobarbital	Give IV, to effect; higher dose is usually required than that required for anesthesia; place animal in warm, quiet room
	Amobarbital	Give by slow IV, to effect; duration of sedation is usually 4 to 6 hours
	Methocarbamol (Robaxin, Robins)	10% solution; average first dose is 149 mg/kg IV (range. 40 to 300 mg); repeat half dose as needed
	Glyceryl guaiacolate (Geocolate, Summit Hill Labs)	110 mg/kg IV, 5% solution; repeat as necessary
	Diazepam (Valium, Roche)	2 to 5 mg/kg, control convulsions,
Thallium	Diphenylthiocarbazone	Dog: 70 mg/kg orally t.i.d. for 6 days; hastens elimination but is partially toxic;
	Prussian blue	0.2 mg/kg orally in three divided doses daily
	Potassium chloride	Give simultaneously with thiocarbazone or Prussian blue, 2 to 6 g orally daily in divided doses

initiated to remove any lead present in the gastro-intestinal tract with saline purgatives, emetics, and gastric lavage. Sedatives may be administered in cases of neurologic overstimulation.

Cholecalciferol

Cholecalciferol (Quintox, Rampage, Rat-Be-Gone) is a new rodenticide advertised as being safer than the second-generation anticoagulant rodenticides. The active ingredient, cholecalciferol, is an active vitamin D_3 derivative. The mechanism of action of cholecalciferol is through mobilization of calcium from the bones into the blood, causing death by hypercalcemic cardiotoxicity. Long-term low-dose exposures could cause vitamin D toxicoses, but this has not been documented.

The oral lethal dose of cholecalciferol to mice is 84 mg/kg and to rats 50 mg/kg. The formulation is supposed to make the material less toxic to domestic animals. Clinical signs are vague and include inappetence, depression, and sudden death. Postmortem examinations show only heart stoppage in systole. Calcium deposits may be found in soft tissues, aorta, tendons, and muscle following long-term exposure.

Treatment is speculative, as there are presently no proven antidotes. Calcitonin, at an initial dosage rate of 4 IU subcutaneously or intramuscularly, may be advantageous, since it is useful for hypercalcemic crises in humans. The slow infusion of sodium EDTA solutions might be useful. Diuresis should be instituted using intravenous furosemide and 0.9% saline to promote Ca^{++} excretion. There is no treatment that will remove soft-tissue calcification.

Methylxanthine poisoning (chocolate and caffeine)

Theobromine, a methylxanthine, is found in chocolate, cocoa beans, cocoa bean hulls, cola, and tea. Milk chocolate contains 44 mg/30 g, and unsweetened baking chocolate contains 390 mg/30 g. Caffeine occurs in coffee, tea, chocolate, colas, and stimulant drugs. Theophylline is found in tea and other medicinals.

The oral median lethal dose of theobromine in dogs is 250 to 500 mg/kg (20 to 40 g of baking chocolate/kg body weight). Deaths have been reported in dogs after ingestion of approximately 115 mg/kg. The lethal dose of caffeine in dogs is approximately 140 mg/kg.

Methylxanthines are rapidly absorbed from the gastrointestinal tract and are excreted in the urine. Some biotransformation occurs in the liver. In dogs, theobromine has a half-life of 17.5 hours and caffeine has a half-life of 4.5 hours. The mechanism of action is through inhibition of cellular phosphodiesterase, causing an increase in intracellular cyclic adenosine monophosphate concentrations. The primary effect of xanthines is to cause the release of catecholamines and to competitively inhibit cellular adenosine receptors. Calcium entry into cells is enhanced, and calcium sequestration by the sarcoplasmic reticulum is inhibited, causing increased muscular contractility.

The clinical signs of caffeine intoxication include vomiting, diuresis, restlessness, and hyperactivity. Tachypnea, ataxia, cyanosis, cardiac arrhythmias, and seizures may occur. Death is not common but may result from cardiovascular collapse. Clinical signs associated with theobromine intoxication include diarrhea, diuresis (sometimes reported as urinary incontinence), abdominal pain, hematuria, muscle weakness, muscle tremors, dehydration, cardiac arrhythmias, hyperthermia, ataxia, central nervous system hyperactivity or depression, seizures, coma, and death. Postmortem lesions with chronic theobromine intoxication include gastroenteritis, congestion of the organs, and a fibrotic cardiomyopathy. The diagnosis of methylxanthine intoxications are based on a history of possible exposures, presence of consistent clinical signs, and identification of xanthines in serum, plasma, tissue, urine, or stomach contents. (Only very small amounts of methylxanthines remain in the feces.)

Treatment of methylxanthine intoxications is primarily supportive and symptomatic, as there are no specific antidotes. Muscle tremors or seizures may be treated with intravenous diazepam. Tachycardias may have to be treated with β-sympatholytics. Xanthines may be reabsorbed from the urinary bladder; therefore, frequent catheterization of the urinary bladder is recommended in order to prevent reabsorption of excreted methylxanthines.

Ethylene glycol (antifreeze)

Antifreeze is 95% ethylene glycol (EG). EG is widely employed as a solvent in the paint and plastics industries. Careless use of EG as antifreeze by animal owners leads to accidental ingestion by pets. Many automobile owners drain their vehicle's radiators onto the ground or into containers where it is available for animals to drink. Thirsty animals will voluntarily drink the fluid because it has a pleasant, sweet taste and causes a warm sensation to the tongue and esophagus. There is a variation in EG toxicity with respect to species. The cat is extremely sensitive, with a median lethal dose of 2 to 4 ml/kg. In the dog, the median lethal dose is 4 to 5 ml/kg.

EG is rapidly absorbed from the gastrointestinal tract. Unmetabolized EG has a toxicity similar to ethanol and is not responsible for all the signs of toxicosis that follow ingestion. Almost all ingested EG is biotransformed or excreted unchanged in the urine within 24 hours.

EG serves as a substrate for alcohol dehydrogenase, an enzyme occurring primarily in the liver. Biotransformation consists of a series of oxidations with each intermediate step forming additional toxic products. The most important intermediates are glycolic acid and glyoxylic acid. Oxalic acid is the primary terminal product of biotransformation of EG. Glycolic acid is the only intermediate to accumulate to any degree. The accumulation of glycolic acid is affiliated with the signs associated with EG toxicosis, including the profound metabolic acidosis. Oxalic acid forms insoluble calcium oxalate crystals in the kidneys 48 to 72 hours following ingestion of EG, producing tubular degeneration and necrosis. The quantity of oxalate crystals deposited is not correlated with the severity of the renal lesions. The cytotoxic effects of the intermediate metabolites of EG appear to be significant in the pathogenesis of renal lesions. The quantity of glycolic acid in the urine may be used as an indicator of disease severity, i.e., the higher the glycolic acid levels, the higher the likelihood of death.

EG produces central nervous system depression and an appearance of intoxication resembling ethanol. The oxidation products of EG are cytotoxic and invariably produce metabolic acidosis. The intermediate products of EG are suspected as possible inhibitors of the citric acid cycle and of oxidative phosphorylation. Two to 4 hours following ingestion of EG there may be a transient exhilaration followed by central nervous system depression with ataxia within 4 to 7 hours, progressing to coma and possibly death within 12 hours. Nausea, vomiting, anorexia, polydipsia, and polyuria resulting in dehydration often occur. Animals may survive the initial intoxication and return to a near normal clinical appearance within 12 hours, but they generally experience a recurrence of the more severe signs within 24 hours following ingestion. A terminal metabolic acidosis (pH approaching 6.9 or 7.0) occurs with congestion of mucous membranes. Heart and respiratory rates are often increased, but the terminal events include bradycardia with ectopic activity. Animals surviving longer than 24 to 36 hours will have signs of uremia with oliguria or complete anuria, primarily as a result of toxic effects of EG metabolites on renal tubular cells. The formation of calcium oxalate and hippurate crystals results in mechanical blockage of the renal tubules and contributes to the acute renal failure, as well. Since dogs can live for 2 to 7 days without kidneys, it is highly unlikely that early deaths are due to kidney failure. There is usually a progressive increase in

blood urea nitrogen, hyperkalemia, and acidosis. Urine sediment may contain small birefringent crystals, best observed under polarized light.

The lesions observed at autopsy will vary, depending on the duration between ingestion of EG and death. Hemorrhages in the gastric mucosa, swollen and congested kidneys, and hyperemic, edematous lungs are often seen, with death occurring within 3 to 4 hours. Microscopically, oxalate crystals may be found in the convoluted renal tubules and perivascular spaces of CNS blood vessels, even in animals succumbing within 24 hours, but are more frequently seen in animal deaths in excess of 72 hours after ingestion.

Diagnosis must be made from history and clinical signs, including detection of the sweet smell of EG on the breath in some cases. Laboratory findings are not specific for diagnosis, but can provide strong presumptive evidence when increased serum osmolality, hypocalcemia, a high anion gap, and metabolic acidosis are present. Differential diagnosis should include acute hepatitis, nephritis, encephalitis, head trauma, and garbage intoxication. There are chemical methods for detecting EG in the body fluids. Glycolic acid may be detected in the urine by high-pressure liquid chromatography and gas chromatography/mass spectroscopy. There is an ethylene glycol test kit available (PRN Pharmacal) for use on blood samples obtained within hours of EG ingestion.

The course of treatment in EG intoxication is threefold. If EG intoxication is diagnosed within 4 to 8 hours of exposure, activated charcoal and a saline cathartic are extremely helpful. Ethanol is administered as a competitive inhibitor of alcohol dehydrogenase. A sterile, 20% solution of ethanol in isotonic saline is administered at a dosage rate of 5.5 ml/kg intravenously every 5 to 8 hours for 48 hours. Animals will often remain stuporous or comatose for more than 48 to 72 hours. Sodium bicarbonate is administered intravenously to correct the severe metabolic acidosis. Base deficits can be calculated from blood gas data or, sterile 5% sodium bicarbonate in isotonic saline can be given empirically at a dosage rate of 8 ml/kg every 5 to 8 hours for 48 or more hours, as needed. Research studies have shown that 1,3-butandiol and 4-methylpyrazole (4-MP) are more effective than ethanol as an alcohol dehydrogenase inhibitors. These treatments are unapproved and not widely available at present (see Chapter 21). An additional benefit of 4-MP, as compared with ethanol, is that this compound will not cause central nervous system signs.

Plants containing insoluble oxalates

These plants are primarily ornamentals, and intoxications associated with them are generally

TABLE 27-4 Plants containing insoluble oxalates

Scientific Name	Common Names	Descriptions
Caladium spp.	Fancy leaf caladium	An ornamental herb that is stemless and has large varicolored heart-shaped leaves and tuberous roots
Colcasia spp.	Elephant ear, dasheen	Herbs that are grown as ornamentals and for their edible tubers; the leaves are large, varicolored, and heart-shaped, up to 65 cm long; the flowers are enclosed in a leafy bract
Dieffenbachia spp.	Dumbcane, elephant ear	A perennial that is a common ornamental with a resemblance to the sugar cane; it is usually 62 to 185 cm tall; the leaves are large, entire margins, oblong, green and variously mottled with white, yellow, light green, or darker green; the stems are straight, and the leaves are clustered on sheathlike petioles; the male and female flowers are produced separately in folded leaflike bracts; The plants have a skunklike odor when bruised
Monstera spp.	Split-leaf philodendron	A climbing or erect ornamental that may have aerial roots; the leaves are triangular or heart-shaped with margins that are entire or lobed and vary in color from green to red to white; the leaf blades may be to 1.5 m in length; flowers, when produced, are enclosed in a leafy bract; the fruit is a white to orange berry
Parthenocissus quinquefolia	Virginia creeper, American ivy	A high-climbing woody vine with tendrils that often have disklike tips; the leaves are palmately divided into five lance-shaped toothed leaflets, and the leaves may turn red in the fall; the flowers are small and greenish, growing in clusters at the tips of branches; fruit is a black or blue-black berry
Philodendron spp.	Elephant ear	A climbing or erect ornamental that may have aerial roots; the leaves are triangular or heart-shaped with margins that are entire or lobed and vary in color from green to red to white; the leaf blades may be to 1.5 m in length; flowers, when produced, are enclosed in a leafy bract; the fruit is a white to orange berry
Rheum raponticum	Rhubarb	A perennial with fleshy acid petioles commonly used for food; the leaves are large on long green or red stalks or stems; the leaves have a radial appearance and grow 25-50 cm tall from thick rootstocks; the flowers are on hollow branched stems and are greenish, white or occasionally red; the fruit is a winged cordate

limited to inflammation and swelling in the pharyngeal region causing respiratory difficulties and gastrointestinal upsets (Table 27-4).

Mycotoxins and mycotoxicoses

Mycotoxins are metabolic products from fungi. Mycotoxicoses are diseases of animals or humans caused by fungal metabolites. Some antibiotics are classified as mycotoxins. Some mycotoxins cause a diminished immune response, and some may be carcinogenic. There are over 100 fungi known to produce toxic metabolites under certain conditions such as in a standing crop or in stored feeds. Twenty to 30 mycotoxins are associated with diseases of humans or animals. Generally, all organ systems may be affected by mycotoxins.

Aflatoxins are the most common cause of mycotoxicoses in dogs, primarily occurring in contaminated dog food. Aflatoxins are produced by *Aspergillus flavus, A. parasiticus,* and *Penicillium puberulum.* These fungi may be found in feed products and on the fruit of plants such as corn, peanuts, pecans, and cottonseed. The main toxins are labeled B_1, B_2, G_1, G_2, and M_1. Mycotoxins' mechanism of action include alterations in cellular RNA and protein synthesis. Dogs are fairly susceptible to aflatoxins, but their effect on cats is unknown.

Clinical signs in dogs include anorexia, dehydration, jaundice, and the development of extensive hemorrhages. Treatment is supportive and nonspecific, including fluid therapy, low-fat diets, administration of lipotropic agents, avoidance of stress, and treatment of any coagulopathy (see Chapters 22, 23, and 28). Adequate protein in the diet aids in resistance to the development of mycotoxicoses.

Mycetismus (mushroom poisoning)

Mushroom poisoning is due to ingestion or inhalation of a potent toxin(s) intrinsically contained in poisonous mushrooms (toadstools). The principle species include *Amanita phalloides* (death angel), *A. virosa* (destroying angel), *A. muscaria* (fly agaric), and *Psilocybe cubensis* (the local "magic mushroom"). Identification of these mushrooms should be done by experts.

The major toxins are phalloidine, phalloin, amanitine, muscarine, tricholomic acid, ibotenic acid, disulfiram, psilocybin, and ergot alkaloids. The clinical signs include mild to violent gastrointestinal disorders, vomiting (often violent), and diarrhea with massive dehydration. Cholinergic and anticholinergic responses have been seen in affected humans. Hallucinogenic responses frequently occur. Death may occur due to hepatic coma or renal failure.

Phosphorus

White (or yellow) phosphorus is extremely toxic. Red phosphorus and most other phosphorus compounds are relatively nontoxic. White phosphorus is employed in "tracer" rounds for weapons, incendiary and fireworks manufacturing, and other industrial purposes. White phosphorus and zinc phosphide are used as rodenticides. The oral toxic dose for dogs is 50 to 100 mg. Secondary poisonings, which are intoxications due to the ingestion of poisoned rodents, may occur in dogs and cats.

The clinical signs are biphasic. Gastrointestinal irritation, vomiting, hemorrhage, abdominal pain, and shock may be evident initially. Vomitus may be luminescent and have a garlic-like odor (smell like wet matches or acetylene). There may be an apparent recovery for a few hours to 3 to 4 days. Clinical signs recur with icterus, nervous signs, convulsions, coma, and death. The convulsions may resemble strychnine convulsions. Postmortem lesions include gastrointestinal hemorrhages, fatty change in the liver and other organs, icterus, and subcutaneous or intramuscular hemorrhages.

Diagnosis is based on history, signs, and lesions. Chemical detection is required to confirm the diagnosis, and gastrointestinal contents are the best sample to use for detection.

Treatment includes evacuation of the stomach by emesis or lavage. Mineral oil may be used to dissolve phosphorus. The administration of milk or digestible fats and oils will promote absorption and is not recommended. Other supportive and symptomatic treatments, including treatment for liver dysfunction, are important considerations (see Chapter 22). Prognosis is generally guarded, and any delay in diagnosis and treatment is often fatal.

Garbage and foodborne intoxications (enterotoxemias)

Garbage intoxication is an ill-defined disease entity in dogs and cats. This intoxication generally occurs in free-ranging animals. Factors predisposing to enterotoxemia include the ingestion of garbage, decomposed food, carrion, and decaying organic substances (compost). Garbage intoxication is problematic in puppies overeating highly fermentable and low-digestible foods or ingesting foreign materials such as bones and large-animal manure. Concurrent achlorhydria results in a small-bowel pH above 6, which allows putrefactive bacterial growth and increased susceptibility to enterotoxemia. Causative agents incriminated in enterotoxemia or garbage intoxications include *Escherichia coli, Salmonella* spp., *Clostridium perfringens, Clostridium botulinum,* and *Staphylococcus aureus.*

Clinical signs in animals with "garbage intoxication" include anorexia, depression, nausea, vomiting, diarrhea (mucoid, watery, bloody), weakness, stiffness, ataxia, nervousness, prostration, and dehydration. Severe signs may be due to endotoxic shock, and death can occur.

Treatment includes fluid therapy and either broad-spectrum antibiotics or enteric sulfonamides in cases of sepsis. Administration of intestinal protectives such as kaolin and pectin is advisable. Over-the-counter preparations containing salicylates may be advantageous in the treatment of any secretory component to diarrhea. In the case of endotoxic shock, large doses of corticosteroids should be administered intravenously.

Zootoxins

Zootoxins (snakes, spiders, etc.)[4] are proteins with enzymatic activity including phosphodiesterases, hyaluronidase, hemolysins, collagenases, and other enzymes. These venoms may be neurotoxic, cytotoxic, necrotizing, or proteolytic.

Snake bites. Poisonous snakes of the United States include coral snakes (*Micrurus fulvius* and *Micruroides euryxanthus)* and pit vipers such as rattlesnakes (*Crotalus* spp. and *Sistrurus* spp.), copperheads *(Agkistrodon mokasen),* and water moccasins or cottonmouths *(Agkistrodon piscivorus).* Other more toxic vipers and sea snakes could escape captivity and may be problematic in some instances.

Factors that contribute to the severity of toxicity following snake bites include the species of the snake, size of the snake, amount of venom present (length of time since the snake has eaten), number of fangs (there can be 1 to 6 puncture wounds in pit viper bites), type of tissue injected, and whether defensive or offensive strikes are involved. As many as 45% to 50% of snake bites are dry with no envenomation. Host factors, including age, weight, general body condition, site of bite (head, body, extremity) amount of physical activity following bite, time between bite and treatment, all play important roles in the development of systemic responses to snake bites. Early in the spring, enzyme fractions in snake venoms are low, causing mild local reactions, but severe systemic reactions following snake bites. Late in the summer, enzyme fractions are high in venoms and severe local reactions to snake bites are common in addition to systemic reactions. There are 26 protein fractions in rattlesnake venoms.

Cats may be more resistant to the effects of snake bites than dogs, but they can be severely affected, too. In cats, 50% of the snake bites are to the head and 40% to the forelimbs. Body bites in cats are generally lethal. Dogs get bitten on the head about 70% of the time, but in general, the snake bites are rarely fatal (<1%).

Clinical signs of snake bite include marked edema and erythema at the site of the bite. This swelling may extend over the entire head, limb, or affected part of the body. The clinician should measure the circumference of the swelling several times within 2 to 3 hours. A rapidly developing swelling indicates probable snake bite. The swelling from pit viper bites is painful to the touch. A blood-stained frothy exudate may come from the animal's nose in a head bite. Affected animals may exhibit excessive thirst, and hypovolemic shock is an extremely important feature in smaller animals. Nausea, vomiting, diarrhea, painful/stiff locomotion, incoordination, and respiratory paralysis (especially, with coral snake bites) may occur. Anaphylaxis is rare. Dyspnea may be present, especially if the bite is in a location that leads to swelling and obstruction of the upper airway. Animals may be unable to eat because of cervical swellings. Hemolytic anemia may be seen in animals that survive for a number of hours. Tissue sloughs and local infection are common sequelae. Laboratory tests of value include white blood cell count, packed cell volume, total serum protein concentration, and creatine kinase activity. Thrombocytopenia is a common finding. A urinary hemoglobin:myoglobin ratio of 4 or more may indicate a pit viper bite.

Differential diagnoses include fractures and cellulitis. Snake bites are common in the spring and fall, as snakes are less active at other times due to extremes (heat and cold) of environmental temperatures.

The proper treatment of snake bites is somewhat controversial. Early transportation to medical treatment is an important aspect of first-aid treatment for snake bites. There are several electronic gadgets sold for the treatment of snake bites, but these have not shown efficacy. Lactated Ringer's solution or phosphate-buffered saline, up to 88 ml/kg, should be administered rapidly in cases of hypovolemic shock. Polyvalent antivenin (equine origin) (Fort Dodge = $75/vial, Wyeth = $110/vial—5- to 10-year shelf life) is most effective if given early (i.e., following rapid swelling of site or detection of thrombocytopenia). The antivenin should be placed into the intravenous fluids and given by slow infusion, and not injected around the bite site. The solutions must *not* be shaken as the mixture will foam and inhibit rapid administration. If hyperemia of the skin or ears develops, administer diphenhydramine, 2 to 4 mg/kg, with half the dose administered subcutaneously and the remainder administered intravenously. If the animal's serum creatine kinase activity is greater than 1000 IU/L, two vials of antivenin should be administered. The dosage of antivenin to be administered depends on the amount of venom injected, not the size of the animal being treated. *Corticosteroids are contraindicated,* but antibiotics and tetanus toxoid may be indicated. Fasciotomies, cold therapy, and tourniquets are of little value.

Toads. Bufo alvarius (Colorado river toad, West Texas to California) and *Bufo marinus* (marine toad, Florida and Hawaii) are toads that contain cardioactive glycosides. All toads, toxic and nontoxic, secrete substances in skin glands that are repulsive to animals that mouth them. Puppies usually do not make the mistake twice.

Clinical signs can occur within minutes of a

dog mouthing a toad. These signs include profuse salivation, prostration, cardiac arrhythmias, pulmonary edema, hypertension, and convulsions. Death can occur in as little as 15 minutes.

Treatment includes flushing the mouth with flowing water and treating for cardiac glycoside overdosage. Atropine is used to control salivation and speed the heart if bradycardia is present. Propranolol (beta-adrenergic blocker), procainamide, or other antiarrhythmics may be used to control cardiac arrhythmias. Electrocardiographic monitoring is essential in order to initiate therapy appropriately. Oral potassium hydrochloride is administered in divided dosages, since intracellular hypokalemia often potentiates cardiac glycoside intoxication.

Arachnids. Tarantula bites (*Eurytelenna* spp.) produce mild poisonings, but may produce a painful bite. Spider bites, on the other hand, can be extremely hazardous to pets.

Black widows *(Lactrodectus mactans)* produce a labile toxin that is most toxic in the fall and least toxic in the spring. The toxin contains five to six active proteins, which increase membrane Ca^{++} permeability, causing a massive release of both norepinephrine and acetylcholine. Exercise slows the onset of clinical signs, but does not prevent them following a bite.

Clinical signs in dogs following a bite by a black widow include regional numbness, muscular fasiculations, and the appearance of an acute abdomen without tenderness. Black widow bites are seldom fatal to dogs. Clinical signs develop rapidly in cats following a bite. Clinical signs include paralysis, evidence of pain, salivation, tremors, ataxia, and death due to respiratory collapse.

Treatment includes administration of antivenin intravenously. This treatment produces relief of clinical signs associated with the black widow spider bite within 15 minutes of administration. Atropine administration, treatment for shock, and ventilatory support may be necessary in some instances.

The brown recluse spider (fiddle-back spider) *(Loxosceles reclusa)* was first recognized in the 1950s as a cause of toxicity in humans. The common clinical sign in cases of severe envenomation is a nonpainful bite, which produces a wound that does not heal for months. Within 8 to 15 hours, the bite area becomes edematous and black. Necrosis develops at the bite within 72 hours. (Fatty areas become very necrotic.) A brown recluse bite may cause systemic signs of hyperthermia, weakness, nausea and vomiting, and a hemolytic anemia with ensuing hemoglobinuria. Hepatic lesions may develop in some cases, leading to hepatic insufficiency and jaundice. Microscopically, lesions are characterized by vasculitis, hemorrhage, and polymorphonuclear leukocyte infiltration. Early changes (within 1 hour) include endothelial swelling, perivascular leukocytic infiltration, and hemorrhage.

Treatment is symptomatic. Dapsone administered at a dosage rate of 1 mg/kg, twice a day for 10 days blocks complement and polymorphonuclear leukocyte infiltration. If Dapsone is ineffective in preventing development of the nonhealing wound, surgical excision should be delayed for 6 weeks. Hyperbaric oxygen therapy has been advocated, but is not practical. Intravenous fluids should be considered.

There are many species of scorpions (*Centruroides* spp.) but only a few produce toxins, and some are very toxic. Clinical signs of scorpion bites include local pain, parasympathetic stimulation, muscular fasiculations, cardiovascular collapse, neuromuscular collapse, and respiratory paralysis. There are no specific treatments. Treatment includes the use of atropine, muscle relaxants, sedatives, and ventilatory support. Epinephrine administration exacerbates the cardiovascular signs.

Insects. Signs of envenomation by insects are primarily anaphylactic in nature. With bees and wasps, a single sting will produce a local swelling and can cause severe anaphylaxis if the animal is sensitized. Multiple stings result in severe swelling and an allergic response and may kill in a few minutes to hours.

Most other insect bites just produce local inflammation and pain. The differential diagnosis includes drug reactions with urticaria and anaphylaxis, atopy, foreign protein reactions, and other shock-inducing conditions. Treatment is directed toward alleviating the anaphylactic reaction with antihistamines, corticosteroids, and sympathomimetic agents.

REFERENCES

1. Gans JH, Mercer PF. The kidneys. In Swenson MJ, ed. Dukes' physiology of domestic animals, ed. 9. Ithaca, NY: Comstock Publishing Associates, 1977;463-492.
2. Gerkin D. American Veterinary Medical Association Annual Meeting, Portland, OR, 1988.
3. Bailey EM. Emergency and general treatment of poisonings. In Kirk RW, ed. Current veterinary therapy X—Small animal practice. Philadelphia: WB Saunders, 1989;116-125.
4. Peterson ME, Meerdink GL. Bites and stings of venomous animals. In Kirk RW, ed. Current veterinary therapy X—Small animal practice. Philadelphia: WB Saunders, 1989;177-186.

28 Avian Emergencies

Gretchen E. Kaufman

The criteria used for evaluation of avian patients presented for emergency treatment differs little from that followed for traditional animal species. A proper and thorough history, physical examination, and the use of basic diagnostic tests are equally important for avian patients. Accurate evaluation of system disorders, hydration status, and cardiovascular integrity are a priority. There are, however, some fundamental differences between birds and mammals that must be acknowledged in order to safely move through the steps of evaluation and treatment of an avian patient.

The metabolic rate of birds is markedly faster than that of mammals. This fundamental difference results in a more rapid progression of disease or deterioration of condition than is commonly associated with similar circumstances in a dog or cat. Another concern relating to an increased metabolic rate is the degree to which stress (physiologic or environmental) can have an impact on the condition of the patient. Excessive handling or inappropriate environmental conditions, including inadequate environmental temperature and extraneous noise, can often mean the difference between life and death for the patient. With these two concepts in mind, evaluation and treatment can safely proceed.

A major investment in specialized equipment, drugs, and supplies is not necessarily required in order to handle most avian emergencies. Some minor adaptations to preexisting veterinary facilities may be necessary. In order to minimize the environmental stress from barking dogs and general activity of a busy practice, it is desirable to designate a semiisolated area for housing birds.

The sick bird has considerable difficulty maintaining its normal body temperature, consequently thermal support is required. If possible a small room, or even an unused storage area, can be adapted to provide a room temperature of 80 to 90°F (26 to 32°C). If a separate climate-controlled room cannot be provided, a variety of solutions are available, such as heat lamps or individual climate-controlled incubator units obtainable from hospitals or from commercial sources (Animal Intensive Care Unit, Animal Care Products, Norco, CA).

An oxygen chamber is another item that is essential in avian emergency practice. Its use can be life saving in many instances. Suitable oxygen chambers used for dogs and cats may already be available in some veterinary clinics, or these chambers can easily be constructed for birds using an incubator or an anesthetic chamber that has an oxygen supply.

Additional smaller items required include a gram scale for accurate weight determinations; a selection of small endotracheal tubes such as Cole tubes, sizes 8, 10, 12, etc.; a selection of gavage tubes or needles (Lafeber); and various medications (see the box on the next page).

With these few supplies available, most emergencies can be handled adequately within the standard small animal practice. A practice specializing in avian medicine and surgery will have made the investment in some additional medications and equipment that also may be applied to emergency situations, but are not essential.

EVALUATION AND BASIC EMERGENCY CARE

History and physical examination

A concerted effort must be made to be as efficient as possible to minimize handling of the patient. An initial visual evaluation of the bird will often give the clinician an idea of how to proceed. Any bird in respiratory distress should be placed in an oxygen-enriched environment (oxygen cage) for 10 to 15 minutes before handling. Preoxygenation will help avoid the unfortunate experience of the

---

BASIC MEDICATIONS REQUIRED FOR AVIAN EMERGENCIES

Tube feeding formula—Emeraid (LaFeber, Odell, IL) or a human non-dairy-based formula

Parenteral fluid solutions—lactated Ringer's, 5% dextrose, saline

Parenteral vitamin/mineral solutions—Injacom (A, D_3), B-Sol, vitamin K_1, vitamin E/selenium (L-Se), iron dextran

Antibiotics—Trimethoprim-sulfa, oxytetracycline, vibramycin, amikacin

Nystatin

Oxytocin

Dexamethasone sodium phosphate

Glucose, 50%

Parenteral calcium solutions—calcium gluconate, Calphosan (Glenwood, Tenafly, NJ)

Calcium disodium edetate

Diazepam

Isoflurane anesthetic gas

---

bird dying in the hand of the doctor during the initial examination. During the preoxygenation period, a complete history can be obtained, while the owner feels that something is being done for the bird. If preoxygenation is not required, and the bird appears stable, a history should be obtained with the bird in the cage or the box, undisturbed.

History taking with avian patients requires particular attention to certain details not often emphasized in canine and feline medicine. The origin of the bird, exposure to other birds, environmental conditions in the home (cage location, temperature, unsupervised flight in the home), and general behavioral information (recent egg-laying activity, tendency to chew on plants and window molding, etc.) may be critical to arriving at a correct diagnosis. An emphasis should be made on dietary management, appetite, water drinking, and examination of the droppings as well as routine questions concerning age, sex (often unknown), coughing, and sneezing.

Wild birds will often arrive for emergency care apparently "without a history." The small amount of historical information available in these cases should not be overlooked. Details such as location, length of time seen on the ground, or length of time in the "Good Samaritan's" possession, may provide insight into the problem at hand (Chapter 30). For example, a hawk found in a field where there has been recent insecticide spraying may demonstrate only clinical signs of nonspecific depression when in fact it is suffering from organophosphate toxicity.

The initial visual evaluation and history should lead the clinician to formulate a list of possible differential diagnoses or system disorders. With this list in mind, all materials required to proceed with examination of the patient, collection of appropriate diagnostic samples, and administration of medications should be assembled. If respiratory distress is involved and preoxygenation is performed, it is not unusual for the examination, collection of samples, and administration of therapy to be performed in stages, with periods of "oxygen rest" in between. It is always better to err on the side of caution in this matter than to push the patient too far with aggressive techniques.

The physical examination should be undertaken in a routine but expedient manner. Physical examination of the bird is well described elsewhere and will not be discussed here.[1] For emergency evaluation, particular attention should be placed on assessing level of hydration, attitude, strength, evidence of blood loss or trauma, and specific body system disorders (dyspnea, diarrhea, etc.).

Diagnostic tests

Some simple diagnostic tests that may need to be performed for initial evaluation are listed in the box below. The first three tests listed in the box can be performed on a very small amount of blood (usually one or two microhematocrit tubes) collected from a brachial or metatarsal vein (Fig. 28-1). A clipped toenail may be used if clotting is a concern or if the practitioner is not proficient at the aforementioned techniques; however, this is not the preferred site.

Microbiologic samples should be obtained if an infectious process is suspected, so that empirical antibiotic therapy may be instituted as soon as possible (see Appendix I). Due to the bird's metabolic rate and potential for rapid deterioration, there is rarely time to wait for culture results before instituting therapy for a bacterial infection. A Gram stain may be helpful in making initial determinations; however, this technique should not be relied upon as the sole microbiologic evaluation.

DIAGNOSTIC TESTS FOR AVIAN EMERGENCY EVALUATION

Packed cell volume and total serum solids evaluation

Blood sugar determination—Chemstrip bG (Boehringer Mannheim, Indianapolis, IN)

Blood smear—examination of cell morphology and relative differential distribution

Radiography

Microbiologic samples

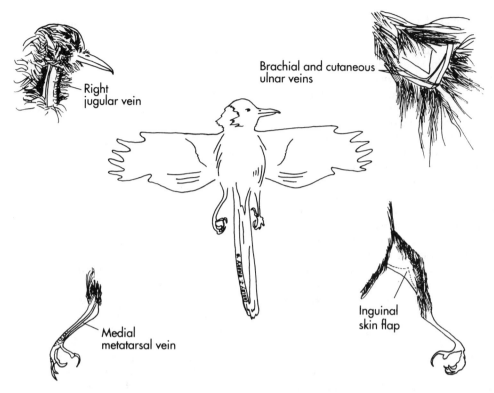

Fig. 28-1 Common sites of venipuncture and administration of subcutaneous fluids in birds.

Basic emergency care

With the history, physical examination, and simple diagnostic tests completed, a preliminary assessment of the patient can be made (see box at right) and steps undertaken to stabilize the bird's condition.

Basic emergency treatments that may be instituted include shock therapy, fluid and electrolyte therapy, nutritional support, thermal and oxygen support, blood transfusions, antibiotic therapy, and wound management. Compromises may have to be made. Delays in obtaining information or in performing what may be considered "optimal care" may be necessary in the unstable patient.

Fluid and electrolyte therapy

Hydration status is evaluated using clinical subjective impression and with the aid of diagnostic tests (packed cell volume and total serum solids). Severe depression rapidly develops in birds suffering from dehydration. These birds will also demonstrate decreased skin turgor, sunken and/or closed eyes, and dry oral mucous membranes. A significantly dehydrated bird will demonstrate thick stringy mucus in the back of its throat. A bird that has been anorectic for several days, has been experiencing vomiting or diarrhea, or a wild bird that has obviously been disabled for some

---

PRELIMINARY ASSESSMENT GUIDELINES

Attitude or degree of depression
Hydration status
Nutritional status
Presence or absence of anemia
Infectious disease potential
Preliminary evaluation of body systems

---

undetermined time, can be assumed to be at least 10% dehydrated. Determination of packed cell volume and total serum solids can be used to help estimate hydration, but must be interpreted with discretion. In certain conditions these parameters can be misleading. A bird that has been starving for some time will have low total serum solids, as indicated on a refractometer. This may occur even in the face of severe dehydration. Consequently, a dehydrated bird does not necessarily have elevated total serum solids. Conversely, an abnormally high total serum solids usually does correlate with dehydration. A severely debilitated bird may demonstrate an anemia of chronic disease or malnutrition in the face of significant dehydration. In this case the packed cell volume will be decreased and will not correlate with the level of dehydration. Packed cell volume and total serum solids must always be used in conjunction with the subjective evaluation of the patient. In addition to aiding in assessment of hydration these measured parameters provide very useful information regarding nutritional status, chronic disease states, and degree of anemia.

The estimation of fluid needs is made based on the bird's daily fluid requirements plus the estimate of fluid deficits and continuing losses. Continuing fluid losses occur with diarrhea, regurgitation, hemorrhage, polyuria, tachypnea, and hyperthermia. As in mammals, fluid deficits in birds may be corrected in 36 to 48 hours. Estimates for daily maintenance requirements range from 40 to 60 ml/kg per day[2] to 66 to 132 ml/kg per day.[3] Alternatively, the individual bird's water requirements may be calculated based on basal metabolic rate. This figure is obtained for nonpasserine birds with the following formula (Sedgwick, personal communication, 1989)

$$1.5[78 (\text{Wt. in kg}^{0.75})] = \text{ml water per day.}$$

Clearly, any of these formulas provide rough estimates for individual fluid requirements and will not account for variability between species of birds.

Severely dehydrated animals require intravenous fluid therapy whenever possible. In larger birds (more than 250 g), the cutaneous ulnar or medial metatarsal veins are used for administration of fluids (see Fig. 28-1). In severely obtunded patients, a 24-gauge intravenous indwelling catheter may be placed in the brachial vein, secured to the skin with tissue glue, and stabilized with a standard figure-8 wing wrap (Fig. 28-2). These birds may be maintained on a continuous infusion or may be given repeated intravenous bolus therapy. Birds have been shown to tolerate easily intravenous fluid rates in excess of 100 ml/kg per hour when needed. Boluses of 20 to 30 ml/kg are well accepted if given slowly over 1 to 2 minutes.[2]

In birds smaller than 250 g, intravenous fluids may be given via the jugular vein if the clinician is proficient in this technique. The potential hazards of jugular laceration make this technique undesirable for the inexperienced.

When intravenous therapy is not possible, fluids may be given alternatively via the intraosseous route. This technique involves placement of a needle catheter in the ulna and allows delivery of fluids nearly as rapidly as with intravenous administration. In larger birds, an 18- to 22-gauge spinal needle is used, and in smaller birds, 25- to 30-gauge hypodermic needles are used. The needle may be secured and left in place for continuous or repeated bolus fluid administration.[4,5]

Subcutaneous fluids may be administered to patients in whom intravenous or intraosseous administration is not possible (or not within the skills of the practitioner), and in instances in which rapid rehydration is not necessary. Unless the bird is in shock, subcutaneous fluid administration is an acceptable route to use. As much as 50 ml/kg may be given at one time to a patient. The most common sites for subcutaneous fluid administration are the inguinal skin flaps and the area over the lumbosacral region (see Fig. 28-1). Caution must be used when giving fluids in the lumbar region. Fluids administered too far cranially and too deeply may result in accidental injection of fluids into the air sacs and subsequent drowning of the bird. Fluids may also be given in the wing web, although this site is difficult to handle because of the very thin membrane making up the patagium. Subcutaneous fluids are readily absorbed by birds and may be administered repeatedly two or three times per day. Glucose solutions greater than 2.5% or any hypertonic solutions should not be given subcutaneously in a dehydrated patient.

Oral fluids may be administered, with caution, to birds as a means of rehydration. Care must be taken when using this method in patients that have been anorectic for some time and are severely dehydrated. Unexplained deaths have been observed as a result of premature administration of oral substances to patients with significant gastrointestinal stasis associated with prolonged anorexia. The administration of hypertonic solutions orally to a dehydrated patient is contraindicated because it will lead to sequestration of body fluids into the gastrointestinal tract and exacerbate dehydration. It is prudent to rehydrate the patient thoroughly through parenteral means before introducing oral substances. When oral substances are introduced, they must be introduced slowly, beginning with an isotonic balanced electrolyte solution. This should be followed by increasing concentrations of a tube-feeding formula and gradual introduction of whole food items. These guidelines are particularly important in starving raptors.

The choice of fluids for administration in emergency situations is usually not critical and often lactated Ringer's solution, Normosol-R, or other balanced electrolyte solutions are used. Glucose supplementation may be required in the severely debilitated or starving patient (blood glucose less than 200 mg/dl). Intravenous glucose administration is preferred. In the dehydrated patient, a mixture of 5% dextrose and lactated Ringer's solution is commonly used as an initial intravenous fluid solution.

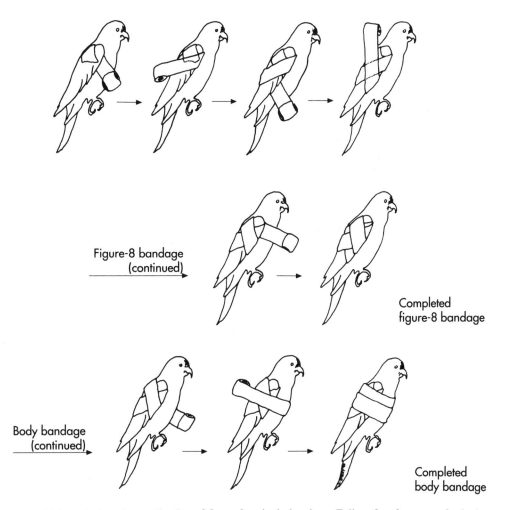

Figure-8 bandage
(continued)

Completed
figure-8 bandage

Body bandage
(continued)

Completed
body bandage

Fig. 28-2 Technique for application of figure-8 or body bandage. Follow first four steps for both bandages.

Acid-base and electrolyte abnormalities are not often diagnosed in birds but undoubtedly are important. Electrolyte imbalances may be expected to occur in cases of diarrhea, regurgitation, and acidosis or alkalosis. In documented cases of acidosis, sodium bicarbonate may be added to the fluid therapy. Sodium bicarbonate may be administered intravenously initially (1 mEq/kg), followed by subcutaneous administration (1 mEq/kg every 15 to 30 minutes up to a maximum of 4 mEq).[2]

Shock therapy

Shock therapy is frequently indicated for treatment of traumatic injuries in wild birds, notably raptors. A serious traumatic injury involving blood loss, followed by several days on the ground subjected to the elements, often leads to a severe shocklike state in these birds. Birds in an advanced state of disease or starvation may also

---

SUGGESTED MATERIALS FOR EVALUATION AND RESUSCITATION OF BIRDS IN SHOCK

Warm lactated Ringer's/5% dextrose (20-30 ml/kg intravenous bolus)
Dexamethasone sodium phosphate (4 mg/kg intravenously)
Broad-spectrum antibiotic (e.g., trimethoprim-sulfa)
Heat lamp or hot water bottles
24-gauge butterfly catheter
Microhematocrit tubes and clay
Blood glucose reagent test strip
Gram scale

---

present in cardiovascular collapse. The patient will appear severely depressed and weak and may be unresponsive. Peripheral veins (such as the cutaneous ulnar vein) appear flat and collapse easily, due to hypovolemia.

The pathophysiology of shock has not been well defined in birds but is presumably very similar to shock in mammals. Consequently, the principles of therapy are the same (see box on p 457). Support and expansion of the cardiovascular system by administration of intravenous fluids is of the utmost importance. Many patients respond within several hours to this therapy, allowing further workup. Others require repeated intravenous fluid therapy, which may be best served with an indwelling intravenous or intraosseous catheter.

Nutritional support

Nutritional support is required in a severely emaciated patient with a blood glucose of <100 mg/dl. Intravenous glucose solutions (5%) may be given initially. Following intravenous therapy, subcutaneous dextrose solutions may be given if oral therapy is not possible, but glucose should not be given subcutaneously at concentrations greater than 2.5%. Very small amounts of Karo syrup or 50% dextrose may be given orally, and will be absorbed across the mucous membranes to elevate blood glucose levels quickly. Semicomatose patients or severely dehydrated patients should not be given any medications orally.

Once a patient is stabilized and rehydrated, enteral nutritional support may be required if the patient remains anorectic. A highly digestible non-dairy-based carbohydrate/protein formula is suggested (see box above). Caloric requirements may be calculated using the following formulas.[6]

Nonpasserine birds $78 (\text{wt. in kg}^{0.75}) = \text{kcal/day}$

Passerine birds $129 (\text{wt. in kg}^{0.75}) = \text{kcal/day}$

Trauma

The principles of trauma therapy in birds are essentially the same as those in mammals. Cessation of bleeding is most important, and it can be accomplished with various techniques: direct pressure and bandaging, the use of hemostatic agents (silver nitrate, ferrous sulfate, thromboplastin), electrocautery, or vessel ligation. Alarming blood loss may occur following damage to a "blood feather." This "emergency" can readily be handled by complete removal of the offending feather. The feather must be firmly grasped with a hemostat or needle forceps at the base and pulled in the direction of the feather. Direct pressure may have to be applied to the empty follicle for a few minutes.

Significant blood loss in birds can occur very quickly, and is often underestimated by the clinician. The very small size of the bird must be kept in mind, as compared to the more familiar dog or cat. Blood volumes are estimated from 60 to 130 ml/kg, depending on species[1] or can be calculated from the following formula (Sedgwick, personal communication, 1989):

$0.0605 (\text{wt. in kg}^{0.99}) = \text{total volume in liters}$
for nonpasserine birds

By way of example, an Amazon parrot weighing 380 g has an estimated blood volume of 23 ml. Loss of 5 ml of blood would be considered significant. In severe blood loss, a blood transfusion must be considered (see below).

Wounds should be assessed according to severity and location. Wounds open to the body cavity must be attended to quickly, especially if they involve the air-sac space. Contamination of internal body cavities clearly conveys a guarded prognosis. Less serious wounds may be treated at the time of presentation, or treatment may be delayed depending on the patient's condition. The degree of handling and/or anesthesia required to repair a wound should be taken into account when making treatment decisions involving a bird in shock or very poor condition.

Repair or support of fractured limbs should also be undertaken with the condition of the patient in mind. The patient must be stabilized before specific treatment can proceed. If the patient is recumbent, temporary fracture stabilization is usually not necessary. In more active birds, simple bandaging techniques can be employed to provide adequate stabilization until definitive treatment is possible.

Bandage materials used should be lightweight and conforming. Vetrap (3M, St. Paul, MN) is ideal for most temporary bandages. White porous tape should never be applied directly to feathered areas. The adhesive is too strong and will result in significant feather damage and difficult removal. Masking tape or nylon tape may be used if an adhesive must be applied.

Fractures of the distal wing (including the radius, ulna, carpal joint, metacarpal bones, or phalanges) can easily be immobilized with a "figure-8" bandage. The wing is held against the body of the bird approximating a natural position, and a lightweight bandage material (Vetrap) is placed alternately around the carpal joint and the elbow joint and primary wing feathers. Care must be taken to include the humerus into the bandage (see Fig. 28-2). This bandage need not be very tight, only snug enough to hold the wing in a natural position. In larger birds, a rigid object, such as a tongue depressor or a cut piece of cardboard, can be incorporated into the bandage for added support. The figure-8 bandage can also be used to fix a sterile dressing over an open wound or fracture, or to stabilize an indwelling intravenous catheter in a wing vein.

Fractures of the humerus or bones of the shoulder girdle (including the coracoid, clavicle, and scapula), and luxations of the shoulder or elbow can be immobilized with a combination of a figure-8 and a "body-wrap." This technique begins with a figure-8, which anchors the bandage material and keeps the wing in position. After a few rotations the bandage continues around the body to cross the sternum. The opposing wing should be left out of the wrap. Often, the bandage need only go below the contralateral shoulder but may alternatively go below and above the contralateral shoulder. Care must be taken not to make the wrap too tight, restricting respiratory movements; allow the lower portion of the bandage to drop below the limitations of the sternum and trap the legs; or allow the bandage to restrict the crop or thoracic inlet (see Fig. 28-2).

Fractures of the leg below the stifle may be temporarily immobilized with a modified lightweight Robert-Jones type of bandage. If more rigid stabilization is needed, a Schroeder Thomas splint can be made to fit the individual bird using coat-hanger material. Fractures of the femur usually cannot be stabilized externally and are not treated by temporary methods. The patient is confined until surgery can be performed.

Antibiotics are indicated in the face of obviously contaminated wounds, open fractures, low-velocity gunshot wounds, or cat-bite wounds. The projectile from a pellet or B-B gun carries particles of feathers and skin into the wound, resulting in contamination and subsequent infection. Cat-bite trauma should be considered an emergency, even if there is minimal visible injury. A life-threatening *Pasteurella* septicemia can develop in birds within 12 hours following a cat bite.

Thermal and oxygen support

The benefits of these two therapies cannot be overemphasized. Thermal support must be provided for any sick bird. Optimally, an environmental temperature of 80 to 90°F (26 to 32°C) is desired.

Oxygen therapy is usually warranted in the face of respiratory disease, and is essential prior to handling compromised individuals.

Blood transfusion

Patients with significant acute blood loss or a markedly depressed packed cell volume (less than

BLOOD TRANSFUSION (SUGGESTED SETUP FOR BLOOD TRANSFUSION)

Healthy donor bird
Isoflurane anesthesia (mask)
Acid-citrate-dextrose solution
22-gauge butterfly catheter (collection)
24-gauge indwelling catheter (administration)
Blood-component infusion set
Warm lactated Ringer's solution
B-Sol
Iron dextran
Dexamethasone sodium phosphate

15%) may require a blood transfusion. Studies have shown that the source of the donor blood may safely come from a species different from the recipient. The use of pigeon, chicken, or raptor blood has proven to be quite safe, and often life saving in psittacines. Administration of blood is no more difficult than administration of intravenous fluids. A life-saving transfusion should be carried out even when cross matching is not readily available (see box above).

Blood donor. Blood may be collected from the donor bird from either the jugular or brachial vein. Isoflurane anesthesia of the donor may make the procedure easier to perform, although it is not always required. Ten milliliters of blood per kilogram of body weight may safely be taken without harm to a healthy donor bird. Blood should be collected in some form of anticoagulant. A syringe coated with heparin, edetate (EDTA), or containing a citrate solution (9 parts blood to 1 part acid-citrate-dextrose solution) will suffice. Heparin anticoagulant is preferred over edetate for smaller recipients in order to avoid adverse effects (hypocalcemia) in the recipient.[1] Following blood collection, the donor bird should receive an equivalent 10 to 30 ml/kg intravenous fluid replacement, as well as intramuscular administration of B vitamins and iron dextran. This supportive therapy is especially important if the donor is used repeatedly.

Blood should be used within hours after collection. Studies have not been conducted to determine the life of stored avian red blood cells.

Recipient. The recipient may be given blood through any available vein (cutaneous ulnar, jugular, or tibiotarsal). The use of an indwelling catheter or a butterfly catheter is prudent. A small blood administration set that includes an inline filter is commercially available (Blood component infusion set, 4C2223, Fenwal Laboratories, Deerfield, IL). Care must be taken to minimize stress in the severely anemic patient. Preoxygenation and/or oxygen administration during the procedure may be required. Anesthesia of the recipient is usually not necessary and may be risky. The recipient should also receive intramuscular iron dextran and B vitamins as supportive therapy.

Studies have shown an increased mortality associated with repeated transfusions given to a patient from the same donor within 10 days of the first transfusion.[8] Reasons for this observation are not understood. It is recommended that repeated transfusions should *not* be given to a patient from the same donor within 10 days, and preferably 3 weeks, of the first transfusion without cross matching.[1] If this is unavoidable, the recipient should be given dexamethasone sodium phosphate

before repeating the transfusion.[9] Cross matching with unwashed red cells is apparently not valid.[8] Cross matching with washed and incubated red cells may be valid, showing either hemolysis or agglutination reactions.[1]

APPENDIX I
Common emergencies by system

The following tables list some commonly seen problems that may present as emergencies affecting one or more systems. The list is by no means complete, and the reader is referred to the suggested reading list for more information. The tables are meant to guide the clinician and suggest some preliminary tests that may be performed to help with differential diagnoses.

Respiratory emergencies

	Clinical Signs	Differential Diagnosis	Diagnostic Tests
Upper respiratory	Anorexia +/− Oculonasal discharge Obstructed nares Coughing +/− Sneezing Choking	Upper respiratory infection Foreign body Thyroid dysplasia	Choanal culture Sinus flush/culture Transilluminate neck
Lower respiratory	Anorexia Dyspnea Severe depression Coughing +/−	Pneumonia Air sacculitis Air sac mites Toxic (Teflon) Heart disease	Choanal culture Radiography Complete blood count (CBC) Serum biochemistry profile
Secondary to abdominal disorders	Anorexia Dyspnea Abdominal distention Lack of droppings +/−	Neoplasia Hepatomegaly Egg binding Ascites/peritonitis	Radiography

+/− = May be present or may be absent.

Gastrointestinal emergencies

	Clinical Signs	Differential Diagnosis	Diagnostic Tests
Upper gastrointestinal tract	Anorexia Dehydration Regurgitation Emaciation Weight loss Palpable crop abnormality	Oral/pharyngeal lesion Crop infection Crop motility disorder Foreign body Proventricular dilation Lead poisoning Behavioral regurgitation Lower intestinal disease (nausea)	Crop swab/flush (culture/cytology) Radiography CBC
Lower gastrointestinal tract	Anorexia Dehydration Diarrhea Emaciation Weight loss Feces color change Lack of feces	Enteritis Hepatitis Pancreatitis Peritonitis Psittacosis Lead poisoning Obstruction Parasitic infestation	Fecal examination Cloacal culture Radiography CBC Serum biochemistry profile Psittacosis titer

Neurologic emergencies

Clinical Signs	Differential Diagnosis	Diagnostic Tests
Seizures	Trauma	Blood lead level
Severe depression/coma	Lead poisoning	CBC
Head tilt, nystagmus	Meningitis/encephalitis	Serum biochemistry profile
Ataxia	Hypoglycemia	Radiography
Blindness	Hypocalcemia	
Anisocoria	Hepatoencephalopathy	
Paralysis	Toxicity	
	Epilepsy	
	Thiamine deficiency	

Reproductive emergencies

Clinical Signs	Differential Diagnosis	Diagnostic Tests
Abdominal distention +/−	Egg binding	Radiography
Straining +/−	Follicular cysts	Abdominocentesis
Depression	Egg peritonitis	Surgical exploration
History of egg laying +/−	Urogenital tumor	

+/− = May be present or may be absent.

Renal emergencies

Clinical Signs	Differential Diagnosis	Diagnostic Tests
Depression	Renal failure (gout, aminoglycosides)	Radiography
Dehydration	Hepatitis (psittacosis)	CBC
Polyuria	Lead poisoning	Serum biochemistry profile
Polydipsia	Diabetes mellitus	Urinalysis (glucose, blood)
Hematuria	Stress	
Green or yellow urates		

APPENDIX II

Common emergency conditions

Condition	Clinical Signs	Diagnostic Tests	Treatment	Comments
Fluffed bird (nonspecific)	Anorexia Depression Fluffed feathers	History/PE PCV/TP Blood glucose	1. Supportive care—fluids and heat 2. Closely monitor for specific symptoms	The "emergency" fluffed bird may be an acute presentation of a chronic disease, usually evident from the history and PE
Lead poisoning	Anorexia Regurgitation Diarrhea GI stasis Paralysis Seizures Hematuria	History/PE Radiography Blood lead CBC Serum biochemistry profile	1. Diazepam (seizures) 2. Remove lead source; cathartics/oral chelators such as $MgSO_4$, peanut butter; endoscopy; proventriculotomy 3. $CaNa_2EDTA$: 35 mg/kg IM b.i.d. for 5 days 4. Supportive care	Consult references for details on therapy[10,11]; begin therapy with any seriously ill patient before blood results are available
Egg binding	Anorexia +/− Straining Abdominal distention	History/PE Radiography	1. Warm, moist heat 2. Lubrication 3. Distal position—oxytocin: 0.2-2.0 U IM; calcium: 50-100 mg/kg IM 4. Treat for shock if warranted 5. Proximal position—laparotomy	There are many variations of egg binding; consult references for details in handling these cases[6,12]; by far most cases respond to moist heat and medical therapy
Hypocalcemia (African gray parrot)	Lethargy Severe weakness Fainting/coma Tetany/seizures	History/PE CBC Serum biochemistry profile Serum calcium	1. Calcium: 50-100 mg/kg IV or IM 2. Follow up with daily calcium supplement—Neocalglucon: 5 ml/30 ml water for 7 days, then 1 ml/30 ml water indefinitely	Give calcium slowly IV or diluted IM[13]
Polytetrafluoroethylene toxicity (burnt Teflon)	Respiratory distress Sudden death	History	1. Oxygen therapy 2. Supportive care	Therapy is usually not successful

PE = physical examination; PCV = packed cell volume; TP = total proteins; GI = gastrointestinal CBC = complete blood count; $MgSO_4$ = magnesium sulfate; $CaNa_2EDTA$ = calcium disodium edetate; IM = intramuscularly; b.i.d. = twice a day; +/− = may be present or may be absent; t.i.d. = three times a day.

Common emergency conditions

Condition	Clinical Signs	Diagnostic Tests	Treatment	Comments
Oil contamination	Hypothermia Anorexia Diarrhea (intestinal malabsorption) Respiratory distress (aspiration pneumonia) Dehydration	History/PE PCV/TP	1. Stabilize with supportive care, including heat, fluid therapy 2. Remove oil first with towel, then with Dawn dishwashing liquid; rinse 3. Dry thoroughly	Wash/rinsing should be repeated until water beads up on feathers. Use water temp. of 103-104°F; consult references[14,15]
Hemochromatosis (mynahs)	Respiratory distress Ascites	History/PE Radiography Abdominocentesis CBC Serum biochemistry profile	1. Abdominocentesis 2. Furosemide. 0.15 mg/kg IM t.i.d. 3. Oxygen therapy	Extremely poor prognosis; may need to repeat treatment; diet change recommended; phlebotomy therapy may help[16-18]

REFERENCES

1. Harrison GJ, Harrison LR. Clinical avian medicine and surgery. Philadelphia: WB Saunders, 1986.
2. Redig PT. Fluid therapy and acid-base balance in the critically ill avian patient. Proceedings of the International Conference on Avian Medicine, Toronto, Canada. 1985;59-73.
3. Evans D. Fluid therapy in birds. WRC J 1984; Spring:3-13, Fall:5-11.
4. Otto CM, Kaufman GM, Crowe DT. Intraosseous infusion of fluids and therapeutics. Compend Contin Educ Pract Vet 1989;11:421-430.
5. Ritchie BW, Otto CM, Latimer KS, Crowe DT. A technique of intraosseous cannulation for intravenous therapy in birds. Compend Contin Educ Pract Vet 1990;12:55-58.
6. Hainsworth FR. Animal physiology. Reading, MA: Addison-Wesley, 1981;162.
7. Schmidt-Neilsen K. Animal physiology. London: Cambridge University Press, 1975;255.
8. Altman RB. Heterologous blood transfusion in avian species. Proceedings of the Annual Meeting of the Association of Avian Veterinarians, San Diego, CA. 1983;28-32.
9. Quesenberry KE, Hillyer E. Hospital management of the critical avian patient. Proceedings of the AAV Basic Avian Medicine Symposium, Seattle, WA: 1989;365-369.
10. McDonald SE. Lead poisoning in psittacine birds. In Kirk RW, ed. Current veterinary therapy IX. Philadelphia: WB Saunders, 1986;713-718.
11. LaBonde J. Pet avian toxicology. Proceedings of the Annual Meeting of the Association of Avian Veterinarians, Houston TX. 1988;159-174.
12. Nye RR. Dealing with the egg-bound bird. In Kirk RW, ed. Current veterinary therapy IX. Philadelphia: WB Saunders, 1986;746-747.
13. Hochleithner M. Convulsions in african grey parrots (Psittacus erithacus (Psittacus erithacus). Proceedings of the Annual Conference of the Association of Avian Veterinarians, Seattle, WA: 1989;78-81.
14. Harris JM. Management of oil-soaked birds. In Kirk RW, ed. Current veterinary therapy VII. Philadelphia: WB Saunders, 1980;687-692.
15. Dein FJ, Frink LS. Rehabilitation of oil-contaminated birds. In Kirk RW, ed. Current veterinary therapy IX. Philadelphia: WB Saunders, 1986;719-722.
16. Gerlach H. The so-called iron storage disease in mynahs. Proceedings of the First International Conference on Zoological and Avian Medicine, Oahu, Hawaii. 1987;79-85.
17. Dorrestein GM, van der Hage MH. Veterinary problems in mynah birds. Proceedings of the Annual Meeting of the Association of Avian Veterinarians, Houston, TX: 1988;263-274.
18. Morris PJ, Avgeris SE, Baumgartner RE. Hemochromatosis in a Greater Indian Hill Mynah (Gracula religiosa). J Assoc Avian Vet 1989;3:87-92.

SUGGESTED READINGS

Harrison GJ, Harrison LR. Clinical avian medicine and surgery. Philadelphia: WB Saunders, 1986.
Jenkins JR. Emergency avian medicine. Proceedings of the First International Conference on Zoological and Avian Medicine, Oahu, Hawaii. 1987;279-285.
Joyner KL. Avicultural emergency medicine. Sixtieth Western Veterinary Conference. 1988;390-398.
McCluggage DM. Avian emergency medicine. Association of Avian Veterinarians Basic Medicine Symposium, Houston, TX: 1988;1-6.
Petrak ML. Diseases of cage and aviary birds. ed. 2. Philadelphia: Lea & Febiger, 1982.

29 Neonatal and Pediatric Emergency Care

M. J. LaRue

Information regarding the science of veterinary neonatology and pediatrics is unfortunately quite scarce. Many physiologic differences exist that clearly separate the neonatal or pediatric patient from an adult. These differences play an important role in the diagnosis and management of the pathologic processes that affect young animals. This chapter will briefly discuss the unique physiologic functions of the juvenile and a spectrum of diseases that may require veterinary care on an emergency basis.

PERIPARTURIENT CARE

Significant physiologic adjustments are made by the neonate in the immediate postnatal period. The initial respiratory efforts of the neonate are critical, as alveolar spaces are collapsed until the first breath. At birth, all membranes should be removed from the newborn's head and stimulation of the entire body should be accomplished by rubbing the neonate with a clean, dry towel. The accumulation of fetal fluid in the pharynx should routinely be aspirated. The neonate should be grasped between the palms of two hands and gently swung in a downward direction while holding the mouth open with a finger. This procedure aids in eliminating fluid from the airways. Blowing gently into the nose and mouth may enhance the initial respiratory efforts. Doxapram (Dopram-V, A-H Robbins, Richmond, VA) can be used to stimulate respirations by placing one to two drops on the tongue or by injection of 0.1 ml intravenously into the umbilical vein. Oxygen supplementation should be administered to newborns demonstrating signs of respiratory distress. Glucose solution, 20%, placed on the tongue of the neonate, can be used when the patient is responding poorly.[1] The neonate should be reunited with the mother as soon as possible.

GENERAL CONSIDERATIONS IN THE NEONATE

There are significant biochemical and physiologic differences from adults that one must consider when handling the young of any species. The rectal temperature of the neonate ranges from 95 to 99°F (35 to 37°C) at birth. The rectal temperature reaches that of an adult dog or cat (100 to 102°F, 38 to 39°C) by 4 weeks of age. Kittens and puppies require a warm environmental temperature. The shivering reflex and vasoconstrictive mechanisms are not functional in the neonate.[1] Environmental temperature control plays an important role in treatment of the newborn. The ambient temperature should be maintained at 85 to 90°F (29 to 32°C) from 1 to 5 days of age; 80°F (27°C) from 5 to 20 days, and then reduced to 70 to 75°F (21 to 24°C) for neonates 20 days or older. If hypothermia should occur, slow warming of the neonate, in an incubator, over 1 to 2 hours is recommended.

The birth weight of a puppy or kitten is the most reliable indicator of ability to survive.[1] The weight of the neonate should be documented at birth and should be monitored daily for the first 7 to 10 days. A loss of up to 10% of birth weight can be expected in the first 24 hours. Normal puppies should gain at a daily rate of 1 to 1.25 g/455 g of anticipated adult weight.[1] A daily weight gain of 7 to 10 g is considered normal for healthy kittens.[2] A lack of weight gain or a decrease in body weight should prompt investigation.

Young animals of most species experience a decrease in hematocrit and hemoglobin during the fourth to sixth week of life. This phenomenon is termed "physiologic anemia of the newborn" and results from several factors, including hemodilution by an expanding blood volume, reduced erythropoiesis, and a shortened red blood cell life span.[3] An increase in the concentration of 2,3-diphosphoglycerate within the red blood cell shifts the oxyhemoglobin-dissociation curve to the right, maintaining oxygen delivery in these animals.[4] Reticulocytosis is usually marked after the sixth week and red blood cell numbers are approaching adult values by 12 weeks of age.

Glomerular filtration rate and renal tubular concentrating mechanisms are decreased below adult capacities in the neonate and juvenile under 8 weeks of age.[5-7] Problems with fluid imbalances can develop quickly following slight deviations in fluid intake and/or elimination. Dehydration, iatrogenic overhydration, and other metabolic derangements are dangers for the sick neonate with immature kidneys. Young animals in an anabolic state produce less urea and creatinine. Therefore, measurements of these parameters on blood samples may be misleading in interpretation of a neonate's renal function.

CARE OF ORPHANS

Orphaned kittens and puppies are a challenge and require a strong commitment from the owner and the veterinarian. The veterinarian must emphasize that basic principles (environmental temperature control, feeding schedules, weight monitoring) must be followed strictly for the first 2 weeks of life. The choice of a milk supplement should approximate the composition of the maternal milk. Esbilac (PetAg, Hampshire, IL) for puppies and KMR (PetAg) for kittens are excellent commercially available formulas for feeding orphaned animals. The feeding schedule should be every 4 hours for the first 4 weeks. During the first week, the stomach capacity is about 50 ml/kg of body weight.[8]

Feeding techniques include bottle feeding and tube feeding. Proper measurement of the feeding tube is important. The length should be measured from the nose to the last rib. The tube should be filled with formula and attached to a syringe containing the proper dosage. The orphan should be adequately aroused and placed in sternal recumbency. The tube is gently inserted (allow the neonate to suckle and swallow the tube) to the premeasured distance and the contents are slowly expelled into the stomach. The tube should be "kinked" and quickly withdrawn to prevent aspiration of formula. Bottle-fed orphans should be burped to expel trapped gas after each feeding. Stimulation of urination and defecation after each meal can be accomplished by gently massaging the anogenital area with a moistened cottonball or warm damp cloth.

Once the orphan has opened its eyes and becomes more mobile, it should be encouraged to lap formula and/or gruel from a bowl. Feedings can be completed with a bottle or tube if necessary. When the orphan is able to take the entire meal from a bowl, the introduction of solid food and water may be initiated. Excellent references for further details on orphan care and nutrition are available.[9]

DRUG DISPOSITION IN THE NEONATE

The disposition of various drugs may be significantly different in the newborn as compared with that in the adult. The physiologic differences relate to the mechanisms by which the neonate absorbs, distributes, or eliminates different drugs. Deficiencies of drug-metabolizing enzyme systems or glomerular filtration and renal tubular secretory mechanisms, low plasma protein concentrations, increased permeability of the blood-brain barrier, and differences in the relative volumes of body fluid compartments may affect drug disposition in the neonate as compared with adult animals.[10] Application of adult dosage regimens to the neonate may be ineffective or even dangerous.

Low plasma albumin concentrations may influence drug disposition by decreasing the fraction of drug that is protein-bound. Differences in body water and fat content of the neonate as compared with adult animals may lead to a greater volume of distribution for drugs and decreased sequestration of lipid-soluble drugs in adipose tissue (barbiturates). Drugs that require metabolic conversion to an active form will have decreased activity and may require higher dosages than those used in the adult animal.

Drugs that have a prolonged effect in the neonate include chloramphenicol, short-acting barbiturates, anticonvulsants, salicylates, sulfonamides, and local anesthetics.[10]

THE SICK NEONATE

The sick neonate may cry continuously and become listless. Weakness may be recognized as an inability to nurse or to remain with the mother and the littermates. These animals usually exhibit weight loss or a failure to gain weight. The demonstration of flexor dominance (abnormal after 3 days of age) is common in the sick neonate. Without prompt medical attention, these animals may succumb to hypothermia, hypoglycemia, and dehydration.

Hypothermia

Neonates are inefficient at body-temperature regulation, and hypothermia can easily occur. Hypothermic puppies and kittens are frequently isolated from the litter and are cool to the touch. Severe hypothermia (85 to 90°F; 29 to 32°C) may result in cardiopulmonary depression. The animals frequently have poor cardiovascular and neurologic responses. Slow rewarming is recommended, and the appropriate environmental temperature depends on the overall status and age of the patient. A general goal is to maintain the ambient temperature at 90 to 95°F (32 to 35°C). This is best accomplished through the use of an incubator. It is not advisable to tube feed formulas to a severely hypothermic individual. Nutritional supplementation may be resumed once the patient has been successfully treated for hypothermia.

Hypoglycemia

The neonate is particularly susceptible to the development of fasting hypoglycemia. Between feedings, the neonate relies on glycogenolysis and gluconeogenesis to maintain glucose homeostasis.[11] Liver glycogen stores are quickly depleted, providing glucose for only 8 to 12 hours in a normal fasting infant.[12] The neonate is deficient in gluconeogenic precursors. The very low body fat content of the neonate reduces the supply of free fatty acids available for energy. The glucose requirements for the neonate are two to four times that of the adult.[13] Factors that increase metabolic demand, decrease glucose intake, or alter endocrine responses may precipitate hypoglycemia. Signs of hypoglycemia include hypothermia, weakness, ineffectual nursing, continuous crying, bradycardia, apnea, convulsions, and death[1,13-15]

Ideally, the blood glucose concentration should be monitored. This may be a difficult task in very small animals. A 25-gauge needle may be introduced into the jugular vein or a peripheral vein and a small amount of blood can be collected for testing from the needle hub with a microhematocrit tube. Significant hypoglycemia may be considered when measurements are less than 40 mg/dl.

Intravenous or intraosseous administration of 20% glucose solutions (0.25 ml/25 g) may be attempted in the neonate. Alternatively, honey, syrup, or concentrated sugar solutions may be rubbed into the buccal mucosal surfaces. Administration of 5% to 10% glucose solution can be administered by tube feeding (0.25 ml/25 g). Concurrent attempts to warm and rehydrate the neonate should be initiated if necessary. Once the patient is stabilized, an appropriate formula or bitch's milk may be given.

Dehydration

Fluid therapy to correct dehydration may be administered by oral, subcutaneous, intravenous, or intraosseous routes. A mixture of lactated Ringer's solution with 2.5% dextrose can be given at a rate of 1 ml/25 g body weight.[1,16] The intraosseous route of administration has become popular because of the difficulty in accessing veins in small patients. A 18 to 25-gauge needle can be inserted into the medullary cavity of long bones.[17] Types of crystalloid fluid solutions and dose rates are similar to those given intravenously.

NEONATAL DISEASES
The "fading" syndrome

"Fading" syndrome is commonly implicated in the deaths of puppies and kittens. This syndrome is characterized by a normal (occasionally low-birth-weight) neonate at birth with anorexia, lethargy, weakness, and emaciation described during the first few weeks of life. Frequently, the apparent cause remains unidentified, and death results. Numerous causes have been suggested, including viral and bacterial infections, nutritional disorders, toxins, and environmental factors.[9] Infectious causes such as canine hepatitis virus in puppies and beta-hemolytic streptococcal infections or feline infectious peritonitis in kittens have been implicated. The role of thymic deficiency has been suggested as playing a role in "fading" syndromes.[9] Treatment should be aimed at the underlying cause when identifiable. Since identification of causative factors is usually impossible, supportive management including nutritional support and prevention of hypothermia, hypoglycemia, and dehydration is of paramount importance.

Toxic-milk syndrome

Incompatibility to a bitch's milk or toxins in the milk may cause "toxic-milk" syndrome. Puppies may show signs of discomfort, excessive vocalization, and bloating. This syndrome is generally seen in pups 3 to 14 days old. Toxic milk has been associated with metritis or subinvolution of the uterus in the bitch.[1]

Affected puppies should be removed from the bitch. Oral dextrose solution should be given until there is resolution of bloating. When this is accomplished, replacement formula should be fed. In cases in which the cause of toxic milk can be identified and eliminated, the pups can be returned to the bitch following treatment.

Hemorrhagic syndrome

Hemorrhage from the nares, petechiae, and ecchymoses of the lips and tongue or hematuria occurring in puppies between 1 and 4 days of age is consistent with "hemorrhagic syndrome." During the first 48 hours of life, the prothrombin time will be prolonged as a result of hypoprothrombinemia.[1] Affected puppies generally demonstrate a rapid onset of lethargy and weakness. Extensive hemorrhage may be noticed in the subcutaneous tissues. Bleeding into the pulmonary parenchyma and also intraperitoneally is common. Evidence of intrapulmonary hemorrhage at autopsy is suspicious for the diagnosis; however, septicemia, severe anoxia, and infectious hepatitis must also be considered. Intraperitoneal hemorrhage may result from the bitch severing the umbilicus too close to the puppies' body, resulting in vessel retraction and fatal hemorrhage.

Low-birth-weight puppies may benefit from prophylactic administration of vitamin K_1. With obvious hemorrhage, 0.01 to 0.1 mg of vitamin K_1 should be given subcutaneously or intramuscularly.[1] Infusions of fresh plasma should also be considered. Clinical evidence of hemorrhage in the neonate carries a poor prognosis.

Prolonged storage of the bitch's diet or storage at improper temperatures may decrease the vitamin K activity in the diet. Fresh, nutritionally balanced diets should be fed to the gestational bitch. When hemorrhagic syndrome occurs in kennels, administration of vitamin K_1 to the bitch (1 to 5 mg per day), during the last half of gestation, may be helpful in prevention of the disorder in subsequent litters.

BACTERIAL INFECTIONS AND SEPTICEMIA IN THE NEONATE
Umbilical infections

A variety of organisms can cause infections at the site of the umbilicus, but most frequently, infections involve *Streptococcus* species. These infections occur most commonly during the first 4 days of life. The neonate will lose vigor, become anorectic, and have abdominal distention. The umbilicus frequently becomes swollen and discolored. Treatment consists of general supportive care, antibiotic therapy and drainage of any abscesses. Prevention of this syndrome may be accomplished through proper cleansing and disinfection of the navel following birth.

Ophthalmia neonatorum

In neonatal puppies, a purulent conjunctivitis may occur prior to the time (10 to 16 days of age) that the eyes open. In kittens, herpesvirus may cause infections after the lids are open. Eyelid swelling and protrusion resulting from exudate accumulation between the eye and eyelid may be the first clinical sign in pups and kittens. This generally occurs bilaterally. Kittens can demonstrate extensive chemosis, third-eyelid protrusion, corneal ulcers, and other signs of upper respiratory tract infection. Prompt therapy should include gentle lid

separation, application of topical antibiotics, and cleansing of the periocular area when necessary. The prognosis is usually fair with appropriate treatment, but corneal scarring can occur.

Septicemia

Neonates that have failed to receive colostrum, that develop umbilical infections, or that nurse from bitchs harboring infections (mastitis, metritis, or dermatitis) show an increased prevalence of sepsis.[1] A wide variety of organisms have been recovered at necropsy including: *Escherichia coli, Streptococcus, Staphylococcus, Proteus,* and *Pseudomonas.*[1] The development of septicemia in the neonate has been associated with improper ventilation and high humidity.[1]

Septicemia can occur in puppies ranging from 1 to 40 days of age. Clinical signs may develop in one neonate, followed by development of disease in littermates within 12 to 24 hours. Common presentations include vocalization, abdominal distention, rapid respirations, dehydration, weakness, incoordination and, death.

Autopsy reveals serosal petechial hemorrhages, gas-filled intestines, congested lungs, and enteritis. Blood cultures must be collected within 4 hours of death in order for results to be considered valid.[1] Cultures of brain or from ocular structures (vitreous) of pups dead for 4 or more hours may identify the causative organism.[1]

Treatment consists of isolating the litter from the bitch (potential source of infection) and aggressive supportive care, including heat and fluid administration. Antibiotics should be administered to all pups in the litter. Chloramphenicol and ampicillin have been recommended.[1] Intermittent introduction of stomach tubes or trochars may relieve severe bloating and improve respiratory capacity and recovery.

Prevention is aimed at improving sanitation and environmental conditions. Proper disinfection of the umbilicus at birth and ensuring the intake of colostrum is essential. Examination of the bitch prior to whelping, with proper treatment of any infections, aids in preventing septicemia in the newborn.

Herpes infection

Herpesvirus infections generally occur in puppies 1 to 3 weeks of age. Previously healthy pups become lethargic, vocalize excessively, become anorectic, and die within 18 hours of the onset of clinical signs.

Clinical signs may appear in a number of pups in a litter. The acquisition of CHV by puppies may occur in utero, during passage through the birth canal, or following birth.[18] Characteristic lesions at autopsy confirm the diagnosis of CHV. Hemorrhagic lesions are present in the kidneys and liver. Intranuclear inclusion bodies can be seen in lesions of the liver, kidney, and the respiratory tract.

Therapy for suspected neonatal herpesvirus infection is primarily supportive. The litter should be placed in an area with an environmental temperature of 100°F (38°C) for several hours, followed by 90 to 95°F (32 to 35°C) for 24 hours. The virus replicates at temperatures ranging from 92 to 98°F (33 to 37°C), and elevation of the environmental temperature may depress virus replication.[1] Hydration status should be monitored closely during this time. Tube feeding a commercial milk-replacement formula should be employed for several days.

The prognosis for recovery from neonatal CHV is poor. Permanent damage to nervous, renal, or lymphoid tissue is possible. Prevention involves quarantine of a previously unexposed bitch for 3 weeks prior to whelping and isolation of the bitch and her litter for 3 weeks postpartum. This prevents direct or indirect (handlers) exposure to dogs that may be carriers.[18]

TRAUMA

Traumatic injuries result from neonates being stepped or laid on, bite wounds, or falls and are relatively common occurrences. The traumatized newborn can be remarkably resilient and often responds well to basic supportive care. Traumatized neonates should be handled in a manner similar to that of an adult.

DISEASES AFFECTING THE PEDIATRIC PATIENT (3 TO 12 WEEKS OF AGE)
Infectious diseases of canine and feline pediatric patient

Numerous infectious agents can affect the pediatric patient. A summary of diseases, causes, clinical signs, and recommendations for therapy and prevention are included in Tables 29-1 and 29-2. Infectious diseases of the respiratory tract will be summarized in the section on the respiratory system.

Metabolic diseases

Juvenile hypoglycemia. Young puppies and kittens (<3 months old) exhibit limitations in their ability to regulate blood glucose and, to varying degrees, have a high glucose requirement. The same mechanisms apply in the juvenile as were previously discussed in the section on neonates. Hypoglycemia is frequently complicated by severe stress, such as cold exposure, infection, starvation, or drug ingestion.[11]

Clinical signs of hypoglycemia include weakness, severe depression, stupor, facial muscle twitching, seizures, and coma.[14] Prompt therapy is of paramount importance. When clinical signs are suggestive of hypoglycemia, blood should be drawn for serum glucose analysis. Glucose test strips are a rapid screening test requiring only a small amount of whole blood. In addition to diagnosis and treatment of predisposing causes for hypoglycemia, initial therapy includes the intravenous administration of 25% dextrose, initiated at a rate of 2 to 4 ml/kg over 30 to 60 seconds.[14] Continuous intravenous infusion using a 10% glucose solution (5 to 10 ml/kg per hour) can be used for maintenance treatment.[1] A large-bore catheter in the jugular vein is preferred for infusion of hypertonic glucose solutions in order to minimize the development of catheter thrombosis. Frequent monitoring of the blood glucose is essential during treatment (every 4 hours). Therapy should continue until clinical signs abate, the animal is euglycemic, and oral intake of nutrients is reestablished. A thorough history and physical examination is important to search for potential underlying processes that may predispose the juvenile to hypoglycemic episodes.

Juvenile puppies and kittens with persistent, recurrent hypoglycemic episodes require a thorough evaluation. Animals with hepatic disease (portosystemic shunts), Addison's disease, and glycogen-storage diseases may present for persistent hypoglycemia.

Digestive system

Intestinal parasites. The primary parasites that cause problems in the pediatric patient include roundworms *(Toxocara canis, Toxascaris leonina)*, hookworms *(Ancylostoma)*, whipworm in dogs *(Trichuris vulpis)*, coccidia, and giardia.

Ascarid infestations can cause significant disease in the pediatric patient. Clinical signs include unthriftiness, distended abdomen, a rough, dry hair coat, vomiting, and diarrhea. Appropriate anthelmintic therapy such as fenbendazole (Panacur, Hoechst-Roussel Agri-vet, Somerville, NJ), 50 mg/kg orally for 3 consecutive days, or pyrantel pamoate (Strongid-T, Pfizer, New York), 5 to 10 mg/kg orally (repeat dose in 3 weeks), combined with supportive care is generally successful in eliminating the parasite.

Hookworm infestation can be a serious problem in the pediatric canine patient. Associated blood loss may lead to severe anemia and hypoproteinemia. Juveniles may present with signs of weakness, depression, and mucoid to melenic stools. Therapy includes anthelmintics (see above), blood

Table 29-1 Infectious diseases in canine pediatrics (3 to 8 weeks of age)

Disease	Causative Agent	Clinical Signs	Diagnostic Tests	Therapy	Prevention
Canine distemper	Paramyxovirus	Early: fever, anorexia, mild conjunctivitis; Late: systemic illness, respiratory, gastrointestinal, CNS signs	History Fundic examination CSF (↑ lymphs, ↑ protein) Fluorescent antibody (conjunctiva, peripheral blood, CSF)	Supportive Antimicrobials Anticonvulsants	Vaccination
Tracheobronchitis	Etiologic complex: Canine adenovirus 2 Parainfluenza virus Reovirus Herpes virus *Bordetella bronchiseptica*	Mild fever Serous nasal/ocular discharge Dry "hacking" cough	History Clinical signs Transtracheal aspirate	Supportive (generally self-limiting) Broad-spectrum antibiotics Antitussives	Parenteral vaccine Intranasal vaccine
Viral enteritis	Canine parvovirus Coronavirus Rotavirus	Mild to severe gastroenteritis Depression, fever Abdominal tenderness Dehydration	History, clinical signs CBC ↑ PCV/TS: dehydration May suggest ↓ PCV/TS:GI blood loss Leukopenia EM of stool* Hemagglutination* ELISA Serologic tests[†]	Supportive IV fluid therapy Closely monitor blood glucose, electrolytes Broad-spectrum antibiotics	Vaccination Disinfection of environment (dilute hypochlorite solution)

*Caution must be used in test interpretation; performed on stool. Only applicable during periods of active shedding.
†False positive results common.
CNS = central nervous system; CSF = cerebrospinal fluid; ↑ = increased; ↓ = decreased; CBC = complete blood count; PCV = packed cell volume; TS = total solids; GI = gastrointestinal; EM = electron microscopy; ELISA = enzyme-linked immunosorbent assay.

replacement, and iron supplementation as dictated by the individual's needs.

Whipworm infestation can present with clinical signs of large-bowel diarrhea. Severe infestations may cause unthriftiness and debilitation. Cecal inversion has been described following therapy for whipworms.[21] Whipworms require an initial treatment with repeat treatment at 3 weeks and 3 months. Fenbendazole is an effective anthelmintic treatment for whipworms.

Giardiasis and coccidiosis occur frequently in young animals, often as a kennel problem. Profuse, watery diarrhea with occasional mucus or blood is usually observed. Dehydration may be an associated secondary problem. The diagnosis is based on visualization of the organisms on a fresh fecal smear or fecal flotations. Zinc sulfide centrifugation or trichome preparations may aid in the identification of *Giardia*. Treatment for coccidia includes the use of sulfadimethoxine (Albon, Hoffmann-LaRoche, Nutley, NJ) at 50 mg/kg once, then 25 mg/kg daily until asymptomatic. Cases of documented giardiasis may be treated with metronidazole (Flagyl, United Research Laboratories, Philadelphia) at 60 mg/kg per day orally for 5 days.

Table 29-2 Infectious diseases in feline pediatrics (3 to 8 weeks of age)

Disease	Causative Agent	Clinical Signs	Diagnostic Tests	Therapy	Prevention
Viral respiratory complex	Feline viral rhinotracheitis Feline calicivirus	Fever Sneezing Ocular/nasal discharge, ulcerative keratitis/glossitis Maybe leukocytosis Maybe lymphopenia	History Clinical signs Complete blood count	Supportive Fluid therapy Systemic antibiotics; ocular antibiotics/antiviral medications Cleansing of nasal and periocular exudates	Vaccination
Panleukopenia	Feline parvovirus	Fever Vomiting/diarrhea Leukopenia Dehydration	History Clinical signs Complete blood count (white-cell count <4,000/µl)	Supportive Fluid therapy Monitor blood glucose and electrolytes Broad-spectrum antibiotics	Vaccination
Feline leukemia virus	Feline leukemia retrovirus	"Fading kitten" syndromes Immunosuppression	IFA ELISA	Supportive care	Vaccination Environmental hygiene Avoid overcrowding Improve ventilation and cleanliness Isolation
Feline infectious peritonitis	Coronavirus	Kitten mortality complex* Reproductive failures Kitten mortality Concurrent feline leukemia virus infection	History Clinical signs Serology[†] Histopathology[‡]	Supportive care	Environmental conditions See section on feline leukemia virus
Bacterial enteritis	*Salmonella sp Campylobacter* sp.	Vomiting Diarrhea Dehydration Fever	Bacterial culture and sensitivity of stool specimen	Supportive Intravenous fluid therapy Antibiotic therapy[§] Chloramphenicol Trimethoprim-Sulfa	Zoonotic potential Environmental hygiene

*An association of this complex with feline infectious peritonitis has been made.[19]
†Not diagnostic as a sole criterion; results must be interpreted with caution.
‡Only means of definitive diagnosis.
§The use of antibiotics should be limited to animals exhibiting signs of septicemia.[20] Choice of antibiotic should be based on results of culture and sensitivity.

Intestinal obstruction. Intestinal obstruction in young puppies and kittens can be caused by foreign objects, intussusception, incarceration of bowel in a hernia or mesenteric tear, and congenital malformations (stenosis or atresia).[22] The playful and curious nature of young animals makes them particularly susceptible to ingestion of foreign bodies, leading to obstruction. Viral gastroenteritis is relatively common in young animals. Small-bowel irritation associated with gastroenteritis may cause increased peristaltic waves predisposing to the development of an intussusception.

The clinical manifestations of a gastrointestinal obstruction depend on the location, completeness and duration of obstruction, and the vascular integrity of the affected bowel.[22] Common clinical signs include anorexia, vomiting, diarrhea, and weight loss. Physical examination may reveal abdominal pain or distention and fever. In smaller animals, the obstruction may be palpable.

The diagnosis may be confirmed by palpation and diagnostic radiography. Radiographic findings suggestive of an obstruction include gas or fluid distention of the bowel, fixation or displacement of gut loops, and delayed transit time or luminal filling defects (foreign material, intussusception) detected during radiographic contrast studies.[22]

Special attention must be paid to the maintenance of fluid and electrolyte imbalances. Severe acid-base deviations can develop secondary to intestinal obstruction. An exploratory laparotomy should be performed once the patient is stabilized. Potential complications of intestinal obstruction include bowel perforation, peritonitis, and endotoxic shock.

Respiratory system

Pneumonia. Pneumonia is a common, serious disease affecting young animals and can be caused by bacteria, viruses, fungi, parasites, or by aspiration of pharyngeal or gastric contents and secretions. A summary of the various types of pneumonia, causative agents, clinical signs, diagnosis, and treatment is included in Table 29-3.

Electric-cord injury. Because of an inherent curious nature and the tendency to chew on objects, injury by chewing electric cords is seen commonly in young puppies and kittens.[23] Electrical stimulation of the neonate's brain results in centrally mediated vasomotor changes.[24,25] These changes may lead to an acute fulminating pulmonary edema.[26,27]

Animals may be presented after the owner has found them, unconscious, with the electric cord in their mouth. Frequently, animals will present for varying degrees of respiratory distress. The owner may be unaware of the animal's having bitten an electric cord, making the diagnosis a challenge.

Oral burns are seen in both dogs and cats with electric cord bites. Heat generated by electrical current flow damages the oral tissues. The lesions may involve the lips, gums, tongue, and hard palate. Prominent findings on examination include dyspnea, tachypnea, and moist pulmonary crackles on thoracic auscultation. Thoracic radiography may demonstrate characteristic changes of diffuse alveolar or mixed alveolar and interstitial patterns, most prominent in the dorsal caudal lung fields.[23]

The pulmonary edema caused by electric-cord shock is most likely due to an increased pulmonary hydrostatic pressure.[23] Therapeutic measures should be aimed at decreasing hydrostatic pressure through the use of furosemide (2 mg/kg intravenously) to decrease plasma volume, morphine (0.1 mg/kg in cats, 0.25 to 2 mg/kg in dogs, intramuscularly or subcutaneously) to relieve anxiety and decrease venous return and a bronchodilator (aminophylline [5 to 10 mg/kg intramuscularly or intravenously]). Cage rest and oxygen therapy are additional beneficial supportive measures. The efficacy of corticosteroid therapy is undetermined in the patient with electric-cord-induced pulmonary edema.[28] Positive-pressure ventilation and positive end-expiratory pressure can be used to maximize gas exchange in the presence of pulmonary edema.[29] Cardiac arrhythmias and seizures can occasionally occur as a result of biting an electric cord, requiring appropriate therapeutic intervention.[30] The oral burns should be treated conservatively, and the majority appear to heal satisfactorily without reconstructive surgical intervention.

In one study, 38.5% of dogs presented for electric-cord-induced pulmonary edema died. Cats in this same report appeared to have lower mortality rates as none of the four cats presented died.[23] Most animals that survive the initial 48 hours will continue to improve and recover completely.

Hemolymphatic system

The most common abnormality of the hemolymphatic system in pediatric patients is anemia. Hematocrit levels of 25% to 30% are common in animals less than 6 months of age.[3] Anemia is a symptom of an underlying disease process. Medical management should be aimed at identifying and removing or treating the primary disorder.

Clinical signs of anemia include weakness and lethargy. Physical examination may reveal pallor, tachycardia, tachypnea, and hypothermia. Systolic murmurs are common findings secondary to

Table 29-3 Respiratory infections of the pediatric patient

Disease	Agent	Clinical Signs	Diagnostics	Therapy
Bacterial pneumonia	Any bacterial pathogen	Depression, anorexia, lethargy Nasal discharge Cough With or without dyspnea, tachypnea	CBC Leukocytosis with or without left shift Radiography Transtracheal aspirate Culture and sensitivity Arterial blood gas analysis	Supportive IV fluids Oxygen supplementation Nebulization with coupage Antibiotic therapy based on culture results Expectorant
Mycotic pneumonia	*Histoplasma capsulatum* *Blastomyces dermatidis* *Coccidioidomyces immitis*	Fever Cough, dyspnea, tachypnea Lymphadenopathy Simultaneous organ involvement Skin Gastrointestinal Ocular Bone	History (geographical) Radiography Hilar lymphadenopathy Mixed interstitial/alveolar/bronchial pattern Identification of organism from Transtracheal aspirate Lymph node aspirate Biopsy Serology	Supportive (see above) Amphotericin B 5-flucytosine Ketoconazole
Viral pneumonia	Canine distemper virus Canine adenovirus Canine parainfluenza virus	Mild fever Serous to purulent ocular/nasal discharge Cough	History Clinical signs Radiography—normal to increased interstitial pattern (not uncommon to have secondary bacterial infections) Transtracheal aspirate	Supportive Specific treatment of overlying bacterial infections
Parasitic pneumonia	*Pneumocystis carinii* (canine) *Aleurostrongylus* (feline) *Paragonimus* sp. *Toxoplasma gondii* Larval migration of *Strongyloides* spp. *Toxocara* *Ancylostoma*	Cough With or without fever With or without dyspnea, tachypnea	Fecal examination Direct smear Flotation/sedimentation Baermann technique CBC With or without eosinophilia Transtracheal aspirate Identification of organism	Supportive Appropriate therapy based on identification of causative organism

a decrease in blood viscosity.

It is important to determine if the anemia is regenerative or nonregenerative. Most cases of anemia in the young animal are regenerative, secondary to blood loss or blood destruction. If chronic blood loss is present, the anemia may become nonregenerative secondary to iron deficiency (microcytic, hypochromic anemia).

Endoparasites and ectoparasites are the most common cause of blood loss anemia in the juvenile. Hypoproteinemia and regenerative anemia are the hallmarks of parasite-induced disease. Gastrointestinal disturbances may be present concurrently in patients with intestinal parasitism. Severe blood loss has been associated with overwhelming flea and tick infestations.

Treatment includes appropriate parasiticide therapy, replacement of fluid volumes, and blood transfusions, if necessary. Iron supplementation with ferrous sulfate (Feosol, Smith-Kline Consumer Products, Philadelphia) should be included for patients with iron deficiency.

Hemolytic anemia in the pediatric patient is less common than blood-loss anemia. Hemolytic anemia may be a result of a pyruvate kinase deficiency in the basenji[21] or neonatal isoerythrolysis.[31] The latter disease has been reported in puppies and kittens.[31,32] Isoantibodies are formed in a sensitized pregnant female and transferred to the neonate via the colostrum. Isoantibodies then recognize antigenic determinants of the surface of the neonatal red blood cell membrane. The red blood cells are destroyed in the intravascular space as well as in the spleen and liver. The source of isoantibodies may be sensitization from a previous incompatible blood transfusion in the bitch[33] or from transplacental hemorrhage accompanying previous pregnancies.[31]

Treatment for hemolytic anemia is primarily supportive care, including the judicious use of blood transfusion therapy. Kittens and puppies are generally transfused with whole blood, as it is difficult to separate small volumes into components. The volume of whole blood to be transfused is 10 ml/455 g of body weight. A 1:10 dilution of anticoagulant (CPD-A$_1$, citrate-phosphate-dextrose-adenine is preferred) to donor blood is recommended. Intravenous administration is preferred, but in situations in which venipuncture is impossible, blood may be given by the intramedullary or intraperitoneal route. A 18- to 25-gauge needle or bone marrow needle may be introduced to the intramedullary canal of the humerus or femur. Approximately 95% of the cells are absorbed within 5 minutes.[34,35] The intraperitoneal route results in approximately 50% of the cells being absorbed into the circulation within 24 hours.[34]

REFERENCES

1. Mosier JE. The puppy from birth to six weeks. Vet Clin North Am 1978;8:79-99.
2. Lawler DF. Care of neonatal and young kittens. Proceedings of the Annual Meeting of the Society for Theriogenology. 1988;250-257.
3. O'Brien RT, Pearson HA. Physiologic anemia of the newborn infant. J Pediatr 1971;79:132-138.
4. Bjerkas E. Eclampsia in the cat. J Small Anim Pract 1974;15:411.
5. Stapleton FB, Arant BS Jr. Ontogeny of renal uric acid excretion in the mongrel puppy. Pediatr Res 1981;15:1513-1516.
6. Horster M, Valtin H. Postnatal development of renal function: micropuncture and clearance studies in the dog. J Clin Invest 1971;50:779-795.
7. Heller J, Copek K. Changes in body water compartments and insulin and PAH clearance in the dog during postnatal development. Physiol Biochem 1965;14:433-438.
8. Anderson AC. The beagle as an experimental dog. Ames, IA: Iowa University Press, 1970;226.
9. Monson WJ. Orphan rearing of puppies and kittens. In Lawler DF, Colby ED, eds. Vet Clin North Am 1987;17:567-576.
10. Short CR. Drug disposition in neonatal animals. J Am Vet Med Assoc 1984;184:1161-1162.
11. Atkins CE. Disorders of glucose homeostasis in neonatal and juvenile dogs: hypoglycemia—Part I. Compend Contin Educ Pract Vet 1984;6:197-204.
12. Pagliara AS, Karl IE, Haymond M, et al. Hypoglycemia in infancy and childhood. Part I. J Pediatr 1973;82:365-379.
13. Aynsley-Green A. Hypoglycemia in infants and children. Clin Endocrinol Metab 1982;11:159-194.
14. Johnson RJ, Atkins CE. Non-neoplastic causes of canine hypoglycemia. In Kirk RW, ed. Current veterinary therapy VII. Philadelphia: WB Saunders, 1980;1023-1027.
15. Milner RDG. Neonatal hypoglycemia. J Perinat Med 1979;7:186-194.
16. Sheffy BE. Nutrition and nutritional disorders. Vet Clin North Am 1978;35:622-628.
17. Otto CM, Kaufman G, Crowe DT. Intraosseous infusion of fluids and therapeutics. Compend Contin Educ Pract Vet 1989;11:421-431.
18. Evermann JF. Clinical and diagnostic perspectives on canine herpesvirus infections. Proceedings for the Annual Meeting of the Society for Theriogenology. 1988;214-221.
19. Scott FC. Viral diseases. In Holzworth J, ed. Diseases of the cat: medicine and surgery, vol. 1. Philadelphia. WB Saunders, 1987;182-211.
20. Lorenz MD. Diseases of the large bowel. In Ettinger SJ, ed. Textbook of veterinary internal medicine: Diseases of the dog and cat. ed. 2. Philadelphia. WB Saunders, 1983;1346-1372.
21. Richardson RC. Diseases of the growing puppy. Vet Clin North Am 1978;8:101-128.
22. Sherding RG. Diseases of the small bowel. In Ettinger SJ, ed. Textbook of veterinary internal medicine: Diseases of the dog and cat. ed. 2. Philadelphia: WB Saunders, 1983;1335-1341.
23. Kolata RJ, Burrows CF. The clinical features of injury by chewing electrical cords in dogs and cats. J Am Anim Hosp Assoc 1981;17:219-222.
24. Ellis CH, Colville KI. Effect of current intensity of cardiovascular response to transcranial stimulation. Dis Nerv Sys 1958;19:54.
25. Colville KI, Ellis CH, et al. Mechanisms involved in the cardiovascular response to transcranial stimulation. AMA Arch Neurol Psych 1958;80:374.
26. Aravinis E. Pulmonary reflexes in pulmonary edema. Am J Physiol 1957;187:132.
27. Sarnoff SJ, Sarnoff LC. Neurohemodynamics of pulmonary edema. II. Circulation 1956;6:51.
28. Staub NC. Pulmonary edema: physiological approaches to management. Chest 1978;74:559.
29. Brendenburg CE, Kazui T, et al. Experimental pulmonary edema: The effect of routine end-expiratory pressure on lung water. Ann Thorac Surg 1978;26:62.
30. Murtaugh RJ. Thermal, electrical, and chemical injuries: An overview—The patient. Scientific Proceedings for the Veterinary Emergency and Critical Care Society, Washington DC: The Society, 1988;78-82.
31. Cain GR, Suzufi Y. Presumptive neonatal isoerythrolysis in cats. J Am Vet Med Assoc 1985;187:46-48.
32. Stormont C. Neonatal isoerythrolysis in domestic animals: a comparative review. Adv Vet Sci Comp Med 1975;19:23-45.
33. Authement JM. Personal communication, 1989.
34. Clark CH, Woodley CH. The absorption of red blood cells after parenteral injections at various sites. Am J Vet Res 1959;20:1062-1066.
35. Corley EA. Intramedullary transfusion in small animals. J Am Vet Med Assoc 1963;142:1005-1006.

30 Wildlife Emergencies

Mark A. Pokras and Rebecca May

This chapter will focus on emergencies involving individual native North American wildlife and will not emphasize the handling of large-scale emergencies such as oil spills or botulism outbreaks. It is apparent from our survey (Appendix I) and from previous reports that traumatic injuries are the most common class of wildlife-related emergencies.[1-9]

The majority of cases involving injury and death to individual wild animals are probably of little significance to the stability of wildlife populations. When dealing with individuals of endangered species, or with mass mortalities from such factors as lead poisoning, botulism, fowl cholera, or oil spills, entire populations or species may be threatened.

The degradation, destruction, and elimination of wildlife habitats for the short-term benefit of a burgeoning human population is by far the most significant cause of death to individual wild animals, and the endangerment of populations.

Veterinarians interested in treating wildlife are encouraged to:

1. Purchase appropriate field guides so that animals presented can be properly identified,
2. Find out which species are endangered or protected in your area, and what permits are required to treat native wildlife,
3. Assemble a library of books and journals on zoo and wildlife medical topics,
4. Identify individuals in your area who are licensed for wildlife rehabilitation, and
5. Encourage interest and education of your staff on issues of wildlife biology and medicine (several pertinent professional organizations are listed in Appendix II).

WILDLIFE—DEFINITION

Wildlife may be considered to be all species of animals not classified as companion animals or livestock.[10] This categorization can be confusing when one considers wild animals maintained and bred in such captive situations as zoos and research facilities. Most "exotic" pets popular in the United States and other developed countries are simply wild animals that were captured in Third-World countries and imported (often illegally).

The ecologists' definition of native wildlife might be the species that existed in a geographic area before humans began to alter the distribution of animal species. From this perspective dogs, cattle, and horses are as "exotic" to the United States as are Amazon parrots.

INDIVIDUALS VERSUS POPULATIONS

Wildlife biologists and conservationists view animals as members of dynamic and interacting populations. This view downplays the role of individual animals and focuses on preservation of quality habitat and genetically viable populations. Conversely, animal welfare/rights advocates and the veterinary community most often focus on animals as individuals. This view often ignores the complex issues of long-term population stability for animals in the wild.

In making treatment decisions regarding free-ranging wildlife, major conflicts arise between these viewpoints. It is axiomatic that there are never enough resources (e.g., money) to meet everyone's goals. Decisions must be made on how limited resources should be used and on prioritizing needs.

In most veterinary practices or wildlife rehabilitation centers it is often impossible to give the best possible care to all the injured or sick wild animals that are presented. Veterinarians must perform triage and decide which animals are likely to live with treatment depending on the skill and technology they have at their disposal. Inevitably, those working with wildlife will become drawn into discussions of why one species is more "important" or "valuable" than another. Importance is a subjective term. Ethical absolutists might contend that each living creature is equally important. Wildlife biologists might assign a low importance to such "pest" species as the pigeon, starling, or herring gull, whose populations have mushroomed thanks to human alterations of the environment. Conservationists might assign a high degree of importance to individuals of endangered species.

Individuals working with wildlife spend a great deal of effort in rehabilitating very common birds of prey, such as red-tailed hawks and screech owls, but relatively little effort working on rarer but less interesting species, such as upland sandpipers or timber rattlesnakes (endangered throughout the northeastern United States). Similarly, the

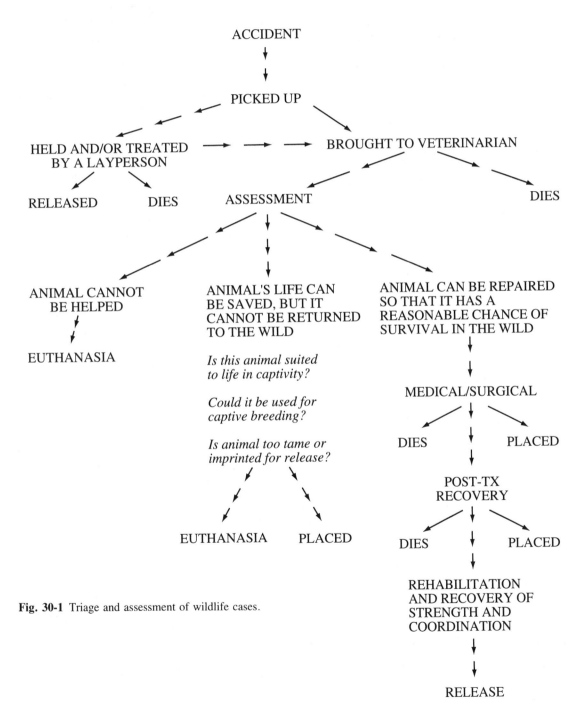

Fig. 30-1 Triage and assessment of wildlife cases.

raccoon is an intelligent, beautiful species that is overly abundant in most urban and suburban areas. The raccoon represents an example of the dilemma of having to decide between euthanasia versus the use of scarce time and money to rehabilitate a member of (what some consider to be) a common pest species. Rehabilitation of game species could arguably be considered an improper use of resources, as successful treatment and release often results in the animals' being shot during the next hunting season. But it can also be argued that by honing one's techniques on more common species, one may develop a high degree of skill that can be applied to rarer animals.

RELEASABILITY

Wildlife are treated with the intent of releasing the animals back into their native habitat. No one wants to condemn a wild animal to life in a cage, nor do we wish to release suboptimal animals that will have little ability to compete and survive in the wild. It is important to constantly balance in your mind the eventual releasability of the animal versus the advisability of prompt euthanasia (Fig. 30-1). The following discussions will help the reader make these difficult, but sometimes necessary, decisions.

Cooper et al.[11] made three suggestions for evaluating the potential for release of birds of prey. These criteria may be applied to the treatment and rehabilitation of any wildlife species. To paraphrase:

1. Consider the health of the animal. It must be able to fly, swim, or run well enough to perform all the functions of a member of its species—find food, escape from predators, reproduce, migrate, etc.;
2. Consider the animal's behavior. Any animal that is tamed or imprinted is unlikely to breed normally and may well become a problem animal due to its lack of fear of people; and
3. Consider the location for release. A wild animal must be released in the proper habitat for any given time of year. It is also important to try to choose a location where competition or aggression from other members of its species will be minimal, to enhance its early survival.

EUTHANASIA VERSUS PERMANENT CAPTIVITY

One of the kindest considerations we can sometimes make for injured wildlife is to opt for euthanasia early in the triage process. Ideally, the purpose of treating wild animals is to release them back to their normal, wild existence. Some nonreleasable animals may be placed in appropriate captive facilities (see Fig. 30-1). We emphasize that the decision to allow an animal to spend the remainder of its life in captivity should not be taken lightly.

The federal Endangered Species Act does not contain guidelines or provisions for the euthanasia of endangered animals. In practice, federal enforcement officials nearly always respect the clinical judgment of licensed veterinary professionals who possess wildlife permits, but it is always safest to check with your local or regional office of the U.S. Fish and Wildlife Service (USFWS) or the National Marine Fisheries Service (NMFS) before euthanizing one of these species. After euthanasia, do not dispose of the body without federal approval. Federal officials may wish to recover the entire cadaver for research purposes.

The decision to place a nonreleasable animal in captivity should be based on three factors:

1. Facility—Can you find a facility that has the space, expertise, etc. to give the animal proper care? Ideally, the animal will become part of an organized educational, breeding, or research effort.
2. Temperament—Is this particular animal suited to a life in captivity? Although this is difficult to assess for amphibians and reptiles, there is a great deal of individual variation among birds and mammals. Some high-strung wild animals will never adjust to life in captivity. They will be continually stressed by confinement and the presence of people and may exhibit stereotypical or self-destructive behaviors. It is not humane to condemn these individual animals to such a fate.
3. Rarity—Most individuals would probably agree that the rarer the species, the greater the effort that should be made to find that individual a suitable captive situation and the more value that animal may have for breeding or research.

HISTORY

A good history is important in the early assessment of injured wildlife. Information on where the animal was found and under what circumstances, how long the people have had it, what they have tried to feed it, and other factors will all play an important role in your assessment. The name, address, and telephone number of the finder should be recorded in case there are later questions regarding the animal. If a zoonotic disease is diagnosed in the animal, the people should be alerted to seek advice from their family physician.

TRIAGE OF WILDLIFE PATIENTS

The majority of individual wildlife emergencies are clearly associated with human activity (Appendix I). The "natural" causes of morbidity and mortality such as parasites and infectious diseases are relatively uncommon reasons for emergency presentation. But one must always have a high index of suspicion—Why did the animal get caught by the cat in the first place? Perhaps it was healthy to start with, or perhaps it was debilitated by poisoning, infection, or parasites and could not escape injury.

The approach to the diagnosis and treatment of wildlife emergencies is similar to the approach used with domestic animals. Issues of respiration and gas exchange, cardiac function, and fluid balance are of immediate importance. You must also be able to restrain the wildlife patient in such a way that danger to you, your staff, and the animal is minimized.

You must always be alert for potential zoonotic disease that could affect the people finding the animal, you and your staff, or domestic animals in your care. Most state fish and wildlife or public health agencies can provide you with information about the prevalent and reportable zoonoses in your area (rabies, tularemia, plague, etc.). The high incidence of canine distemper in wild canids and raccoons, echinococcosis in foxes in some regions, and cerebral larval migrans in children (and other warm-blooded species) from the raccoon roundworm *Baylisascaris procyonis* are examples of ailments that might be transmissible to your staff or domestic animal patients (Table 30-1).

Cat-bite wounds in any small birds or mammals should be considered emergencies. Punctures go considerably deeper than they first appear, and secondary infections are often rapidly fatal. Small animals should have puncture wounds cleaned and debrided. Broad-spectrum systemic antibiotic therapy should be initiated. In the absence of microbiologic culture and antibiotic sensitivity information we prefer to use trimethoprim-sulfa combination antibiotics (at a minimum energy cost [MEC] dose of 0.5 mg/kcal). Parenteral antibiotics are often preferred in rabbits and rodents because of the possibility of altering normal gastrointestinal flora with oral antibiotics leading to gram-negative overgrowth and fatal consequences.

KNOW YOUR LIMITS

In receiving wildlife patients, the first question one must address is "What does this animal have that can hurt me?" This question implies an index of suspicion for zoonoses and a healthy respect for "weapons" that animal species may possess (e.g., talons of owls, beaks of herons).

An important consideration is to identify the species you *cannot* handle. There should be no shame in advising callers that you are not equipped to handle adult bison, deer, bears, or cougar, for example. You should be prepared to refer these callers to another agency or facility.

A wild animal cannot be examined or treated if you cannot handle it. In addition to the normal armamentarium of medical and surgical supplies, you need some specialized items. These items might include very small or large endotracheal tubes (pediatric Cole tubes are good for birds and small mammals, and Teflon IV catheters can be used to intubate even the smallest patients), rabies poles, a pole or projectile syringe, a squeeze cage, heavy leather gloves, a snake pole or tongs, ad infinitum (Appendix III). Welders' gloves, available at most welding supply companies, are very useful for animal handling. Do not become overconfident; large raptors or even rodents, such as squirrels, can easily penetrate thick leather. Caution must be used when handling small animals with heavy gloves as it is easy to apply excessive force and cause further damage to the patient. You will need caging that is appropriate and that will isolate wildlife from your domestic patients, both to reduce stress and to avoid the spread of infectious diseases.

Veterinarians are frequently injured by their patients.[12] The potential dangers of the claws of felids or birds of prey are readily apparent. The beak of fish-eating birds, often set on a long neck, can move faster than a striking snake and inflict considerable damage. It is essential that you be able to identify the animal's species, or at least taxonomic group, to have some insight into these factors.

Unless the animal is unconscious, in shock, has arterial bleeding, tracheal obstruction, or other problems requiring immediate intervention, it is best to let the animal sit in a darkened, quiet place for a few minutes while you obtain a history and gather your thoughts and equipment. This gives you time to observe the animal's behavior and to begin to make judgments concerning how to catch, restrain, and examine the patient.

With a modicum of experience, staff can manually restrain most native birds and reptiles for physical examination and minor procedures. For many smaller mammals various "tricks of the trade" exist for handling. For example, even though most small native rodents can inflict a deep and painful bite with their incisors, most can be immobilized with a firm hold on the scruff of the neck. Good information on restraint and handling of many wild species can be found in references 13 and 14.

TABLE 30-1 Zoonotic diseases in North American wildlife

Disease	Cause	Species*	Transmission†	Occurrence‡	Clinical Syndrome§	Geographic Distribution
Bacterioses						
Arizona infection	*Arizona hinshawi*	Birds, mammals reptiles	Fecal-oral	Not well known	Gastroenteritis	Possible worldwide
Botulism	*Clostridium botulinum*	Freshwater birds, mink	Ingestion, wound infection	Sporadic	Neurologic, often fatal	All continents
Brucellosis	*Brucella* spp.	Hoofed mammals, lagomorphs, rodents, canids	Direct contact	Occasional	Septicemia, fever	Worldwide
Campylobacteriosis	*Campylobacter jejuni*	Hoofed mammals, birds	Fecal-oral	Occasional (probably underreported)	Gastroenteritis	Worldwide
Colibacillosis	*Escherichia coli* subspp.	Mammals, birds	Fecal-oral	Rare	Enteritis	Worldwide
Erysipeloid	*Erysipelothrix rhusiopathiae*	Marine mammals, swine, birds	Wound infection	Occasional	Skin lesions	Worldwide
Leptospirosis	*Leptospira interogans* serovars	Hoofed mammals, carnivores, rodents	Contact with infected urine	Sporadic	Septicemia, many organs affected	Worldwide
Listeriosis	*Listeria monocytogenes*	Mammals, birds	Oral (airborne?)	Rare	Septicemia, abortion, meningitis	Worldwide
Pasteurellosis	*Pasteurella multocida*	Mammals, birds	Bite wounds, aerosol	Occasional	Infected wounds, respiratory disease	Worldwide
Plague	*Yersinia pestis*	Rodents/fleas	Fleas, infected wounds	Occasional	Septicemia, pneumonia, lymphadenopathy	Worldwide, except Australia
Rat-bite fever	*Streptobacillus moniliformis*	Rodents	Bite wounds	Occasional	Influenza-like symptoms	Worldwide
Salmonellosis	*Salmonella* spp.	Mammals, birds, herps	Fecal-oral	Common	Gastroenteritis	Worldwide
Tickborne relapsing fever (Lyme disease)	*Borrelia* spp.	Small mammals	Tick bites	Rare	Relapsing fever	Worldwide, except Australia
Tuberculosis	*Mycobacterium* spp.	Hoofed mammals, birds	Aerosol	Occasional	Pulmonary disorders	Worldwide

Disease	Agent	Reservoir	Transmission	Occurrence	Signs	Distribution
Tularemia	*Francisella tularensis*	Rodents, lagomorphs, ticks	Tick bites, wound infection	Occasional	Ulcer, lymphadenopathy, pneumonia, gastroenteritis	Northern hemisphere
Yersiniosis	*Yersinia* spp.	Mammals, birds	Fecal-oral	Common	Mesenteric lymphadenitis, enteritis	Worldwide
Mycoses						
Aspergillosis	*Aspergillus fumigatus*	Mammals, birds	Airborne	Rare	Pulmonary disorders	Worldwide
Dermatophytosis (ringworm)	*Microsporum* and *Trichophyton* spp.	Mammals, birds	Contact	Common	Dermatitis	Worldwide
Chlamydioses and Rickettsioses						
Chlamydiosis	*Chlamydia psittaci*	Birds	Aerosol	Sporadic	Respiratory disease	Worldwide
Fleaborne typhus fever	*Rickettsia typhi*	Rodents	Flea bites	Sporadic	Fever, macular eruption	Worldwide
Q fever	*Coxiella burnetti*	Bovids, other mammals	Aerosol, handling infected tissues	Rare	Fever, headaches, pneumonitis	Worldwide
Rocky Mountain spotted fever	*Rickettsia rickettsii*	Rodents, lagomorphs, marsupials	Tick bites	Sporadic	Fever, macular lesions	Western hemisphere
Viruses						
California encephalitis, Colorado tick fever, Eastern equine encephalitis, St. Louis encephalitis, Western equine encephalitis, Venezuelan encephalitis	Arboviruses	Mammals, birds, reptiles	Mosquitoes	Sporadic	Influenza-like symptoms, encephalitis	Worldwide

Continued.

TABLE 30-1 Zoonotic diseases in North American wildlife—cont'd

Disease	Cause	Species*	Transmission†	Occurrence‡	Clinical Syndrome§	Geographic Distribution
Influenza	Myxovirus	Swine	Aerosol	Not known	Fever, respiratory disorders, myalgia	Worldwide
Lymphocytic choriomeningitis	RNA arenavirus	Rodents	Contact with animals, excreta or bite wounds	Sporadic	Influenza, meningitis	Worldwide
Newcastle disease	Paramyxovirus	Birds	Aerosol, contact	Occasional	Conjunctivitis	Worldwide
Rabies	RNA virus	Mammals (birds?)	Bite wounds	Sporadic	Neurologic signs, fatal	All continents except Australia
Rotaviral enteritis	Rotavirus	Young hoofed animals, suckling mice, and rabbits	Fecal-oral	Not known	Enteritis	Worldwide
Vesicular stomatitis	Rhabdovirus	Hoofed mammals, other mammals	Contact	Sporadic	Influenza-like symptoms	Western hemisphere
Parasitoses						
Hydatid disease	*Echinococcus* spp.	Carnivores	Fecal-oral	Sporadic	Space-occupying lesion	Worldwide
Cerebral larval migrans	*Baylisascaris procynis*	Raccoons	Fecal-oral	Rare?	Central nervous system signs	North America
Scabies	*Sarcoptes* spp.	Mammals	Contact	Common	Pruritic dermatitis	Worldwide
Strongyloidiasis	*Strongyloides* spp.	Carnivores	Infected soil	Sporadic	Dermatitis, enteritis, pneumonia	Worldwide
Toxoplasmosis	*Toxoplasma gondii*	Felids, all warm-blooded animals	Ingestion	Infection common, disease uncommon	Congenital toxoplasmosis lymphadenopathy	Worldwide
Visceral larval migrans	*Toxocara* spp., *Baylisascaris* spp.	Carnivores	Fecal-oral (soil)	Sporadic	Hepatomegaly, pneumonitis, ocular granuloma	Worldwide
Zoonotic filariasis	*Dirofilaria* spp.	Canids, procyonids	Mosquitoes	Rare	Nodular lung lesions	Worldwide

*Major nonhuman species affected.
†Route of infection for people.
‡Relative occurrence of disease transmission from animals to people.
§Major clinical syndrome in people.
Modified with permission from Siemering H. Zoonoses, In: Fowler ME, ed. Zoo and wild animal medicine, Philadelphia: WB Saunders, 1986:65-67.

AVOID STRESSING THE PATIENT

Each time you disturb or handle a wild animal for diagnostic work the animal is subjected to a great deal of stress. It is crucial to perform all examinations and treatments as rapidly and accurately as possible. Bright lights and loud noises are additional stressors, and should be limited to those that are a necessary part of the examination.

Frequently, the presence of a wildlife patient will bring curious staff and friends. Such visits should be firmly discouraged, as the stress is harmful to the patient, and there is always the risk of human injury.

If the wild patient requires medication and is eating, oral medications are frequently preferred because one can reduce the stress of unnecessary handling.

CHEMICAL RESTRAINT

When dealing with wild mammals of any size you must be prepared for early and prompt chemical restraint. If inhalation anesthesia is an option, most birds can be simply administered an anesthetic by mask (masked down). Dim light and quiet surroundings will facilitate this process. Isoflurane is clearly the agent of choice because of its rapid induction and recovery times, lack of sensitization of the myocardium, and low toxicity. Halothane, methoxyflurane, and other agents can be safe in experienced hands. Paying attention to maintaining body temperature and cardiac monitoring will result in many more successful procedures. Smaller mammals can often be anesthetized by using an anesthetic induction box, fish tank, or other closed container for induction. However, these animals must be watched closely, as they can quickly reach undesirable depths of anesthesia. Following anesthesia induction, intubation should be performed, if possible. This is a straightforward procedure in most reptiles and birds, in which the glottis is rostral in the oral cavity (Fig. 30-2). But this can be difficult in some mammals, notably rabbits and rodents, in which the mouth does not open widely and the glottis is far to the rear. With practice, laboratory animal veterinarians can often intubate these animals blindly once they have been masked down. But for visual intubation, the stylet method works well. The glottis is visualized with a very small laryngoscope or rigid endoscope and a tube (stylet) of small enough diameter that it does not obstruct the lumen is threaded into the trachea (a small-gauge urinary catheter works well). The endotracheal tube is then placed over the stylet and is gently rotated into place in the glottis. Once the endotracheal tube is seated, the stylet is removed.[15]

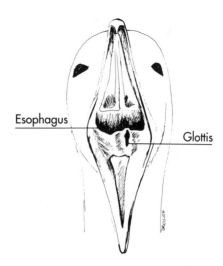

Fig. 30-2 Appearance of avian glottis.

In many situations, injectable tranquilizers or anesthetics are desirable. In the discussions of various taxonomic groups, Fowler[14] gives specific recommendations on injectable agents. Telazol is increasingly popular for immobilizing a variety of species. Ketamine or combinations of ketamine with xylazine, acepromazine, or diazepam have been used successfully in most animal groups. Ketamine or the combination of ketamine-diazepam is absorbed well across the oral mucosa and can be squirted into the mouths of fractious animals in the same dosages that one would use for intramuscular or intravenous administration.

Table 30-2 contains guidelines for the dosage of a 50:50 (by volume) mixture of ketamine (100 mg/ml) and xylazine (20 mg/ml) for intramuscular

TABLE 30-2 Immobilization doses for a 50:50 mixture (by volume) of ketamine (100 mg/ml) and xylazine (20 mg/ml)*

Body Weight of Animal	Volume of Ketamine-Xylazine (ml) to Immobilize	Volume Required per Kilogram Body Weight
30 g	0.01-0.02ml	0.33 ml/kg
100 g	0.03-0.06ml	0.3 ml/kg
1kg	0.15-0.30ml	0.15 ml/kg
10kg	0.9-2.0 ml	0.1 ml/kg
100kg	4.75-10 ml	0.04 ml/kg
1000kg	25-50 ml	0.025ml/kg

*In general, birds will use doses at the high end of the recommended volumes.

Volumes can be decreased by using xylazine sold in concentrations of 100 mg/ml. Then the xylazine is used in only one fifth the volume of the ketamine.

immobilization purposes. As with many drugs there is some variation in species sensitivity. For example, barred owls *(Strix varia),* are very sensitive to this mixture and must be dosed at about one fourth of the recommended rate. On the other hand, pigeons *(Columba livia)* are resistant and must often be given two to three times the expected dose. Rabbits and rodents are notoriously tolerant of ketamine and must often receive at least twice the expected dose (or roughly 35 to 60 mg of ketamine/kg). Millichamp[16] gives an excellent review of chemical immobilization for reptiles. When using ketamine in crocodilians he recommends a rate of 12 to 25 mg/kg, while 50 or more mg/kg may be needed in other reptile taxa.

DIAGNOSTIC—DATA BASE

Once the decision has been made to begin treatment, a clinical data base should be obtained as rapidly as possible with minimum stress to the patient. This data base should include a thorough physical examination, basic laboratory evaluations (packed cell volume/total serum proteins, blood glucose concentration, and complete blood count) and lateral and dorsoventral whole-body radiography.

Even large wounds can be difficult to find beneath feathers and fur, so a diligent search is often in order. Radiography is an important early step in the assessment of injured wildlife and will often reveal lead shot or other foreign materials, fractures, and changes in position or morphology of the viscera due to trauma, parasites, and disease. It is not unusual to find old, partially healed fractures that may contribute to an animal's debility. Low-velocity projectiles (B-Bs, lead pellets, etc.) often carry a plug of skin, fur, or feathers into visceral structures. This will serve as a major nidus of infection.

Injured animals may survive in the wild for extended periods before being found. In these cases the initial injury may be much less significant than secondary effects of starvation, dehydration, and hypothermia or hyperthermia.

NEUROLOGIC ASSESSMENT

Assessing the neurologic status of wildlife patients is difficult. Wild animals, when in captivity and the presence of people, are acutely stressed. Each species tends to behave in a predictable manner. Some animals become aggressive, while others curl up and try to remain inconspicuous. Captive wildlife may exhibit misleading neurologic signs, including muscular rigidity; lack of response to visual, auditory, or tactile cues; and blunted pupillary light response, limb withdrawal, or deep pain recognition caused by the animal's fear and elevated sympathetic tone. It is a mistake to assume that a wild animal that is immobile is paralyzed or unaware of your presence.

Birds and most other nonmammalian vertebrates demonstrate only the direct pupillary light response. Absence of the consensual response is normal. The pupillary muscles of birds are made up of striated rather than smooth muscle. Mydriatics typically used in mammals will have no ophthalmic effect, but may have undesirable systemic sequelae. Snakes have a clear scale covering the eyes (the spectacle), which mydriatics and ophthalmic medications cannot normally penetrate.

Often, the only way to assess vision or other neurologic function accurately is to observe the activity of the animal in a large outdoor enclosure. It is important that observers cannot be seen, heard, or smelled by the animal.

PAIN ASSESSMENT

It is common for wildlife patients to be presented with massive injuries and yet still be alert and functional. You should not assume that these animals are not in pain. Because predators selectively prey on animals that are sick or injured, wild animals have evolved a remarkable ability to mask pain and injury. Wild animals should be appropriately anesthetized for any planned procedures that can be anticipated to produce pain.

The alleviation of "invisible" pain can be of major therapeutic benefit in treatment of these animals. This therapy can make the difference between an animal that eats and one that does not. Narcotic analgesics, salicylates, and other nonsteroidal antiinflammatory drugs (NSAIDs) can be used at dosages similar to those used for related taxa of domestic animals. Although effective dosages of NSAIDs appear to scale in accordance with metabolic rate this is *not* true of the opioids. Dosage of the narcotics cannot be effectively extrapolated and must be arrived at through laboratory or clinical trials. Care must also be taken with opioids to avoid undesirable effects on the respiratory and gastrointestinal systems. It is common for animals in pain to become anorectic when given opiates. In addition, most opioids have too short a half-life to make their use as analgesics practical for wildlife species. However, buprenorphine is reported to possess good analgesic properties and a significantly longer (6 to 12 hours) duration of action in some mammalian species.[17,18] Wild feline species should be assumed to have all the drug sensitivities of their domestic counterparts.

METABOLISM AS RELATED TO TAXONOMIC GROUP AND BODY SIZE

Physiologists noted over a century ago that animals' resting metabolic rates vary according to the size of the animal and to its taxonomic group. In addition, it has been found that within a taxonomic group small animals use energy proportionally faster than larger animals. Energy utilization has been shown to be related to body mass to the 0.75 power.[19,20]

For the vast majority of terrestrial vertebrates this resting metabolism, or minimum energy cost (MEC), may be calculated with the following formula:

$$MEC \text{ (kcal/24 hours)} = K (W_{kg})^{0.75}$$

where W_{kg} = the animal's body weight in kilograms; K = a taxonomically specific constant derived from research data (10 for reptiles, 49 for marsupials, 70 for placental mammals, 78 for non-passerine birds and 129 for passerine birds).[19,20]

Rates of metabolism can critically influence the uptake, distribution, and excretion of drugs as well as nutrients. Some researchers have therefore begun extrapolating drug dose and treatment interval or frequency for nondomestic animals based on calculated metabolic rates rather than the traditional extrapolation based on body mass.[21,22] The dose rates for ketamine/xylazine as shown in Table 30-2 were derived by this method. Note that the dose per kilogram body weight decreases rapidly with an increase in animal size. Appendix IV contains a sample calculation for deriving a drug dose based on metabolic rate.

METABOLIC TIME

Calder[19] states "that there are two kinds of time scales, absolute time and size-dependent relative time (physiological time)." If one looks at groups of similar animals that vary only in size (e.g. felines, raptors, etc.), certain generalizations can be made:

1. Smaller species have higher heart rates and respiratory rates,
2. Smaller species have higher basal metabolic rates and consume a higher percentage of their body weight in food daily,
3. Smaller species mature faster, have shorter gestation periods, reproduce more frequently, and have shorter lifespans,
4. Smaller species have shorter induction and recovery times from anesthesia, and
5. Smaller species become hypothermic more rapidly during anesthesia.
6. Large species are more prone to malignant hyperthermia and capture myopathy.

One way to unify all these concepts is to consider that smaller species are living at a faster rate and have a greater relative surface area than larger ones. The challenge for clinicians treating a broad taxonomic diversity of animals is to appreciate and quantify this variation.

One of the most useful indicators for measuring depth of anesthesia is heart rate. The resting heart rate of placental mammals can be estimated from the equation $241 M^{-0.25}$ (M = mass in kilograms) and that of birds scales according to $156 M^{-0.23}$.[19] These formula allow us to calculate the resting heart rates for most species. A functional definition of bradycardia can be considered as any heart rate more than 20% below the calculated rate.

A knowledge of metabolic time is critical for successful anesthetic technique. It is said that humans can live for about 5 minutes without oxygen before sustaining brain damage[23] and dogs can survive for about 4 minutes under the same conditions.[24] According to metabolic time, this indicates that any vertebrate should be able to live for about 500 heartbeats before serious central nervous system damage occurs (Sedgwick, personal communication). We know that birds have slower heart rates than mammals of the same mass. Calculating the heart rate for a 6-kg raptor reveals that it should have a resting heart rate of around 100 beats per minute. A 50-g raptor, on the other hand would have a calculated heart rate of 310 beats per minute. The large raptor should survive about 5 minutes without oxygen, but our smaller patient would suffer irreversible damage in 2 minutes or less. Physiologically then, every minute on the surgical table for our 6-kg raptor is metabolically equivalent to 3 minutes of surgical time for the 50-g bird. Therefore, in planning the length of stressful procedures with small patients we must remember to pay attention to the metabolic clock, not the one on the wall. A 1-hour surgery on the tiny bird could be expected to cause the same amount of physiologic stress as subjecting the larger raptor to a 3-hour procedure.

Our smaller patients have proportionately more surface area from which to lose heat than our larger patients. Anesthesia eliminates our patients' ability to generate heat by movement, shivering, or other adaptive actions. In addition, we often ventilate these small patients with relatively cool, dry gases. Thus, before we make our initial incision these small animals may be hypothermic and rapidly losing water from respiratory surfaces. Surgical incision eliminates the insulative protection of an animal's fur or feathers and drastically increases the surface area available for cooling and evaporative water loss. It is apparent that the provision of external sources of heat and moisture are especially critical to surgical success with small patients. Most manufacturers of anesthesia equipment sell modules for the provision of warmed, humidified inspired gases.

FLUID THERAPY

Fluids are often a critical component of emergency therapy for wildlife patients. Routes of fluid administration are no different for wildlife species than for domestic animals. However, since wildlife patients are much less tolerant of handling and often will not retain catheters or intravenous lines, the clinician must often resort to bolus or depot methods of fluid administration. Advances in the use of intraosseus fluid administration[25] may provide a new tool for treating critical wildlife patients. Caution must be taken to avoid using this technique in fractured bones or any of the pneumatic bones that connect to the respiratory system of many birds.

Fluid requirements vary dramatically across taxonomic lines. As a generalization, one can say that small species or species with higher metabolic rates have higher fluid requirements per unit mass. Quantitatively, most species have a daily water requirement of between 0.75 and 1.5 ml of water for each kilocalorie of basal energy required.[26] Thus, a 250-kg bear would require about 4.5 L of water daily ($\pm$0.02% of body weight), a 500-g turtle would require about 6 ml ($\pm$1% of body weight) per day, a 150-g owl would require about 20 ml of water daily ($\pm$13% of body weight), while a 30-g mouse would require about 6 ml ($\pm$20% of body weight). Note that these water requirements include not only liquid water, but preformed water (contained in food) and metabolic water as well.[26]

In birds, intravenous fluids can be given in a number of locations depending on the species anatomy. With practice the (right) jugular vein is readily accessible and large volumes of fluids may be given rapidly. The medial metatarsal vein running on the inside of the leg between the ankle and the toes is convenient in many species. The cutaneous ulnar (or basilic) vein runs subcutaneously on the ventral aspect of the elbow and is easy to identify, but it is thin walled and subject to hematoma formation. These three sites are also useful for blood sample collection (see Chapter 28).

Birds are very tolerant to rapid rates of fluid administration.[27] As a rule of thumb, birds can be given up to 5% of their body weight in intravenous emergency fluids in 1 to 2 minutes (50 ml/kg)—almost as rapidly as the plunger can be depressed. In less than critical situations, or when a bird's cardiac or respiratory status may be in doubt, 2.5% of the body weight in intravenous emergency fluids is indicated. With such rapid rates of administration, careful observation of the patient is essential. Monitoring the regularity of respiratory and cardiac rate and rhythm will give valuable clues. Restlessness or rapid movements

of the head or eyes may signal circulatory collapse or overhydration. Although pulmonary edema is a potential danger, it rarely occurs. In the absence of acid-base information, lactated Ringer's solution is generally considered to be the fluid of choice.

In many cases, intravenous fluid therapy may not be necessary. In our experience, birds absorb water, electrolytes, and simple sugars very rapidly from the upper gastrointestinal tract. So for cases in which intravenous therapy may not be desirable, because of the bird's temperament or because veins are not readily accessible, gavage may be the preferable technique (Fig. 30-3). Published volumes for gavage of psittacines tend to be much larger than most wild birds will tolerate without regurgitation and aspiration. On first attempt, it is reasonable to attempt to gavage 5 ml into a 100-g bird and 15 to 20 ml into a 1000-g species. If this is well tolerated, volumes can be gradually increased during later treatments.

Subcutaneous fluids can be readily given to birds by using the relatively loose skin dorsally between the scapulae, in the wing web (patagium), or just craniodorsal to the patella.

It can be difficult to administer intravenous fluids to reptiles. If adequate restraint is possible, most reptiles can be readily gavaged (although many species readily regurgitate). Luckily, many reptiles that are mildly to moderately dehydrated will self-rehydrate if provided a large pan of water in which to soak. For parenteral use, Jarchow[28] recommends a slightly hypotonic solution to facilitate intracellular diffusion (2 parts 2.5% dextrose in 0.45% sodium chloride and 1 part Ringer's or the equivalent electrolyte solution). He also describes techniques for administering in-

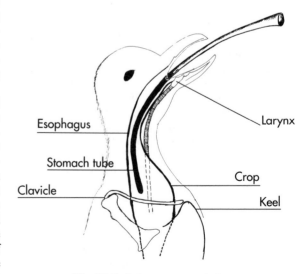

Fig. 30-3 Avian gavage technique.

traperitoneal fluids to reptiles. Fluids administered as an intracolonic bolus (rectal administration) are absorbed rapidly and may be life saving.

AVIAN BLOOD TRANSFUSION

It is considered relatively safe to perform single, unmatched transfusions in avian emergencies. Blood can be taken in heparinized syringes from pigeons, or from large donors such as geese, and given as a slow intravenous injection. This procedure can be life saving. Although reactions to a single transfusion are rare, patients should be observed for any adverse signs (see Chapter 28).

ORPHANS

A wildlife rehabilitator's definition of an orphan is, "any young animal that couldn't run faster than the person trying to catch it." The vast majority of baby animals that the public "rescues" during the spring and summer are not in need of help. They are usually normal young animals that were doing just what they were supposed to be doing. In 99% of the cases, the right approach is to put the baby animal back exactly where it was found and go away. Almost certainly, if left alone the parents will return to feed the young. The finders may assure you that they watched for wildlife parents, but that no adult animals appeared. Adult animals will typically hide until the intruders leave.

What about the situation in which a tiny baby bird (unfeathered, eyes closed, unable to hop around) has fallen out of the nest? Assuming that it is active and not hypothermic, it is prudent to put the orphan right back into the nest as soon as possible (it is a myth that birds will smell your scent and reject the baby).

Certainly, there are times when young animals are injured or are genuinely orphaned. In these situations, rapidly get the orphan to a licensed wildlife rehabilitator who is experienced with baby wildlife.

If it will be an hour or more until the orphan gets to the rehabilitator, you (or the finders) need to ensure its proper care. The two critical factors are warmth and food.

A baby bird can be kept warm for a short period with a hot water bottle, heating pad, or overhead lamp. Room temperature is inadequate unless the bird is quite well feathered and almost big enough to fly. These birds have normal body temperatures of 104 to 108°F. Maintaining a moderate humidity can also help to prevent problems of dehydration.

There are many diets described for nestling passerines. Finely ground, canned dog food (or dog kibbles broken up and soaked in water until they soften) provide adequate short-term nutrition. Small bits of food are placed far back in the birds mouth when they gape. Typically, passerines need to be fed all they will consume about every 15 to 20 minutes from dawn to dusk.

If young birds do not gape for food, the likelihood is either that you are dealing with a species that does not normally gape (such as a dove), or that the baby is hypothermic or ill. If hypothermia is the problem, 15 to 20 minutes of gentle warming should markedly improve the activity and attitude of the nestling.

Do not give nestlings any oral liquids. They will invariably aspirate and develop a fatal pneumonia. Baby passerines obtain their water from metabolism of food.

Doves, swifts, woodpeckers, and some other birds do not beg (gape), and have very different dietary requirements. Species identification is critical in devising proper diets; local nature centers and Audubon societies will be able to provide help if you need it.

In emergency situations most orphan carnivores may be given artificial milk products designed for puppies or kittens until a more suitable diet is determined. For herbivorous orphans, goat's milk is often well tolerated.

REGULATORY AGENCIES GOVERNING THE HANDLING OF WILDLIFE

It is important for veterinarians to be familiar with the laws governing the species with which they work. In many areas of the country Good Samaritan regulations allow any licensed veterinarian to administer emergency aid to injured wildlife. However, if you wish to work on wildlife on a regular basis it is strongly advised that you obtain the appropriate state and federal permits. Most agencies are interested in encouraging veterinary assistance, and you will find them straightforward and cooperative.

Federal regulations protect many species. The U.S. Fish and Wildlife Service (USFWS, Department of the Interior) issues permits for anyone working with migratory birds (except pigeons, starlings, and house sparrows) and most federally endangered animals. All marine mammals and sea turtles are protected by the National Marine Fisheries Service (NMFS, National Oceanographic and Atmospheric Administration), and you should contact them for treatment and permit information. Appendix V contains a listing of federal wildlife agencies. Garbe[29] contains an excellent review of U.S. laws regarding wildlife species.

In addition to federal regulations, most states have their own regulations and statutes protecting various species. These may vary significantly from state to state.

CONCLUSION

In summary, there is no reason that veterinary clinicians interested in treating wildlife emergencies should not be encouraged to do so. The training and expertise that veterinarians have developed in their professional careers can be an important supplement to efforts to preserve and rehabilitate our native wildlife species.

APPENDIX I

Causes for emergency presentation of wildlife species at rehabilitation centers: results of a survey of 50 centers in the United States, Canada, and Great Britain.*†

Taxa	Cause of Injury	Type of Injury	Comments
Amphibians and reptiles	Trauma H, P	Fx	Many lawnmower injuries
Marine birds (loons, alcids, cormorants, pelicans, etc.)	Trauma H, G, P, Pl/F[1] Medical T, O, D, Ps[2]	Fx, ST, Pouch L[1] Erysipelas, E[2]	[1]Only trauma (cormorant and pelican) [2]Only medical (cormorant and pelican)
Waterfowl	Trauma F, G, P, H Medical Pl, O, T, D Juveniles and orphans	ST, Fx Avian cholera, aspergillosis, botulism Starvation	
Shorebirds	Trauma W, H, P Medical D, Ps, T Juveniles and orphans	Fx, ST Avian botulism, E	
Raptors	Trauma H, G, W, Tr, Fi, F Medical T, Ps, D Juveniles and orphans	Fx, ST E, trichomoniasis	
Gulls, terns, herons, ibises, etc.	Trauma G, H, Pl/F, Tr[3] Medical Ps, T, D, O	ST, Fx, gastrointestinal E, aspergillosis, septicemia	[3]Herons and ibises only
Passerines, galliformes, pigeons, and doves	Trauma H,[4] P, G[5] Medical T,[6] Ps,[6] D[6]	Fx, ST E, septicemia, trichomoniasis, avian pox	[4]Includes window impact [5]Passerines not affected [6]Galliformes not affected, order in pigeons: Ps, T, D
Marsupials, procyonids, and artiodactyls	Trauma H, P, G, F Medical E[7] D,[8] Ps[8] Juveniles and orphans[11]	Fx, ST Distemper,[9] rabies, parvovirus (bluetongue, EHDV, pasteurellosis, cerebrospinal parelaphostrongylosis[10])	[7]Artiodactyls only, before gunshot [8]Marsupials excepted [9]In procyonids [10]Artiodactyls only [11]Before medical in artiodactyls
Bats	Trauma P, G Medical T, D	Wing Fx Rabies	
Rodents and rabbits	Trauma P, H Juveniles and orphans, Fall[12] Medical D, Ps	ST, Fx Spinal trauma Myxomatosis, mange	[12]Squirrels only, from nest

Causes for emergency presentation of wildlife species at rehabilitation centers: results of a survey of 50 centers in the United States, Canada, and Great Britain.*†

Taxa	Cause of Injury	Type of Injury	Comments
Canids, felids, and mustelids	Trauma H, Tr, P,[13] G[14] Medical S,[15] D, T,[16] Ps[17] Juveniles and orphans	Fx, ST, eye trauma[14] Distemper, rabies, parvovirus,[18] mange[18]	[13]Felids excepted [14]Felids only [15]Felids only [16]Felids excepted [17]Canids only [18]Mustelids excepted
Seals, other marine mammals	Juveniles and orphans Medical Ps, D Trauma G, Boats, Fi, nets	 Seal pox, pneumonia, liver disease, lung worms, leptospirosis ST	Seals primarily

H = hit by machine (usually car); P = predation by house pets; Fx = fractures; G = gunshot; Pl = plastic entanglement; ST = soft-tissue injury (lacerations); pouch L = pouch laceration; T = toxicity; O = oil covered; D = disease; Ps = parasites; W = hit overhead wires; E = emaciation; Tr = trapped; Fi = fighting, EHDV = epizootic hemorrhagic disease virus; F = fishhook; S = starvation.

*Animal taxa are grouped according to the similarity of injury categories reported. Within each taxonomic grouping causes of injury are listed beginning with most common types of injuries. For example, in water fowl, traumatic injuries were more common than medical problems and within the category Trauma, fishhook injuries were the most common, followed in decreasing frequency by gunshot, predation, and hit by car.

†Due to the enormous range of species, differences in location and public awareness, and variations in the method of reporting by survey participants, this listing should be used primarily as an indication of what the wildlife veterinarian may see. The experience of individual organizations may differ from the compiled data. Only the most common types of injury reported for each taxon could be included for reasons of space. Please note that when a particular family or species is excepted from a category, the implication is that the category is not the most common for that animal, not that it never occurs. Not all families are represented, due to infrequency of presentation for treatment.

APPENDIX II
Wildlife-related organizations

American Association of Wildlife Veterinarians
Dr. Elizabeth Williams
c/o Wyoming State Diagnostic Lab
Box 950
Laramie, WY 82070

American Association of Zoo Veterinarians
c/o Dr. Wilbur Amand
34th St. and Girard Ave.
Philadelphia, PA 19104

Association of Avian Veterinarians
P.O. Box 299
East Northport, NY 11731
International Association for Aquatic Animal Medicine
c/o Dr. M. Solangi
Institute for Marine Mammals
P.O. Box 4078
Gulfport, MS 39502

Wildlife Disease Association
P.O. Box 886
Ames, IA 50010

National rehabilitators organizations:

National Wildlife Rehabilitators Association
Treehouse Wildlife Ctr.
RR 1 Box 125 E
Brighton, IL 62012

International Wildlife Rehabilitation Council
P.O. Box 3007
Walnut Creek, CA 94598

APPENDIX III
Sources of equipment and supplies
Capture equipment

Addison Biological Laboratories, Inc. (blowguns)
Rte. 3, Box 16
Fayette, MO 65248

Kay Research Products (pole syringes)
1525 E. 53rd St., Suite 503
Chicago, IL 60615

Palmer Chemical Equipment Co. (dart guns)
Palmer Village
P.O. Box 8671
Douglasville, GA 30134

Paxarms Ltd. (dart guns)
P.O. Box 317
Timaru, New Zealand

Zoolu Arms of Omaha (dart guns, pole syringes)
10315 Wright St.
Omaha, NB 68124

Capture and handling tools

Animal Care Equipment and Services (wide range of capture and handling equipment)
22895 Valley View Dr.
P.O. Box 3275
Crestline, CA 92325

Animal Technology (squeeze cages)
23655 San Fernanado Rd.
Newhall, CA 91321-3189

Furhman Diversified (heavy gloves, capture nets, reptile handling equipment)
905 S. 8th St.
La Porte, TX 77571

J.A. Cissel (capture nets, cage netting)
P.O. Box 339
Farmingdale, NJ 07727-0339

Ketch-All Co. (heavy gloves)
Department of VMA
2537 University Ave.
San Diego, CA 92104

NASCO (wide range of restraint equipment)
901 Janesville Ave.
Fort Atkinson, WI 53538

One of a Kind (gloves)
327 E. Lake St.
Horicon, WI 53032

Research Equipment Co., Inc. (squeeze cages)
P.O. Box 1151
Bryan, TX 77801

Live traps

Safe-N-Sound Live Traps
116 Main St.
Garrison, IA 52229

Tomahawk Live Trap Co.
P.O. Box 323 W
Tomahawk, WI 54487

Heating units

Animal Spectrum Inc. (infra-red heaters)
P.O. Box 6307
Lincoln, NB 68506-0307

Animal Technology (heated sleeping platforms)
23655 San Fernanado Rd.
Newhall, CA 91321-3198

Gorman-Rupp Industries Div. (circulating water blankets)
Belleville, OH 4813

Broad-spectrum lighting

SunBox Co. (Vitalite)
1037 Taft St.
Rockville, MD 20850

Sylvania Corp. (Gro-lux light)
Danvers, MA 01923

Cole endotracheal tubes

Rusch, Inc.
New York, NY 10000

APPENDIX IV
Scaling drug dosages

Assume that you would like to administer a drug to an unusual species, say, a 450-g turtle.

1. Find a model species in the literature, one for which laboratory pharmacokinetic studies of this drug have been performed. For example, in 10-kg dogs it was determined that this drug needed to be administered twice a day at 15 mg/kg to maintain effective blood levels.

2. Convert the typical (mg/kg) dose to a metabolically based dose (mg/kcal), remembering that the constants (K) are 129 for passerine birds, 78 for nonpasserines, 70 for placental mammals, 49 for marsupials, and 10 for reptiles at their optimal body temperature and that minimal effective concentration (MEC) = K × mass $(kg)^{0.75}$.

   a. Calculate MEC for 10-kg dogs: $70(10)^{0.75}$ = 393.6 kcal/day, where 70 is the constant for placental mammals and 10 is the animal's weight in kilograms

   b. Dose for 10-kg dog = 15 mg × 10 kg = 150 mg/treatment.

   c. *MEC dose* = 150 mg ÷ 393.6 kcal = 0.38 mg/kcal.

3. Determine required periodicity of dosing.

   a. Calculate MEC for patient (turtle): $10(0.45)^{0.75}$ = 5.4 kcal/day.

   b. Calculate the mass specific metabolic rate (SMEC) for both control (c) species (dog) and subject (s) species (turtle):

   Dog: $SMEC_c$ = 393.6 *kcal/day*

   10 *kg* = 39.4 *kcal/kg*

   Turtle: $SMEC_s$ = 5.4 *kcal/day*

   0.45 *kg* = 12 *kcal/kg*

   c. The treatment interval for the dog (T_c) was 12 hours. Therefore, the treatment interval for the turtle (TS) is

   $$T_s = T_c \times (SMEC_c \div SMEC_s)$$
   $$= 12 \ hr \times (39.4 \div 12)$$
   $$= 39.4 \ hours$$

We would then dose this 450-g turtle a total of 5.4 kcal × 0.38 mg/kcal = 2 mg once every ± 36 hours

NOTE: This method for calculating drug dosages can in no way predict metabolic peculiarities of particular species.

APPENDIX V
Federal wildlife agencies
U.S. fish and wildlife service regional offices (U.S. Department of the Interior)

Northwest Regional Office—Region 1
(CA, HI, ID, NV, OR, WA)
Multnomah St., Suite 1692
Portland, OR 97232
503-231-6118

Southwest Regional Office—Region 2
(AZ, NM, OK, TX)
500 Gold Ave. SW, Rm. 3018
Albuquerque, NM 87102
505-766-2321

Great Lakes Regional Office—Region 3
(IA, IL, IN, MI, MN, MO, OH, WI)
Federal Bldg.
Fort Snelling
Twin Cities, MN 55111
612-725-3563

Southeast Regional Office—Region 4 (AL, AR,
FL, GA, KY, LA, MS, NC, PR, SC, TN, VI)
Richard B. Russell Federal Bldg.
75 Spring St. SW, Rm. 1200
Atlanta, GA 30303
404-331-3588

Northeast Regional Office—Region 5 (CT, DC, DE,
MA, MD, NH, NJ, NY, PA, RI, VA, VT, WV)
One Gateway Ctr., Suite 700
Newton Corner, MA 02158
617-965-5100

Rocky Mountain Regional Office—Region 6
(CO, KS, MT, ND, NE, SD, UT, WY)
134 Union Blvd.
P.O. Box 25486, Denver Federal Ctr.
Denver, CO 80225
303-236-7920

Alaska Regional Office—Region 7 (AK)
1011 E. Tudor Rd.
Anchorage, AK 99503
907-786-3542

National marine fisheries service (NMFS) regional offices (U.S. Department of Commerce, National Oceanic and Atmospheric Administration)

Northwest Regional Office NMFS
7600 Sand Point Way, NE
BIN C15700, Bldg. 1
Seattle, WA 98115-0070
206-526-6150

Southwest Regional Office NMFS
300 South Ferry St.
Terminal Island, CA 90731
213-514-6196

Northeast Regional Office NMFS
14 Elm St.
Federal Bldg.
Gloucester, MA 01930
617-281-3600

Southeast Regional Office NMFS
9450 Koger Blvd.
St. Petersburg, FL 33702
813-893-3141

Alaska Regional Office NMFS
P.O. Box 1668
Juneau, AK 99802
907-586-7221

REFERENCES

1. Frink L, Frink J. A new approach to records analysis in a wild bird rehabilitation center. In Beaver P, Mackey DM. Wildlife rehabilitation, vol. 5. Brighton, IL: National Wildlife Rehabilitators, 1986.
2. Barten SL. Common problems among reptiles presented to rehabilitation centers. In Beaver P, Mackey DM. Wildlife rehabilitation, vol. 5. Brighton, IL: National Wildlife Rehabilitators, 1986.
3. May RM. Control of feline delinquency. Nature 1988;332:392-393.
4. Kenward RE. Mortality and fate of trained birds of prey. J Wildl Manage 1974;38:751-756.
5. Macdonald JW. Mortality in wild birds. Bird Study 1965-66;11-12:181-195.
6. Jackson DD. Nobody counts squashed skunks. Audubon. 1986;March:78-81.
7. Jennings AR. An analysis of 1000 deaths in wild birds. Int Ornithol Congr Proc 1963;61:353-357.
8. Terres JK. Diseases of birds—how and why some birds die. Am Birds 1981;35:255-260.
9. Durham K. Injuries to birds of prey caught in leghold traps. Int J Study Anim Probl 1981;2:317-328.
10. Franzmann AW. Wildlife medicine. In Fowler M, ed. Zoo and wild animal medicine. Philadelphia: WB Saunders, 1986;8-11.
11. Cooper JE, Gibson L, Jones CG. The assessment of health in casualty birds of prey intended for release. Vet Rec 1980;106:340-341.
12. Landercasper J, et al. Trauma and the veterinarian. J Trauma 1988;28:1255-1259.
13. Fowler ME. Restraint and handling of wild and domestic animals. Ames, IA: Iowa State University Press, 1978.
14. Fowler ME, ed. Zoo and wild animal medicine. Philadelphia: WB Saunders, 1984.
15. Sedgwick CJ. Anesthesia for small nondomestic mammals. In Jacobson ER, Kollias GV. Exotic animals. New York: Churchill Livingstone, 1988;223-228.
16. Millichamp NJ. Surgical techniques in reptiles. In Jacobson ER, Kollias GV. Exotic animals. New York: Churchill Livingstone, 1988;49-74.
17. Flecknell PA. Laboratory animal anesthesia. San Diego: Academic Press, 1987;84-88.
18. Hall LW, Clarke KW. Veterinary anesthesia, ed. 8. East Sussex, England: Bailliere Tindall, 1983;65.
19. Calder WA III. Size, function and life history. Cambridge, MA: Harvard University Press, 1984.
20. Schmidt-Nielsen K. Scaling: why is animal size so important? New York: Cambridge University Press, 1984.
21. Gibbons G, Pokras MA, Sedgwick CJ. Allometric scaling and veterinary medicine. Aust Vet Pract 1989;18:160-164.
22. Pokras MA, Karas A, Kirkwood J, Sedgwick CJ. An introduction to allometric scaling and its uses in raptor medicine. Proceedings of the International Symposium on the Status of Biomedical Research on Raptors. In press.

23. Guyton AC. Textbook of medical physiology, ed. 6. Philadelphia: WB Saunders, 1981;342.

24. Hall LW, Clarke KW. Veterinary anesthesia, ed. 8. East Sussex, England: Bailliere Tindall, 1983;378.

25. Otto CM, Kaufman GM, Crowe DT. Intraosseus infusion of fluids and therapeutics. Compend Contin Educ Pract Vet 1989;11:421-431.

26. Robbins CT. Wildlife feeding and nutrition. New York: Academic Press. 1983.

27. Redig PT. Fluid therapy and acid-base balance in the critically ill avian patient. Proceedings of the International Conference on Avian, Medical Association of Avian Veterinarians. 1984;59-73.

28. Jarchow JL. Hospital care of the reptile patient. In Jacobson ER, Kollias GV. Exotic animals. New York: Churchill Livingstone, 1988;19-34.

29. Garbe JAL. Wildlife Law. In Wilson JF, ed. Law and ethics of the veterinary profession. Yardley, PA: Priority Press, 1988;376-410.

SUGGESTED READINGS

Barnard SM, Frank NCA. The role of the wildlife rehabilitator in the captive care of insectivorous bats. In Mackey DM, ed. Wildlife rehabilitation, vol. 6. Brighton, IL: National Wildlife Rehabilitators, 1987.

Cooper JE, Eley JT, eds. First aid and care of wild birds. North Pomfret, VT: David & Charles, 1979.

Friend M, ed. Field guide to wildlife diseases, vol. 1—General field procedures and diseases of migratory birds. Washington, DC: Government Printing Office, 1987. (US Fish and Wildlife Service resource publication no. 167.1987.)

Harkness JE, Wagner JE. The biology and medicine of rabbits and rodents, ed. 3. Philadelphia: Lea & Febiger, 1988.

SECTION THREE

Selected Topics in Critical Care

31 Wound Management in Small Animal Practice

Michael M. Pavletic

A wound is a break or loss of tissue continuity by violence or trauma. The severity of the injury is dependent on the strength and nature of the energy source, how it is dispersed, and the tissues absorbing it. Wounds involving the skin are the most common injuries seen by the veterinarian. Lacerations, shearing wounds, bite wounds, thermal injuries, and penetrating/perforating wounds are among the common forms of trauma. In essence, all wounds are the result of energy transfer to the body. The principles of healing and wound management are basically the same for all of these injuries. It is essential to understand the basic components of this vital process.

WOUND-HEALING PRINCIPLES

Following injury, the healing process can be divided into three phases: the inflammatory phase, the proliferative phase and the remodeling phase, occuring in conjunction with epithelialization and wound contraction. These divisions of healing are used for descriptive purposes only; the processes of healing are continuous under optimum conditions.[1]

Inflammatory phase

Inflammation is a cellular and vascular response to wounding, foreign debris, bacteria, and nonviable tissue. The degree of inflammation generally is proportional to the severity of the wound incurred and the ability of the body to respond. The classic signs of inflammation (redness, swelling, heat, and pain) are the result of vasodilation, fluid escape, and obstruction of local lymphatic channels. Transudation increases in magnitude for approximately 72 hours after injury.[1,2]

Polymorphonuclear cells and macrophages pass through gaps in venules by diapedesis and migrate into the wound. In an uncomplicated wound, the large population of polymorphs begins to subside by the fifth day as the longer-lived macrophages begin to dominate in numbers. It is now known that tissue macrophages play a critically important role in modulating wound healing.[1,2]

Macrophages engulf bacteria and macromolecules and are capable of surviving in the low-pH, hypoxemic environment of the wound. This environment stimulates the release of potent proteolytic enzymes from the lysosomes of granulocytes. These enzymes and collagenase break down damaged connective tissue. While the macrophage is operating in this infection-prone environment, it releases factors that promote fibroplasia and angiogenesis. The lactic acid released by macrophages in turn stimulates fibroblast proliferation (Fig. 31-1).[1,2]

Proliferative phase

In the above uncomplicated wound, fibroplasia begins 3 to 5 days after injury as the inflammatory phase winds down.[1,3] Fibrin and fibronectin form a filamentous scaffold for the fibroblasts to attach to as they begin to deposit collagen. As collagen is deposited, this fibrin-fibronectin network disappears. In all, the proliferative phase lasts for 2 to 4 weeks depending on the magnitude of the wound. The end of this phase is heralded by a decline of capillaries and fibroblasts as collagen fills the defect.[1]

Remodeling phase

Over the weeks and months following injury, collagen undergoes continuous remodeling. Older collagen is resorbed and new collagen is deposited and woven into a pattern for improved tensile strength. Collagen fibers align parallel to line of tension in the wound.[1,2]

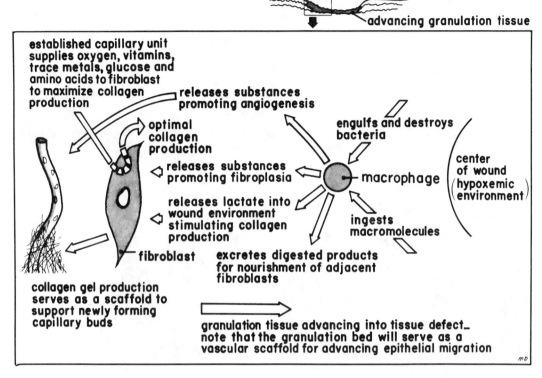

Fig. 31-1 The wound module. Summary of the basic components of wound healing and their interrelationship. (Pavletic MM. Introduction to wound healing and wound management. Proceedings of the American Animal Hospital Association. Orlando, Florida, 1985:655.)

Epithelialization

The marginal basal cells from the adjacent skin border mobilize and migrate downward over the exposed dermal border and adjacent healthy granulation bed.[1,2,4] Migrating epithelial cells travel under the clot or scab present by secreting proteolytic enzymes to cleave a path for their migration. In sutured wounds with a small dermal gap, epithelial cells can bridge the gap by 48 hours.[1,2] In moderate-sized wounds, epithelial migration may take weeks or may never completely cover the open wound. The surface of epithelialized wounds (scar epithelium) under these circumstances is thin and fragile and is prone to reinjury from exposure or by constant licking by the animal. Only a limited number of hair follicles and sebaceous glands may regenerate by differentiation of migrated epithelial cells. As a result, a skin graft or skin flap may be required for better function and cosmetic results for large wounds.[5,6]

Wound contraction

Most veterinarians have seen large skin wounds heal with surprisingly small epithelialized scars as compared with the magnitude of the original defect. The normal bordering skin appears to have been pulled toward the center of the wound. This centripetal movement of the skin is termed "wound contraction."[1,2,4] Wound contraction occurs remarkably well in loose skin areas in the dog and cat, independent of the process of epithelialization previously discussed.

Specialized fibroblasts possessing the contractile properties of smooth muscle are likely responsible for the stretching or pulling of the normal adjacent skin.[1,2,4] These cells are called myofibroblasts and appear to attach to the underlying dermis of the bordering skin margin and the underlying fascia or panniculus muscle of the wound bed.[1,2] Square wounds contract more readily than circular wounds because the straight sides are drawn inward unimpeded, whereas the force of contraction in a circular wound is not evenly distributed along a linear border. Open wounds no longer able to contract must rely on the process of epithelialization or surgical intervention (Fig. 31-2).

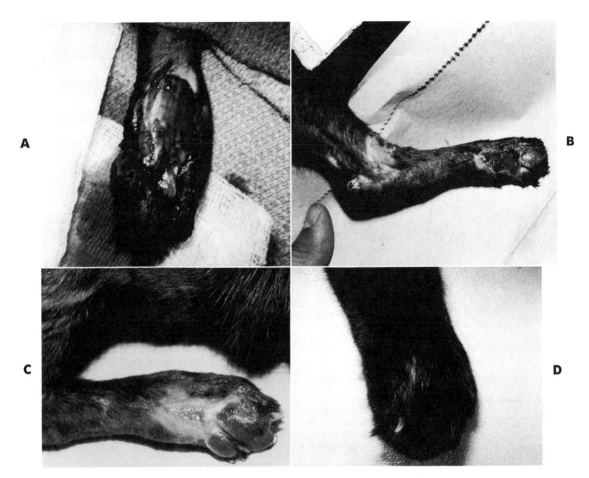

Fig. 31-2 A, Large avulsion wound overlying the metatarsal surface. **B,** Conservative management promoted granulation tissue formation. The flat granulation bed serves as a vascular scaffold for the advancing epithelial cells during second intention healing. **C,** Wound contraction and significant epithelialization was noted within 4 weeks after the initial injury. **D,** On completion of hair growth, the scar could not be detected without separation of the fur overlapping the healed wound.

WOUND CLASSIFICATION

Wounds should be examined closely for extent, depth, underlying tissue involvement, the degree of contamination, and signs of infection. These factors can be used to classify wounds in increasing order of severity. Wound classification can be used to decide on the proper course(s) of action. In all, there are four categories: clean, clean-contaminated, contaminated, and dirty and infected.[1]

On occasion it is difficult to decide in which of two categories a given wound should be classified. When in doubt the injury should be downgraded and treated as a more serious wound.

Clean wound

A clean wound is a nontraumatic, uninfected op-

erative wound in which neither the respiratory, alimentary, or genitourinary tracts nor the oropharyngeal cavities are entered. Clean wounds are made under aseptic conditions. They usually are primarily closed without drains.[1]

Clean-contaminated wounds

Clean-contaminated wounds are operative wounds in which the respiratory, alimentary, or genitourinary tract is entered without unusual contamination. Minor contamination of a clean wound due to a break in sterile surgical technique may be classified in this category.[1]

Contaminated wounds

Contaminated wounds include open traumatic

wounds, operations with a major break in sterile technique and incisions encountering acute non-purulent inflammation, or wounds made in or near contaminated or inflamed skin. Unless the procedure is very clean, wounds made for access to the lumen of the colon belong in this category.[1]

Dirty and infected wounds

Dirty and infected wounds include old traumatic wounds and those involving clinical infection or perforated viscera. The definition of this classification suggests that the organisms causing postoperative infection are present in the operative field before the operation or that pus contaminates the wound.[1]

OPTIONS FOR WOUND CLOSURE

There are five options available for wound closure depending on the wound classification after its initial assessment: primary closure, delayed primary closure, secondary closure, closure by second-intention healing, and closure by adnexal reepithelialization.

Primary closure

Primary closure or healing by first intention is reserved for wounds created under aseptic conditions. Wounds with minor contamination can be converted to "surgically clean" wounds with judicious debridement and copious lavage with sterile isotonic solutions.[1,2,4]

Delayed primary closure

Wounds with borderline contamination may be left unsutured and covered with a sterile dressing. Delayed closure allows for adequate drainage and time for improved tissue resistance to infection prior to suturing. If no devitalized tissue or infection is noted on wound inspection on the fourth or fifth day, primary closure may be attempted. Quantitative bacterial cultures may be used to determine the optimal time for safe closure.[1]

Secondary closure

Secondary closure is generally reserved for wounds with superficial contamination or invasive infection. This would include wounds that become infected during delayed primary closure.[1] Secondary closure can be attempted between the 5th and 10th day with two methods: direct suture apposition of the two granulation surfaces (healing by third intention) or granulation tissue excision and primary closure. The latter technique is preferred by many surgeons because of the relative ease in mobilization of the wound edges for closure, the better cosmetic results, and the lower incidence of postoperative infection after excision of the granulation tissue.[1]

Closure by second-intention healing

Healing by second intention, or contraction and epithelialization, is a technique commonly employed in veterinary medicine.[6,7] It generally is reserved for dirty and infected wounds in which closure by the previous three techniques is not advisable. Large cutaneous defects that cannot be sutured closed may be left open to contract and epithelialize. As noted, two processes occur independently in the open wound to promote closure: epithelialization and wound contraction (Fig. 31-3).

In many cases, healing by second intention is a practical and economical method of affecting closure if adequate wound care is administered. However, not all wounds will heal properly by second-intention healing. Some wounds will not contract and epithelialize to completion. Excessive scarring and contraction may result in restricted motion to a limb or other body region (wound contracture) (Fig. 31-4). Cosmetic results may be unsatisfactory. The occasionally prolonged process of healing combined with the cost of hospital visits, bandage materials, and medications may end up costing the owner more time, money, and "aggravation" as compared with early closure with a skin flap or grafting technique.[6]

Closure by adnexal reepithelialization

Cutaneous burns and abrasions may be categorized as superficial, partial-thickness, and full-thickness according to the depth of injury. Superficial cutaneous loss includes loss of epithelium but preservation of the germinal layer. Reepithelialization originates from this epithelial layer and a variable portion of the dermal adnexa. A partial-thickness loss results in the removal of the entire epithelial layer and a variable portion of the dermis. Reepithelialization in this case arises from adnexal structures (hair follicles, sebaceous glands, sweat glands).[1,2] As previously discussed, a full-thickness skin loss results in complete loss of the epidermis and dermis. Ultimate coverage of this cutaneous defect must occur from the viable cutaneous epithelium peripheral to the wound unless surgical intervention or graft coverage is instituted. The donor site from which a split-thickness graft is harvested will heal as a partial-thickness wound. Healing of the donor site, however, has the advantage of minimal tissue injury because the wound is made under aseptic conditions with minimal trauma involved. One must remember that any partial-thickness injury may be con-

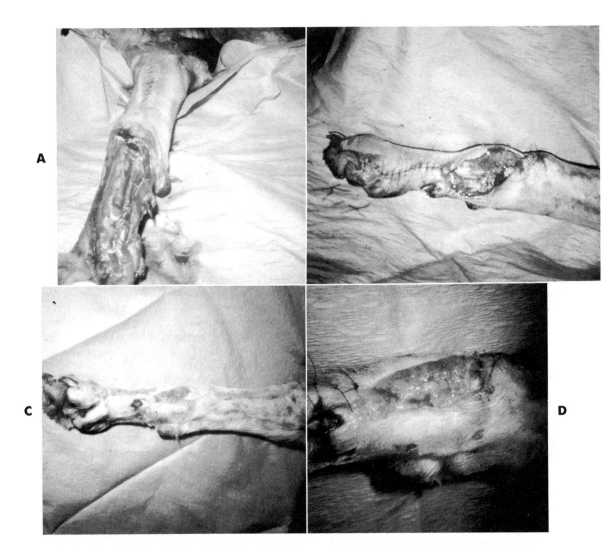

Fig. 31-3 A, Shearing wound involving the carpal and metacarpal surfaces. **B,** Partial closure accomplished after copious lavage and debridement. **C,** After 2 weeks of bandaging and splint support, swelling had subsided revealing a small wound filled with granulation tissue. **D,** A close-up view of the carpal wound demonstrating a granulation bed elevated above the skin margin. A scalpel blade was used to trim the "proud flesh" to facilitate epithelialization.

verted to a full-thickness loss by infection and improper, abusive wound management.

WOUND MANAGEMENT

The principles of wound management to be discussed have not significantly wavered from the principles advocated by Esmarch and Halsted decades ago despite the increased severity of wounds seen in 20th century society. It is fortunate that many of the wounds seen by the emergency clinician are *not* life threatening. The clinician's initial assessment and management of the wounds will have a significant impact on out-

come. Many smaller wounds can heal despite the misguided efforts of a disinterested clinician. Careless wound management of more serious injuries can promote multiple wound complications (infection, dehiscence, seromas, etc.). More importantly, further trauma by the veterinarian may be the "death" blow to a body region barely able to survive with a seriously compromised circulation. The tissue necrosis that follows may result in amputation of the affected limb or the death of the animal. The veterinary clinician must strive for consistency. Consistently successful results require practice, attention to small details and ad-

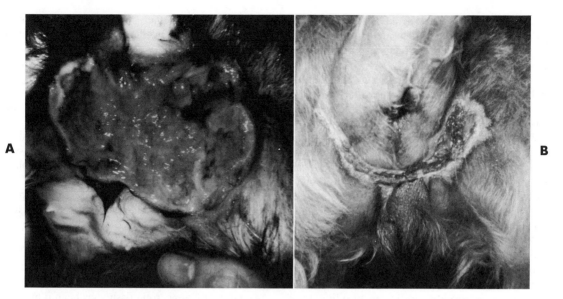

Fig. 31-4 A, Debridement of a large segment of necrotic skin between the anus and vulva of an 8-week-old Lhasa apso (cause unknown). **B,** Dramatic wound contraction was noted 2 weeks later. Note the dorsal displacement of the vulva as a result of myofibroblastic activity. No clinical problem was noted. Young dogs and cats have a remarkable ability to heal by second intention.

herence to the basic principles of wound management discussed.

While clean wounds and wounds with minor contamination received within 6 hours of occurrence pose less of a problem to the surgeon, wounds with gross contamination or infection can become a major challenge in treatment and closure. In selected areas of the dog or cat, small wounds of this nature can be excised completely and the surgical defect closed primarily. Larger wounds generally require management in a stepwise fashion before closure can be safely accomplished. The primary goal in managing all wounds is to establish a healthy vascular wound bed that is free of necrotic tissue, foreign debris, and infection. The six basic steps in the management of contaminated, dirty or infected wounds include: (1) prevention of further contamination; (2) debridement of dead and dying tissue; (3) removal of foreign debris and contaminants; (4) adequate wound drainage; (5) promotion of a viable vascular bed; and finally (6) selection of the appropriate method of closure.[8]

Prevent further contamination

On admission, wounds should be protected temporarily from desiccation and further contamination with debris and resistant strains of hospital organisms by the temporary application of a sterile dressing with an antimicrobial agent. Water-

miscible ointments are preferred over heavier oil-based agents, which are difficult to rinse out of the wound. Wet saline dressings (sterile gauze soaked with saline) that include an antibiotic or nonirritating antimicrobial agent are useful.[7,8] A povidone iodine solution of 0.5%, a benzalkonium chloride solution of 1:2500, and a chlorhexidene solution of 0.5% to 1.0% proved to be useful in reducing bacterial populations in one study, with the chlorhexidine solution being the most effective for wound irrigation.[9] These agents also could be incorporated into wet dressings. In general, the more serious infected wounds should be cultured (aerobic, anaerobic) prior to the institution of systemic antibiotics. Ideally, animals should be anesthetized for optimal wound preparation and debridement. On removal of the bandage, the open wound is covered with sterile gauze pads impregnated with sterile K-Y Jelly (Johnson & Johnson), sterile saline, or an antimicrobial solution prior to liberally clipping the skin peripheral to the defect. Water-impermeable drapes are used to drape off the surgical site, and the wound cover is removed.[5]

Debridement

Necrotic tissue is excised. Areas of questionable viability may be excised if the tissue is not essential to healing or function. However, staged (daily) debridements may be advisable over a single aggressive surgical debridement. Contaminated and injured fat overlying exposed skeletal muscle can be excised safely to remove debris. However, aggressive excision of subcutaneous fat and portions of panniculus muscle attached to exposed skin segments should be avoided to preserve the skin's blood supply (subdermal plexus and associated direct cutaneous vessels). Skin can be excised "liberally" in areas where ample loose skin prevails, whereas a more conservative "wait and reassess" approach is justified with skin of questionable viability involving the extremities where skin is "at a premium." Although bleeding along the skin margins is considered a desirable intraoperative clinical sign of adequate cutaneous arterial circulation, it does not give any information about venous drainage.[6] Vasospasm may cause a temporary drop in local cutaneous circulation with a misleading decline in bleeding from the wound edge. The presence of bleeding from the subdermal plexus is no guarantee that blood is not being shunted from the nutrient circulation of the skin. Furthermore, the presence of circulation within a skin area also is no assurance that trauma, edema, infection, venous compromise, or progressive thrombosis will not destroy the circulation present at the time of the initial examination.[6]

Various enzymatic debriding agents are available on the market and can be employed successfully for debridement.[1,2,7] I restrict their use to small areas or pockets where surgical debridement is likely to cause unnecessary trauma and bleeding. However, these agents generally are not a substitute for surgical debridement of large areas of necrosis.[5] Wet-to-wet and wet-to-dry dressings can facilitate removal of necrotic tissue in the first few days of wound management (see "Dressing and Bandage Techniques").

Removal of debris and contaminants

Dirt, clay particles, and organic debris promote infection and delay wound healing.[1,2] Manual removal of gross debris followed by pressure lavage with an isotonic solution can remove most contaminants remaining after the initial debridement. "Moderate-sized" wounds generally are lavaged with 500 to 1000 ml of saline or lactated Ringer's solution. Additional lavage solution can be employed if necessary. The addition of chlorhexidene, povidone iodine solution, and benzalkonium chloride can reduce significantly the bacterial count of the wound.[1] I have had excellent clinical results with the use of isotonic solutions in contaminated wounds under pressure using a 18- or 19-gauge needle attached to a 35-ml syringe. Full force of the plunger will effectively deliver 8 lb per square inch (PSI) to the wound surface when the needle is placed immediately perpendicular to the wound surface.[1,8] The addition of a three-way stopcock attached to a sterilized intravenous fluid line will enable the surgeon to rapidly refill the syringe. The surgeon can cup his/her hand around the area to minimize overspray. Alternatively, pressure lavage units are available for clinical use, but these are expensive.

It is important for the surgeon carefully to separate and elevate the wound edges and explore adjacent fascial planes likely to be harboring debris. However, indiscriminant dissection is to be avoided to prevent additional tissue trauma and contamination to uninvolved areas.

Drainage

Wound drainage is critical to the treatment of grossly contaminated wounds. Unless the surgeon is confident that necrotic tissue has been removed, all debris was removed, and bacterial contamination has been minimized, primary closure is best avoided. Even then, a Penrose drain or closed suction unit is best inserted to drain tissue fluid to minimize postoperative infection. When possible, the drain should be covered with a sterile protective bandage to minimize the danger of an ascending infection.[5]

Delayed primary closure is a more conservative approach to the care of the wound postoperatively. My current preference is to pack the wound open with a wet dressing, employing several layers of gauze pads soaked in saline solution with or without a nonirritating antimicrobial agent, followed by layers of adherent roll gauze and an outer elastic tape covering. Packing the wounds open maximizes wound drainage, while the saline bandage maintains tissue hydration, thins out any tenacious discharge, and absorbs and stores drainage material. In difficult areas, a "tie-over" dressing can be used by placing a series of interrupted suture loops around the periphery of the wound and "lacing" suture material through the loops to retain the underlying dressing. Bandages are changed under aseptic conditions one to three times daily, allowing the surgeon to reinspect the wound for additional necrotic tissue requiring debridement. The wound is generally in a healthy enough condition in 3 to 5 days to permit selection of an appropriate closure technique.[5]

Promotion of a viable vascular bed

Removal of necrotic tissue, debris, and contaminants minimizes infection and the hazards of delayed healing. Similarly, adequate postoperative drainage provides a route for the escape of debris and discharge, further reducing the likelihood of abscess formation. Postoperative wound bandaging and support protects the wound from additional contamination and trauma. Under these circumstances, circulation to the remaining viable tissues can improve and support the development of a granulation bed. Although exposed bone stripped of periosteum cannot support a granulation bed, the adjacent viable soft tissue often will form healthy granulation tissue, which creeps over its surface. Small holes drilled into the medullary cavity can assist in promoting granulation coverage of exposed cortical bone if care is used to select cases in which their creation does not predispose the bone to fracture formation.[2]

As discussed, granulation tissue forms a barrier that discourages bacteria from invading underlying tissues, fills in defects, and provides a vascular scaffold capable of supporting epithelialization and grafts. Thus, the veterinarian's major effort in the management of the dirty and infected wound is to promote a healthy vascular (granulation) bed. From this point, the doctor can decide on the appropriate method to close the wound.[5]

Selection of the method of closure

The true magnitude of the defect is best determined once tissue swelling subsides and the wound is devoid of necrotic tissue. At this stage (generally 7 to 10 days after the initial injury) the surgeon may note that the wound is considerably smaller than originally ascertained and may heal by contraction and epithelialization without further surgical intervention. Such wounds may be closed secondarily if there is adequate skin. Similarly, the clinician may promote second-intention healing and reserve surgical intervention when contraction and epithelialization slows or early complications are recognized (e.g., contracture). Local or distant flap techniques or free grafts should be considered for larger defects, where healing by second intention may take a considerable period of time (if it occurs at all), and these techniques can economically bypass the prolonged wound care required. Pedicle grafts and free grafting techniques also are advisable when excessive scarring or wound contraction may result in restricted function (contracture) to the area involved.

UNDERMINING SKIN

The loose elastic skin over the neck and trunk in the dog and cat permits the veterinary surgeon to close many skin defects by undermining alone (Fig. 31-5). The key to the successful surgical elevation of skin is preserving its blood supply. This requires the preservation of the direct cutane-

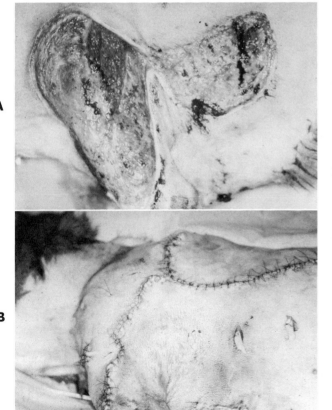

Fig. 31-5 A, Shoulder and lateral thoracic skin loss in a dog accidentally tied to a truck bumper and dragged. Other wounds included shearing injuries of both elbows, the sternum, and left stifle area. **B,** Loose skin was "directed" toward the center of the major defects by carefully undermining and advancing the skin.

ous arteries and associated subdermal (deep) plexus. The following six points can be employed by the clinician as general guidelines for undermining skin in small animals.[10]

1. Skin should be undermined below the panniculus muscle layer when present to preserve the subdermal plexus and associated direct cutaneous vessels.
2. Skin without an underlying panniculus muscle layer (middle and distal portion of the extremities) should be undermined in the loose areolar fascia beneath the dermis to preserve the subdermal plexus.
3. Preserve direct cutaneous arteries and veins whenever possible during undermining.
4. Skin closely associated with an underlying muscle should be elevated by including a portion of the outer muscle fascia with the dermis rather than undermining between these structures. This may help minimize injury to the subdermal plexus.
5. Avoid direct injury to the subdermal plexus by using atraumatic surgical technique.
6. Avoid or minimize the surgical manipulation of skin recently traumatized until circulation improves as noted by the resolution of contusions, edema, and infection.

OINTMENTS

Veterinarians are frequently "bombarded" by pharmaceutical companies with a variety of topical agents that are reported to promote healing and control infection. With variable spectrums of activity, different vehicles, and variable concentrations it is reasonable to assume they have a variable influence on the wound environment. Topical agents can have a variety of desirable effects, including the prevention of tissue desiccation, stimulation of epithelialization, promotion of granulation tissue formation, wound contraction, and collagen formation; facilitation of debridement, and inhibition of infection. Unfortunately, some agents can have the opposite effect to a greater or lesser degree. For example, topical agents such as neosporin ointment, bacitracin zinc, silver sulfadiazine, and benzoyl peroxide (10% and 20%) have been noted to speed epithelialization whereas U.S.P. petrolatum and nitrofurazone slow epithelialization. The antimicrobial properties may play a lesser role as compared with the vehicle or base of the ointment or lotion.[11-14]

A healthy granulation bed is surprisingly resistant to infection because of the presence of white cells, antibodies, and a surface transudate that has a "flushing" function to accumulating surface contaminants. A variable bacterial flora routinely can be cultured from its surface. Despite the presence of these factors wounds do contract and epithelialize. Overuse of topical antibiotics can select for undesirable resistant organisms. As a result, antibiotics are not advocated for routine use on granulation beds. I reserve their use to suppress bacterial growth 36 to 48 hours before secondary closure or the use of skin grafts or skin flaps. Systemic antibiotics are not indicated. It is essential for clinicians to keep current with the literature on new agents and their use and misuse.

DRESSING AND BANDAGE TECHNIQUES

A dressing is a protective covering in contact with a wound. A bandage is a wrap used to hold dressings in place, to support or immobilize a body part, to apply pressure to control hemorrhage, or to obliterate cavities. The terms are occasionally used interchangeably.

Bandages have three basic layers: the primary (contact dressing) layer, the secondary (intermediate) layer, and the tertiary (outer) layer. The primary layer lies in direct contact with the wound.[5,15,16] A nonadherent dressing is generally applied over wounds to facilitate bandage removal without disturbing the underlying tissue. I find Telfa nonadherent strips (Kendall, Boston) and Adaptic dressings (Johnson & Johnson, New Brunswick, NJ) the most useful of the nonadherent dressings. Adherent dressings are useful in wound debridement. Dry, coarse or wide-mesh gauze can be applied over moist wounds with loose necrotic tissue. The dry gauze absorbs the discharge and adheres to pieces of dead tissue. The gauze is removed "dry." Lifting off the dry-to-dry bandage strips the necrotic tissue from the underlying viable tissue. A variation of this technique is the wet-to-dry dressing. Gauze pads soaked with sterile saline or water can be applied to wounds to soften tenacious necrotic tissue and thin the viscous exudates on the wound. Again, removal of the dry gauze facilitates debridement.[5,15,16] Wet-to-wet dressings are those that are periodically moistened until the next bandage change. This serves to flush or bathe the wound and accelerate the softening of necrotic tissue. I insert sterile tubing between gauze layers to inject additional fluid into the bandage in order to maintain the moisture level.[5,15,16]

Adherent dressings are not advisable for healthy wounds, because bandage removal can strip off epithelial cells attempting to migrate over the wound surface. Soaking the gauze with warm saline will reduce patient discomfort on their removal. Topical lidocaine also may be used, although sedation may be necessary during subsequent bandage changes. For these reasons I rarely use wet-to-dry dressings for more than 3 days.[5]

The secondary layer of a bandage is an absorptive layer, usually composed of cotton fiber and/or gauze. The secondary layer wicks fluids and exudate from the wound surface. Moisture in this intermediate layer can evaporate depending on the composition of the outer layer of the bandage. The frequency of bandage changes in part depends on the volume of wound discharge and the storage capacity of the absorptive layer. For this reason, wounds in the early stages of healing generally require more frequent bandage changes, one to three times daily. As a healthy granulation bed forms, the bandage replacement can generally be reduced to a bandage change every 2 to 4 days depending on the condition of the wound.[5,15,16]

The outer or tertiary layer serves as a binding or security layer for the contact and absorptive layers of the bandage.[5,15,16] Stretch gauze followed by a layer of tape or elastic bandage are commonly used. Porous surgical tape facilitates aeration and moisture passage from the absorptive layer. However, moisture from the environment also can pass into this layer and contaminate the bandage. Occlusive (nonporous) tapes may be advisable if this is a significant concern, only if the veterinarian remembers that the tape will also restrict evaporation from the secondary layer, necessitating more frequent bandage changes in order to avoid tissue maceration from prolonged moisture contact. I generally limit the use of occlusive tape to those bandage areas prone to fluid contamination, with porous tape for the remaining bandage area.

Elastic or self-adhering tapes have the advantage of strength, support, and ease of conforming to the underlying bandage area. They are considerably more expensive than surgical tape. Their use is limited to bandages requiring a durable support covering and when infrequent bandage changes are anticipated.[5]

A variety of occlusive and semiocclusive dressings have been evaluated within the past few years to promote epithelialization and dermal healing in the moist wound environment created.[17-23] Other advantages reported include reduced pain and tenderness, better cosmetic results, ease of application, and reduction in bandage changes.[17-23] Occlusive dressings can limit contamination to the wound but also provide a favorable environment for bacterial proliferation. Accumulation of pus and promotion of pathogenic bacteria are potential complications warranting close assessment during their use.[18] Some occlusive dressings include a hydrocolloid gel. This hydroactive layer contacts the wound surface and absorbs wound fluid, forming a moisture-laden gel favorable to epithelialization. On removal, the semipaste retained on the wound may have the alarming appearance of pus. It is important to warn owners of this fact. Dermaheal (Squibb) hydroactive dressings have been employed to promote epithelialization on granulation beds in animals but do not adhere satisfactorily to fresh wounds. Tape strips are required to secure the pads onto the affected area. Because the pads require application to the skin bordering the wound for adherence, they are best employed for small wounds on the limbs. However, the rigidity of this dressing may impede wound contraction by splinting the wound borders.[5,15]

SPLINTS, CASTS, AND REINFORCED BANDAGES

The bandage is the most common method of protecting and supporting the affected area. However, inappropriately applied bandages can be detrimental to wound healing. Tight bandages can restrict circulation. Loosely fitting bandages, however, may rub over the wound and abrade the wound surface, especially wounds involving the joints and mobile areas (flank, axilla, neck, etc.).[5] Additional immobilization is required under these circumstances. Partial casts, Mason metasplints, tongue-depressor splints, and heat malleable plastic (Orthoplast, Johnson & Johnson, New Brunswick, NJ) are effective for immobilizing lower-limb wounds when applied to the outside of the bandage. Shroeder-Thomas splints provide excellent immobilization to the limbs, using aluminum rods or sturdy coat hangers (smaller dogs and cats). The Shroeder-Thomas splint will immobilize the elbow, carpus, knee, and tibiotarsal joint and allow the veterinarian to change the bandage without the need to remove the splint. Spica bandages or splints also are effective in immobilizing the upper extremities. The spica bandage envelops the limb and trunk, restricting motion of the shoulder and hip joint. They can be reinforced with an aluminum bar or a plywood silhouette of the affected limb to increase bandage rigidity.[5]

COMPLICATIONS IN WOUND HEALING
The nonhealing wound

Chronic problem wounds are open ulcers with the loss of epidermis and dermis.[24] Failure to heal may be due to a single major factor or a series of events that cascade into an indolent condition. Factors that impede key steps in the three phases of wound healing can impede the repair process. For example, irradiation of wounds, administration of anticancer drugs, prolonged use of corticosteroids at pharmacologic dosages, and defi-

ciencies of essential nutrients can directly interfere with the steps of healing outlined. Successful
management requires eliminating the factor(s) that
precipitated the delay in healing.

As previously noted, the surgeon has the ability
to minimize or eliminate many of the complications noted in wound healing by adhering to the
basic surgical principles outline by Halsted and
Esmarch. Healthy tissue is surprisingly resistant
to infection. The surgeon can reduce the incidence of infection significantly simply by excising
necrotic tissue and preserving the circulation of
the bordering viable tissue. Injuries heal more
slowly when destruction of the blood supply is a
primary feature.

Tissues wounded by chemical, mechanical, or
thermal insults may have insufficient circulation
to survive. Ischemic tissues may recover from the
initial insult but lack circulation to support formation of a granulation bed. Fibroblasts, leukocytes,
and epithelial cells require blood supply to survive. Compromised tissues require protection to
promote healing. The formation of a granulation
bed serves as a vascular scaffold for supporting
the migrating epithelial cells. Myofibroblasts

within the granulation bed anchor themselves
along the wound borders to promote contraction.
Unfortunately, granulation beds can become fibrotic in time as collagen deposition increases and
the numbers of capillaries and fibroblasts declines. If sufficient time has progressed without
natural closure of the wound, the wound bed becomes unsatisfactory for healing by second intention. Excessive fibrosis can form a restrictive barrier to myofibroblastic contraction by immobilizing the skin margins (Fig. 31-6). Similarly, in
body regions containing insufficient loose skin peripheral to the wound to accommodate to the pull
of the myofibroblast, countertension offsets the
force of wound contraction. Once contraction is
halted, the body's only option to close the wound
is epithelialization from the skin bordering the
full-thickness defect (Fig. 31-7). If complete epithelialization occurs, the fragile epithelial surface
may not tolerate external trauma. This is particularly evident over bony prominences, the foot
pads, and body regions subject to repeated motion. Improperly applied bandages and dressings
can abrade migrating epithelial cells from the
wound bed. Without proper surgical and/or medi-

A

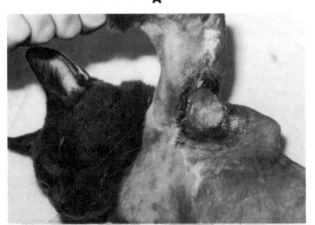

Fig. 31-6 A, Nonhealing ulcer of the axilla as a result
of a wound dehiscence after laceration repair. Wound
contraction was impeded by restrictive fibrosis of the
skin margins. Epithelialization was impaired by a
chronic granulation bed unable to support migrating epithelial cells. Chronic motion, licking and improper
bandaging abraded the wound surface. **B,** Complete
wound excision was performed. **C,** Primary closure
was easily accomplished. A Penrose drain was inserted
to control deadspace.

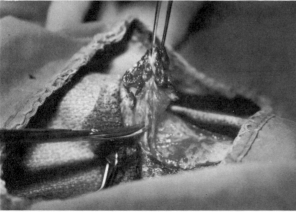

B

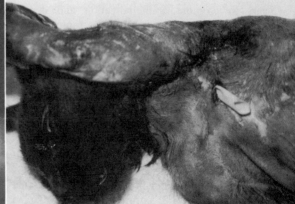

C

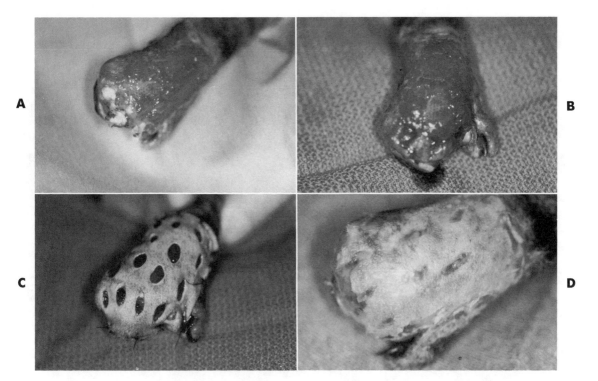

Fig. 31-7 A, Degloving wound of a feline front paw. Conservative management promoted development of a healthy granulation bed. A portion of the metacarpal pad survived. **B,** Necrotic phalanges were removed below the granulation surface with rongeurs. **C,** A full-thickness mesh graft was applied to the wound surface. **D,** By Day 7 the graft successfully covered the wound.

cal intervention, the optimal period for a wound to heal is finite; repeated interference or the lack of the basic components of wound healing can promote formation of an indolent ulcer.[8]

The presence of necrotic tissue can have a devastating effect on the wound environment. Dead tissue promotes bacterial infection and delays healing. A thickened eschar can splint the wound margins and halt contraction. Surgical debridement should be instituted as early as possible to prevent these complications.[1,2,8,24,25]

On occasion, skin wounds fail to contract and epithelialize despite the presence of a healthy granulation bed surrounded by loose skin. The surrounding skin is separated from the underlying muscle fascia despite the formation of granulation tissue on opposing surfaces. Normal wound contraction and epithelialization cannot occur properly because the elevated skin does not attach to the margins of the defect. This indolent ulcer more commonly seen in the cat, becomes a large flat granulation-lined cavity in which the granulation bed covering the dermal surface fails to cross link with the underlying granulation bed covering the muscle fascia. Epithelial cells from the skin migrate beneath its margin onto the dermal surface. Myofibroblastic contraction cannot advance the skin; instead the skin margins curl under. The pocket supports bacterial growth, movement, and fibrinolysis within the wound to prevent the opposing granulation beds from uniting. In time, the granulation bed matures and collagen deposition increases. Successful closure requires controlling the infection, excision of the scar border, and incising the restrictive "dermal scar" carefully to preserve cutaneous circulation yet allow the skin to be advanced over the wound with these release incisions. Skin margins must be sutured directly to each other or firmly anchored to the granulation bed to promote wound closure. Dead space must be managed with carefully placed evacuation drains (Fig. 31-8).[7,8,25]

Proper nutritional support is essential to normal healing and prevention of infection. Protein depletion and longstanding nutritional deficiencies are particularly harmful to healing (see Chapter 37). This is most evident in the young growing animal and the geriatric patient. A vital compo-

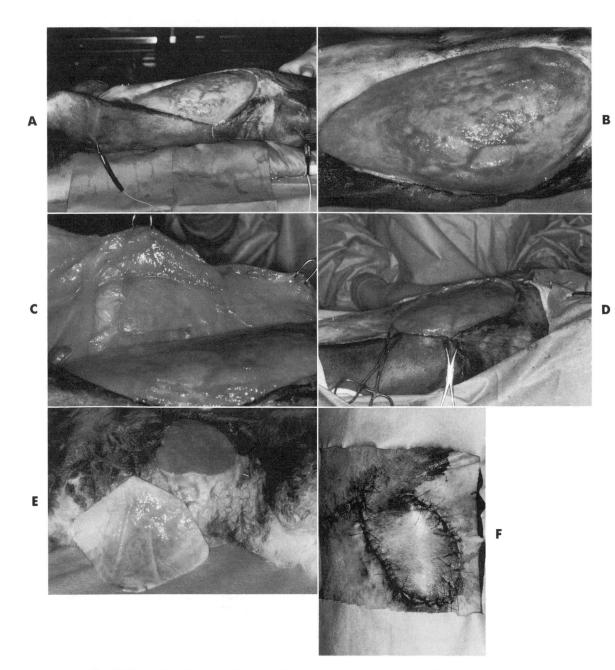

Fig. 31-8 A, Chronic nonhealing wound involving the lower thorax and abdomen in a cat, the result of a dog bite. Previous attempts at closure were unsuccessful. **B,** A close-up view of this wound of several months' duration. Skin edges were not attached to the underlying granulation bed. Instead, a large pocket was present. **C,** After wound management with chlorhexidine wet dressings for 48 hours, the restrictive scar overlying the dermal surface of the skin was carefully incised with "grid" incisions. Care was taken to preserve the vascular supply to the skin. **D,** Towel clamps facilitated skin apposition and subsequent closure with a continuous subcuticular pattern and simple interrupted sutures alternated with a vertical mattress pattern. Penrose drains were used to control dead space. **E,** Partial dehiscence occurred on the craniolateral aspect of the defect. Buried 3-0 chromic catgut sutures were used to attach the dermal borders to the granulation bed. The wound failed to contract and epithelialize despite the use of occlusive dressings and the regional availability of loose skin. **F,** Final closure was accomplished with the use of a 90-degree transposition flap adjacent to the defect.

nent to the management is nutritional support of the patient (see Chapter 37). Nasogastric tubes, gastrostomy tubes, jejunostomy tubes or pharyngotomy tubes may be required if the injured patient is incapable of eating or unwilling to eat. Intravenous fluid and caloric support may be vital to the successful recovery of the patient. Hypovolemia and poor perfusion are especially harmful to wound healing.[1,2,7,8,24,25]

A necessary component to wound management is proper assessment of the injury and the history of the patient to determine whether closure with a skin flap or skin graft is necessary. In many cases wound excision and immediate closure with a skin flap can bypass the difficulties associated with managing a chronic open wound.[6]

It is important to remember that neoplasms frequently have the appearance of an open wound depending on its location and stage of growth. Chronic nonhealing wounds can become malignant as noted in the development of squamous-cell carcinoma (Margolin's ulcer) in chronic nonhealing burn wounds in humans. When in doubt, biopsy.[25]

Scarring

Scar tissue is a normal response to healing. While scarring is beneficial in some injuries, its formation in other wounds is undesirable. For example, the formation of the granulation tissue and collagen deposition is desirable for many shearing injuries involving the carpal or tarsal points to improve joint stability and close the defect. Excessive scarring in other areas may restrict motion or function to an area. To minimize scar tissue, meticulous atraumatic surgical technique, physical therapy, traction, pressure, and control of infection is essential. Infection has the added undesirable effect of diverting components required for healing and promoting the unsatisfactory deposition of scar tissue to wall off the microorganisms.[1,2,5,24,25] Lastly, a fragile epithelialized scar may not withstand external trauma even as mild as occasional licking (Fig. 31-9).

The term "wound contracture" implies a loss or restriction of function to an adjacent joint, usually as a result of excessive scarring. Excessive wound contraction may contribute to contracture formation. Positioning of the affected areas in a more comfortable flexed position by the injured patient can favor collagen deposition, which "locks" the area into this position. Prevention of wound contracture requires early recognition of the developing problem with the appropriate steps to combat it. In veterinary medicine, early appropriate coverage of open wounds with skin flaps and related Z-plasty techniques or by free grafts followed by physical therapy can prevent contrac-

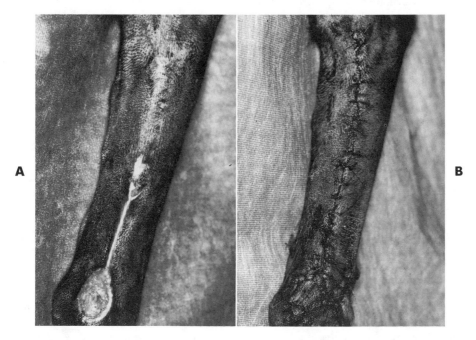

A **B**

Fig. 31-9 A, A large wound involving the forelimb of a 1-year-old Labrador healed by second intention except for a small ulcer overlying the carpal joint. Licking of the epithelized scar resulted in recurrent ulcerations. **B,** The epithelialized linear scar was excised and closed primarily; a transposition flap, developed parallel to the limb, was rotated 90 degrees and successfully sutured over the carpal defect.

ture development. Scar excision, partial myotomies, flap or free graft coverage, and physical therapy may be required once contracture has developed. Traction to the area may be required temporarily to combat recurrence until healing is complete and physical therapy can be implemented. Physical therapy can be effective in modifying collagen deposition and cross linking to improve mobility.[1,2,5,7,8,24,25]

Infection

Although a laceration and a puncture wound both may have the same degree of tissue injury, the environment of each wound is vastly different. Open wounds rarely are the source of invasive infection. A puncture wound lacking drainage forms a closed pocket that provides an ideal environment for bacterial proliferation. As a result, puncture wounds (such as bite wounds) should be opened wider, gently explored, debrided, lavaged, and allowed to heal as an open wound unless the surgeon is confident that his or her techniques have converted the wound into a "surgically clean" wound that will tolerate closure.[1,2,5,7,8,24,25]

Abscess formation is more common in the cat, usually as a result of previous bite wounds from other cats. The small puncture holes readily seal and promote abscessation. *Pasteurella multocida* is a common oral contaminant in small animals and frequently is responsible for bite-wound infections. Areas of cellulitis eventually coalesce to form the abscess cavity. Abscesses are drained ventrally once they have "pointed." Warm compresses can facilitate their formation. Many abscesses in small animals readily respond to this regimen followed by gentle exploration, flushing, debridement, and systemic broad-spectrum antibiotic support for 7 to 10 days. Large abscess cavities occasionally are packed open for 2 or 3 days with moistened medicated gauze packs changed one or more times daily. Partial drying of the pack facilitates the absorption of the discharge and helps to strip out necrotic tissue adhered to the cotton fibers. Thereafter, periodic warm compresses (three times daily for 10 to 15 minutes) is followed by the application of nonirritating topical agents to protect the developing granulation bed from desiccation until second-intention healing is complete. Microbiological culture and antibiotic sensitivity testing and Gram stains usually are not warranted for many of the abscesses seen in small animal practice. Deep abscesses, recurrent infections, persistent or recurrent draining tracts, and potentially life-threatening infections do warrant their use. These clinical observations

should alert the clinician that the condition is not a "minor" local infection and warrants a detailed diagnostic evaluation and surgical exploration.[1,2,5,7,8,24,25]

Draining tracts

Persistent or intermittent draining tracts have been seen with the presence of large pockets of necrotic tissue that cannot be expelled by the body; underlying bone infection, bone sequestra, or bone chips harboring bacteria; bacterial or fungal organisms resistant to the routine treatment regimens; foreign bodies, especially plant material (grass fragments, wood, grass awns, etc.); surgical implants or braided nonabsorbable suture material (silk, vetafil, cotton, polyester, etc.); and neoplastic conditions (with or without the presence of microorganisms) that mimic infection. Animals immunosuppressed by various therapeutic measures or underlying disease (e.g., feline leukemia, feline infectious peritonitis) may explain the patient's susceptibility to infection or poor healing and should be investigated.

Radiography of these draining areas occasionally reveals radiopaque objects amenable to removal. Fistulograms occasionally are useful to highlight foreign bodies, determine the magnitude of the tract(s), and examine their relationship with neighboring structures. Cannulation and injection of dyes such as sterilized methylene blue can stain the tracts, facilitating their removal. Deep-wound tissue or exudate should be obtained for aerobic, anaerobic, and fungal culture. Small foreign bodies can be elusive by migrating through tissue planes or by being hidden by layers of scar tissue and necrotic debris. Whenever feasible, I cannulate each tract, dissect around each tract, and completely excise the entire area while avoiding the spillage of contaminated material into the neighboring tissues. On completion of the surgical procedure, the excised tissue is open and examined, culture samples are taken, and the tissue submitted for histopathologic examination.[5]

Seromas

Seroma formation may be noted beneath the skin in areas traumatized accidentally or surgically. Inflammation and lymphatic injury result in the formation of serum pockets in areas where dead space prevails. Traumatic surgical technique, harsh wound-cleansing techniques, the presence of foreign debris and irritants, and areas subject to constant movement also contribute to seroma formation. Small seromas beneath skin are of no major consequence and resolve in time. Larger pockets usually require drainage. Aspiration of large seromas generally is unrewarding, although the application of a firm compression bandage after aspiration may help to eliminate dead space to promote healing of the separated tissue planes. On occasion, intermittent seroma aspiration every 3 to 5 days and the continued application of a compression bandage can be successful.

Drains are usually required to prevent/treat seromas. The insertion of a Penrose drain for 2 to 5 days generally is necessary with an overlying compression bandage when possible. Alternatively, closed suction units can be effective in removing fluid and obliterating dead space. Closed suction units have less likelihood of developing an ascending infection but have the major drawback of expense. They will occasionally obstruct with tissue debris. Compression bandages, Penrose drains, or closed suction units should be employed any time the surgeon feels that the accumulation of fluid is likely in an area where dead space is present. Buried "tacking" sutures also can be employed to discourage seroma formation in small sterile dead space areas. However, large areas of dead space may be impossible to tack down completely. Excessive use of buried sutures may promote wound infection and cannot be advocated for routine use in contaminated wounds. Buried sutures also may result in the formation of smaller seroma pockets, which do not communicate with one another for simple drainage.[5]

REFERENCES

1. Peacock EE. Wound repair, ed. 3. Philadelphia: WB Saunders, 1984.
2. Hunt TK, Dunphy JE. Fundamentals of wound management. New York: Appleton-Century-Crofts, 1979.
3. Schilling JA. Wound healing. Surg Clin North Am 1976;5:859-874.
4. Johnston DE. The process in wound healing. J Am Anim Hosp Assoc 1977;13:185-196.
5. Pavletic MM. Surgery of the skin and management of wounds. In Sherding RG, ed. The cat: diseases and clinical management. New York: Churchill Livingstone, 1989:1601-1629.
6. Pavletic MM. Pedicle grafts. In Slatter D, ed. Textbook of small animal surgery. Philadelphia: WB Saunders, 1985:458-486.
7. Swaim SF. Surgery of traumatized skin: management and reconstruction in the dog and cat. Philadelphia: WB Saunders, 1980.
8. Pavletic MM. Introduction to wound healing and wound management. Proceedings of the American Animal Hospital Association. Orlando, Florida 1985:655-663.
9. Amber EI, Henderson RA, Swaim SF, Gray BW. A comparison of antimicrobial efficacy and tissue reaction of four antiseptics of canine wounds. Vet Surg 1983;12:63-68.
10. Pavletic MM. Undermining the skin in the dog and cat. Mod Vet Pract 1986;67:13-16.
11. Geronemus RG, Mertz PM, Eaglstein WH. Wound healing. Arch Dermatol 1979;115:1311-1314.
12. Eaglstein WH, Mertz PM. "Inert" vehicles do affect wound healing. J Invest Dermatol 1980;74:90-91.
13. Alvarez OM, Mertz PM, Eaglstein WH. Benzoyl peroxide and epidermal wound healing. Arch Dermatol 1983;119:222-225.
14. Eaglstein WH, Mertz PM, Alvarez OM. Effect of topically applied agents on healing wounds. Clin Dermatol 1984;2:112-115.
15. Swaim SF, Wilhalf D. The physics, physiology and chemistry of bandaging opening wounds. Compend Contin Educ Pract Vet 1985;7:146-156.
16. Bojrab MH. A handbook of veterinary wound management. Boston: Kendall, 1981.
17. Alvarez OM, Mertz PM, Eaglstein WH. The effect of occlusive dressings on collagen synthesis and re-epithelialization in superficial wounds. J Surg Res 1983;35:142-148.
18. Mertz P, Eaglstein WH. The effect of semiocclusive dressing on microbial population in superficial wounds. Arch Surg 1984;119:287-289.
19. Alvarez OM, Hefton JM, Eaglstein WH. Healing wounds: occlusion or exposure. Infect Surg 1984;3:173-184.
20. Eaglstein WH. Effect of occlusive dressings on wound healing. Clin Dermatol 1984;2:107-110.
21. Eaglstein WH. Experiences with biosynthetic dressings. J Am Acad Dermatol 1985;12:434-440.
22. Mertz PM, Marshall DA, Eaglstein WH. Occlusive wound dressings to prevent bacterial invasion and wound infection. J Am Acad Dermatol 1985;12:662-668.
23. Eaglstein WH, Mertz PM, Falanga V. Occlusive dressings. Am Fam Physician 1987;35:211-216.
24. Rudolph R, Noe JM. Chronic problem wounds. Boston: Little, Brown, 1983.
25. Pavletic MM. Complications of soft tissue injuries. Proceedings of the American Animal Hospital Association. Orlando, Florida, 1985;639-644.

32 Cardiopulmonary Resuscitation

Bradley L. Moses

The nationally organized study of cardiopulmonary resuscitation (CPR) can be traced back to the 1960s. The American Heart Association, American Medical Association, American Red Cross, National Academy of Sciences, and National Research Council focused efforts on the problem of prehospital sudden deaths.[1,2] As a result of those efforts, the original and revised standards for CPR in humans have been published in 1974, 1980, and 1986.[2] As research provides findings that warrant changes in basic life support and advanced cardiac life support protocols, new standards are proposed, reviewed, and instituted by the national organizations. The veterinary profession has not unified efforts of appropriate disciplines for the purpose of defining standards for cardiopulmonary resuscitation.

This chapter reviews well-established principles of prevention and therapy for cardiopulmonary arrest (CPA), but also introduces new concepts important to management of CPA in the veterinary patient. A number of controversial areas in which changes in standards for CPR have been proposed will be reviewed. Veterinarians should be careful about modifying standard CPR procedures on the basis of anecdotal reports or results from experimental studies with limited applicability. Modifications in CPR procedures should be made after careful review of all pertinent studies with elimination of ineffective procedures and introduction of new protocols of proven value.

CPR IN THE VETERINARY POPULATION

The need for CPR in animals is largely limited to hospitalized patients. The success rate for CPR varies greatly depending on the patient population studied. The success in resuscitation of the terminally ill animal is very low. In these cases, the option to attempt resuscitation of the animal should CPA occur should be discussed with the owner (Chapter 7). If one considers the group of patients experiencing CPA under general anesthesia, there should be a very high rate of successful resuscitation. In one veterinary study four of seven intubated, anesthetized cats in which CPA developed survived to discharge after CPR.[3] None of four cats without an endotracheal tube in place at the time of CPA survived to discharge following CPR. In this study, only 1 cat out of 11 with chronic disease and CPA was successfully resuscitated.

PREDISPOSING FACTORS AND PREVENTION

There are a variety of circumstances in which respiratory or cardiac arrest may occur in the veterinary patient (see box below and box on p. 509). Disorders of the respiratory system can precipitate CPA.[4] Many of these disorders are readily cor-

---

POTENTIAL CAUSES OF RESPIRATORY FAILURE IN THE SMALL ANIMAL PATIENT

Neuromuscular disorders (anesthetics and other drugs, central nervous system disorders, peripheral neuromuscular disorders)

Structural disorders of the chest wall or diaphragm (flail chest, diaphragmatic hernia)

Disorders of the pleural space (pneumothorax, pleural effusion)

Airway obstruction (aspiration, foreign bodies, bronchoconstriction [asthma, bronchitis], extraluminal compression)

Disorders of the pulmonary parenchyma (pneumonia, edema, fibrosis, contusion)

Disorders of pulmonary vasculature (vasoconstriction, obstruction, obliteration)

I wish to thank Drs. WW Muir and PM Henricks for reading this manuscript and providing criticisms and suggestions.

CAUSES OF CARDIAC ARREST

Hypoxia due to respiratory failure, anemia or
  circulatory failure
Cardiac disease
Anesthetics and other drugs
Toxemia/septicemia
Central nervous system trauma or disease
Electrical shock
Drowning
Hypothermia
Sympathetic-parasympathetic imbalances
Acid-base abnormalities
Electrolyte abnormalities

rectable or preventable (airway obstruction, pneumothorax, aspiration, or anesthetic overdose).

The administration of anesthetic agents produces complex alterations of heart rate, blood pressure, myocardial contractility, peripheral vascular resistance, and baroreceptor responsiveness that can precipitate CPA.[5] Administration of barbiturates produces peripheral vasodilation and often a significant decrease in mean arterial blood pressure and their use in a volume-depleted patient can be fatal.[6] Halothane and isoflurane impair left ventricular systolic performance; the heart rate decreases with increasing levels of halothane and can increase or decrease with increasing levels of isoflurane administration.[5] Increases in heart rate with isoflurane appear to be due to preservation of baroreflex responsiveness to isoflurane-induced hypotension.[5]

In 1985 Keenan and Boyan reported 27 CPAs due solely to anesthetic administration in a human population undergoing 163,240 anesthetic procedures over a 15-year period.[7] Fourteen of the patients died. Twelve of the 27 arrests occurred because of failure to provide adequate ventilation. Nine of the CPA patients received an absolute overdose of inhaled anesthetic, and six patients who had hemodynamic instability received relative overdoses. The authors observed that 26 of 27 CPA patients exhibited progressive bradycardia prior to CPA. When atropine was administered it was generally ineffective. It is suggested that anesthetists learn to respond to progressive bradycardia by quickly discontinuing inhalation anesthetics and "directing attention to adequate ventilation." It is interesting that none of these CPAs were initiated by development of ventricular tachycardia or ventricular fibrillation.

The feline patient population is similar to the human pediatric patient population with respect to the potential for anesthetic arrest. Injected drug dosages become more critical in smaller individuals. Achieving intravenous access and restraint in these patients is a challenge. Laryngospasm and airway reactivity may be precipitating factors in the development of CPA in felines.[7-9]

The prevalence of anesthetic-related cardiac arrest in the veterinary population is difficult to measure. In 1977 a study was conducted in Scotland in which a group of 29 practices responded to a questionnaire.[9] The number of deaths reported was 35 in 10,000 procedures. Several conclusions were made, which still serve as useful suggestions: (1) it is important to know the patient's exact weight for calculation of dosages for anesthetics administered; (2) endotracheal intubation is essential, as it provides control of the airway; and (3) premedication practices make induction of anesthesia safer for the patient.

Selection of preanesthetic agents should be done with proper regard to inhibition or preventing potentiation of cardiac arrhythmias that may be anticipated with intravenous induction agents. Xylazine administration has been shown to potentiate arrhythmias in some settings, whereas acetylpromazine administration inhibited the development of cardiac arrhythmias.[10]

SIGNS AND PATHOPHYSIOLOGY OF THE DEVELOPING ARREST

The specific presentation of incipient CPA in veterinary patients can take many different forms. There may be a change in an electrocardiogram that is readily and specifically interpreted. Observations of a subjective nature such as "the heart rate seems low," "the patient's color seems cyanotic," "the respirations seem delayed," or "the patient seems disoriented and dyspneic" suggest developing CPA. Such warnings should quickly be followed by checking the animal's pulse, ventilation, and perfusion. The more quickly these assessments are made, the better the chance of correctly interpreting the finding(s) and preventing CPA.

Heart rate is one of the most commonly monitored vital signs in veterinary patients. Moderate hypoxemia increases heart rate. This increase in heart rate is carried out by indirect reflexes involving the brain, pulmonary inflation reflexes, and peripheral chemoreceptors.[11] Stimulation of the chemoreceptors located in the carotid bodies occurs when blood pH decreases, blood partial pressure of carbon dioxide (P_{CO_2}) increases or blood partial pressure of oxygen (P_{O_2}) falls below 80 mm Hg. The strongest stimuli altering heart rate are changes in blood pH and P_{CO_2}.[12] The net change in heart rate depends on an interplay between an inhibitory primary reflex (lowering heart rate) and a facilitative secondary response to increased respirations (elevating heart rate). If respirations are controlled or eliminated, bradycardia ensues. This bradycardia may occasionally be reversed by atropine.[11] Hypoxemia can activate the cardioinhibitory center of the brain directly, causing a decrease in heart rate. Increases in intracranial pressure similarly induce bradycardia.[12]

In the asphyxiated dog model, respiratory efforts subside 2 to 4 minutes after occlusion of the endotracheal tube. Progressive hypotension and bradycardia lead to an absence of measurable systemic arterial blood pressure within 7 to 11 minutes. At this point, if atropine is administered in conjunction with opening the airway and initiating CPR, there is minimal change in heart rate. If, on the other hand, an alpha-adrenergic drug is administered in conjunction with CPR, heart rate and blood pressure rapidly return to normal levels[13] (see "Drugs"). The clinician who assumes that bradycardia in a CPA is due to a vagal reflex may waste valuable time administering atropine to the animal instead of looking for a ventilatory problem.[7]

VETERINARY CARDIOPULMONARY RESUSCITATION

The objectives of cardiopulmonary resuscitation are as follows[14]: (1) airway, (2) breathing, (3) circulation, (4) drugs, (5) electrocardiographic monitoring, (6) treatment of arrhythmia, and (7) postresuscitation monitoring and support. There have been extensive revisions in some of these steps in the past 10 years, but many of the basics remain unaltered.

Airway

In animals experiencing airway obstruction related to anesthesia or loss of consciousness, the airway can often be opened by simply pulling the tongue forward. If vomitus is present it must be removed from the oral cavity digitally or by suctioning of the oropharynx. Unless aspiration is an immediate danger, the head should be positioned at the same level as the rest of the body. In patients with airway obstruction due to a foreign body, subdiaphragmatic thrusts can be used in a similar manner to the Heimlich maneuver performed in humans. Important seconds can be saved in cases presenting with upper-airway foreign-body obstructions by keeping Forrester sponge forceps, used for removal of the material, in or near the emergency kit.[15]

Intubation is preferable to face-mask or mouth-to-nose insufflation for the purpose of providing a patent airway and ventilation during CPR. Following intubation, digital pressure can immediately be applied around the trachea to provide the seal needed for initial ventilations. If mouth-to-nose or face-mask techniques are used, avoid

rapid puffs and high airway pressures, which tend to cause gastric distention. The use of an endotracheal tube avoids gas distention of the stomach and its associated risks of vomition and aspiration.

If the glottis is obstructed, an emergency tracheostomy should be performed. Increased survival time in these animals can be obtained by inserting a large-caliber needle or catheter percutaneously through the tracheal wall and administering oxygen at a rate of 2 to 3 L per minute.[15]

Breathing

Once an airway has been established, two to four rapid breaths should be given. Ventilations can be administered using an ambu bag attached to an oxygen source (100% oxygen). Anesthetic machines may be more cumbersome, but are satisfactory alternatives, provided anesthetic residues have been flushed out of the rebreathing circuit. T adapters attached directly to the oxygen line are not a safe means of providing ventilation. Animals should be ventilated at a rate of 30 to 35 breaths per minute with tidal volumes of 10 to 15 ml/kg.[15] The inhalation:exhalation ratio should be 1:2. If metabolic acidosis was present or suggested before the CPA, higher ventilation rates are recommended.

The use of simultaneous ventilation/chest compression CPR is under investigation. With this technique, airway pressures of 80 to 100 mm Hg are generated.[15] It appears that ventilation/chest compressions can be given on independent timing cycles with little concern about avoiding simultaneous deliveries.

Any adjustments to ventilation during CPR, based on monitoring blood gases, should recognize that measured arterial blood gases are not an appropriate guide for acid-base management during CPR.[16] Mixed venous blood has been found to reflect better the patient's acid-base status at the level of peripheral tissues.[16] End-tidal carbon dioxide is favored as a measure of the patient's effective circulatory status during CPR,[17] but it is not commonly measured in veterinary clinical medicine. Arterial blood gases are useful when evaluating oxygenation of the CPR patient. The resuscitation effort can be started with 100% oxygen, but there is some evidence that once spontaneous circulation resumes, oxygen supplementation should be reduced to levels necessary to maintain normoxia (Chapter 36).[18,19]

Circulation

Prior to 1960, the human medical community relied on open-chest cardiac massage to provide circulation for the CPA victim. A few historical accounts of successful closed-chest cardiac massage

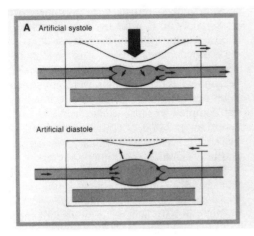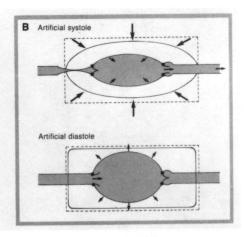

Fig. 32-1 Two theoretical mechanisms have been proposed to explain blood flow during cardiopulmonary resuscitation. **A,** Direct cardiac compression may be the prominent mechanism in cats and dogs under 20 kg in body weight. **B,** The "thoracic pump" mechanism relies on collapse of the jugular veins to provide carotid blood flow during chest compressions. (Reprinted with permission from Babbs EF. Crit Care Med 1980;8:191-5.)

in humans and animals date back to the 19th century.[20] In 1969 Kouwenhoven et al. showed that closed chest cardiac compression could be used successfully in CPR.[21] The development of external defibrillation and mouth-to-mouth ventilation techniques occurred concomitantly. Laboratory investigations since the 1960s have helped clarify how closed-chest cardiac massage CPR works, what limitations are inherent with it, and how to optimize it in human and veterinary patients.[15,22-24]

In 1976 Criley et al. demonstrated that humans with ventricular fibrillation could maintain circulation and consciousness for brief periods by repeated forceful coughing.[25] This "thoracic pump" concept was extended in an effort to explain how the external application of force to the chest wall could sustain circulation when the heart has stopped. Coughing and closed-chest massage both generate an increase in arterial and venous pressures within the chest. There are functional venous valves that block pressure waves from ascending central veins. In addition, collapse of these veins prevents retrograde blood flow in closed-chest-massage CPR[20] (Fig. 32-1). The carotid arteries are more rigid and less likely to collapse. Carotid and cerebral blood flows are provided by a difference in arterial and venous pressures.[23] With the thoracic pump, myocardial blood flow appears to be less satisfactory than cerebral blood flow.[26] This limitation is not eliminated by the use of adjunct procedures such as abdominal binding, military antishock trousers, synchronous ventilation or fluid loading.[27-31] Some experimental models have shown an actual decrease in coronary perfusion pressure with adjunct procedures applied during closed-chest massage.[28-30] Adjunct procedures elevate right atrial pressures as well as aortic pressures, and consequently, the gradient that provides coronary flow is not improved. This limitation is especially important in larger animals, in which the thoracic pump is most active.[15,30]

Studies have been cited in support of interposed or constant abdominal compression in closed-chest CPR[15,32,33] (Fig. 32-2). These studies used abdominal compressions for 3 to 5 minutes in small dogs and then removed the adjuncts for 3 to 5 minutes. When reinstituted, the adjuncts improved blood flow measurements. This improvement may be related to increased cardiac filling brought about by augmented venous return increasing coronary perfusion and systemic arterial blood pressure. Interposed abdominal compression may enhance these factors by directing blood flow away from abdominal organs as well.[15] The authors do discuss the possibility that this improvement in "pump priming" might not have been seen if their experimental subjects had been treated with epinephrine. It would also be easier to put these studies into perspective if they had been performed on dogs heavier than 20 kg so that the thoracic pump would have been the dominant mechanism. The result of these studies appear to support the use of intermittent interposed abdominal compression early in CPR, prior to the distribution of administered epinephrine to the peripheral vasculature. One very simple and readily available aid to cardiac filling, which is occasion-

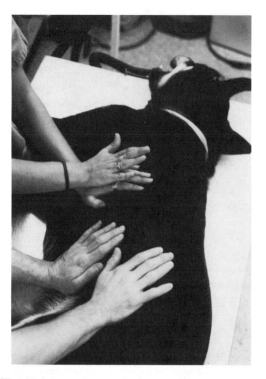

Fig. 32-2 Intermittent or constant abdominal compression can be applied by an assistant's hands pressing on the patient's abdomen. This pressure may augment venous return early in the resuscitation effort before administered epinephrine has taken effect.

ally used in humans, is the elevation of the patient's legs. Currently, adjunct procedures such as abdominal binding, military antishock trousers, synchronous ventilation, and fluid loading are not recommended in human CPR procedures.[31,34,35] Clinically, I have used adjuncts such as intravenous fluids or constant abdominal pressure very early in resuscitation, when cardiac filling may be inadequate and other measures such as epinephrine have not yet been administered.

Studies can be cited supporting either the thoracic pump or the cardiac pump as being the more active pump mechanism during closed-chest-compression CPR.[36-38] It is probable that within our patient population undergoing CPR, some are aided by cardiac compression (cardiac pump) and others are aided primarily or exclusively by the thoracic pump mechanism.[15,29] The cardiac pump is least likely to be effective in patients in which the heart cannot be effectively compressed between the walls of the thoracic cavity.[15,30] This population includes dogs over approximately 20 kg in body weight, obese dogs, or dogs with barrel-shaped chests. Attempted external cardiac compressions may be ineffective or create fractured ribs in dogs with noncompliant thoracic walls.[39]

Optimization of closed-chest massage. A com-

pression rate of 80 to 120 per minute with approximately 50% of the cycle spent in release and a 30% compression of the chest-wall circumference is recommended.[15,40,41] In one study, 8 of 13 dogs supported at 120 manual compressions per minute for 30 minutes were conscious at 24 hours, and only 2 of 13 that had received 60 manual compressions per minute survived and were conscious at 24 hours. The dogs weighed 17 to 30 kg and received high-velocity, moderate-force, and brief-duration (high-impulse) compressions.[40]

Henik et al. studied the effects of body position and ventilation/compressions ratios in cats.[24] They found significantly higher arterial oxygen tensions in cats in left lateral recumbency when compared with cats in dorsal recumbency. Preliminary work done by Crowe, and others, favors right lateral or ventral recumbency for the animal undergoing CPR.[15] CPR on veterinary patients is most commonly performed with the animal in either left or right lateral recumbency. The distinguishing features, if any, of the ideal positioning of the quadriped thorax during CPR have yet to be established.

Compressive forces should initially be applied directly over the precordium in small patients with narrow and compliant thoracic walls. In larger patients, the compressions may need to be shifted dorsally on the animal's thorax to provide for effective thoracic-pump CPR.[15] Techniques used (rate, force of compression, hand position) must be "individualized" in each instance to optimize indicators of effective closed-chest cardiac massage CPR.

Clinical monitoring and evaluation of the patient must be used during CPR to determine efficacy of the measures being taken to provide airway, breathing, and circulation. The most basic evaluations include observation of lung inflation and palpation of an arterial pressure wave. Since

Fig. 32-3 This algorithm can be used to help organize the clinician's approach to cardiopulmonary arrest. *a,* Extend head, pull tongue forward, remove foreign material, and place endotracheal tube. *b,* Ambu bag or anesthesia machine (100% oxygen), 2 full breaths, then 35 bpm. *c,* 80 to 120 cycles per minute, 50% compression, 50% release, within 1 minute check for return of spontaneous circulation. *d,* 2 to 10 J/kg (external). *e,* May be preferred in presence of arrhythmogenic drugs. *f,* Defibrillator and trained personnel should be available. *g,* 0.02 mg/kg intravenously (atropine). *h,* 1 ml/5 to 10 kg intravenously (calcium) if within 5 minutes after cardiopulmonary arrest. *i,* 1 mEq/kg intravenously at 10 minutes of CPA and for every additional 10 minutes of CPR (bicarbonate). *j,* 2 mg/kg, dog; 0.5 mg/kg, cat (lidocaine). *k,* 0.2 J/kg (internal). *, Return of spontaneous circulation; **, development of asystole or electromechanical dissociation.

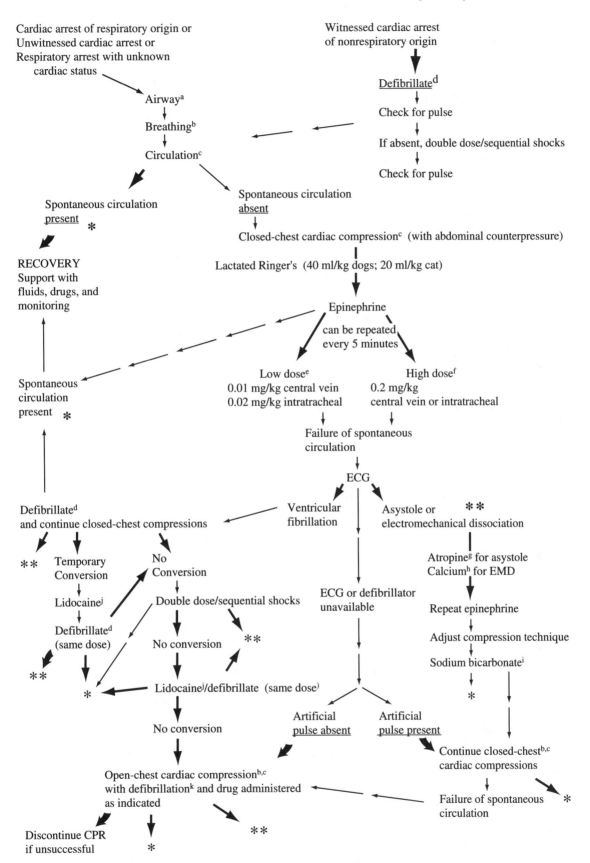

Fig. 32-3 For legend see opposite page.

arterial diastolic blood pressure is crucial to successful CPR (see "Epinephrine") the clinician must understand that adequate circulation is not guaranteed by the palpation of a systolic pulse. Initial indicators of effective CPR can include the return of spontaneous respiratory efforts or cranial nerve reflexes. The return of pupillary light responses is an excellent sign. Direct blood pressure measurements or Doppler measurements of arterial blood flow are very specific indicators of adequate cardiac massage. Improvement in the electrocardiographic wave form may predict successful resuscitation.

Open-chest cardiac-massage CPR. Open-chest cardiac massage produces greater perfusion of critical structures than does closed-chest massage with or without adjunctive procedures.[20,30,42-44] Cardiac output in dogs in cardiac arrest receiving closed-chest CPR was found to be 22% of control, while open-chest cardiac massage provided 2.5 times more blood flow, or 56% of control.[44] After 1 minute of cardiac arrest, cerebral blood flow was 30% of control in dogs with closed-chest massage but nearly normal in dogs with open-chest cardiac massage.[44]

In small patients the efficacy of CPR provided by closed-chest massage incorporating the cardiac pump may negate the need for thoracotomy.[45] For the majority of animals with CPA the question commonly becomes one of when, not whether, to perform thoracotomy.

One author recommends a decision about thoracotomy as early as 2 minutes after CPA.[15] Many authors suggest these interventions can be performed successfully following a longer interval of closed-chest massage. In a study by Sanders et al., 75% of the experimental dogs returned to spontaneous circulation when open-chest massage was instituted after 15 minutes of closed-chest massage.[45] The resuscitation rate dropped to 38% when a 20-minute period of closed-chest massage was used. Inadequate closed-chest massage of 15 minutes' duration has been followed by successful (improved 7-day survival) open-chest massage.[46] A 5- to 10-minute period of closed-chest-massage CPR and assessment of efficacy may be most appropriate, provided the animal has an intact thoracic wall/diaphragm and no pleural or pericardial effusions, i.e., an "effective" thoracic pump.[43,47]

During this 5- to 10-minute period the staff will have administered epinephrine at least once (see "Epinephrine" and Fig. 32-3) and will have started electrocardiographic monitoring and fluid administration. If there are no signs of patient response, especially when the patient is over 20 kg, emergency thoracotomy is usually indicated. If the patient is under 20 kg and there are no signs of response following 5 minutes of CPR, then the closed compression technique should be adjusted in an effort to improve the cardiac/thoracic pump. Thoracotomy is indicated in any patient that has not shown return of spontaneous circulation within 10 minutes of closed chest compression CPR or immediately following recognition of CPA in animals without an "effective" thoracic pump.

Reluctance to invade the thorax and expose the patient to the risks of infection or trauma to the thoracic viscera is not supported by retrospective studies. The prevalence of infection ranges from 0% to 9.1%, and the prevalence of iatrogenic cardiac injury ranges from 0% to 1.4% in humans following open-chest cardiac massage.[43] These results would seem to encourage an aggressive approach.

Emergency thoracotomy can be performed quickly with a minimum of equipment.[15] The hair can be left in place or a few quick passes can be made with clippers. A scalpel incision is made over the left fourth or fifth intercostal space. Mayo scissors can be used to quickly incise muscle layers down to the pleura. The pleural space is entered by blunt dissection (fingertips or closed Mayo scissors) to avoid injury to underlying viscera. A Balfour retractor or Finochetto rib spreader is applied. The pericardium is quickly opened near its apex by lifting and cutting the pericardial-diaphragmatic ligament. Direct cardiac massage can be done using one or two hands. The heart should not be rotated or kinked. Compressive forces should be applied from apex to base of the heart with good palmar and digital distribution to the surfaces of the left and right ventricles. The descending aorta can be cross clamped temporarily to maximize coronary and carotid blood flow (see Chapter 10).

After successful resuscitation the thorax should be thoroughly lavaged with warm sterile saline. Closure of the pericardium is not indicated. A chest tube is placed before routine closure of the thoracotomy; patient condition and character/volume of material obtained on repeated chest-drain aspiration will determine the length of time the chest tube is left in place (commonly, 24 to 36 hours). Broad-spectrum antibiotic administration may be selected perioperatively and the patient is monitored closely for evidence of infection (e.g., fever, leukocytosis).

Trickle flow theory. The critical cerebral and coronary blood flows required to sustain viability of tissues appears to be approximately 20% of normal. This generally requires an effective mean perfusion pressure of approximately 30 mm Hg.[48] Results with some experimental models have been cited in support of the concept that periods of no flow may actually be better than periods of severe incomplete ischemia (trickle flow).[47,49] Low flow may be detrimental because the continued supply of glucose allows brain lactate levels and therefore hydrogen ion levels to rise and participate in neuronal injury. Other studies have suggested that compared to no flow, low cerebral blood flow associated with a normal blood glucose concentration is advantageous,[50] but in association with a high blood glucose concentration it is harmful.[51] In the clinical setting the trickle flow theory should not be used as an argument to delay aggressive CPR. Improved neurologic outcome in fibrillated dogs receiving immediate closed-chest massage as compared with dogs receiving 5 minutes of no flow has been demonstrated.[52] The trickle flow theory appears to heighten the need for early, effective circulatory support and continued development of cytoprotective treatment agents.

Drugs

Pharmacologic agents may be classically considered the fourth step in CPR, but often drug interventions such as epinephrine administration should be among the first responses of the clini-

Table 32-1 Pharmacologic agents used in CPR

Drug	Major Indications	Dosage
Epinephrine	Cardiopulmonary arrest	Use 1:1000 if defibrillation available: 0.2 ml/kg (0.2 mg/kg) IV or IT; use 1:10,000 dilution if defibrillation is not available: 0.10 ml/kg (0.01 mg/kg) IV or 0.2 ml/kg IT
Dopamine	Shock, bradycardia, hypotension	Use 20 mg in 250 ml D/W; 2.0-25.0 µg/kg per minute IV; start at approximately 0.1 ml per 5 kg per minute for diuresis; increase to effect blood pressure; monitor for toxicity (tachycardia or hypertension)
Dobutamine	Cardiogenic shock	Use 25 mg in 250 ml D/W; 2.0-40.0 µg/kg per minute IV; start at approximately 0.1 ml per 5 kg per minute; Titrate to effect monitoring electrocardiogram for toxicity (tachyarrhythmia)
Isotonic intravenous fluids	Relative or absolute hypovolemia	Dogs: 40 ml/kg IV; cats: 20 ml/kg IV
Hypertonic saline (3% to 7.5%)	Hemorrhagic shock	3-5 ml/kg IV
10% calcium chloride or calcium gluconate	Hyperkalemia, hypocalcemia, calcium channel blocker toxicity	1 ml/9.1 kg IV of 10% calcium chloride; 1 ml/2.27 kg IV of calcium gluconate
Sodium bicarbonate	Metabolic acidosis; hyperkalemia; addisonian crisis	1 mEq/kg IV after 10 minutes of arrest; give immediately if preexisting acidosis or hyperkalemia
Atropine	Vagally mediated bradycardia with hypotension	0.02 mg/kg IV or IM
Glycopyrrolate	Vagally mediated bradycardia with hypotension	0.005-0.01 mg/kg IV or IM
Lidocaine	Ventricular tachycardia, recurrent or resistant ventricular fibrillation	Dog: 2-4 mg/kg IV, repeat up to maximum 8 mg/kg; cat: 0.25-0.75 mg/kg IV over 5 minutes, once
Procainamide	Ventricular tachycardia	Dog: 6-8 mg/kg IV over 5 minutes; 25-40 µg/kg per minute
Propranolol	Tachyarrhythmias	0.04-0.06 mg/kg slowly IV
Mannitol	Cerebral edema	1-2 g/kg IV
Dexamethasone	Cerebral edema, shock	1-3 mg/kg IV
Methylprednisolone, sodium succinate	Cerebral edema, shock	5-10 mg/kg IV
Doxapram	Apnea	1-2 mg/kg IV over 5-10 minutes

IV = intravenously; IT = intratracheally; D/W = 5% dextrose in water; IM = intramuscularly.
(Adapted from Haskins SC. Cardiopulmonary resuscitation In: Kirk RW, ed. Current veterinary therapy VIII. Philadelphia: WB Saunders, 1983:382. Reprinted with permission.)

Table 32-2 Use of epinephrine* and countershock in CPR

Body Weight (kg)	Low-Dose† Epinephrine, 1:10,000 (0.01 mg/kg)	High-Dose‡ Epinephrine, 1:1,000 (0.2 mg/kg)	Countershock, Internal§ (J)	Countershock, External§ (J)
2	0.2ml	0.4ml	0.4	4
5	0.5ml	1.0ml	1	10
10	1.0ml	2.0ml	2	50
15	1.5ml	3.0ml	3	75
20	2.0ml	4.0ml	4	100
25	2.5ml	5.0ml	5	125
30	3.0ml	6.0ml	6	150
35	3.5ml	7.0ml	7	175
40	4.0ml	8.0ml	8	200
45	4.5ml	9.0ml	9	300
50	5.0ml	10.0ml	10	300

*Epinephrine should be given by central venous injection. If given by peripheral IV injection, delivery to arterial circulation may be less than ideal. Intratracheal administration route has been proven effective (see Table 32-1). Use a sterile urinary catheter of adequate length to reach distal major airways. Dilute and/or flush drug for airway delivery. Drug administration should be repeated every 5 minutes. If no response occurs when using low-dose epinephrine, consider progressively doubling the dose at intervals shorter than 5 minutes.
†This dose is favored if defibrillator and trained personnel are *not* available.
‡This dose may fibrillate the heart.
§Initial dose may be doubled when initial defibrillation is ineffective.

cian to CPA in a patient (Tables 32-1 and 32-2).

Drug administration (endotracheal, intravenous, intracardiac). The current standards for human CPR and emergency cardiac care[2] state that if an endotracheal tube is in place, before an indwelling intravenous line is established, epinephrine should be given into the patient's tracheobronchial tree. With intravenous administration of epinephrine, central-vein injections are preferable to peripheral-vein injections.

When the tracheobronchial route is selected, a higher dose of pressor agent may be needed than for intravenous administration. One study in dogs, in which epinephrine was aerosolized 3 in. past the tip of the endotracheal tube, found that the median effective dose required (0.130 mg/kg) was 10 times that required for the intravenous route (0.014 mg/kg).[53]

Several techniques may be used to improve absorption of drugs from airways following endotracheal drug administration. Endotracheal injection can be accomplished over a larger surface by using a long catheter (sterile urinary catheter) and gently moving the tip back and forth over several inches of the airway during injection. Elevation of the animal's head during injection and dilution or flushing of the agent with saline may be helpful techniques as well. Forceful ventilations following drug administration may help disperse the agent.[53] Epinephrine is the drug most commonly administered into the trachea, but this route can be used for other emergency drugs (atropine, calcium, and lidocaine) as well. Sodium bicarbonate should not be given into the airways because it inactivates surfactant.[54]

Intracardiac administration should be used only if the other sites are unavailable. The risks associated with attempted intracardiac injection include hemorrhage, coronary artery laceration, cardiac tamponade, and pneumothorax.[2] One study of the accuracy of intracardiac injections in humans who died following CPA found that only 11% of attempted injections pierced the left ventricle. Structures that were entered included the right ventricle (28%), the pulmonary trunk, the aorta, and the lungs.[55]

Epinephrine. In the asphyxiated dog model of CPA, successful resuscitation correlated with the use of epinephrine and alpha-adrenergic stimulation.[56] Cerebral and myocardial perfusion is augmented when epinephrine is used to constrict peripheral vascular beds. Detrimental systolic pressure gradients between the aorta and the carotid arteries are reversed by the use of epinephrine, which helps to avoid collapse of the carotid arteries.[57] Aortic diastolic pressure, as enhanced by epinephrine administration, has been heralded as a prognostic and therapeutic aid in CPR.[58] The clinical efficacy of epinephrine administration in CPR has long been recognized.[59-61] Epinephrine may have less action in patients with acidosis.[62] Based on clinical and experimental response rates, there have been suggestions that traditional protocols (0.01 mg/kg) be modified to use high-dose regimens (0.2 mg/kg).[15,54,61,62] The dose-response curve appears to support a dosage range between 0.03 and 0.2 mg/kg[61] (see Table 32-2).

The arrhythmogenicity of epinephrine used in CPR can be influenced by vagal tone, dose, anesthetic agents, and blood pressure.[10,63-65] Parasympathetic tone appears to provide antiarrhythmic activity by depressing catecholamine-induced increases in spontaneous electrical activity of cardiac tissues.[63] In Redding and Pearson's 1963 study,[59] 2 of the 10 dogs receiving 1 mg of epinephrine went into fibrillation. Muir et al. demonstrated that the mean fibrillatory dose of epinephrine in halothane-anesthetized dogs was 57.2 μg.[10] That dose dropped to 20.5 μg in dogs having also received xylazine. The arrhythmogenic potential of epinephrine suggests that the more aggressive CPR regimens with this drug should probably be reserved for settings in which the personnel, training, and equipment are available for defibrillation.

Phenylephrine and epinephrine administration have been compared in resuscitation studies.[56,60,62] These studies do not indicate that administration of any agent is more successful than epinephrine. Since phenylephrine may have arrhythmogenic potential because of alpha$_1$-adrenergic activity,[65] there does not appear to be any advantage to its use. Brown et al. state that the alpha$_1$-receptors stimulated by epinephrine are located near the vessel lumen and that helpful vascular responses may be superior with epinephrine administration for this reason. Methoxamine administration has been found to be less effective than epinephrine administration in resuscitation from ventricular fibrillation in a swine model.[62]

Calcium. The use of calcium during CPR was commonplace prior to 1986.[2] Evidence supporting its efficacy is lacking,[66-68] and its administration has been associated with myocardial necrosis and reperfusion injury.[69] For these reasons, calcium administration during CPA is recommended only when hypocalcemia is proven or suspected, when hyperkalemia is present, or when calcium-channel-blocker administration may be responsible for the CPA (see boxes at right).[2]

The dosage of calcium to be administered when indicated in CPR is 1 ml/9.1 kg when using 10% calcium chloride and 1 ml/2.27 kg when using calcium gluconate[70] (see Table 32-1).

Ionized intracellular calcium is responsible for triggering the contraction of myocardium and vascular smooth muscle.[11] Without adequate ionized calcium, ventricular performance declines and the measurable hemodynamic response to catecholamines is reduced.[71] Most of the calcium used for excitation/contraction coupling in the myocardium comes from intracellular storage sites on the sarcoplasmic reticulum. The total calcium content in the myocardial cells is several hundred times the amount necessary for myocardial contraction; in normal myocardial cells this excess calcium is safely sequestered. Energy is required to return calcium to the sarcoplasmic reticulum and to

transport it out of the cell following activation of the excitation/contraction process. When energy supplies are disrupted by CPA, the myocardial cells are no longer able to control calcium movement properly. This leads to an increase in ionized calcium concentration within the cytosol.[69] Additionally, normal relaxation of the contractile elements (an important factor in effective myocardial function) requires lowering the ionized calcium levels in the cytosol, an event that is disrupted by CPA.

There are several mechanisms through which calcium administration may be harmful to the patient experiencing CPA and reperfusion.[66,69] Reperfusion of the heart after a period of ischemia leads to dramatic increases in calcium uptake by myocardial cells. This event is accompanied by microscopic evidence of intracellular damage and an accumulation of calcium phos-

---

PROPOSED INDICATIONS FOR THE EMERGENCY USE OF PARENTERAL CALCIUM THERAPY

Severe hypocalcemia
  Eclampsia
  Hypoparathyroidism
  Potential causes of ionized hypocalcemia
    (pancreatitis, renal failure, ethylene glycol
    poisoning, excess citrate in transfused blood)
Severe hyperkalemia
  Urinary obstruction/acute renal failure
  Hypoadrenocorticism
  Severe metabolic acidosis
Cardiopulmonary arrest or symptomatic bradycardia
  associated with calcium-channel-blocker
  administration
Cardiopulmonary arrest with the following features
  Electromechanical dissociation of less than 5
    minutes' duration associated with wide QRS
    complexes unresponsive to high doses of
    epinephrine
  Cardiopulmonary arrest in the patient with septic
    shock

PROPOSED CONTRAINDICATIONS FOR THE EMERGENCY USE OF PARENTERAL CALCIUM THERAPY

Asystole
Sustained CPA of greater than 5 minutes unless
  hypocalcemia is known to be present

---

phate deposits within mitochondria.[72] Administration of calcium during CPR could increase the influx of calcium during this reperfusion period and aggravate the cellular injury. Vascular smooth muscle responds to increases in serum ionized calcium content and the postresuscitation patient receiving calcium administration could suffer cerebrovascular spasm disrupting critical cerebral blood flow[69] (see "Postresuscitation Treatment").

The use of ionized calcium measurements may lead to a better understanding of which patients, if any, are deficient in ionized calcium and therefore are in need of calcium administration. One study found that patients with out-of-the-hospital CPA had ionized blood calcium levels at admission that were below normal, while patients who had an arrest in the hospital had normal levels when measured within 3 minutes.[71] Ionized hypocalcemia was found to be common in pediatric arrests in which the patient was in septic shock.[73] Electromechanical dissociation was not associated with ionized hypocalcemia in a canine model.[74] However, in a prospective study in humans with short-term electromechanical dissociation and wide QRS complexes (more 0.12 second) a higher resuscitation rate was found with the administration of calcium chloride.[75]

Sodium bicarbonate. Sodium bicarbonate is not recommended for use during the first 10 minutes of a resuscitation effort unless the patient is known to have had metabolic acidosis before arrest occurred.[2] Adequate or augmented alveolar ventilation is the mainstay of acid-base homeostasis during CPR. Sodium bicarbonate administration does not improve outcome from ventricular fibrillation in dogs.[76] Hyperosmolarity, hypernatremia, and paradoxical cerebrospinal fluid acidosis are the potential negative effects of sodium bicarbonate therapy in the arrest victim.[2] If given after the first 10 minutes, the empirical dose is 1 mEq/kg intravenously.[2] Further dosing should be based on mixed venous blood gas measurements. Sodium bicarbonate inactivates adrenergic agents such as epinephrine and should therefore not be mixed with fluids that are being used to carry those drugs.

Atropine. Atropine administration is useful in treating sinus bradycardia accompanied by hypotension or frequent ventricular ectopic beats (overdrive suppression).[2] Atropine may be useful for treatment of atrioventricular block as it enhances atrioventricular nodal conduction. One study showed marginal efficacy of atropine administration in reversing CPA-associated asystole.[77] A number of cases of ventricular fibrillation have occurred in conjunction with intravenous atropine administration to the patient with bradycardia.[2,78,79]

Atropine should be administered cautiously, selectively, and at the proper dosage to achieve an increased heart rate. The dosage is 0.02 mg/kg intravenously or intramuscularly.[70] Low intravenous dosage of atropine (under 0.015 mg/kg) cause slowing of the heart and occasional dysrhythmias, such as first- and second-degree atrioventricular block.[80] At higher dosages (over 0.015 mg/kg) there is a transient bradycardia followed by a sustained tachycardia. The initial bradycardia results from stimulation of vagal efferent activity.[80,81]

Glycopyrrolate administration has been suggested as an alternative to atropine administration.[5] Ventricular ectopic beats can occur but are less frequent when glycopyrrolate administration is titrated to effect.[82]

In veterinary patients, severe bradycardia that may precipitate CPA occurs commonly in two settings. The first is the patient in which an acidotic, hypercarbic crisis (hypoventilation) is developing. The therapy of choice is discontinuation of any anesthetic administration and implementation of ventilatory support. Bradycardia in this setting may actually have protective effects by decreasing oxygen consumption of the myocardium (see "Predisposing Factors and Prevention"). Administration of parasympatholytic agents is contraindicated in this setting.[7] If routine preoperative atropine administration is avoided, problems such as hypoventilation may be recognized earlier. The second setting for severe bradycardia in veterinary patients is found with surgical manipulations triggering vagal reflexes. Manipulations of the eye, vagus nerve or larynx are especially prone to triggering bradycardia. Pretreatment with atropine or glycopyrrolate may prevent the development of this form of bradycardia.[5]

Bradycardia has been observed during gastric insufflation, commonly required for endoscopy of the upper digestive tract. It is not clear whether this is due to induction of visceral reflexes or hypoventilation. Bradycardia is infrequent if care is taken to avoid overdistention of the patient's stomach and if the endoscope is properly sized for the patient's pylorus (Tams TR, personal communication).

Bradycardia can be associated with excessive anesthetic depth; hypoxia; administration of narcotics, xylazine, anticholinesterases, and digitalis; hypothermia; endocrine disorders; electrolyte abnormalities; and cardiac conduction defects.[5] The clinician should be familiar with causes of bradycardia-induced CPA in order to treat the specific condition effectively.

Dopamine and dobutamine. Many post-resuscitation patients will have exogenously administered epinephrine influence systemic arterial blood pressure and myocardial contractility for a period of minutes after spontaneous circulation returns.[48] In patients in which myocardial performance deteriorates, dopamine or dobutamine can be given in an effort to maintain blood pressure and heart rate (see Table 32-1) (dopamine, 2 to 10 μg/kg per minute; dobutamine, 5 μg/kg per minute). Cardiac patients who have required resuscitation may need not only positive inotropes but also vasodilator and diuretic administration (see Chapter 17).

Fluid therapy. Fluid therapy in CPR should be guided by the patient's prearrest status. Selection and dosing of intravenous fluids should not be arbitrary. Hypovolemic patients need to receive crystalloid solutions, dextran solutions, or if indicated, blood transfusions rapidly. Patients with congestive heart failure or pulmonary edema should receive judicious administrations of fluids.[2] There is an increase in capillary permeability to plasma proteins during CPA.[83] This factor predisposes the subject with CPA to pulmonary edema. The adverse effects of volume loading during CPR have been discussed in a study that demonstrated that coronary and cerebral blood flows decreased when dogs weighing 20 to 50 kg rapidly received 1 L of fluid intravenously. This effect occurred because right atrial and intracranial pressures increased disproportionately.[84]

The use of dextrose-containing fluids before and after CPA in dogs increased the morbidity and mortality associated with attempted CPR.[85] This phenomenon is probably related to the availability of substrate in an anaerobic environment and the production of lactic acid.

Hypertonic saline administration may have a direct negative inotropic effect in dogs with poor contractility and should not be administered until normal cardiac function has returned (Muir W, personal communication). Controlled studies are needed to define the effect of hypertonic saline administration on postresuscitation survival. Dosages that have been suggested are 3 to 5 ml/kg of a 3% to 7.5% hypertonic saline with or without dextran-70.[86]

Electrocardiogram and treatment of arrhythmias

Several electrocardiographic findings represent common syndromes in the patient with CPA: asystole, ventricular fibrillation, and electromechanical dissociation.

Asystole. Asystole (the absence of electrocardiographic activity) is usually due to extensive myocardial ischemia and carries with it a poor prognosis for resuscitation.[2] The clinician should search for reversible abnormalities such as hyperkalemia, severe acidosis, or (rarely) high levels of parasympathetic tone. A precordial thump can be administered (see "Ventricular Fibrillation"). If a precordial thump is unsuccessful, CPR should be continued, and epinephrine, atropine, and sodium bicarbonate should be administered sequentially (see Fig. 32-3). Transvenous or transthoracic pacing can be attempted (see Chapter 41).

Ventricular fibrillation. Ventricular fibrillation can be defined as the disordered depolarization of the ventricular myocardium (Fig. 32-4) (see Chapter 17). It can have the electrocardiographic appearance of asystole if the fibrillatory waves are perpendicular to the electrocardiographic-lead configuration.[87] This phenomenon can and should be ruled out by using a different lead arrangement, since two-thirds of the time, one frontal lead shows no electrical activity during CPA with ventricular fibrillation. Fine ventricular fibrillation waves carry a poorer prognosis than coarse ventricular fibrillation waves.[88] Epinephrine can be used in an effort to increase wave amplitude, but Weaver et al. were unable to demonstrate any "coarsening" of fine ventricular fibrillation waves following epinephrine administration.[88]

Approximately 35% of small animal patients

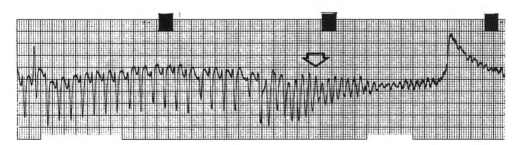

Fig. 32-4 During cardiopulmonary arrest this patient progressed from ventricular tachycardia to ventricular flutter (*arrow*) to ventricular fibrillation (recorded at 25 mm per second). (Reprinted by permission from Moses BL. Cardiac arrhythmias and cardiopulmonary arrest. In Morgan RV, ed. Handbook of small animal practice. New York: Churchill Livingstone, 1988:88.)

with CPA in a university hospital presented with ventricular fibrillation (Muir W, personal communication). The sudden loss of heartbeat and peripheral pulses (witnessed CPA), is likely the result of ventricular fibrillation, and immediate defibrillation is indicated in these cases.[89] Following defibrillation in these cases, electrocardiography will be needed to assess response and the need for additional interventions.

Once a decision to defibrillate has been made, the following steps should be undertaken. Electrode (electrocardiography) paste or saline should be used to enhance electrical contact of the animal to the surface of the paddles. Alcohol or ultrasound coupling gel should not be used. The largest paddles that can be applied should be used. They should be positioned in an effort to maximize current flow through the myocardium. For external defibrillation the initial setting should be 2 J/kg (under 7 kg), 5 J/kg (8 to 40 kg) and 5 to 10 J/kg (over 40 kg) (see Table 32-2). During open-chest resuscitation, if the electrodes are applied directly to the heart, energy settings should start at 0.2 J/kg.[2,14,15,54,90] If initial shocks are unsuccessful, the energy level should be doubled and two countershocks delivered in rapid succession (see Fig. 32-3). Do not exceed 50 J with internal defibrillation.[15] If the ventricular fibrillation is converted, but then deteriorates again to fibrillation, the previously effective energy level should be used again to attempt defibrillation. Lidocaine (1 to 2 mg/kg) is indicated following successful defibrillation to raise the threshold for redeveloping ventricular fibrillation.[2] Bretylium given 5 minutes before, immediately after, or 75 seconds after ventricular fibrillation has been shown to be ineffective in treatment of canine ventricular fibrillation.[91] In one prospective study in humans, lidocaine was more effective than bretylium in treatment of human patients with potential for recurrent ventricular fibrillation.[92] Bretylium's antifibrillatory effect often takes several hours to become prominent in humans.[93]

There have been reports of felines spontaneously recovering from ventricular fibrillation.[94] Heart size influences fibrillatory potential, and the small heart of the cat may explain this phenomenon. I recommend following the normal protocol for defibrillation in the cat rather than waiting for the chance of spontaneous recovery.

The development of ventricular tachyarrhythmias after CPR is not uncommon. Management of those arrhythmias is discussed in Chapter 17.

Precordial thump has been advocated for conversion of ventricular fibrillation and ventricular tachycardia with electrocardiographic monitoring.[2] In order to deliver a precordial thump, the hand is held 8 to 12 in. above the patient's chest and a blow is delivered with the fleshy part of the palm. Continuous electrocardiographic monitoring is imperative throughout this procedure. The delivery of energy to the heart by using a precordial thump has been successful in converting ventricular tachycardia, complete atrioventricular block and ventricular fibrillation to sinus rhythm.[95] There are documented cases of nonlethal arrhythmias deteriorating into ventricular fibrillation following precordial thump. The procedure should not be considered benign and should be attempted only after an electrocardiographic rhythm has been determined.

Hazards of defibrillators. Safety should be everyone's first concern when working with defibrillators. Newer machines use direct-current (DC) impulses. Decades ago alternating current (AC) was used. Since AC instruments are more likely to fibrillate the operator, veterinarians should make certain that they do not use this type of unit. Even with up-to-date, serviced equipment, improper usage can be fatal to the operator or attending staff. The defibrillator should only be used by individuals who have received instruction in its use and who are practiced in the technique. The operator should be familiar with the controls and should regularly check the wires and paddles for defects. The operator should be the person to hold the paddles and to issue verbal instructions to the resuscitation team. Only one person should be in charge during the use of the defibrillator. This person should keep his or her hands dry. The animal can be tipped up on its back by several assistants. Electrode paste is applied to the surfaces of the paddles and the paddles are placed firmly against the chest wall crossing the cardiac area. The operator should then instruct someone to remove the electrocardiographic cable from the machine and loudly say "Clear the table." Once everyone is clear of the patient and any conductive structures the operator defibrillates the patient. If the equipment in use requires a second person to press the control button he/she should be trained to wait until told to press the button.

Electromechanical dissociation. The term "electromechanical dissociation" (EMD) has been used to describe the generation of organized electrical depolarizations of the heart without concurrent mechanical (pumping) activity.[96] The QRS wave form is often wide and bizarre, and atrial activity may be present or absent; however, normal QRS morphology is possible with EMD. Pulseless idioventricular rhythms at rates exceeding 100 bpm in humans are typically classified as ventricular tachycardias, although they are also examples of EMD.[91] One echocardiographic study demonstrated subtle wall motion in 86% of humans with EMD.[96] This reveals that mechanical activity may be more correctly described as inadequate rather than absent in EMD. Hypovolemia, pulmonary embolism, tension pneumothorax and pericardial tamponade are potential causes of "apparent" EMD.[97] The clinical implication is that every effort should be made to assess and treat the entire circulatory system not just the myocardium as represented by the electrocardiogram.

Isoproterenol was administered to dogs with EMD, in the presence of an alpha-adrenergic blocker, and electrical complexes improved, but only 27% of the animals were resuscitated.[56] When alpha-adrenergic stimulation was provided, improving coronary circulation, 100% of the dogs were resuscitated.[56] The qualitative appearance of the electrocardiogram during cardiac arrest and resuscitation had no prognostic value.[56]

Endocardial and transcutaneous cardiac pacing, calcium chloride, and epinephrine administration were studied in one canine model in which asystole or EMD was induced by countershock after 2 minutes of ventricular fibrillation.[98] The only intervention that was associated with measurable mechanical activity was infusion of epinephrine.

High-dose corticosteroids have been advocated for treatment of pulseless idioventricular rhythms,[15] but a prospective clinical trial did not confirm any beneficial effect.[99]

I recommend management of confirmed EMD with basic CPR and high-dose epinephrine administration. In cases with very wide QRS complexes, calcium administration can be attempted (provided the CPA is less than 5 minutes in duration). High-dose corticosteroids and sodium bicarbonate administration can also be attempted (see Fig. 32-3).

POSTRESUSCITATION TREATMENT

Specific steps taken at the time of restoration of spontaneous circulation in patients resuscitated successfully can influence long-term outcome and prevent postresuscitation disease (reperfusion injury).

In 1970, animal research programs were initiated to study cerebral resuscitation after cardiac arrest.[48] Laboratory studies have shown that cerebral neurons and myocardial cells can tolerate 30 to 60 minutes of ischemic anoxia.[100] Survival of the patient for more than 5 minutes of CPA is frustrated by secondary derangements, including perfusion failure (increased vascular resistance and decreased cardiac output), cerebral reoxygenation injury, and cerebral "intoxication" from derangements of extracerebral organs such as the liver and bowel.[48] The release of chelated iron

from ferritin, altered cellular calcium homeostasis, and presence of xanthine oxidase appear to cause oxygen radical production and subsequent damage (peroxidation) to cell-membrane lipids, structural proteins, and cell enzymes following reperfusion of ischemic tissue.[100]

The impact of administration of antioxidants, calcium antagonists, heparin, ibuprofen, deferoxamine, lidoflazine, and other agents on treatment and prevention of cerebral postresuscitation (reperfusion) disease are being evaluated.[18,19,48,101-105] There is evidence that once spontaneous circulation resumes, oxygen supplementation should be reduced to levels sufficient to maintain normal Pao_2.[18,19]

One study in monkeys failed to demonstrate any benefit to neurologic recovery resulting from altered head position following ischemic injury.[106] The same study showed negative effects on neurologic function in animals receiving infusion of 5% dextrose before ischemic insult.

A large multicenter study in humans having experienced cardiac arrest failed to show any advantage with barbiturate loading.[107]

Postresuscitation life-support protocols to preserve cerebral integrity have been established in humans and may prove useful in veterinary patients (see the box on the next page). Practitioners should keep in mind that species differences in response to therapy may occur.

Postresuscitation monitoring includes serial measurement of pulse, respirations, indexes of tissue perfusion, body temperature, electrocardiography, urine production, blood gases, serum electrolytes, and neurologic status. In humans, constricted pupils or pupils that were dilated initially and subsequently constrict following CPR are favorable findings.[109] Persistently dilated pupils or pupils that dilate subsequent to CPR are less favorable findings (11% recovery rate).[109] Absent pupillary light reflexes, 6 to 24 hours after CPR are an ominous sign.[109] It is important to note that atropine administration during CPR will alter pupillary response to light.

Seizure activity during the postresuscitation period is relatively common in many species. Krumholz et al. studied the significance of seizures and myoclonus in humans following CPR.[110] They found that isolated seizures and myoclonus were not related to failure to recover consciousness. The development of status epilepticus and myoclonic status epilepticus were correlated with failure to recover consciousness.[110] Patients who are alert or arousable within 12 hours of resuscitation usually recover neurologically.[108] Barring any sedative or postictal induced neurologic depression, humans who are likely to do well will arouse within 72 hours.[111]

BRAIN-ORIENTED LIFE SUPPORT FOR POST-CPR PATIENTS

1. Mild hypertension is common (mean arterial pressure between 120 and 140 mm Hg) and desirable after epinephrine administration during CPR. After this brief hypertension (1 to 5 minutes), blood pressure (mean arterial pressure, 90 mm Hg) and capillary refill time (1 to 2 seconds) should be maintained with vasopressors, vasodilators, and fluid administration
   a. Epinephrine: 0.1 to 1.0 μg/kg per minute
   b. Dopamine: 0.5 to 5 μg/kg per minute
   c. Dobutamine: 5 to 15 μg/kg per minute[2]
   d. Volume expansion using 10 ml/kg of 0.9% saline should be considered.
2. Oxygen supplementation as needed (maintain normal Pa_{O_2})[18,19]
3. Insert urinary, central venous pressure, and arterial catheters
4. Control ventilation as needed to maintain arterial P_{CO_2} at 25 to 35 mm Hg (20 to 40 mm Hg with spontaneous breathing)
5. Turn patient from side to side every 2 hours
6. Control restlessness or seizures with intravenous valium or pentobarbital administration
7. Provide analgesia with intravenous narcotic administration
8. Maintain arterial pH at 7.3 to 7.6 with ventilation and sodium bicarbonate administration
9. Consider intravenous corticosteroid administration—dexamethasone (0.2 mg/kg intravenously, followed by 0.1 mg/kg every 6 hours intravenously for 48 to 72 hours)
10. Maintain normothermia
11. Maintain hydration; administer lactated Ringer's solution or 0.9% saline—30 to 50 ml/kg per 24 hours (add potassium as needed)
12. Monitor blood constituents: hematocrit, electrolytes, serum albumin, serum osmolality, and glucose.
13. Take steps to keep intracranial pressure at or below 15 mm Hg
   a. Controlled hyperventilation (Pa_{CO_2} to 20 mm Hg), if needed
   b. Mannitol administration (2 g/kg) may have detrimental effects on cerebral blood flow.[107] When used at 0.1 g/kg it may act as a free radical scavenger[16]
   c. Loop diuretic (0.5 to 1.0 mg furosemide/kg intravenously)
   d. Corticosteroid (see no. 9)
   e. Short term hypothermia (30 to 32°C), with controlled ventilation and muscle relaxant
14. Assess neurologic progress

Modified from Safar P. Cerebral resuscitation after cardiac arrest: A review. Circulation 1986;74(suppl IV):138-153, by permission of the American Heart Association.

CONCLUSION

In veterinary medicine the standard of care constantly improves. The incidence of anesthetic-related cardiopulmonary arrest appears to be decreasing, and the success rate for cardiopulmonary resuscitation appears to be increasing. In both areas, improvement relies on the training and preparedness of our staffs and ourselves and on the proper equipping and maintenance of our hospitals. While perfection may be beyond our reach, we can all try consciously to improve.

REFERENCES

1. Moss AJ. Prediction and prevention of sudden cardiac death. Annu Rev Med 1980;31:1-14.
2. Standards and guidelines for cardiopulmonary resuscitation (CPR) and emergency cardiac care (ECG). JAMA 1986;255:2905-2989.
3. Gilroy BA, Dunlop BJ, Shapiro HM. Outcome from cardiopulmonary resuscitation in cats: laboratory and clinical experience. J Am Anim Hosp Assoc 1986;23:133-139.
4. West JB. Pulmonary pathophysiology—the essentials, ed. 2. Baltimore: Williams & Wilkins, 1982.
5. Short CE, ed. Principles & practice of veterinary anesthesia. Baltimore: Williams & Wilkins, 1987.
6. Maier GW, Tyson GS, Olsen CO, et al. The physiology of external cardiac massage; high-impulse cardiopulmonary resuscitation. Circulation 1984;70:86-101.
7. Keenan RL, Boyan P. Cardiac arrest due to anesthesia. JAMA 1985;253:2373-2377.
8. Eisenberg M, Bergner L, Hallstron A. Epidemiology of cardiac arrest and resuscitation in children. Ann Emerg Med 1983;12:672-674.
9. Dodman NH. Feline anaesthesia survey. J Small Anim Pract 1977;18:653-658.
10. Muir WW, Werner LL, Hamlin RL. Effects of xylazine and acetylpromazine upon induced ventricular fibrillation in dogs anesthetized with thiamylal and halothane. Am J Vet Res 1975;36:1299-1303.
11. Berne RM, Levy MN. Cardiovascular physiology, ed. 5. St. Louis: CV Mosby, 1986.
12. Shepherd JT, Vanhoutte PM. The human cardiovascular system—facts and concepts. New York: Raven Press, 1979.
13. Redding JS, Haynes RR, Thomas JD. Drug therapy in resuscitation from electromechanical dissociation. Crit Care Med 1983;11:681-684.

14. Haskins SC. Cardiopulmonary resuscitation. Compend Contin Educ Pract Vet 1982;4:170-182.
15. Crow DT. Cardiopulmonary resuscitation in the dog: a review and proposed new guidelines (Parts 1 & 2). Semin Vet Med Surg Small Anim 1988;3:321-348.
16. Weil MH, Rackow EC, Trevino R, Grundler W, Falk JL, Griffel MI. Difference in acid-base state between venous and arterial blood during cardiopulmonary resuscitation. N Engl J Med 1985;315:153-156.
17. Gudipati CV, Weil MH, Bisera J, Deshmakh HG, Rrackow EC. Expired carbon dioxide: a noninvasive monitor of cardiopulmonary resuscitation. Circulation 1988;77:234-239.
18. Mickel HS. Successful resuscitation of an elderly patient following cardiac arrest: possible role of reduction of reactive oxygen. Am J Emerg Med 1988;6:31-34.
19. Mickel HS, Vaishar YN, Kempski O, et al. Breathing 100% oxygen after global brain ischemia in Mongolian gerbils results in increased lipid peroxidation and increased mortality. Stroke 1987;18:426-430.
20. Jackson RE, Freeman SB. Hemodynamics of cardiac massage. Emerg Med Clin North Am 1983;1:501-513.
21. Kouwenhoven WB, Jude JR, Knickerbocker GG. Closed chest cardiac massage. JAMA 1969;173:1064-1067.
22. Criley JM, Niemann JT, Rosborough JP, Hausknecht M. Modifications of cardiopulmonary resuscitation based on the cough. Circulation 1986;74(suppl IV):42-50.
23. Halprin HR, Tsitlik JE, Guerci AD, et al. Determinants of blood flow to vital organs during cardiopulmonary resuscitation in dogs. Circulation 1986;73:539-550.
24. Henik RA, Wingfield WE, Angleton GM, et al. Effects of body position and ventilation/compression ratios during cardiopulmonary resuscitation in cats. Am J Vet Res 1987;48:1603-1606.
25. Criley JM, Blaufuss AH, Kissell GL. Cough-induced cardiac compression. JAMA 1976;236:1246-1250.
26. Niemann JT. Differences in cerebral and myocardial perfusion during closed-chest resuscitation. Ann Emerg Med 1984;13:849-853.
27. Niemann JT, Rosborough JP, Criley JM. Continuous external counterpressure during closed-chest resuscitation: a critical appraisal of the military antishock trouser garment and abdominal binder. Circulation 1986;74(suppl IV):102-107.
28. Niemann JT, Rosborough JP, Ung S, Criley JM. Hemodynamic effects of continuous abdominal binding during resuscitation. Am J Cardiol 1984;53:269-274.
29. Ewy GA. Alternative approaches to external chest compression. Circulation 1986;74(suppl IV):98-101.
30. Raessler KL, Kern KB, Sanders AB, Tacker WA, Ewy GA. Aortic and right atrial systolic pressures during cardiopulmonary resuscitation: a potential indicator of the mechanism of blood flow. Am Heart J 1988;115:1021-1029.
31. Howard M, Carrubba C, Foss F, Janiak B, Hogan B, Guinness M. Interposed abdominal compression—CPR: its effects on parameters of coronary perfusion in human subjects. Ann Emerg Med 1987;16:253-259.
32. Voorhees WD, Niebauer MJ, Babbs CF. Improved oxygen delivery during cardiopulmonary resuscitation with interposed abdominal compressions. Ann Emerg Med 1983;12:128-135.
33. Harris LC, Kirimli B, Safar P. Augmentation of artificial circulation during cardiopulmonary resuscitation. Anesthesiology 1967;28:730-734.
34. Kern KB, Carter AB, Showen RL, et al. Twenty-four hour survival in a canine model of cardiac arrest comparing three methods of manual cardiopulmonary resuscitation. J Am Coll Cardiol 1986;7:859-867.
35. Babbs CF, Tacker WA. Cardiopulmonary resuscitation with interposed abdominal compression. Circulation 1986;74(suppl IV):37-41.
36. Paraskos JA. External compression without adjuncts. Circulation 1986;74(suppl IV):33-36.
37. Deshmukh HG, Weil MH, Rackow EC, Trevino R, Bisera J. Echocardiographic observations during cardiopulmonary resuscitation: a preliminary report. Crit Care Med 1985;13:904-906.
38. Feneley MP, Maier GW, Gaynor JW, et al. Sequence of mitral valve motion and transmitral blood flow during manual cardiopulmonary resuscitation in dogs. Circulation 1987;76:363-375.
39. Weisfeldt ML, Halperin HR. Cardiopulmonary resuscitation: beyond cardiac massage. Circulation 1986;74:443-448.
40. Feneley MP, Maier GW, Kern KB, et al. Influence of compression rate on initial success of resuscitation and 24 hour survival after prolonged manual cardiopulmonary resuscitation in dogs. Circulation 1988;77:240-250.
41. Maier GW, Newton JR, Wolfe JA, et al. The influence of manual chest compression rate on hemodynamic support during cardiac arrest: high-impulse cardiopulmonary resuscitation. Circulation 1986;74(suppl IV):51-59.
42. Weiser F, Adler L, Kuhn L. Hemodynamic effects of closed and open chest cardiac resuscitation in normal dogs and those with acute myocardial infarction. Circulation 1962;10:555.
43. Bircher N, Safar P. Manual open-chest cardiopulmonary resuscitation. Ann Emerg Med 1984;13:770-773.
44. Alifimoff JK. Open versus closed chest cardiac massage in nontraumatic, cardiac arrest. Resuscitation 1987;15:13-21.
45. Sanders AB, Kern KB, Ewy GH. Time limitations for open-chest cardiopulmonary resuscitation from cardiac arrest. Crit Care Med 1985;13:897-898.
46. Kern KB, Sanders AB, Badylak SF, et al. Long-term survival with open-chest cardiac massage after ineffective closed-chest compression in a canine preparation. Circulation 1987;75:498-503.
47. Indrieri RJ, Evans AT, Krause GS, et al. Cardiac arrest and resuscitation: The lights are on but nobody's home. Proceedings of the American College of Veterinary Internal Medicine, 1986, Washington DC., 1986:11-3 to 11-14.
48. Safar P. Cerebral resuscitation after cardiac arrest: a review. Circulation 1986:74(suppl IV):138-153.
49. Nordstrom CH, Rehncrona S, Siesjo BK. Restitution of cerebral energy state, as well as of glycolysic metabolites, citric acid cycle intermediates and associated amino acids after 30 minutes of complete ischemia in rats anesthetized with nitrous oxide or phenobarbital. J Neurochem 1978;30:479-486.
50. Steen PA, Michenfelder JD, Milde JH. Incomplete versus complete cerebral ischemia: improved outcome with a minimal blood flow. Ann Neurol 1979;6:389.
51. Rehncrona S, Mela L, Siesjo BK. Recovery of brain mitochondrial function in the rat after complete and incomplete cerebral ischemia. Stroke 1979;10:437-446.
52. Sanders AB, Kern KB, Bragg S, et al. Neurologic benefits from the use of early cardiopulmonary resuscitation. Ann Emerg Med 1987;16:142-146.
53. Ralston SH, Tacker WA, Showen L, Carter H, Babbs CF. Endotracheal versus intravenous eipinphrine during electromechanical dissociation with CPR in dogs. Ann Emerg Med 1985;14:1044-1048.
54. Henik RA, Wingfield WE. Cardiopulmonary resuscitation in cats. Semin Vet Med Surg Small Anim 1988;3:185-192.
55. Sabin HI, Coghill SB, Khunti K, McNeill GO. Accuracy of intracardiac injections determined by a post-mortem study. Lancet 1983;2:1054-1055.

56. Yakaitis RW, Otto CW, Blitt CD. Relative importance of alpha and beta adrenergic receptors during resuscitation. Crit Care Med 1979;7:293-296.

57. Michael JF, Guerci AD, Koehler RC, et al. Mechanisms by which epinephrine augments cerebral and myocardial perfusion during cardiopulmonary resuscitation in dogs. Circulation 1984;69:822-835.

58. Sander AB, Ewy GA, Taft TV. Prognostic and therapeutic importance of the aortic diastolic pressure in resuscitation from cardiac arrest. Crit Care Med 1984;12:871-873.

59. Redding JS, Pearson JW. Evaluation of drugs for cardiac resuscitation. Anesthesiology 1963;24:203-207.

60. Brillman J, Sanders A, Otto CW, Fahmy H, Bragg S, Ewy GA. Comparison of epinephrine and phenylephrine for resuscitation and neurologic outcome of cardiac arrest in dogs. Ann Emerg Med 1987;16:11-17.

61. Koscove EM, Paradis NA. Successful resuscitation from cardiac arrest using high-dose epinephrine therapy. JAMA 1988;259:3031-3034.

62. Brown CG, Taylor RB, Werman HA, Luu T, Ashton J, Hamlin RL. Myocardial oxygen delivery/consumption during cardiopulmonary resuscitation: a comparison of epinephrine and phenylephrine. Ann Emerg Med 1988;17:302-308.

63. Bednarski RM, Muir WW. Arrhythmogenicity of dopamine, dobutamine, and epinephrine in thiamylal-halothane anesthetized dogs. Am J Vet Res 1983;44:2341-2343.

64. Muir WW, Werner LL and Hamlin RL. Antiarrhythmic effects of diazepam during coronary artery occlusion in dogs. Am J Vet Res 1975;36:1203-1206.

65. Maze M, Hayward E, Gaba DM. Alpha-1-adrenergic blockade raises epinephrine-arrhythmia threshold in halothane-anesthetized dogs in a dose-dependent fashion. Anesthesiology 1985;63:611-615.

66. Thompson BM, Steuven HS, Tonsfeldt DJ, et al. Calcium: limited indications, some danger. Circulation 1986;74(suppl IV):90-93.

67. Stueven HA, Thompson B, Aprahamian C, Tonsfeldt DJ, Kastenson EH. Lack of effectiveness of calcium chloride in refractory asystole. Ann Emerg Med 1985;14:630-632.

68. Blecic S, DeBacker D, Huynh CH, et al. Calcium chloride in experimental electromechanical dissociation: placebo-controlled trial in dogs. Crit Care Med 1987;15:324-327.

69. Stempien A, Katz AM, Messineo FC. Calcium and cardiac arrest. Ann Intern Med 1986;105:603-606.

70. Moses BL. Cardiac arrhythmias and cardiopulmonary arrest. In Morgan RV, ed. Handbook of small animal practice. New York: Churchill Livingstone, 1988:71-90.

71. Urban P, Scheidegger D, Buchmann B, Barth D. Cardiac arrest and blood ionized calcium levels. Ann Intern Med 1988;109:110-113.

72. Shen AC, Jennings RB. Myocardial calcium and magnesium in acute myocardial ischemic injury. Am J Pathol 1972;67:417.

73. Zaritsky A, Nadkarmi V, Gaston P, et al. CPR in children. Ann Emerg Med 1987;16:1101-1107.

74. Best R, Martin GB, Carden DL, Tomlanovich MC, Foreback C, Nowak RM. Ionized calcium during CPR in the canine model. Ann Emerg Med 1985;14:633-635.

75. Stueven HA, Thompson B, Aprahamian C, et al. The effectiveness of calcium chloride in refractory electromechanical dissociation. Ann Emerg Med, 1985;14:626-629.

76. Guerci AD, Chandra N, Johnson E, et al. Failure of sodium bicarbonate to improve resuscitation from ventricular fibrillation in dogs. Circulation 1986;74(suppl IV):75-79.

77. Stueven HA, Tonsfeldt DJ, Thompson BM, Whitcomb J, Kastenson E, Arahamian C. Atropine in asystole: human studies. Ann Emerg Med 1984;13:815-817.

78. Cooper MJ, Abinader EG. Atropine-induced ventricular fibrillation: case report and review of the literature. Am Heart J 1979;97:225-228.

79. Lazzari JO, Benchuga EG, Elizari MV, Rosenbaum MB. Ventricular fibrillation after intravenous atropine in a patient with atrioventricular block. Pace 1982;5:196-200.

80. Muir WW. Effects of atropine on cardiac rate and rhythm in dogs. J Am Vet Med Assoc 1978;172:917-921.

81. Rardon, DP, Bailey JC. Parasympathetic effects on electrophysiologic properties of cardiac ventricular tissue. J Am Coll Cardiol 1983;2:1200-1209.

82. Mirakhur RK. Premedication with atropine or glycopyrrolate in children—effects on heart rate and rhythm during induction and maintenance of anaesthesia. Anaesthesia 1982;37:1032-1036.

83. Grundler WG, Weil MH, Miller M, Rackow EC. Observations on colloid osmotic pressure, hematocrit, and plasma osmolality during cardiac arrest. Crit Care Med 1985;13:895.

84. Ditchey RV, Lindenfeld J. Potential adverse effects of volume loading on perfusion of vital organs during closed-chest resuscitation. Circulation 1984;69:181-189.

85. D'Alcey LG, Lundy EF, Barton KJ, Zelenock GB. Dextrose containing intravenouse fluid impairs outcome and increases death after eight minutes of cardiac arrest and resuscitation in dogs. Surgery 1986;100:505-511.

86. Muir WW. Comparative aspects of hypertonic saline resuscitation. In Proceedings of the Seventh Annual Veterinary Medical Forum. San Diego: American College of Veterinary Internal Medicine, 1989:836-839.

87. Ewy GA. Ventricular fibrillation masqueradting as asystole. Ann Emerg Med 1984;13:811-812.

88. Weaver WD, Cobb LA, Dennis D, Ray R, Hallstrom AP, Copass MK. Amplitude of ventricular fibrillation waveform and outcome after cardiac arrest. Ann Intern Med 1985;102:53-55.

89. Sisson DD. The clinical management of cardiac arrhythmias in the dog and cat. In Fox PR, ed. Canine and feline cardiology. New York: Churchill Livingstone, 1988:289-308.

90. Geddes LA, Tacker WA, Rosborough JP, et al. Electrical dose for ventricular defibrillation of large and small animals using precordial electrodes. J Clin Invest 1974;53:310.

91. Breznock EM, Kagan K, Hibser NK. Effects of bretylium tosylate on the in vivo fibrillating canine ventricle. Am J Vet Res 1977;38:89-94.

92. Olson DW, Thompson BM, Darin JC, Milbrath MH. A randomized comparison study of bretylium tosylate and lidocaine in resuscitation of patients from out-of-hospital ventricular fibrillation in a paramedic system. Ann Emerg Med 1984(Part 2);13:807-810.

93. Sobel BE, Braunwald E, Pasternak, RC. Acute myocardial infarction. In Braunwald E, ed. Heart disease: A textbook of cardiovascular medicine, ed. 3. Philadelphia: WB Saunders, 1988:1222-1313.

94. Coulter DB, Duncan RJ, Sander PD. Effects of asphyxia and potassium on canine and feline electrocardiograms. Can J Comp Med 1975;39:442-449.

95. Miller J, Tresch D, Horwitz L, et al. The precordial thump. Ann Emerg Med 1984;13:791-794.

96. Bocka JJ, Overton DT, Hauser A, Oak R. Electromechanical dissociation in human beings: an echocardiographic evaluation. Ann Emerg Med 1988;17:450-452.

97. Sutton-Tyrrell K, Abramson NS, Safar P, et al. Predictors of electromechanical dissociation during cardiac arrest. Ann Emerg Med 1988;17:572-575.

98. Niemann JT, Adomian GE, Garner D and Rosborough JP. Endocardial and transcutaneous cardiac pacing, calcium chloride, and epinephrine in postcountershock asystole and bradycardias. Crit Care Med 1985;13:699-704.

99. Carden DL. High-dose corticosteroids in the treatment of pulseless idioventricular rhythm. Ann Emerg Med 1984;13:817-819.

100. Weaver WD. Calcium-channel blockers and advanced cardiac life support. Circulation 1986;74(suppl IV):94-97.

101. Babbs CF. Reperfusion injury of posischemic tissues. Ann Emerg Med 1988;17:1148-1157.

102. Grice SC, Chappel ET, Prough DS, et al. Ibuprofen improves cerebral blood flow after global cerebral ischemia in dogs. Stroke 1987;18:787-791.

103. Vaagenes P, Cantodore R, Safar P, et al. Amelioration of brain damage by lidoflazine after prolonged ventricular fibrillation cardiac arrest in dogs. Crit Care Med 1984;12:846-855.

104. Kuhn, JE, Steimle CN, Zelenock GB, et al. Ibuprofen improves survival and neurologic outcome after resuscitation from cardiac arrest. Resuscitation 1986;14:199-212.

105. Fleischer JE, Lanier WL, Milde JH, et al. Failure of deferoxamine, an iron chelator, to improve neurologic outcome following complete cerebral ischemia in dogs.Stroke 1987;18:124-127.

106. Lanier WL, Stangland KJ, Scheithauer BW, et al. The effects of dextrose infusion and head position on neurologic outcome after complete cerebral ischemia in primates: examination of a model. Anesthesiology 1987;66:39-48.

107. Brain Resuscitation Clinical Trial I Study Group. Randomized clinical study of thiopental loading in comatose survivors of cardiac arrest. N Engl J Med 1986;314:397-403.

108. Arai T, Tsukahara I, Nitta K, et al. Effects of mannitol on cerebral circulation after transient complete cerebral ischemia in dogs. Crit Care Med 1986;14:634-637.

109. Steen-Hansen JE, Hansen NN, Vaagenes P, Schreiner B. Pupil size and light reactivity during cardiopulmonary resuscitation: a clinical study. Crit Care Med 1988;16:69-70.

110. Krumholz A, Stern BJ, Weiss HD. Outcome from coma after cardiopulmonary resuscitation: relation to seizures and myoclonus. Neurology 1988;38:401-405.

111. Snyder BD, Tabbaa MA. Assessment and treatment of neurological dysfunction after cardiac arrest. Curr Concepts Cerebrovasc Dis Stroke 1987;22:1-6.

33 Anesthesia for Compromised Patients

David C. Seeler

GENERAL CONSIDERATIONS

Anesthesia for the compromised patient, or any patient with multisystemic disorders including trauma, requires meticulous attention to detail, rapid evaluation of changes in the patient's status, and therapeutic intervention by the clinician when deemed necessary.

The successful outcome of an anesthetic procedure for a compromised patient is intricately related to the preoperative and postoperative care provided (see also Chapter 12). The clinician must use anesthetic protocols and techniques with which he or she is familiar. Anesthetic protocols provide guidelines for action that enable the practitioner to

1. Ensure adequate preanesthetic preparation of the patient;
2. Identify potential risks to the patient associated with the administration of specific anesthetic agents;
3. Standardize techniques in order to reduce the incidence of technical errors;
4. Detect patient abnormalities by adequate monitoring;
5. Provide optimal intraoperative supportive therapy; and
6. Ensure adequate postoperative care.[1]

The clinician must develop predefined anesthetic regimens based on the diseases encountered in the veterinary patient. When the clinician must anesthetize a compromised patient, selection of the basic regimen is based on knowledge of the interrelationships of the technique(s) involved, the pharmacologic effects of the drugs being considered, the pathophysiologic effects of the patient's disease processes, and the possible occurrence of an unanticipated event.

Adherence to specific protocols during the anesthetic procedure will reduce the incidence of technical errors that often occur in the emergency situation. While defined anesthetic regimens will improve the clinician's ability to handle difficult procedures efficiently, in terms of time and effort it is essential that a flexible attitude be maintained. Induction, surgical and recovery rooms must be well organized, with functional equipment and emergency supplies readily available in order to avoid the frustration of being forced to leave the room to retrieve emergency equipment when it is acutely needed. All personnel must learn where the equipment is and how to use it properly. This familiarization process must occur before the need to use the equipment arises. Implementation of untried techniques or new technology in the emergency situation can only jeopardize the chance of a successful outcome.

PREOPERATIVE PATIENT ASSESSMENT

There are a number of potential complications that can be encountered in emergency cases. These may include inadequate time to stabilize the patient completely, alteration of central nervous system function, respiratory abnormalities, cardiovascular disturbances, and other unrecognized injuries possibly unrelated to the primary disease process. It is possible that under certain circumstances, the patient will not have been stabilized prior to induction of anesthesia, and this reduces the chance of a successful outcome.

Preoperative assessment and preparation of the patient for anesthesia is based on a critical clinical assessment and assignment of priorities. The physical examination must be completed with particular attention directed to the body systems adversely affected during general anesthesia. It is not uncommon for traumatized patients to have concurrent functional alterations in many of these body systems.

Trauma patients may suffer traumatic myocar-

Table 33-1 Pulmonary causes of respiratory impairment in compromised patients

Obstructive	Restrictive	Ventilation/Perfusion Mismatch
Excessive secretions	Pulmonary contusion	Pulmonary atelectasis
Allergic asthma	Hyaline membrane disease	Pulmonary contusion
Pulmonary edema	Pneumonia	Pulmonary cysts
	Pulmonary edema	Pneumonia
	Infiltrative disease	Pulmonary neoplasia
		Pulmonary embolism

Adapted from Dodman NH, Seeler DC, Norman WM, Court MH. General anesthesia for small animal patients with respiratory disease. Br Vet J 1987;143:291-305.

ditis as the result of direct injury to the myocardium or indirectly due to neurovascular injury. These patients may present with posttraumatic dysrhythmias such as premature ventricular contractions, ventricular tachycardia, or nonspecific ST-segment elevations on electrocardiography.[2-4] These dysrhythmias may occur spontaneously up to 48 hours after injury. Similarly, the clinician must expect that dysrhythmias secondary to gastric dilatation/volvulus can occur up to 72 hours postoperatively.[5] The clinician must ensure that such rhythm disturbances are not present, or are controlled prior to administration of a general anesthetic.

Pulmonary disorders commonly seen in the traumatized patient include pulmonary contusions, edema, atelectasis, and cysts.[6-8] These disorders of the lung will have varying negative impact on the overall ventilatory and physiologic status of the patient (Table 33-1). Extrapulmonary disorders may also have a negative influence on respiratory function[8,9] (Table 33-2). It is important to note that a disorder with significant anesthetic implications such as a mild pneumothorax, may not be clinically obvious in the conscious animal.[10] The degree of risk associated with administration of a general anesthetic to the patient is related to the degree of respiratory dysfunction. Oxygen supplementation of the inspired gas mixture may be provided by the use of a face mask or other means prior to induction of anesthesia,[11] and where necessary, ventilatory support should be provided.

Traumatic injury to the abdominal and pelvic regions may result in rupture or laceration of abdominal viscera such as kidney, liver, or spleen.[12] Subclinical to clinical alterations in cardiovascular function or electrolyte and acid-base status should be suspected in the above situations.

The compromised patient may exhibit diminished levels of consciousness, which has an impact on the choice of anesthetic agents and how they are administered. There would be minimal requirement for the administration of a general

Table 33-2 Extrapulmonary causes of respiratory impairment in the compromised patient

Obstructive	Restrictive
Larynx	Intrapleural
Stenosis	Diaphragmatic hernia
Spasm	Pleural effusion
Foreign body	Pneumothorax
Everted lateral ventri-	Thoracic wall
cles	Rib fracture
Extralaryngeal mass	Flail chest
Collapsed arytenoids	Body bandages
Laryngeal paralysis	
Trachea	Abdominal
Collapse	Ascites
Foreign body	Hemoperitoneum
Edema	Gastric dilation

Adapted from Dodman NH, Seeler, DC, Norman WM, Court MH. General anaesthesia for small animal patients with respiratory disease. Br Vet J 1987;143:291-305.

anesthetic to the comatose patient. The clinician should be prepared to administer a general anesthetic or a local analgesic if the patient regains consciousness during the surgical procedure.

In the acute situation in which the patient must undergo surgery to correct a life-threatening disorder, it is imperative that blood samples be obtained and submitted for laboratory analysis in order to obtain information necessary for the selection of an appropriate anesthetic technique. Laboratory data, which will aid the clinician in assessing the patient's status and allow for the selection of an optimal anesthetic protocol, would include hematocrit, hemoglobin concentration, total serum protein concentration, white blood cell and platelet counts, blood urea nitrogen, creatinine, glucose, serum sodium and potassium levels, and where possible, serum lactate concentrations and a coagulation profile. The value of these tests to the clinician is improved immeasurably when each is rapidly and accurately obtained. Ancillary diagnostic tests such as radiography, contrast radiography, ultrasonography, electrocardiography, and abdominocentesis or thoracocentesis must be considered for each patient.

PREOPERATIVE PATIENT TREATMENT

It is incumbent on the clinician to ensure that, when possible, abnormalities detected during the preoperative preparation period are attended to prior to the induction of anesthesia. In situations in which patient stabilization is not possible due to a life-threatening emergency, clinical management of the disorder(s) must occur intraoperatively.

An attempt should be made to restore vascular volume, preload, and blood pressure if deficiencies exist, in order to ensure adequate cardiovascular function and organ perfusion in the perioperative period. Acute reductions in packed cell volume to levels less than 25% or hemoglobin values to levels less than 7 g/dl should be corrected by administration of fresh packed cells or fresh whole blood. Such reductions in packed cell volume and hemoglobin levels are compensated for in the normal patient by a decrease in systemic vascular resistance and an increase in cardiac output, thus maintaining organ perfusion and oxygen delivery. Compromised patients may not be able to compensate for acute reductions in packed cell volume. The packed cell volume would be reduced during general anesthesia by an additional 3% to 5%, further diminishing oxygen delivery to peripheral tissues. Once a general anesthetic is administered, these patients would be put at further risk because of reduction in cardiac output and redistribution of peripheral blood flow.

Pneumothorax or pleural effusions in the traumatized patient adversely affect cardiopulmonary function. Volumes of air equivalent to 175% of the lung volume introduced into the pleural space of healthy, conscious dogs was required to cause respiratory distress.[10] Respiratory dysfunction was evidenced by pulmonary collapse, impairment of oxygen diffusion, ventilation/perfusion abnormalities and intrapulmonary shunting of blood.[10] Since it is unlikely that a compromised patient could withstand similar changes in respiratory function, a pneumothorax must be corrected by thoracocentesis prior to induction of anesthesia. A tube thoracostomy should be seriously considered. Ventilatory disturbances may occur intraoperatively, and if positive-pressure ventilation is applied, pneumothorax may recur. Without a tube thoracostomy in place, the patient's status could be rapidly compromised.

Hypovolemic animals, or patients who have suffered trauma to the urinary system may have reduced renal function. Reductions in renal function can lead to numerous metabolic disturbances, including acid-base and serum electrolyte abnormalities. Volume replacement in hypovolemic patients will improve renal blood flow and glomerular function. A urinary catheter should be placed in order that urine production can be monitored throughout the perioperative period. This preoperative treatment will help support renal function, particularly during the intraoperative period, when general anesthetics may reduce renal blood flow and glomerular filtration by 40%.[13] It should be remembered that systemic disturbances resulting from urinary system dysfunction will directly affect the pharmacologic actions of commonly used anesthetic drugs.[14]

Acid-base and electrolyte disturbances should be corrected prior to induction of anesthesia. In many instances in the compromised patient, acidemia is present. Acidosis should be corrected prior to induction of anesthesia if the pH is less than 7.1. When the pH is less than 7.1, myocardial responses to cardioactive agents are reduced.[15] Serum potassium levels greater than 6.0 mEq/L can result in significant alterations in cardiac bioelectricity,[16] further compromising the patient.

Central nervous system dysfunction may profoundly affect the type of anesthetic technique employed or pharmacologic agents administered. Increases in intracranial pressure (ICP), if present, should be reduced by proper application of positive-pressure ventilation and by the intravenous administration of mannitol at a dose of 1.0 to 2.0 g/kg. Mannitol should be administered only after vascular volume and mean systemic arterial blood pressure have been restored to appropriate levels. Bradycardia can occur in animals with increased ICP, and it often self-corrects once the pressure has been reduced to normal.

ANESTHETIC PLAN

Once the patient has been stabilized, the clinician must assess the anesthetic risk to the patient.[1] Classification of the patient's physical status using standardized criteria will enable the clinician to handle problems in a consistent manner. Class I patients are considered to be at minimal risk. Animals classified as Class II, or low-risk, patients show slight to mild systemic disturbances. Class III patients present moderate systemic disease or disturbances. Animals with severe preexisting systemic disease or disturbances are considered to be high-risk patients and are considered Class IV. Animals in the Class V category are at grave risk and include moribund animals that may not survive 24 hours. If the anticipated procedure is considered an emergency, then an E is added to the classification (Class IVE).

Assessment of risk to the patient, the degree to which the patient has been stabilized, the clinician's familiarity with various anesthetic techniques, and the pharmacologic properties of the agents contemplated all play a role in the selection of the anesthetic technique. Primary consideration, in terms of anesthetic regimens, must be given to optimizing oxygen transport to tissues, reducing oxygen consumption, ensuring unconsciousness, providing analgesia, and providing the conditions necessary for the procedure to be carried out. In many instances, airway control, supplemental oxygenation, and ventilatory support will be required in the perioperative period. In order for care of the endangered patient to be optimized, some form of balanced anesthetic technique using either a single agent, a combination of inhalational or injectable agents, or both, should be considered. This type of anesthetic regimen will produce the desired level of central nervous system depression and analgesia while minimizing depression of cardiovascular function. If the animal is depressed or comatose, local analgesia may be all that is required. With this technique, the ability of the clinician to control the airway or implement positive-pressure ventilation, if required, is limited.

Venous access is mandatory in these patients prior to the induction of anesthesia, and consideration should be given to the placement of two large-bore catheters. If significant intraoperative blood loss occurs, fluid or whole blood can be administered rapidly when two patent catheters are available. Any catheter that has been placed previously must be checked to ensure that it is patent and has not been dislodged. If the catheter is not functional or is smaller than 18-gauge in diameter it should be replaced or supplemented by placement of another larger-bore catheter. The second catheter also provides an intravenous access for therapeutic agents that are incompatible with the fluid being administered for vascular volume support. Sodium bicarbonate, for example, is incompatible with dextrose, lactated Ringer's, and calcium salt solutions.[16] No therapeutic agents should be administered mixed with whole blood. Emergency drugs, such as the sympathomimetics should be diluted to clinically useful concentrations using normal saline or 5% dextrose.

A central venous catheter should be placed in animals that present with cardiovascular instability or that require substantial fluid therapy. The central venous catheter should not be relied on for rapid volume replacement due to its small diameter. The primary purpose of the central venous

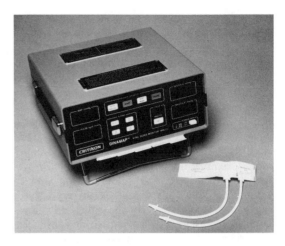

Fig. 33-1 An indirect blood pressure monitor may be used to monitor systolic, mean, and diastolic blood pressures and peripheral pulse rate.

catheter is to provide the clinician with information regarding trends in cardiovascular function.

An intraarterial catheter can be placed in the dorsal pedal artery or femoral artery to monitor blood pressure directly. The arterial access enables the clinician to collect arterial blood samples for measurement of blood gas partial pressures. If the catheter cannot be placed until after the induction of anesthesia, it is important to ensure that the time required for its placement does not unnecessarily extend total anesthesia time. If there is delay or difficulty in placing the arterial catheter, the attempt should be abandoned in favor of indirect methods of monitoring blood pressure (Fig. 33-1).

PREMEDICATION

The induction of, and recovery from, general anesthesia tends to be smoother when a premedicant has been used. The dosages required to induce and maintain anesthesia are reduced as well. Excitement, either as a result of restraint or fear, may cause an increase in circulating catecholamine levels. This could have a substantial impact on cardiovascular stability in the compromised patient. For these reasons, premedication of the compromised patient prior to induction of anesthesia may be desirable. Appropriate or selective use of a premedication agent will ensure that the animal is free from pain and apprehension. If the physical status of the patient is critical, administration of a premedicant may not be warranted. If such is the case, care should be taken throughout the induction period to ensure that the patient is not excessively stressed or overdosed with the induction agent.

The premedicant chosen varies according to the

physical status and temperament of the patient, the type and duration of the procedure, and the anesthetic regimen being considered. It is desirable to use drugs that have pharmacologic properties that can be reversed. The clinician should consider using an analgesic such as a narcotic or a partial opioid agonist in the compromised patient. Narcotic analgesics do cause ventilatory depression, but this effect can be minimized by careful selection of the agent and dosage used. Narcotics have a minimal impact on the cardiovascular system, particularly if used in conjunction with an anticholinergic. While dosages used vary according to the health status of the small animal patient, common dosages for narcotic analgesics are meperidine, 2.0 to 4.0 mg/kg intramuscularly, oxymorphone, 0.05-0.1 mg/kg intramuscularly, and morphine, 0.1 mg/kg intramuscularly. If systemic effects of the narcotic analgesic are more profound than originally anticipated, the clinician may reverse the narcotic's action by administering an antagonist. Partial opioid agonists such as butorphanol may be used as a preoperative analgesic for the compromised patient. While butorphanol (0.1 to 0.2 mg/kg) has moderate sedative effects in the dog or cat it does have minimal impact on cardiovascular performance.[17,18] An anticholinergic such as glycopyrrolate should also be administered when a narcotic analgesic or a partial agonist is used for premedication of the compromised patient. Glycopyrrolate (0.01 mg/kg intramuscularly) will prevent the parasympathomimetic action of the narcotic analgesics and does not normally cause as significant a change in heart rate as does atropine.[13]

Acepromazine (0.05-0.1 mg/kg intramuscularly) is one of the more commonly used premedicants in small animal practice. It is an alpha-adrenergic antagonist and can cause significant hypotension in hypovolemic animals that are maintaining systemic arterial blood pressure through enhanced sympathetic nervous system activity. Acepromazine will also reduce the seizure threshold, which could be an important consideration in an animal with a history of central nervous system trauma or seizures. Acepromazine does protect the myocardium to some extent from adrenergic-induced dysrhythmias, and its mild sedative effects do facilitate smooth induction of anesthesia.[13] Its use, however, is not generally warranted in the compromised patient.

Diazepam, at a dose of 0.2 to 0.4 mg/kg may be used for premedication of the compromised patient. While it has minimal sedative effects in the healthy small animal patient, its effect in compromised patients may be adequate. Diazepam has minimal effects on cardiopulmonary performance.

The drug may be given intravenously, thus maximizing its pharmacologic effects.

Diazepam and acepromazine both have a synergistic effect with analgesics, resulting in enhanced sedation and a prolonged duration of analgesia. Such combinations of tranquilizers or sedatives and analgesics are known as neuroleptanalgesics. These combinations can be used either for premedication or for induction of anesthesia in the compromised patient.

Premedicants are generally administered intramuscularly, except in cases in which time constraints exist due to the patient's status. When the premedicant is given intramuscularly, a period of at least 15 minutes should be allowed to elapse before anesthesia is induced. This ensures that peak pharmacologic effects of the drug or drugs are reached prior to administration of an induction agent. If a premedicant is given intravenously, it must be given slowly, so that the potential adverse reactions are minimized.

INDUCTION

The induction of anesthesia in the compromised patient should occur rapidly and smoothly. It is important to ensure, prior to inducing anesthesia, that the patient has been denitrogenated by breathing oxygen through a face mask.[19] A key goal during induction is rapid intubation of the patient, ensuring control of the airway. If the clinician is uncertain that he or she can gain control of the airway, especially when ventilatory abnormalities exist, then a tracheostomy (using local anesthesia) should be done prior to inducing anesthesia.

The physical status of the compromised patient plays a key role in the selection of an induction agent, particularly if the patient has not been stabilized. Injectable agents permit rapid inductions with minimal struggling, thus ensuring smooth transition to the anesthetized state. Unfortunately, most of the induction agents commonly used in small animal practice do alter neurocirculatory control, and these effects may last longer than is desirable in the compromised patient.[20] In addition, once administered, there is little the clinician can do to alter the drug's pharmacologic course of events, except to provide supportive therapy.

Injectable agents that could be considered for use in compromised patients include the sedative hypnotic etomidate or a neuroleptanalgesic combination. Etomidate may be administered at a dosage of 0.5 to 1.0 mg/kg intravenously and has minimal cardiopulmonary effects.[20-22] If etomidate is used as an induction agent, the clinician may consider using diazepam as a premedicant. Barbiturates alter cardiopulmonary function in the induction and postinduction periods and are not indicated for inducing anesthesia in compromised patients. Ketamine or drug combinations that include ketamine may also have a significant and undesirable impact on cardiovascular function in the compromised patient.[20,23-27] If the patient has primary cardiac disease or is maintaining cardiovascular function through enhancement of the sympathetic nervous system, ketamine should not be used as an induction agent.[15]

Narcotics can be combined with a tranquilizer or sedative for induction of anesthesia. Such combinations would include diazepam and oxymorphone or a commercial preparation such as Innovar (fentanyl/droperidol). Innovar may be used to induce anesthesia at a dosage of 1.0 ml per 15 to 25 kg, administered intramuscularly. It is important that an anticholinergic be administered in conjunction with the neuroleptanalgesic. Oxymorphone (0.1 to 0.2 mg/kg intravenously) may also be used as an induction agent in the compromised patient.

Anesthesia may also be induced by face mask, using an inhalational agent that has a low blood gas partition coefficient. Isoflurane and halothane are suitable for face-mask inductions. On occasion, the patient may become excited or struggle, particularly if a premedicant has not been used. The addition of nitrous oxide to the inspired gas mixture, if safe to do so (e.g., no pneumothorax), may minimize this potential problem. This approach is particularly effective when nitrous oxide is added to a mixture containing 1.5 to 2.0 volumes percent of the inhalational agent. The patient should be intubated rapidly following induction, the cuff inflated, and the endotracheal tube connected to an anesthetic circuit.

Patients weighing less than 7 kg are connected to a Bains circuit or similar nonrebreathing system. Partial rebreathing of expired gases occurs when fresh gas flow to the Bains system is set at 130 ml/kg per minute. Arterial carbon dioxide levels are not significantly altered by the system with this flow rate. Fresh gas flow rates ranging from 400 to 600 ml/kg per minute ensure that the system is a nonrebreathing circuit. If the patient is to be artificially ventilated, the fresh gas flow to the Bains circuit is set at 100 ml/kg per minute in order to prevent significant hypocapnia.

Animals weighing more than 7 kg should be placed on a circle system. Initially, the fresh gas flow should be at least 30 ml/kg per minute in order to ensure denitrogenation of the patient. Subsequently, the fresh gas flow being delivered to the system may be set such that the oxygen flow ranges between 20 and 30 ml/kg per minute.

The clinician's attention is then directed toward maintaining anesthesia and instituting positive-pressure ventilation if ventilatory support is to be provided. Continual monitoring of the patient remains critical as alterations in the patient's physiologic status must be attended to in a timely fashion.

MAINTENANCE

Injectable techniques using combinations of narcotics, nitrous oxide, and positive-pressure ventilation are viable alternatives to standard inhalational techniques for maintenance of anesthesia.

Anesthesia may be maintained by administering oxymorphone (0.1 mg/kg) or fentanyl (0.01 mg/kg) intravenously every 20 minutes or as needed. Bradycardia, hypoventilation, lack of muscle relaxation, and the degree of narcosis present are concerns with these techniques. Bradycardia may be prevented by use of an anticholinergic. The use of diazepam intraoperatively (0.2 mg/kg) may be considered if the level of narcosis is insufficient. Nitrous oxide administration or the inclusion of low levels of an inhalational agent in the inspired gas mixture may also be required. When using balanced narcotic techniques it is important that the patient is mechanically ventilated due to the degree of ventilatory depression that occurs with this technique.

Inhalational agents are commonly used for maintenance of general anesthesia. Isoflurane or halothane are preferred due to their low blood gas partition coefficients. This characteristic enables the clinician to respond quickly to changes in the patient's physiologic status. Isoflurane has pharmacologic properties that, when compared with those of halothane, are more desirable for use in compromised patients.[28] Cardiovascular function is better maintained with isoflurane, and there is minimal, if any, sensitization of the myocardium to the effects of circulating catecholamines. Isoflurane has been recommended for use in traumatized patients or those that present with or develop ventricular dysrhythmias.[29,30] In the unstimulated anesthetized animal, ventilatory depression can be significant. However, in the surgically stimulated patient, particularly when nitrous oxide is being used as an adjunct, ventilatory parameters can approach normal values. While there have been no studies to demonstrate that the long-term outcome for surgical procedures in compromised patients treated with isoflurane is superior to that in patients treated with halothane, isoflurane is considered the agent of choice.

Nitrous oxide administration may be useful during maintenance of anesthesia in the compromised patient if the effective oxygen delivery to the peripheral tissues is not compromised and no other contraindications exist.[13] Nitrous oxide, when delivered at a concentration of 66%, reduces the dosage requirement of the volatile anesthetic in use.[31] The reduction in dose of the inhalational agent administered to the patient can result in improved physiologic function. When the inspired gas mixture contains 66% nitrous oxide, the minimal flow rate for oxygen to the circle system is 30 ml/kg per minute.[32] Care should be taken in the postoperative recovery period to ensure that the patient is allowed to breath oxygen for at least 5 minutes in order to prevent the occurrence of diffusion hypoxia.

Ventilatory support in the form of mandatory positive-pressure ventilation (MPPV) is an integral part of a balanced anesthetic technique. If it is to be employed as part of the anesthetic regimen, MPPV should be instituted immediately after induction of anesthesia. Care must be taken to ensure that airway pressure is applied correctly to the compromised patient. Increased intrathoracic pressures resulting from improperly applied MPPV reduces venous return and cardiac output. This is of particular concern in the compromised patient, who would be unable to compensate for these increases in mean thoracic pressure. The ventilator is initially set for a ventilatory rate of 8 to 10 breaths per minute and a tidal volume equivalent to 20 ml/kg. Pressure-cycled ventilators can be adjusted in order that the peak inspiratory pressure ranges from 15 to 20 cm H_2O. In this instance use of a respirometer is recommended in order for tidal volumes to be known.

If atelectasis or pulmonary collapse is present, the clinician may increase the tidal volume or peak inspiratory pressure in an attempt to improve ventilation. It is important in this instance that improvements in ventilatory parameters are balanced against the adverse effects of increased mean intrathoracic pressure on cardiovascular function. The cardiopulmonary system must be closely monitored in order to ensure that ventilatory support of the patient is effective and safe. Postoperatively, the patient should be gradually weaned from ventilatory support, ensuring that transition from controlled to spontaneous ventilation occurs without compromising the patient's cardiopulmonary status.[13]

Muscle relaxants can be used to facilitate control of ventilation and for muscle relaxation. Nondepolarizing muscle relaxants such as pancuronium or vecuronium may be used in the compromised patient. These neuromuscular blocking agents have minimal effects on the cardiovascular system, and their pharmacologic activities can be reversed by an anticholinesterase such as neostigmine or edrophonium.[13] Factors that can exist in the compromised patient and that could affect the duration of action of a muscle relaxant include hypothermia, acid-base disturbances, electrolyte imbalances, and the concurrent use of an aminoglycoside.

MONITORING

During the intraoperative period, it is necessary to closely observe and record changes in the patient's status. There are two main purposes for such intensive monitoring of the compromised patient. First, it enables the clinician to maintain the lightest possible plane of anesthesia for the procedure being performed. Secondly, it enables the clinician to identify adverse trends or changes in the patient's status, allowing timely and appropriate interventions. There are a number of parameters that the clinician should monitor.[15]

Heart rate and rhythm disturbances are common in the compromised patient.[33] Bradycardia can be considered significant if the heart rate is less than 70 or if the resultant mean arterial blood pressure is less than 70 mm Hg. Atropine may be used to correct the bradycardia. If there is no response to the anticholinergic and if anesthetic depth is not excessive and requiring adjustment, then an intravenous infusion of dopamine may be used to increase the heart rate.[33]

Commonly, premature ventricular contractions are seen in the compromised patient (see Chapter 17). If the incidence of the premature contractions is greater than six per minute or if they are multiform in appearance, then therapeutic intervention is warranted.[33] In the dog, lidocaine (1.0 to 2.0 mg/kg) may be administered slowly intravenously. If the rhythm is successfully converted to a normal sinus rhythm and the rhythm disturbance recurs, a lidocaine infusion (25.0 to 80.0 μg/kg per minute) is indicated. In cats, propranolol (0.05 to 0.1 mg/kg) may be slowly administered intravenously to correct ventricular dysrhythmias. Cats are sensitive to the toxic effects of lidocaine and if lidocaine is to be used, the dose is 0.5 to 0.75 mg/kg. Infusion rates for lidocaine in the cat range from 2.0 to 6.0 μg/kg per minute.[33]

Blood pressure may be measured directly or indirectly. There are some disadvantages to the direct measurement of blood pressure, but the information obtained is accurate and continuous. Indirect methods may not provide the information required in a timely fashion, but they may be more applicable in the practical situation.[15] Indirect blood pressure measurement has become easier to use in the clinical setting. Equipment utilizing an oscillometric method of blood pressure determination has been shown to be accurate and reliable[34,35] (see Fig. 33-1). This unit is capable of measuring systolic, diastolic, and mean blood pressures either manually or automatically. Accuracy is dependent on the use of a proper size cuff and its proper application over the dorsal pedal artery (Chapter 40).

Mean systemic arterial blood pressure may be indirectly estimated by measuring urine production. Reduction of mean arterial pressure to values less than 60 mm Hg results in reduced renal perfusion and urine production. Normally, urine production ranges from 1.0 to 2.0 ml/kg per hour and values less than this indicate renal dysfunction, possibly due to hypoperfusion. It is desirable to maintain mean arterial pressure above 60 mm Hg and systolic pressures above 80 mm Hg in order to ensure adequate organ perfusion intraoperatively.

Central venous pressure (CVP) measurement provides the clinician with information regarding cardiovascular function. The monitoring system should be zeroed at the level of the right atrium since it is right atrial pressure that is to be monitored. In the healthy anesthetized animal the CVP ranges from 2.0 to 7.0 cm H_2O. Minor alterations from normal values may not indicate cardiovascular instability, but serial measurements allow the clinician to determine if a trend exists. Severe alterations in CVP indicate cardiovascular dysfunction or blood-volume abnormalities. It is necessary to determine the probable causes and to act accordingly.

Ventilatory function must be monitored during general anesthesia of the compromised patient to ensure that adequate oxygenation and removal of carbon dioxide from blood occurs. When the patient is not being mechanically ventilated, arterial carbon dioxide levels should not be allowed to exceed 60 mm Hg. Carbon dioxide levels exceeding 60 mm Hg are an indication that the spontaneously breathing patient should be mechanically ventilated. If the facilities do not exist to measure blood gas values, the clinician may use a respirometer to monitor ventilatory function. The normal tidal volume of a small animal patient ranges from 10 to 15 ml/kg. Minute ventilation ranges from 150 to 250 ml/kg per minute. Reductions of 33% in either tidal volume or minute ventilation generally indicate hypoventilation and the need for ventilatory support.

Oxygen saturation of arterial blood can be accurately determined by using a pulse oximeter (Fig. 33-2).[36,37] Measurements may be taken by placing a standard ear probe on the patient's tongue. It is important to be aware that such units only provide information related to hemoglobin saturation and not arterial oxygen tension. Thus, in the presence of a shift in the oxyhemoglobin dissociation curve due to changes in temperature or pH, oxygen delivery to peripheral tissues is not accurately reflected by a pulse oximeter.

Intraoperative fluid administration should take

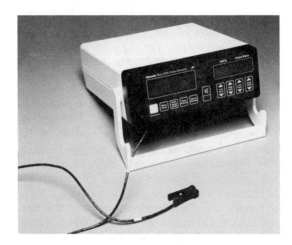

Fig. 33-2 Pulse oximetry provides information regarding arterial oxygen saturation of hemoglobin.

into account perioperative blood loss and fluid translocation from the vascular system due to surgical trauma. If volume deficits do not exist, then a balanced electrolyte solution is administered at a rate of 10-15 ml/kg per hour. In some instances of fluid loss and hypotension, lightening the plane of anesthesia and correcting the underlying cause may be all that is necessary. If 10% of the blood volume is lost, it may be replaced with a balanced electrolyte solution. The volume of fluid administered should be three times that of the volume of blood lost from the vascular system. In severe cases of hypotension, the rate of fluid administration should be increased so that volumes up to 40 ml/kg are administered quickly. The packed blood cell volume and total serum solids must be closely monitored and fresh whole blood, packed red blood cells, or colloids administered as indicated.

If blood losses exceed 10% or if the packed cell volume is less than 20% then A⁻ or typed, cross matched, fresh whole blood should be administered.[13] Plasma may be used in situations in which the packed cell volume is adequate, but in which total plasma protein levels are below 3 g/dl. Alternatively, packed red blood cells or dextran-70 may be used, respectively.[13]

If the cardiovascular system is unresponsive to the initial measures taken to replace fluid loss and improve systemic arterial blood pressure, an intravenous infusion of dopamine or dobutamine (1.0 to 10.0 μg/kg per minute) may be considered. If oliguria exists in conjunction with vascular hypotension, dopamine may be administered at a rate of 1.0 to 3.0 μg/kg per minute in an attempt to improve renal perfusion and urine production.

Hypothermia is a common intraoperative problem, which reduces body metabolism 7% for each degree Celsius drop in core temperature. Such reductions in body temperature and metabolism delay distribution of drugs and prolong recovery from the anesthetic. The dose of anesthetic required to maintain anesthesia is also reduced. Bradycardia occurs as the result of the depressant effect of hypothermia on the sinoatrial node. This bradycardia is often unresponsive to the administration of an anticholinergic agent.[33] Postoperatively, excessive shivering on the part of the patient in an attempt to increase core body temperature dramatically increases oxygen demand. In this instance, supportive therapy by oxygen enrichment of the inspired gases is required.

Finally, the clinician should monitor acid-base and serum electrolyte levels and, where necessary, take the required therapeutic measures (see Chapter 38).

RECOVERY

The clinician's primary responsibility is to facilitate recovery of the patient from anesthesia and stabilize its physiologic condition. Intense monitoring of the patient must continue in order for ongoing systemic disturbances to be managed. Common postoperative problems include cardiovascular instability, ventilatory depression, hypothermia, fluid and electrolyte imbalances, and postoperative pain (see Chapter 12). Medical management of these disturbances ceases only when the patient's physiologic status has been stabilized and the patient has recovered from the anesthesia.

REFERENCES

1. Dodman NH, Seeler DC, Court MH. Recommended techniques in small animal anesthesia: an update. Br Vet J 1984;140:505-516.
2. MacIntire DK, Snider TG. Cardiac arrhythmias associated with multiple trauma in dogs. J Am Vet Med Assoc 1984;184:541-545.
3. Tamas P, Paddleford RR, Krahwinkel, DJ. Incidence of thoracic trauma in conjunction with limb fractures following motor vehicle injuries in dogs and cats. In Proceedings of the Scientific Meeting of the American College of Veterinary Anesthesiologists. Atlanta: American College of Veterinary Anesthesiologists, 1983:1-2.
4. Alexander JW, Bolton GR, Koslow GL. Electrocardiographic changes in non-penetrating trauma to the chest. J Am Anim Hosp Assoc 1975;11:160-166.
5. Muir WW, Lipowitz AJ. Cardiac dysrhythmias associated with gastric dilation-volvulus in the dog. J Am Vet Med Assoc 1978;172:683-689.
6. Spackman CJA, Caywood DD, Feeney DA, Johntson GR. Thoracic wall and pulmonary trauma in dogs sustaining fractures as a result of motor vehicle accidents. J Vet Med Assoc 1984;185:975-977.
7. Aron DN, Kornegay JN. The clinical significance of traumatic lung cysts and associated pulmonary abnormalities in the dog and cat. J Am Anim Hosp Assoc 1983;19:903-912.
8. Dodman NH, Seeler DC, Court MH. General anesthesia for small animal patients with respiratory insufficiency. Br Vet J 1987;143:291-305.
9. Roudebush P, Burns J. Pleural effusion as a sequela to traumatic diaphragmatic hernias: a review of four cases. J Am Anim Hosp Assoc 1979;15:699-706.
10. Bennett RA, Orton EC, Tucker A, Heiller, CL. Cardiopulmonary changes in conscious dogs with induced progressive pneumothorax. Am J Vet Res 1989;50:280-284.
11. Court MH, Dodman NH, Seeler DC. Inhalational therapy: oxygen administration, humidification and aerosol therapy. In Spaulding G, ed. Veterinary clinics of north america: small animal practice: Symposium on respiratory disease. Toronto: WB Saunders, 1985:1041-1059.
12. Pechman RD. Urinary trauma in dogs and cats. A review. J Am Anim Hosp Assoc 1982;18:33-40.
13. Paddleford RR, ed. Manual of small animal anesthesia. New York: Churchill Livingstone, 1988.
14. Dodman NH, Seeler DC, Court MH, Norman WM. Anaesthesia for small animal patients with disease of the hepatic, renal or gastrointestinal system. Br Vet J 1989;145:3-22.
15. Seeler DC, Dodman NH, Court M. Recommended techniques in small animal anaesthesia. IV. Anaesthesia and cardiac disease. Br Vet J 1988;144:108-122.
16. Seeler DC, Thurmon JC. Fluid and electrolyte disturbances. In Davis LE, ed. Handbook of small animal therapeutics. New York: Churchill Livingstone, 1985:21-43.
17. Trim CM. Cardiopulmonary effects of butorphanol tartrate in dogs. Am J Vet Res 1983;44:329-331.
18. Sawyer DC, Rech RH. Analgesia and behavioural effects of butorphanol, nalbuphine and pentazocine in the cat. J Am Anim Hosp Assoc 1987;23:438-446.
19. Carmichael FJ, Cruise CJE, Crago RR, Paluk S. Preoxygenation: a study of denitrogenation. Anesth Analg 1989;68:406-409.
20. Priano LL, Bernards C, Marrone B. Effect of anesthetic induction agents on cardiovascular neuroregulation in dogs. Anesth Analg 1989;68:344-349.
21. Nagel ML, Muir WW, Nguyen K. Comparison of the cardiopulmonary effects of etomidate and thiamylal in dogs. Am J Vet Res 1979;40:193-196.
22. Wauquier A. Profile of etomidate—a hypnotic, anticonvulsant and brain protection compound. Anaesthesia 1983;38:26-33.
23. Waxman K, Shoemaker WC, Lippman M. Cardiovascular effects of anesthetic induction with ketamine. Anesth Analg 1980;59:355-358.
24. White PF, Way WL, Trevor AJ. Ketamine—its pharmacology and therapeutic uses. Anesthesiology 1982;56:119-136.
25. Farver TB, Haskins SC, Patz JD. Cardiopulmonary effects of acepromazine and of the subsequent administration of ketamine in the dog. Am J Vet Res 1986;47:631-635.
26. Bednarski RM, Sams RA, Majors LJ, Ashcroft S. Reduction of the ventricular arrhythmogenic dose of epinephrine by ketamine administration in halothane-anesthetized cats. Am J Vet Res 1988;49:350-354.
27. Ingwersen W, Allen DG, Dyson DH, Black WD, Goldberg MT, Valliant AE: Cardiopulmonary effects of ketamine/acepromazine combination in hypovolemic cats. Can J Vet Res 1988;52:423-427.
28. Wade JG, Stevens WC. Isoflurane: an anesthetic for the eighties? Anesth Analg 1981;60:666-682.
29. Harvey R, Short CE. The use of isoflurane for safe anesthesia in animals with traumatic myocarditis or other sensitivities. In Proceedings of the Scientific Meeting of the American College of Veterinary Anesthesiologists. Las Vegas: American College of Veterinary Anesthesiologists, 1982:3-4.
30. Hubbell JAE, Muir WW, Bednarski RM, Bednarski LS. Change of inhalational anesthetic agents for management

of ventricular premature depolorization in anesthetized cats and dogs. J Am Vet Med Assoc 1984;185:643-646.

31. DeYoung DJ, Sawyer DC. Anesthetic potency of nitrous oxide during halothane anesthesia in the dog. J Am Anim Hosp Assoc 1980;16:125-128.

32. Dohoo SE, McDonell WN, Dohoo IR. A comparison of fresh gas flows during anesthesia with nitrous oxide in the dog. J Am Anim Hosp Assoc 1982;18:900-904.

33. Seeler DC, Dodman NH, Court MH. Recommended techniques in small animal anesthesia. II. Intraoperative cardiac dysrhythmias and their treatment. Br Vet J 1987;143:97-111.

34. Geddes LA, Chaffe V, Whistler SJ, Bourland JD. Indirect mean blood pressure in the anesthetized pony. Am J Vet Res 1977;38:2055-2057.

35. Hamlin RL, Kittleson MD, Rice D, Knowles G, Seyffert R. Non-invasive measurement of systemic arterial pressure in dogs by automatic sphygmomanometry. Am J Vet Res 1982;43:1271-1273.

36. Alexander CM, Teller LE, Gross JB. Principles of pulse oximetry: theoretical and practical considerations. Anesth Analg 1989;68:368-376.

37. Tremper KK, Barker SJ. Pulse oximetry. Anesthesiology 1989;70:98-108.

34 Transfusion Medicine

Marjory Brooks

The mainstay of transfusion therapy in veterinary medicine has been the administration of fresh whole blood.[1,2] In contrast, human transfusion medicine has increasingly relied on the use of specific components of whole blood. Blood component therapy allows more efficient utilization of each unit of whole blood by taking advantage of differential storage properties of various blood elements. It also reduces the recipient's exposure to unnecessary cellular elements and plasma proteins.[3-5] These advantages are directly applicable to veterinary medicine.[6-8] Problems common to veterinary and human transfusion medicine include limited blood donor availability and transmission of bloodborne diseases.[6-10] Development of synthetic blood components could ultimately solve these problems, but synthetic products are unlikely to be readily available in the near future.[11] The "best" transfusion medicine at present is the timely use of selected blood components.

COMPOSITION OF WHOLE BLOOD

Components unique to whole blood include certain plasma proteins and the cellular elements of red blood cells, white blood cells, and platelets.[2-4,6-8] Proteins involved in normal hemostasis include factors and cofactors of the clotting cascade, von Willebrand factor, anticoagulants such as antithrombin III and proteins C and S, and the fibrinolysin plasminogen. Additional critical proteins are albumin and the globulin fractions. Cross-species (heterologous) transfusions of any of these blood components are contraindicated because these transfusions can cause adverse reactions to foreign cells or proteins in recipients.[1,12]

PATIENT EVALUATION

Blood transfusions are temporary tissue transplants. While a patient's clinical status may necessitate immediate transfusion therapy, it is only by identifying and correcting underlying disorders that further transfusion support can be minimized or avoided. Ancillary laboratory testing may be required if initial history, physical examination, and complete blood count do not reveal the underlying disease process. For maximum diagnostic yield blood samples must be drawn prior to transfusion. These samples should include whole blood in edetate, plasma from citrated whole blood, and serum.[13] Benefits of transfusion are immediate, but a rational treatment plan and prognosis can only be established after accurate diagnosis.

INDICATIONS FOR TRANSFUSION
Replacement of red blood cells

Most blood transfusions are given to increase oxygen-carrying capacity of the recipient's blood, by increasing the supply of viable red blood cells.[1-5] Clinical status of the patient, and not hematocrit per se, is the best guideline for determining when to transfuse.[3,4] Clinical indications for red blood cell transfusion in anemic patients include prolonged capillary refill time, tachycardia and tachypnea at rest, and exercise intolerance. A sudden drop in hematocrit is likely to cause clinical signs. In contrast, if anemia has had a gradual onset, many dogs and cats have no signs at rest with hematocrits as low as 15%. As a rule of thumb, most patients with acute anemia and hematocrit below 20% to 25% will benefit from transfusion. Most patients with chronic anemia will benefit from transfusion if the hematocrit has fallen below 12%. If the donor's hematocrit is 40%, transfusing 2 ml per kilogram of body weight of whole blood will raise the recipient's hematocrit 1%.[2,6,8]

Anemia. Classifications of anemia include blood-loss anemia, nonregenerative anemia, and

536

hemolytic anemia. A careful physical examination and evaluation of a complete blood count, including red blood cell indices, and red blood cell morphology will often enable classification. Based on these findings, more specific tests can be pursued.[13] It must be emphasized that samples for initial hematologic evaluation should be drawn prior to transfusion.

Blood-loss anemia. Blood-loss anemia can be subclassified as acute or chronic. The source of hemorrhage for patients with acute blood-loss anemia can usually be found on physical examination. If signs of severe hypoxia and hypovolemia are present, then red blood cell transfusion and additional volume support should be administered. Patients with hematocrits above 20% to 25% on presentation, who respond to volume support alone, require red blood cell transfusion only if prolonged anesthetic procedures or significant additional blood loss is anticipated.

In patients with chronic blood-loss anemia, signs of hypoxia and hypovolemia are usually not present, and the source of hemorrhage may not be obvious. In these cases initial efforts can be directed toward diagnosis, rather than emergency transfusion. Red blood cell transfusion may be needed if signs of hypoxia develop during hospitalization, diagnostic evaluation, or blood sampling (removal of considerable volume).

Nonregenerative anemia. Nonregenerative anemia requires diagnostic efforts directed at evaluating the bone marrow for primary or secondary causes of suppression.[14] Requirements for red blood cell transfusion are dictated by patients' clinical status and likelihood for restoration of effective erythropoiesis. Some nonregenerative disorders involve lengthy treatment and ultimately prove irreversible.[14] The owners' commitment and patients' prognosis must be considered when deciding whether multiple red blood cell transfusions are warranted.

Hemolytic anemia. Hemolytic anemia can be subclassified as immune or nonimmune mediated. Macroagglutination in saline or edetate (EDTA), spherocytosis, and a positive antiglobulin (Coombs') test, suggest immune-mediated red blood cell destruction. Diagnostic tests to uncover underlying disease processes causing secondary immunohemolytic anemia and polysystemic immune disorders are indicated in these cases (Chapter 23).[15] Whether anemia is due to primary (idiopathic) or secondary immune-mediated destruction, red blood cell transfusions should be avoided, because transfused red cells are destroyed along with autologous cells. If, in spite of specific treatments and immunosuppressive drugs, severe signs of hypoxia develop or persist, small

volumes of red cells may be transfused. The potential burden of red blood cell breakdown products increases with transfusion in these patients and may increase the predisposition to acute renal failure, thrombosis, and disseminated intravascular coagulation (DIC). The goal in transfusing these patients is not to restore hematocrit to the normal range, but to increase the oxygen-carrying capacity of blood. In general, transfusion to a hematocrit of 15% to 20% is adequate.

Hemolytic anemia that is not immune mediated is caused either by inherited or acquired red-cell membrane or enzyme abnormalities (Chapter 23).[16,17] In these cases transfused red blood cells are more "normal" than the recipients' cells. Transfusion of red blood cells to restore hematocrit to the normal range is an appropriate management strategy. At the same time, reversible causes of hemolysis should be identified and corrected.

Replacement of hemostatic proteins

Animals that are affected with either acquired or inherited bleeding disorders may require specific transfusion of activated clotting factors and other hemostatic proteins.[6-8] Red-cell transfusions are indicated in these cases only when significant anemia (signs of hypoxia) is present.

Animals with clinically significant coagulation factor deficiencies will have a variable prolongation of activated partial thromboplastin time (APTT) (the intrinsic system screening test) and prothrombin time (PT) (the extrinsic system screening test). Individual factor analysis can document specific deficient factors. Inherited or acquired dysfibrinogenemia can be detected by abnormalities in thrombin clotting time (TCT) and fibrinogen measurements.[13,18] Clotting assays should be performed prior to transfusion or 5 to 7 days following any transfusion, so that only the patient's endogenous clotting factor activity is measured. Accurate coagulation assays require species-specific reagents. Plasma samples for coagulation screening tests and individual factor analysis should be submitted to established veterinary diagnostic laboratories.[19]

Inherited disorders. Inherited bleeding disorders caused by plasma factor deficiencies include hemophilias A and B, other specific coagulation factor deficiencies, and von Willebrand's disease.[18]

Inherited factor deficiencies. Hemophilia and other coagulation factor deficiencies are characterized by severe, often spontaneous, bleeding in young animals.[18] The breeds at risk and inheritance patterns vary with the specific factor deficiency (Chapter 23). Hemophilia A (factor VIII deficiency) is the most common form of hemophilia in dogs and cats. Inheritance pattern is sex-linked recessive and males are affected while females are usually asymptomatic carriers. There is relatively high prevalence of hemophilia A in German shepherds. Hemophilia B (factor IX deficiency) is also sex-linked recessive, but is much less common than hemophilia A. Deficiencies of clotting factors VII, X, XI, fibrinogen, and prothrombin complex have also been documented in dogs as autosomal traits associated with bleeding diatheses.[18] Replacement of active clotting factors requires transfusion of fresh or fresh frozen plasma (FP, FFP) or specific plasma concentrates (cryoprecipitate). Fresh whole blood transfusions can be administered if red blood cells are also required, or if plasma components are not available.

von Willebrand's disease. von Willebrand's disease (vWD) is the most common canine inherited bleeding disorder.[18,20] Bleeding is due to a deficiency of functional von Willebrand factor (vWF), a plasma protein necessary for normal platelet function. Bleeding is generally observed in affected animals following surgery and/or trauma or may occur spontaneously from mucosal surfaces of the nose, mouth, digestive, reproductive, and urinary tracts. Stress conditions including infections, hormonal fluctuations associated with estrus and parturition, and endocrinopathies can exacerbate signs of vWD in some affected dogs. von Willebrand's disease is inherited as an autosomal trait and both males and females are affected. Breeds with a high prevalence of the vWD trait include Doberman pinschers, Scottish terriers, Shetland sheepdogs, golden retrievers, standard poodles, and Pembroke Welsh corgis.[18,20]

Diagnosis of vWD requires specialized assays of vWF protein. The most widely used test measures the concentration of plasma vWF as von Willebrand factor antigen (vWF:Ag). This test is only quantitative and does not provide a functional assessment of vWF protein. Some dogs with a low concentration of vWF:Ag never experience abnormal hemostasis. Further complicating the clinical spectrum of vWD is the fact that acquired deficiencies or dysfunctions of vWF are associated with concurrent endocrine disorders, including thyroiditis and Addison's disease. In these cases, hormonal replacement therapy may reverse the observed bleeding diathesis.[20] Thyroid insufficiency, due to immune-mediated thyroiditis, is common in many breeds having a high prevalence of the vWD trait.[20,21] Institution and maintenance of appropriate thyroid hormone supplementation can prevent or reverse significant bleeding episodes in some dogs affected with concomitant vWD and thyroid insufficiency. Desmopressin acetate (DDAVP, USV Laboratories, Tarrytown, NY), has shown some efficacy when ad-ministered preoperatively to Dobermans affected with vWD, at a dose of 1 μg/kg subcutaneously.[22] Response is variable between dogs and duration of action transient, so routine use of desmopressin in all affected dogs is not recommended.[20] Dogs with vWD, who fail to respond to symptomatic or nontransfusional support, need transfusion with fresh whole blood, FP, FFP, or plasma cryoprecipitate to receive active vWF.[6,7,20]

Animals with inherited clotting factor deficiencies or vWD are at lifelong risk for abnormal hemostasis and may require periodic transfusion to supply the missing factors. Symptomatic treatment alone will not control all hemorrhagic episodes.

Acquired coagulation disorders. Acquired coagulation defects can be due to decreased clotting factor production secondary to liver dysfunction, abnormal clotting factor activation due to vitamin K deficiency, or increased consumption of clotting factors as in DIC.[19]

Hepatic dysfunction. Severe acute or chronic intrahepatic disease causes decreased clotting factor production.[23] Deficiencies of clotting factors should be suspected if concomitant signs of severe liver dysfunction such as hypoalbuminemia or hepatic encephalopathy are present. Multiple factors are affected, including fibrinogen, and APTT, PT, and TCT tests are prolonged. These patients may not exhibit spontaneous bleeding, but often experience severe hemorrhage following invasive procedures. To prevent intraoperative bleeding in these patients, FP or FFP transfusions can be administered immediately before and during liver biopsy or other surgical procedures.[6-8,23]

Vitamin K deficiency states. A continuous supply of vitamin K is required for activation of the prothrombin group of coagulation factors (II, VII, IX, and X).[23] Posthepatic bile-duct obstruction and infiltrative bowel disease decrease intestinal absorption of this fat-soluble vitamin. Antibiotic administration decreases gastrointestinal bacterial production of vitamin K. These conditions may result in vitamin K deficiency, but the most common cause of vitamin K deficiency in small animal medicine is anticoagulant rodenticide toxicity.[24] These rodenticides prevent recycling of endogenous stores of vitamin K. Newer poisons that cause severe bleeding due to increased potency and long duration of action, include diphacinone, pindone, bromadiolone, and brodifacoum. The PT assay is prolonged earliest after rodenticide ingestion due to the short plasma half-life of factor VII (an extrinsic system factor). The APTT and PT tests are both prolonged when most animals present with signs of bleeding due to vitamin K deficiency. In severe toxicities, transfusion of fresh whole blood or fresh plasma products, in addition to parenteral (subcutaneous) vitamin K therapy, will optimize the patient's response. When treating long-acting rodenticide toxicities, vitamin K_1 can be administered in a tapering dosage schedule with an initial dose of 2.2 mg/kg per day in divided doses for the first week, followed by 1.1 mg/kg per day for the second week, 0.5 mg/kg per day for the third and fourth week, and finally 0.5 mg/kg every other day for an additional 2 weeks, for a total of 6 weeks of therapy.[25] Preparations containing vitamin K_1, but not vitamin K_3, are effective for treating rodenticide toxicity.[24,25] The poor clinical response to vitamin K_3 is related to its slow intrahepatic conversion to menaquinone (vitamin K_2).[24]

Consumptive coagulopathies. Disseminated intravascular coagulation causes clinical signs of hemorrhage via secondary consumption of clotting factors, and systemic fibrinolysis. Disease states that cause tissue trauma, damage endothelial surfaces, or release thromboplastic substances to the systemic circulation can all trigger DIC.[26] Conditions associated with DIC in veterinary medicine include neoplasia (especially hemangiosarcoma, prostatic and mammary carcinoma, and lymphoma) intravascular hemolysis, severe burn wounds, sepsis, heartworm disease, and liver failure.[27] While bleeding is a common clinical sign of DIC, preceding microvascular thrombosis and activation of the clotting cascade can cause significant organ dysfunction and death independent of hemorrhage.[26] The critical factor for successful treatment of DIC is identification and correction of the underlying disease process. Transfusion of FP or FFP to supply active clotting factors may be indicated when hemorrhage due to factor depletion is evident.[26,28] Fresh or fresh frozen plasma transfusion replenishes antithrombin III (ATIII), a natural anticoagulant often deficient in DIC states. Antithrombin III modulates the coagulation cascade to favor reduced factor activation. In cases in which persistence of thromboplastic substances in the systemic circulation is expected, low-dose subcutaneous heparin therapy may prevent ongoing activation of the coagulation cascade (Chapter 23). A dose that has been recommended in human medicine is 80 U/kg every 6 hours.[26] Heparin is contraindicated in any patient with signs of central nervous system hemorrhage.[26,28] Administration of drugs, like aspirin, that inhibit platelet function may be appropriate for treatment of patients with chronic forms of DIC.[26,27]

Replacement of platelets

If platelets have normal function, characteristic clinical signs of thrombocytopenia are not present until platelet count falls below 50,000/μl.[29] These signs include petechiae of skin and mucous membranes and mucosal surface bleeding. In some patients, platelet counts below 25,000/μl do not cause spontaneous bleeding.[29,30] If the hematocrit is stable, and there are no signs of bleeding into the central nervous system, platelet transfusion is rarely indicated. The goal of platelet transfusion is to raise recipients' numbers of functional platelets above the minimum critical level needed to provide adequate primary hemostasis. The underlying cause of thrombocytopenia must be identified and specifically treated early in the course of therapy, because benefits of transfusion for platelet support are transient, lasting from hours to at most a few days.[30,31]

Thrombocytopenia. Thrombocytopenia can be caused by decreased production of platelets, increased sequestration or consumption of platelets, or immune-mediated destruction of platelets. Immune-mediated thrombocytopenia (IMT) is common.[29,30,32] In primary, or idiopathic IMT, the immune response is specifically directed against platelets, and there is no identifiable cause for this lack of "self" recognition. Secondary IMT implies an underlying disease process that alters immune tolerance or changes the platelet membrane, resulting in an antibody response directed against platelets. Whether the patient has primary or secondary IMT, platelet transfusions are rarely of benefit. Transfused platelets are destroyed rapidly.[32] In these patients, initial efforts should be directed at identifying and treating causes of secondary IMT and initiating immunosuppressive therapy. If signs referable to shock or hypoxia are present, intravenous fluids and red blood cell transfusion can be administered.

Thrombopathia. Platelet dysfunction (thrombopathia) can cause petechiae and mucosal bleeding characteristic of thrombocytopenia in patients with normal or only slightly decreased platelet counts.[33] Acquired causes of platelet dysfunction include metabolic disorders (uremia and hyperproteinemia) and drug administration (nonsteroidal antiinflammatory drugs). Inherited platelet function defects are less common, but are significant problems in otterhounds and basset hounds. Cuticle or buccal mucosal bleeding time are in vivo screening tests that detect inherited or acquired platelet function defects.[19,34] Animals with abnormal screening tests can then undergo more specific platelet function testing.

Transfusions to supply active platelets may benefit patients whose bleeding is due to platelet dysfunction.[33] In cases with acquired disorders, temporary stabilization via transfusion provides time for correction of underlying disorders and production of new, active platelets. Patients with inherited disorders may benefit from periodic transfusions to control hemorrhagic episodes.

Platelets in whole blood must be administered within 6 hours of collection. Certain platelet concentrates can be stored for up to 3 days. For optimal activity, platelets should be maintained at room temperature until transfused.[7,8]

Replacement of nonhemostatic proteins

Transfusions to supply plasma proteins, other than hemostatic proteins, are not commonly administered in small animal medicine.[8] Diseases that compromise the liver's synthetic capacity or cause significant protein loss through the urinary tract, digestive tract, skin, and pleural or peritoneal linings can result in hypoproteinemia. Unless these disorders are reversible, maintenance of adequate plasma protein levels through repeated transfusion of whole blood or plasma is impossible. The concentration of albumin in plasma is about 3 g/dl.[8] The volume of plasma that can be transfused at one time limits the expected increase in a recipient's albumin concentration to at most 1 g/dl. Some examples of reversible disorders in which plasma transfusion can minimize temporary protein losses include bacterial pleuritis or peritonitis with repeated drainage of effusion, parvovirus enteritis in young puppies, and acute hepatic necrosis in which subsequent hepatic regeneration restores adequate protein synthesis.

Replacement of white blood cells

Neutropenia may be secondary to bone marrow aplasia, myelophthisis, and increased peripheral utilization or sequestration. The efficacy of granulocyte transfusions in treating these disorders has not been proven in human medicine.[35] After donation, neutrophils are viable for only a few hours and require special temperature and storage conditions. White blood cell transfusions can cause multiple adverse immunologic reactions in the recipient.[35,36] Because of the questionable efficacy, limited availability, and adverse reactions, granulocyte transfusions are not recommended.

BLOOD COLLECTION AND PROCESSING
Equipment and supplies

Anticoagulants. The best available anticoagulants for blood collection and storage are acid-citrate-dextrose (ACD) and citrate-phosphate-dextrose-adenine (CPDA).[2,8,37] Citrate in these solutions acts as an anticoagulant by inhibiting calcium-dependent steps of the clotting cascade. The other additives act as buffers and energy sources to prolong red blood cell viability. Canine red blood cells are viable for up to 3 weeks when stored in ACD and for up to 4 weeks when stored in CPDA.[2,7] Feline red blood cells stored in ACD are viable for up to 30 days.[38] CPDA is used in a 1:10 dilution with blood, and a collection unit (in dogs) usually consists of 450 ml of blood collected into 50 ml of CPDA, for a total unit volume of 500 ml. ACD is used in a dilution of 1:6 with blood and a common unit volume (in cats) is 50 ml of blood collected into 10 ml of ACD for a total volume of 60 ml.

Heparin is not recommended for routine use as an anticoagulant.[2,6,8,37] Heparin contains no preservatives; blood must be used within 48 hours of collection. Heparin activates platelets, and it should not be used as an anticoagulant when transfusing thrombocytopenic patients or animals with platelet dysfunction. Platelet aggregates that form in the recipient after heparin-anticoagulated transfusions may cause undesirable circulatory effects. If heparin is the only available anticoagulant, 250 to 625 units per 50 ml of whole blood is used.

Collection containers. Small volumes of blood (up to 75 ml) can easily be drawn into plastic syringes containing anticoagulant. For collecting large volumes of blood from dogs, it is advisable to use either glass vacuum bottles or plastic bags. Advantages of plastic bags include less hemolysis and minimal platelet and coagulation factor activation during collection and storage. Commercial plastic blood bags with a selection of attached satellite bags (Baxter/Fenwal) allow collection and subsequent separation of blood components within a closed system. Whole blood can be divided into smaller, more convenient, unit sizes or centrifuged to separate packed red cells from other components. Several 2-ml aliquots of blood or packed cells can be sealed in the inlet tubing attached to commercial blood bags for later use in cross matching without entering the main unit container.[7]

Blood donor selection and management

Canine donors. Dogs designated for use as blood donors should weigh at least 25 kg, have a hematocrit of at least 40%, be in good physical condition and have a calm disposition. Although either sex can be blood donors, males tend to be heavier and have higher hematocrits than females. Female blood donors should be spayed to prevent the hematologic effects of hormonal fluctuations associated with heat cycles. Blood donors should be of known blood type. The ideal blood donor is negative for blood groups dog erythrocyte antigen (DEA) 1.1, DEA 1.2, and DEA 7, and has a normal plasma concentration of vWF.

Greyhounds are often chosen as donors because they are large, docile dogs with accessible veins, and a high percentage of them are DEA 1-negative. Many greyhounds have low concentration of vWF:Ag (Veterinary Hematology Laboratory, NYS Department of Health, unpublished data).

All canine blood donors should also be screened for bloodborne diseases. Serologic tests for brucellosis, borreliosis, ehrlichiosis, and Rocky Mountain spotted fever should be performed. In addition, a blood smear should be carefully examined for the presence of trypanosomiasis, babesiosis, and hemobartonellosis. Blood donor dogs should be negative for dirofilariasis. Routine splenectomy of donors is not advised. Screening tests should be repeated at 6- to 12-month intervals.

Collection techniques. Dogs can donate a maximum volume of 22 ml/kg at one time. This volume can be drawn once every 3 to 4 weeks from dogs that are used for repeated donations. The femoral artery or the jugular vein can be used for collection. Collection from the femoral artery requires anesthesia or heavy sedation of the donor. Most dogs tolerate blood collection from the jugular vein without sedation. The skin over the artery or vein is clipped and scrubbed, and venipuncture using the needle connected to the collection bag or bottle is performed. Commercial plastic blood bags and bottles utilize 17-gauge needles. Bags and bottles contain sufficient anticoagulant to collect 450 to 500 ml of whole blood and should be gently rotated during collection to mix blood and anticoagulant.

Feline donors. Feline donors should weigh at least 5 kg, have a hematocrit of at least 30%, and be in good physical condition. Male cats are preferred, as they are larger, leaner, and have higher hematocrits than females. Routine blood typing of domestic shorthair blood donor cats is not necessary, since most individuals of this breed in the United States are type A, and incompatibility between feline donor and recipient pairs can be detected in cross matching (see section on Blood Typing and Cross Matching). Blood donor cats should be negative for feline leukemia virus antigen and for feline immunodeficiency virus antibodies. A stained blood film and buffy coat smear should be examined for *Hemobartonella* and white blood cell parasites. Cats with persistently elevated or rising antibody titers to coronaviruses or *Toxoplasma* should not be used as blood donors. Serologic monitoring for bloodborne diseases should be performed at 6- to 12-month intervals.

Collection techniques. Cats maintained as blood donors, can safely donate a maximum of 15 ml/kg once a month. A unit volume of blood collected is usually between 50 and 75 ml. Adequate restraint for blood collection in cats requires sedation. Acepromazine and barbiturates should be avoided because they cause hypotension.[8] For most blood donor cats 1 to 2 mg/kg of ketamine (with or without 0.1 mg/kg diazepam) given intravenously is sufficient for sedation. Atropine or glycopyrrolate administration will prevent hypersalivation and bradycardia associated with ketamine sedation. Replacement fluids are not routinely required for donors when using low-dose drug combinations and suggested volumes of blood per donation. In cats, jugular veins are the only accessible veins large enough for donation of more than a few milliliters of blood. The skin over both jugulars should be clipped and scrubbed with antiseptic and alcohol. Use of large 19-gauge butterfly catheters for venipuncture will minimize clot formation and hemolysis during collection. An average unit of blood can be collected, over 5 to 10 minutes, directly into 35-ml syringes containing anticoagulant. Collecting into two small syringes rather than one large syringe prevents the vein from collapsing. Blood collected in syringes can be transfused immediately or stored in closed-end syringes. Commercially available blood transfer packs (Baxter/Fenwal) hold up to 150 ml of blood and are ideal for storing and later administering feline blood.

If the donor animal (canine or feline) is to be exsanguinated, the carotid artery can be cannulated and blood collected directly into a plastic bag containing anticoagulant. Expected volume of blood that can be collected without administering replacement fluids, is the fluid equivalent of 5% of the donor's body weight in kilograms.

Component processing and storage of blood products

Red blood cells in whole blood and packed cell units should be stored at temperatures between 1 and 6°C. Daily gentle agitation to mix cells and plasma will maintain red-cell viability.[2]

Whole blood transfused to supply active platelets or clotting factors should be administered within 6 hours of collection. Platelets become inactivated if blood is refrigerated.[6,7,31]

Blood components. Separation of canine whole blood to produce packed red blood cells and plasma is performed by collecting blood in commercial plastic units with attached satellite bags and then spinning the bags in large, swinging-bucket, cold centrifuges.[6-8]

Packed red cells. After centrifugation, red cells settle to the bottom of the bags and supernatant plasma can be expressed into satellite bags. The hematocrit of packed red blood cells is about 80%. Transfusion of 1.0 ml/kg body weight of recipient of packed red cells is expected to raise the recipients' hematocrit about 1%.

Plasma products. Fresh frozen plasma is produced by separating whole blood within 3 to 4 hours of collection and freezing supernatant plasma at low temperature. Plasma stored at $-70°C$ preserves activity of hemostatic proteins for up to 1 year after collection.[39] Small aliquots of plasma can be frozen in inlet tubing segments and stored with plasma units for cross matching. The dose of fresh frozen plasma is 6 to 10 ml/kg.

Cryoprecipitate is a plasma concentrate prepared from fresh frozen plasma. It contains fibrinogen, fibronectin, and the factor VIII complex (factor VIII and von Willebrand factor). Expected activity of factor VIII in cryoprecipitate is about 50% of that in starting plasma, in one tenth the volume of that plasma. Cryoprecipitate formed from 150 to 200 ml of starting plasma is administered per 10 kg of recipient body weight. The optimal dosage interval depends on severity and cause of the bleeding episode. In general, patients with hemophilia A and von Willebrand disease are treated at 8- to 12-hour intervals, and patients with fibrinogen deficiency are treated at 12- to 24-hour intervals.[6-8]

Supernatant plasma left after cryoprecipitation, (cryosuper), contains active prothrombin complex factors (II, VII, IX, X), ATIII, and albumin and globulin.[6] The amount of cryosuper to administer per dose is 6 to 10 ml/kg. Cryoprecipitate and cryosuper can be stored at $-70°C$ for 1 year. Cryosuper can be stored at $0°C$ for at least 1 month with no significant loss in activity.[7]

Platelet products. Platelet concentrates are prepared by centrifugation of whole blood within 6 hours of collection.[31] Blood should be stored at room temperature until centrifugation. Superna-tant plasma contains about 75% of the platelets in that volume of whole blood and is administered as platelet-rich plasma (PRP). A second centrifugation of PRP causes further concentration of platelets to produce packed platelet units (platelet concentrate). PRP and packed platelet units should be used as soon as possible after separation. The maximum storage time at room temperature with frequent agitation is 72 hours. Platelets concentrated from 500 ml of whole blood would be expected to raise platelet count of a 30-kg recipient by about $10,000/\mu l$.[8]

ADMINISTRATION OF BLOOD PRODUCTS
Products and dosage

Table 34-1 presents guidelines for selecting blood products and dosages to transfuse.

Routes of administration

Intravenous transfusion. Small volumes of whole blood (<100 ml) and blood products may be administered from a syringe through an intravenous butterfly catheter. Relatively large (21-, 20-, or 19-gauge) catheters are preferred for administration of blood products in order to minimize red-cell hemolysis and platelet aggregation caused by turbulent flow through a small-bore catheter. Whenever more than 100 ml of whole blood or blood component is administered, an aseptically placed indwelling catheter and a commercial blood administration set with filter should be used. Blood filters with 170-μm pore size are designed to remove fibrin clots and platelet aggregates formed during blood collection and storage.

Table 34-1 Guidelines for transfusing blood products

	Rate	Volume to Transfuse	Frequency
Products that supply red blood cells			
Fresh whole blood	6 ml/min	12-25 ml/kg	Every 24 hours
Stored whole blood	6 ml/min	12-25 ml/kg	Every 24 hours
Packed red cells	6 ml/min	6-10 ml/kg	Every 24 hours
		for treating hemorrhagic shock maximum dosage and rate = 22 ml/kg/hr	
Products that supply hemostatic proteins			
Fresh whole blood	6 ml/min	12-25 ml/kg	Every 24 hours
Fresh/fresh frozen plasma	6 ml/min	6-10 ml/kg	Every 8-12 hours
Cryoprecipitate*	10 ml/min	1 unit/10 kg	Every 8-12 hours
Cryosupernatant†	10 ml/min	6-10 ml/kg	Every 8-12 hours
Products that supply platelets			
Fresh whole blood	6 ml/min	12-25 ml/kg	Every 24 hours
Platelet-rich plasma	6 ml/min	6-10 ml/kg	Every 8-12 hours
Platelet concentrate‡	10 ml/min	1 unit/10 kg	Every 8-12 hours

*Cryoprecipitate supplies active factor VIII, vWF, and fibrinogen. One unit of cryoprecipitate is derived from 150 ml of plasma.
†Cryosupernatant supplies active prothrombin group factors, albumin and globulin.
‡One unit of platelet concentrate is derived from 500 ml of whole blood.

Administration of these substances can cause adverse transfusion reactions.[6,7] More specialized filters are also available that reduce the number of white blood cells administered.[40] When blood products are transfused to supply active platelets, polypropylene or polyvinyl chloride plastic equipment should be used. Latex plastic or glass equipment will cause platelet adhesion and aggregation.[31] Peripheral veins should be used for placement of intravenous catheters in patients with hemostatic disorders. Significant bleeding can occur at catheter sites before adequate response to replacement therapy occurs.

Autotransfusion. Autotransfusion of blood drawn from body cavities can be used to replace intravascular red cells.[41] This blood does not supply active platelets or hemostatic proteins. Microaggregates and red blood cell fragments in autotransfused blood can cause dyspnea, respiratory insufficiency, and DIC. Commercial blood filters will reduce the size of transfused particles, but use of hemolyzed blood, or blood that has been extravasated for several days should be avoided.

Intraosseous transfusion. In small puppies and kittens or other animals in which intravenous catheterization is difficult, whole blood or packed red blood cells can be administered via intraperitoneal or intraosseous route. Intramedullary cavities of femur, ilium, humerus, and tibia are most often used. Intraosseous transfusion provides faster absorption and allows more red blood cells to gain access to the peripheral circulation.[42]

BLOOD TYPING AND CROSS MATCHING
Blood group systems

Canine and feline blood group systems are determined by the presence of species-specific antigens on the surface of red blood cell membranes.

Canine. The canine blood group system is relatively well defined.[1,6,37,43] There are eight major blood group antigens known as DEA (dog erythrocyte antigen) 1 through 8. The DEA 1 antigen system is involved in virtually all clinically significant transfusion reactions. There are two alternate alleles at the DEA 1 locus. Dogs that have either DEA 1.1 or DEA 1.2 antigen on the surface of their red blood cells are designated DEA 1 positive (or A^+). About 60% of dogs selected from a random population are A^+ and the remaining dogs are A^- recipient.[37]

Immediate hypersensitivity reactions are rarely seen during first transfusion of incompatible red blood cells in dogs, because most dogs have no preformed antibodies against canine blood group antigens.[1,6,37] Following transfusion of A^+ cells into an A^- recipient, sensitization with antibody formation against foreign A antigens will occur.

Once formed, these antibodies can shorten survival of incompatible donor red blood cells in recipients. Immediate hypersensitivity reactions, including anaphylaxis, can occur following single or multiple transfusions of incompatible blood to previously sensitized recipients. Hemolysis of neonatal red blood cells can occur in the offspring of sensitized dams.[37]

Feline. Feline blood groups consist of relatively few antigens. Three blood types have been described: A, B, and AB.[43,44] Prevalence of these three blood types is apparently dependent on breed and geographic location. Type A is by far the most common blood type in the United States, being present in over 90% of all American domestic shorthairs.[8] The proportion of blood type B individuals is greater in most exotic breeds. Blood type B cats generally have naturally occurring antibodies against the A antigen. Acute transfusion reactions occur during a first transfusion of type A blood to type B feline recipients. Cats with blood type A generally do not have acute transfusion reactions after transfusion with type B cells, but survival of transfused cells is reduced.[44] Blood typing cats is useful to establish the cause of adverse transfusion reactions and the presence of neonatal isoerythrolysis.

Blood typing

Blood-typing techniques are based on detection of hemolysis and agglutination when red cells are combined with specific typing antisera. Reagents used in canine and feline blood typing are not commercially available, and some expertise is needed to evaluate the typing reactions. A list of centers that currently offer canine blood typing includes veterinary schools (Tufts University, Michigan State University, Kansas State University, University of Tennessee); and veterinary laboratories (Stormont Laboratories, Vacaville, CA). Feline-blood-typing services are offered by the veterinary school at Tufts University and the University of Pennsylvania or Stormont Laboratories. Each laboratory should be contacted for specific instructions on sampling and shipping conditions.

Cross matching

Blood cross matching tests will detect preformed antibodies to foreign cells. The major cross match detects preformed antibodies in the recipient to donor red-cell antigens and is the most clinically significant reaction.[6,37,44] Compatible cross matches, however, do not imply that sensitization to transfused red blood cells will not occur. Antibodies against foreign-donor red blood cell antigens are detectable in sensitized recipients within 5 to 7 days after incompatible transfusion. These

CROSS MATCHING

I. Recipient samples
1. Collect 1 to 2 ml of recipient blood in a serum tube and in an EDTA or heparin tube.
2. Separate the supernatant serum and plasma from red blood cells by centrifugation for 10 minutes, or by allowing samples to stand for at least 30 minutes.
3. Make a 4% recipient red blood cell suspension (0.2 ml packed red blood cells in 4.8 ml 0.9% saline).

II. Donor samples
1. Collect 1 to 2 ml of donor blood in a serum tube and in an EDTA or heparin tube, (a separate 2-ml aliquot of blood from a red blood cell unit can substitute for EDTA and serum samples).
2. Separate the supernatant serum or plasma from red blood cells by centrifugation for 10 minutes, or by allowing samples to stand for at least 30 minutes.
3. Make a 4% donor red blood cell suspension (0.2 ml packed red blood cells in 4.8 ml 0.9% saline).

III. Major cross match
1. Place 0.1-ml aliquots of donor red blood cell suspension in three tubes.
2. Add 0.1 ml of recipient serum to each tube.
3. Incubate for 15 minutes: one tube at 7°C, one at room temperature, and one at 37°C.
4. Centrifuge the tubes for 1 minute, then check for hemolysis and/or red blood cell agglutination in each tube.
5. The presence of hemolysis or agglutination in any tube indicates an incompatible major cross match.

IV. Minor cross match
1. Place 0.1-ml aliquots of recipient red blood cell suspension in three tubes.
2. Add 0.1 ml of donor serum (or plasma) to each tube.
3. Incubate and centrifuge the tubes as in Steps 3 and 4 of the major cross match.
4. The presence of hemolysis or agglutination in any tube indicates an incompatible minor cross match.

V. Controls
1. Place 0.1 ml of donor red blood cell suspension in three tubes, add 0.1 ml of donor serum or plasma to each tube.
2. Place 0.1 ml of recipient red blood cell suspension in three tubes, add 0.1 ml of recipient serum to each tube.
3. Incubate and centrifuge the tubes as in Steps 3 and 4 of the major cross match.
4. The presence of hemolysis or agglutination in any tube invalidates the major and minor cross match performed at that temperature.

antibodies may be hemolysins or agglutinins, warm or cold reacting, and complement dependent. Cross-matching tests should be performed under conditions that will detect all these antibodies (see box). If incompatibilities are noted in any of the cross-match tubes, an alternate donor should be tested. Animals with immune-mediated hemolytic anemia may show incompatibility with all donors, because antibodies directed against antigens common to all red blood cells are present.

RESPONSE TO TRANSFUSION THERAPY
Therapeutic monitoring

Appropriate responses to red blood cell transfusions include improvement in mucous membrane color, capillary refill time, pulse quality, respiratory rate, and overall patient strength. Onset of response is rapid and should occur during or within hours of transfusion. Hematocrit should be measured 2 to 4 hours after transfusion to establish a base line for further comparisons. Half-life of transfused compatible red blood cells is about 20 days in dogs and 30 days in cats.[6] There may be a transient fall or temporary stabilization of the hematocrit before effects of the recipient's regenerative response is apparent. If the hematocrit progressively falls below base line, then ongoing blood loss, hemolysis, or failure of hematopoiesis is present.

Response to hemostatic protein transfusion can be monitored directly by cessation of blood loss and a subsequent increase in hematocrit. Cuticle or buccal mucosal bleeding time can be used as an in vivo indication of platelet function.[34] Laboratory measurements of specific hemostatic factors can also be performed.[19]

Most thrombocytopenic disorders can be adequately monitored by checking a platelet count at 24- to 48-hour intervals. If petechiae or mucosal bleeding are present, direct response to therapy can be observed as these signs disappear. Positive response should be seen within 1 to 3 days of initiating effective therapy.[30]

Adverse reactions

Immunologic reactions. Immunologic reactions involve specific antibodies in recipients reacting to foreign antigens in transfused blood products. The antigens may be associated with red cells, white cells, or plasma proteins. Signs of immunologic transfusion reactions include urticaria, edema, fever, hypotension, and intravascular or extravascular hemolysis. Nonfebrile urticaria or edema reactions should be managed by temporarily discontinuing the transfusion and administering an immunosuppressive dose of a short-acting corticosteroid. Additionally, diphenhydramine chloride can be administered subcutaneously, intramuscularly, or intravenously to dogs at a dose of 1 to 2 mg/kg. Intravenous administration of antihistamine may cause hypotension. Transfusions can be resumed, at a slower rate, after urticaria and edema resolve.[6-8] Patients that are newly sensitized to transfused red blood cells may have fever, falling hematocrit, and signs of hemolysis 7 to 10 days after the incompatible transfusion.

Acute hemolytic reactions occur within minutes of transfusion, and may be accompanied by tremors, vomiting, collapse, shock, or DIC.[37,44] These reactions are seen in animals sensitized by prior transfusion, in blood type B cats transfused with type A blood, and in neonatal isoerythrolysis (the dam's colostrum contains anti-fetal-red-cell antibodies). Cross matching a previously transfused female with a potential mate can detect isoantibodies present in the female directed against the male's red blood cells.

Most immunologic transfusion reactions can be prevented by using only donors of known compatible blood type, and cross matching previously transfused animals.[37,44]

Nonimmunologic reactions. Improper processing, storage, or administration of blood products, contamination of blood products with infectious agents, or circulatory overload are causes of nonimmunologic reactions.[6-8]

Bacterial contamination. Bacteria introduced during collection or processing, will survive in refrigerated blood products. An indication of bacterial growth in stored blood is a dark brown supernatant layer overlying red blood cells. Prevention of bacterial contamination includes aseptic technique when collecting and processing blood, storage at well-regulated temperatures, and discarding blood products that have been open or warmed to room temperature for over 6 hours. If bacterial contamination of transfused products is suspected, transfusion should stop immediately, and an aliquot of the blood product examined with Gram stain and culture. Blood cultures of the recipient can document sepsis. Appropriate selection of donors and serologic monitoring can prevent most cases of bloodborne transmission of viral, bacterial, or rickettsial infections.

Circulatory overload. Overtransfusion can result from administering blood products too quickly or giving too large a total volume.[1,6-8] Signs of circulatory overload include vomiting, retching, coughing, dyspnea, tachycardia, and ultimately death. Cats, small dogs, and animals with cardiac insufficiency are most likely to show signs of circulatory overload.

Hypocalcemia. Hypocalcemia is a potential complication if large volumes of citrated blood products are given rapidly, or if recipients have impaired liver function.[6-8] Patients undergoing systemic anticoagulation for procedures such as plasmapheresis are at risk of citrate toxicity. Signs of calcium chelation include tetany, muscle tremors, hyperthermia, and cardiac arrhythmia. These signs are alleviated by slow intravenous calcium administration (see Chapter 18).

Improper administration. Coagulation and agglutination can result if anticoagulated blood products come in contact with solutions containing calcium or dextrose.[6-8,44] Hemolysis results if red blood cells come in contact with hypotonic solutions, if blood is heated above 37°C, or if cells are forced through small-gauge needles or catheters. These complications are preventable by transfusing blood through infusion sets and catheters separate from those used for crystalloid fluid administration. *Sterile 0.9% saline is the only solution that can be mixed with blood products or infused through an administration set used for blood products.*

Advantages of blood components. Component therapy eliminates the risk of many immunologic reactions, reduces the number of nonimmunologic reactions due to circulatory overload, and increases the utilization of limited blood resources. The availability of blood components will become more widespread through development of blood banks by private commercial companies and veterinary institutions. Use of these components, rather than whole blood, will greatly enhance the practice of veterinary transfusion medicine.

ACKNOWLEDGMENT

From the Wadsworth Center for Laboratories and Research, New York State Department of Health, PO Box 509, Albany, NY, 12201; Supported in part by NIH grant HL 09902 from the NHLBI PHS/DHHS.

REFERENCES

1. Tangner CH. Transfusion therapy for the dog and cat. Compend Contin Educ Pract Vet 1982;4:521-527.
2. Pichler ME, Turnwald GH. Blood transfusion in the dog and cat. Part I. Physiology, collection, storage, and indications for whole blood therapy. Compend Contin Educ Pract Vet 1985;7:64-71.
3. Consensus development conference. Perioperative red cell transfusion. Transfusion Med Rev 1989;111:63-68.
4. Sacher RA, Luban NLC, Strauss RG. Current practice and guidelines for the transfusion of cellular blood components in the newborn. Transfusion Med Rev 1989;111:39-54.
5. Crowley JP, Guadagnoli E, Pezzullo J, Fuller J, Yankee R. Changes in hospital component therapy response to reduced availability of whole blood. Transfusion 1988;28:4-7.
6. Turnwald GH, Pichler ME. Blood transfusion in dogs and cats. Part II. Administration, adverse effects and component therapy. Comp Cont Ed 1985;7:115-122.
7. Authement JM, Wolfsheimer KJ, Catchings S. Canine blood component therapy: product preparation, storage and administration. J Am Anim Hosp Assoc 1987;23:483-493.
8. Cotter S. Blood banking I and II. In Pidgeon G, ed. ACVIM Proceedings sixth annual veterinary forum. Washington, DC, 1988:45-50.
9. Haugen RK, Hill GE. A large-scale autologous blood program in a community hospital. JAMA 1987;257:1211-1214.
10. Rock A, Maker MJ. Inside the billion dollar business of blood. Money 1986;32-40.
11. Greene CE. Blood substitute therapy. In Kirk RW, ed. Current veterinary therapy IX. Philadelphia: WB Saunders, 1986:107-109.
12. Gordon DS. Intravenous immunoglobulins: historical perspectives. Am J Med 1987;83(suppl 4A):1-3.
13. Madewell BR. Sample preparation for the lab. In Kirk RW, ed. Current veterinary therapy X. Philadelphia: WB Saunders, 1989:410-419.
14. Harvey JW. Canine bone marrow: normal hematopoiesis, biopsy techniques, and cell evaluation. Compend Contin Educ Pract Vet 1984;6:909-925.
15. Dodds WJ. Immune mediated blood diseases in dogs. Part 2. Mod Vet Pract 1983;69:453-456.
16. Giger U. Hereditary disorders of canine erythrocytes. In Kirk RW, ed. Current veterinary therapy X. Philadelphia: WB Saunders, 1989:429-436.
17. Harvey JW. Canine hemolytic anemias. J Am Vet Med Assoc 1980;176:970-974.
18. Dodds WJ. Inherited bleeding disorders. Curr Pract 1978;5:49-58.
19. Johnstone IB. Diagnostic approach to the bleeding patient. In Kirk RW, ed. Current veterinary therapy X. Philadelphia: WB Saunders, 1989:436-442.
20. Dodds WJ. Acquired von Willebrands disease. In: Proceedings of the 56th annual meeting. St. Louis: American Animal Hospital Association, 1989:614-619.
21. Haines DM, Lording PM, Penhale WJ. Survey of thyroglobulin antibodies in dogs. Am J Vet Res 1984;45:1493-1497.
22. Kraus K, Turrentine MA, Jergens A, et al. Effect of desmopressin acetate on bleeding times and plasma von Willebrand factor in doberman pinscher dogs with von Willebrands disease. Vet Surg 1989;18:103-109.
23. Badylak S. Coagulation disorders in liver disease. Vet Clin North Am Hemost 1988;18:87-93.
24. Mount ME. Diagnosis and therapy of anticoagulant rodenticides. 1988;18:115-130.
25. The professional's guide to managing poisoning by anticoagulant rodenticides. New York: Chempar Chemical, 1985.
26. Bick RL. Disseminated intravascular coagulation and related syndromes: a clinical review. Semin Thromb Hemost 1988;14:299-338.
27. Slappendel RJ. Disseminated intravascular coagulation. Vet Clin North Am Hemost 1988;18:169-184.
28. Feinstein DI. Treatment of disseminated intravascular coagulation. Semin Thromb Hemost 1988;14:351-362.
29. Davenport DJ, Breitschwerdt EB, Carakostas MC. Platelet disorders in the dog and cat. Part I. Physiology and pathogenesis. Compend Contin Educ Pract Vet 1982;4:762-772.
30. Feldman BF, Thomson KJ, Jain NC. Quantitative platelet disorders. Vet Clin North Am Hemost 1988;18:35-49.
31. Sibinga C. Platelets for transfusion: collecting, processing and preservation aspects. Blut 1987;55:475-481.
32. Kelton JG. Immune thrombocytopenia. ISI Atlas Sci Immunol 1988;1:265-271.
33. Catalfamo JL, Dodds WJ. Hereditary and acquired thrombopathias. Vet Clin North Am Hemost 1988;18:185-193.
34. Forsythe LT, Willis SE. Evaluating oral mucosa bleeding times in healthy dogs using a spring-loaded device. Can Vet J 1989;30:344-345.
35. Quie PG. The white cells: use of granulocyte transfusions. Rev Infect Dis 1987;9:189-193.
36. Schiller CA, Wide JC. Supportive care: issues in the use of blood products and treatment of infection. Semin Oncol 1987;14:454-467.
37. Dodds WJ, Bull RW. Canine blood groups and blood banking. Pure Bred Dogs Am Kennel Gaz 1979;68-70.
38. Manion RS, Smith JE. Post transfusion viability of feline erythrocytes stored in acid citrate dextrose. J Am Vet Med Assoc 1983;183:1459-1460.
39. Greene CE, Beck BB. Coagulation properties of fresh frozen canine plasma during prolonged storage. Am J Vet Res 1980;41:147-150.
40. Schiffer CA, Patten E, Reilly J, Patel S. Effective leukocyte removal from platelet preparations by centrifugation in new pooling bag. Transfusion 1987;27:162-164.
41. Zenoble RD, Stone EA. Autotransfusion in the dog. J Am Vet Med Assoc 1978;172:1411-1414.
42. Otto CM, Kaufman GM, Crowe ST. Intraosseous infusions of fluids and therapeutics. Compend Contin Educ Pract Vet 1989;11:421-430.
43. Stormont CJ. Blood groups in animals. J Am Vet Med Assoc 1982;181:1120-1124.
44. Auer LA, Bell K. Feline blood transfusion reactions. In Kirk RW, ed. Current veterinary therapy IX Philadelphia: WB Saunders, 1986:515-521.

35 Critical Care Imaging

Lawrence J. Kleine and Dominique G. Penninck

GENERAL CONSIDERATIONS

Trauma, acute abdominal disorders, and respiratory problems account for the major share of imaging indications for animals in the intensive care environment. These cases are often presented for imaging with a nonspecific diagnosis and an ambiguous constellation of clinical signs. Life-threatening conditions must be attended to prior to undertaking most diagnostic imaging procedures on critical care patients. Fractures should be immobilized, if possible, to prevent unnecessary pain to the animal and to minimize further soft-tissue or bone injury.

Radiologic imaging often serves several roles: as base-line data regarding the initial clinical situation, as an aid in triage to identify animals that need treatment urgently, as an indication of the need for specific tests or treatment, and in some cases as a means of establishing an etiologic diagnosis.

X-ray and ultrasound equipment should be in close proximity to the intensive care area to increase both its utility and efficiency in an intensive care setting. The diagnostic imaging area or portable imaging equipment should accommodate the monitoring equipment, oxygen, and intravenous fluid stands that often accompany acutely ill animals. A "crash cart," must be easily accessible (Chapters 1 and 3). Frequently used contrast agents, ultrasound coupling gel, syringes, needles, and intravenous sets should be within reach. Vinyl-covered table pads, restraint devices, and cleaning supplies should be convenient.

Preparation of the area will reduce the time needed for the imaging procedure and increase diagnostic efficiency. Rehearsing the handling of an emergency or urgent situation will determine what specific supplies are needed and where they best can be stored for easy accessibility.

Except in extreme cases, supportive care, including fluid administration and routine electrocardiographic (ECG) monitoring, can continue simultaneously with diagnostic imaging procedures.

With ingenuity, most intensive care imaging can be carried out in a manner similar to that employed in the routine setting, although the animal's clinical state may mandate a compromise in regard to the desired number of radiographic views or the accuracy of positioning. Such examinations, while often valuable, also usually yield less diagnostic information than examinations performed in a more optimal setting. Imaging studies that are by necessity compromised must be interpreted cautiously and with the intention of repeating the examination if and when the animal's health will permit.

GENERAL INDICATIONS

Imaging is most effective and efficient when it is used to answer a specific question or to confirm a suspicion based on the clinical examination or history. Those imaging procedures, which are done to see "what's going on," have a much lower diagnostic yield. Survey radiographic examinations should nearly always precede any other imaging procedure such as radiographic contrast study or ultrasound examination.

While a specific etiologic diagnosis based on the correlation of the clinical examination and imaging findings is the clinician's objective, in the intensive care situation, an exact diagnosis is often not possible following the initial examination. Correct classification of the disorder by correlating imaging results with other clinical findings is often sufficient to direct the initial therapy rapidly toward restoration of homeostasis. Imaging findings are often valuable in determining whether surgery should be performed and which diagnostic procedures or laboratory tests are indicated.

A recent history of any of the following injuries to an animal should lead to radiography of the thorax or abdomen or both in two planes: automobile accident, fall of more than 10 ft, gunshot wound, foreign-body ingestion, and animal-bite wounds or other penetrating wounds to the thorax or abdomen.

Physical examination findings in animals with a history of trauma or suspected trauma that suggest the need for abdominal and thoracic radiography include fractures involving the ribs, sternum, pelvis, or spinal column; the presence of peritoneal or pleural fluid, blood in the urine or feces, substantial abdominal- or thoracic-wall bruising, subcutaneous emphysema, and abdominal tenderness. Dyspnea, coughing, asymmetric or other abnormal lung or heart sounds, and muffled heart sounds are other indications for thoracic radiography. In addition, any evidence of internal organ malfunction, pain, or other unexplained clinical signs relating to the animal's thorax or abdomen should be investigated radiographically.

SURVEY RADIOGRAPHY

Findings on survey radiography are usually an accurate reflection of the pathologic changes that occur secondary to trauma. Rupture, displacement, or tearing of viscera (or their attachments) and hemorrhage or thrombosis may be suspected by radiographic findings that demonstrate alterations of size, position, margin, or opacity of the structure in question. Initially, normal radiographic findings provide base-line data from which subsequent changes can be assessed. A systematic evaluation of thoracic and abdominal radiographs in both planes will minimize the possibility of overlooking a significant injury. Soft tissues external to the ribs and spine should be examined for swelling and increased or decreased opacity that might occur with the presence of bruising, laceration, hernia, or subcutaneous emphysema. Skeletal structures should be examined for fractures, displacements, or preexisting disease. Displacement of viscera and accumulation of gas or fluid within the thorax or abdomen are important findings, which should lead to further investigation. Intrathoracic viscera should be specifically assessed for the following:

1. Gas or fluid in the thoracic cavity and mediastinum,
2. Airway obstruction,
3. Pulmonary hemorrhage/contusion/consolidation/bullae,
4. Pericardial effusion or other cause of cardiac enlargement, and
5. Diaphragmatic discontinuity.

Specific observations to be made when evaluating abdominal radiographs are:

1. The presence of air or fluid and the nature of contrast in the peritoneum and retroperitoneum,
2. The location, size, margins, opacity, and continuity of each viscus, and
3. The presence of intraperitoneal or retroperitoneal mass(es).

If the physical examination or the survey radiographic findings indicate that abdominal or thoracic fluid are present, centesis should be considered. The fluid obtained should be subjected to laboratory evaluation.

Radiographic contrast examinations are a necessity in cases of suspected urinary tract trauma, and gastrointestinal contrast studies may be indicated in intensive care patients with suspected gastrointestinal disorders.

CERVICAL SOFT TISSUES

Survey radiography of the cervical region may provide evidence of tracheal collapse or rupture or tracheal obstruction caused by foreign body, hemorrhage, edema and intraluminal or extraluminal neoplasm or granuloma. Fractured hyoid bones, penetrating foreign bodies lodged in soft tissues, and subcutaneous emphysema are often recognized in survey radiography. Since the cervical fascia is anatomically continuous with the mediastinum, emphysema of cervical soft tissues may lead to pneumomediastinum.

Cervical soft-tissue wounds may be evaluated for potential radiolucent foreign bodies or a nidus of infection by fistulography. Fistulography is a low-yield diagnostic procedure. Greatest success is found in visualizing the source of the problem when the fistula is well defined. Spreading, multiple, ill-defined tracts are seldom clearly visualized. A viscous agent such as diatrizoate meglumine (Renografin, Squibb) and diatrizoate sodium (Hypaque-90, Winthrop Laboratories, New York) or propyliodone (Dionosil Oily, Glaxo, Greenford, England), although difficult to infuse, may provide better definition of tissue tracts by not spreading as rapidly through the tissues as the less viscous contrast agents such as 60% diatrizoate meglumine (Hypaque Meglumine 60%, Winthrop Laboratories, New York). If there is reason to suspect that an external fistula connects with the trachea or pleural cavity, a non-ionic contrast agent such as iopamidol (Isovue-200, Squibb, Princeton, NJ) is preferred, since it is less irritating to tissues than the oil-based or conventional aqueous ionic media.

Tracheal collapse can best be confirmed by making two lateral radiographs that include both the cervical and thoracic portions of the trachea: one at full inspiration, another at expiration. The

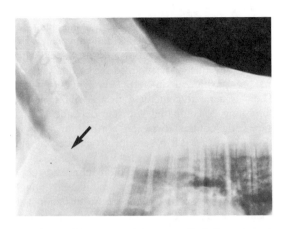

Fig. 35-1 This 11-year-old toy poodle had severe episodes of coughing. The radiograph made on inspiration shows tracheal collapse *(arrow)* at the thoracic inlet.

collapse is seen on expiration in the case of intrathoracic collapse and on inspiration in the case of cervical collapse (Figs. 35-1 and 35-2). Fluoroscopic visualization can be exceptionally valuable in evaluating suspected tracheal collapse in tachypneic animals when radiographs cannot be reliably exposed on expiration.

Tracheal foreign bodies can usually be identified , even when the foreign body is relatively radiolucent, because of the contrast provided by the surrounding air in the trachea (Fig. 35-3).

Tracheal perforation can be confirmed by instillation of aqueous contrast medium into the trachea, followed by conventional radiographic evaluation.

Pharyngeal foreign bodies, hematomas, and edema can ordinarily be identified without the aid of special imaging methods or contrast media.

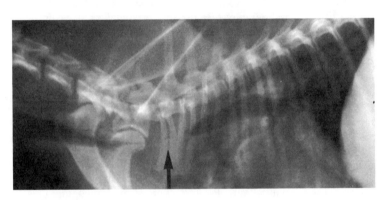

Fig. 35-2 This 8-year-old Yorkshire terrier had severe stress-induced coughing and tachypnea. Intrathoracic tracheal collapse *(arrow)* is prominent in the radiograph made on expiration.

A **B**

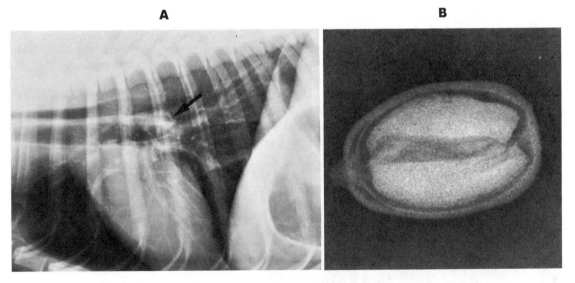

Fig. 35-3 A, A 1-year-old German shepherd had become acutely dyspneic and collapsed. The radiographic findings included microcardia, aerophagia, and an oval opacity at the carina surrounded by a concentric shell of gas *(arrow)*. **B,** The foreign body (acorn) removed from the carina.

Such disorders compromise the pharyngeal lumen and are usually associated with aerophagia, which may enhance contrast, making visualization of the area more clear.

Pharyngeal swallowing disorders such as cricopharyngeal achalasia generally are not associated with survey radiographic abnormalities. Swallowing disorders can only be recognized during the act of swallowing, and pharyngeal functional abnormalities can be characterized only by using motion imaging combined with a contrast medium such as barium paste. These real-time motion-imaging techniques include direct visualization with an image amplifier, various types of video recording, rapid-sequence spot filming, or cineradiography.

THORAX
Survey radiography

Survey thoracic radiography is always indicated in animals that suffer a serious injury or any time respiratory distress is recognized clinically. Subcutaneous emphysema, swelling, opaque foreign bodies, and mineralization of the thoracic wall can be recognized and characterized. Draining tracts may be investigated by fistulography (see "Cervical Soft Tissues"). Fractures and dislocations of sternebrae and ribs can be identified. These injuries may lead to additional intrathoracic or extrathroacic lesions such as perforation or laceration of the surrounding soft tissues, including the lung and blood vessels.

Conventional radiography is a highly successful imaging technique for identifying and characterizing infectious, allergic, and granulomatous pneumonia; pulmonary atelectasis, hemorrhage, bullae, and edema; and neoplastic, bacterial, and granulomatous lung masses. In some instances the radiographic findings will strongly suggest a specific cause for the clinical signs in the acutely ill animal (Fig. 35-4). Unilateral nodular lung lesions are best seen in the lateral view when the affected side is positioned away from the cassette; a right lung mass is visualized best when the animal is positioned in left lateral recumbency. There is a relative increase in air volume in the "up" lung as compared with the dependent lung, increasing contrast between normal lung parenchyma and the soft-tissue opacity created by the lung nodule(s).

The fenestrated nature of the canine and feline mediastinum typically results in bilateral though not necessarily symmetrical pleural effusion and pneumothorax. Trapped air and fluid sometimes pose a diagnostic dilemma by being difficult to characterize and distinguish from other lesions. For example, trapped fluid in the caudal pleural cavity can mimic diaphragmatic hernia and localized pneumothorax may not be easily distinguished from bullous emphysema. In these cases, radiography that uses a horizontal x-ray beam or radiography done with the animal in several different positions may help to clarify the situation (Fig. 35-5). Gravity will always cause free fluid to fall to a dependent position, while masses and viscera displaced through a diaphragmatic tear tend to remain in a more constant position, allowing one to determine whether fluid or a mass is causing a particular opacity. Ventrodorsal radiography of the thorax with the animal in lateral recumbency and using a horizontal beam will permit accurate visualization of a small volume of pleural air. Positive-contrast peritoneography is sometimes indicated when diaphragmatic rupture is suspected, but the survey radiographic findings are inconclusive (Fig. 35-6).

The heart and pulmonary vasculature is examined radiographically in critical care imaging, not only to assess primary cardiovascular disease, but also to evaluate the animal's cardiovascular sta-

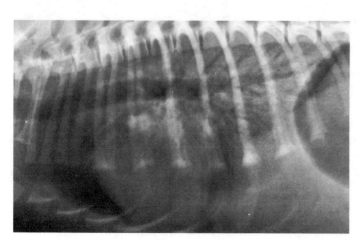

Fig. 35-4 A puppy underwent radiography within 2 hours of having bitten through a live electrical cord. The puppy was weak and faintly cyanotic. Prominent air bronchograms in the dorsocaudal lung lobes are a radiographic manifestation of the pulmonary edema that accompanies electrocution.

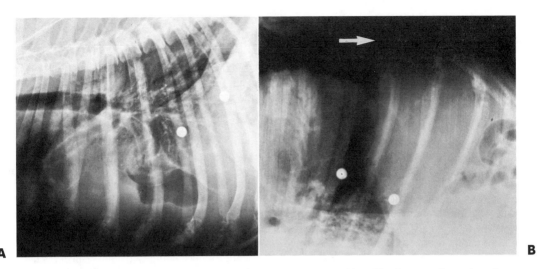

Fig. 35-5 A, A 10-year-old Irish setter was struck by an automobile. The dog was dyspneic and had several rib fractures. Based on the inability to visualize the ventral aspect of the diaphragm, diaphragmatic rupture was a diagnostic consideration. **B,** Lateral, dorsal recumbency horizontal beam radiography demonstrated an intact ventral diaphragmatic silhouette *(arrow)*, pneumothorax, and lung consolidation.

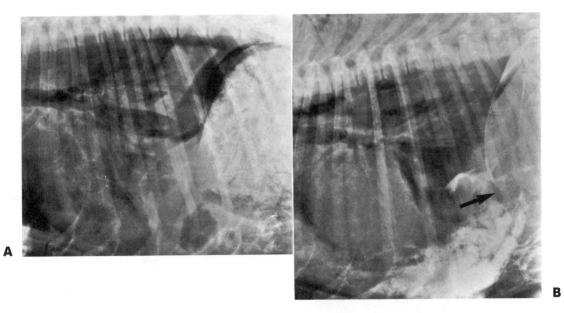

Fig. 35-6 A, Diaphragmatic rupture was suspected in this dog, based on the survey radiographs, but was difficult to verify because of pneumohemothorax. **B,** Intraperitoneal injection of positive contrast medium clearly demonstrated the diaphragmatic rupture *(arrow)*.

tus, regardless of the cause of the acute condition. An enlarged cardiac silhouette can be associated with cardiac dilatation or hypertrophy as well as with pericardial effusion or mass. In cases of primary cardiac enlargement, generally, focal chamber enlargements are recognized along with pul-

monary congestion, appropriate to the degree of enlargement. With significant pericardial effusion, the cardiac silhouette assumes a more circular configuration. These are useful general guidelines but there are many exceptions, and often echocardiography is necessary for definitive diagnosis. A small cardiac silhouette with small and attenuated pulmonary vessels indicates reduced cardiac output and underperfusion of the lung. These changes are associated with adrenocortical hypofunction, polymyositis, myasthenia gravis, emaciation, dehydration, and shock.

Ultrasonography

Ultrasonographic examination of the thorax is indicated in animals suspected of having cardiac disease, mediastinal masses, pleural masses, or mediastinal, pleural, or pericardial effusions. Air-filled lung is a barrier to ultrasonic transmission, therefore, a solid tissue or fluid interface or fluid (acoustic window) must be interposed between the ultrasound transducer and the area imaged. The heart at the cardiac notch, a mass lesion, and pleural effusion are acoustic windows adequate to allow visualization of other non-air-filled normal and pathologic structures in the thorax.

Echocardiography is frequently useful to diagnose both cardiac and pericardial disorders (see Chapter 17). This noninvasive technique uses two-dimensional and M-mode methods to study heart chambers, wall thickness, heart-valve motion and morphology, papillary muscles, chordae tendineae, and endocardial and pericardial surfaces. Doppler studies provide additional quantitative information on blood flow, velocity, and direction. Pulmonary, mediastinal, and heart-base masses can be located and characterized using vascular landmarks such as the venae cavae and aorta as well as by examining the base of the mass. However, anatomic differentiation of masses is challenging, especially in the cranial thorax. The location, ultrasonographic characteristics (relative echogenicity) and the approximate volume of pleural fluid accumulation can be assessed by ultrasound examination. This information is useful in the performance of ultrasound-guided thoracocentesis.

Lung masses, consolidation, and atelectasis or collapse are tentatively differentiated on ultrasound primarily by the shape and echogenicity of the structure being examined. A pulmonary mass has irregular to rounded borders with a variable echogenicity (often mixed), pulmonary consolidation appears as a "filled" convex, triangular structure with a homogeneous or mixed echogenicity (Fig. 35-7). The presence of bright echoes may indicate incomplete consolidation with pockets of air or a lung abscess. Pulmonary atelectasis appears as a flat or concave, triangular structure. If the atelectasis is complete, the lung lobe is homogeneous. If the collapse is partial, there is evidence of gas bubbles (bright "speckles") irregularly located throughout the lung. Specific and uncommon conditions such as fetal lung lobe sequestration have been reported in humans.[1]

Scintigraphy

Masses in the thoracic wall, ribs, and sternebrae can be evaluated by means of nuclear scintigraphy if the lesion is associated with increased resorption, vascularization, or deposition of bone. Nuclear scintigraphy has considerable potential for evaluating suspected perfusion defects associated with pulmonary thromboembolism (Fig. 35-8) and ventilation abnormalities due to bronchial or alveolar disease.

Computed tomography

The anatomical boundaries of infiltrating lesions of the pleura or thoracic wall can be clearly identified by computed tomography, even in the presence of pleural effusion due to the far greater contrast resolution in computed tomography as compared with conventional radiography.

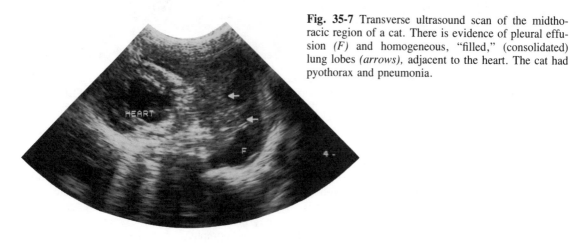

Fig. 35-7 Transverse ultrasound scan of the midthoracic region of a cat. There is evidence of pleural effusion *(F)* and homogeneous, "filled," (consolidated) lung lobes *(arrows)*, adjacent to the heart. The cat had pyothorax and pneumonia.

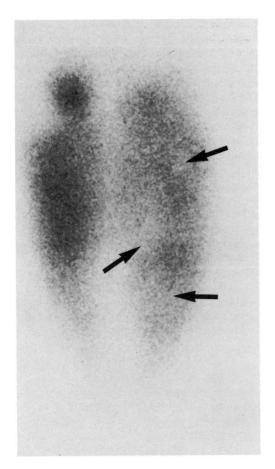

Fig. 35-8 A 7-year-old collie was presented with a coagulopathy, tachypnea and a partial pressure of arterial oxygen of 65mm Hg. The radiographic findings were nonspecific, with a moderate, increased interstitial opacity in the right middle lung lobe area.

The lung-perfusion scan shows overall reduced isotope uptake in the right lung and focal areas of almost no uptake *(arrows)*. The clinical and radiographic findings indicate reduced right lung perfusion and probable thromboembolism due to coagulopathy. The final diagnosis was immunohemolytic anemia.

ESOPHAGUS
Dilatation

Motility disorders are the commonest cause of esophageal dilatation. Animals with motility disorder may be acute-care problems when the disorder is secondary to adrenocortical insufficiency, lead poisoning, myasthenia gravis, or trauma. Aspiration pneumonia, which often accompanies regurgitation, can also cause acute signs.

The commonest esophageal disorders may be recognized on survey radiography. Megaesophagus, whether congenital or acquired, consists of esophageal dilatation due to reduced or absent motility. Radiographically, the entire esophagus will contain air and variable quantities of fluid and ingesta. The trachea and the heart may be deviated ventrally by the enlarged esophagus, and there is often radiographic evidence of aspiration pneumonia. A vascular ring such as a persistent right fourth aortic arch incarcerates the esophagus, producing dilation proximal to the ring. Esophageal motility is normal early in the disease, but increasing dilation of the esophagus proximal to the vascular ring may result in progressive loss of motility. Esophageal dilatation can also occur proximal to a point of extrinsic compression. An example is the dilation of the cervical esophagus produced by a mediastinal mass at the thoracic inlet compressing the esophagus between itself and the paraspinal muscles. An esophagram may be done to confirm esophageal motility disorders by making a gruel of canned pet food or baby food mixed with barium powder and feeding the mixture to the animal. Dogs and cats will often eat the mixture readily. If the animal is allowed to gorge on the barium mixture there is a potential for regurgitation and the risk of subsequent aspiration of the mixture into the trachea and lungs. Lateral and oblique radiographic views that include the entire esophagus usually show the degree and location of distention satisfactorily.

Foreign bodies

Even esophageal foreign bodies that are radiolucent are often visualized on survey radiography because they are outlined by the esophageal air that accompanies an animal's repeated attempts at swallowing. A commercial barium paste (Esophatrast, barium sulfate esophageal cream, Armour Pharmaceuticals, Kankakee, Il) is the contrast agent of choice for radiographic investigation of suspected esophageal foreign bodies. The paste will adhere to the esophageal mucosa for several minutes, allowing time for radiographs to be obtained. This contrast agent also facilitates visualization of mucosal erosions, ulcers, and filling defects.

Perforation

Esophageal perforation may result in radiographic manifestations of pneumomediastinum, pneumothorax, and pleural effusion. If suspected perforation is to be confirmed by an esophagram, the contrast medium (Dionosil Oily, propyliodone suspended in peanut oil, Glaxo, Greenford, England) will minimize further problems such as aspiration pneumonia or chemical irritation that might follow leakage of the agent into the pleural cavity.

DIAPHRAGM

Diaphragmatic tears are one of the common injuries seen in intensive care imaging. Fortunately most such injuries are readily diagnosed by survey radiography, but when extensive pleural effusion obscures the displaced viscera, ultrasound examination is an effective diagnostic procedure. Alternatively, radiography performed following thoracocentesis and drainage of the pleural cavity may also be diagnostic. Occasionally, orally administered barium may help to clarify an otherwise puzzling situation by outlining gastrointestinal displacement associated with the diaphragmatic rupture. The presence of a normal diaphragmatic silhouette on survey radiography does not necessarily eliminate the diagnosis of diaphragmatic tear. For example, when the stomach is distended with ingesta at the time of the injury, the opening in the diaphragm may be occluded temporarily, preventing visceral displacement through the opening until the stomach empties (Fig. 35-9).

Gastrodiaphragmatic herniation is a surgical emergency that must be recognized radiographically. When the stomach passes through a small tear in the diaphragm and the stomach distends with swallowed air, lung capacity is reduced and major thoracic blood vessels are compressed. The potential for rapid death must be considered, and the need for surgical intervention is urgent.

Gastroesophageal intussusception resembles hiatal hernia radiographically. The survey radiographic findings are nonspecific; however, acute vomiting or regurgitation, possibly hemorrhagic, accompanied by a tubular, tissue-dense protrusion from the cranial aspect of the diaphragm at the level of the esophagus may be indicative of gastroesophageal intussusception. Although an esophagram may clarify the diagnosis by showing the characteristic coiled spring appearance of intussusception, usually the serious nature of the clinical disease limits further diagnostic tests.

Animals with pericardioperitoneal hernias are seldom seen as intensive care or emergency medicine problems. These hernias usually create min-

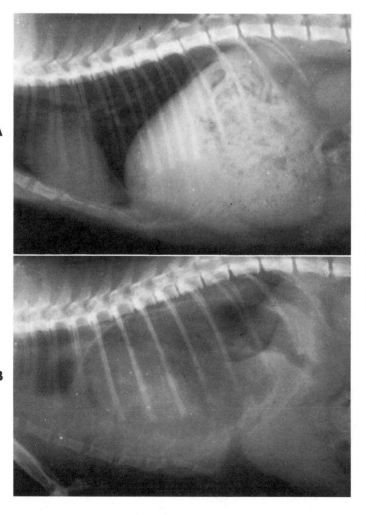

A

B

Fig. 35-9 A, This cat was examined within 2 hours after it was struck by an automobile. Initially, no radiographic abnormality was seen. **B,** The next day dyspnea developed. In the follow-up radiograph a diaphragmatic rupture is apparent. (Courtesy of Dr. Richard Roberts, Hanover, MA.)

imal or vague clinical signs, but a loop of bowel may become incarcerated or twisted in the hernia, resulting in an acute intestinal obstruction. These pericardiodiaphragmatic hernias are generally recognized in survey radiographs by the gaseous and fluid distention of the intestinal loops within the pericardium. If the liver or other abdominal viscera are contained within a pericardioperitoneal hernia, ultrasound evaluation can be diagnostic.

Ultrasound

Ultrasonographic evaluation of the diaphragm in traumatized animals, although accurate, may be physically difficult because of the discomfort and dyspnea that accompanies the injury. Diaphragmatic tears are diagnosed ultrasonographically by the identification of cranial displacement of the abdominal viscera and less commonly by imaging the diaphragmatic tear directly. Liver, stomach, spleen, mesentery, and intestines are commonly observed passing through a traumatic diaphragmatic tear (Fig. 35-10). Mirror image artifact of the liver, associated with the highly reflective surface of the diaphragm, may cause a false positive diagnosis of a diaphragmatic tear (Fig. 35-10).

Scintigraphy

Scintigraphic evaluation using technetium-99m mixed with saline and administered in the perito-

neal space is possibly the most sensitive technique to rule out small diaphragmatic tears. The only site of normal tracer uptake in the thorax is the sternal lymph node in animals with an intact diaphragm. Therefore, the scintigraphic detection of any quantity of free isotope, cranial to the diaphragm, following abdominal infusion, is diagnostic of a diaphragmatic tear.

ABDOMEN
Survey radiography

In acute abdominal disorders the survey radiographic findings are exceptionally important because contrast examinations may be impossible to perform because of the animal's deteriorating condition and the need for rapid diagnosis. When the roentgen findings are correlated with the findings from the history, the physical examination, and laboratory tests, the clinician can decide whether a contrast examination is indicated. Survey radiography also indicates whether the initial roentgen technique was appropriate for use in further imaging studies and whether findings such as effusion exist, which will prevent adequate visualization of abdominal structures during contrast examinations.

Abdominal radiography must include the entire dome of the diaphragm and the pelvis through the level of the acetabula in both the lateral and ven-

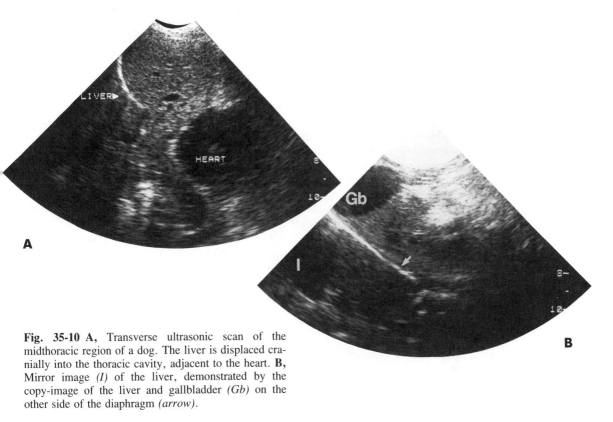

Fig. 35-10 A, Transverse ultrasonic scan of the midthoracic region of a dog. The liver is displaced cranially into the thoracic cavity, adjacent to the heart. **B,** Mirror image *(I)* of the liver, demonstrated by the copy-image of the liver and gallbladder *(Gb)* on the other side of the diaphragm *(arrow).*

trodorsal views. The rear legs should be pulled caudally to prevent the soft tissues of the quadriceps muscles from overlapping the caudal abdomen and obliterating detail. The exposure should permit evaluation of soft tissue, the lumbar spine, and the caudal ribs. Large dogs, especially those with a large dorsoventral depth may require two separate ventrodorsal radiographic exposures because the abdomen is much thicker cranially than caudally.

Each radiograph should be evaluated systematically and thoroughly to ensure that technical quality is adequate and that no abnormality will be overlooked. Clinical judgment is used to assess the proper significance of abnormalities detected. When examining abdominal radiographs one should first visualize structures external to the abdomen, including the spinal column, the ribs, and the ilia. Next, the abdominal wall should be evaluated for any disruption of its integrity, changes in opacity, or the presence of foreign bodies. The diaphragmatic contour should be examined. The overall serosal detail and the general abdominal shape are then evaluated. A search should be made for evidence of gas within the peritoneal cavity. Gas that is free to migrate tends to accumulate in the subdiaphragmatic area between the liver and the diaphragm in both the ventrodorsal and the lateral radiographs. Horizontal-beam radiography in a recumbent position may be useful in further delineating small amounts of peritoneal gas. Gas may also be trapped within the mesentery, forming small bubbles, which may be difficult for the inexperienced observer to discern. These bubbles will tend to occupy a central position in the abdomen and may have a stippled appearance similar to hemorrhage in the omentum or mesentery in the midabdomen. Intraabdominal fat provides a less opaque image than the solid portions of the other viscera, permitting visualization of solid, water-dense organs such as the liver, spleen, kidneys, and urinary bladder. Intraabdominal masses have a nearly solid tissue opacity and may or may not be clearly associated with typically seen viscera. For example, granulomas due to peritoneal foreign bodies or lymphadenopathy may be seen as masses. Any situation in which intraabdominal or mesenteric fat is reduced or obliterated will result in poor abdominal contrast and detail. Emaciation or the lack of intraabdominal fat development such as occurs in immature individuals results in uniformly reduced contrast. Peritoneal effusion obliterates fat planes and reduces abdominal contrast. Any infiltrating neoplastic or inflammatory lesion that invades the fat planes produces a nonuniform, focal, or diffuse reduction in contrast.

The retroperitoneum should be searched for masses that may involve the adrenal glands, kidneys, or lymph nodes. Uneven contrast in the retroperitoneum can result from extravasation of fluids such as blood or urine, or neoplastic or inflammatory infiltration.

Survey radiography is sensitive in detecting reduced abdominal and retroperitoneal contrast, but the findings are often nonspecific as to cause.

Ultrasound and computed tomography

The importance of evaluating the peritoneum and retroperitoneum in the critical care setting and the difficulty in doing so by conventional radiographic methods has led to widespread acceptance of ultrasound and computed tomography as alternative imaging methods in this area by medical radiologists.

Gas within the gastrointestinal tract is a limiting factor to ultrasonographic evaluation of the abdomen. However, in suspected proximal small intestinal mechanical obstruction or pancreatic abnormality, instillation of water into the gastrointestinal tract through a stomach tube will reduce this impediment by providing a suitable acoustic window for ultrasound imaging. The morphology and thickness of the layers of the intestinal wall as well as gastrointestinal motility can be assessed ultrasonographically. Intraperitoneal fluid, whether due to a disease process or introduced to enhance ultrasound visualization, may be an aid to the ultrasound imaging of abdominal contents.

Computed tomography has contrast resolution that is an order of magnitude better than that available by conventional radiography. This factor allows abdominal viscera and masses to be readily identified when emaciation or effusion would otherwise render the radiographs nondiagnostic.

Although changes in size, margins, and opacity of the liver, spleen, kidneys, and prostate are usually observed on survey radiography, computed tomography and ultrasound offer dramatically improved diagnostic sensitivity and specificity. The internal architecture of viscera can be evaluated. Guided fine-needle aspiration or percutaneous biopsies can also be performed as part of the imaging procedure. The utility of such a combined procedure is especially valuable in the evaluation of the liver and spleen for suspected metastases and other masses and in differentiating the causes of hepatic and splenic enlargement.

STOMACH

The most common causes of caudal gastric displacement are impingement by hepatic neoplasms, displacement by pancreatic or hepatic lymphadenopathy, hepatic enlargement, and a caudal diaphragmatic location due to increased respiratory effort. An inflammatory or neoplastic pancreatic mass may displace the pylorus of the stomach to the left of the midline, increase the gastric-duodenal angle, and produce focally diminished contrast along the pylorantral portion of the greater curvature of the stomach. The pylorus is seen radiographically to be displaced cranially when the liver or duodenum pass forward through a pericardioperitoneal hernia or a diaphragmatic rupture.

Trauma

Direct trauma to the stomach is seldom recognized radiographically. Traumatic bruising of the stomach is probably infrequent because of the protection given by the ribs. Gastric hemorrhage can sometimes be recognized by a granular radiographic appearance of the gastric contents. Gastric hemorrhage can be the result of trauma, gastric ulceration, inflammatory disease, or neo-

plasm. Gastric foreign bodies are often identified by survey radiography or pneumogastrography, the introduction of air into the stomach through an orogastric tube (Fig. 35-11).

Distention

Aerophagia, regardless of its cause, may result in considerable gastric and small-intestine distention. Situations in which substantial air swallowing occurs in animals include upper respiratory disorders, congestive heart failure, conditions associated with regurgitation or vomiting, shock, and pain due to any cause. Gastric distention with fluid or ingesta may occur in animals with gastric hypomotility disorders or gastric-outflow obstruction.

Volvulus (see also Chapter II)

Volvulus of the stomach results from twisting of the pylorus craniodorsally and to the left of the midline. When this displacement occurs neither air nor fluid can easily leave the stomach, and progressive gastric distention occurs. The pres-

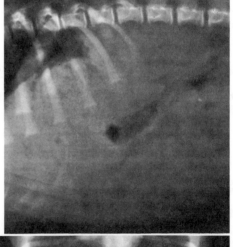

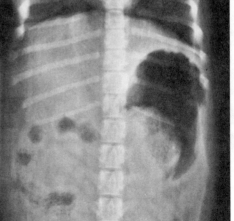

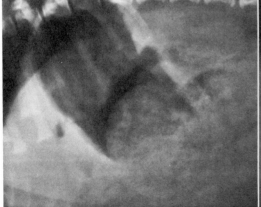

Fig. 35-11 **A,** This 5-month-old cairn terrier was presented for acute vomiting. The lateral survey radiograph shows a circular mass that leads one to suspect a foreign body. **B** and **C,** The pneumogastrogram helps to identify the circular gastric foreign body. A rubber ball was removed from the stomach.

ence of gastric torsion is recognized on survey radiographs by the dorsal displacement of the pylorus and by an opaque line along the cranial dorsal third of the gastric silhouette, resulting from the folding of the pylorus on the body of the stomach.

When the gastric ischemia that usually accompanies gastric torsion is severe enough, gastric-wall necrosis will occur. Initially, small gas bubbles will be seen radiographically within the gastric wall. If the gastric wall perforates, a large quantity of gas will be seen radiographically in the peritoneal cavity. This gas accumulation is best recognized in the ventrodorsal radiograph immediately caudal to the diaphragm and cranial to the liver, creating a clear silhouette of the diaphragm between the air-filled lung and the gas in the peritoneum. Small amounts of free air in the peritoneum are best seen radiographically by making a radiographic exposure with the animal in lateral recumbency using a horizontal x-ray beam.

Ulcers

Gastric ulcers may be idiopathic or associated with the administration of medication, but are most frequently seen as a complicating factor in animals with gastric neoplasia or gastric foreign body. Ulcers are recognized in the upper gastrointestinal contrast examination as defects in the gastric wall that fill with and retain barium (see Chapter 22). Double-contrast gastrography and pharmacologically aided gastrography, using glucagon, may be

helpful in cases in which conventional barium-contrast examination is equivocal.[9-11]

A few cases of gastric ulceration in animals have been diagnosed by ultrasound.[12] A specific diagnosis of gastric ulceration requires appropriate ultrasound equipment and expertise.

SMALL INTESTINE
Trauma

Injury to the small intestine due to blunt trauma is uncommon because the intestines are more readily displaced than lacerated or bruised by external force. Bruising of the intestine may not produce any radiographic abnormality. The degree of radiographic change is usually dependent on the loss of contrast associated with hemorrhage. An abdominal mass may develop with fibrinous or fibrous adhesions between an injured portion of intestine and the mesentery or omentum. Additionally, an organizing intramural hematoma may rarely cause small-bowel obstruction.

Duodenal hematoma has been recognized by ultrasound examination in abused children[13] and presumably could be imaged in small animal patients.

A small perforation may be identified by contrast radiography (Fig. 35-12). A large perforation of the intestine liberates a large amount of free gas which is readily seen radiographically within the peritoneal cavity. When small tears occur the gas may only appear as small bubbles trapped within the mesentery and omentum.

Infarction of large areas of intestine produces

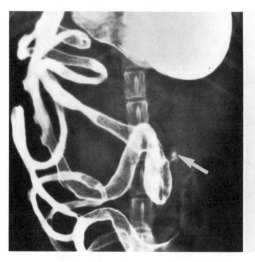

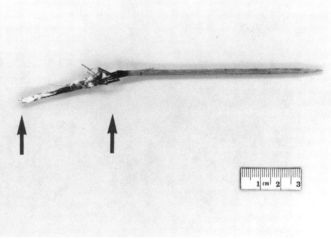

A　　　　　　　　　　**B**

Fig. 35-12 Foreign-body ingestion was suspected by the owner of this dog. Survey radiographs were normal. **A,** The upper gastrointestinal radiograph depicts the site of perforation *(arrow)* in the midjejunum. **B,** Only the portion of the stick coated with barium (between the *arrows*) was within the lumen of the small intestine. The remainder of the stick extended into the peritoneal cavity.

gaseous and fluid distention of the small intestine due to reduced peristalsis and diminished absorptive ability in the infarcted intestinal segment. Small intramural infarcts may not produce any radiographic or clinical findings initially, but days later perforation can cause focal or diffuse peritonitis. Fibrosis is a rare complication, which may occur in the healing phase of infarction without perforation, and can lead to intestinal stricture and obstruction weeks after the original injury.

Paracostal, abdominal, and inguinal hernias contain small intestine less commonly than do diaphragmatic tears. Incarceration of the intestine in a hernia, with or without volvulus, may result in obstruction and vascular compromise.

Obstruction

Foreign bodies are the most common cause of intestinal obstruction in dogs and cats. The size and nature of ingested objects defy the imagination. The most common complication of foreign-body ingestion is obstruction of the intestinal lumen. The radiographic signs are those of distention of the intestine proximal to the point of obstruction, with delayed transit of material through the gastrointestinal tract (see Chapter 22). Proximal small-bowel obstruction generally results in a relatively greater volume of intraluminal gas and less fluid accumulation than obstructions that are more distal. Obstructive radiographic patterns in the small intestine can also be seen in animals with benign and malignant intestinal neoplasms.

Linear foreign bodies that are firmly attached in the gastrointestinal tract or at the frenulum of the tongue, present additional radiographic features such as plication of the small bowel, which results from hypermotility. The small intestine may appear "stacked," with a combination of both gas and fluid contents, but not necessarily distended. In some cases, eccentrically placed, intraluminal gas pockets are also seen. The radiographic features are more clearly identifiable in the upper gastrointestinal contrast examination. A "sawing" action of the foreign body on the mesenteric border of the intestine may cause intestinal perforation, creating a variable degree of reduced serosal detail due to leakage of intestinal contents. Initially, small gas bubbles in the mesentery may be recognized radiographically. As the perforation becomes larger, other viscera may be outlined by larger amounts of free peritoneal air. Barium administration is contraindicated in cases of perforation. Barium and intestinal contents leaking into the peritoneal cavity may cause a severe foreign-body-induced inflammatory response in the peritoneum. In cases of suspected perforation, an aqueous organic iodine such as diatrizoate solution (Hypaque sodium, oral solution, Winthrop Laboratories, New York) may be used instead of barium to reduce the risk of worsening the peritonitis associated with intestinal perforation. However, the aqueous organic iodides have a rapid and unpredictable transit time through the gastrointestinal tract, are readily diluted by intestinal secretions, coat the gastrointestinal mucosa poorly, and can be absorbed from the gastrointestinal tract. These features limit the diagnostic use of this class of contrast agents in gastrointestinal contrast radiography.

Ultrasound is an effective technique for detecting the cause of intestinal obstruction. Common foreign bodies such as balls are clearly identified by their shape and the strong acoustic shadowing associated with the foreign body.[12] The characteristic "accordion" pleating of the intestine is seen ultrasonographically with linear foreign bodies and the foreign body itself is imaged in some cases.

Gastrointestinal obstruction due to intussusception is usually not complete initially, but vascular compromise can produce infarction and necrosis. A tubular structure of fluid density may be visualized radiographically in the midabdomen along with intraluminal gas accumulation proximal to the point of obstruction.

Although seldom necessary for establishing the diagnosis, a barium enema will often provide a specific diagnosis of intussusception. The characteristic radiographic finding in intussusception is a spiral configuration of the barium column caused by the telescoping bowel segment. Barium enema is usually performed with the animal under general anesthesia. Large-bore tubing with an inflatable cuff surrounding the tubing is inserted into the terminal colon. The cuff is inflated to prevent leakage of barium. Approximately 10 ml/kg of 100% (weight/volume) commercial barium sulfate suspension is instilled into the colon by gravity flow. The tubing is clamped and radiographs are made in the ventrodorsal, dorsoventral, right lateral, and left lateral positions. After draining the barium suspension from the large bowel, air may be insufflated through the tubing to produce a double-contrast effect. Radiography is repeated in the same views as for the positive contrast enema.

Ultrasound findings are highly sensitive and specific for intussusception,[14] making ultrasound the preferred method for diagnosing this condition. A multilayered appearance of the bowel is pathognomonic of intussusception (Fig. 35-13). Fluid accumulation is often seen in the proximal intestinal segment. Associated signs such as peritoneal effusion, lymphadenopathy, and intestinal mass may also be seen by ultrasound, helping to define the cause of the intussusception. However,

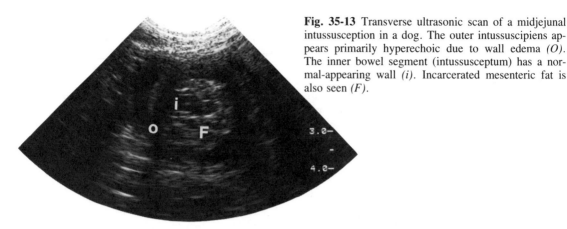

Fig. 35-13 Transverse ultrasonic scan of a midjejunal intussusception in a dog. The outer intussuscipiens appears primarily hyperechoic due to wall edema *(O)*. The inner bowel segment (intussusceptum) has a normal-appearing wall *(i)*. Incarcerated mesenteric fat is also seen *(F)*.

the specific site of the intussusception may not be determined by ultrasound because of the lack of specific anatomical landmarks identifying different parts of the gastrointestinal tract.

Adynamic (paralytic) ileus is associated with peritonitis, shock, and intestinal obstruction, but may also be mimicked by the administration of anticholinergic drugs. Difficulty may arise in determining whether loops of intestine that contain gas are small bowel or colon. As a rule of thumb, the small bowel is expected to occupy a more central position in the ventrodorsal radiograph than the laterally located loops of the colon. Distention of the small intestine with fluid and gas accompanied by the presence of an empty or nearly empty colon is highly suggestive of obstruction of the small intestine.

Intestinal obstruction may be either simple or strangulated. In simple obstruction an intestinal loop is partially or totally occluded, without significant interference with the blood supply to the bowel wall, whereas when strangulation is present, there are two obstructed ends and the intestinal blood supply is compromised. When the ischemic segment becomes infarcted, perforation rapidly follows. The use of horizontal-beam radiography to demonstrate air fluid interfaces at different heights in the same intestinal loop may be an invaluable technique in the diagnosis of strangulated obstruction particularly when contrast medium cannot be administered or a rapid diagnosis is essential.

Nuclear scintigraphy and computed tomography have been shown to be useful in the diagnosis of small-intestine infarction.[15-17]

Inflammatory diseases

Few inflammatory small intestinal disorders require emergency imaging. However, some acute conditions, especially those associated with vom-

iting and abdominal pain, produce rapid morbidity and may be a diagnostic challenge that requires imaging to determine the best course of action.[18,19]

Inflammatory disease of the small intestine is common in dogs and cats, but the radiographic signs are not consistent (Fig. 35-14). The findings may include mild to moderate dilation of the small intestine with varying volumes of fluid and gas, thickening of intestinal loops, evidence of hyperperistalsis, rapid transit of contrast medium, and dilution of barium during radiographic contrast examination. Early in its course, parvovirus enteritis may be difficult to distinguish radiographically from intestinal obstruction. Gaseous distention of the small intestine is sometimes severe with parvovirus and may be accompanied by delayed gastric emptying in the upper gastrointestinal contrast examination. However, when the barium enters the small intestine, transit time is rapid, and frequently there is substantial dilution of barium by excessive intestinal secretions.

Thickening of the small intestinal wall, with or without loss of the normal intestinal layers is the most common ultrasound finding in enteritis.

Rarely, abscesses of the small intestine complicate inflammatory disease. Abscesses may protrude into the lumen of the small intestine and cause obstruction.

Ulceration of the small intestine is usually associated with a neoplasm or foreign body, but inflammatory lesions also have the potential to cause ulceration (Fig. 35-15). The potential of nuclear scintigraphy to localize small-bowel bleeding has been demonstrated.[20-22]

Ultrasound examination may be useful in the detection and as an aid in the drainage of intestinal abscesses and trapped or free intraperitoneal fluid accumulations. Ultrasound may also be used to assess the architecture and size of the abdomi-

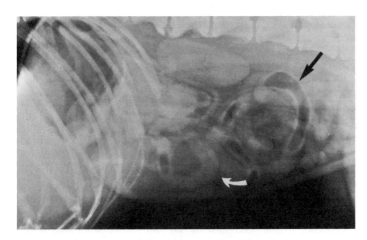

Fig. 35-14 This 11-year-old German shepherd had an acute onset of vomiting. The absence of distention in the gastrointestinal tract and the alternating regions of gas *(arrow)* and fluid *(curved arrow)* in the small intestine suggest enteritis rather than obstruction. Later, the dog developed diarrhea. The clinical diagnosis was nonspecific enteritis.

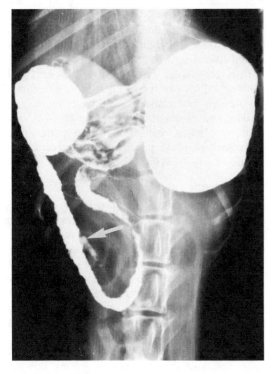

Fig. 35-15 Hemoptysis and weakness associated with blood loss were the main clinical signs in this 4-year-old terrier. Extensive irregularity of the descending duodenum with spiculation of the barium column persisted throughout the upper gastrointestinal study. There is evidence of perforation *(arrow)*. The cause of the perforating ulcer was not identified.

nal lymph nodes and to guide abscess drainage and fine-needle aspiration of lymph nodes, which may be enlarged in inflammatory small-bowel disease.

Adhesions and strictures

Adhesions and strictures that occur as a sequela to a surgical procedure, previous inflammatory disease, or external trauma can produce obstruction of the small intestine weeks or months after resolution of the original insult.

CECUM AND COLON

Blunt abdominal trauma seldom produces any radiographic abnormality in the cecum or colon. Abdominal injury caused by penetrating objects may be associated with perforation of either of these structures, resulting in pneumoperitoneum and bacterial contamination of the peritoneal cavity.

Intraluminal foreign bodies in the cecum and colon cause clinical signs much less commonly than those located in the stomach or small intestine. Malicious insertion of foreign bodies into the rectum of an animal can also cause perforation. Such foreign bodies are occasionally detected by radiographic examination of animals presented to emergency clinics.

Intussusception of the cecum is a difficult condition to diagnose clinically but is recognized by barium enema examination. A "coiled spring" filling defect is produced by the invagination of the cecum into the ascending colon. Occasionally, the diagnosis can be strongly suspected based on survey radiographic findings of a filling defect (invaginated cecum) in the gas-filled ascending or transverse colon. Volvulus of the cecum or colon may occur secondary to tears or neoplastic erosion of the mesentery. Tumors in the cecum and colon may produce acute clinical signs due to ulceration and massive bleeding or perforation and peritonitis.

GALLBLADDER AND LIVER

The liver, bile ducts, and gallbladder are infrequently injured severely in animals that suffer blunt abdominal trauma because of the protection afforded by the rib cage. Liver lacerations may be associated with displaced rib fractures. Rupture of the bile ducts or gallbladder results in abdominal pain associated with bile peritonitis. These injuries may be occult immediately following traumatic injury. Liver lacerations and bleeding neoplasms produce the nonspecific radiographic findings of reduced serosal definition due to abdominal effusion. Acute abdominal signs may also be associated with bleeding tumors of the liver, bile ducts, and gallbladder. Cholelithiasis may cause bile-duct obstruction and acute abdominal pain.

Hepatitis, cholecystitis, and choledochitis are difficult to diagnose clinically or radiographically. An enlarged liver may be seen radiographically in the acute phase of hepatic disease in which edema and congestion are the predominant pathologic changes. Acute hepatitis may also create a blunt, rather than the usual sharply angular caudal hepatic margin. In the chronic phases of disease the liver may be shrunken, due to fibrosis.

In rare instances, lucent pockets of emphysema may be recognized radiographically within the liver parenchyma, in association with severe gas-forming infections (Fig. 35-16).

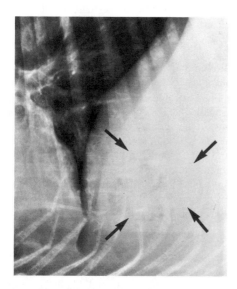

Fig. 35-16 A 10-year-old male German shepherd had lethargy and severe weakness for one day. In the caudal aspect of a lateral thoracic radiograph, a circular pattern of gas bubbles *(arrows)* was seen. The gas was associated with hepatic abscesses.

Emphysematous cholecystitis is also a rare lesion, recognized radiographically by the reduced opacity of the gallbladder lumen or wall. Emphysematous cholecystitis sometimes complicates acute necrotizing pancreatitis or diabetes mellitus. Oral or intravenous administration of cholegraphic agents may be helpful procedures to allow differentiation of cholecystitis from intrahepatic bile-duct obstruction or in ruling out the gallbladder as the source of acute abdominal disease.

Ultrasound is routinely used to evaluate the hepatic parenchyma, biliary system, and vasculature. Hepatitis may not produce any abnormality in the ultrasound examination, but in some cases the liver is enlarged and has reduced echogenicity. Hepatic parenchymal masses such as abscesses, hematomas, lacerations (Fig. 35-17) and neoplasms are readily detected by ultrasound (Fig. 35-18). Ultrasound-guided biopsy is recommended to aid in the differential diagnosis of suspected liver disorders of many types.

Ultrasonographic evidence of a thickened gallbladder wall can be seen with ascites, a collapsed gallbladder, and cholecystitis. An enlarged gallbladder and common bile duct can be associated with hyperechoic gallstones or an extrahepatic mass such as acute pancreatitis, pancreatic neoplasm, or hepatic lymphadenopathy.

Portosystemic vascular shunts

Portal venous anomalies in animals are rarely emergencies requiring diagnostic imaging, but these animals may be intensive care cases because of the clinical abnormalities associated with the metabolic upset caused by portosystemic shunting. Although there are no specific radiographic findings, typically the liver is small. Contrast portography, ultrasonography, and nuclear scintigraphy can be used to provide more specific data, which will confirm the diagnosis.

Operative portography is effective in anatomically demonstrating the portal venous flow. A small catheter is passed into a jejunal vein via a minilaparotomy. The abdomen is surgically closed, leaving a section of the catheter extending from the abdominal closure. Approximately 600 mg of iodine/per kilogram in the form of a sterile aqueous organic triiodinated solution (diatrizoate meglumine 60%, Hypaque 60M, Winthrop) is injected through the catheter. Radiographs of the abdomen are made in the lateral and ventrodorsal planes at the rate of 1 exposure per second for 15 seconds, with an automatic film changer. The pattern of contrast flow outlines the portal venous system and any vascular shunts that may be present. The contrast procedure may be repeated intraoperatively to verify shunt ligation and the change in portal blood flow.

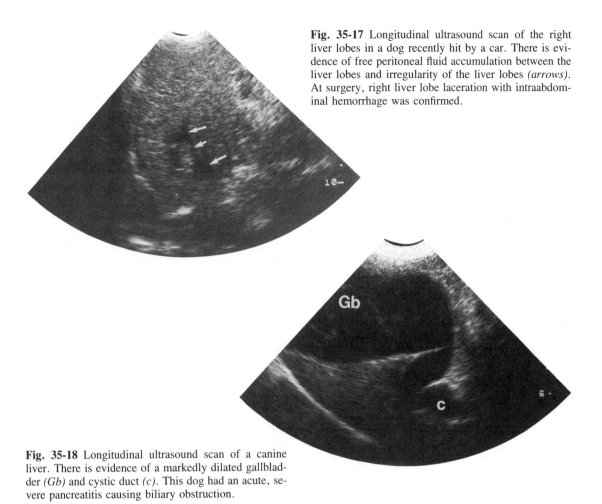

Fig. 35-17 Longitudinal ultrasound scan of the right liver lobes in a dog recently hit by a car. There is evidence of free peritoneal fluid accumulation between the liver lobes and irregularity of the liver lobes *(arrows)*. At surgery, right liver lobe laceration with intraabdominal hemorrhage was confirmed.

Fig. 35-18 Longitudinal ultrasound scan of a canine liver. There is evidence of a markedly dilated gallbladder *(Gb)* and cystic duct *(c)*. This dog had an acute, severe pancreatitis causing biliary obstruction.

Ultrasound is an effective and noninvasive method of evaluating portal venous drainage, especially by using duplex Doppler techniques. However, ultrasound evaluation of suspected portosystemic shunts is often limited by microhepatica and air within the gastrointestinal tract and in the lungs. Therefore, the intercostal approach is most often used.

Positive-pressure ventilation (under general anesthesia) can be applied to the animal to displace the diaphragm and liver caudally, thereby increasing access to the liver and increasing the sensitivity of the ultrasound examination to the detection of intrahepatic vascular anomalies.[23] Few or no portal vessels are seen in the small liver, and when the shunt is imaged by ultrasound, a turbulent flow can be detected by Doppler sampling. However, the presence of normal portal branches in the liver does not rule out a portosystemic shunt. Extrahepatic shunts are extremely difficult to assess by ultrasound because of overlying gas-filled intestines.

Nuclear medicine is a highly sensitive technique to detect portosystemic shunts and quantitate portal-vein blood flow. Scintigraphy can serve as a screening test in suspected cases of portal venous anomalies.[24,25] This imaging method can also be used after a corrective surgical procedure to quantify the change in portal blood flow produced by shunt ligation. The scintigraphic image does not usually provide the specificity needed to classify portal venous anomalies anatomically in individual animals.

SPLEEN

The spleen is often injured in animals with abdominal trauma and may also be affected by a variety of other processes that result in acute disorders that require diagnostic imaging. Tumors of the spleen may bleed acutely either spontaneously or as the result of vigorous abdominal palpation or other abdominal trauma. The most common radiologic finding in splenic trauma is loss of peritoneal contrast associated with hemorrhage due to splenic laceration and intraabdominal hemorrhage. Volvulus, infarction and infection are rare splenic lesions that can cause acute abdominal signs. Volvulus of the spleen may produce toxemia due to vascular compromise. The abdominal pain that occurs in volvulus and the infectious disorders of the spleen is due to increased intracapsular pressure created by acute swelling, hemorrhage, or both. Infection caused by gas-forming bacteria creates the survey radiographic findings of splenic irregularity with numerous gas pockets throughout the splenic parenchyma.

Ultrasound is often used to assess the spleen in animals suffering from abdominal trauma. Splenic hematomas produce inhomogeneous, echoic, variably sized masses with or without anechoic or hypoechoic cavities and may be associated with a variable quantity of peritoneal fluid. Splenic hematoma may not be distinguishable from splenic neoplasm or abscess. An enlarged spleen with regular, anechoic stripes is pathognomonic for splenic torsion.[26] Occasionally, peritoneal effusion and a splenic thrombus may also be seen in association with splenic torsion and can be detected by ultrasound (Fig. 35-19).

PANCREAS

The pancreas is protected from direct trauma by the rib cage, but traumatic pancreatitis may accompany a fall or an automobile accident.[27] Acute traumatic pancreatitis cannot be distinguished radiographically from other types of acute pancreatitis. The survey radiographic findings may be normal or may consist of a granular, uneven opacity and reduced contrast immediately caudal to the pyloric antrum that extends along the medial aspect of the proximal descending duodenum. These changes are associated with pancreatic and parapancreatic edema and hemorrhage. In addition, the usually acute gastroduodenal angle may be widened, due to shifting of the thickened, distended proximal descending duodenum toward the right flank and the pylorus to the left of the midline.(Fig. 35-20).[2,3,28]

Primary or secondary pancreatic neoplasms may produce acute clinical signs of upper gastrointestinal obstruction if these masses reach sufficient size or invade the small intestine.

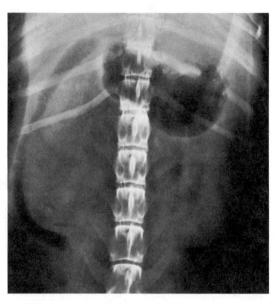

Fig. 35-20 An 8-year-old dog was presented with an acute onset of vomiting and abdominal tenderness that could not be localized. The survey radiographic findings included widening of the gastroduodenal angle and displacement of the descending duodenum toward the right flank (*arrow*). Gas retention in the duodenum persisted in later radiographs.

The subsequent laboratory and clinical findings confirmed the clinical diagnosis of acute pancreatitis.

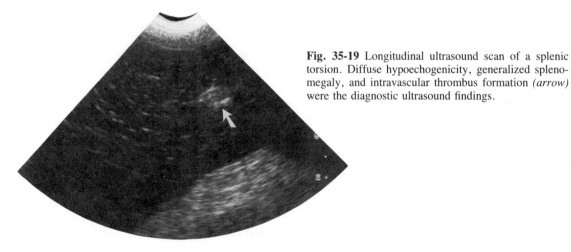

Fig. 35-19 Longitudinal ultrasound scan of a splenic torsion. Diffuse hypoechogenicity, generalized splenomegaly, and intravascular thrombus formation (*arrow*) were the diagnostic ultrasound findings.

Ultrasonographic and computed tomographic imaging of the pancreas are useful and may provide a more specific diagnosis. Either procedure may be helpful in guiding a fine-needle aspiration or core biopsy of the lesions identified by imaging. Pancreatic neoplasms, such as adenocarcinoma, tend to create a large complex mass, which markedly deforms the contour of the pancreas.

The normal pancreas is not visualized by survey radiography and is often not seen by ultrasound examination. Uniformly hypoechoic areas along the greater curvature of the stomach or the mesenteric border of the duodenum, or both, are seen by ultrasound imaging in acute pancreatitis. Edema and hemorrhage cause pancreatic swelling reducing the echogenicity of the pancreas, making it hypoechoic, in contrast to the surrounding hyperechoic fat (Fig. 35-21)). The ability to recognize the changes associated with acute pancreatitis and pancreatic masses by radiographic and ultrasound evaluation has been described.[2,3]

Chronic pancreatitis has a similar ultrasound pattern associated with irregular and patchy foci of hyperechogenicity, probably representing fibrosis or mineralization, or both (Fig. 35-22). Occasionally, dilatation of the pancreatic duct can be observed in either acute or chronic cases of pancreatitis.[29]

Ultrasound is a routinely useful diagnostic tool for the evaluation of the pancreas and provides a reliable assessment of response to medical or surgical treatment.

Computed tomography, because of cost and the need for the use of deep sedation or general anesthesia in dogs and cats, has not been used frequently in small-animal intensive care for the diagnosis of acute pancreatitis. Computed tomography has been shown to be the most sensitive imaging method to confirm the diagnosis of acute pancreatitis, determining the prognosis and predicting the need for surgical intervention in the human being with acute pancreatitis.[4-8]

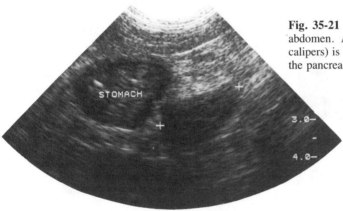

Fig. 35-21 Longitudinal ultrasound scan of the cranial abdomen. A diffusely hypoechoic pancreas (between calipers) is seen adjacent to the stomach. Both limbs of the pancreas were inflamed.

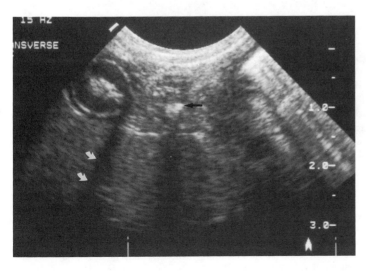

Fig. 35-22 Transverse ultrasound scan of the descending duodenum and pancreas. The duodenum is thickened (6 mm) but the wall layers are clearly identified. The pancreas is thickened and inhomogeneous with some hyperechoic areas *(arrow)* associated with clean acoustic shadowing. This represents focal mineralization. Note the edge shadowing produced by the rounded border of the descending duodenum *(curved arrows)*.

ABDOMINAL WALL, PERITONEUM, AND RETROPERITONEUM

Abdominal-wall trauma occurs frequently in dogs and cats, but the radiographic findings are usually limited to changes in the soft-tissue opacity or thickness due to bruising or emphysema secondary to skin lacerations or the presence of foreign bodies such as gravel, other road debris, and metallic fragments associated with a gunshot wound. Radiographic findings of fractures of the last few ribs or transverse processes of lumbar vertebrae suggest the possibility of lacerations of the liver, spleen, or kidneys.

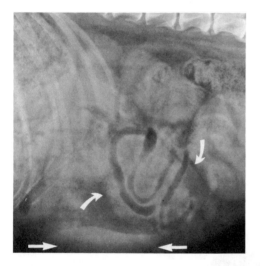

Fig. 35-23 A 10-year-old spayed female collie dog had a fever, weakness, and a palpable abdominal mass. The ventral mass *(curved arrows)* is radiographically distinct from the spleen *(straight arrows)*. Mesenteric lymph-node abscess was the microscopic diagnosis.

Peritoneal effusion is recognized on survey radiography by loss of serosal detail and has diverse causes, including pancreatitis; ruptures of prostatic or mesenteric abscesses, bile ducts, gallbladder, or urinary bladder; liver failure or laceration, heart failure, feline infectious peritonitis, penetrating abdominal wounds, bowel perforation, intestinal obstruction with strangulation, and hypoproteinemia. Unfortunately, there are no diagnostic features that permit pus, blood, bile or transudate to be distinguished from one another based on their radiographic appearance.

Tumors, abscesses, and granulomas involving the omentum, mesentery, and associated lymph nodes may produce a radiographically recognizable mass (Fig. 35-23) and sometimes a stippled opacity in the midventral abdomen due to diffuse involvement and obliteration of the fat planes, which usually provide contrast between the abdominal viscera.

Ultrasound examination can assist in determining the origin and characteristics of most pathologic processes in the peritoneum or retroperitoneum. Examples of such conditions in which ultrasound examination is valuable include lacerations of the liver, spleen, kidney, and urinary bladder as well as prostatic or mesenteric abscesses.

Lacerations of the solid viscera are seen ultrasonographically as hypoechoic or anechoic regions in the parenchyma, associated with loculated or free effusion, or both, due to hemorrhage. Multiple small echoes in the fluid suggest blood clots or fibrin tags.

Computed tomography allows far greater contrast discrimination than conventional x-ray techniques; therefore, the various types of effusion

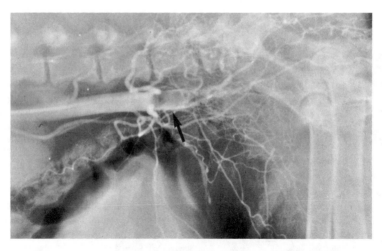

Fig. 35-24 A 5-year-old dog was presented because of rear leg paresis after being hit by a descending overhead door. Femoral pulses were faint to absent and the rear legs were cool. Terminal aortic occlusion was confirmed by the aortogram. The filling defect *(arrow)* in the terminal aorta represents the thromboembolus.

can sometimes be distinguished by computer measurements of x-ray absorption.

Aortic thromboembolism may occur secondary to cardiac disease, especially feline cardiomyopathy, or blunt external trauma. In such cases, the retroperitoneum may be enlarged, displacing the kidneys ventrally, but no specific survey radiographic signs are produced. Aortography will depict the site and degree of aortic occlusion (Fig. 35-24). In cases of aortic laceration, contrast extravasation will be produced. Nuclear scintigraphy has been used in the diagnosis of canine aortic thomboembolism.[30] Duplex or color-flow Doppler ultrasound provides a noninvasive method to determine the presence and character of blood flow in the aorta.[31]

UROGENITAL TRACT
Perineum and urethra

Bruising, fluid accumulation, or pain in the perineal area is an indication for investigation of the integrity of the urethra by means of positive-contrast, retrograde urethrography (Chapter 21). Negative-contrast urethrography (pneumourethrography) is usually not as discriminating diagnostically and carries with it the hazard of air embolism.[32]

Urethrography is necessary to evaluate the integrity of the urethra, since a normal cystogram does not rule out a urethral tear. The urethrovesicular junction is the most common site for urethral tears. Survey radiographs may be normal in these cases, but more often, peritoneal effusion is seen radiographically due to blood and urine accumulation in the peritoneal cavity. Similarly, when positive contrast medium is introduced into the urethra, the medium will spill from the lumen of the urethra into the adjacent tissues, readily identifying the site of the rent. Urethral tears occurring during catheterization and postoperative stricture formation are common examples of iatrogenic trauma. These too, are clearly observed with the use of positive-contrast urethrography.

Acute urethral obstruction may occur when a cystic calculus or blood clot lodges in the urethra. Opaque calculi are readily recognized in survey radiographs, but lucent calculi and blood clots require positive-contrast urethrography for radiographic diagnosis. Obstruction associated with the feline urologic syndrome does not produce specific radiographic signs and is largely diagnosed by clinical signs, not by imaging procedures. Positive-contrast urethrography will identify the site of obstruction.

Urinary bladder

Blunt trauma. Blunt trauma of the urinary bladder due to automobile accidents is common in small animals. Lesions produced by this type of injury include laceration, contusion, herniation, and rarely, volvulus of the urinary bladder. The typical survey radiographic findings in laceration of the urinary bladder include reduced abdominal contrast and a small or absent urinary bladder silhouette. Urinary-bladder contusions can be recognized radiographically only by contrast examination. Focal bladder-wall thickening along with intraluminal or extraluminal hematomas are best identified by double-contrast cystography. Contrast urography clearly identifies mucosal herniation (Fig. 35-25), or a urinary bladder contained within an abdominal or inguinal hernia. Urinary bladder volvulus is a rare event, which may occur in blunt abdominal trauma after transection of the median ligament of the bladder.

Iatrogenic trauma. An inflexible catheter may lacerate and penetrate the wall of the urinary bladder, while a flexible catheter can be knotted within the bladder if it is inserted too deeply. Overinflation of the bladder during pneumocystography can cause focal mucosal tears or even rupture the wall of the urinary bladder. Overinflation can be avoided by carefully monitoring the pressure exerted on the syringe barrel. When sufficient gas has been instilled in the bladder to cause the plunger to recoil, no further gas should be introduced. Special caution should be exercised when a cuffed catheter of the Foley type is used, because excessive intraluminal pressure can easily be produced.

Fatal air embolism may be associated with pneumocystography performed with room air. Air that enters the venous system by way of a bleeding lower urinary tract lesion can form a bubble large enough to occlude the caudal vena cava or fill the right heart, preventing circulation to the pulmonary arteries and causing death. The use of a more soluble gas such as carbon dioxide is recommended for pneumocystography to minimize this potential hazard.

Additionally, the urinary bladder may be accidentally traumatized during an ovariohysterectomy as the uterine stump is ligated.

Cystitis. No survey radiographic abnormality is expected in acalculus cystitis. In chronic cases, mineralization of the wall of the urinary bladder may be seen in association with granulomatous or necrotic lesions. Negative- or double-contrast cystographic evaluation may also result in normal findings, but more often, a uniformly circumferential thickening or focal cranioventral thickening is found. In acute cystitis, the signs may be functional (straining and spasticity), rather than anatomic. However, filling defects, associated with blood clots are sometimes found in both acute and chronic cystitis.

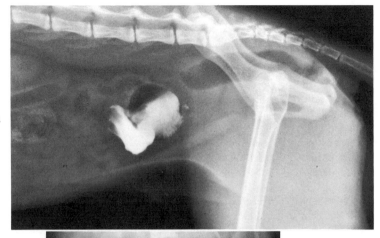

A

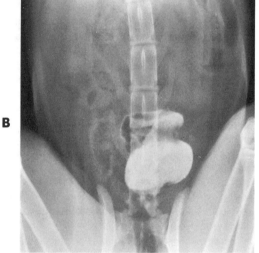

B

Fig. 35-25 A and **B,** The positive-contrast cystogram demonstrates mucosal herniation through the cranial aspect of the urinary bladder caused by an automobile accident.

A urachal remnant is recognized on the cystogram as a diverticulum on the cranioventral aspect of the urinary bladder. This lesion may accompany acute recurrent or chronic cystitis.

Emphysematous cystitis is recognized on survey radiography by the presence of gas bubbles in the wall and lumen of the bladder. Urinary bladder infection in the presence of glucosuria is the most common condition predisposing to emphysematous cystitis.[34]

Urinary bladder tumors. Benign or malignant tumors of the urinary bladder in animals may be associated with acute clinical signs of hematuria or urethral obstruction. Survey radiographs of the urinary bladder are usually normal, but double-contrast cystography and ultrasound examination may provide information specific to the diagnosis. Ultrasound-guided biopsy or fine-needle aspiration may yield a cytologic or histologic diagnosis.

Kidneys and ureters

Trauma. The primary survey radiographic signs associated with rupture of the kidneys or

ureters are accumulation of fluid in the abdominal cavity or retroperitoneal space. These lesions tend to obscure the kidneys, but in some cases renal enlargement or renal displacement may be recognized. Fractures of the last few ribs or the transverse processes of lumbar vertebrae, especially when associated with radiographic evidence of a retroperitoneal mass, should lead to a search for evidence of ureteral or renal trauma. Intravenous urography and ultrasonography are the favored imaging techniques for evaluating suspected or known cases of renal and ureteral trauma (Fig. 35-26).

Inflammatory diseases. Acute inflammatory diseases of the kidneys include pyelitis, pyelonephritis, and nephritis. While pyelitis and pyelonephritis are ordinarily caused by infection, nephritis may be either infectious or toxic. Although renal enlargement may be present, the survey radiographic signs are more often subtle or nonexistent, and these disorders are best imaged by intravenous urography and ultrasound. In nephritis, there may be enlargement of the paren-

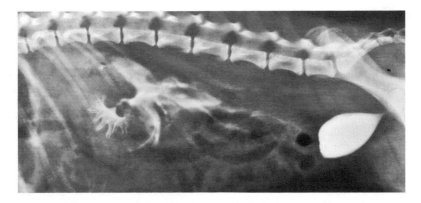

Fig. 35-26 Abdominal pain was the major clinical finding in this dog, which was suspected of having been struck by an automobile. The survey radiograph showed an uneven opacity in the retroperitoneum. Twenty minutes after intravenous injection of 3 ml/kg of diatrizoate meglumine, contrast medium is accumulating in the retroperitoneum because of rupture of the proximal left ureter.

chymal portion of the kidney with or without hydronephrosis, and the kidneys may appear more opaque due to edema and inflammation of parenchyma. As these diseases progress, distortion of the renal pelvis, a prolonged pyelogram, a variable degree of hydronephrosis, and blunting of the pelvic diverticula are seen. Corticomedullary junction distortion occurs with acute nephritis and can best be defined ultrasonographically.

Calculi. While formation of renal calculi is a chronic phenomenon, the clinical signs may be acute because of passage of a renal calculus into a ureter, causing obstruction and extreme abdominal pain or an acute infection accompanying the stone(s). Radiolucent renal stones cannot be visualized except by intravenous urography or ultrasound.

Neoplasms. When tumors of the kidneys and ureters rupture, the acute blood loss may produce retroperitoneal or intraperitoneal masses and loss of radiographic contrast, along with clinical signs of shock. Intravenous urography is diagnostic. The location of the spillage of medium is readily seen, as in traumatic renal and ureteral rupture. Renal arteriography and ultrasound will indicate the size and degree of invasiveness of kidney neoplasms. If the bleeding has a focal origin, the focus may be visualized by arteriographic examination.

The ultrasound appearance of renal neoplasms varies[33]; they may be focal, multifocal, or diffuse. The corticomedullary ratio and the renal pelvis can also be variably affected and the echogenicity of renal masses varies from hypoechoic to hyperechoic. While there is no clear ultrasound feature that distinguishes malignant from benign renal tumors, the presence of neoplastic invasion, such as to the opposite kidney, to blood vessels, or to lymph nodes may assist in the diagnosis. An assessment of Doppler characteristics and ultrasound-guided biopsy are necessary for a definitive diagnosis.

Prostate

Trauma. The prostate gland is generally protected by the pelvic bones and is seldom seriously injured by external force, unless the pelvis is crushed. Occasionally, a large prostatic cyst may be ruptured by external trauma or by traumatic passage of a urethral catheter into a cyst that communicates with the prostatic urethra, causing acute hemorrhage, and radiographic signs of diminished peritoneal serosal contrast may then occur.

Infection. Prostatitis and abscess formation cause acute signs due to stranguria, obstruction, pain, infection, and sepsis. Prostatic enlargement is recognized in survey abdominal radiography and positive-contrast retrograde cystourethrography, but is a nonspecific finding. Cysts, causing prostatic enlargement, may be associated with benign prostatic hyperplasia, cystic prostatitis, prostatic abscesses, or prostatic adenocarcinoma. Prostatic cysts that communicate with the urethra may be seen radiographically by injecting positive contrast medium through a urethral catheter whose orifice is placed at or immediately distal to the prostatic urethra.

Ultrasonographic evaluation of the prostate gland is complex and should include information concerning the size, shape, symmetry, and the echogenic properties of the gland and visualization of the regional structures, including the lymph nodes. The prostatic parenchyma should be uniformly echoic and any local or generalized changes is echogenicity may assist the diagnosis. Canine prostatic disease has been classified, based on the changes in echogenicity, into cavitating bacterial, noncavitating bacterial, noncavitating nonbacterial, paraprostatic, and neoplastic disease.[35] Real-time ultrasound is a sensitive method to evaluate the prostate. Most authors believe that ultrasound contributes more information about the nature of prostatic disease than radiography and urethrography.[35] One of the most valuable features of ultrasound is its use in guiding a transabdominal fine-needle aspiration or biopsy of the prostate gland.

Neoplasms. Prostatic neoplasms that metastasize to the lumbar spine and pelvis may produce acute lameness, paresis, and pain. The most common survey radiographic findings in cases of bone metastases are mixed proliferative and lytic lesions, with proliferation predominating, in the middle of the ventral aspect of the last few lumbar vertebrae. Less commonly, the transverse processes of the lumbar vertebrae and the pelvis may also be involved.

Enlargement of the retroperitoneal iliac lymph nodes that compress the colon and rectum ventrally is also sometimes observed in survey radiograms in various types of prostatic disease.

Ovary and testis

Volvulus of an ovary or a retained testis causes abdominal pain due to vascular compromise and swelling of the parenchyma of the organ. Such lesions can sometimes be recognized radiographically as an oval abdominal mass in the caudal abdomen (testis) or midabdomen (ovary). Torsion of an ovary or intraabdominal testis occurs most often in association with a neoplasm of the affected gonad.

Ultrasonographic evaluation may be a substantial aid in making a more definitive evaluation by further characterizing the nature of the mass.

Uterus

Trauma. Occasionally the uterus may be traumatized directly by a blunt force such as an automobile accident, especially if pyometra or pregnancy is present. A uterine laceration is accompanied by peritoneal bleeding and spilling of uterine contents, which produces loss of abdominal contrast. Laceration of the gravid uterus may allow a fetus to enter the peritoneal cavity. Uterine rupture also occurs as a rare complication of dystocia. When the gravid uterus enters an inguinal or abdominal hernia, the possibility of vascular compromise and accompanying toxemia must be anticipated. Volvulus of the gravid uterus is a rare occurrence and has no specific radiographic findings.

Uterine stump inflammation, infection, abscess, and granuloma formation may occur as complications of ovariohysterectomy. Occasionally, a radiographically or ultrasonographically recognizable mass dorsal to the neck of the urinary bladder and ventral to the rectum may be seen in these cases. In the cystographic examination, the dorsal aspect of the urinary bladder may be displaced ventrally.

Infection. In endometritis the uterus has a turgid, nodular appearance on radiography and is usually two to three times larger than normal. Whereas with pyometra, the uterus is usually not as lobulated in its radiographic appearance, but instead has a smooth configuration and may be five to eight times its normal diameter.

Ultrasonographic evaluation of the pelvic canal is indicated to assist in the anatomic differentiation of the involved intrapelvic structures and when a satisfactory evaluation cannot be made by routine clinical, laboratory, or radiographic techniques. Ultrasound examination of the uterus often provides the best diagnostic data in animals suspected of having endometritis, pyometra, or other types of uterine enlargement.

Fetal abnormalities. Dystocia caused by fetal head-maternal pelvis incompatibility is easily diagnosed radiographically.

Gas within a fetus or the uterus and fetal skull fractures are radiographic manifestations of fetal death. Mummified fetuses, whether ectopic or uterine, are sometimes recognizable radiographically by disorganization and compression of the skeleton.

Ultrasound imaging and Doppler techniques may be used to assess the fetal heartbeat as an indication of living fetuses.

AXIAL SKELETON
Skull

The complex anatomy of the skull requires meticulous attention to positioning of the animal for radiography and to the technical details of the radiographic examination. Interpretation requires careful evaluation and a through knowledge of the anatomy of the skull. An animal must be under general anesthesia to enable a complete radiographic examination of the skull. The use of high-detail intensifying screens and film or nonscreen film technique will aid in visualizing subtle changes. Multiple views are essential for a thorough radiographic evaluation.

Linear tomography is occasionally useful in more clearly defining skull fractures and temporomandibular joint abnormalities.

Computed tomography is exceptionally useful for anatomic demonstration of neoplastic, inflammatory, or traumatic lesions of the brain (Figs.

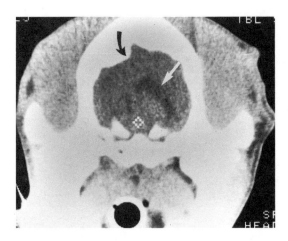

Fig. 35-27 A 6-month-old Rottweiler had been bitten by another dog 4 months earlier. The current clinical presentation was for seizures. Computed tomographic examination of the skull was performed. There is asymmetric hydrocephalus, as indicated by a dilatation of the right lateral ventricle *(arrow)*, with deformity of the calvarium *(curved arrow)* secondary to the previous trauma.

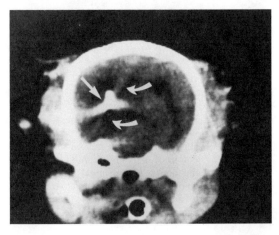

Fig. 35-28 This 3-year-old Maltese had a sudden onset of seizures. In a survey radiograph of the thorax and cervical region, the tip of a linear metallic foreign body (needle) was seen. Subsequent skull radiography failed to localize the needle conclusively to an intracranial or extracranial location. The computed tomographic image proves the needle *(arrow)* is within the left lateral ventricle. The ill-circumscribed hyperdense areas lateral and medial to the needle *(curved arrows)* are caused by beam hardening associated with the metallic foreign body.

35-27 and 35-28), skull, jaws, tympanic bullae, and nasal cavity. Computed tomographic imaging has proved valuable in diagnosis and in planning surgical and radiation therapy. Generally, administration of an intravenous contrast medium is required in computed tomographic imaging to demonstrate lesions such as brain tumors, which cause a breakdown in the blood-brain barrier. Contrast medium tends to accumulate in focal neoplastic lesions, thereby enhancing visualization of the tumor. Diffuse contrast enhancement is a nonspecific finding and may occur in widespread neoplastic or inflammatory brain disorders.

In human medicine, magnetic resonance imaging has gained widespread acceptance for the evaluation of central nervous system disorders, as the overlying bone opacity is eliminated and subtle morphologic changes not seen by other imaging methods are revealed. Increased diagnostic utility is also attributed to superior contrast rendition and the ability to manipulate the image data to provide optimal tissue characteristics. Narrow tissue slices (2 mm) are depicted as in computed tomography. The expense, availability, and degree of expertise required currently limits its role in veterinary imaging.

Three-dimensional computed reconstruction of magnetic resonance imaging and computed tomographic images and the subsequent computer manipulation of the images represents a new and exciting radiologic method that may prove valuable, especially in radiotherapy and surgical planning and in the evaluation of the response to treatment (nasal adenocarcinomas and intracranial lesions). The cost and requisite computer skills for three-dimensional techniques have limited its application in veterinary imaging.

Spine

Imaging of the vertebral column and intervertebral disk spaces of animals is often required in the intensive care environment. Multiple lesions are often found in animals with traumatic injuries.[36] Conventional radiography is the primary imaging method used in evaluating suspected cases of spinal fractures, dislocations, neoplasms, disk herniation, and infectious disorders (Figs. 35-29 and 35-30). In some intensive care situations spinal radiographs *must* be made without anesthesia because of the animal's critical state, but the limitations of radiography in these conditions must be taken into account in interpretation. Identification of all but the most obvious lesions requires general anesthesia for adequate radiographic evaluation of the spine. Previous comments regarding attention to details in imaging the skull apply equally to the imaging procedures used in spinal column imaging.

Myelography is indicated when the subarachnoid space is to be visualized. The most common example for the use of myelography is in the evaluation of an animal suspected of having extradural compression associated with disk herniation

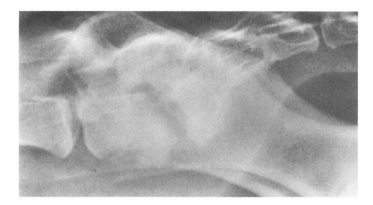

Fig. 35-29 Poorly marginated proliferation of dense, nontrabecular bone with ill-defined lucency in the enlarged L7-S1 disk space and partial destruction of the caudal aspect of L7 (especially dorsally), strongly indicates diskospondylitis.

Fig. 35-30 This 2-year-old mastiff had obscure back pain and acute recurrent urinary tract infection. A lucency separates the caudal end plate from the body of L4. The caudal half of L4 is sclerotic. Extensive, ill-defined bone proliferation bridges the ventral aspect of L4-5. The clinical and radiographic diagnosis was L4 physitis.

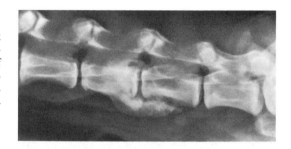

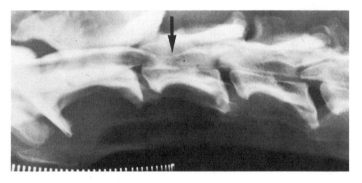

Fig. 35-31 Acute tetraparesis occurred in this 8-year-old German shepherd. No abnormalities were seen on survey radiographs of the spine. Ventral deviation of the dorsal subarachnoid space contrast column (arrow) in the myelogram is due to an extradural lesion. The histologic diagnosis was metastatic carcinoma.

Fig. 35-32 This 8-year-old English setter had an acute onset of neck pain and rear limb ataxia. The survey radiographs were normal. The filling defect on the ventral aspect of the contrast column (arrow) strongly suggests an intradural lesion, probably involving the nerve root. The histologic diagnosis was neurofibrosarcoma.

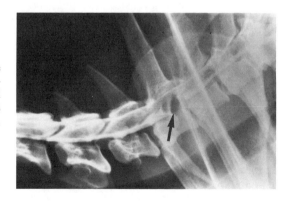

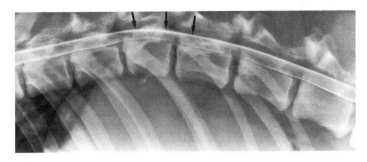

Fig. 35-33 This 1½-year-old German shepherd had hindlimb paresis after being struck by an automobile. A compression fracture of T12 was diagnosed from the survey radiographs. The myelogram demonstrates ventral deviation of the dorsal subarachnoid space *(arrows)*. Extradural hemorrhage and edema caused the deviation of the contrast medium column. Satisfactory surgical stabilization was accomplished.

(Chapter 11). Whenever a laminectomy is considered, myelography is probably indicated to localize the affected area with greater certainty. Myelography is especially useful in distinguishing extradural, intradural, and intramedullary causes of spinal cord disease (Figs. 35-31, 35-32, and 35-33).

The technique used to introduce the contrast medium varies with the individual case. The cervical (cisterna magna) approach is preferred when a cerebrospinal fluid sample is needed, cerebrospinal fluid pressure is to be measured, a cervical spinal lesion is suspected, or the lumbar approach to a suspected caudal thoracic or lumbar lesion has not been successful. The lumbar approach using the L4-5 or L5-6 interspace is preferred when a caudal thoracic or lumbar lesion is suspected.

The availability of non-ionic contrast agents such as iopamidol (Isovue-200, Squibb) has dramatically increased the safety of myelography. The dosage of contrast agent used varies from 0.35 to 0.5 ml/kg, with the lower dosage being used in large dogs and the higher dosage being used in small dogs and cats or when a considerable length of the subarachnoid space must be opacified.

Imaging of the caudal epidural space may be indicated in cases of suspected lumbosacral instability, pelvic canal neoplasms and infections, and proliferative osteoarthritis of the spine. The space may be visualized by the injection of 0.3 to 0.45 ml/kg of non-ionic myelographic contrast medium into the epidural space through the lumbosacral junction or the sacrococcygeal space.[37,38]

Diskography may be used to assess the integrity of the fibrous dorsal portion of the intervertebral disks in animals that have the cauda equina syndrome and suspected intervertebral disk herniation.[37] Approximately 0.5 ml of a non-ionic contrast agent is introduced into the disk by a dorsolateral approach using a spinal needle with fluoroscopic guidance. Less than 0.5 ml (often none) can be introduced into a normal disk. Lateral radiography of the area performed after injection of medium will show spilling of the contrast agent into the area of herniation. When the dorsal annulus is intact, and contrast medium that has been injected will outline the extent of the disk in its normal location.

Magnetic resonance imaging has become the primary spinal imaging method at some medical centers because of the exquisite contrast, the spatial resolution, and the ability to depict tissue differences that are characteristic of the method. Another special advantage of magnetic resonance imaging in the spine and skull is that the relatively immobile protons in the overlying bone do not produce a signal and therefore do not interfere with the visualization of the underlying soft tissues. These features of magnetic resonance imaging greatly enhance the radiologist's ability to visualize small, otherwise undetected abnormalities.

REFERENCES

1. Buntain WL, Isaacs H, Payne VC, et al. Lobar emphysema, cystic adenomatoid malformation, pulmonary sequestration, and bronchogenic cyst in infancy and childhood. A clinical group. J Pediatr Surg 1974;9:85.
2. Nyland TG, Mulvany MH, Strombeck DR. Ultrasonic features of experimentally induced, acute pancreatitis in the dog. Vet Rad 1983;24:260-266.
3. Johnson ML, Mack LA. Ultrasonic evaluation of the pancreas. Gastrointest Radiol 1978;3:257-266.
4. Hessel SJ, Siegelman SS, McNeil BJ, et al. A prospective evaluation of computed tomography and ultrasound of the pancreas. Radiology 1982;143:129-133.

5. Clark LR, Jaffe MH, Choyke PL, Grant EG, Zeman RK. Pancreatic imaging. Radiol Clin North Am 1985;23:489-501.

6. White EM, Wittenberg J, Mueller PR, et al. Pancreatic necrosis: CT manifestations. Radiology 1986;158:343-346.

7. Vernacchia FS, Jeffrey RB, Federle MP, et al. Pancreatic abscess: predictive value of early abdominal CT. Radiology 1987;162:435-438.

8. Balthazar, EJ, Robinson DL, Megibow AJ, Ranson JAC. Acute pancreatitis: value of CT in establishing prognosis. Radiology 1990;174:331-336.

9. Evans SM, Laufer I. Double contrast gastrography in the normal dog. Vet Radiol 1981;22:2-9.

10. Evans SM, Biery DN. Double contrast gastrography in the cat: technique and normal radiographic appearance. Vet Radiol 1983;24:3-5.

11. Evans SM. Double versus single contrast gastrography in the dog and cat. Vet Radiol 1983;24:6-10.

12. Penninck DG, Nyland TG, Kerr LY, Fisher PE. Ultrasonographic evaluation of gastrointestinal diseases in small animals. Vet Radiol 1990;31:134-141.

13. Orel SG, Nussbaum AR, Sheth S, Yale-Loehr A, Sanders RC. Duodenal hematoma in child abuse: sonographic detection. Am J Roentgenol 1988;151:147-149.

14. Montali C, Croce F, DePra L, et al. Intussusception of the bowel: a new sonographic pattern. Br J Radiol 1983;56:621-623.

15. Federle MP, Chun G, Jeffrey RB, et al. Computed tomographic findings in bowel infarction. Am J Roentgenol 1984;142:91-93.

16. Gray H, Richards J. Clinical imaging with indium-111 labeled leukocytes: uptake in bowel infarction. J Nucl Med 1981;22:701-702.

17. Coleman R, Black R, Welch D, et al. Indium-111 labeled leukocytes in the evaluation of suspected abdominal abscesses. Am J Surg 1980;139:99-103.

18. Kleine LJ. Radiology of acute abdominal disorders in the dog and cat. Part II. Compend Contin Educ Pract Vet 1979;1:580-589.

19. Kleine LJ. Radiology of acute abdominal disorders in the dog and cat. Part II. Compend Contin Educ Pract Vet 1979;1:614-623.

20. Denham JS, Becker GJ, Siddiqui AR, et al. Detection of acute gastrointestinal bleeding by intra-arterial Tc-99m sulfur colloid scintigraphy in a canine model. Invest Radiol 1987;22:37-40.

21. Thorne DA, Datz FL, Remley K, Christian PE. Bleeding rates necessary for detecting acute gastrointestinal bleeding with technetium-99m labeled red blood cells in an experimental model. J Nucl Med 1987;28:514-510.

22. Vasquez TE, Bridges RL, Braunsten P, Jansholt AL, Meshkinpour H. Gastrointestinal ulcerations: detection using a technetium-99m labeled red blood cells in an experimental model. J Nucl Med 1983;148:227-231.

23. Wrigley RN, Konde LJ, Park RD, Lebel JL. Ultrasonographic diagnosis of portacaval shunts in young dogs. J Am Vet Med Assoc, 1987;191:421-424.

24. Koblik, PD, Yen, CK, Komtebedde, J, Hornof, WJ, Moore PF, Fisher PE. Comparison of transcolonic 123-iodoamphetamine and portal vein injection of 99m Tc-macroaggregated albumin shunt fraction calculations in experimental dogs with acquired portosystemic shunts. Vet Radiol 1990;31:170-174.

25. Daniel GB, Bright R, Monnet E, Ollis P. Comparison of per-rectal portal scintigraphy using 99m-technetium pertechnetate to mesenteric injection of radioactive microspheres for quantification of portosystemic shunts in an experimental dog model. Radiology 1990;31:175-181.

26. Konde LJ, Wrigley RN, Lebel JL, Park RD, Pugh C, Finn S. Sonographic and radiographic changes associated with splenic torsion in the dog. Vet Radiol 1989;30:41-45.

27. Suter PF, Olsson, SE. Traumatic hemorrhagic pancreatitis in the cat: a report with emphasis on the radiological diagnosis. J Am Vet Radiol Soc 1969;10:4-11.

28. Kleine LJ, Hornbuckle WE. Acute pancreatitis: the radiographic findings in 182 dogs. J Am Vet Radiol Soc 1978;14:102-106.

29. Lamb CR. Abdominal ultrasonography in small animals: examination of the liver, spleen and pancreas. J Small Anim Pract 1990;31:6-15.

30. Daniel GB, Wantschek L, Bright R, Silva-Krott I. Diagnosis of aortic thromboembolism in two dogs with radionuclide angiography. Vet Radiol 1990;31:182-185.

31. Reneman RS, Van Merode T, Hoeks APG. Noninvasive assessment of arterial flow patterns and wall properties in humans. News Physiol Sci 1989;4:185-190.

32. Ackerman, N, Wingfield W, Corley EA. Fatal air embolism associated with pneumourethrography and pneumocystography in a dog. J Am Vet Med Assoc 1972;160:1616-1618.

33. Konde LJ. Renal sonography. Semin Vet Med Surg 1989;4:32-43.

34. Sherding RG, Chew DJ. Nondiabetic emphysematous cystitis in two dogs. J Am Vet Med Assoc 1979;174:1105-1109.

35. Feeney DA, Johnston GR, Klausner JS, Bell FW. Canine prostatic ultrasonography—1989. Semin Vet Med Surg Small Anim 1989;4:44-57.

36. Feeney DA, Oliver JE. Blunt spinal trauma in the dog and cat: insight into radiographic lesions. J Am Anim Hosp Assoc 1980;16:885-890.

37. Hathcock JT, Pechman RD, Dillon AR, Knecht CD, Braund KG. Comparison of three radiographic contrast procedures in the evaluation of the canine lumbosacral spinal canal. Vet Radiol 1988;29:4-15.

38. Feeney DA, Wise M. Epidurography in the normal dog: technic and radiographic findings. Vet Radiol 1981;22:35-39.

36 Respiratory Support of the Critically Ill Small Animal Patient

Michael H. Court

Successful treatment of animals with advanced pulmonary disorders often entails intensive support of pulmonary function in addition to treatment of the primary disease process. Hypoxemia, hypoventilation, and ineffective clearance of material from the airway are abnormalities that are commonly associated with advanced respiratory disease. Oxygen therapy, positive-pressure ventilation and aerosol therapy are used to correct these deficits. The indications, equipment, and clinical application of these respiratory support methods are discussed in this chapter. Techniques of airway humidification commonly used in conjunction with oxygen therapy and ventilatory support are also described.

OXYGEN THERAPY

Oxygen therapy is indicated in conditions in which there is inadequate oxygenation of tissues within the body (hypoxia). Hypoxia may result from inadequate inspired partial pressure of oxygen, impaired pulmonary function, ineffective or inefficient transport of oxygen through the blood, or increased tissue oxygen consumption not matched by increased oxygen delivery.[1] Hypoxia is associated with many detrimental effects causing dysfunction of vital organs, particularly those with a high metabolic demand. Administration of supplemental oxygen to patients with the dysfunction(s) will help to prevent or reverse these changes and decrease the ventilatory and myocardial work required to maintain adequate tissue oxygen levels. Conditions in which oxygen therapy would be beneficial are listed in the following box.

One of the more definitive methods to ascertain the need for oxygen therapy is analysis of blood gases. Techniques of anaerobic collection and analysis of blood gas samples have been described.[2] Values for partial pressure of arterial oxygen (Pa_{O_2}) as low as 60 mm Hg (normally, 90 to 100 mm Hg) are generally well tolerated. Below this level, compensatory mechanisms, including increases in cardiac output and ventilation are initiated. This is a point commonly selected at which to initiate oxygen therapy.[3] An increase in partial pressure of arterial carbon dioxide (Pa_{CO_2}) above 55 mm Hg (normally, 35 to 40 mm Hg) indicates inadequate pulmonary ventilation for the level of carbon dioxide production and should be treated primarily by positive-pressure ventilation (PPV).

There are limitations in the usefulness of Pa_{O_2} to determine the need for oxygen therapy, particularly in situations in which there is altered affin-

---

EXAMPLES OF CONDITIONS THAT MAY BENEFIT FROM OXYGEN THERAPY

Inadequate inspired oxygen
  High-altitude sickness
  Following cessation of nitrous oxide administration ("Fink effect")
Impaired pulmonary function
  Pneumonia
  Pulmonary edema
  Respiratory distress syndrome
Decreased oxygen delivery
  Congestive heart failure
  Shock
  Anemia
Increased oxygen consumption
  Seizures
  Postanesthetic shivering
  Malignant hyperthermia

---

ity of hemoglobin for oxygen (methemoglobinemia), reduced hemoglobin concentration in the blood (anemic or hemodiluted animals), or reduced delivery of blood to the tissues (low cardiac output states, shock). In these cases, the Pao_2 may be normal, but oxygen delivery to the tissues is inadequate since there is a reduction in absolute or effective hemoglobin content or reduced physical oxygen transport. In these situations, measurement of jugular (or central) partial pressure of venous oxygen (Pvo_2) may be useful. PvO_2 indicates the degree of extraction of oxygen that has occurred from the blood by the tissues. Normal PvO_2 is approximately 50 mm Hg. As an index of adequate tissue oxygenation, PvO_2 should be no less than 30 mm Hg.[4]

Additional criteria that can be used to evaluate the need for oxygen therapy included knowledge of the pathophysiology of the animal's primary condition and the presence of clinical signs related to hypoxia (cyanosis, dyspnea, tachypnea, tachycardia, and anxiety). Animals with conditions such as diaphragmatic hernia, pneumonia, and shock are likely to benefit from oxygen administration. Cyanosis is a clinical sign that indicates the need for oxygen therapy. On the other hand, hypoxic animals do not always appear cyanotic. The appearance of cyanotic membranes is dependent on the presence of at least 5 g/dl of reduced hemoglobin in the blood.[5] Anemic animals or animals with carbon monoxide poisoning, for instance, may not be cyanotic but will benefit from oxygen therapy. Many clinical signs related to hypoxia are not specific for hypoxia when present individually, but when they occur in combination they are highly suggestive and indicate the need for more definitive tests. In the absence of blood gas analysis or if blood gas results are equivocal, then the clinical response to administration of 100% inspired oxygen should be used to assess an animal's need for oxygen therapy.

Techniques of oxygen administration

Selection of an appropriate oxygen administration system depends on the expected duration of therapy, the concentration of oxygen required, the demeanor of the patient, and equipment availability. Oxygen administration is usually initiated using 100% oxygen to determine the response to therapy, but should then be reduced to the lowest concentration that maintains arterial oxygenation within normal limits. As a general rule, the delivered oxygen concentration should not exceed 50% for more than 24 hours, or complications associated with oxygen toxicity may ensue.[3] If a high inspired oxygen concentration is required, other forms of respiratory support, such as PPV, positive end-expiratory pressure (PEEP) or continuous positive airway pressure (CPAP), should be considered.

There are four main techniques commonly used for oxygen administration in small animals. The indications for and advantages and disadvantages of each of these techniques are given in Table 36-1.

Face mask. Face masks are used for short-term administration of oxygen either in an emergency situation, during induction of anesthesia, or to evaluate the need for oxygen therapy in equivocal cases. Existing equipment, such as an anesthetic machine with a circle system or a nonrebreathing circuit may be attached to the mask to provide an oxygen source. High inspired concentrations of oxygen (up to 100%) are possible with a well-fitted mask. Poorly fitting face masks should be avoided, since leakage of air around the

Table 36–1 Methods of oxygen administration

Technique	Indications	Advantages	Disadvantages
Mask	Emergencies, initial therapy, anesthetic induction	Readily available with existing equipment; rapid application; 100% oxygen possible	Poor patient acceptance unless obtunded; requires supervision
Nasal catheter	Prolonged oxygen therapy	Good access to patient; minimal restraint required; inexpensive	Irritating to nasopharyngeal mucosa; possible gastric dilation
Intratracheal catheter	Prolonged oxygen therapy	Good access to patient; minimal restraint required; inexpensive.	Invasive; may induce tracheitis
Oxygen cage	Prolonged oxygen therapy	Provides a controlled environment.	Minimal access to patient; expensive; high oxygen usage for inspired oxygen >50%

mask will limit the delivered oxygen concentration, while excessive dead space within the mask will increase the animal's work of breathing. Unfortunately, some animals may struggle when a mask is applied to their face, thereby increasing oxygen consumption and negating the beneficial effects of the mask. In these cases, although less than ideal, the mask or oxygen outlet may be held close to the face using high oxygen-flow rates. Insertion of a nasal oxygen catheter should be considered, particularly if therapy is likely to be required for any length of time. Prolonged use of a mask is usually only possible in a comatose patient, since most animals will remove the mask when left unattended. A bland eye ointment should be applied periodically in these patients to prevent corneal desiccation, particularly if there is leakage around the mask.

Nasal catheter. The use of a nasal catheter is probably one of the more efficient, convenient, and least expensive ways to provide oxygen therapy for prolonged periods in small animals (see Chapter 25). Inspired oxygen concentrations of up to 90% are possible, while the animal is allowed to ambulate and be treated with minimal restrictions.

Purpose-designed nasal catheters are preferred but may not be available in sizes suitable for small dogs and cats. Alternatively, soft, flexible pediatric feeding tubes with fenestrations cut in the end to prevent mucosal jetting damage can be used. Before insertion, the nasal mucosa should be desensitized by instilling approximately 1 ml of 2% lidocaine or proparacaine into the nostril with the head elevated. A 10% metered lidocaine spray could also be used for this purpose. Following desensitization, the premeasured catheter is then passed up the ventral meatus of the nostril so that the tip is level with the carnassial tooth. The catheter is anchored in place at the nostril and forehead using sutures, cyanoacrylate adhesive, or a combination of the two. The proximal end of the catheter is connected to a metered oxygen source. The flow rate of oxygen required will be proportional to the size of the animal and the desired inspired oxygen concentration, but will vary with changes in the ventilatory pattern. Table 36-2 gives approximate flow rates, which have been determined experimentally.[6] The minimum flow rate to achieve the desired effect (based on clinical response and blood gases) should be used. High flow rates may be associated with complications such as jetting damage of the nasopharyngeal mucosa or gastric dilation. Humidification of the inspired gases using a commercial in-line bubble humidifier or by bubbling the oxygen through an intravenous fluid bottle filled with warm sterile water is recommended, to reduce the damage re-

Table 36-2 Approximate oxygen flow rates for nasal catheter administration*

	Oxygen flow rates (liters/minute) required to achieve an inspired O_2% of:		
Weight (kg)	30-50%	50-75%	75-100%
0-10	0.5-1	1-2	3-5
10-20	1-2	3-5	>5
20-40	3-5	>5	?

*Data derived from Fitzpatrick RK, Crowe DT, nasal oxygen administration in dogs and cats: Experimental and clinical investigations. J. Am Anim Hosp Assoc 1986;22:293–300.

sulting from mucosal drying. It is also recommended that the catheter be replaced with a new one using the opposite nare every 24 to 48 hours to avoid problems with pressure necrosis, jetting damage, and mucus accumulation.

Intratracheal catheter. Intratracheal catheters tend to be less irritating than nasal catheters but are more invasive and technically more difficult to insert. With this technique, a long, flexible intravenous catheter is inserted percutaneously into the trachea through the cricothyroid membrane or between tracheal rings close to the larynx.[7] The catheter should be a large-gauge, over-the needle type. The end of the catheter should be fenestrated with a sterile scalpel blade before use to minimize jetting damage to the tracheal mucosa. (The edges of the fenestrations should be "smoothed" prior to insertion to prevent difficulty with subsequent removal.) Aseptic technique should be followed during insertion. Desensitization of the overlying skin using local anesthetic will assist atraumatic introduction of the catheter. The tip of the catheter should come to lie in the region of the carina. Oxygen flow rates and humidification procedures similar to those used for a nasal catheter are recommended.

Oxygen cage. Oxygen cages designed for use in small animals are available commercially or may be custom built. An effective oxygen therapy cage should incorporate methods to regulate oxygen concentrations with minimal oxygen flows, eliminate expired carbon dioxide, and control ambient temperature and humidity.[1] These cages tend to be expensive to purchase. Less expensive systems that do not provide all of these features may be detrimental to the critically ill patient. Most oxygen cages can only achieve an inspired oxygen concentration of 40% to 50% at economical oxygen flow rates (<10 L per minute). Ambient temperature and humidity should be maintained at about 22°C (70°F) and 40% to 50% relative humidity, respectively. The major disadvantage of using an oxygen cage is that the patient is isolated from the clinician. In order to evaluate the patient adequately it is necessary to remove it from the cage and expose it to room air, where the oxygen concentration is only 21%. Clinical signs observed upon removal of the animal from the cage (mucous membrane color, blood gases) do not accurately reflect the condition of the animal in the cage. The use of newer noninvasive techniques, such as pulse oximetry to allow remote monitoring of arterial oxygen saturation (Sao_2), may help to overcome this deficit (see Chapter 4).

Alternative techniques. Oxygen may be administered through an endotracheal or tracheostomy tube. Endotracheal tubes are readily available and are most often used in the anesthetized or comatose patient to maintain a patent airway and facilitate PPV. The tube can be connected to an oxygen source, such as a nonrebreathing anesthetic circuit, which will deliver the desired oxygen concentration. Conscious patients are unlikely to accept an endotracheal tube unless heavily sedated. In these patients, placement of a tracheostomy tube is the preferred technique (Chapter 25). Soft, flexible tubes with high-volume, low-pressure cuffs should be used to minimize tracheal mucosal damage.

Monitoring

In order to avoid the complications associated with prolonged hyperoxia, it is desirable to maintain an inspired oxygen concentration of 50% or less and yet sustain adequate tissue oxygen delivery. It is often difficult or impractical to determine the exact concentration of delivered oxygen with most methods of oxygen therapy. Various approaches are used to monitor the efficacy of oxygen therapy and therefore determine the most appropriate concentration or flow rate of oxygen to use.

The simplest and most practical of these techniques is to monitor the animal frequently for clinical signs related to hypoxia (cyanosis, dyspnea, tachypnea, tachycardia, hypertension, or anxiety) and to determine the lowest concentration of oxygen that abolishes these signs. If the animal is showing these signs, then the inspired oxygen concentration should be increased. If the animal is already receiving 100% oxygen, other forms of therapy, such as PPV, PEEP, or CPAP, may be required.

Arterial blood gas analysis provides one of the more definitive and valuable methods with which to monitor the progress of oxygen therapy in the critically ill small animal patient. Unfortunately, in some practices, this technique may be unavail-

able, impractical, or uneconomical for repeated use. If a blood gas machine is unavailable within the practice, clinicians should investigate the possibility of analyzing samples at a nearby human or other equipped veterinary hospital. Although the frequency of sampling is dictated by the severity and rate of change in the condition of the animal, blood gas analysis should be attempted at least twice a day. More frequent sampling would be facilitated by placement of an intraarterial line, which could also be used to monitor blood pressure (Chapter 4). This would minimize the stress to the animal associated with frequent percutaneous blood collection.

Therapy should aim to maintain Sao_2 close to 100%. In most instances this can be achieved with a Pao_2 of 90 to 100 mm Hg. Pao_2 values greater than 100 mm Hg generally will not substantially increase the oxygen content of the blood but will increase the patient's susceptibility to oxygen toxicity. For instance, a patient receiving 100% oxygen may have a Pao_2 of 500 mm Hg; however, the oxygen content of the blood is only 7% greater than a patient with a Pao_2 of 100 mm Hg. Fig. 36-1 describes the normal relationship between Po_2, oxygen bound to hemoglobin, dis-

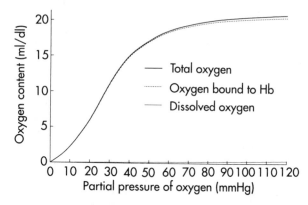

Fig. 36-1 The oxyhemoglobin dissociation curve *(dashed line)* derived from dog's blood, showing the relationship between partial pressure of oxygen (Po_2) and content of oxygen in the blood bound to hemoglobin (Hb). The effect of Po_2 on the amount of dissolved oxygen *(thin line)* and total oxygen content within the blood (dissolved plus bound: *thick line)* is also illustrated. Temperature, partial pressure of carbon dioxide, pH, and 2,3-diphosphoglycerate content are assumed to be normal. It is also assumed that there is 15 g of Hb per 100 ml of blood, that 1.39 ml of oxygen binds to every gram of Hb when 100% saturated, and that 0.003 ml of oxygen per millimeter of mercury of Po_2 is dissolved for every 100 ml of blood. (Data derived from Rossing RG, Cain SM. A nomogram relating Po_2, pH, temperature and hemoglobin saturation in the dog. J Appl Physio 1966;21:191-201.)

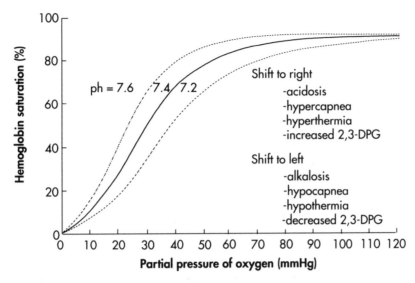

Fig. 36-2 The effect of changes in pH, partial pressure of carbon dioxide (PCO_2), temperature, and 2,3-diphosphoglycerate content on the relative position of the oxyhemoglobin dissociation curve. The position of this curve at a range of pH values (7.2, 7.4, and 7.6) with other factors maintained at normal values is also illustrated. (Data derived from Rossing RG, Cain SM. A nomogram relating PCO_2, pH, temperature and hemoglobin saturation in the dog. J Appl Physiol 1966;21:195-201.)

solved oxygen, and total oxygen content of the blood.[8] Factors such as pH, $PaCO_2$, body temperature, and 2,3-diphosphoglycerate content will alter this relationship. Attempts should be made to normalize acid-base balance and body temperature in the critically ill patient. Fig. 32-2 illustrates the effect of these factors on the normal oxyhemoglobin dissociation curve.[8] Since the vast majority of oxygen carried within the blood is bound to hemoglobin, it is also important to optimize the concentration of hemoglobin within the blood, by administration of whole blood or packed red blood cells when necessary (Chapter 34). The recent development of purified, polymerized bovine hemoglobin may also prove valuable as a means of increasing the oxygen-carrying capacity of blood in the critically ill small animal patient.

Technologic advances have provided compact portable instruments that enable continuous, noninvasive, and relatively reliable monitoring of SaO_2.[9] Pulse oximeters are now commonly used in human neonates with respiratory distress syndrome and are currently being evaluated for use in veterinary patients. These instruments measure the SaO_2 of the blood by determining the relative absorbance of hemoglobin at specified wavelengths of light. By using nonvisible wavelengths it is also possible to measure SaO_2 through pigmented skin. Unfortunately, since these instruments rely on the pulsatile flow of arterialized blood through the tissue being measured, correlation of SaO_2 as measured by a pulse oximeter with arterial blood gas values will be suboptimal in animals with reduced peripheral perfusion. In humans, the most common sites for measurement are the ear lobe and finger, whereas in veterinary patients, the tongue has been used for monitoring animals during anesthesia. The ear lobe and skin folds in the flank are potential sites available for use in awake dogs and cats. Other methods of noninvasive oxygen monitoring in animals (measurement of transcutaneous oxygen tension using polarographic techniques) have proved either inaccurate or impractical.[10,11]

Weaning from oxygen therapy

The duration of oxygen therapy will be dictated by the progress of the animal's primary disease. Trial cessation of oxygen therapy may be attempted when there is significant improvement in the patient's condition. This may be indicated, for example, by favorable changes in the radiographic appearance of the lungs in an animal with bronchopneumonia. Collection and analysis of arterial blood gases while the animal is breathing room air is beneficial for determining whether there is a continued need for oxygen therapy, and could also be used to monitor the progress of treatment of the animal's disease. The animal should be observed closely during this time for signs of respiratory distress, and oxygen therapy should be reinstituted if these signs become apparent.

Complications of oxygen therapy

Prolonged exposure of the lungs to high oxygen tensions can result in a syndrome known as pulmonary oxygen toxicity.[12] Symptoms of this disease include pulmonary edema, atelectasis, consolidation, congestion, hemorrhage, fibrosis, and associated functional impairment. Microscopic lesions seen with oxygen toxicity are indistinguishable from respiratory distress syndrome. The pathogenesis of these lesions is thought to be associated with production of highly reactive and cytotoxic peroxides and free radical products of oxygen within exposed pulmonary tissue. The occurrence of this syndrome appears to be a function of Pao_2 rather than inspired oxygen concentration. For example, astronauts may safely breathe 100% oxygen at reduced atmospheric pressure, while air containing 21% oxygen (normal room air) is lethal when administered at elevated atmospheric pressures to laboratory rats.

Microscopic changes and initial signs of pulmonary dysfunction become apparent in dogs within 24 hours of breathing 100% oxygen (at 1 atm). Further exposure to 100% oxygen results in further deterioration in lung function and has been reported to cause death from respiratory failure in 2 to 3 days. There is considerable variation between species and individuals in susceptibility. In studies with dogs, prolonged exposure to oxygen tensions less than 0.5 atm (50% oxygen at 1 atm pressure) failed to produce significant clinical or histopathologic changes.[13]

Oxygen therapy may be associated with other clinically important pathophysiologic changes, including absorption atelectasis, suppression of ventilatory drive, decreased erythropoiesis, pulmonary vasodilation, and systemic arteriolar vasoconstriction.[14] Administration of high concentrations of oxygen will result in progressive lung collapse and increased intrapulmonary shunting as the small airway "splinting" effect of the inert gases (especially nitrogen) is lost. Animals with severe, chronic respiratory disease may become apneic when administered oxygen, as pulmonary ventilation may be triggered in these animals by low arterial oxygen tensions (hypoxic ventilatory drive). These animals will require PPV in addition to oxygen therapy.

It should be remembered that hypoxia will kill an animal much more rapidly than will oxygen toxicity. Therefore, if there is doubt as to the adequacy of tissue oxygenation in an animal and

ventilatory support techniques (PPV, PEEP, CPAP) are not available, the clinician should not hesitate to administer oxygen at concentrations greater than 50%.

POSITIVE-PRESSURE VENTILATION

Apart from relatively short periods in anesthetized animals, PPV of the critically ill patient for more than a few hours is an infrequent undertaking in veterinary practice. The most likely reason for this reluctance is the time and labor commitment required for such a venture. Ventilators and respiratory care equipment, in general, tend to be expensive. With a little ingenuity, however, it may be possible to adapt existing anesthetic equipment or obtain surplus human respiratory care equipment for little capital outlay. In some cases, short periods of ventilatory support may be all that is needed to at least halt or even reverse deterioration in the patient's condition.

The three main indications for PPV include support of animals with ventilatory failure, treatment of pulmonary conditions in which oxygen therapy has failed to reverse hypoxia, and as an adjunct in the treatment of intracranial hypertension.[15] Table 36-3 lists conditions in which ventilatory support would be beneficial.

Ventilatory failure describes a condition in

Table 36-3 Examples of conditions that may benefit from positive-pressure ventilation

Ventilatory failure
Primary failure
Anesthetic overdose
Head trauma
Cervical spinal cord disease
Peripheral neuropathies
Flail chest
Open pneumothorax
Obstructive condition
Bronchospasm
Pneumonia
Restrictive condition
Diaphragmatic hernia
Gastric torsion
Pleural or pulmonary fibrosis
Failure to respond to oxygen therapy
Respiratory distress syndrome
Smoke inhalation injury
Pulmonary edema
Pneumonia
Atelectasis
Pulmonary contusion
Intracranial hypertension
Brain tumor
Head trauma
Cerebral edema

which there is inadequate gas transport into and out of the lungs.[16] The result of this is insufficient excretion of carbon dioxide from the blood and increased $Paco_2$. Oxygen uptake into arterial blood is also severely affected. Criteria that are used to determine the need for PPV include measurement of minute ventilation and arterial blood gases. Minute ventilation may be determined by attaching a volumometer (respirometer, ventilometer) to a face mask, in the conscious patient, or to an endotracheal tube, in the anesthetized patient. The volume of gas the animal breathes in (or out) in 1 minute is then measured. Normal minute ventilation for a dog or cat is 150 to 250 ml/kg.[3] Measurement of arterial blood gases may be easier to accomplish, if a blood gas analyzer is available, and also gives additional information regarding the oxygenation and acid-base status of the animal. $Paco_2$ is normally 35 to 45 mm Hg.[3] A $Paco_2$ greater than 55 mm Hg or minute ventilation less than 100 ml/kg indicates the need for ventilatory support.[3] Ventilatory support is also indicated in patients administered greater than 50% oxygen who have normal or subnormal $Paco_2$ and Pao_2 less than 60 mm Hg.

Cerebral blood flow, intracranial blood volume, and intracranial pressure respond to changes in $Paco_2$ through a direct influence of carbon dioxide on cerebral vascular tone. Elevation in $Paco_2$ causes dilation of intracranial vessels and increased blood flow to the brain, while decreased $Paco_2$ results in vasoconstriction and reduced blood flow. An acceptable technique to treat or at least to palliate acute increases in intracranial pressure is to reduce intracranial blood flow and volume by hyperventilating the patient.[17] Beneficial effects usually become evident at a $Paco_2$ of between 20 and 30 mm Hg. Excessive hyperventilation should be avoided since $Paco_2$ values less than 20 mm Hg may cause inordinate cerebral vasoconstriction resulting in cerebral ischemia.

Techniques and equipment

General principles. Techniques of artificial ventilation attempt to mimic normal gas transport within the lung. In this regard, there are general principles that apply when one is attempting to initiate and maintain effective PPV in a patient, regardless of the method or equipment used.

Minute ventilation directly determines the rate of excretion of carbon dioxide through the lungs. Minute ventilation (MV) is calculated as the product of tidal volume (TV) and respiratory rate (RR):

$$MV = TV \times RR.$$

An increase (or decrease) in either tidal volume or respiratory rate will increase (or decrease)

minute ventilation and therefore alter carbon dioxide removal. In most animals a tidal volume of 20 ml/kg with a respiratory rate of 8 to 10 breaths per minute will maintain a normal $Paco_2$.[15] Occasionally, larger breaths, on the order of 25 to 30 ml/kg every 15 minutes, may be needed to reexpand atelectatic areas of the lung, which form as a result of recumbency and breathing high concentrations of oxygen.[7] This process is termed "sighing."

The pressure reached in the airway at the end of inspiration is termed the "peak airway pressure." In most animals a peak airway pressure of approximately 15 to 20 cm H_2O is reached when a normal tidal volume is delivered. This value is commonly used during manual ventilation using an anesthetic machine or with a pressure-cycled ventilator to determine the end point of inspiration. Unfortunately, if the compliance of the lungs changes, the pressure required to deliver the same volume also changes. Stiff, edematous lungs, for instance, will require higher inflation pressures to achieve delivery of the same tidal volume than will normal lungs. Therefore, peak airway pressure should not be used as the sole guide to adequacy of ventilation.

Inspiration during PPV should only last long enough to deliver an adequate tidal volume. In most animals this takes from 1 to 2 seconds, with larger animals requiring more time. Longer inspiratory times also may be needed to achieve full expansion of the lungs in animals with airway narrowing.

Unlike spontaneous breathing in which pleural pressure is consistently subatmospheric, PPV elevates pressure within the lungs and pleural space during inspiration, thereby impeding thoracic blood flow. Specific mechanisms for this reduction in blood flow include decreased venous transmural pressure that impedes venous return, stretching and compression of pulmonary vessels that increases pulmonary vascular resistance, and restriction of cardiac diastolic filling.[7] The overall effect is a reduction in cardiac output and systemic arterial blood pressure. The degree of cardiovascular impairment is dependent on the magnitude of pressure applied (peak airway pressure), the duration of application (inspiratory time), and the time allowed for recovery (expiratory time). It is therefore desirable to use the minimum pressure and inspiratory time necessary to provide adequate ventilation. In animals with concomitant cardiovascular impairment or when high airway pressures are used, it may be necessary to support cardiovascular function by administration of intravenous fluids or inotropic agents.

Manual ventilation. It is possible to ventilate

an animal effectively for short periods using either an anesthetic circuit or self-inflating Ambu bag. With this method there is a tendency to hyperventilate the patient, particularly if delivered tidal volume or airway pressure cannot be measured, as is often the case when using an Ambu bag. This method of ventilatory support is very tedious and labor intensive when used for more than a short period.

The advantage of manual ventilation is that it is possible, with some experience, to qualitatively evaluate airway inflation resistance and lung compliance. The Ambu bag has an additional advantage of being portable, which is of value when transporting an animal or in emergency situations.

Conventional mechanical ventilation. Mechanical ventilators are designed either to work in combination with an anesthetic circuit (anesthesia ventilators) or to be attached directly to the patient (dedicated intensive care ventilators). Modern intensive care ventilators, although providing comprehensive control of ventilation, tend to be bulky, complex, and expensive. Anesthesia ventilators are more reasonably priced, tend to be more compact, and can be used for ventilating anesthetized patients. An additional benefit of this versatility and increased usage is that the operator is more likely to be familiar with the correct operation of this type of ventilator. Table 36-4 describes the characteristics of a number of available anesthesia and intensive care ventilators.

Mechanical ventilators may either generate a constant flow or constant pressure of gas to effect inspiration. The majority of ventilators in North America are of the constant-flow-generator type.[17] Termination of inspiration may be determined by reaching either a preset pressure limit (pressure-cycled) or volume limit (volume-cycled). Some volume-cycled ventilators actually determine delivered volume by applying a constant flow for a measured period and are termed "flow-time-cycled ventilators."[18] As compared with pressure-cycled ventilators, volume-cycled ventilators have the advantage of consistently delivering a preset volume regardless of changes in thoracic compliance. Problems arise if a leak develops in the ventilator or delivery apparatus, as most volume-cycled ventilators continue to deliver the same volume, regardless of whether the gas is being delivered to the patient or the atmosphere. Pressure-cycled ventilators in this circumstance will usually continue to attempt to deliver an adequate tidal volume with a prolonged inspiratory time or else fail to cycle, thereby alerting the operator of a problem. Some ventilators employ more than one cycling technique to overcome some of the problems associated with any single method. For example, a ventilator that is

volume-cycled with an upper pressure limit setting would ensure accurate volume delivery while avoiding risks of overinflation.

It should be remembered that while the use of a mechanical ventilator significantly reduces the labor commitment involved in ventilating a patient, it does increase the risks to the patient associated with equipment failure.

Assisted ventilation. Some ventilators are able to monitor airway pressure and initiate inspiration when a sudden drop in airway pressure is detected. In this fashion, the patient is able to determine its own respiratory rate and pattern; however, the delivered tidal volume will still be determined by the ventilator settings. This is termed "assisted ventilation." The advantage of using this technique is that if the animal has a condition in which the responsiveness to $Paco_2$ is maintained, then the need for monitoring blood gases to determine $Paco_2$ is diminished. Such situations may include animals with hypoventilation as a result of muscular fatigue or chest-wall defects. Assisted ventilation should not be used in patients with depressed responsiveness to $Paco_2$, such as hypoventilation resulting from central nervous system dysfunction.

PEEP and CPAP. Parenchymal lung disease, pulmonary trauma, hypoventilation, abnormal posture, or administration of high concentrations of oxygen can be associated with formation of areas of alveolar collapse, known as atelectasis. Atelectasis results in increased intrapulmonary blood flow shunting and therefore hypoxia unresponsive to oxygen administration. One technique that can be used to reinflate these collapsed areas is to apply a small amount of positive pressure to the airway. In the spontaneously breathing patient this may be done in either of two ways. With the first technique, some form of resistance device is attached to the expiratory limb of a breathing circuit so that airway pressure is maintained slightly positive during the expiratory phase (positive end-expiratory pressure [PEEP]). Airway pressure usually becomes negative during inspiration. The simplest way to apply PEEP is to place the expiratory hose of the breathing circuit in a container of water. The distance to which the end of the hose is submerged reflects the amount of PEEP applied (e.g., 5 cm under the surface = 5 cm H_2O PEEP). Simple PEEP valves that are somewhat less cumbersome are also commercially available. The second technique involves maintaining the airway pressure fairly constant, during both inspiration and expiration, at a low positive value (continuous positive airway pressure [CPAP]). To achieve this usually requires some form of pressurizing device on the inspiratory side of the breathing circuit. The Bird Mark 4A anes-

Table 36-4 Features of some available ventilators

Ventilator	Manufacturer	Type	Cycling Method	Assist Mode	PEEP/CPAP	Basic Controls	Other Features
Bird Mark 4A	Bird Corporation Palm Springs, CA	Anesthesia	Pressure	Yes	Yes	Pressure limit, inspiratory flow, expiratory time	Inspiratory trigger
Frazer/Harlake Model 701	Frazer Sweatman, Inc. and Harlake Cyprane Inc. 145 Mid County Drive Orchard Park, NY	Anesthesia	Volume	No	No	Minute volume, respiratory rate, inspiration:expiration	Sighing
Metomatic	Ohio Medical Products 3030 Airco Dr. Madison, WI	Anesthesia	Volume (pressure limit)	Yes	No	Tidal volume, inspiratory flow, expiratory time	Excess pressure limit, inspiratory trigger, inspiratory plateau, expiratory resistance
Bird Mark 7 and Mark 9	Bird Corporation Palm Springs, CA	Intensive care (anesthesia with optional bellows)	Pressure	Yes	Optional	Pressure limit, inspiratory flow, expiratory time	Inspiratory trigger, 50-100% inspired oxygen, negative end-expiratory pressure (Mark 9 only)
Bennett MA-1	Puritan-Bennett Corp. 12655 Beatrice St. Los Angeles, CA	Intensive care	Volume (pressure limit)	Yes	Yes	Tidal volume, respiratory rate, inspiratory flow	Excess pressure limit, inspiratory trigger, expiratory resistance, 21-100% inspired oxygen, sighing, spirometer, heated humidifier, nebulizer
Bear 1	Bourns Medical Systems Inc. 9335 Douglas Drive Riverside, CA	Intensive care	Volume (pressure limit)	Yes	Yes	Tidal volume, respiratory rate, inspiratory flow	Express pressure limit, inspiratory trigger, inspiratory plateau, 21-100% inspired oxygen, sighing, nebulizer

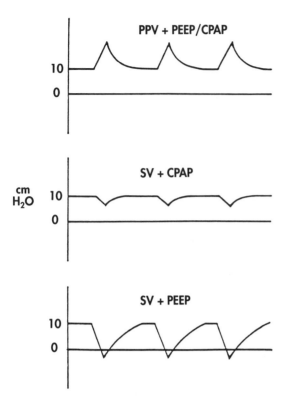

Fig. 36-3 Changes in airway pressure versus time for positive-pressure ventilation (PPV) or spontaneous ventilation (SV) with application of positive end-expiratory pressure (PEEP) or continuous positive airway pressure (CPAP). (Reprinted with permission from Pascoe PJ. Short-term ventilatory support. In Kirk RW, ed. Current veterinary therapy IX. Philadelphia: WB Saunders, 1986:269-277.)

thesia ventilator provides this feature. The advantage of CPAP over PEEP is that there is reduced work of breathing when the airway is continuously pressurized. When either PEEP or CPAP is applied during controlled ventilation the differences between these techniques become inapparent. Fig. 36-3 illustrates the changes in airway pressure associated with each of these special techniques.

Optimal values for PEEP/CPAP are generally between 5 and 10 cm H_2O. The exact setting will be determined by Pao_2 values obtained from the patient following initiation of therapy. Since PEEP/CPAP raises the mean airway pressure, the minimal setting that elevates the Pao_2 to within acceptable values should be used, to avoid undue circulatory depression.

High-frequency ventilation. High-frequency ventilation is any method of mechanical ventilation that uses higher respiratory rates and lower tidal volumes than those used during conventional PPV.[19] In its most extreme form, respiratory frequency may reach 1200 breaths per minute and tidal volume may only be a fraction of respiratory dead-space volume. Transfer of gases (oxygen and carbon dioxide) is thought to occur primarily via facilitated diffusion along concentration gradients rather than by bulk transfer along pressure gradients. The advantage of using this technique over conventional ventilation is that lower mean airway pressures can be used; therefore, there is less cardiovascular depression. This advantage is negated, though, if it becomes necessary to use significant levels of PEEP or CPAP during high frequency ventilation.[20] A multicenter study investigated the efficacy of high frequency ventilation as compared with conventional ventilation for the treatment of preterm human infants with respiratory failure.[21] The results showed that there was no advantage of using one technique over the other. In fact, high frequency ventilation was associated with a higher incidence of serious complications related to machinery failure than was conventional mechanical ventilation.

Ventilating the veterinary patient

Establishment of an airway. Following the decision to initiate PPV in an animal, the next step is to establish and secure a patent airway. In the comatose or mentally obtunded patient, this is most easily achieved using an orotracheal tube. In responsive patients, it will be necessary to use sedation and perhaps paralytic agents to allow continued endotracheal intubation. In this case, it is probably less stressful to perform a tracheostomy and ventilate through a tracheostomy tube. Both endotracheal and tracheostomy tubes should be composed of soft pliable material and have high-volume, low-pressure cuffs to minimize pressure necrosis associated with prolonged placement. Some larger tracheostomy tubes have two separate cuffs that can be alternately inflated and deflated every couple of hours to minimize focal pressure-related problems. Additional features of available tracheostomy tubes that are desirable for prolonged placement include a removable inner stylet for atraumatic insertion; a removable inner cannula for easy cleaning of the interior of the tube without necessitating tube removal; and a swivel connector to allow movement of the animal without kinking or disconnection of the tube. Endotracheal and tracheostomy tubes should be securely fastened to the animal by suture, tape, or preferably both. The ventilator delivery tubing should also be securely attached to the airway connector and to the animal to prevent accidental disconnection.

Ventilator setup. Before any animal is connected to a ventilator, the patency and operation of the ventilator need to be checked and adjustments made to provide the approximate ventilator settings for the size of the particular patient. This setup procedure helps to ensure safe, leak-free ventilator operation and also reduces the risk of dangerous lung hyperinflation on initiation of PPV.

The easiest way to perform this procedure is to attach an "artificial lung," such as a rebreathing bag, to the breathing circuit of the ventilator. The ventilator settings are then approximated based on the weight of the patient: 20 ml/kg tidal volume (volume-cycled ventilators) or 20 cm H_2O inspiratory pressure (pressure-cycled ventilators), 1 to 2 seconds inspiratory time, 4 to 5 seconds expiratory time, and 8 to 10 breaths per minute respiratory rate. If using an anesthesia ventilator attached to a circle circuit, the popoff valve should be closed and oxygen flow initiated at this point. The delivery circuit is attached to the artificial lung. The ventilator is then switched on and the settings readjusted with the ventilator in operation.

With both pressure- and volume-cycled ventilators, tidal volume should be checked using a ventilometer attached to the expiratory limb of the breathing circuit. An approximation of tidal volume may be made in some ventilators by observing the excursion of the bellows of the ventilator. It should be remembered that the delivered volume to the artificial lung or patient is often less than that indicated by excursion of the bellows because of expansion of the tubing within the breathing circuit. Volume settings on the machine should not be relied on to deliver exact volumes, but should be double-checked by measurement.

Small leaks within the system will usually become evident as a gradual collapse of the bellows of the ventilator or prolongation of inspiratory time. Large leaks will cause failure to fill the artificial lung. Common areas to check for leaks include the seals around the soda lime canister (if a circle anesthetic circuit is used) and around the cuff of the endotracheal or tracheostomy tube during PPV.

Following operational checks, the ventilator can then be attached to the patient. The ventilator settings commonly need to be readjusted following initiation of PPV, especially with pressure-cycled ventilators, because of the higher compliance of an animal's chest as compared with an artificial lung.

Controlling ventilation. Several methods may be used to abolish spontaneous ventilation and therefore establish control over the ventilatory pattern. If the patient is mentally obtunded such that there is reduced responsiveness to an elevated $Paco_2$, spontaneous efforts should cease immediately following initiation of PPV. Some patients, though, may maintain a normal response to $Paco_2$. These patients can either be hyperventilated to reduce the $Paco_2$ to subnormal levels, administered drugs to reduce carbon dioxide responsiveness, or paralyzed to ablate the ventilatory response. Sedation may also be required in these patients to improve ventilator acceptance.

Drugs that have been used to abolish spontaneous ventilation and provide sedation include small doses of pentobarbital or opioids (morphine or oxymorphone) alone or in combination with a benzodiazepine (diazepam or midazolam). Low concentrations of inhalant gases such as halothane, enflurane, isoflurane, or methoxyflurane may be used if an anesthetic machine is being used for ventilation.[17] Pancuronium or intravenous infusions of atracurium are used to paralyze patients for PPV, but must be given in combination with heavy sedation or light anesthesia in conscious animals.[17]

Monitoring. Ventilation may be monitored by arterial blood gas analysis, capnometry, or volumometry. Arterial blood gas analysis provides definitive information regarding both the adequacy of ventilation and efficiency of oxygen uptake by the lungs. In most animals, the aim should be to maintain the $Paco_2$ between 35 and 45 mm Hg and the Pao_2 between 90 and 100 mm Hg. As with patients undergoing oxygen therapy, the frequency of sampling will be dictated by the severity of disease and rate of change in the condition of the animal. Sampling twice each day should be adequate for most animals. More frequent sampling may require placement of an indwelling arterial line.

Capnometry involves measurement of carbon dioxide concentrations in the expired air of the patient, providing an indirect measurement of $Paco_2$. With this technique, small amounts of gas are continuously aspirated for measurement from the breathing circuit, usually at the level of the endotracheal or tracheostomy-tube connector. An end-tidal (or peak) carbon dioxide concentration of 5% represents a $Paco_2$ of approximately 40 mm Hg. Capnography provides a graphic representation of changes in carbon dioxide concentration over time, including both inspiratory and expiratory phases. Problems such as airway occlusion, circuit leakage, disconnection and soda lime exhaustion can be relatively easily detected and diagnosed using capnography.[22]

Volumometry provides one of the easiest and least expensive methods to monitor ventilation. Respiratory volumes may be measured in a number of ways. The crudest method is to estimate tidal volume from the excursion of the ventilator bellows. This method tends to overestimate tidal volume because of expansion of the tubing within the breathing circuit, and it will not account for circuit leakage. Some ventilators, such as the Bennett MA series of intensive care ventilators, have a set of bellows attached to the expiratory limb of the breathing circuit that inflate on exhalation, giving a rough, but more reliable guide to delivered tidal volume. The most accurate method is to attach a volumometer between the tracheostomy (or endotracheal) tube and the breathing circuit and measure either tidal volume or minute ventilation directly. Although volumometry provides information regarding the quantity of gas the animal is receiving, it does not determine whether this degree of ventilation is adequate for the metabolic state of the animal. Problems may arise in cases in which carbon dioxide production is elevated (pyrexic patients) or depressed (hypothermic patients). Volumometry also does not provide a means of evaluating the adequacy of blood oxygenation.

In addition to the respiratory system, cardiovascular and renal function should be closely monitored in the ventilated patient. Circulatory impairment manifested as poor peripheral pulses and reduction in systemic arterial blood pressure may become evident during PPV. Animals with reduced cardiovascular reserve are particularly susceptible to ventilation-induced cardiovascular impairment. Methods used to treat cardiovascular depression include minimizing peak airway pressure and inspiratory time, administration of intravenous fluids, use of plasma volume expanding agents (dextran-70), and administration of inotropic agents (dopamine or dobutamine). Renal function is depressed by PPV, as evidenced by a reduction in glomerular filtration rate, sodium excretion, and urine output associated with an increase in vasopressin levels in patients ventilated for prolonged periods.[23] The rate of fluid administration and urine output should be carefully balanced in these patients to avoid overhydration.

Airway and general patient treatment. Patients ventilated for extended periods will require intensive nursing care. Airway hygiene is probably the most important aspect of this care. Endotracheal and tracheostomy tubes bypass the normal filtration and humidifying effects of the nasal passages. They also deny normal removal of material from the airway by blocking effective coughing and swallowing reflexes. Inspiration of dry gases increases the viscosity of airway secretions and adversely affects mucociliary transport. Thick mucoid secretions containing cellular and foreign debris accumulate within the airway and eventually obstruct airflow to portions of the lung. These effects can be minimized by humidifying the inspired gases using a humidifier or nebulizer in the breathing circuit.[1] The viscosity of airway secretions can also be decreased by ensuring patient hydration. Accumulation of excess secretions and other material, as evidenced by coarse crackles on auscultation of the upper airway, should be treated by aseptic tracheal suctioning. Postural drainage and chest percussion prior to suctioning will help in removal of this material from the lower airways.[7] The inner cannula of the tracheostomy tube should be removed and cleaned every 1 to 6 hours to prevent obstruction of the tube by accumulation of inspissated airway secretions.

Management practices should include frequent repositioning of the patient to prevent lung atelectasis and formation of decubital ulcers, as well as daily inspection and cleaning of the tracheostomy wound. Nutritional support should be provided in the form of a balanced, high-caloric-density, liquid diet through a nasogastric, pharyngostomy, intragastric, or jejunostomy feeding tube (Chapter 37). Parenteral nutrition should be considered in patients with gastrointestinal dysfunction (Chapter 37). Intravenous fluid requirements should be monitored closely by assessing daily changes in the animal's packed cell volume, total solids, and body weight.

Personnel should be readily available to the ventilated patient in the event an emergency develops. Emergency equipment in the form of an Ambu bag, spare tracheostomy or endotracheal tube, suctioning apparatus, and emergency drugs (epinephrine, atropine, and lidocaine) should be located in close proximity to the patient in the event of ventilator failure, airway obstruction, or other emergency. Measurement of physiologic parameters should be recorded on flow sheets in order to monitor the progress of the animal and assist in the early detection of potentially life-threatening changes in the animal's condition.

The warm, humid environment within the ventilator and breathing circuits tends to promote the growth of bacterial contaminants. For this reason, breathing circuits should be replace with sterilized ones every 48 hours. All respiratory equipment should be sterilized with either steam, ethylene oxide, or, less ideally, cold sterilization techniques, before being used on another patient.

Weaning from ventilatory support. Because of the attendant risks of PPV, weaning from ventilatory support should be contemplated as soon as there is evidence of significant improvement in the animal's condition. Weaning should be considered when spontaneous respiratory efforts are observed in patients that were ventilated because of reduced carbon dioxide sensitivity (anesthetic overdose or head trauma), and in animals being ventilated for impaired pulmonary oxygenation (smoke inhalation or respiratory distress syndrome) when a Pao_2 greater than 60 mm Hg is achieved with inspired oxygen concentrations close to that of room air. In patients with surgical lesions (flail chest), weaning may be possible immediately following correction of the primary condition. Weaning should be attempted in ventilated patients with prior intracranial hypertension when there is significant improvement in the animal's neurologic function. Respiratory depressant effects of sedative and neuromuscular relaxant drugs should be allowed to wear off or be pharmacologically antagonized before weaning is attempted.

Weaning from ventilatory support involves a gradual reduction in minute ventilation to allow an increase in $Paco_2$ that provides the stimulus for spontaneous ventilation by the animal. This process is achieved most easily by reducing respiratory rate to approximately two to four breaths per minute while maintaining the same tidal volume. This procedure is continued for about 15 minutes while monitoring the animal for signs of spontaneous breathing. Abrupt cessation of PPV ventilation is potentially dangerous because the Pao_2 may fall to dangerous levels before there is adequate stimulus for the animal to breath. If breathing is weak or irregular, or if apnea continues after 15 minutes then PPV should be reinstituted. If the patient's breathing is deep and regular, PPV may be terminated. The animal's ventilation should be monitored closely to detect signs of respiratory muscle fatigue, such as rapid, shallow breathing. Respiratory muscle fatigue may develop following cessation of PPV in patients that have been ventilated for prolonged periods. Minute ventilation should be monitored periodically using a volumometer to ensure adequacy of airflow. Arterial blood gases should be measured after about 30 minutes and again several hours following discontinuation of ventilatory support to ascertain the effectiveness of the animal's spontaneous ventilation.

HUMIDIFICATION

Humidification of the inspired gases is indicated in tracheostomized or intubated patients that are being ventilated or in patients receiving oxygen therapy.[1] Inspired air is normally heated and humidified by the nasopharynx and tracheobronchial tree so that alveolar air is 100% humidified at body temperature and contains approximately four to six times the water vapor content of room air.[24] Administration of dry medical gases and inspiration of gases that bypass the upper airways (endotracheal intubation or tracheostomy) will increase the humidifying requirements of the mucosal surfaces of the trachea and lower airways. If these surfaces are unable to provide adequate quantities of water vapor, then mucosal drying will occur. Detrimental effects of mucosal drying include an increase in the viscosity of mucosal secretions; impairment of mucociliary transport function; retention of thickened, tenacious secretions; inflammation and degeneration of respiratory epithelium; small airway closure, atelectasis, and increased pulmonary blood flow shunting; decreased functional residual capacity; reduced pulmonary compliance; and increased risk of infection.[25,26] These effects will be compounded by the presence of respiratory disease.

Since vaporization of liquids results in cooling of the surface of the liquid, increased vaporization of fluid from the respiratory mucosal surfaces will result in increased heat loss from the patient. Humidification of the inspired air has the additional advantage of reducing whole-body heat loss, which can be of particular benefit in the smaller patient.

Principles of humidification

It is important to understand that the maximum quantity of water vapor that any gas can contain is dependent on temperature. Warmer gases can contain more water vapor than colder gases. The term "relative humidity" is commonly used to describe the percentage of water vapor that a gas contains, relative to its maximum capacity at that temperature:

Relative humidity (%)
$$= \frac{\text{Actual water vapor content of gas}}{\substack{\text{Maximum water vapor content} \\ \text{possible at this temperature}}} \times 100.$$

When gases are 100% humidified and then cooled down, a proportion of the water vapor condenses into liquid water, thereby reducing the water vapor content and yet maintaining humidity at 100%. This phenomenon occurs when heated humidifiers are located in a regular breathing circuit at a distance from the patient. When the heated and humidified gases travel through the cooler delivery tubes en route to the patient, the gases cool down and moisture condenses on the interior of the tubes resulting in "rainout." Less than optimal water vapor content of inspired gases results. The solution is to locate the humidifier closer to the patient, which is often impractical, or to use heated delivery tubing.

Equipment

Four types of humidifiers are commonly used. These include simple bubble humidifiers, heated bubble humidifiers, humidity exchange filters, and nebulizers.

Simple bubble humidifiers function by bubbling the inspired gases through a container of water. Since the water is not heated, the water vapor content is only marginally above that of room air. These devices are usually employed to humidify oxygen prior to administration through a nasal or intratracheal catheter. An economical bubble humidifier can be made using a sterile intravenous fluid bottle filled with sterile water. With the bottle upright, the oxygen inlet is attached to the vent port while the patient oxygen line is attached to the infusion-line port. Commercial bubble humidifiers that attach directly to the oxygen tank regulator or to the oxygen wall outlet are also available.

Heated bubble humidifiers are able to produce inspired gases at low flows that are 100% humidified at body temperature. They are usually incorporated into the delivery tubing of the breathing circuit of a mechanical ventilator or anesthesia machine. Efficient humidifiers of this type include heated delivery tubing and monitor the temperature of the proximal airway. For effective humidification without risking thermal injury to the respiratory mucosa, proximal airway temperature is normally maintained between 32 and 37°C.

Humidity exchange filters are disposable devices that attach directly to an endotracheal or tracheotomy tube (Humid-Vent and Trach-Vent: Portex Inc., Wilmington, MA). They trap moisture on exhalation and release it during inhalation, functioning much like the nasopharynx. The manufacturer claims that use of these devices provides a means of achieving a relative humidity of 70% to 80% at the tracheal level, which is close to that associated with spontaneous breathing through the nose. One disadvantage of this system is that airway resistance is elevated by the filter, which may become clinically important with usage, as the filter becomes clogged with dust and respiratory secretions. These filters are also potential sites for bacterial colonization. For these reasons, filters should be replaced every 24 hours.

Nebulizers may be used to administer a fine mist of water particles into the inspiratory side of the breathing circuit. An inspired humidity close to 100% may be achieved without the need for heating inspired gases. Overzealous use of nebulization may result in patient overhydration, airway flooding, and maceration of the respiratory mucosa.

AEROSOL THERAPY

An aerosol is a fine suspension of liquid droplets contained within a carrier gas, usually air or oxygen. These droplets may be composed of water, saline, or pharmaceutical solutions. Aerosols are used to deliver these substances directly to respiratory mucosal surfaces to prevent desiccation of these surfaces (water), to loosen tenacious secretions and stimulate coughing (saline), or to treat respiratory disease directly (drugs).

Aerosol deposition

The site of aerosol deposition within the respiratory tract is dependent on the physical characteristics of the aerosol and the ventilatory pattern of the animal.[27] Therapeutic aerosols are designed to be deposited in the lower airways. In general, larger dense particles (>20 μm diameter) tend to impact in the nasopharynx and upper airways. Slightly smaller particles (5 to 20 μm diameter) deposit in the larger lower airways, including bronchi and bronchioles, while small particles (0.5 to 5 μm diameter) settle in the peripheral airways. Inspired particles less than 0.5 μm in diameter are usually exhaled. It should be noted that aerosolized particles tend to decrease in size through evaporation en route to the patient's airways.

The rate and depth of breathing influences the site of aerosol deposition.[27] Rapid, shallow breathing results in impaction of particles in the upper airways, while slow, deep breathing promotes a more peripheral distribution of the aerosol. Open-mouth breathing also reduces the loss of aerosol to the nasopharyngeal regions. Patients with respiratory disease often have narrowed airways and breathe rapidly and shallowly. Aerosol deposition is enhanced by instructions to human patients to breathe deeply and slowly during therapy. Since it is not possible to achieve a voluntary change in respiratory pattern in veterinary patients, less than ideal aerosol distribution is obtained.

Equipment

Aerosols are generated by devices known as nebulizers. Three types of nebulizers are commonly used for aerosol therapy. These include the jet, Babbington, and ultrasonic nebulizers.

The jet nebulizer uses a narrow, high-velocity stream of gas directed over the end of a capillary tube. The other end of this tube is immersed into a reservoir containing the liquid to be aerosolized. The fluid is drawn up the tube by the Bernoulli effect and then shattered by the gas stream into fine particles. The resultant mist is commonly baffled to produce smaller particles of more uniform size. Nebulizers of this type are capable of producing aerosol densities of 10 to 20 µL/L of carrier gas with particle diameters averaging 3 to 6 µm.[27] Different types of jet nebulizers are available for specific purposes. Jet nebulizers with large reservoirs (over 250 ml) allow nebulization, usually of bland liquids, for prolonged periods. Jet nebulizers with small reservoirs are designed to administer accurate quantities of medications.

Babbington nebulizers consist of a hollow glass sphere, about 1 cm in diameter, which contains a small slit in the side that emits a jet of pressurized gas. The fluid to be nebulized is dripped over the sphere, forming a thin film, which is shattered by the high-velocity gas jetting out of a side slit. Larger particles are usually baffled by a sphere or other object placed in the path of the gas flow. This type of nebulizer produces particles similar in size to a jet nebulizer, but in greater quantities for a given carrier gas flow. Aerosol densities average 30 µL/L of carrier gas.[27]

Ultrasonic nebulizers use an entirely different system of liquid comminution. These nebulizers contain a piezoelectric crystal in close proximity to a fluid reservoir. This crystal transforms electrical energy into high-frequency oscillations that eject aerosol particles from the surface of the liquid. Aerosolized particles are carried away by a stream of gas directed over the surface of the liquid. These nebulizers are capable of producing very-high-density aerosols (50 to 150 µL/L of carrier gas) of fairly uniform particle size with an average diameter of 5 µm.[27]

Aerosol administration

Aerosols may be administered through a mask, into an enclosure (oxygen cage, mist tent, or other enclosed space), or directly into the breathing circuit of a ventilator or anesthetic machine. Continuous administration of high-density mists to patients is not recommended because overhydration of the airway will result. In general, therapy with water or saline aerosols for 15 to 30 minutes every 4 to 8 hours is sufficient to humidify the respiratory tract and loosen viscid secretions. Patient hydration must be maintained in order for nebulization of bland fluids to be effective in treating animals with respiratory disease. Chest physiotherapy (postural drainage, chest percussion, and induction of coughing) should be used in conjunction with nebulization to optimize the beneficial effects.[7] If coughing is not possible, such as in the unconscious, intubated, or tracheostomized patient, then sterile suctioning of the airway to remove loosened material should be performed following nebulization therapy. Bronchodilators, such as salbutamol or terbutaline, may be administered orally, intramuscularly, intravenously, or as an aerosol before nebulization therapy. These agents aid in the dispersion of the aerosol within the lungs, removal of airway secretions, and minimization of aerosol-induced bronchospasm.

Aerosol pharmacology

The direct administration of drugs to the respiratory tract by aerosol appears to offer advantages over extrapulmonary routes of medication administration during treatment of animals with pulmonary disease. There are, however, disadvantages associated with aerosol therapy. Compared with oral or other routes of systemic administration, it is more difficult to regulate the exact amount of drug that an animal receives with aerosolization. Some drugs when aerosolized are locally irritant and can stimulate severe bronchospasm. Because of these potential side effects, there is no advantage in administering drugs by aerosol when these drugs are equally effective following administration by other routes. The use of aerosolized medicants should be limited to agents that are only effective topically (mucolytics) or agents that produce severe side effects when administered by other routes (nephrotoxic antibiotics). Aerosolization of other drugs may be attempted if administration of these drugs by other routes has failed to provide an effective therapeutic response in the animal.

The following sections discuss some of the more commonly used agents that are administered as aerosols.

Drugs

Mucolytics and proteolytics. Aerosolized mucolytic and proteolytic agents function to depolymerize mucoid secretions and cellular proteins, thereby decreasing viscosity and promoting mobilization of accumulated airway secretions.[28]

Acetylcysteine is a mucolytic agent that has been used widely for this purpose. This agent works by reducing disulfide bonds in mucoproteins and mucopolysaccharides. Nebulization of 3 to 10 ml of a 10% solution every 6 to 8 hours has been recommended.[7] Immediately prior to tracheal suctioning 0.25 to 2 ml of a 10% solution may also be administered directly into the trachea.[7] Concentrations of acetylcysteine greater than 10% should not be used, as higher concentrations cause irritation of airway tissues. Acetylcysteine has an unpleasant sulfurlike odor and inactivates several antibiotics, including penicillin and its derivatives, when administered in combination.

Proteolytic agents such as deoxyribonuclease, trypsin, chymotrypsin, and streptokinase may be of benefit in degrading purulent secretions that contain increased amounts of DNA and protein.[28] Unfortunately, there are increased risks of bronchial irritation and spasm associated with aerosol administration of these agents, and immune sensitization may occur following repeated use.

Bronchodilators. Nonselective sympathomimetic agents, such as epinephrine, isoproterenol, and ephedrine, have been used for many years as bronchodilators. Selective β_2 agonists, including salbutamol (albuterol), terbutaline, isoetharine, metaproterenol, rimiterol, and fenoterol, are now preferred for this purpose, as these agents minimize the undesirable cardiovascular and neurologic side effects associated with administration of the nonselective agents.[7,28] Additionally, many β_2 agonists provide longer duration of action than nonselective sympathomimetics, are associated with minimal development of tolerance, and are effective by extrapulmonary as well as inhalational routes of administration.

The side effects associated with administration of β_2 agonists relates to residual β_1 effects of the drugs (tachycardia and hypertension with high doses) or are a function of β_2 effects elsewhere in the body (skeletal muscle tremors, hypotension, and uterine relaxation).

Antibiotics. Treatment with aerosolized antibiotics may be indicated if extrapulmonary administration has failed (poor penetration of the drug from the blood to the site of pulmonary infection) or if the effective drug, as demonstrated by culture and sensitivity, is highly toxic when administered by other routes. Drugs that may meet these criteria include amphotericin B, nystatin, bacitracin, polymixin B, and the aminoglycosides.[29]

Aerosol antibiotic therapy may be of particular benefit in birds with air sac infections since the poor blood supply of the avian air sacs limits the efficacy of treatment by other routes.[30]

Prolonged or inappropriate antibiotic therapy should be avoided because there is a risk of opportunistic fungal infections and resistant bacterial overgrowth. In one study, involving human burn patients with inhalation injury, it was found that aerosolized gentamicin had no effect on mortality rate, time of death, prevalence of sepsis, or pulmonary complications.[31] In fact, continued use of gentamicin by aerosol resulted in increased detection of resistant bacterial strains in both sputum and burn wounds.

Miscellaneous drugs. Many therapeutic agents have been administered via aerosol; however, there is little or no clinical data in the veterinary literature to recommend their use.

Antifoaming agents such as 25% to 50% ethanol have been used to treat fulminant pulmonary edema, but their use is controversial.[28] Corticosteriods with minimal absorption from the respiratory tract, such as beclomethasone dipropionate, are used in human patients to treat refractory allergic pulmonary disease. These drugs are administered by the inhalational route to minimize induction of systemic side effects, such as adrenal suppression.[32] Therapeutic effects of these corticosteriods may take up to 3 weeks to develop, and prolonged use may be associated with development of mycotic pneumonia.

Dosage. The exact dosage will vary depending on the agents used, individual patient response,

Table 36-5 Approximate dosages of drugs that can be administered by aerosol*

Drug	Action	Dosage	Interval
Water/saline	Airway hydration Mobilize secretions	15-30 minutes of nebulizations	4-8 hours
N-acetylcysteine	Mucolytic	Nebulize 3-10 ml of 10% solution or give 0.25-2 ml intratracheal	6-8 hours; hourly
Salbutamol	β_2 bronchodilator	AER: 20-40-μg/kg	6-8 hours
		IV: 2-5μg/kg	4-6 hours
		IM: 3-10 μg/kg	4-6 hours
		Oral: 60-70 μg/kg	8 hours
Terbutaline	β_2 bronchodilator	AER: 30-70μg/kg	6-8 hours
		IV: 3-5 μg/kg	4-6 hours
		IM: 5-10 μg/kg	4-6 hours
		Oral: 70 μg/kg	8 hours
Amphotericin B	Antimycotic	AER: 0.1-0.3 mg/kg	6 hours

AER = aerosol; IV = intravenous; IM = intramuscular.
*Data derived from Haskins SC. Management of pulmonary disease in the critical patient. In: Zaslow IM, ed. Veterinary trauma and critical care. Philadelphia: Lea & Febiger, 1984:339-384.

route of delivery, and efficiency of the nebulization apparatus. Table 36-5 lists dosages, based on human data, that have been suggested for a number of drugs.[3] In general, drugs to be aerosolized should be diluted to 5 ml with saline and administered every 6 to 8 hours. The lowest dosage should be used initially, and the dosage increased until the desired effect is obtained or until signs of toxicity appear.

Complications. Aerosol therapy may adversely affect pulmonary function, particularly with prolonged use of high-output nebulizers. Detrimental effects include a decrease in functional residual capacity and pulmonary compliance and an increase in intrapulmonary shunting and resistive work of breathing.[33,34] Bronchospasm may be a problem, especially when irritating medicants or cold aerosols are used. Heated nebulizers should be used judiciously because of the risk of causing thermal injury to respiratory mucosa.

Respiratory care equipment can support the propagation of bacteria. For this reason, daily and between-patient cleaning and sterilization of this equipment is recommended to prevent cross contamination and spread of nosocomial infections. Nebulizers should not be shared between patients. Humidifiers and nebulizers should be filled only with sterile solutions, which should be replaced daily. The internal parts of the nebulizer should be cleaned and disinfected following use by nebulizing a cold sterilizing solution, such as glutaraldehyde, for about 30 minutes. Residual sterilizing solution should be flushed out of the nebulizer with sterile water before the next use. Between patient uses, all detachable equipment should be either steam or ethylene oxide sterilized. Other equipment should be disassembled, cleaned with detergent and water, and thoroughly dried. Formal guidelines are available for the control of contamination in inhalation therapy devices.[35]

REFERENCES

1. Court MH, Dodman NH, Seeler DC. Inhalation therapy: oxygen administration, humidification, and aerosol therapy. Vet Clin North Am 1985;15:1041-1059.
2. Haskins SC. Sampling and storage of blood for pH and blood gas analysis. J Am Vet Med Assoc 1977;170:429-433.
3. Haskins SC. Management of pulmonary disease in the critical patient. In Zaslow IM, ed. Veterinary trauma and critical care. Philadelphia: Lea & Febiger, 1984:339-384.
4. Haskins SC. Blood gases and acid-base balance: clinical interpretation and therapeutic implications. In Kirk RW, ed. Current veterinary therapy VIII. Philadelphia: WB Saunders, 1983:201-215.
5. Nunn JF. Applied respiratory physiology, ed. 2. London: Butterworths, 1977:437-439.
6. Fitzpatrick RK, Crowe DT. Nasal oxygen administration in dogs and cats: experimental and clinical investigations, J Am Anim Hosp Assoc 1986;22:293-300.
7. Haskins SC. Physical therapeutics for respiratory disease. Semin Vet Med Surg Small Anim 1986;1:276-288.
8. Rossing RG, Cain SM. A nomogram relating PO_2, pH, temperature and hemoglobin saturation in the dog. J Appl Physiol 1966;21:195-201.
9. Kagle DM, Alexander CM, Berko RS, Giuffre M, Gross JB. Evaluation of the Ohmeda 3700 pulse oximeter: steady-state and transient response characteristics. Anesthesiology 1987;66:376-380.
10. Warren RG, Webb AI, Kosch PC, Coons L. Evaluation of transcutaneous oxygen monitoring in anaesthetised pony foals. Equine Vet J 1984;16:358-361.
11. Webb AI, Daniel RT, Miller HS. Kosch PC. Preliminary studies on the measurement of conjunctival oxygen tension in the foal. Am J Vet Res 1985;46:2566-2569.
12. Frank L, Massaro D. The lung and oxygen toxicity. Arch Intern Med 1979;139:347-350.
13. Frank L, Bucher JR, Roberts RJ. Oxygen toxicity in neonatal and adult animals of various species. J Appl Physiol 1978;45:699-704.
14. Fisher AB. Oxygen therapy: side effects and toxicity. Am Rev Respir Dis 1980;122:61-69.
15. Pascoe PJ. Oxygen and ventilatory support for the critical patient. Semin Vet Med Surg Small Anim 1988;3:202-209.
16. Amis TC, Haskins SC. Respiratory failure. Semin Vet Med Surg Small Anim 1986;1:261-275.
17. Pascoe PJ. Short-term ventilatory support. In Kirk RW, ed. Current veterinary therapy IX. Philadelphia: WB Saunders, 1986:269-277.
18. Muir WW, Hubbell JAE. Ventilation and mechanical assist devices. In Muir WW, Hubbell JAE, eds. Handbook of veterinary anesthesia. St Louis: CV Mosby 1989:153-164.
19. Bjorling DB. High frequency ventilation: a review. Vet Surg 1986;15:399-406.
20. Bednarski RM, Muir WW. Hemodynamic effects of high-frequency oscillatory ventilation in halothane-anesthetized dogs. Am J Vet Res 1989;50:1106-1109.
21. The HIFI Study Group. High-frequency oscillatory ventilation compared with conventional mechanical ventilation in the treatment of respiratory failure in preterm infants. N Engl J Med 1989;320:88-93.
22. Swedlow DB. Capnometry and capnography: an anesthesia disaster warning system. Semin Anesth 1986;5:194-205.
23. Marquez JM, Douglas ME, Downs JB. Renal function and cardiovascular responses during positive airway pressure. Anesthesiology 1979;50:393-398.
24. Dery R. Humidity in anesthesiology. IV. Determination of alveolar humidity and temperature in the dog. Can Anaesth Soc J 1971;18:145-151.
25. Marfatia S, Donahue PK, Hendren WH. Effect of dry and humidified gases on the respiratory ephithelium of rabbits. J Pediatr Surg 1975;10:582-592.
26. Noguchi H, Takumi Y, Aochi O. A study of humidification in tracheotomized dogs. Br J Anaesth 1973;45:844-848.
27. Swift DL. Aerosols and humidity therapy: generation and respiratory deposition of therapeutic aerosols. Am Rev Respir Dis 1980;122:71-77.
28. Lourenco RV, Cotromanes E. Clinical aerosols. II. Therapeutic aerosols. Arch Intern Med 1982;142:2299-2308.
29. Wanner A, Rao A. Clinical indications for and effects of bland, mucolytic and antimicrobial aerosols. Am Rev Respir Dis 1980;122:79-87.
30. Miller TA. Nebulization for avian respiratory disease. Mod Vet Pract 1984;65:309-311.
31. Levine BA, Petroff PA, Slade CL. Prospective trials of dexamethasone and aerosolized gentamicin in the treat-

ment of inhalation injury in the burned patient. J Trauma 1978;18:188-193.

32. Kass I, Nair SV, Patil KD. Beclomethasone diproprionate aerosol in the treatment of steroid-dependent asthamatic patients. Chest 1977;71:703-707.

33. Malik SK, Jenkins DE. Alteration in airway dynamics following inhalation of ultrasonic mist. Chest 1972;62:660-664.

34. Modell JH, Moya F, Ruiz BC. Blood, gas and electrolyte determinations during exposure to ultrasonic nebulized aerosols. Br J Anaesth 1968;40:20-26.

35. Nett LM. General recommendations for control of contamination of inhalation therapy devices. In Petty TL, ed. Intensive and rehabilitative respiratory care. Philadelphia: Lea & Febiger, 1974:372-378.

37 The Metabolic Response to Injury: Enteral and Parenteral Nutritional Support

Aunna C. Lippert

The care of the critically ill small animal patient will be enhanced if the clinician has a good understanding of the organism's metabolic response to injury and the systemic consequences of this response. Critically ill animals are frequently unable or unwilling to eat in the face of diseases that produce significant increases in their protein and energy requirements. Early nutritional support of critically ill patients is standard practice in human medicine, but it has only recently drawn attention in veterinary medicine as a means of decreasing the morbidity and mortality associated with many diseases. After a brief review of the metabolism of simple fasting and stressed starvation, this chapter will discuss techniques of providing nutrients to patients in the intensive care unit.

NORMAL METABOLIC RESPONSE TO STARVATION

This topic has been well reviewed in both the human[1] and veterinary[2] literature. Energy in the form of glucose must be supplied to obligate glucose-consuming tissues such as the central and peripheral nervous systems, red and white blood cells, fibroblasts participating in wound healing, and renal medullary cells. During the initial postabsorptive period, decreased insulin and elevated glucagon levels stimulate hepatic glycogenolysis in order to maintain normoglycemia. After 12 to 24 hours, glycogen stores are depleted and gluconeogenesis, occurring primarily in the liver and to some extent in the kidney, becomes the main source of endogenous glucose production. Muscle and visceral proteolysis supplies alanine and other glucogenic amino acids to the liver. These amino acids undergo deamination to provide three carbon skeletons for gluconeogenesis. Lactate, pyru-

vate, and adipose tissue-derived glycerol are additional substrates for this process. Concurrently, hormone-sensitive lipase-induced lipolysis supplies free fatty acids for the energy needs of other tissues. Adipose tissue is the only significant and disposable source of stored energy in mammals.

After 24 to 48 hours of fasting, maximum hepatic production of ketone bodies from fatty acids provides tissues with an alternate energy source. With adaptation, even the brain can use ketones to some extent in place of glucose. Amino acid mobilization decreases as the fast is prolonged. Urinary excretion of nitrogen derived from proteolysis falls to 25% to 33% of that seen in the immediate postabsorptive state (Fig. 37-1). This is an adaptive response essential to conservation of body protein and prolonging survival during simple starvation. The 30% to 40% decline in the basal metabolic rate (Fig. 37-2), accompanied by decreased oxygen consumption and triiodothyronine levels, is an additional adaptation of the body to prolonged starvation.[3] These mechanisms prolong the calculated time to lose 50% of body cell mass from 69 days to 232 days.[4]

METABOLISM DURING STRESSED STARVATION DUE TO TRAUMA, SURGERY, OR SEPSIS

The metabolic state of an animal undergoing starvation accompanied by stress is quite different from that of simple starvation. Although some quantitative differences exist between physical insults such as hypovolemia, trauma, surgery, cancer, sepsis, and the ultimate stress, a major thermal burn, the cascade of events precipitated by injury is qualitatively similar. The magnitude of the metabolic aberration is directly proportional to the severity of the insult; that is, it proportional to

593

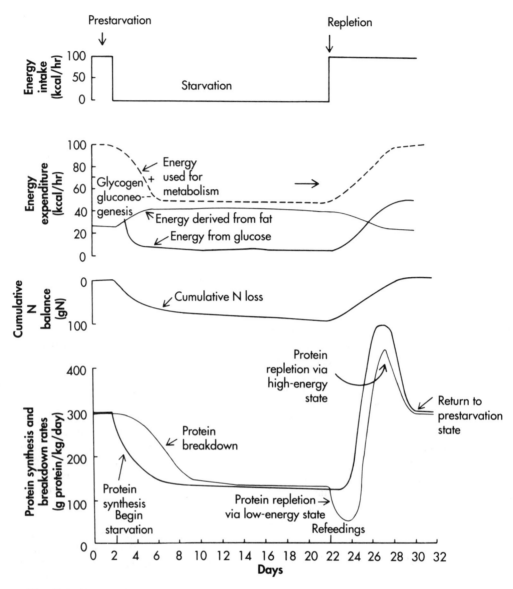

Fig. 37-1 Changes in energy and protein metabolism during starvation and the response to refeeding. (From Stein TP. Protein metabolism and parenteral nutrition. In Rombeau JL, Caldwell MD, eds. Clinical nutrition, vol. 2. Parenteral nutrition. Philadelphia: WB Saunders, 1986:117).

the amount of tissue damaged. This complex protective phenomenon was first described over 60 years ago,[5] and has been the subject of research and clinical investigation since. Originally, the response to injury was described as having two phases—"ebb" and "flow," but actually, three and sometimes four distinct periods are observed.[6] Initially, manifestations of hypovolemic shock, depressed metabolic rate, hypothermia, and associated hemodynamic instability are seen, corresponding to the classic "ebb" phase. Without

intervention, this may progress to a state of refractory shock characterized by lactic acidosis, oliguria, and death. Cardiopulmonary support is critical during the "ebb" phase. If hemodynamic resuscitation is successful, an acute period of elevated metabolic rate, cardiac output, and body temperature accompanied by catabolism follows (the classical "flow" phase), which peaks at about 3 days postinjury. Metabolic and nutritional support are indicated during the "flow" phase. Under favorable conditions, a restorative period of anab-

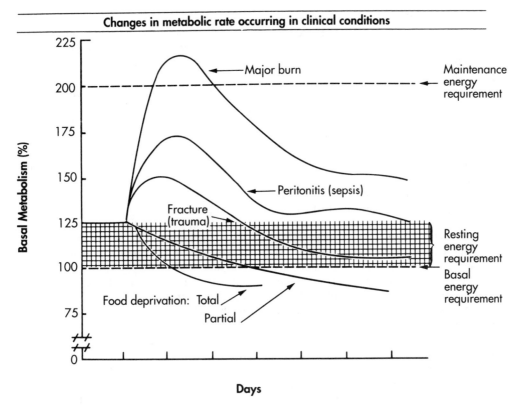

Fig. 37-2 Changes in metabolic rate occurring in clinical conditions. (From Lewis LD, Morris ML, Hand MS. Small animal clinical nutrition, ed. 3. Topeka: Mark Morris, 1987:5-11.)

olism ensues, during which hypermetabolism subsides. If sepsis develops or persists or multiple-organ failure intervenes, chronic hypermetabolism and catabolism often lead to the death of the organism. Well-characterized neuroendocrine and biochemical alterations accompany each phase of the stress response.[6-8] Descriptions of this response are based primarily on studies performed on humans in clinical situations or experimental animals under research conditions; few observations have been made of clinically affected small animals.

With tissue injury, nociceptive impulses reach the brainstem, hypothalamus, and pituitary. Another major initiating stimulus is a decrease in effective circulating volume, which activates baroreceptors and atrial stretch receptors. The central nervous system sends afferent signals via the sympathetic nervous system to the adrenal medulla, which secretes the catecholamines epinephrine and norepinephrine. The latter is also secreted by sympathetic nerve endings in adipose tissue, liver, and other tissues. Catecholamines trigger hemodynamic changes such as selective vasoconstriction, increased cardiac contractility,

tachycardia, and splenic contraction, designed to maintain blood pressure and preserve cerebral and myocardial perfusion acutely. Metabolic effects of catecholamines include accelerated glycogenolysis, gluconeogenesis, lipolysis, and the stimulation of glucagon release, which magnifies these effects and enhances proteolysis.

Hypothalamic and pituitary stimulation result in adrenocorticotropic hormone (ACTH) secretion, which leads to adrenocortical release of corticosteroids. Cortisol has a permissive effect on peripheral proteolysis, hepatic amino acid uptake, gluconeogenesis, and protein synthesis. Muscle proteolysis with visceral manufacture of acute-phase proteins important for coagulation, immune function, and healing appears to have adaptive value in the response to injury. Infusion of hydrocortisone, glucagon, and epinephrine into normal humans reproduces the state of hypermetabolism, glucose intolerance, negative nitrogen balance, and other changes typical of the physiologic response to trauma.[9]

Circulating blood volume is supported by extracellular fluid redistribution from the interstitial and intracellular compartments to the vascular space. Stimulation of the renin-angiotensin-aldosterone system and antidiuretic hormone release promote sodium and water retention and enhance vasoconstriction.

More recently, attention has been directed away from the "classic" hormonal mediators of the stress response and toward newly discovered biochemical mediators such as lymphokines, monokines, prostaglandins, and leukotrienes.[10-12] Interleukin-1, a lymphokine, stimulates ACTH and subsequent glucocorticoid release and causes the pancreatic secretion of insulin and glucagon. It appears to work synergistically with a potent monokine, cachectin, or tumor necrosis factor (TNF), to increase muscle proteolysis, induce fever and hepatic acute-phase protein synthesis, and suppress lipoprotein lipase activity resulting in elevated plasma triglycerides. Prostaglandins and leukotrienes play important roles in the inflammatory and immune responses. A complete discussion of this complex and changing topic is beyond the scope of this publication; the reader is referred to other sources.[11-15]

The metabolic alterations discussed above have important implications regarding energy expenditure, changes in body composition, and substrate utilization in stress states. Injury induces an increase in energy expenditure proportional to the severity of the insult (see Fig. 37-2). Protein catabolism results in loss of muscle mass and increased urinary nitrogen losses, which, if persistent, would result in the loss of 50% of the body cell mass in just 34 days.[4] Hyperglycemia induced by catecholamines, glucagon, and corticosteroids is accompanied by normal or even elevated insulin concentrations. The increase in glucose production ensures an adequate energy supply for wound healing and host defense. However, insulin-dependent tissues, especially muscle and adipose tissue, become partially resistant to insulin's effects, resulting in a decreased peripheral clearance of glucose.[16,17] These tissues retain some ability to clear and oxidize glucose. The liver becomes resistant to the normal suppression of gluconeogenesis by hyperglycemia and insulin release.[16,17]

Significant alterations in fat metabolism occur during the response to injury.[17,18] Catecholamine- and glucagon-induced lipolysis, during stress, causes an increase in plasma free fatty acids. This is accompanied by an elevated rate of fatty acid oxidation by most tissues, as free fatty acid uptake by cells does not require an enzymatic mechanism. In the liver, free fatty acids are incorporated into triglycerides and exported in the form of very-low-density lipoproteins (VLDLs). The VLDLs provide energy to tissues possessing lipoprotein lipase. During stress, lipoprotein lipase activity is increased in cardiac and skeletal muscle, but decreased in adipose tissue. Fat oxidation appears to be the major energy source in the hypermetabolic phase, accounting for 70% to 90% of the energy expenditure. Hyperglycemia fails to inhibit lipolysis and fat oxidation, as would occur normally. Ketone bodies appear to be less important sources of energy during stress than during simple starvation. In shock and severe sepsis, lipid oxidation for energy appears to be limited by adipose tissue perfusion as well as cytokine production, which suppresses the activity of lipoprotein lipase. Intriguing possibilities exist for enhancing lipid utilization through the use of medium-chain fatty acids, which are transported passively into mitochondria without requiring the carnitine transferase system.[18,19] Modifying the inflammatory and metabolic response to injury by the administration of fish oils is another potential method of altering fat metabolism during stress.[20]

The effects of injury on protein metabolism must be considered; protein breakdown and synthesis are both stimulated.[21] Muscle catabolism occurs in stress in order to provide glucogenic precursors and other amino acids to the liver for glucose and acute-phase protein production. Protein synthesis and the activities of white blood cells in the wound require an additional availability of amino acids. Increased urinary nitrogen excretion is primarily a result of increased gluconeogenesis; the extent of negative nitrogen balance is proportional to the severity of the injury. Amino acid profiles performed on septic and traumatized human patients reveal a decrease in the level of the branched-chain amino acids leucine, isoleucine, and valine.[10,22] These amino acids appear to be an important energy source for muscle during stress, and they provide the nitrogen and the carbon skeletons for alanine synthesis in muscle.[23] Alanine is exported to the liver and becomes a primary substrate for gluconeogenesis. Administration of branched-chain enriched amino acid solutions to stressed patients may reduce weight loss and muscle protein catabolism and improve nitrogen retention.[10,22,23]

IMPACT OF MALNUTRITION ON ORGAN SYSTEMS, AND CLINICAL CONSEQUENCES

Malnutrition has a major impact on all organ systems through loss of cell mass and function.[2,4,7,8,24] In skeletal muscle, early loss of strength occurs prior to any measureable loss of mass, implying some degree of myopathic change secondary to even brief periods (less than 1 week) of nutritional deprivation.[25] With the development of obvious muscle wasting, recovery of health may be delayed due to inactivity and fatigue. Fortunately, refeeding improves function before skeletal muscle mass is regained.

The diaphragm and muscles of the thoracic wall are not spared, and parameters of pulmonary function deteriorate, including the response to hypoxia and hypercapnia. Abnormalities of pulmonary function may be apparent after as little as 7 days of semistarvation.[26-28] With progressive nutritional depletion, the ability to cough effectively and protect the airway may be compromised; the respiratory pattern becomes rapid and shallow with a marked reduction in the number of "sighs." These changes, in combination with the immune function abnormalities discussed below, make pneumonia a major complication and cause of death in malnourished patients.

Renal concentrating ability is decreased by chronic malnutrition,[29] as well as the capacity to excrete an acid load.[30] Metabolic acidosis and a diuresis inappropriate to the state of hydration may result.

Hepatic synthesis of albumin and other plasma proteins is often depressed in states of chronic malnutrition.[2,4,24] Acute starvation of 36 hours' duration depletes microsomal enzyme activity and may result in deranged drug metabolism.[31]

With chronic malnutrition, cardiac muscle mass is reduced, leading to reduced contractility and responsiveness to inotropic agents.[32] Electrocardiographic changes may occur, and congestive heart failure may be precipitated by overzealous refeeding.[32]

Mucosal thinning, villous atrophy, alterations in bacterial flora, and loss of brush-border enzyme activity occur in the gastrointestinal tract with malnutrition. The subsequent malabsorption and gastric and colonic ileus may hinder initial attempts to refeed. Gut atrophy also compromises its barrier function against bacterial invasion and endotoxin absorption.[2,4,24]

Protein-calorie malnutrition is the most common cause of secondary immunodeficiency, and the effects of malnutrition and stress on immune function are synergistic.[33,34] Immunologic abnormalities include a peripheral lymphopenia, involution of lymphoid organs, and suppression of cell-mediated immunity as evidenced by loss of delayed cutaneous hypersensitivity and response to mitogens. Humoral immunity and serum immunoglobulin levels appear to be less affected. The macrophage is very vulnerable to the effects of protein deficiency.[33] Important plasma factors such as fibronectin and complement, which play roles in chemotaxis, opsonization, and phagocytosis, decrease rapidly with starvation.[33,35] Anes-

thesia, aging, and chemotherapeutic drug administration represent additional immunosuppressive influences that may confront critically ill patients.[36]

The clinical consequences of malnutrition in the critically ill patient appear obvious, and have been well documented in human medicine. As early as 1936, preoperative weight loss was recognized as an adverse effect in people undergoing surgery for peptic ulcer disease.[37] The association between deteriorating nutritional status and an increase in perioperative morbidity, especially sepsis and poor wound healing, and mortality has been demonstrated repeatedly.[4,24,38] In patients with cancer, the presence of weight loss may have more prognostic importance than tumor type or histology.[39] It has been more difficult to demonstrate statistically in many diseases that nutritional support either improves outcome or is cost effective.[38,40,41] In spite of this fact, some degree of specialized nutritional support is part of the routine standard of care in most human intensive care units.

PATIENT SELECTION FOR NUTRITIONAL SUPPORT

Nutritional support is rarely a primary or definitive type of therapy in veterinary patients, with the possible exception of cats with idiopathic hepatic lipidosis. Nutritional support plays an important role as a secondary or supportive therapy, which sustains the patient, allowing time for primary therapy to work or healing to take place. Nutritional support therapy is seldom contraindicated, as long as the method of administration is chosen with the individual patient's needs in mind. The challenge in critical care nutrition is establishing criteria for the selection of recipients that anticipates the demands of those at nutritional risk and prevents the development of malnutrition. There will always be animals presented for therapy in advanced states of debilitation; our energies should be directed toward protecting the patients under our care from a similar fate. Criteria for selection should ensure the maximum provision of benefits while balancing the risks and expense of the various methods available for providing nutritional support.

Candidates for nutritional support are selected using subjective (experience and intuition) and objective nutritional assessment data. The art and science of nutritional assessment are well described in human medicine. Criteria examined include physical, anthropometric, biochemical, immunologic, and nutrition history analyses, as well as the measurement of energy expenditure using indirect calorimetry.[42-44] Controversy exists over which assessments are valid in the critically ill patient, which are cost effective, and which, if any, best predict outcome.[45,46] A technique (subjective global assessment) based on easily collected historical information (degree and pattern of weight loss, changes in oral intake, presence of gastrointestinal signs, depression of functional capacity) and changes present on physical examination (loss of subcutaneous fat, muscle wasting, presence of edema or ascites) predicts nutrition-associated complications better than more complex and costly methods of nutritional assessment.[47]

Objective methods of assessment such as body composition measurement and biochemical and immunologic testing have not been adequately investigated in clinically ill small animal patients. Serum albumin, a commonly used index of nutritional status in human medicine, did not correlate with nutritional status assessed by history and physical examination in a group of critically ill dogs and cats receiving total parenteral nutrition.[48] Hydration status, blood or plasma losses, and specific disease processes involving the liver, kidney, and gastrointestinal tract will influence the serum albumin, unrelated to the effects of malnutrition.

A technique similar to subjective global assessment would be a useful way to interpret the history and physical examination findings. General recommendations regarding the selection of patients for specific nutritional support may be made.[2,49-51] If oral intake has been or will be interrupted for 3 to 5 days, depending on initial nutritional status, nutritional support should be considered. There may be a documented acute weight loss of 5% or more, excluding losses due to dehydration, or a more chronic weight loss of 10% or more. Asking the owner what the animal normally weighs, or referring to weights previously recorded in the medical record may be helpful. Physical examination may reveal a lack of subcutaneous fat or generalized muscle wasting. The animal may be suffering from a disease process known to cause increased protein losses, induce hypermetabolism, suppress the appetite, or interfere with nutrient ingestion, transit, or absorption. Any of these historical or clinical findings should raise the clinician's index of suspicion that the patient is at nutritional risk.

CALCULATION OF NUTRITIONAL REQUIREMENTS

In veterinary patients, nutritional requirements must be estimated, since the measurement of energy expenditure using indirect calorimetry, commonly employed in human medicine, is generally unavailable. Estimates of protein and caloric re-

ENTERAL NUTRITION WORKSHEET FOR DOGS AND CATS

1. Basal energy requirement (BER):
   = 70 × weight in $kg^{0.75}$ (for all patients) or
   = (30 × weight in kg) + 70 (for patients weighing >2kg)
   = _____ kcal/day
2. Illness energy requirement (IER):
   Healthy animal, cage rest = 1.25 × BER
   Trauma or major surgery = 1.3 to 1.6 × BER
   Sepsis or major burns = 1.5 to 2.0 × BER
   Cats up to 1.4 × BER
   IER = _____ × BER = _____ kcal/day
3. Volume of liquid diet required:
   Diet selected _____
   Energy density of diet = _____ kcal/ml
   Volume to be administered/day = _____ ml
4. Protein requirement:
   = 2 to 4 g/kg in adult dogs
   = 6 g/kg in dogs with extraordinary protein loss
   = 1.5 g/kg in dogs with renal or hepatic failure
   = 4 to 6 g/kg in adult cats
   = 3.5 g/kg in cats with renal or hepatic failure
   Protein requirement = _____ g/day
5. Protein provided by diet selected:
   = _____ ml of diet × _____ g of protein per milliliter
   = _____ g of protein/day
6. Supplemental protein required:
   = _____ g/day protein requirement − _____ g/day protein provided by diet = _____ g/day supplemental protein
   One scoop of ProMod provides 5 g of supplemental protein.
   Add _____ scoops of ProMod to each day's diet.
7. Transition to gastrostomy or nasogastric feeding:
   If patient has had prolonged anorexia, begin with one third of total requirement and increase by thirds until total volume administered on Day 3. If patient has been taking some food orally, begin with half of total requirement and increase to full amount on Day 2.
8. Bolus feeding schedule for gastrostomy and nasogastric tubes:
   Total of _____ ml to be administered in _____ feedings/day results in _____ ml/feeding
   On Day 1 feed _____ ml of diet _____ times/day
   On Day 2 feed _____ ml of diet _____ times/day
   On Day 3 feed _____ ml of diet _____ times/day
9. Continuous feeding schedule for enterostomy tubes:
   total of _____ ml to be administered in 24 hour results in goal administration rate of _____ ml/hr
   On Day 1 administer half at this rate and use diet prepared at half strength.
   On Day 2 administer at goal rate and use diet prepared at half strength.
   On Day 3 administer at goal rate and use diet prepared at full strength.

PARENTERAL NUTRITION WORKSHEET FOR DOGS

1. Basal energy requirement (BER):
   = $70 \times$ weight in $kg^{0.75}$ (for all patients) or
   = $(30 \times$ weight in kg$) + 70$ (for patients weighing >2 kg)
   = _____ kcal/day
2. Illness energy requirement (IER):
   Healthy animal, cage rest = $1.25 \times$ BER
   Trauma or major surgery = 1.3 to $1.6 \times$ BER
   Sepsis or major burns = 1.5 to $2.0 \times$ BER
   IER = _____ $\times$ BER = _____ kcal/day
   (provide as nonprotein calories)
3. Protein requirement:
   = 2 to 4 g/kg in adult dogs
   = 6 g/kg in dogs with extraordinary protein loss
   = 1.5 g/kg in dogs with renal or hepatic failure
   Protein requirement = _____ g/day
4. Volumes of nutrient solutions required:
   a. 8.5% amino acid solution = 85 mg protein per milliliter
      To supply _____ g of protein, need _____ ml
   b. 20% lipid solution = 2 kcal/ml
      To supply 40% to 60% of IER (_____ kcal), need _____ ml
   c. 50% dextrose solution = 1.7 kcal/ml
      To supply 40% to 60% of IER (_____ kcal), need _____ ml (use half this volume on first day and increase to full volume on second if no glucosuria)
5. Total volume of total parenteral nutrition solution
   = _____ ml
   Extra fluids added: _____ ml of _____
   Administer at _____ ml/hr
6. Electrolyte requirement:
   Dependent on patient status and parenteral products selected.
7. Vitamin requirement:
   Administer 0.5 mg/kg vitamin K_1 subcutaneously on first day and weekly.
   Add 2.5 ml/10 kg per day multivitamin (up to 10 ml) to total parenteral nutrition solution.

From Lippert AC, Armstrong PJ. Parenteral nutritional support. In Kirk RW, ed. Current veterinary therapy X. Philadelphia: WB Saunders, 1989:26.

PARENTERAL NUTRITION WORKSHEET FOR CATS

1. Basal energy requirement (BER):
   = $70 \times$ weight in $kg^{0.75}$ (for all patients) or
   = $(30 \times$ weight in kg$) + 70$ (for patients weighing >2 kg)
   = _____ kcal/day
2. Illness energy requirement (IER):
   = $1.4 \times$ BER = _____ kcal/day (provide as protein and nonprotein calories)
3. Protein requirement:
   = 4 to 6 g/kg in adult cats
   = 3.5 g/kg in cats with renal or hepatic failure
   Protein requirement = _____ g/day
   Protein calories = 4 kcal/g = _____ kcal
   Nonprotein calories = IER − protein calories
   = _____ kcal
4. Volumes of nutrient solutions required:
   a. 8.5% amino acid solution = 85 mg protein per milliliter
      To supply _____ g of protein, need _____ ml
   b. 20% lipid solution = 2 kcal/ml
      To supply 50% of nonprotein calories (_____ kcal), need _____ ml
   c. 50% dextrose solution = 1.7 kcal/ml
      To supply 50% of nonprotein calories (_____ kcal), need _____ ml (use half this volume on first day and increase to full volume on second if no glucosuria)
5. Total volume of total parenteral nutrition solution
   = _____ ml
   Extra fluids added: _____ ml of _____
   Administer at _____ ml/hr
6. Electrolyte requirement:
   Dependent on patient status and parenteral products selected.
7. Vitamin requirement:
   Administer 0.5 mg/kg vitamin K_1 subcutaneously on first day and weekly.
   Add 1.5 ml/5 kg per day multivitamin to total parenteral nutrition solution.

From Lippert AC, Armstrong PJ. Parenteral nutritional support. In Kirk RW, ed. Current veterinary therapy X. Philadelphia: WB Saunders, 1989:26.

quirements are made more useful if animals receiving nutritional support are carefully monitored. Overfeeding critically ill patients may be detrimental,[2] especially if parenteral nutrition is being administered, so it is best to begin conser-vatively and increase the amount fed gradually as dictated by individual tolerance. Nutrition worksheets (see boxes above and on previous page) are a convenient method of including nutritional support information in the medical record, as well as being a useful teaching tool.

The calculation of nutritional requirements begins with the estimation of the basal energy requirement (BER). This is the amount of energy needed by an animal resting quietly, in a thermoneutral environment, and in a postabsorptive state.[52] BER is estimated using body weight in kilograms according to one of two equations:

$70 \times$ (body weight in kg)$^{0.75}$

(for any size dog or cat)[53]

or

$(30 \times$ body weight in kg$) + 70$

(for dogs and cats weighing greater than 2 kg)[52]

The fractional exponent in the first equation is easily calculated by cubing the body weight, then taking the square root of the result twice.

Maintenance energy requirement (MER) estimates the energy needs of a moderately active, healthy, adult animal, also in a thermoneutral environment. For dogs, MER is 2.0 times BER; for cats, MER is 1.4 times BER, since they are generally less active.[52]

Critically ill animals require less than MER in most instances, due to a lack of physical activity, but require more than BER due to the increased energy demands of their hypermetabolic state (see Fig. 37-2). The term illness/injury/infection energy requirement (IER) expresses the energy requirements of sick animals, using data extrapolated from indirect calorimetry studies in sick humans.[2,49,50] For dogs, IER is 1.25 to 2.0 times BER, depending on the extent of hypermetabolism imposed by the disease state. Using 1.4 times BER to estimate the energy requirements of sick cats appears adequate under most circumstances.

The protein requirements of critically ill humans are frequently individually determined based on nitrogen balance studies. Nitrogen balance is not easily measured in diseased small animals, so protein needs are based on those of healthy dogs and cats (Table 37-1).[52] These figures may underestimate the protein requirements of animals suffering extensive protein losses in urine, diarrhea, or inflammatory exudates. Studies in critically ill humans, especially those suffering from sepsis, indicate that protein requirements are considerably higher under these circumstances.[10,21-24] Renal or hepatic failure will reduce the amount of protein that can be tolerated by affected patients. Whenever possible, feeding a dog or cat food appropriate for the individual (Prescription Diet Canine p/d or k/d or Feline p/d or k/d, Hill's Pet Products, Topeka, KS) ensures a balanced diet; for custom-designed enteral diets, or parenteral nutrition, suggested allowances of protein are made in the nutrition worksheets (see boxes on pp. 598 and 599). Modifications in the amount of protein provided are often made on the basis of clinical response and changes in biochemical parameters.

Table 37-1 Minimal protein requirements

Animal	Ideal Protein		In Nondietary Pet Foods*	
	% in Diet	% of Gross Energy	% in Diet	% of Metabolizable Energy
Kitten	16	22	35	30
Adult cat	8	9	25-30	25
Puppy	11	12	29	29
Adult dog	4	4	18	18

From Lewis LD, Morris ML, Hand MS. Small animal clinical nutrition, ed. 3. Topeka: Mark Morris, 1987, pp. 1-16.
*Based on a diet providing 4 kcal of metabolizable energy/gram. For diets with different caloric contents, multiply the percent protein in the diet by the quotient of (the caloric density of the diet divided by 4).

ENTERAL NUTRITIONAL SUPPORT

The gastrointestinal tract should be used for nutritional support if it is functional, which it is in the majority of clinical situations in which nutritional support is indicated, and if it can be safely used. Enteral techniques are simple, economical, and more physiologic as compared with parenteral methods. Providing at least a proportion of the nutrient requirements via the gut has beneficial effects on intestinal structure and function and may decrease the tendency for bacterial invasion and endotoxin absorption.[2,49-51,54-57] Enterally administered nutrients are essential for adaptive hyperplasia to occur subsequent to small-bowel resection.[58] There is evidence to suggest that the intestine plays a more active role in the metabolic response to injury than was formerly believed—another justification for using enteral nutrition to help maintain gastrointestinal integrity.[59]

ENTERAL NUTRITION—METHODS OF ADMINISTRATION

Enteral nutritional support consists of methods designed to induce voluntary consumption of food, methods for force feeding, and methods of feeding by tube.[2,49-51,57] The technique is chosen after considering the following: (1) the animal's clinical and nutritional status; (2) the degree of anorexia; (3) the anticipated duration of nutritional support; (4) the animal's ability to protect its airway against aspiration; (5) the animal's ability to tolerate anesthesia; (6) the animal's ability to tolerate the method of feeding; (7) the facilities available; (8) the need for abdominal surgery due to the primary disease process; (9) cost considerations; and (10) the experience of the clinician. Simple techniques to encourage spontaneous feeding may be successful in animals who are only partially anorexic.[2,60] Methods of increasing the palatability of food include offering a variety of foods (especially of varying textures), warming the food, and ensuring that the animal can smell by cleaning the nostrils and using decongestant nose drops if necessary. Feeding small amounts frequently, hand feeding accompanied by petting, feeding in a quiet environment, and having the owner feed the animal while it is hospitalized are other ways to increase food intake.

Appetite stimulation

Appetite stimulation using pharmacologic means is another simple, short-term approach to the animal unwilling, but able, to eat.[2,50,60] Many drugs are reported to stimulate appetite, but only a few work consistently enough to be useful. The benzodiazepine tranquilizers are proven to induce food consumption in dogs and especially in cats.[60,61] Their effect is generally more potent but of shorter duration after intravenous administration, as compared with oral or intramuscular routes. Diazepam (Valium, Roche Laboratories, Nutley, NJ) is most commonly used, at a dose of 0.1 to 0.2 mg/kg intravenously, intramuscularly, or orally, once or twice daily, with a maximum single dose of 5 mg. Oxazepam (Serax, Wyeth Laboratories, Philadelphia) is another benzodiazepine proven effective at stimulating the appetite, but is available only in oral form. The dose used in cats is 0.2 to 0.4 mg/kg once daily. These drugs may also be used to ease the transition from long-term methods of nutritional support such as gastrostomy tubes. Disadvantages of these agents include their failure to work in some cases; sedative side effects, especially in debilitated patients; and the potential for abuse (by clients).

Glucocorticoids, anabolic steroids, and progestational compounds have side effects that tend to outweigh their inconsistent effectiveness as short-term appetite stimulants in critically ill animals.

Potassium and B vitamin supplementation is justified. Deficiencies may develop with even short periods of anorexia. These deficiencies may perpetuate anorexia due to skeletal and smooth-muscle weakness, poor intestinal motility (potassium), and depression or other neurologic abnormalities (thiamine).[2,60]

Force feeding

Forced oral feeding of canned dog or cat food, liquid pet food gruels or supplements, or vitamin-calorie pastes is frequently attempted,[2,57] but it often results in more nutrients being applied topically, to the patient and person feeding, than are actually ingested. Critically ill animals are easily stressed by force feeding,[50] and some cats appear to develop a psychologic aversion to food after repeated attempts to force feed. This method is only feasible for very short-term nutritional support (1 or 2 days) and can be very time consuming. The amount of nutrients actually administered is often overestimated; for example, over 2 ft of a popular paste supplement (Nutri-cal, EVSCO Pharmaceuticals Immunogenetics, Buena, NJ) would be required to meet the caloric requirements of a 4-kg cat.[49]

Repeated orogastric intubation is equally stressful, with the added dangers of pharyngeal or laryngeal trauma, vomiting associated with feeding, tracheal intubation, and aspiration pneumonia.

Feeding tubes

For animals requiring nutritional support for more than 2 days, an indwelling feeding tube avoids the struggle associated with force feeding or repeated orogastric intubation. Indwelling tubes are usually well tolerated by critically ill patients, and are a much more efficient way of providing nutrients.

Nasogastric tubes. The nasogastric tube ranks highest with respect to ease of placement and simplicity[2,49,50,57,62]; it is also the least invasive and least expensive type of indwelling tube. A nasogastric tube may be used for the nutritional support of hospitalized dogs and cats for up to 1 week. Absolute contraindications to nasogastric tube placement include vomiting, functional or mechanical gastrointestinal obstruction, and depressed consciousness. Dyspnea due to upper airway obstruction, pneumonia, or other cardiac or pulmonary disease; facial trauma; and esophageal disease are relative contraindications to their use. Tubes made of polyurethane (Travasorb Feeding Tube, Travenol Laboratories, Deerfield, IL), or (Peditube, Biosearch Medical Products, Somerville, NJ) are less irritating than those made of polyvinylchloride (Infant Feeding Tube, Argyle Division of Sherwood Medical, St Louis) or red rubber (Sovereign Feeding Tube, Monoject Division of Sherwood Medical, St Louis). In cats and dogs, less than 10 kg, a 5 or 6 French tube is appropriate. In larger dogs, an 8 French tube, preferably with a stylet, is indicated.

Placement of the nasogastric tube[2,49,50,57,62] does not require general anesthesia; local anesthesia of the nasal mucosa with 0.5 to 1.0 ml of 2% lidocaine or mepivicaine (Carbocaine-V, Sterling Animal Health Products, New York) is usually sufficient for dogs. If a dog will not tolerate placement with local anesthesia alone, chemical restraint with diazepam may be considered, but this patient may not be sick enough to tolerate the tube and the method of nutritional support should be reconsidered. Nasogastric tube placement is facilitated in most cats if a small dose of ketamine (1 to 2 mg/kg) is given intravenously in addition to intranasal instillation of a local anesthetic. The end of the tube may be located in the distal esophagus or stomach; to estimate the length of tube to be inserted, measure from the nose to the 9th or 13th rib, respectively. After lubrication with water-soluble jelly, the tube is inserted into the external nares; it is directed dorsomedially initially in dogs, in order to pass a ventral tissue prominence, and then ventrally into the ventral meatus. In cats, no prominence is present so a ventromedially directed tube will result in ventral meatal placement. If resistance is felt, withdraw the tube partially and try again. Atraumatic nasogastric tube placement may not be possible in some normal dogs,[49] but it is usually successful in cats. The animal's head should be allowed to remain in a normal position to prevent intratracheal passage. This complication is still possible in debilitated or depressed patients. Verification of tube position is best made with radiography. Other techniques include aspiration of the tube yielding gastric contents (tip in stomach) or negative pressure (tip in caudal esophagus) rather than air. A small amount of sterile saline may be administered; if the animal coughs, the tube is likely malpositioned. Injection of air through the tube may result in an auscultatable gurgle heard over the left cranial abdomen. In thin animals, the tube may be palpable in the cervical esophagus. Using an adhesive (Superglue, Loctite Corp, Cleveland) to secure the tube as it emerges from the nostril, and to the side of the face or top of the head, prevents the discomfort associated with sutures (Fig. 37-3).

One of the disadvantages of nasogastric tubes is that an Elizabethan collar is required to prevent tube removal in all but the most depressed animals; cats especially resent these collars, and may also not eat voluntarily with the tube in place, so it is difficult to tell when removal is indicated. It is usually necessary to administer enteral nutrition products designed for humans, since cat or dog food gruels will occlude the small-diameter lumen of nasogastric tubes. Other complications include vomiting or regurgitation of the meal or tube, rhinitis, dacryocystitis, reflux esophagitis with intragastric tube placement, and aspiration pneumonia.[2,49,50,57,62]

Pharyngostomy tubes. Pharyngostomy tubes are still widely recommended and used for enteral nutritional support,[2,63-65] and placement modifi-

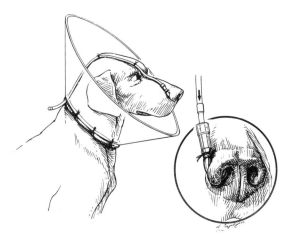

Fig. 37-3 The nasogastric tube is secured as close as possible to its exit from the nostril with suture or adhesive. An Elizabethan collar is necessary to prevent removal by the patient. (From Crowe DT. Enteral nutrition, J Vet Crit Care 1982;5:8-31.)

cations have been suggested to reduce the risk of complications.[65-67] In many institutions, pharyngostomy tubes have been replaced by percutaneous endoscopic gastrostomy tubes, considered a superior method of long-term enteral nutritional support.[49,50] The increasing availability of endoscopic equipment will likely make pharyngostomy tubes obsolete, and referral to veterinarians with this capability should be considered. Complications, occasionally fatal, associated with pharyngostomy tubes and leading to their decline in popularity include upper airway obstruction, stoma infection, aspiration pneumonia, reflux esophagitis, vomiting of the tube, and patient reluctance to eat voluntarily with the tube in place.[49,50,66,67]

Gastrostomy tubes. The innovative adaptation of a percutaneous method of gastrostomy tube placement to dogs and cats[68] solves many of the problems associated with nasogastric and pharyngostomy tube feeding. This is considered by many the technique of choice for long-term (longer than 1 week) enteral nutritional support and/or when bypass of the oral cavity, pharynx, and esophagus is necessary. It is also the best-tolerated type of feeding tube to use in anorexic animals.[49,50,69,70] Percutaneous endoscopic gastrostomy (PEG) tube placement requires a brief period of general anesthesia, but it is a safe, simple, and easily learned technique that can be performed in less than 10 minutes with practice. The larger diameter of the tube allows the feeding of dog or cat food put through a blender, and superior patient tolerance allows prolonged use at home if necessary. As anorexia resolves, there is no interference with normal feeding, and the amount of food provided through the tube can be tapered. The tube can be left in place for up to 1 year, certainly long enough in most cases to ensure adequate voluntary consumption of food. The major limitation of the technique is the availability of endoscopic equipment. Gastrostomy tubes are contraindicated in animals with persistent vomiting or functional/mechanical gastrointestinal obstruction. Caution should be exercised in patients with depressed consciousness or megaesophagus, since regurgitation and aspiration may occur.[70] Severe ascites or extensive adhesions within the abdominal cavity that alter the normal anatomy may make safe PEG tube placement difficult or impossible.

The technique of PEG tube placement has been well described (Figs. 37-4 to 37-12).[2,68,69] Use of a 14 or 16 French mushroom tip urologic catheter (Pezzer Model Drain, Bard Urological Division of CR Bard, Murray Hill, NJ) and a 16- or 18-gauge plastic intravenous catheter with a metal stylet (Argyle Medicut Intravenous Cannula, Sherwood Medical Industries, St Louis, or Sovereign Indwelling Catheter, Monoject Division Sherwood Medical, St Louis) is much less expensive than using a kit marketed for humans (E-Z PEG, Mill-

Rose Laboratories, Mentor, OH). Difficulties encountered in obtaining the correct intravenous catheter may be overcome by using an 18-gauge needle for placement of the suture in the stomach, and a plastic pipette tip (200 µL MLA Disposable Pipette Tip, Medical Laboratory Automation, Pleasantville, NY) to pull the tube out through the body wall.[69] Preparation of the feeding tube includes cutting off the small closed end of the mushroom tip to reduce resistance to flow. The flared open end is also removed, and two 2-cm lengths of the narrow part of the tube are cut off, punctured with a number 11 scalpel blade, and used for the inner and outer flanges. The tube end is beveled, and threaded through the inner flange so the mushroom tip rests against the inner flange.

The procedure may be performed using injectable anesthesia, but inhalation anesthesia is indicated for critically ill dogs and cats. I recommend perioperative antibiotics. The placement of a PEG tube is illustrated in Figs. 37-4 to 37-11. A light bandage is applied to cover the stoma and incorporate the free end of the tube, which is cut perpendicularly and plugged with an injection cap. The bandage is changed 48 hours after tube place-

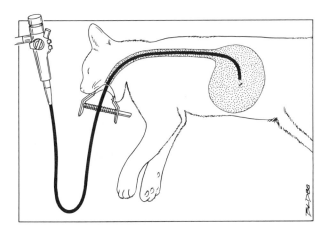

Fig. 37-4 The anesthetized patient is placed in right lateral recumbency and a generous area surrounding the ventral tip of the last rib is shaved and prepared for surgery. The area is draped, and the operator, wearing sterile gloves, makes a 2-mm stab incision through the skin just caudal to the 12th rib and level with the tip of the 13th (incomplete) rib. In medium and large dogs, it is recommended that the incision be made prior to gastric distention in order to avoid anatomic distortion that would change the location of tube emergence. The endoscopist passes the scope into the stomach and insufflates until the stomach is taut and palpable through the body wall. The finger of the operator should be visible through the endoscope indenting the stomach. (From Armstrong PJ, Hardie EM. Percutaneous endoscopic gastrostomy. Vet Med Rep. In press.)

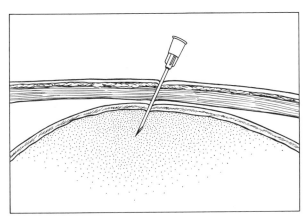

Fig. 37-5 An 18-gauge 1.5-in. needle is "popped" into the distended gastric lumen. (From Armstrong PJ, Hand MS, Frederick GS. Enteral nutrition by tube. Vet Clin North Am Small Anim Pract. In press.)

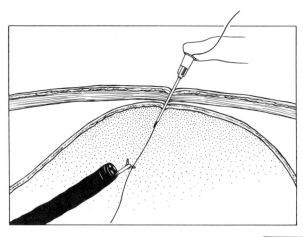

Fig. 37-6 A length of 0 nonabsorbable suture (100 to 150 cm long, depending on the size of the animal) is threaded through the needle into the gastric lumen. The suture is grasped with endoscopic biopsy forceps and withdrawn, with the endoscope, through the mouth. (From Armstrong PJ, Hand MS, Frederick GS. Enteral nutrition by tube. Vet Clin North Am Small Anim Pract. In press.)

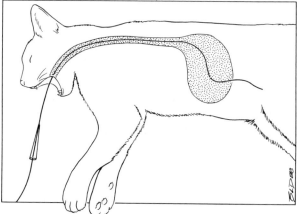

Fig. 37-7 The endoscopist threads the pipette tip, narrow end first, over the suture emerging from the animal's mouth. (From Armstrong PJ, Hand MS, Frederick GS. Enteral nutrition by tube. Vet Clin North Am Small Anim Pract. In press.)

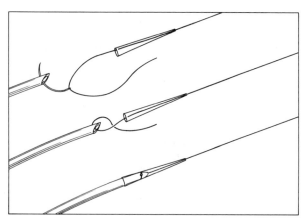

Fig. 37-8 The suture is passed once or twice through the beveled end of the feeding tube. Tension is applied to the suture to wedge the beveled end of the feeding tube into the flared end of the pipette tip, which acts as a tapered guide to stretch the hole made in the stomach and body wall and allow passage of the feeding tube. From Armstrong PJ, Hand MS, Frederick GS. Enteral nutrition by tube. Vet Clin North Am Small Anim Pract. In press.)

Fig. 37-9 The operator applies the aboral end of the suture, pulling the pipette tip and attached feeding tube with inner phlange down the esophagus. (From Armstrong PJ, Hand MS, Frederick GS. Enteral nutrition by tube. Vet Clin North Am Small Anim Pract. In press.)

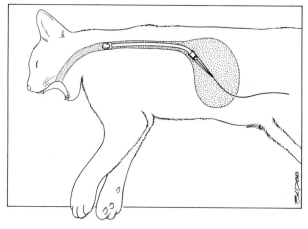

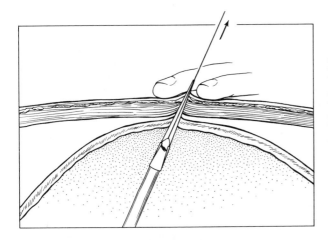

Fig. 37-10 The operator pulls the pipette tip out through the body wall, applying counterpressure against the body wall to aid the process. Steady traction is applied to the suture (do not pull on the pipette tip or it may be separated from the feeding tube), pulling the feeding tube out through the body wall. (From Armstrong PJ, Hand MS, Frederick GS. Enteral nutrition by tube. Vet Clin North Am Small Anim Pract. In press.)

Fig. 37-11 The feeding tube is pulled out until the inner flange is resting against the gastric mucosa without indenting it—this must be verified by the endoscopist. The outer flange is threaded onto the feeding tube so that it rests against the skin. If the external flange is too tightly apposed to the skin, pressure necrosis may develop. Swelling of the area in larger dogs may require loosening of the external flange 24 to 48 hours after tube placement. The external flange is adequate to secure the tube; no tape butterfly or sutures are required. (From Armstrong PJ, Hardie EM. Percutaneous endoscopic gastrostomy. Vet Med Rep. In press.)

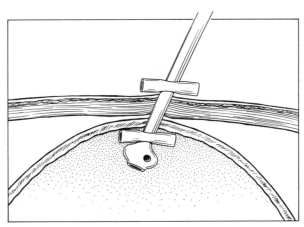

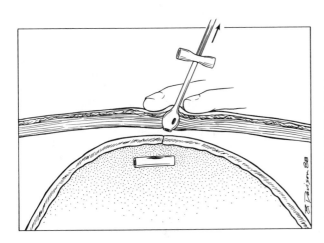

Fig. 37-12 Removal of the tube is accomplished by steady traction, which collapses the mushroom tip and allows it to be pulled through the inner flange, which falls back into the stomach and is passed in the feces. (From Armstrong PJ, Hardie EM. Percutaneous endoscopic gastrostomy. Vet Med Rep. In press.)

ment and subsequently as needed if soiled or displaced.

Whether they are used or not, PEG tubes should be left in place for at least 5 days; and even longer in debilitated animals, since adhesion formation may be delayed by malnutrition. Removal of the tube is accomplished by steady traction, which collapses the mushroom tip and allows it to be pulled through the inner flange (Fig. 37-12). It is rarely necessary to retrieve this small piece of plastic endoscopically, because it will fall back into the stomach and be passed in the feces. Even cats will tolerate this procedure without much restraint. In larger dogs, the tube may be transected level with the skin, and the mushroom tip and inner flange are passed without difficulty. Withholding food and water for 12 hours following tube removal has been recommended.[70] The gastrocutaneous fistula closes within a few days and does not require suturing.

If abdominal surgery is required because of the primary disease process, or if PEG-tube placement is not an option, gastrostomy tubes may be placed surgically.[50,65,71] A left flank approach is used if gastrostomy-tube placement alone is necessary. Balloon-tipped urethral catheters (Foley Catheter, Bard Urological Division of CR Bard, Murray Hill, NJ), varying from 16 to 30 French sizes, are generally recommended for the procedure. Unfortunately, gastric acid will dissolve the balloon within 5 to 7 days; when the catheter loses its self-retaining ability, tube dislodgement frequently occurs. For this reason, the use of a mushroom-tipped catheter as is used for a PEG tube yields better long-term results, since the self-retaining tip is more resistant to acid damage.

The patient is anesthetized, and the left paracostal area clipped and surgically prepared. The area is draped and a 3- to 5-cm skin incision is made just caudal and parallel to the last rib, beginning 2 to 4 cm below the ventral extent of the epaxial muscles. The external and internal oblique muscles are bluntly separated in the direction of their fibers, and the transverse abdominal muscle and parietal peritoneum are incised. Location of the stomach at this point is facilitated by insufflation with air by the anesthetist, using an orogastric tube. The stomach is brought up to the incision, packed off with laparotomy pads, and stay sutures placed at the 6 and 12 o'clock positions relative to the anticipated gastrostomy site located in the gastric body. Two concentric purse-string sutures of 2-0 nylon, polypropylene (Prolene®, Ethicon), polydioxane (PDS) are placed through all tissue layers encircling the gastrostomy site. The small closed nipple of the mushroom tip is removed, the tube is inserted into the stomach through a stab incision, and the purse-string sutures are tightened and tied, starting with the inner suture. The stomach is then sutured to the body wall using simple interrupted or continuous 2-0 nylon, polypropylene, or PDS sutures placed around the ostomy site, being sure to incorporate the submucosal layer.[65] Alternatively, attachment of the stomach to the body wall is ensured by using the ends of the inner purse-string suture to close the muscle layers of the abdominal incision and the ends of the outer purse-string suture to close the subcutaneous tissues.[50] Routine closure of the skin follows, and the tube is secured to the skin using a friction suture and a tape butterfly. The tube is plugged and an abdominal bandage is applied and changed as needed. If a mushroom-tipped catheter is used, tube removal is accomplished by cutting the tip off flush with the body wall and allowing it to fall back into the stomach

and be passed in the feces. If a Foley catheter is used, an attempt should be made to deflate the balloon prior to removal, but it has likely ruptured if the tube has been in place for more than a week.

Complications encountered in a series of PEG placements[70] include splenic laceration, benign pneumoperitoneum, aspiration pneumonia occurring in animals with esophageal disease, tube displacement or migration, and intolerance to feeding. Peritonitis and cellulitis at the gastrostomy site are possible specific complications for both percutaneous and surgically placed tubes, but problems are unlikely if the tubes are properly placed, secured, and maintained.[70] Most animals tolerate the tubes extremely well, but an Elizabethan collar may be required in the occasional canine patient.

Enterostomy tubes. Enterostomy tubes are another option for providing enteral nutritional support for animals who have undergone abdominal surgery.[49,50,65,72] They are particularly well suited for procedures involving the stomach and duodenum, since bypass of these portions of the gastrointestinal tract may be necessary postoperatively, but the function of the distal bowel is intact. A 5 French polyvinylchloride tube (Infant Feeding Tube, Argyle Division of Sherwood Medical, St Louis) or 6 French polyurethane tube (Entron Nasogastric Feeding Tube, Biosearch Medical Products, Somerville, NJ) is recommended for use. A loop of the distal duodenum or proximal jejunum, distal to any site of surgery, is chosen for enterostomy placement. After a skin nick is made, hemostats are used to pass the tip of the tube through the body wall at a site adjacent to the selected bowel loop. A purse-string suture of 3-0 nylon, polypropylene, PDS, or polyglactin 910 (Vicryl®, Ethicon) is placed in the antimesenteric border of the bowel (Fig. 37-13). A stab incision is made in the center of the purse-string, the feeding tube is inserted and advanced aborally along the lumen of the small intestine for 20 to 30 cm, and the purse-string suture is tightened and tied. The bowel loop is secured to the body wall using four to six simple interrupted sutures of 3-0 nylon, prolene, PDS, or polyglactin 910. The tube is secured to the skin at its exit site with a friction suture and a tape butterfly. Alternatively, a 12-gauge needle may be used to introduce the feeding tube through the body wall and into the intestinal lumen.[50,72] The enterostomy site is covered with an abdominal bandage postoperatively, which is changed as needed. Cutting the external sutures allows the tube to be withdrawn when it is no longer required. Complications associated with enterostomy tubes include diarrhea, stomal cellulitis, and localized or generalized peritonitis.

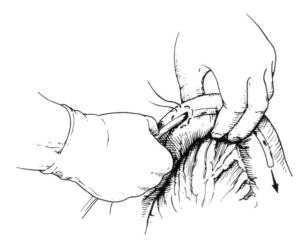

Fig. 37-13 Enterostomy-tube placement. A purse-string suture is placed in the antimesenteric border of the bowel loop. A stab incision is made in the center of the purse-string, the feeding tube is inserted and advanced aborally along the lumen of the small intestine, and the suture is tightened and tied. (From Crowe DT. Enteral nutrition of critically ill or injured patients—Part II. Compend Contin Educ Pract Vet 1986; 8:727.)

Table 37-2 Diet prepared in a blender for tube feeding dogs and cats

	Analysis	
	As fed	**Dry matter**
Moisture (%)	83	0
Protein (%)	7.4	44.2 or 33% of calories
Fat (%)	5.0	29.6 or 55% of calories
Carbohydrate (%)	2.8	17.0 or 12% of calories
Calcium (%)	0.19	1.1
Phosphorus (%)	0.13	0.8
Sodium (%)	0.10	0.6
Metabolizable energy (%)	0.8 kcal/ml	4.76 kcal/g

(1) 0.5 can (224 g) Prescription Diet Feline p/d (Hill's Pet Products, Topeka, KS). (2) 0.75 cup (180 ml) warm water. (3) Blend for 1 minute at high speed. Strain twice through a kitchen strainer (approximately 1-mm mesh). Yield: 390 ml. (From Lewis LD, Morris ML, Hand MS. Small animal clinical nutrition. ed. 3. Topeka: Mark Morris, 1987:5-29.)

What to feed

Once a route of administration of enteral nutritional support is established, a decision must be made regarding what diet to feed. If force feeding, using pharmacologic enhancement of appetite, or using orogastric, pharyngostomy, or gastrostomy tube feeding, the best diet is one specifically designed for the species and physiologic state of the patient. A calorically dense product is preferred to reduce the volume necessary to fulfill the animal's nutritional needs; easy digestibility is also an advantage. A diet of cat food prepared in a blender (Prescription Diet Feline p/d, Hill's Pet Products, Topeka, KS) has been analyzed (Table 37-2), passes easily through tubes of 14 French size or larger, and is well tolerated by both cats and dogs with normal renal and hepatic function.[2,49] If organ function is compromised, reduced protein diets may be substituted (Prescription Diet Canine or Feline k/d, Hill's Pet Products, Topeka, KS).

Diets appropriate for feeding through the smaller-bore nasogastric and enterostomy tubes and marketed specifically for dogs and cats have become available (Clinical Care Feline and Canine Liquid Diets, Pet Ag Inc, Hampshire, IL). My experience with them is limited. Human products are frequently utilized in critically ill dogs and cats. A wide variety of products are available for human enteral support, with the number expanding continually; detailed reviews are available in both the human [73] and veterinary[2,74] literature. Becoming familiar with a few products that are well tolerated by the majority of patients is the recommended approach. Enteral products are available in liquid or powder forms; this affects the ease of preparation as well as the cost. Powdered formulas may become contaminated with bacteria during reconstitution, which may contribute to gastrointestinal complications.[73] Several classification systems for enteral nutritional products have been described (see first box, next page).[73] Considering major criteria and selected minor criteria for choosing an enteral nutrition product (see second box, next page) lends some degree of logic to decision making when the clinician is confronted with the large number of options available. The first box categorizes several commonly used enteral feeding formulas in therapeutically comparable groups.[73]

Caloric density is important because it determines the number of calories the animal will receive as well as the amount of other nutrients. If the higher-density products are used without additional fluids, dehydration may result.

Protein content merits special consideration, since these diets are designed for human use, and the protein requirements of veterinary patients may differ. It is recommended to calculate the amount of protein required by the individual (box, pp. 598 and 599) and the amount of protein supplied by the enteral product; the difference may

CATEGORIZATION OF ENTERAL FEEDING FORMULAS IN THERAPEUTICALLY COMPARABLE GROUPS

Lactose-free formulas
  1 kcal/ml
    Standard protein
      Polymeric
        Ensure, Travasorb, Renu, Nutri-Aid, Ensure HN, Osmolite,
        Isocal, Osmolite HN, Compleat Modified, Vitaneed, Precision
        Isotonic Diet, Travasorb MCT, Entrition Entri-Pak, Portagen,
        Precision HN, Resource, Precision LR
      Oligomeric
        Travasorb STD, Criticare HN, Standard Vivonex, Vital HN,
        Travasorb HN, Vivonex HN, Vivonex TEN, Peptamen
      Fiber containing
        Enrich, Jevity
    High protein
      Sustacal, Isotein HN
  1.5 kcal/ml
    Standard protein
      Ensure Plus, Sustacal HC, Ensure Plus HN
    High protein
      TraumaCal
  2 kcal/ml
    Standard protein
      Magnacal, Isocal HCN, TwoCal HN
Specialized formulas
  Hepatic encephalopathy
    Hepatic-Aid, Hepatic-Aid II, Travasorb Hepatic
  Renal failure
    Amin-Aid, Travasorb Renal
  Trauma (44-50% branched-chain amino acids)
    Traum-Aid HBC, Stresstein
  Respiratory failure
    Pulmocare
Modular products
  Protein
    Propac, Pro-Mix, Casec, Gevral, Nutrisource amino acids, Nutrisource amino acids—high branched-chain, Nutrisource protein, ProMod
  Carbohydrate
    Polycose, Moducal, Sumacal, Cal Plus, Nutrisource carbohydrate, Hycal, Pro-Mix Carbohydrate
  Fat
    Medium-chain triglycerides
      MCT Oil, Nutrisource lipid—medium-chain triglycerides
    Long-chain triglycerides
      Microlipid, Lipomul oral, Nutrisource lipid—long-chain triglycerides

Modified from Heimburger DC, Weinsier RL. Guidelines for evaluating and categorizing enteral feeding formulas according to therapeutic equivalence. J Parenter Enter Nutr 1985;9:61-67.

CRITERIA FOR EVALUATION OF ENTERAL FEEDING FORMULAS

Major criteria
  Caloric density (kcal/ml)
    1.0, 1.5, or 2.0
  Protein content (expressed as % of total kcal)
    Standard, <20%
    High protein, >20%
  Cost
Minor criteria
  Osmolality (mOsml/kg water)
    Isotonic, <350
    Moderately hypertonic, 350-550
    Markedly hypertonic, >550
  Complexity
    Polymeric
    Oligomeric
  Fat content (expressed as % of total kcal)
    Standard, >20%
    Low, 5-20%
    Free, <5%
  Fat source
    Long-chain triglycerides only
    Long-chain and medium-chain triglycerides
  Residue content
    Fiber-containing
    Low residue
  Lactose content
  Form
    Ready-to-use
    Powder

Modified from Heimburger DC, Weinsier RL. Guidelines for therapeutic evaluating and categorizing enteral feeding formulas according to therapeutic equivalence. J. Parenter Enter Nutr 1985;9:61-67.

be provided by adding a powdered protein supplement (ProMod, Ross Laboratories, Columbus, OH—each 6.6-g scoop provides 5 g of whey protein) to each day's enteral formula.[50] The standard products (<20% of total calories as protein) are more suitable for veterinary patients requiring protein restriction; the high-protein products (>20% of total calories as protein) are generally appropriate for dogs with normal renal and hepatic function, but supplemental protein is required by cats as well as dogs with extraordinary protein losses. Cost varies with the manufacturer, supplier, local circumstances (for example, state contracts), and type of formula. In general, oligomeric products will be more expensive than polymeric, and those intended for use in specific disease states will be most expensive.

The osmolality of a product may not be an important consideration in every case, but there is evidence to suggest an association between gastrointestinal complications and hyperosmolality.[47,73,74] Isotonic products are preferred, especially for enterostomy feeding.

The complexity of the nutrients in enteral formulas is of debatable significance. Those containing crystalline amino acids are high in osmolality and cost; studies have demonstrated that the absorption of single amino acids is less efficient than that of dipeptides and tripeptides in protein hydrolysates.[75] Both crystalline amino acid and peptide-containing formulas are classified as oligomeric; they also contain carbohydrates in the form of oligosaccharides and monosaccharides. Diets containing higher-molecular-weight forms of proteins, fats, and carbohydrates are termed "polymeric." Oligomeric formulas (also the only products available that are low in fat) are recommended for maldigestive and malabsorptive states, but no significant clinical superiority over polymeric diets has been demonstrated in human trials.[76] However, the fat content and fat source are significant factors in patients with maldigestion, malabsorption, or hyperlipidemic disorders. Long-chain triglycerides are often partially replaced by medium-chain triglycerides in products designed for these disease states; absorption into the portal blood instead of the intestinal lymphatics make them preferable as an energy source. Products containing medium-chain triglycerides should be used with caution in cats, since they may result in hepatic lipid accumulation.[77] Medium-chain triglycerides are not a source of essential fatty acids. Energy could alternatively be provided primarily as carbohydrate, but this often results in a hypertonic formulation.

The necessity for supplementation of human enteral diets fed on a short-term basis to cats with taurine and arachidonic acid, two essential nutrients not likely included in these products, has not been determined. The addition of 250 mg of taurine (Taurine Tablets, Pet-Ag Inc, Hampshire, IL) to each day's enteral formula is recommended. Arachidonic acid deficiency is unlikely to develop in the short-term feeding of diets lacking this nutrient.[77]

Several products have been introduced that contain dietary fiber, consisting of soy polysaccharide, unlike the majority of enteral nutrition products, which are low in residue (examples include Enrich and Jevity, Ross Laboratories, Columbus, OH). They may be useful in patients experiencing constipation or diarrhea with the standard formulas, but experience with these products is limited in veterinary patients.

Lactose-free formulas are generally preferable in both human and veterinary patients. Lactose intolerance manifested as diarrhea and cramping is common in mature individuals,[73,74] and there is no beneficial effect peculiar to lactose as an energy source.

Specialized formulas must be considered for specific disease states. These diets are more expensive and may be nutritionally incomplete. Those designed for hepatic encephalopathy have increased amounts of branched-chain amino acids but are aromatic amino acid restricted. Their composition is intended to correct the abnormal plasma amino acid profile of affected patients, resulting in an improvement in their neurologic status.[78,79] Renal failure formulas contain only essential amino acids; theoretically, the body should use these as a nitrogen source for the manufacture of nonessential amino acids. The resultant recycling of nitrogen reduces the load of nitrogenous wastes, which must be eliminated by the failing kidneys.[80] Formulas marketed for the nutritional support of trauma victims or septic patients are branched-chain amino acid-enriched with adequate aromatic amino acids. Their use may stimulate protein synthesis and reduce proteolysis, allowing an earlier return to a positive nitrogen balance and attenuating muscle catabolism.[10,22,23] Finally, patients suffering from respiratory insufficiency or failure may benefit from a high-fat, low-carbohydrate formulation designed to reduce carbon dioxide production.[27,28] Experience with these products in veterinary patients is limited, and their cost effectiveness even in humans is controversial.[73]

The modular nutritional products are another unique category. These single-nutrient preparations may be used to supplement enteral diets on an individual basis with additional protein, carbohydrate, or fat. Addition of protein to human enteral products, as described previously, is often necessary to provide balanced diets for dogs and cats. A complete modular feeding system (Nutrisource Modular System, Doyle Pharmaceutical, Minneapolis) may be used to custom-design enteral diets.

How to feed

The administration of enteral nutrition is by intermittent bolus (every 4 to 8 hours) or continuous feeding techniques. The method chosen depends on the route of feeding selected, facilities available, and individual patient tolerance. The "small amounts often" approach is applicable in most critically ill animals, whether they are force-fed, pharmacologically induced to eat, or fed via orogastric, nasogastric, pharnygostomy, or gastrostomy tube. Feeding in an upright position may prevent problems with regurgitation and aspiration.[49] Enterostomy feeding must be continuous, since there is no reservoir capacity in the small intestine. In addition, occasionally patients with nasogastric and gastrostomy tubes will tolerate continuous feeding, but will vomit if bolus-fed. An enteral pump (Flo-Gard 2000 Enteral Pump, Clintec Nutrition, Deerfield, IL) marketed for human use is appropriate for medium and large dogs; a syringe pump (Auto Syringe, Auto Syringe, Hooksett, NH) works well for cats and small dogs.

Feeding through nasogastric tubes may begin immediately after placement. If using a pharyngostomy tube, the patient should be completely recovered from anesthesia prior to feeding. A 12-hour (PEG tube) to 24-hour (surgically placed tube) delay is recommended before feeding by gastrostomy tube, in order for gastric motility to return and a fibrin seal to form at the tube site.[50] Enterostomy feeding may begin after recovery from anesthesia as long as peristaltic movements were noted at the time of tube placement.

Prior to bolus feeding into the stomach, residual volume should be measured by negative pressure with an empty syringe; the liquid should then be returned to the stomach. Feeding may proceed if the residual volume is one third or less of the bolus volume.[65] Slow (over 5 to 10 minutes) administration of a room to body temperature meal is recommended. Tubes should be flushed with 5 to 10 ml of warm water after each bolus feeding. Intermittent (every 6 hours) irrigation of enterostomy tubes is also recommended. If feeding continuously into the stomach, residual volume measurement is performed every 6 hours; in dogs, there should be less than twice the volume infused hourly; in cats, there should be less than one half the volume infused hourly.[50]

When feeding pet foods prepared in a blender, begin with one third to one half of the calculated requirement and increase the volume fed over 2 to 3 days, depending on patient tolerance. At this point, the frequency of feeding may be reduced and the bolus volume increased accordingly.

When feeding human enteral diets, dilute the product to half strength and begin with one third to one half the calculated volume (bolus feeding) or hourly rate (continuous feeding). Advance feeding over the next 2 to 3 days, depending on patient tolerance, increasing first volume administered and then formula concentration.

Monitoring and complications

Careful monitoring during the administration of nutritional support is vital to its success; patient response and tolerance may be determined and complications may be detected before they become serious. Monitoring in these animals is seldom more intense than that recommended for critically ill animals in general. Twice-daily assessment of attitude, hydration status, mucous membrane color, capillary refill time, body temperature, heart rate, and respiratory rate are recommended. The animal should be weighed each morning (on the same scale), and packed cell volume, total serum solids, urine glucose, and urine specific gravity should be measured daily. Additional laboratory monitoring may be required depending on the animal's primary problem and condition. Feeding records (concentration and volume administered, residual volumes, observation of vomiting, abdominal discomfort, or diarrhea) should be reviewed prior to formulating the day's feeding plan.

Complications associated with enteral nutritional support are categorized as gastrointestinal, mechanical, or metabolic. Problems in the first category are the most commonly encountered, but are rarely of a serious nature.[81] Gastrointestinal complications observed in veterinary patients include diarrhea, delayed gastric emptying, abdominal discomfort, vomiting, and constipation; in addition, abdominal distention and gastrointestinal hemorrhage have been observed in humans. If gastrointestinal problems occur, it will likely be during initiation of therapy, especially if a prolonged period of anorexia preceded feeding. Diarrhea is uncommon in animals fed blenderized pet food, but is frequent when human enteral products are fed (especially to cats) or when enterostomy tubes are used.

Diarrhea caused by hypertonicity of the formula, too rapid administration, and lactose or other nutrient intolerance may be remedied by alterations in method or rate of administration, or enteral product chosen. Enterally administered antibiotics may alter intestinal flora and induce diarrhea. Malabsorptive diarrhea may occur subsequent to prolonged anorexia and villous atrophy. Reduced colloidal osmotic pressure due to hypoalbuminemia may exacerbate diarrhea. Treatment with parenterally administered antibiotics, short-term adjunctive parenteral nutrition, or plasma may be necessary. The use of supplemental fiber or drugs to modify gastrointestinal motility may be considered.

Bacterial contamination of enteral diets is a well-recognized cause of diarrhea in human patients, and has led to the increased popularity of marketing enteral products in a ready-to-use form. Factors contributing to this complication are prolonged exposure to warm temperatures, careless preparation and handling, and lack of exposure to gastric acid by bacterial contaminants as a result of enterostomy feeding or the use of H_2 antagonists or antacids. Although the importance of this problem has not been determined in veterinary patients, care in preparation and administration of enteral feedings is recommended.

Delayed gastric emptying, abdominal discomfort associated with feeding, and vomiting are commonly observed problems in the first days of gastrostomy feeding after prolonged periods of anorexia. Cats with idiopathic hepatic lipidosis are particularly prone to these complications, often associated with constipation. Possible solutions include continuous feeding, giving smaller volumes more frequently, slower infusion of bolus feedings, and promotility therapy with metaclopramide given subcutaneously at 0.2 to 0.4 mg/kg every 6 to 8 hours. If constipation is present, enemas, stool softeners, additional fiber, or laxatives may be required. Lactulose given through the tube at 1 to 3 ml every 6 to 8 hours may be effective in cases of feline hepatic lipidosis. Ensuring adequate hydration and encouraging ambulation may also be beneficial in stimulating or maintaining gastrointestinal motility.

Mechanical complications peculiar to each method of enteral feeding have been discussed. Tube obstruction is most likely to occur with the smaller-bore nasogastric and enterostomy tubes. Preventive tactics include using a product specifically designed for tube feeding, only administering medications through the tube in a liquid form, continuous feeding techniques, and flushing the tube regularly with water. Obstructed tubes may be cleared by irrigation with cola[82] or a solution prepared by crushing one Viokase tablet with one sodium bicarbonate tablet and adding 5 ml of water to the resulting powder.[83]

Metabolic complications are not commonly encountered in animals receiving enteral nutritional support. Possibilities include dehydration, hyperglycemia, azotemia, and electrolyte abnormalities.[84] They may be avoided with careful monitoring and choosing a diet appropriate to the physiologic state of the patient. Correction of metabolic imbalances may require the administration of intravenous fluids, electrolytes, or insulin.

PARENTERAL NUTRITIONAL SUPPORT

Although most critically ill patients can be maintained using enteral nutrition, a few are temporarily unable or have a very limited capacity to assimilate nutrients administered into the gastrointestinal tract. Parenteral nutrition is appropriately chosen as the method of nutritional support in these animals, as well as in selected patients when withholding or restricting enteral intake allows time for the resolution of disease.[2,24,49,85,86] Parenteral nutrition can be used when the gastrointestinal tract is nonfunctional, which is its princi-

ple advantage over enteral nutrition. In most cases a shorter transition to a full nutrient load is achieved when compared to enteral methods. The requirements for comparatively expensive specialized products, meticulous asepsis in preparation and administration, and experienced personnel remain disadvantages of the parenteral route of nutritional support. There is some risk of septic and metabolic complications, and animals receiving total parenteral nutrition (TPN) with nothing orally may suffer compromises in gastrointestinal integrity.

Parenteral nutrition should be considered in any animal with an anticipated inability to absorb enterally administered nutrients for more than 3 to 5 days, depending on initial nutritional status. Animals undergoing massive small-bowel resection, and those with impaired small intestinal motility or function, severe diarrhea, or intractable vomiting are candidates for TPN.[87] Total parenteral nutrition may also be indicated in severe prolonged pancreatitis[50] and severe malnutrition or catabolism in the presence of a temporarily nonfunctional gastrointestinal tract. Alternative justification for the use of TPN may exist in the clinical situation of patients judged to be unable to tolerate anesthesia for placement of a indwelling feeding tube, as well as being poor candidates for nasogastric, repeated orogastric, or force-feeding.

Components

The three basic components of parenteral nutrition are dextrose, amino acids, and lipids. Dextrose has traditionally been the major source of calories in TPN, but hyperglycemia and hyperosmolality may occur if large volumes of concentrated dextrose solution are given without an adequate transition period.[16,24,49,85,86] Some patients may require exogenous insulin to improve glucose tolerance. Hypoglycemia may occur if the administration of high-dextrose TPN with added insulin is discontinued abruptly. Providing 100% of nonprotein calories as dextrose may be associated with increased metabolic complications.[16,88] Dextrose is the least expensive component of TPN; it is available in concentrations of 2.5% to 70% with corresponding osmolalities of 126 to 3530 mOsm/L and caloric contents of 85 to 2390 kcal/L.

Crystalline amino acid solutions, available in concentrations of 3% to 15% with osmolalities of 405 to 1388 mOsm/L, are the protein and nitrogen source in TPN. Solutions are available with or without added electrolytes. The nonspecialized solutions (Travasol, Clintec Nutrition, Deerfield, IL) contain all essential amino acids for dogs and cats, with the exception of taurine.[46,85,86,89] The necessity for taurine supplementation for cats on TPN has not been determined. Specialty formulations for use in renal failure, hepatic encephalopathy, severe trauma or stress, and in neonates are available but are much more expensive and have not been used extensively in veterinary patients.

Lipid emulsions represent a concentrated energy source that is isotonic and may be given through peripheral or central veins; separately, or mixed with the other TPN components in an all-in-one total nutrient admixture.[49,85,86,90-92] Commercially available lipid emulsions are made of soybean (Intralipid, Clintec Nutrition, Deerfield, IL) or safflower oil (Liposyn, Abbott Laboratories, North Chicago, IL), in concentrations of 10% or 20%, with caloric contents of 1.1 and 2.0 kcal/ml, respectively. No transition period is required for the administration of lipids, and hyperglycemia is less likely to occur when lipids provide some of the nonprotein calories. Lipid emulsions can be included in TPN in order to provide the essential fatty acid linoleic acid, but they do not contain arachidonic acid, which is required preformed in the feline diet. Their use is contraindicated in the presence of pathologic hyperlipidemia. Conditions such as pancreatitis may reduce lipid clearance.[93]

Using amino acid solutions with added electrolytes is the most convenient approach to providing electrolytes in TPN solutions. Their composition will be appropriate for the majority of patients; calcium gluconate may be added if not included in the amino acid solution. The amount that is safely added without danger of precipitation (less than 10 mEq/L)[92] will not fulfill the animal's requirement for calcium. If amino acid solutions without electrolytes are used, electrolytes may be added in the form of a concentrated electrolyte mixture (TPN Electrolytes, Abbott Laboratories North Chicago, IL) or as multiple individual electrolyte solutions. Recommended electrolyte concentrations in the final TPN solution (Table 37-3) will maintain normal electrolyte status in most patients not experiencing deficiencies or extraordinary ongoing losses.[49,85,86].

Multivitamin preparations for TPN (Multivitamin 12, Clintec Nutrition, Deerfield, IL) usually provide all fat- and water-soluble vitamins with the exception of vitamin K, which may be given subcutaneously once weekly.[49,85] Trace elements such as zinc, iron, copper, chromium, manganese, selenium, cobalt, and iodine are not added routinely unless the duration of TPN administration exceeds 1 to 2 weeks. Heparin may be added (1 IU/ml) for its antithrombotic effect; it will also help maintain catheter patency and enhance lipid clearance.[91] Crystalloids may be added to the

Table 37-3 Routine electrolyte concentrations in final TPN solution

Sodium = 35-45 mEq/L	Chloride = 35-45 mEq/L
Potassium = 35-45 mEq/ L	Phosphate = 10-15 mmole/l
Calcium = 4-5 mEq/L	Magnesium = 4-5 mEq/L

From Lippert AC, Armstrong PJ. Parenteral nutritional support. In Kirk RW, ed. Current veterinary therapy X. Philadelphia: WB Saunders, 1989:27.

TPN solution or given through a separate catheter if there are continuing excessive fluid losses due to vomiting, diarrhea, exudation, or diuresis. Total parenteral nutrition solutions generally provide maintenance water requirements.

Compounding solutions

Before compounding, the novice should contact a local hospital pharmacist or manufacturer's representative regarding solution compatibility. The all-in-one or total nutrient admixture method of compounding TPN is economical, simple, and convenient in most veterinary settings. Dextrose, amino acids, and lipids are pooled in a sterile container and additives made just prior to administration.[49,85,92] Ethylene vinyl acetate pooling bags equipped with three lead transfer sets and filtered vents (All-In-One Bag, Clintec Nutrition, Deerfield, IL) facilitate compounding, and the admixture may be stored at 4°C for up to a week. Alternatively, less expensive polyvinylchloride bags (Dextrose Solution in Underfilled Viaflex Container, Clintec Nutrition, Deerfield, IL) may be used for pooling, as long as the solution is administered immediately on compounding[94]; storage may result in the leaching of diethylhexylphthalate (DEHP), a potential carcinogen, into the solution. Transfer sets with filtered vents (Transfer Set, Abbott Laboratories, North Chicago, IL) may be used to add the amino acid solution and lipid emulsion to the dextrose. Total parenteral nutrition components should be mixed in the sequence (1) dextrose, (2) amino acids, and (3) lipids, since mixing the lipids directly with the dextrose may break the emulsion.[85,92] Compounding under a laminar flow hood is desirable, but not practical for most veterinarians; asepsis may be maintained by compounding in a clean, low-traffic area, such as a surgery suite. Swabbing injection ports with 70% isopropyl alcohol or povidone iodine solution prior to penetration with needles and transfer sets, and venting bottles only through bacterial filters is recommended. Air should not be injected into vials to facilitate withdrawal of their contents.

Administration

Parenteral nutrition may be administered into a central or peripheral vein. Total parenteral nutrition—the provision of all essential nutrients by an intravenous route—must be administered centrally because of the hypertonicity of the solutions. Partial parenteral nutrition (PPN) supplies some portion of the nutritional requirements, often when the remainder is supplied enterally, as occurs in transition feeding.[95] Partial parenteral nutrition may be administered into a peripheral vein; a solution appropriate for short-term peripheral use is described in the box below.[85] Intravenous hyperalimentation is the practice of administering parenteral nutrients in excess of individual requirements in order to promote anabolism. This is not the goal in adult small animal patients, as it carries a greater risk of metabolic complications in both humans[88] and animals.[89,96] Parenteral nutrition should be used to prevent further deterioration in the nutritional status until weight gain may be more safely achieved by enteral intake.

Nutritional requirements should be calculated as described previously. Dogs may be given the calculated IER as nonprotein calories, with 40% to 60% provided as lipid, if desired, and the remainder as dextrose. This approach may be associated with metabolic complications in cats due to overfeeding,[89] so the protein calories are calculated (4 kcal/g) and the result subtracted from the

---

COMPOSITION OF A PARENTERAL NUTRITION SOLUTION FOR SHORT-TERM PERIPHERAL USE

---

100 ml 20% lipid emulsion*
200 ml 8.5% amino acids with electrolytes†
400 ml 10% dextrose
300 ml lactated Ringer's solution
20 mEq potassium chloride

Provides 337 nonprotein calories (59% as lipid) and 17 g of protein in 1 L of solution
Calculated osmolality = 546 mOsm/L

Electrolyte concentrations:
Sodium = 53 mEq/L	Chloride = 67 mEq/L
Potassium = 33 mEq/L	Phosphate = 6 mmol/L
Calcium = 0.9 mEq/L	Magnesium = 2mEq/L

---

*20% Intralipid, Clintec Nutrition, affiliated with Baxter Healthcare Corp, Deerfield, IL.
†8.5% Travasol with electrolytes, Clintec Nutrition, Deerfield, IL.
From Lippert AC, Armstrong PJ. Parenteral nutritional support. In Kirk RW, ed. Current veterinary therapy X. Philadelphia: WB Saunders, 1989:28.

IER. The remaining calories may be provided as a 50:50 mixture of lipid and dextrose. The administration of nonprotein calories as a mixed fuel source of lipid and dextrose is considered by many to be metabolically desirable.[88]

Establishment of a protocol and supervision by experienced and interested clinicians, technicians, and pharmacists are key features to a successful TPN program. Meticulous central venous catheter placement and care cannot be overemphasized.[49,85,86,97-99] Total parenteral nutrition administration is never an emergency procedure—aseptic and atraumatic catheter insertion by an experienced operator is vital to reduce septic and mechanical complications to a minimum. A single lumen polyurethane (L-Cath, Luther Medical Products, Santa Ana, CA) or silicone elastomer catheter (Centrasil, Baxter Healthcare, Deerfield, IL) may be placed percutaneously in the external jugular vein of most dogs and cats, with the tip of the catheter located in the cranial vena cava. Alternatively, a longer silicone elastomer catheter (Intrasil, Baxter Healthcare, Deerfield, IL) may be threaded into the caudal vena cava from the lateral saphenous vein in dogs weighing more than 10 kg. Catheters made of silicone elastomer and polyurethane are less thrombogenic and subsequently less likely to result in mechanical complications than the less expensive catheters (Intracath, Deseret, Sandy, UT) commonly used in veterinary patients for fluid administration.[97] The catheter is changed as indicated by mechanical or septic problems, not at predetermined times. It is "dedicated" to TPN administration, and is not used for blood sampling, medication administration, or central venous pressure monitoring. The catheter bandage and intravenous sets used for TPN administration are changed every other day. Application of a povidone iodine antiseptic to the catheter placement site is recommended.

When the total nutrient admixture system is used, the initiation of TPN is simplified[49,85,92]; one half of the calculated volume of dextrose is included in the TPN solution on the first day, while other components are present in their full amounts. If glucosuria is minimal, the dextrose is increased to the full amount on the second day. If dextrose provides all of the nonprotein calories, 25% of the anticipated load is given initially, and the administration rate is increased gradually over the next 24 to 48 hours based on urine and blood glucose monitoring. Use of an intravenous infusion pump is considered mandatory for TPN, unless supervision is continuous. Each day's infusion may extend over 24 hours if constant observation is available. If not, cyclic TPN may be administered over 15 hours of the day,[100] with a heparin lock used to prevent catheter occlusion when not in use. Care must be taken to avoid hyperglycemia and hypoglycemia with cyclic TPN, and there may be an increased risk of volume overload as well as septic complications, since the catheter is being violated more frequently.

When enteral intake has increased to provide more than 50% of the IER, TPN may be discontinued by decreasing the rate of the infusion gradually over 2 hours. Alternatively , dilute (5% to 10%) dextrose solutions may be administered. Symptomatic hypoglycemia is rarely seen, even when TPN infusions are abruptly discontinued.[101]

Monitoring and complications

As with enteral nutritional support, the administration of TPN adds little to the routine monitoring of critically ill patients. To the schedule suggested for monitoring patients receiving enteral support may be added an electrolyte determination 24 to 48 hours after the initiation of TPN, and twice weekly performance of a complete blood count and complete biochemical profile.[49,85] Other laboratory and critical care monitoring are indicated by the patient's disease and condition (see Chapter 4). Alterations in the TPN solution composition are often made on the basis of laboratory results or clinical response.

Mechanical complications, including inadvertent catheter removal, catheter occlusion, line disconnection or breakage, and venous thrombosis, are the most commonly encountered problems occurring during TPN administration,[48,98] but they rarely result in patient morbidity. Their occurrence may be reduced by meticulous catheter placement/maintenance and close patient supervision. With active animals or those likely to chew their intravenous lines, all connections should be taped, and adhesive tape may also be applied to the line and sprayed with a bitter-tasting deterrent (Bitter Apple, Valhar Chemical Corp, Greenwich, CT). An Elizabethan collar is rarely required.

Catheter or solution-related sepsis has the potential to induce serious morbidity or mortality in patients receiving TPN. Septic complications occur infrequently when catheter placement/maintenance and solution compounding/administration are strictly supervised and performed according to an established protocol.[48,49,85,86,97-99] If pyrexia or leukocytosis, not attributable to another septic process and/or associated with the primary disease, develops in an animal receiving TPN, the TPN catheter should be suspected as their source. Hyperglycemia or glucosuria appearing in a previously stable patient may also indicate impending sepsis. The bandage is removed and the vein is examined for evidence of phlebitis; if phlebitis is present, the catheter is removed, and the tip is collected aseptically for bacterial culture, preferably with semiquantitative technique.[102] If the vein appears normal, clinical circumstances such as the availability of other venous access may indicate whether catheter removal is desirable, but in most cases the catheter is removed and cultured. If the catheter remains in place, a blood culture should be performed. The animal usually becomes afebrile within hours after catheter removal and antibiotic administration if the catheter was the source of pyrexia or sepsis; TPN may be resumed after 24 hours of normothermia.

Metabolic complications may also be associated with TPN administration,[48,49,85,86,98] but they are generally minimized with careful patient monitoring. Glucose intolerance rarely occurs in dogs unless there is a predisposing cause such as pancreatic disease or hyperadrenocorticism, but is seen commonly in cats with any disease process. A species susceptibility to stress-induced hyperglycemia is the likely explanation.[89] Hyperglycemia, if uncorrected, may result in dehydration due to osmotic diuresis or lead to the development of hyperglycemic, hyperosmolar coma. If a persistent glucosuria of greater than 500 mg/dl occurs on the first day of TPN administration, continued inclusion of only one half the dextrose calories is indicated on the second day. If significant glucosuria persists, insulin therapy is initiated. Ten units of regular insulin is added to each liter of TPN solution, and the amount adjusted according to blood and urine glucose monitoring. Provision of fewer nonprotein calories as dextrose and more as lipid may also be considered.

Most electrolyte imbalances encountered during TPN administration are easily corrected by adjusting the composition of the solution. Hypokalemia is seen most commonly, since glucose and insulin accelerate the intracellular movement of potassium. When administering high concentrations of potassium intravenously, the rate should not exceed 0.5 mEq/kg per hour.

Mild elevations in the blood urea nitrogen may occur occasionally after the initiation of TPN. Absence of hypovolemia and a normal creatinine make a prerenal origin associated with protein administration most likely. The calculated protein requirement is reduced by 1 g/kg per day and the blood urea nitrogen reassessed in 24 hours. Patients suffering from renal failure are usually receiving restricted-protein TPN, but the calculated protein requirement is reduced by 0.5 g/kg per day if the blood urea nitrogen rises in association with a stable or falling creatinine.

Moderate lipemia is expected for 1 or 2 days after initiating a TPN solution containing lipids, but if other than mild lipemia persists, or if the serum triglyceride concentration exceeds 300 mg/dL after 3 days, the nonprotein calories provided by lipid are partially replaced by dextrose calories. Preexisting hyperlipidemia is a contraindication to the use of lipids in TPN.

Reversible hepatic abnormalities and thrombocytopenia have been reported in clinically normal cats given TPN for 2 weeks.[89] Duration of TPN administration is unlikely to exceed 2 weeks in most clinical situations encountered in small animal critical care medicine.

CONCLUSION

After consideration of what is known about the injured animal's response to injury, metabolic support, including nutritional support, becomes an obvious, rational extension of the cardiopulmonary support vital to the survival of the critically ill animal. Attention to the nutritional status of hospitalized patients will bring rewards associated with decreased morbidity and mortality, as well as reducing the duration of patient stay.

REFERENCES

1. Aoki TT, Finley RJ. The metabolic response to fasting. In Rombeau JL, Caldwell MD, eds. Clinical nutrition, vol. 2. Parenteral nutrition. Philadelphia: WB Saunders, 1986:9-28.
2. Lewis LD, Morris ML, Hand MS. Small animal clinical nutrition, ed. 3. Topeka: Mark Morris, 1987: pp. 5-1 to 5-44,
3. Meguid MM, Collier MD, Howard LJ. Uncomplicated and stressed starvation. Surg Clin North Am 1981;61:529.
4. Orr JW, Shingleton HM. Importance of nutritional assessment and support in surgical and cancer patients. J Reprod Med 1984;29:635-650.
5. Cuthbertson DP. The disturbance of metabolism produced by bony and non-bony injury, with notes on certain abnormal conditions of bone. Biochem J 1930;24:1244-1266.
6. Kirkpatrick JR. The neuroendocrine response to injury and infection. Nutrition 1987;3:221-227.
7. Bright RM, Lantz GC. Metabolism of the surgical patient. In Slatter DH, ed. Textbook of small animal surgery; vol. I. Philadelphia: WB Saunders, 1985:82-96.
8. Stamp G. Metabolic response to trauma. In Zaslow IM, ed. Veterinary Trauma and Critical Care. Philadelphia: Lea & Febiger, 1984:25-63.
9. Bessey PQ, Watters JM, Aoki TT, et al. Combined hormonal infusion simulates the metabolic response to injury. Ann Surg 1984;200:264-281.
10. Gilder H. Parenteral nourishment of patients undergoing surgical or traumatic stress. J Parenter Enter Nutr 1986;10:88-99.
11. Pomposelli JJ, Flores EA, Bistrian BR. Role of biochemical mediators in clinical nutrition and surgical metabolism. J Parenter Enter Nutr 1988;12:212-218.
12. Fong Y, Lowry SF, Cerami A. Cachectin/TNF:. a macrophage protein that induces cachexia and shock. J Parenter Enter Nutr 1988;12:72S-77S.
13. Dinarello CA. Interleukin-1 and the pathogenesis of the acute phase response. N Engl J Med 1984;311:1413-1418.
14. Nathan CF. Secretory products of macrophages. J Clin Invest 1987;79:319-326.
15. Robinson DR, Tateno S, Patel B, et al. Lipid mediators of inflammatory and immune reactions. J Parenter Enter Nutr 1988;12:37S-42S.
16. Wolfe RR. Carbohydrate metabolism in the critically ill patient—implications for nutritional support. Crit Care Clin North Am 1987;3:11-24.
17. Spitzer JJ, Bagby GJ, Meszaros K, et al. Alterations in lipid and carbohydrate metabolism in sepsis. J Parenter Enter Nutr 1988;12:53S-58S.
18. Wiener M, Rothkopf MM, Rothkopf G, et al. Fat metabolism in injury and stress. Crit Care Clin North Am 1987;3:25-56.
19. Bach AC, Storck D, Meraihi Z. Medium-chain triglyceride-based fat emulsions: an alternative energy supply in stress and sepsis. J Parenter Enter Nutr 1988;12:82S-88S.
20. Mascioli EA, Babayan VK, Bistrian BR, et al. Novel triglycerides for special medical purposes. J Parenter Enter Nutr 1988;12:127S-132S.
21. Elwyn DH. Protein metabolism and requirements in the critically ill patient. Crit Care Clin North Am 1987;3:57-69.
22. Siegel JH. Physiologic and nutritional implications of abnormal hormone-substrate relations and altered protein metabolism in human sepsis. In Rombeau JL, Caldwell MD eds. Clinical nutrition, vol. II. Parenteral nutrition. Philadelphia: WB Saunders, 1986:555-574.
23. Freund HR. Parenteral nutrition in the septic patient. In Rombeau JL, Caldwell MD eds. Clinical nutrition, vol. II. Parenteral nutrition. Philadelphia: WB Saunders, 1986:533-554.
24. Cerra FB. Pocket manual of surgical nutrition. St Louis, CV Mosby, 1984.
25. Jeejeebhoy KN. Bulk or bounce—the object of nutritional support. J Parenter Enter Nutr 1988;12:539-549.
26. Doekel RC, Zwillich CW, Scoggen CH, et al. Clinical semistarvation: depression of the hypoxic ventilatory response. N Engl J Med 1976;295:358-365.
27. Weissman C, Hyman AI. Nutritional care of the critically ill patient with respiratory failure. Crit Care Clin North Am 1987;3:185-203.
28. Askanazi J, Weissman C, Rosenbaum SH, et al. Nutrition and the respiratory system. Crit Care Med 1982;10:163-172.
29. Klahr S, Tripathy K, Garcia FT, et al. On the nature of the renal concentrating defect in malnutrition. Am J Med 1967;43:84-96.
30. Klahr S, Tripathy K, Lotero H. Renal regulation of acid-base balance in malnourished man. Am J Med 1970;48:325-331.
31. Dixon RL, Shultice RW, Fouts JR. Factors affecting drug metabolism by liver microsomes. IV. Starvation. Proc Soc Exp Biol Med 1960;103:333-335.
32. Quinn T, Askanazi J. Nutrition and cardiac disease. Crit Care Clin North Am 1987;3:167-184.
33. Garre MA, Boles JM, Youinou PY. Current concepts in immune derangement due to undernutrition. J Parenter Enter Nutr 1987;11:309-313.
34. Sheffy BE. Nutrition, infection, and immunity. Compend Contin Educ Pract Vet 1985;7:990-996.
35. Feldman BF, Thomson DB. Fibronectin: its diagnostic and therapeutic implications. J Am Anim Hosp Assoc 1983;19:1027-1030.
36. Forley BG. Protein-calorie malnutrition, immunologic function, and total parenteral nutrition in the surgical patient. Mt Sinai J Med 1985;52:148-157.
37. Studley HO. Percentage of weight loss: a basic indicator of surgical risk in patients with chronic peptic ulcer. JAMA 1936;106:458.

38. Meguid MM, Mughal MM, Meguid V, et al. Risk-benefit analysis of malnutrition and perioperative nutritional support: a review. Nutr Int 1987;3:25-34.

39. Costa G, Donaldson S. The nutritional effects of cancer and its therapy. Nutr Cancer 1980;2:22.

40. Albina JE, Koruda MJ, Rombeau JL. Perioperative total parenteral nutrition. In Rombeau JL, Caldwell MD, eds. Clinical nutrition, vol. II. Parenteral nutrition. Philadelphia: WB Saunders, 1986:370-379.

41. Twomey PL, Patching SC. Cost-effectiveness of nutritional support. J Parenter Enter Nutr 1985;9:3-10.

42. Buzby GP, Mullen JL. Nutritional assessment. In Rombeau JL, Caldwell MD, eds. Clinical nutrition, vol. I. Enteral and tube feeding. Philadelphia: WB Saunders, 1984:127-147.

43. Hooley R, Williams CS, Muray RL, et al. Identifying the patient at nutrition risk. In Krey SH, Muray RL, eds.: Dynamics of nutrition support. Norwalk, CT: Appleton-Century-Crofts, 1986:51-181.

44. Cox JH, Hohenbrink K, Lang CE, et al. Nutritional assessment in critical care. In Lang CE, ed. Nutritional support in critical care. Rockville, MD: Aspen, 1987:1-90.

45. Baker JP, Barrocas A, Eliades J, et al. Open forum: nutritional assessment, present and future. Nutr Supp Serv 1988, November 7-11, 23, 24.

46. Jensen TG. Determination of nutritional status in critical care. J Am Diet Assoc 1984;84:1345-1348.

47. Detsky AS, Baker JP, O'Rourke K, et al. Predicting nutrition-associated complications for patients undergoing gastrointestinal surgery. J Parenter Enter Nutr 1987;11:440-446.

48. Lippert AC. Total parenteral nutrition in dogs and cats. In Proceedings of the American College of Veterinary Internal Medicine, San Diego: American College of Veterinary Medicine, 1987:905.

49. Armstrong PJ, Lippert AC. Selected aspects of enteral and parenteral nutritional support. Semin Vet Med Surg Small Anim 1988;3:216-226.

50. Wheeler SL, McGuire BH. Enteral nutritional support. In Kirk RW, ed. Current veterinary therapy X. Philadelphia: WB Saunders, 1989:30-37.

51. Crowe DT. Understanding the nutritional needs of critically ill or injured patients. Vet Med 1988;83:1224-1249.

52. Lewis LD, Morris ML, Hand MS. Small animal clinical nutrition, ed. 3. Topeka: Mark Morris, 1987: pp. 1-12 to 1-17.

53. Kleiber M. The fire of life. Huntington, NY: Krieger, 1975:179-222.

54. ASPEN Board of Directors. Guidelines for the use of enteral nutrition in the adult patient. J Parenter Enter Nutr 1987;11:435-439.

55. Ingram WJ. Current issues in nutritional support. Nutr Supp Serv 1987;May:11.

56. Koruda MJ, Guenter P, Rombeau JL. Enteral nutrition in the critically ill. Crit Care Clin North Am 1987;3:133-153.

57. Crowe DT. Enteral nutrition for critically ill or injured patients—Part I. Compend Contin Educ Pract Vet 1986;8:603-613.

58. Bristol JB, Williamson RCN. Nutrition, operations, and intestinal adaptation. J Parenter Enter Nutr 1988;12:299-309.

59. Souba WW. The gut as a nitrogen-processing organ in the metabolic response to critical illness. Nutr Supp Serv 1988;May:15-22.

60. Macy DW, Ralston SL. Cause and control of decreased appetite. In Kirk RW, ed. Current veterinary therapy X. Philadelphia: WB Saunders, 1989:18-24.

61. Macy DW, Gasper PW. Diazepam-induced eating in anorexic cats. J Am Anim Hosp Assoc 1985;21:17-20.

62. Crowe DT. Clinical use of an indwelling nasogastric tube for enteral nutrition and fluid therapy in the dog and cat. J Am Anim Hosp Assoc 1986;22:675-682.

63. Bohning RH, DeHoff WD, McElhinney A, et al. Pharyngostomy for maintenance of the anorectic animal. J Am Vet Med Assoc 1970;156:611-615.

64. Lantz GC. Pharyngostomy tube installation for the administration of nutritional and fluid requirements. Compend Contin Educ Pract Vet 1981;3:135-142.

65. Crowe DT. Enteral nutrition of critically ill or injured patients—Part II. Compend Contin Educ Pract Vet 1986;8:719-732.

66. Lantz GC, Cantwell HD, VanVleet JF, et al. Pharyngostomy tube induced esophagitis in the dog: an experimental study. J Am Anim Hosp Assoc 1983;19:207-212.

67. Crowe DT, Downs MO. Pharyngostomy complications in dogs and cats and recommended technical modifications: experimental and clinical investigations. J Am Anim Hosp Assoc 1986;22:493-503.

68. Mathews KA, Binnington AG. Percutaneous incisionless placement of a gastrostomy tube utilizing a gastroscope: preliminary observations. J Am Anim Hosp Assoc 1986;22:601-610.

69. Armstrong PJ, Hardie EM. Percutaneous endoscopic gastrostomy. Vet Med Rep. In press.

70. Armstrong PJ, Hardie EM. Percutaneous endoscopic gastrostomy: a retrospective study of 54 clinical cases in dogs and cats. J Vet Intern Med. In press.

71. Crane SW. Placement and maintenance of a temporary feeding tube gastrostomy in the dog and cat. Compend Contin Educ Pract Vet 1980;2:770-780.

72. Orton EC. Enteral hyperalimentation administered via needle catheter-jejunostoma as an adjunct to cranial abdominal surgery in dogs and cats. J Am Vet Med Assoc 1986;188:1406-1411.

73. Heimburger DC, Weinsier RL. Guidelines for evaluating and categorizing enteral feeding formulas according to therapeutic equivalence. J Parenter Enter Nutr 1985;9:61-67.

74. Crowe DT. Enteral nutrition for critically ill or injured patients—Part III. Compend Contin Educ Pract Vet 1986;8:825-838.

75. Silk DBA, Fairclough PD, Clark ML, et al. Use of a peptide rather than free amino acid nitrogen source in chemically defined "elemental" diets. J Parenter Enter Nutr 1980;4:548-553.

76. Koretz RL, Meyer JH. Elemental diets—facts and fantasies. Gastroenterology 1980;78:393-410.

77. MacDonald ML, Anderson BG, Rogers QR, et al. Essential fatty acid requirements of cats: pathology of essential fatty acid deficiency. Am J Vet Res 1984;45:1310-1317.

78. Fischer JE, Funovics JM, Aguirre A, et al. The role of plasma amino acids in hepatic encephalopathy. Surgery 1975;78:276-290.

79. Fischer JE, Rosen HM, Ebeid AM, et al. The effect of normalization of plasma amino acids on hepatic encephalopathy in man. Surgery 1976;80:77-91.

80. Takala J. Nutrition in acute renal failure. Crit Care Clin North Am 1987;3:155-166.

81. Breach CL, Saldanha LG. Tube feeding complications. Part I: gastrointestinal. Nutr Supp Serv 1988;March:15-19.

82. Breach CL, Saldanha LG. Tube feeding complications. Part II: mechanical. Nutr Supp Serv 1988;May:28-32.

83. Marcuard SP, Stegall KL, Trogdon S. Clearing obstructed feeding tubes. J Parenter Enter Nutr 1989;13:81-83.

84. Breach CL, Salhanha LG. Tube feeding complications. Part III: metabolic. Nutr Supp Serv 1988;June:16-19.

85. Lippert AC, Armstrong PJ. Parenteral nutritional support. In Kirk RW, ed. Current veterinary therapy X. Philadelphia: WB Saunders, 1989:25-30.

86. Raffe MR. Total parenteral nutrition. In Slatter DH, ed. Textbook of small animal surgery, vol. I. Philadelphia: WB Saunders, 1985:225-241.

87. ASPEN Board of Directors. Guidelines for the use of total parenteral nutrition in the hospitalized adult patient. J Parenter Enter Nutr 1986;10:650-658.

88. Sax HC, Bower RH. Hepatic complications of total parenteral nutrition. J Parenter Enter Nutr 1988;12:615-618.

89. Lippert AC, Faulkner JE, Evans AT, et al. Total parenteral nutrition in clinically normal cats. J Am Vet Med Assoc 1989;194:669-676.

90. Adamkin DH, Gelke KN, Andrews BF. Fat emulsions and hypertriglyceridemia. J Parenter Enter Nutr 1984;8.563-567.

91. Pelham LD: Rational use of intravenous fat emulsions. Am J Hosp Pharm 1981;38:198-208.

92. Brown R, Quercia R, Sigman R. Total nutrient admixture: a review. J Parenter Enter Nutr 1986;10:650-658.

93. Das JB, Joshi ID, Philippart AI. Intralipid tolerance in pancreatitis: the role of hepatic triglyceride lipase in plasma clearance of the lipid emulsion. J Pediatr Surg 1981;16:1021-1028.

94. Mazur HI, Stennett DJ, Egging PK. Extraction of diethylhexylphthalate from total nutrient solution containing polyvinyl chloride bags. J Parenter Enter Nutr 1989;13:59-62.

95. Wade J. Parenteral and enteral transition techniques. In Krey SH, Murray RL, eds. Dynamics of nutrition support: Assessment, implementation, evaluation. Norwalk, CT. Appleton-Century-Crofts, 1986:489-496.

96. Mashima Y. Effect of calorie overload on puppy livers during parenteral nutrition. J Parenter Enter Nutr 1979;3:139-145.

97. Murphy LM, Lipman TO. Central venous catheter care in parenteral nutrition. J Parenter Enter Nutr 1987;11:190-201.

98. Wolfe BM, Ryder MA, Nishikawa RA, et al. Complications of parenteral nutrition. Am J Surg 1986;152:93-99.

99. Krajden S. Cannula sepsis prevention in intravenous therapy. Nutr Supp Serv 1988;September:14-16.

100. Caprile KA, Spears KE. Long-term, cyclic total parenteral nutrition in the growing canine. In Proceedings of the American College of Veterinary Internal Medicine. San Diego: American College of Veterinary Internal Medicine, 1987:906.

101. Wagman LD, Miller KB, Thomas RB, et al. The effect of acute discontinuation of total parenteral nutrition. Ann Surg 1986;204:524-529.

102. Maki DG, Weise CE, Sarafin HW. A semiquantitative culture method for identifying intravenous catheter-related infection. N Engl J Med 1977;296:1305-1309.

38 Conventional and Hypertonic Fluid Therapy: Concepts and Applications

Matthew W. Miller, Eric R. Schertel, and Stephen P. DiBartola

The concept of the milieu interieur proposed by Claude Bernard in an 1859 lecture forms the basis of our understanding of the fluid environment of the body and its role in homeostasis.[1] Bernard described the complex interaction of the environment with blood and body fluids in simple and lucid terms: "Blood, driven to every region of the body, is returned to the center and, at once, sent back again. In this way blood is constantly coming into contact with every organic molecule of our tissues; at the same time, by means of certain special mechanisms, it is brought into close relationship with the external environment from which it obtains materials for the maintenance of the tissues and to which it gives up waste substances ... blood forms a true organic environment, intermediary between the external environment in which the individual as a whole lives and the molecules of the living cells." As clinicians, our management of fluid and electrolyte disorders must be based on a detailed knowledge of the physiologic processes that govern the fluid, electrolyte, and acid-base homeostasis that Bernard envisioned. We must not only understand the basic concepts of body fluid compartment volumes, composition, distribution, and their critical control mechanisms, but also understand the pathologic alterations that occur in various disease states. We must also know how to assess the degree of homeostatic alteration as well as to treat these alterations in an expedient and efficient manner.

Water is the solvent in which the inorganic and organic solutes of the body are dissolved. Water makes up about 60% of total body weight in the adult animal. This value varies considerably with age, sex, and the percentage of body weight made up by fat. Total body water (TBW) in the neonate may be as much as 75% of body weight, whereas in the severely obese adult, TBW may be only 35% of body weight. Females, because of an average higher percentage of body fat, have less TBW. The relation between the weight of fat-free tissue (lean body mass) and TBW, however, is remarkably constant—73% in the adult and 82% in the neonate (Fig. 38-1).

Total body water is anatomically compartmentalized into extracellular and intracellular fluid compartments, which each make up 50% of TBW (30% of body weight). The extracellular fluid (ECF) compartment is further subdivided into plasma volume (8% of TBW) and interstitial fluid volume (37% of TBW). A transcellular fluid volume makes up the balance (5%) of the ECF volume. The interstitial fluid compartment forms the fluid continuum between plasma and intracellular fluid, i.e., fluid between and around the cells of the body. Transcellular fluids are those produced in the gastrointestinal, biliary, and urinary tracts and the cerebrospinal system.

Sodium and potassium are the predominant cations of the body fluids. Calcium and magnesium are divalent cations that are present in much lower concentrations. Chloride and bicarbonate are the most important anions, with proteins and organic acids contributing the remainder of negative charges. It is important to consider not only the ion concentration of plasma, but also the total body stores of the major ions and the factors that affect their distribution.

Sodium is the predominant extracellular cation. Because of this, and because the extracellular fluid (particularly blood) is in constant exchange with the external environment through the urinary, gastrointestinal, respiratory, and integumentary systems, sodium plays the major role in

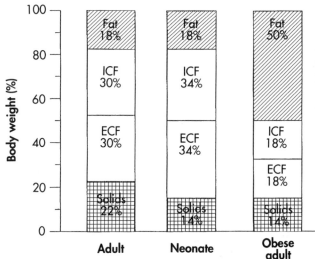

Fig. 38-1 Total body water makes up approximately 60% of body weight in the average adult animal *(Adult)*. In the neonate TBW ranges up to 75% of body weight *(Neonate)*. These values are in contrast to the *Obese Adult* in whom TBW may be only 35% of body weight.

maintaining extracellular and total body water constant. Alterations in plasma volume cause the body to either retain or excrete sodium. Only 75% of total body sodium is exchangeable; the nonexchangeable sodium is in the crystalline phase of bone. Approximately 85% of the exchangeable sodium is in extracellular water, the remainder is in intracellular and transcellular sites. The concentration of sodium in the extracellular fluid (serum sodium) reflects the tonicity of the ECF and the tonicity of the ECF reflects that of the entire body fluid. Since the most common clinical form of water imbalance is dehydration, measurement of the serum sodium concentration will indicate whether the loss has been in the form of hypotonic, isotonic, or hypertonic fluid. The extent of volume loss is more difficult to determine, but often can be estimated by clinical signs, for example, the degree of diminished skin turgor. The most common forms of fluid loss are isotonic and hypotonic, leaving the patient dehydrated with normal or elevated serum sodium concentration, respectively. Knowing the form of fluid imbalance guides replacement therapy with respect to the relative amounts of solute and water necessary to restore volume and tonicity to normal.

The majority of the body's potassium is intracellular and only 2% to 5% is present in the extracellular fluid. Potassium is almost entirely exchangeable. Since sodium is predominantly extracellular, measurement of its serum concentration provides an excellent assessment of total body sodium stores, whereas measurement of serum potassium concentration does not necessarily reflect total body potassium stores. Potassium loss in dehydrated patients can be significant despite normal serum potassium concentrations. Therefore, administration of fluids deficient in potassium may result in hypokalemia. Potassium depletion should be anticipated in dehydration and administered fluids should be supplemented with potassium.

The major forces responsible for water movement between body compartments are hydrostatic and osmotic. Hydrostatic pressure is provided by the mechanical contraction of the heart and the vasomotor tone of the peripheral vasculature. At the capillary level, where the greatest surface area for exchange occurs, the hydrostatic and osmotic forces balance to favor net movement of water and solutes to the interstitial space. As hydrostatic pressure falls along the capillaries, this net force is reversed returning the majority of fluid to the vascular space. The osmotic forces that balance the hydrostatic forces, described by Starling's law, are mainly the result of the relatively high plasma protein concentration. While all solutes provide osmotic forces along any concentration gradient, those that are least permeant to the endothelial membrane of the capillary contribute to the greatest extent.

The extracellular fluid and electrolyte distribution between vascular and interstitial spaces is strongly influenced by the difference in protein concentrations and the relative impermeability of the endothelium to protein. The colloid osmotic force created by the high concentration of protein in plasma is responsible in part for the basic filling pressure of the vasculature. The large impermeant negative charge of protein also contributes to an asymmetric distribution of ions between serum and interstitial fluid termed the "Gibbs-Donnan equilibrium." Changes in the permeability of the vascular endothelium to protein, diminished protein production, or active states of protein loss markedly affect the function of the cardiovascular and other organ systems. Organ dysfunction occurs with increased accumulation of interstitial fluid. Maintenance of adequate protein concentrations in the serum can be as important to homeostasis as adequate water and electrolytes. Albumin is the protein providing the dominant osmotic force.

The distribution of administered fluids in the body fluid compartments is dependent on the ionic composition of the fluids and the rate of administration. Administration of isosmotic solutions such as 0.9% sodium chloride produces no net movement of water across the cell membrane; thus, they expand primarily the extracellular space. An isosmotic solution of 5% glucose or 0.45% sodium chloride in 2.5% dextrose acts differently by expanding both the intracellular and extracellular spaces. These fluids are relatively low in sodium concentration and dilute the ECF sodium concentration. The metabolism of the glu-

cose contained in these fluids accentuates the hypotonicity of these fluids making the ECF hypotonic as compared to the ICV (intracellular fluid). The result is that water moves intracellularly. In acute fluid loss states (e.g., hemorrhage, diarrhea, vomiting), expansion of the vascular volume and the extracellular space is critical for restoration of normal hemodynamic function. This is best accomplished by fluids such as 0.9% sodium chloride or lactated Ringer's solution because Na^+ is distributed almost entirely within the extracellular space. Expansion of the extracellular space can be accomplished relatively quickly because of the rapid movement of water and Na^+ across the endothelium. Maximal recommended rates of fluid administration (shock doses) are 60 to 90 ml/kg per hour. At this rate, the entire extracellular volume can be replaced in 4 hours. An equivalent, or more rapid, means of expanding the extracellular and vascular space can be achieved by administering hyperosmotic sodium chloride solutions (Fig. 38-2). These solutions expand the vascular space initially by drawing fluid from the interstitial

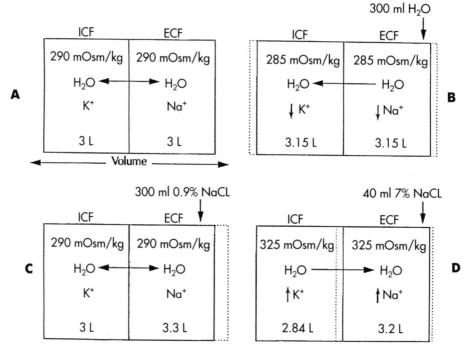

Fig. 38-2 A, Distribution of total body water between intracellular *(ICF)* and extracellular *(ECF)* fluid compartments, flux of water between compartments, relative Na^+ and K^+ concentrations and compartment volumes for an average 10-kg canine. **B,** Addition of 300 ml of H_2O expands ICF and ECF volumes equally, decreasing osmolality and electrolyte concentrations. **C,** Addition of 300 ml of isotonic saline (290 mOsm/kg) expands just the ECF volume. **D,** Addition of 40 ml of 7% sodium chloride (2400 mOsm/kg) expands the ECF volume by a translocation of H_2O from the ICF compartment. This raises osmolality and respective electrolyte concentrations in both compartments when equilibrium occurs.

spaces and then from the intracellular space to expand the entire extracellular space. The use of these solutions is discussed further at the end of the chapter.

ACID-BASE BALANCE

Acid-base balance is normally in a steady state because of constant production of carbon dioxide and fixed acids and their continuous removal by the respiratory system, metabolism, and renal excretion. Marked alterations in pH in response to the normal activities (exercise, eating, etc.) are almost entirely avoided by a very efficient buffering system. Hydrogen ions (H^+) from carbonic acid (H_2CO_3) are buffered by hemoglobin and bicarbonate (HCO_3^- carried in the plasma). This system enables the body to respond quickly to metabolic acid challenges by alterations in minute ventilation and blood carbon dioxide concentration. The kidneys are ultimately responsible for maintaining normal electrolyte and acid-base balance. Their influence is slow, requiring hours to days, but is generally very effective.

Acid-base balance is influenced by a multitude of factors, and therefore, it is very difficult to predict the pH accurately in any given patient. Metabolic acidosis and respiratory acidosis are the most common acid-base disorders in small animals, however, the degree of imbalance is not as easily predicted.[2] Blood pH measurement is critical to accurate assessment and treatment of acid-base imbalances. Measurement of partial pressure of carbon dioxide is helpful in determining the adequacy of a respiratory compensatory response or the presence of a mixed (respiratory and metabolic) acid-base disorder. Except in some extreme cases of pH imbalance, correction of the underlying disease process is often adequate for the body to reestablish pH balance.

Cardiac output and oxygen delivery have tremendous influence on acid-base balance. Anaerobic metabolism resulting from poor oxygen delivery to tissues initiates an excessive production of metabolic acids such as lactic acid and carbon dioxide. Increased production of acids combined with inadequate removal contribute to the lowered pH. Therefore, fluid administration to improve oxygen delivery and correct maldistribution of tissue perfusion plays a critical role in correction of this component of pH imbalance. The only major exception to this general rule is congestive heart failure, in which fluid therapy may be inappropriate; in this circumstance enhancing cardiac function plays the crucial role in resuscitation and pH stabilization.

Electrolyte disturbances are at least secondary effects of pH imbalance and are thought by some to have a primary role in influencing pH balance.[3] Potassium abnormalities are the most commonly seen electrolyte disturbance. Low blood pH is associated with an intracellular production of H^+ that is responsible for a redistribution of intracellular K^+ to an extracellular location, resulting in increased serum potassium concentration. Hyperkalemia generally occurs only secondary to metabolic acidosis. In general, a plasma pH change of 0.1 unit produces an inverse change in serum K^+ of 0.4 to 0.6 mEq/L. The other common acid-base imbalance in which electrolyte abnormalities occur is metabolic alkalosis secondary to chronic vomiting. The alkalosis is due to loss of hydrochloric acid from the stomach, and hypochloremia is a consequence.

When blood gas analysis is not available, there are indirect methods for clinical evaluation of acid-base status. Urine pH provides a crude indicator of severe derangements. In general, when urine pH is less than 5.0 there is an acidemia and when urine pH is greater than 8.0 there is an alkalemia. Hypochloremia is the condition that most commonly complicates the use of urine pH as an indicator of acid-base status. Volume depletion associated with alkalosis and hypochloremia will produce a paradoxical aciduria, thus limiting the usefulness of urine pH measurement under these conditions.

ALTERATIONS OF HYDRATION STATUS

The vast majority of alterations of hydration status involve conditions of fluid deficit. Knowledge of the classic hydration alterations associated with given metabolic abnormalities will aid the clinician in the establishment of logical fluid therapy strategies. The reader is directed to chapters dealing with specific disease states for further discussion of specific fluid, electrolyte and acid-base abnormalities.[4-7] Although there are typical metabolic derangements associated with certain disease states, there is no substitute for accurate serial evaluation of serum electrolytes, other serum biochemistries, and acid-base status in the optimal management of fluid disorders.

Conditions involving fluid excess states are uncommonly encountered in veterinary medicine as compared with fluid deficit situations. They occur when capillary hemodynamics favor movement of fluid into the interstitial space and when sodium and water are retained by the kidney.[8] Edema, or venous congestion, is the most important sequela to fluid excess and may be life threatening if the fluid accumulation is in the form of pulmonary or central nervous system edema. There are several causes of edema formation, including congestive heart failure, hepatic cirrhosis, and nephrotic syndrome. It is important to remember that iatrogenic overhydration is often associated with inappropriate fluid therapy and constitutes one of the most common fluid excess states.

ASSESSMENT AND MONITORING

The most reliable way to assess the extent of dehydration in a patient is to compare the patient's current weight to a weight obtained prior to the onset of dehydration. Acute weight loss is most commonly caused by fluid loss, and every kilogram reduction in body weight corresponds to 1 L of fluid loss. The patient's previous weight frequently is not available for comparison, therefore the clinician must rely on less-accurate estimates of hydration status.

Evaluations of skin turgor, mucous membrane moistness, heart rate, and eye position within the orbits to estimate dehydration are inaccurate estimations of hydration. Animals that have been panting excessively may have dry mucous membranes, which may lead to an overestimation of the degree of dehydration. Emaciated animals may have sunken eyes and alterations in skin elasticity that will lead to overestimation of the severity of dehydration. Obesity usually results in an underestimation of dehydration when based on skin turgor or eye position. Although clinical estimates have inherent potential for error, careful physical examination coupled with laboratory data can provide the clinician with valuable information concerning hydration status.

Laboratory tests that are commonly used to evaluate animals for evidence of dehydration include hematocrit, total serum protein, blood urea nitrogen and creatinine concentrations, and urine specific gravity. It is important to obtain samples for these tests prior to initiating fluid therapy. In the severely dehydrated animal, values for all of the aforementioned tests should be increased, assuming no concurrent problems exist. It should be stressed that these laboratory values do not give a quantitative estimate of dehydration and are influenced by concurrent disease states (anemia, hypoproteinemia, renal disease, drug administration, etc.). Serial evaluation of these tests will provide important information regarding adequacy of fluid therapy. Frequent measurement of body weight is one of the best ways to monitor the patient during fluid therapy.

Central venous pressure (CVP) is the pressure within the intrathoracic cranial vena cava. The CVP is a measure of the filling pressure of the right heart and an indication of the ability of the heart to pump the quantity of blood being returned to it. The CVP will increase with right-heart failure, venoconstriction, and hypervolemia

and decrease with venodilation and hypovolemia. Phase of respiration affects CVP (inspiration causes a decrease), as will application of positive-pressure ventilation (increase), necessitating that the CVP always be measured at end expiration.

Normal CVP ranges from 0 to 5 cm H_2O. Values below 0 suggest inadequate cardiac filling pressures and, most commonly, hypovolemia. During fluid administration an increase of more than 4 cm H_2O warrants consideration for a reduction in rate or temporary cessation of fluid administration. Sudden elevations of CVP may represent cardiac pump failure and may be a harbinger of congestive heart failure (edema formation). Elevated CVP is not always a contraindication to fluid administration but fluid administration in the face of elevated CVP must be performed with great caution. In conditions of severe dehydration or reduced cardiac output, marked increases in sympathetic tone may cause venoconstriction and elevated CVP in the face of hypovolemia.[9,10] Evaluation of all available data (physical examination, laboratory values, measurement of systemic arterial blood pressure) may suggest administration of fluids in the face of an elevated CVP. If the initial fluid load leads to increased cardiac output and withdrawal of excessive sympathetic tone the CVP will fall. If the CVP continues to climb during fluid administration, fluids should be discontinued and the cause for the elevated CVP pursued.

FLUID VOLUME AND COMPOSITION

Once a fluid deficit state has been identified, the volume and composition of fluid to be administered must be determined. Fluid requirements can be broken down into three general categories: existing deficit, maintenance requirements, and contemporary or ongoing losses. The existing deficit is usually based on an estimation of percent dehydration determined by clinical parameters (Table 38-1). Maintenance requirements vary from 40 to 60 ml/kg per day. Small dogs, cats, puppies, and kittens require higher maintenance volumes than do larger mature animals. These requirements can be further divided into sensible and insensible fluid needs. Sensible fluid loss is comprised of urine output (25 to 45 ml/kg per day), while the insensible portion is due to respiratory and fecal loss (15 to 20 ml/kg per day).[2,11]

Contemporary losses are the most frequently overlooked portion of a fluid therapy regimen. Fluid loss secondary to polyuria, vomiting, and diarrhea are commonly underestimated or disregarded. Contemporary fluid loss is frequently significant, and its omission from calculated fluid needs can be the difference between therapeutic

Table 38-1 Clinical signs of dehydration

Percent Dehydration	Clinical Signs
<5	Not detectable
5 to 6	Subtle loss of skin elasticity
6 to 8	Definite delay in return of skin to normal position; slight prolongation of capillary refill time; eyes possibly sunken in orbits; possibly dry mucous membranes
10 to 12	Tented skin stands in place;definite prolongation of capillary refill time; eyes sunken in orbits; dry mucous membranes; possibly signs of shock (tachycardia, cool extremities, rapid and weak pulses)
12 to 15	Definite signs of shock; death imminent

From Cornelius LM. Fluid therapy in small animal practice, J Am Vet Med Assoc 1980;176:110-123.

success and failure. Estimation of contemporary fluid loss can be difficult when it is due to burns, drains, panting, or large wounds. Several general rules are helpful in quantifying ongoing loss: each saturated 4-by-4-in. gauze sponge contains 15 ml of blood, the volume of urine in milliliters equals 0.84 times the radius^2 (inches) of the spot of urine, the volume of diarrhea in milliliters equals 0.52 times the radius^2 (inches) of the spot of diarrhea.

Example
A 20-kg dog is estimated to be 8% dehydrated and during the initial hospitalization period produces 175 ml of diarrhea:

Existing deficit: 20 kg × 0.08 × 1000 ml/kg	= 1600 ml
Maintenance: 50 ml/kg/day × 20 kg	= 1000 ml
Contemporary loss: 175 ml	= 175 ml
Total 24-hour fluid needs	2775 ml

Once the existing fluid deficit is replaced, normal hydration status can be maintained by providing maintenance needs coupled with contemporary fluid losses. Not only do fluid volumes need to be adjusted throughout therapy but fluid composition must also be altered.

Table 38-2 Available Fluid Solutions (mEq/L)

	Na	Cl	K	Ca	Mg	Lactate/Acetate	Osm/L	pH	Cal/L
Plasma (dog)	142	105	4.5	5	2	24	280-300	7.4	3.4
Lactated Ringer's solution	130	109	4	3	0	28	272	6.5	N.D.
Ringer's solution	147	157	4	5	0	0	314	N.D.	0
0.85% saline ("normal")	145	145	0	0	0	0	290	N.D.	0
0.9% saline	154	154	0	0	0	0	308	5.0	0
3% saline	513	513	0	0	0	0	1026	N.D.	0
0.45% saline in 2.5% dextrose	77	77	0	0	0	0	280	4.5	85
5% dextrose in water	0	0	0	0	0	0	252	4.0	170
10% dextrose in water	0	0	0	0	0	0	505	4.0	340
Lactated Ringer's with 5% dextrose	130	109	4	3	0	28	524	5.0	170
5% dextrose in 0.45% saline	77	77	0	0	0	0	406	4.0	170
Normosol-M	40	40	13	0	3	16	115	N.D.	N.D.
Normosol-R	140	98	5	0	3	27 acetate	299	6.2	N.C.
Normosol-M in 5% dextrose in water	40	40	13	0	3	16	365	5.5	170
50% dextrose	0	0	0	0	0	0	2520		1700
10% mannitol	0	0	0	0	0	0	549	N.D.	0
15% mannitol	0	0	0	0	0	0	823	N.D.	0
20% mannitol	0	0	0	0	0	0	1097	N.D.	0
7.5% N$_a$HCO$_3$	892	0	0	0	0	892 HCO$_3$	1784	N.D.	0

ND = not determined.

There are a wide variety of fluids commercially available (Table 38-2). The type of fluid chosen should be based on the underlying disease process and resultant metabolic alterations. The clinician should attempt to replace losses with fluids of similar volume and composition. Knowledge of the disease process combined with electrolyte and biochemical evaluations will aid in selection of the correct fluid solution for replacement or maintenance fluid therapy.

The composition of the various fluid solutions is significantly different, and knowledge of these differences is imperative to enable the clinician to provide optimal care. Maintenance fluids differ substantially from replacement fluids in their concentration of sodium and potassium. Maintenance fluids have much less sodium and more potassium than replacement fluids. Long-term administration of replacement fluids will cause hypernatremia and hypokalemia.[12] Maintenance fluids, on the other hand are poor choices for volume restoration because of their low sodium concentration. Most fluid balance alterations can be adequately handled with administration of lactated Ringer's solution, 0.9% sodium chloride, 5% dextrose in water, or 0.45% sodium chloride and 2.5% dextrose.[11]

POTASSIUM AND SODIUM

Potassium is primarily an intracellular electrolyte; therefore, serum potassium concentrations do not always reflect total body potassium stores. Knowledge of disease states associated with increases or decreases in potassium stores will aid in anticipating potassium requirements.

Severe hyperkalemia represents a potentially life-threatening electrolyte disturbance and requires prompt, aggressive therapy. It is most commonly associated with oliguric renal failure, hypoadrenocorticism, urinary tract rupture, urinary tract obstruction or severe metabolic acidosis. Several treatment methods have been advocated for hyperkalemia, including aggressive saline diuresis, intravenous administration of 1 to 2 mEq/kg sodium bicarbonate and infusion of glucose-containing fluids with or without concurrent administration of insulin. Saline diuresis increases renal excretion of potassium, while sodium bicarbonate as well as glucose and insulin infusions lead to intracellular translocation of potassium. Slow intravenous infusion of 0.3 to 0.5 ml/kg of 10% calcium gluconate will not lower serum potassium levels but will protect the heart from the effects of hyperkalemia.[13] These treatment methods are short-term measures to lower serum potassium acutely and must be combined with therapy directed at the underlying cause.

Hypokalemia is probably the most common electrolyte abnormality encountered in veterinary medicine. Depending on the severity of hypokalemia clinical signs can be absent or range from cardiac arrhythmias to severe weakness including respiratory or cardiovascular failure. Mild to moderate reductions in serum potassium concentrations may result in no clinical signs, but they may have a profound influence on the response to some therapeutic interventions. Hypokalemia markedly reduces the efficacy of some cardiac drugs, most notably the Class I antiarrhythmic drugs (e.g., lidocaine, procainamide). Hypokalemia also predisposes animals to digitalis intoxication. This becomes very important because among the myriad of causes of hypokalemia (vomiting, diarrhea, anorexia, metabolic alkalosis, glucose and insulin administration, renal disease) is the use of certain diuretics such as furosemide, a drug commonly used in concert with digitalis and antiarrhythmics.

Therapy for hypokalemia will depend on the severity of the deficit as well as the animal's underlying disease(s). Mild deficits in animals that are eating and drinking will frequently correct themselves or can be managed with oral supplementation. In severely hypokalemic animals or in those who cannot tolerate oral potassium supplementation, intravenous or subcutaneous administration is indicated. Recommendations for potassium supplementation can be found in Table 38-3. Potassium infusion is a very safe practice as long as the infusion rate does not exceed 0.5 meq/kg per hour.

Sodium is the major extracellular cation. Vascular fluid volume is determined primarily by renal resorption of sodium and water. Serum sodium concentration may be increased, normal, or decreased in the dehydrated patient, depending on the relative amounts of sodium and water lost. Like serum potassium concentration, serum sodium concentration is not always an accurate indicator of total body sodium stores. Serum sodium concentration reflects the tonicity of the body fluids.

Table 38-3 R.C. Scott's scale for gradual K^+ replacement

Serum K^+ (mEq/L)	No. of mEq K^+ to Add to 250 ml Fluids	Maximal Infusion Rate (ml/kg/hr)
<2.0	20	6
2.1-2.5	15	8
2.6-3.0	10	12
3.1-3.5	7	16

From Dr. R.C. Scott, Animal Medical Center, New York.

Therapy for hyponatremia consists of infusion of sodium-rich fluids. Isotonic solutions such as 0.9% sodium chloride most commonly are employed. Correction of hypernatremic conditions requires administration of sodium-poor fluids such as 5% dextrose in water or 0.45% sodium chloride with 2.5% dextrose (see Chapter 18). Rapid reduction in extracellular sodium concentrations and therefore osmolality may lead to the development of cerebral edema. This is especially true in animals that have had chronic hyperosmolal states. Gradual lowering of serum sodium concentrations (1 to 2 mEq/L per hour) is prudent; suggesting the use of 0.45% sodium chloride with 2.5% dextrose in most cases.[11] The water deficit in a hypernatremic animal can be estimated from the following formula:

Water deficit (milliliters of dextrose in water) = 0.4 × body weight (kg) × (plasma $[Na^+]$/140 − 1).

HYPERTONIC SALINE/DEXTRAN SOLUTIONS

Over the past 10 years there has been a resurgence of interest in the use of hypertonic sodium chloride solutions as an alternative form of therapy for the treatment of shock. Before 1980, mildly hypertonic solutions (600 to 1800 mOsm/L) were found to be useful in the treatment of burn and hemorrhagic shock, but no real advantages over other forms of therapy involving isotonic solutions had been demonstrated. In 1980, investigators from Brazil demonstrated that small volumes of hypertonic saline solution were adequate to produce dramatic resuscitative effects in dogs in severe hemorrhagic shock.[14] In a shock model with blood loss approximating 40% of the blood volume, 4 ml/kg of 7% sodium chloride (2400 mOsm/L) injected as a slow intravenous bolus produced rapid and sustained improvements in cardiac output, arterial blood pressure, splanchnic blood flow and acid-base status. While similar results can be obtained with isotonic fluids, the efficacy and economy of this form of therapy drew immediate attention, particularly for its potential use in the field management of trauma victims and for its relative ease and speed of administration.

Subsequent studies in dogs by the same group of investigators suggested that the resuscitative effects of hypertonic saline were dependent on the stimulation of a lung afferent nerve-mediated reflex that traveled up the vagus nerves.[15-17] These studies also suggested that hypertonic saline did not induce a significant expansion of blood volume and, therefore, the reflex changes were critical to its resuscitative effects. The reflex-induced changes responsible for resuscitation were thought to include venoconstriction and a redistribution of cardiac output to favor splanchnic and renal blood flow.[16,17] The primary evidence for this theory was based on the findings that dogs vagotomized prior to treatment with hypertonic saline were not successfully resuscitated.

More recent studies in dogs and sheep have suggested that plasma volume expansion does indeed play a principal role in the resuscitative effects of hypertonic saline. The 4 ml/kg dose induces a plasma volume expansion in the dog of approximately 20 ml/kg[18] and in sheep approximately 8 ml/kg.[19] In a study of the effects of 7% sodium chloride on the mechanical properties of the systemic circulation, hypertonic saline administration to hypovolemic dogs did not induce significant venoconstriction or other changes in the mechanical properties of the systemic circulation that influenced venous return.[20] This study concluded that hypertonic saline administration improves venous return and cardiac output by plasma volume expansion. The involvement of a vagal reflex induced by hypertonic saline has also been questioned.[21] Evidence suggests that the vagus nerves are critical to circulatory control during hypovolemia in the dog, and therefore, previous studies involving the influence of vagotomy on the resuscitative effects of hypertonic saline must be reconsidered. Thus, the majority of the current evidence points to plasma volume expansion as the principal mechanism by which hypertonic saline solutions enhance circulatory function.

The addition of 6% dextran-70 to 7% sodium chloride solution has been demonstrated in sheep[22] and, in dogs[18] to potentiate and sustain the resuscitative effects of hypertonic saline. The addition of dextran stabilizes the plasma volume expansion of hypertonic saline by providing an oncotic force to replace that lost during hemorrhage.

The use of hypertonic saline fluids in experimental *Escherichia coli* endotoxic shock in dogs has also been investigated.[23,24] In one study, a moderately hypertonic saline solution (1200 mOsm/L sodium chloride) was compared with isotonic saline; both solutions being given as needed to maintain atrial filling pressures at control level.[23] Atrial pressures were similar in the two groups, but cardiac output and oxygen consumption were significantly higher in the hypertonic group. The volume of hypertonic solution necessary to produce these effects was 25% less than that needed of the isotonic solution. In a second study, equal sodium loads of a hypertonic and isotonic fluid produced similar hemodynamic responses.[24] The volume of hypertonic fluid used in this study was just 12% of the isotonic volume.

Resuscitation from hemorrhagic shock by infusion of isotonic saline is accompanied by elevations in intracranial pressure. In studies of experimental hemorrhagic shock in dogs, resuscitation with hypertonic saline was found to limit or prevent the elevation of intracranial pressure above control levels.[25] Resuscitation with isotonic solutions of colloid (10% dextran-40) did produce elevations in intracranial pressure. While these elevations may not lead to cerebral edema in all shock patients, patients with head injury may be more likely to develop cerebral edema when resuscitated with isotonic saline or colloid solutions. In a study in dogs in whom head injury was mimicked by inflation of an epidural balloon and combined with hemorrhagic shock, hypertonic saline limited cerebral edema as compared with isotonic or colloid resuscitation.[26]

Hypertonic saline resuscitation of hemorrhagic shock does not increase extravascular lung water and does not compromise pulmonary function or respiratory system mechanics.[27] When hypertonic saline was given in a canine model of oleic acid-induced lung injury, oxygen delivery was improved and there were minimal changes in pulmonary function.[28]

In an experimental study comparing small volumes of 7% sodium chloride in 6% dextran-70 solution to conventional large-volume isotonic solution therapy of experimentally induced gastric dilatation-displacement-induced shock, the hypertonic solution given at 5 ml/kg over 5 minutes followed by maintenance fluid therapy produced a more effective and sustained resuscitation than did 60 ml/kg of lactated Ringer's solution given over 60 minutes followed by maintenance fluid therapy.[29] The dogs were monitored for 3 hours after initiation of treatment and dogs in the hypertonic-solution-treated group were found to have significantly better cardiac outputs and suffered less hemodilution than the isotonic-solution-treated group. No adverse effects were observed in this study.

In human clinical studies of use of hypertonic saline solution, beneficial effects have been demonstrated over conventional forms of therapy. In the first report of the use of 7% sodium chloride in humans, patients in various forms of shock and unresponsive to conventional therapy were treated with hypertonic saline. The patients responded well with no adverse effects, and 9 of 11 patients recovered.[30] In a better-controlled study, 7% sodium chloride in 6% dextran-70 was compared in a blind fashion to equal-volume isotonic fluid therapy of trauma patients being transported to the hospital.[31] On arrival at the hospital, patients receiving the hypertonic solution had significantly higher arterial pressures and ultimately higher survival rate. In a hospital study in which a mildly hypertonic solution (500 mOsm/L) was compared to isotonic fluid therapy for management of surgically induced hypovolemia related to abdominal aortic aneurysm repair, systemic arterial blood pressures, atrial filling pressures, and cardiac output were appropriately sustained with less total fluid administration in the hypertonic fluid treated groups of patients.[32] No veterinary clinical trials have been reported to date.

Serum sodium and osmolality are increased as a result of hypertonic saline administration. When small volumes (4 to 5 ml/kg) of 7% sodium chloride are given, osmolality rises approximately 28 mOsm/L by 10 minutes after administration, but returns to 12 mOsm/L above control by 4 to 12 hours.[33] Underlying the osmolality change are the increased serum sodium and chloride, which average approximately 13 mEq/L at 10 minutes postinfusion. No deleterious effects of these mild elevations in osmolality and sodium concentrations have been reported. Serum potassium has been found to fall in multiple studies after hypertonic saline administration.[19,32,33] This finding was initially thought to be a characteristic of this form of therapy, but more recently it has been shown that equal volume expansion with isotonic fluids produces similar decreases in serum potassium. The drop in serum potassium concentrations is generally mild, averaging approximately 0.8 mEq/L,[33] and has not been reported to be of significance in clinical studies.[29,31,33]

The available literature and our clinical experience with hypertonic saline and dextran solutions suggest that the primary indications for clinical use are treatment of hypovolemic, nonhemorrhagic shock, (traumatic shock, surgical shock, gastric dilatation-displacement-induced shock) and endotoxic shock. These hypertonic solutions should only be used as an adjunctive therapy directed at rapidly reestablishing circulatory function. The use of these fluids should be combined with other standard resuscitative measures to effect recovery of the patient from the signs of shock (Chapters 14 and 15).

The dosage for 7% saline or 7% saline in 6% dextran-70 is 3 to 5 ml/kg of body weight. These solutions should be infused slowly through a peripheral or central vein over 3 to 5 minutes. Treatment can be repeated if serum sodium values are not elevated significantly above normal.

The contraindications for the use of hypertonic saline/dextran solutions in small animal patients at this time should include hypernatremic or hyperosmotic states (e.g., moderate to severe dehydration of diabetic ketoacidosis). Dextrans and hypertonic saline solutions are known to diminish platelet function, and therefore, the combination may not be advisable in thrombocytopenia or in conditions in which blood loss is secondary to coagulopathy.[34] Cardiogenic and possibly hemorrhagic shock, anuric renal failure, and seizures are contraindications for the use of these fluids.

Certain precautions should be exercised in the use of these solutions. The importance of slow infusion must be stressed. Rapid infusion of hypertonic solutions results in reflex bradycardia, hypotension, and bronchoconstriction that, although transient, can be devastating to an animal in shock. Extravasation should be avoided, but otherwise, the effects of these solutions on the veins (i.e., thrombosis and phlebitis) are not significant. Recurrent hemorrhage has been the concern of some investigators; the rationale being that the rapid increases in arterial pressure and blood flow may act to break down early clot formation. This potential disadvantage must be weighed against the deleterious effects of prolonged shock resulting from slower resuscitative measures, but must be considered. Red blood cell lysis has not proved to be of concern; this is likely due to the greater resistance of red blood cells to hyperosmotic than to hyposmotic solutions. Caution should be exercised when considering the use of hypertonic solutions in the presence of cardiac arrhythmias, since the arrhythmogenic effects of hypertonic saline have not been investigated.

Sodium chloride solutions of 7% concentration and sodium chloride and dextran solutions are not yet available commercially. Sodium chloride solutions can be made up at 7% concentration using available sodium-rich fluids. One means of making a 7% solution is to add 60 ml of a commercially available 23.4% sodium chloride solution (LyphoMed, Rosemont, IL) to a 500-ml bag of 5% sodium chloride (Baxter Labs; Chicago). To make up 7% sodium chloride in 6% dextran-70, 33.0 gm of sodium chloride crystal is added to a 500-ml bag of 6% gentran-70 (Baxter Labs; Chicago). This procedure is accomplished by placing half of the crystals into the barrel of a 35-ml syringe and withdrawing in a sterile manner an adequate amount of Gentran to allow dissolution of the crystals. This solution is then infused back into the bag through a 0.22 μ filter to ensure sterility and removal of particulates. The remaining sodium chloride crystals are similarly treated. The shelf life of the mixed solution is approximately 3 months from the time of compounding.

It is our opinion that hypertonic saline and dextran solutions have great potential as adjunctive therapy for shock resuscitation in the veterinary patient. However, until clinical studies are completed to define the indications, contraindications, and precautions required for the administration of these solutions, caution should be exercised in their use. Our clinical experience suggests that these solutions can be used safely in dogs and cats by following the guidelines we have described.

REFERENCES

1. Bernard C. Lecons sur les Propriété Physiologiques et les Altérations Pathologiques des Liquides de l'Organisme, vol. 1. Paris: JB Balliere, 1859.
2. Cornelius LM. Fluid therapy in small animal practice. J Am Vet Med Assoc 1980;176:110-123.
3. Stewart PA. How to understand acid-base. A quantitative acid-base primer for biology and medicine. New York: Elsevier North-Holland, 1981.
4. Feldman EC, Nelson RW. Canine and feline endocrinology and reproduction. Philadelphia: WB Saunders, 1987:200-204, 274-301.
5. Peterson, ME. Hyperadrenocorticism. Vet Clin North Am Small Anim Pract 1984;14:735-737.
6. Ross LA. Fluid therapy for acute and chronic renal failure. Vet Clin North Am Small Anim Pract 1989;19:343-359.
7. Chew DJ, Carothers M. Hypercalcemia. Vet Clin North Am Small Anim Pract 1989;19:265-287.
8. Rose BD. Clinical physiology of acid-base and electrolyte disorders, ed. 2. New York: McGraw-Hill, 1984.
9. Haskins SC. A simple fluid therapy planning guide. Semin Vet Med Surg Small Anim 1988;3:227-236.
10. Allen JW, Teplick R. Assessment and management of the hypotensive patient. Semin Anesth 1989;3:195-204.
11. Muir WW, DiBartola SP. Fluid therapy. In Kirk RW, ed. Current veterinary therapy VIII. Philadelphia: WB Saunders, 1983:28-40.
12. Bell FW, Osborne CA. Maintenance fluid therapy. In Kirk RW, ed. Current veterinary therapy X. Philadelphia: WB Saunders, 1989:37-43.
13. Willard MD. Treatment of hyperkalemia. In Kirk RW, ed. Current veterinary therapy IX. Philadelphia: WB Saunders, 1986:94-101.
14. Velasco IT, Pontieri V, Rocha-e-Silva M, et al.. Hyperosmotic NaCl and severe hemorrhagic shock. Am J Physiol 1980;239:H664-H673.
15. Lopes OU, Pontieri V, Rocha-e-Silva M. et al. Hyperosmotic NaCl and severe hemorrhagic shock: role of the innervated lung. Am J Physiol 1981;241:H883-H890.
16. Lopes OU, Velasco IT, Guertzenstein PG, et al. Hypertonic sodium chloride restores mean circulatory filling pressure in severely hypovolemic dogs. Hypertension 1986;8(Suppl 1):I195-I199.
17. Rocha-e-Silva M, Negraes GA, Soares AM, et al. Hypertonic resuscitation from severe hemorrhagic shock: Patterns of regional circulation. Circ Shock 1986;19:165-175.
18. Velasco IT, Oliveisa MA, Oliveisa MA, et al. A comparison of hyperosmotic and hyperomcotic resuscitation from severe hemorrhagic shock in dogs. Circ Shock 1987;21:338.
19. Smith GJ, Kramer GC, Perron P, et al. A comparison of several hypertonic solutions for resuscitation of bled sheep. Surg Res 1985;39:517-528.
20. Schertel ER, Valentine AK, Rademakers AM, et al. Influence of 7% NaCl on the mechanical properties of the systemic circulation in the hypovolemic dog. Circ Shock. In press.

21. Schertel ER, Valentine AK, Allen DA, et al. Isotonic saline and hemorrhagic shock: role of the vagus. FASEB J 1989;3:A713.

22. Kramer GC, Perron PR, Lindsey G, et al. Small-volume resuscitation with hypertonic saline dextran solution. Surgery 1986;100:239-246.

23. Luypaert P, Vincent JL, Domb M, et al. Fluid resuscitation with hypertonic saline in endotoxic shock. Circ Shock 1986;20:311-320.

24. Mullins RJ, Hudgens RW. Hypertonic saline resuscitates dogs in endotoxin shock. J Surg Res 1987;43:37-44.

25. Gunnar WP, Merlotti GJ, Jonasson O, et al. Resuscitation from hemorrhagic shock. Alterations of the intracranial pressure after normal saline, 3% saline and dextran-40. Ann Surg 1986;204:686-692.

26. Gurrar W, Jonasson O, Merlotti G, et al. Head injury and hemorrhagic shock: Studies of the blood brain barrier and intracranial pressure after resuscitation with normal saline solution, 3% saline solution, and dextran-40. Surgery 1988;103:398-407.

27. Martins MA, Youres RN, Lin CA, et al. Hypovolemic shock resuscitation with hyperosmotic 7.5% NaC1: effects on respiratory system mechanics. Circ Shock 1988;26:147-155.

28. Johnston WE, Alford PT, Prough DS, et al. Cardiopulmonary effects of hypertonic saline in canine oleic acid-induced pulmonary edema. Crit Care Med 1985;13:814-817.

29. Allen DA, Schertel ER, Muir WW. Hypertonic saline/dextran resuscitation of experimental gastric dilatation displacement shock in the dog. Am J Vet Res. In press.

30. de Felippe J, Timoner J. Velasco IT, Lopes OU, Rocha e Silva M: Treatment of refractory hypovolaemic shock by 7.5% sodium chloride injections. *Lancet* 1980;2:1002-1004.

31. Rocha-e-Silva M, Velasco IT, Nogueira da Silva RI, et al. Hypertonic sodium salts reverse severe hemorrhagic shock: other solutes do not. Am J Physiol 1987; 253:H751-H762.

32. Reed RL, Johnston TD, Chen Y, et al: Hypertonic saline allers clotting times and plalelet aggregation. J Trauma 1991;31:8-14.

33. Shackford SR, Sise MJ, Fridlund PG, et al. Hypertonic sodium lactate versus lactated Ringer's solution for intravenous fluid therapy in operations on the abdominal aorta. Surgery 1983;94:41-51.

34. Reed RL, Johnston TD, Chen Y, et al: Hypertonic saline alters clothing times and platelet aggregation. J Trauma 1991;31:8-14.

39 Peritoneal Dialysis

Dennis J. Chew and M. Susan Crisp

Dialysis is the movement of water and solute (ionized and non-ionized molecules) across a semipermeable membrane in either direction between two compartments. This process is governed by diffusion, ultrafiltration, and solute drag.[1-7] Diffusion is the random motion of molecules from regions of high concentration to areas of low concentration.[5] This results in equal distribution of the solute and water on both sides of a membrane if the membrane is permeable to water and the solute, provided that enough time is allowed for equilibration. Diffusion occurs for each solute and for water according to individual concentration or activity gradients.[7,8] The rate of diffusion into the fluid compartment with initially low solute concentration progressively declines as the solute concentration in that compartment increases. The rate of diffusion into the initially low solute concentration compartment can be increased by stirring fluid in that compartment or by draining and adding fresh fluid that is free of solute. Increased temperature of fluid in either compartment increases diffusion following increased random molecular motion. Convective forces enhance solute movement when fluid moves rapidly from one compartment to another according to osmotic or hydrostatic pressure and is referred to as "solute drag."[6,9,10] This effect allows solute to be removed in addition to that moving by diffusion along a favorable concentration gradient, and can allow some solute movement against a concentration gradient. These convective forces do not result in the removal of all solutes in exact proportion to their individual compartment concentration because of sieving of charged particles across a semipermeable membrane. "Ultrafiltration" refers to the volume per unit time of water that has moved across a membrane as the result of osmotic or hydrostatic pressure.

The peritoneum is a semipermeable membrane between fluid of the peritoneal cavity and fluid of extracellular water. Water and solute can move either from blood to peritoneal cavity or from peritoneal cavity into blood. Normally, there is very little fluid within the peritoneal cavity; however, fluid can easily be administered there. The fluid type and volume that is instilled into the peritoneal cavity is called dialysate. The process of fluid infusion into the peritoneal cavity, dwell time within the peritoneal cavity, and drainage of fluid from the peritoneal cavity (effluent) is referred to as an "exchange." Clinical peritoneal dialysis includes a prescription for volume, chemical composition, and physical properties for dialysate, as well as the time allotment for infusion, dwell, and drainage. The direction and magnitude of solute and water movement can be manipulated to the patient's advantage by modifying the dialysis methods.

The main objective of peritoneal dialysis is to transfer uremic solutes from blood into dialysate as a partial substitute for failed renal excretory function. Urea nitrogen, creatinine, and phosphorus are such solutes that are easily measured, but many other uremic solutes also exist that may be removed during dialysis. Solutes can be transferred from dialysate to blood as commonly occurs with bicarbonate buffer (lactate, acetate, or bicarbonate) and calcium, but this transfer can also occur with glucose and potassium. Water can either be removed from or added to blood, depending on dialysis methods. Dialysis does not replace failed endocrine or metabolic functions of the kidneys.

Peritoneal dialysis has emerged as the most practical form of dialysis for veterinary patients. Hemodialysis is available at some referral centers, but high costs, need for technical expertise, and difficulty in its performance in animals weighing less than 13.6 kg limit its routine use.[11] Hemodialysis is more efficient than peritoneal dialysis in the removal of low-molecular-weight substances from the blood, but is less efficient in the removal of so-called middle molecules (molecular weight, 500 to 5000),[7] which may be important in the manifestation of uremia.

Peritoneal dialysis has been said to be available in some form to every veterinarian,[1] but this procedure can be complex and time consuming. Dialysis can be successfully instituted and followed in private practice, but it is advisable to refer these cases to centers with dialysis expertise and 24-hour critical care facilities. Unfortunately, dialysis in clinical veterinary medicine is often not considered until the patient is near death.

TYPES OF PERITONEAL DIALYSIS

Dialysis can be characterized both by the flow pattern for dialysate and by the time period in which dialysis occurs.[6,7,12] Continuous-flow dialysis occurs when fluid is constantly infused during a dialysis session through one catheter while simultaneously draining through another, dependent, catheter (peritoneal lavage). This technique is not commonly used presently. Intermittent-flow dialysis occurs when dialysate is infused and allowed to dwell for a variable period of time before drainage. Intermittent peritoneal dialysis entails a series of successive exchanges followed by a period when dialysate has been drained between sessions and no dialysis is occurring. Continuous peritoneal dialysis occurs when dialysate is always present within the peritoneal cavity except for a short period following drainage of old dialysate and infusion of fresh dialysate.[3,12] Dwell time during chronic continuous dialysis ranges from 4 to 10 hours.[12] (See below for more specific explanation of this technique.) This technique is called "chronic ambulatory peritoneal dialysis" (CAPD). Dwell time may be less than 1 hour during acute continuous dialysis. Tidal peritoneal dialysis maintains a reservoir of fluid within the peritoneal cavity at all times, from which only a part of the fluid is drained and fresh fluid reinfused periodically. This technique is considered a hybrid of intermittent and continuous dialysis techniques[12] and may have advantages over either technique alone. This technique has not been evaluated in veterinary patients.

Acute peritoneal dialysis is usually prescribed for 1 to 4 days for conditions that can quickly be managed (see indications below). Chronic peritoneal dialysis is prescribed for 4 to 30 days for animals with conditions that require a longer time for potential intrarenal healing to occur. Chronic peritoneal dialysis in humans provides maintenance of chronic renal failure lifelong or until renal transplantation can be performed (not often attempted in veterinary medicine).

EXPERIENCE WITH PERITONEAL DIALYSIS IN EXPERIMENTAL DOGS

Surgically anephric dogs survive 2 to 5 days if untreated.[13] Average survival increases to 5 days when a protein- and salt-restricted diet is fed. Continuous peritoneal irrigation and drainage through separate catheters (20 hours each day at a rate of 25 to 35 ml per minute) in 15 nephrectomized dogs resulted in a decline from an initial blood urea nitrogen concentration of 100 to 250 mg/dl to 20 to 50 mg/dl.[14] Subsequently, continuous peritoneal lavage was performed for 8 to 10 hours daily for maintenance. The three longest-living dogs in this experiment survived 6, 9, and 13 days; death was attributed to infection and not to inadequate control of uremia. Survival from 30 to 70 days was achieved when two daily exchanges of hypertonic dialysate were given to nephrectomized dogs using an intermittent technique.[13] Repeated 17-gauge needle punctures were used in this study, and the dialysate was allowed to remain in the peritoneal cavity for at least 3 hours. Serum creatinine concentrations ranged from 4.7 to 9.7 mg/dl, blood urea nitrogen concentrations from 58 to 93 mg/dl, and serum phosphate concentrations 6.0 to 9.0 mg/dl, while sodium, potassium, chloride, and bicarbonate concentrations were near normal following dialysis. Nitrogenous waste products could be reduced to near normal levels by using 8 to 16 exchanges daily.

Equilibration for urea and potassium in dialysate was 90% complete by 40 minutes and 98% complete by 60 minutes in a model of uremia induced by bilateral ureteral ligation in dogs. In the same study, equilibration for creatinine and phosphate was only 65% complete at 40 minutes, 80% complete at 60 minutes, and complete equilibration did not occur until after 2 hours; these longer periods were attributed to the larger molecular size of creatinine and phosphate.[1,2] Two hours were required for urea equilibration in another study of dogs.[13] A dwell time of 40 to 60 minutes was recommended for optimal solute removal in the first study since the most rapid diffusion for all these solutes occurred within the first 30 minutes.[1,2] It was possible to reduce the blood urea nitrogen from 250 mg/dl to 100 mg/dl and the creatinine from 15 mg/dl to 6 mg/dl at the end of seven consecutive hourly exchanges and to reduce serum potassium from about 8 mEq/L to below 5.0 mEq/L after five hourly exchanges in this same study using the Parker dialysis cannula. A dwell time of 30 to 60 minutes for at least four consecutive exchanges was considered necessary to improve significantly the metabolic condition of anuric dogs in this study.[1]

Five nephrectomized dogs that underwent dialysis using the column disk catheter (see "Chronic Access—Surgically Placed Catheters") survived from 37 to 83 days (mean ±SD, 54±19) with maintenance of blood urea nitrogen concentrations at 70 to 90 mg/dl, serum creatinine concentrations at 5 to 10 mg/dl, and serum phosphorus concentrations of 6 to 9 mg/dl (without use of intestinal phosphorus-binding agents). Three exchanges of 2 L each were performed daily, and the dextrose concentration was varied to prevent hypotension or weight gain. Dialysate effluent volume was greater than the infusion volume when the dwell time was 10 hours or less for both 1.5% and 4.5% dextrose dialysate solutions. Dialysate effluent volume was less than that infused when dwell times of 12 to 16 hours were employed. Protein loss in dialysate increased with longer dwell time in the same study, approaching an average of 5 g per day with the 1.5% solutions and 7.5 g per day with the 4.5% solutions.[15] Specific single amino acids (dl-serine, l-lysine, dl-alanine) added to dialysate were able to reduce daily losses of total amino acids and proteins into dialysate of dogs.[16]

Blood urea nitrogen concentration was maintained at 80 to 90 mg/dl and serum creatinine concentration at 8 to 9 mg/dl in one bilaterally nephrectomized dog maintained for 51 days on CAPD using the column disk catheter and three to four exchanges per day.[17] Chronic ambulatory peritoneal dialysis employing the column disk catheter resulted in survival for 54 days in another report of a bilaterally nephrectomized dog. Six exchanges of dialysate per day were administered to maintain a blood urea nitrogen concentration of 26 mg/dl to 53 mg/dl, a serum creatinine of 3.4 mg/dl to 7.0 mg/dl, and serum phosphate concentration of 2.7 mg/dl to 6.4 mg/dl (while the animal was on intestinal phosphate binders).[18]

Chronic ambulatory peritoneal dialysis employing the column disk catheter and four daily exchanges of dialysate resulted in the survival of two dogs for 49 and 67 days following bilateral ureteral ligation. Blood urea nitrogen concentration was maintained from 20 to 70 mg/dl and serum creatinine concentration from 4 to 8 mg/dl.[16]

The effects of dextrose in dialysate during CAPD using the column disk catheter were studied in four nephrectomized dogs.[19] Five daily exchanges of either 1.5% or 4.5% dextrose in Dianeal (Baxter; Deerfield, IL) were administered. Dialysate osmolality progressively declined over an 8-hour period for both 1.5% and 4.5% solu-

tions. This effect was attributed to dilution of glucose in the dialysate by ultrafiltrate and by the absorption of glucose from the dialysate. Ultrafiltration rate was nearly zero when the dialysate osmolality approached that of serum. Glucose concentration and osmolality steeply declined from the 4.5% dextrose dialysate during the first two to three hours, while that for the 1.5% dextrose was more gradual. Four exchanges of 1.5% dextrose solution with a 4-hour dwell and one exchange of 4.5% dextrose solution with an 8-hour dwell were estimated to result in 457.4 kcal absorbed from the dialysate and 1134 ml of ultrafiltrate added to the dialysate.[19] In another study of dogs, glucose disappeared from the dialysate over 2 to 6 hours, depending on the original concentration of dextrose (1, 2, or 3%).[13]

CLINICAL VETERINARY EXPERIENCE WITH DIALYSIS

The first clinical report concerning dialysis in uremic dogs involved the use of intermittent peritoneal dialysis. Treatment involved a dwell time of 2 hours during two or three exchanges per day of 400 to 2000 ml.[20] Dialysate was infused through a 16- or 18-gauge needle and drained with a 13-gauge 3-in. needle containing perforations at the tip. Another clinical report on peritoneal dialysis in uremic dogs described the successful use of a 12-gauge 1.5-in. needle for infusion and drainage. The catheter was kept in place throughout the exchange and was inserted 2 to 3 in. caudal and to the right of the umbilicus. During one or two daily exchanges, 700 to 1500 ml were infused for a dwell time of 30 minutes.[21] Dialysis in the animals in these reports was usually continued for 3 or 4 days; most of the dogs had acute renal failure due to nephritis, but prerenal azotemia was not ruled out. It is unlikely that these dogs would have had such complete and rapid resolution of azotemia following a minimal number of exchanges per day if the underlying renal lesions were severe.

A dog with nonoliguric acute intrinsic renal failure caused by ethylene glycol poisoning was dialyzed using the column disk catheter for 5 days. Exchanges were performed every 2 hours for the first 36 hours and then maintained at three exchanges per day for the next 3.5 days. Blood urea nitrogen concentration declined from approximately 200 mg/dl to 90 mg/dl and serum creatinine concentration from 9.0 mg/dl to 6.0 mg/dl after the first day of exchanges.[22]

A dog with oliguric, acute intrinsic renal failure associated with hypoadrenocorticism was supported by 21 consecutive 1.5-L hourly exchanges using the column disk catheter. Blood urea nitrogen concentration decreased from 188 to 106 mg/dl, serum creatinine concentration from 12.0 to 9.4 mg/dl, and serum phosphorus concentration from 15.0 to 12.2 mg/dl.[23]

Clinical peritoneal dialysis was reviewed in 25 dogs and 2 cats.[24] The column disk catheter was used in 15 patients, while a variety of chest tubes and "home-made" catheters were used in the others. Six to 24 exchanges per day were performed using an approximate volume of 40 ml/kg. Median values for serum creatinine concentration decreased by 28% to 64% while those for blood urea nitrogen decreased by 36% to 75% after 1.5 to 3.0 days of dialysis.

The use of CAPD has recently been described in a small dog (8 kg) in which a single large bag of dialysate (2 L) was used for multiple small-volume exchanges of 250 ml for four consecutive exchanges. The peritoneal effluent is drained back into the original reservoir bag, effectively diluting the uremic toxins. Dialysate is not wasted in this technique and there is less chance for bacterial contamination since bags are less frequently changed.[4]

Pleural dialysis using chronically indwelling commercial thoracic catheters and the pleura as the semipermeable membrane has been successfully used as an alternative to peritoneal dialysis in two dogs for 7 and 25 days[25]; this technique may deserve further consideration.

FACTORS AFFECTING PERITONEAL DIALYSIS

Characteristics of a specific solute and the peritoneum, composition of dialysate, and the methods for dialysis interact to determine the efficiency of solute and water clearance. Solute and fluid transport across the peritoneum can change with bacterial or chemical peritonitis, altered hydrostatic or interstitial pressures, and the systemic or local administration of hormones or drugs.

Molecular size, charge, steric configuration, and degree of protein-binding influence the kinetics of peritoneal dialysis. High-molecular-weight substances are not as readily cleared as those with lower molecular weight, nor are charged particles handled the same as those without charge. Solute with extensive plasma protein binding is not readily removed during peritoneal dialysis.[1,3,6,7]

The peritoneum: barriers to diffusion and ultrafiltration

The peritoneum is a continuous membrane that covers the internal abdominal organs (visceral peritoneum) and the abdominal wall (parietal peritoneum) and forms the mesentery.[6,26] The surface area of the peritoneum is very large but the area available for solute or fluid exchange is small because exchange only occurs across peritoneal capillaries and possibly terminal arterioles.[6] Less than 0.2% of the peritoneal surface area has been estimated to have functional area (pores) for exchange. Blood flow to peritoneal vessels far exceeds the maximal clearance for small solutes such as urea during peritoneal dialysis, suggesting that diffusion barriers rather than solute delivery are more important in limiting clearances.[6,7] Peritoneal blood flow becomes limiting during peritoneal dialysis when severe hypotensive shock exists.[6,7,27] Omentectomy, mesenterectomy, and abdominal evisceration did not alter acute peritoneal dialysis dynamics for glucose, urea, or inulin in a study of dogs.[26] The important portion of the peritoneal membrane used during dialysis remains to be definitively identified but it appears from these studies that the parietal peritoneum is likely.

The role of lymphatics in peritoneal dialysis has received little attention but could be important if lymphatic drainage is substantial. Peritoneal lymphatics are responsible for the isosmotic absorption of fluid, macromolecules, cells, bacteria, and particles.[28,29] Reduced ultrafiltration and solute clearance during CAPD in some human patients has been attributed to excessive lymphatic absorption.[28] End-lymphatics in the diaphragm (stomata) are responsible for most of the lymphatic drainage from the peritoneal cavity, while omental and mesenteric lymphatics make minor contributions. Unlike peritoneal capillaries, lymphatics exhibit one-way return of fluid to the circulation. Increased peritoneal lymphatic flow can follow increased intraperitoneal hydrostatic pressure (overfilling), exaggerated diaphragmatic movements (hyperventilation), and after chemical peritonitis. Lymphatic contractility is increased by several mediators of inflammation as occur in peritonitis.[28]

Diffusion and ultrafiltration from the peritoneal capillaries to peritoneal fluid is opposed by layers of fluid within the capillary lumen, capillary endothelial cells, capillary basement membrane, interstitium, mesothelial cells, and peritoneal cavity.[6,7,29] Transport of water and solute across endothelial or mesothelial cells may occur via vesicles, intercellular junctions, and/or transcytoplasmic routes. Additionally, transport through endothelial fenestrae may occur but there are few fenestrae in peritoneal capillaries.[6] The interstitium represents the longest individual component distance for solute and water to traverse from blood to peritoneal fluid and poses a barrier of extracellular fluid, connective tissue, lymphatics, and both gel-phase and free-phase mucopolysaccharides. The capillary basement membrane offers little resistance to all but the largest of molecules, while the mesothelium poses a barrier to molecules greater than 500,000 molecular weight.[6]

Junctions between endothelial cells or between mesothelial cells of the peritoneum can be tight or wide. The proportion of tight or wide junctions may determine how much fluid and solute travels across or between cells, but it is unclear for both cells which type of junction predominates and whether differences exist within different locations within the peritoneal cavity. Intercellular gaps in peritoneal capillary endothelium may be relatively large but few in numbers and are referred to as "pores."[6]

Mesothelial cells are covered with microvilli, which greatly increase surface area. Fluid may be trapped between microvilli normally to prevent friction between surfaces, but this feature may also promote stagnation of fluid and solute exchange during dialysis. The role of microvilli during peritoneal dialysis has not been clarified; microvilli may be important if transcellular fluid movement is more important than intercellular movement.[6] Surfactant properties of the surface of mesothelial cells repel fluid, which favors the one-way movement of fluid from capillaries into the peritoneal cavity.[29]

Peritonitis alters peritoneal blood flow, effective peritoneal surface area, or peritoneal permeability. Peritonitis can also result in the loss of mesothelial microvilli and increased diameter of intercellular gaps.[6] Chronic peritoneal dialysis during peritonitis in humans increases clearances of urea and creatinine, increases glucose absorption from dialysate, increases protein loss into dialysate, and decreases effluent drainage.[30] Acute peritoneal dialysis during acute bacterial or chemical peritonitis in normal dogs did not alter the clearance of urea or potassium, though protein loss increased into dialysate.[31] It appears that peritonitis does not reduce clearance of uremic solute during peritoneal dialysis.

The nature of the peritoneal membrane and efficiency of peritoneal dialysis in dogs may change with age. Puppies less than 1 month old exhibit greater peritoneal membrane permeability and increased functional peritoneal membrane surface area relative to body weight as compared with adult dogs.[32]

Composition of dialysate

Solute and water transport across the peritoneum is dependent on the type of dialysate solution to which the peritoneum is exposed.[33] Hypertonic dialysate is much more efficient than isotonic solutions in the removal of uremic solute.[9,10,34] So-

dium and attendant anions along with dextrose account for most of the osmolality within dialysate. Osmolality during standard dialysis is altered by varying the amount of dextrose in dialysate from a minimum of 1.5% to a maximum of 4.5%. Hypertonic dialysate increases solute clearance by a combination of solute drag following ultrafiltration, capillary vasodilation, increased pore diameter,[3] and dehydration of the peritoneal interstitium that alters interstitial aqueous channels.[6] Increased solute clearance following use of 4.25% dialysate may persist into subsequent exchanges using 1.5% dextrose or hypotonic dialysate.[10,33,35] Sequential exchanges using 4.25% dextrose dialysate can result in severe patient dehydration.[33,35] Consequently, alternating 4.5% dextrose with 1.5% dextrose dialysate has been suggested[35] as a method to increase dialysis efficiency without causing patient dehydration.

To avoid the problems of hyperglycemia, hypertriglyceridemia, obesity, and inappetence encountered in humans on CAPD,[6,36] alternatives to glucose as a hyperosmotic agent have been sought. An improved hyperosmotic agent would allow sustained ultrafiltration, prolonged dwell time (due to less absorption), and minimal side effects and would not require insulin for metabolism. Amino acids added to dialysate can increase osmolality as well as provide nutrition for human patients undergoing CAPD.[36] A 2% amino acid solution can result in as much ultrafiltration as observed from using a 4.25% dextrose solution, but is very expensive.[36] Dialysate containing glucose polymers, glycerol, and gelatins may be considered for use in the future, but there is presently no alternative to hypertonic dextrose dialysate.[36]

Commercial dialysate is acidified to a pH of 5.2 to 6.2 to prevent carmelization of glucose during preparation. Pain during infusion of these acid solutions has been encountered in humans,[6,36] but this effect has not been noted in dogs.

Alkali precursors (lactate or acetate) are added to commercial dialysate. Acetate and lactate promote vasodilation of peritoneal vessels in addition to their systemic alkalinizing effects.[6,37] Commercial solutions do not contain bicarbonate due to potential problems with calcium and magnesium salt precipitation and increased pH that favors glucose carmelization.[6,7,36] Following metabolism to bicarbonate, acetate, or lactate at 35 mEq/L to 45 mEq/L in dialysate is adequate to correct most uremic acidosis in human patients on dialysis.[6] Though advantages have been described for either acetate or lactate, it appears that there is no difference between the two solutions with respect to protein loss, solute clearances, or correction of metabolic acidosis during routine dialysis.[6,38] The amount of alkali precursor may need to be individually altered to maintain the total carbon dioxide concentration on the serum biochemistry panel or bicarbonate concentration from blood gases at an acceptable level (>15 mEq/L bicarbonate). Techniques to proportion bicarbonate directly at the time of automated dialysate delivery have been developed.[36]

Shock or hypotension can reduce the metabolic conversion of acetate or lactate to bicarbonate. Alkalis in dialysate are designed for the chronic correction of metabolic acidosis and should not be relied on for rapid correction of acidosis or correction of severe metabolic acidosis. The systemic administration of alkali is necessary in these instances. Equilibration for bicarbonate between dialysate and blood required about 12 hours in one study of human subjects.[36]

Many vasodilatory drugs (e.g., isoproterenol) and hormones (e.g., glucagon) given intraperitoneally or intravenously have been studied for their ability to enhance solute clearance into dialysate. It appears that in general vasodilators only modestly increase clearance of small and middle molecules while substantially increasing clearance of high-molecular-weight substances (proteins).[6,37,39] Hypertonic dextrose dialysate (4.25%) has a much greater effect on increasing small solute clearance than does administration of vasodilators.[37] One investigator concluded that vasodilators given intravenously or intraperitoneally to enhance dialysis do not have a large clinical role at this time.[3]

The surface-active agents trisaminomethane and dioctyl sodium sulfosuccinate increase urea clearances in dogs through poorly understood mechanisms,[6,35] but their use has been limited because of toxicity.

MANAGEMENT OF SEVERE AZOTEMIA AND UREMIA PRIOR TO DIALYSIS

Death prior to dialysis can occur from severe metabolic derangements related to uremia (especially hyperkalemia and metabolic acidosis), dehydration, overhydration following fluid therapy, infections, and malnutrition.[40] Every attempt should be made to improve glomerular filtration and other renal functions by standard medical or surgical therapy before considering treatment with dialysis. Dialysis may not be necessary if the magnitude of azotemia, other metabolic abnormalities, fluid imbalances, and uremic signs can be sufficiently reduced by these treatments.

Reduced glomerular filtration and subsequent accumulation of uremic solutes can result from a variety of prerenal, intrarenal, and postrenal factors that may not be obvious on initial examination of the animal. Reduced renal perfusion (prerenal azotemia) commonly contributes to azotemia, either alone or in combination with intrarenal or postrenal lesions.

Fluid therapy

A combination of fluids administered for rehydration, maintenance, and mild volume expansion along with diuretic administration can be used in an attempt to increase glomerular filtration, renal blood flow (RBF), and the rate of renal tubular fluid flow in animals with apparent primary (intrinsic) renal failure. Blood urea nitrogen, serum creatinine, and serum phosphorus concentrations will decline if this therapy successfully increases glomerular filtration rate. When increased renal tubular flow rate reduces the passive tubular reabsorption of urea, blood urea nitrogen levels can also decline without a change in glomerular filtration rate.

Initial therapy is directed toward correction of all potential prerenal factors for the azotemia. The intravenous route is used for fluid administration to ensure rapid access to the circulation and to maximize support of renal perfusion. The volume of fluids administered must be chosen and monitored carefully, since animals that remain oliguric or anuric can become overhydrated from excessive fluid infusion, and it may be difficult to administer adequate fluid volumes to correct dehydration in animals with polyuria.

Mild volume expansion with fluids administered at 3% to 5% body weight can be given in addition to maintenance fluids following correction of dehydration if azotemia or oliguria have not improved. The rationale for this additional fluid administration is that dehydration of 3% to 5% of body weight may be clinically undetectable, and renal function may improve when further fluid is administered. Since the animal with severely diseased kidneys may not be able to tolerate this volume expansion, and overhydration may result, this fluid administration must be closely monitored (see Chapter 4).

Intensive diuresis with 10% to 20% dextrose, mannitol, furosemide, dopamine, or combinations may increase glomerular filtration rate, renal blood flow, and tubular flow rate (see Chapter 21). Success with these agents includes a decreased magnitude of azotemia and/or conversion from oliguria or anuria to increased urine flow. Effects on glomerular filtration and urine flow rate may be independent of each other.

Diet

The magnitude of blood urea nitrogen and serum phosphorus elevations and metabolic acidosis is influenced by the catabolism of dietary and endogenous proteins in addition to the level of renal dysfunction. Dietary intake is not indicated for patients initially until the magnitude of azotemia and vomiting are reduced by medical management. Intake of a restricted quantity of high-quality protein accompanied by adequate nonprotein calories can reduce the accumulation of some uremic solutes.

Control of vomiting

Fluid loss from vomiting is common in uremic states, making it difficult to maintain hydration during fluid therapy. The administration of cimetidine or ranitidine (H_2-receptor antagonists) is often helpful in reducing the severity of vomiting. Phenothiazine-derivative tranquilizers, metoclopramide, and trimethobenzamide act centrally to decrease vomiting if H_2-receptor antagonist administration alone is not effective. Reduction in the magnitude of azotemia is often associated with reduced vomiting.

Anemia

Severe anemia can be apparent initially in animals with advanced chronic renal failure or can develop later in those with acute intrinsic renal failure. Transfusion with whole blood or packed red cells is indicated if the packed cell volume is less than 15% and may be of benefit in some patients with packed cell volume from 15% to 25% (see Chapter 34).

Electrolyte abnormalities

Electrolyte and acid-base disorders commonly develop in uremic patients with severe reductions in glomerular filtration rate. Hyperkalemia, hypokalemia, hypernatremia, hyponatremia, hyperphosphatemia, hypocalcemia, and metabolic acidosis are the abnormalities most likely to be discovered. Depending on their severity, specific treatment for these metabolic abnormalities may be necessary (see Chapters 18 and 38).

Life-threatening hyperkalemia is likely to be encountered in severely oliguric patients, especially when metabolic acidosis is severe. Serial or continuous electrocardiographic monitoring is recommended in these patients. Hyperkalemia can temporarily be reduced in severity following volume expansion with 0.9% sodium chloride and intravenous sodium bicarbonate infusion (1 to 4 mEq/kg slowly). Polystyrene sulfonate (Kayexylate; 25 to 50 g three times a day orally or by retention enema) can reduce the magnitude of chronic hyperkalemia by binding potassium within the gut.

Hypokalemia can occur in patients with polyuric renal failure, especially when anorexia persists. Potassium supplementation should be added

cautiously to daily fluids and serial potassium concentration measured to ensure that hyperkalemia does not develop (see Chapter 38).

Severe metabolic acidosis (blood pH less than 7.2 or total carbon dioxide less than 15 mEq/L) usually requires treatment with alkali. Hypernatremia and seizures can result from sodium bicarbonate replacement that is too rapid or excessive.

Hypernatremia commonly develops in patients with primary renal failure that receive fluids high in sodium (lactated Ringer's, 0.9% saline) for several days. Hypotonic fluids (e.g., 0.45% in 2.5% dextrose) should be considered for maintenance after initial rehydration of these patients in order to avoid development of hypernatremia.

Hyperphosphatemia may be of consequence in the development of further primary renal injury in both acute and chronic intrinsic renal failure.[41] Additionally, hyperphosphatemia contributes to the development of hypocalcemia. Intestinal phosphorus-binding agents (e.g., aluminum hydroxide, calcium carbonate, or calcium acetate) should be administered in an attempt to maintain the serum phosphorus concentration below 5.5 mg/dl. Phosphorus binders are much more effective when given with meals, but may lower serum phosphorus in anorexic patients, presumably by binding secreted phosphorus in gut water.

Symptomatic hypocalcemia (tremors, seizures) is not common, but may require administration of intravenous calcium salts when it does occur (see Chapter 18). Administered calcium may interact with elevated serum phosphorus levels, resulting in metastatic mineralization of various soft tissues, including the heart and kidneys.

Postrenal obstruction should be relieved by surgical means or by hydropulsion when applicable (see Chapter 21). Indwelling urinary catheters that bypass the obstruction allow adequate drainage of urine until more permanent corrective surgery can be performed following resolution of azotemia. Rarely, cystostomy or nephrostomy tube drainage may be needed.

Intrarenal lesions are not immediately reversible following acute injury, whereas chronic lesions are irreversible. The correction of hypercalcemia, hypokalemia/potassium depletion, or upper urinary tract infection will facilitate resolution of azotemia as reversible renal lesions heal. Severe acute lesions of nephrosis or nephritis may heal over weeks to months. Animals with chronic renal failure (CRF) may require at least 3 to 5 days of medical support before recompensation occurs. Some animals may be unable to compensate.

INDICATIONS FOR PERITONEAL DIALYSIS

Animals with acute intrinsic renal failure (AIRF), acutely decompensated CRF, and postrenal azotemia that cannot undergo immediate surgical correction are candidates for peritoneal dialysis. Tube cystostomy drainage may be preferable for acute management of urethral obstruction prior to surgical correction. Dialysis is prescribed when severe clinical signs and laboratory abnormalities of uremia cannot be managed by medical or surgical means alone. Peritoneal dialysis is most indicated when there is potential for reversal of underlying renal lesions (acute intrinsic renal failure) or lessening of uremic signs such that life can be maintained without dialysis in the future. Unfortunately, it may not be obvious whether the underlying renal disease is potentially reversible or irreversible at a time that dialysis may need to be instituted to maintain life. Animals often undergo peritoneal dialysis while awaiting results of renal biopsy (see boxes at right).

Peritoneal dialysis is not indicated for the treatment of prerenal azotemia or for chronic renal failure (irreversible renal lesions) in general. Some animals with CRF may benefit from a few days of peritoneal dialysis (repeated puncture or acute catheter technique) to lessen uremic signs such that clinical recompensation could occur, but this approach is not often attempted.

Aggressive medical therapy is continued until it is clear that renal function will not further improve without dialysis. Clinical signs, urine output, and hematologic and serum biochemical results must be integrated to make the decision to euthanize or to institute dialysis. It is not indicated to dialyze a patient based solely on the magnitude of azotemia. Rapidly rising blood urea nitrogen or serum creatinine concentrations, severe oliguria or anuria, overhydration, hyperkalemia, hypernatremia, hyperphosphatemia, hypocalcemia, and metabolic acidosis despite medical treatments may be indications to start dialysis in an animal regardless of the level of azotemia. It is difficult to manage medically animals who are normally hydrated and have clinical signs of uremia and blood urea nitrogen concentrations greater than 100 mg/dl and serum creatinine concentrations greater than 10 mg/dl. It is not worthwhile to initiate dialysis in animals with moderate-grade azotemia since a blood urea nitrogen level of 40 to 80 mg/dl and serum creatinine concentration from 4 to 7 mg/dl are expected results following dialysis using current CAPD techniques.

Peritoneal dialysis has been most successful for both short- and long-term management when a

---

INDICATIONS FOR PERCUTANEOUS PERITONEAL DIALYSIS*

Awaiting surgical catheter placement
Acute overhydration (nonresponsive to diuretics)
Hyperkalemia/severe metabolic acidosis
Acute decompensation of chronic renal failure
Ethylene glycol and metabolite intoxication (<24 hour duration)
Hypercalcemic crisis
Hypothermia
Hyperthermia
Barbiturate intoxication

---

*Less than 4 days and few exchanges per day anticipated; considered after standard medical and surgical treatments have been instituted with inadequate resolution of uremia. Techniques include repeat needle puncture or Cohen acute pediatric peritoneal dialysis catheter systems (Cook, Bloomington, IN).

INDICATIONS FOR PERITONEAL DIALYSIS WITH SURGICALLY PLACED CATHETER*

Reversible intrarenal lesions
  Nephrosis
  Nephritis
  Early hydronephrosis (before and after surgery)
Awaiting results of renal biopsy
Chronic overhydration
Hyperkalemia/severe metabolic acidosis

---

*Two to 30 days of dialysis anticipated with multiple exchanges per day; not generally recommended for maintenance of animals with chronic renal failure; considered after standard medical and surgical treatments have been instituted with inadequate resolution of uremia.

---

column disk catheter has been placed (see procedures below). Acute dialysis using intermittent puncture for two to four exchanges per day over 2 to 3 days may help alleviate uremic signs if a dialysis catheter is unavailable. This approach may allow recompensation in some patients with chronic renal failure or may "buy time" for an animal awaiting chronic peritoneal dialysis with a surgically placed catheter. Repeat-puncture peritoneal dialysis for longer periods will be difficult or impossible because of patient trauma, time factors, and mechanical difficulties with this technique.

Rare indications for acute peritoneal dialysis include hypothermia,[42,43] hyperthermia,[6] hypercalcemic crisis,[6,44] and dialyzable intoxication such as with barbiturates or early ethylene glycol poisoning.[45] Occasionally, life-threatening overhydration that is not responsive to diuretics can be managed with a few exchanges of hypertonic dialysate.

TECHNIQUES OF PERITONEAL DIALYSIS

Aseptic technique is imperative with any type of peritoneal dialysis.[3,46] This includes the use of surgical scrub and sterile surgical technique during catheter placement, as well as the use of sterile gloves, disinfectants, and the careful handling of dialysate fluids, catheters, and catheter lines during dialysis.

Alcohols are the preferred substances for disinfection of dialysis connections because of their broad range of antimicrobial activity, activity in the presence of organic matter, and rapid evaporation.[47] It has been found that both chlorhexidine and iodophores are inadequate for disinfection in the dialysis environment; both have been associated with preparations that are contaminated with bacteria. Additionally, chlorhexidine is largely bacteriostatic, while iodophores have poor effect on *Staphylococcus aureus* and are inactivated by blood and glucose.[47]

Access to the peritoneal cavity

Several types of catheters, cannulas, or needles are available for performing peritoneal dialysis. Selection of a particular catheter will depend on the duration of dialysis anticipated and the number of daily exchanges of dialysate prescribed to manage an animal's uremia. Animals with severe adhesions along the midline or those with ileus will require a surgically placed catheter.

Acute access—percutaneous peritoneal dialysis

Acute (short-term, temporary) dialysis can be most simply accomplished using a multiple-intermittent-puncture technique with large-gauge hypodermic needles for infusion and drainage of dialysate. An 18- or 20-gauge needle puncture along the ventral midline 2 cm caudal to the umbilicus can be used to infuse dialysis fluids. Drainage of dialysate may require a 16-, 14-, or 12-gauge needle or plastic cannula. Prior dialysate infusion distends the abdomen, which minimizes possible trauma to abdominal viscera associated with needle puncture for drainage. A sterile intravenous extension set and collection bag (empty parenteral fluid bag) is attached to the drainage needle during outflow. Trauma from multiple punctures and difficulty in consistent outflow of dialysate limit the long-term usefulness of this technique. To reduce trauma, large-gauge needles or plastic cannulas may be secured in

place during each dwell period. Obstruction of dialysate outflow is common with this technique, and frequent postural adjustments or repeated punctures are necessary to encourage continued drainage. Hydropulsion with dialysate or mechanical dislodgment of the obstruction via a small-gauge urinary catheter introduced through the needle may also be helpful.

Peritoneal lavage (continuous peritoneal dialysis) is an alternative technique. A 14 French tube is percutaneously placed (Brunswick sterile disposable feeding tube and urethral catheter, Sherwood Medical Instruments, St. Louis) in the flank for infusion of dialysate. One or more outflow drains is placed inside a fenestrated Penrose drain and then inserted along the ventral abdomen (tube or sump, Shirley wound drain, ANPRO, HN Anderson Products, Oyster Bay, NY). Infection with this technique can be a problem because this is an open drainage system.[48]

A commercially available human peritoneal dialysis stylet catheter (Trocath, McGraw Laboratories, Division of American Hospital Supply, Glendale, CA) is composed of a multifenestrated stiff plastic tube with an internal stylet. The advantage to this catheter is that it can be inserted percutaneously using only local anesthesia. It is difficult to obtain a good seal at the point of entry that can lead to dialysate leakage and/or infection. This catheter is free-floating in the abdominal cavity, and migration toward the omentum and plugging of the small holes in the catheter are problems frequently encountered. This catheter frequently becomes obstructed during chronic dialysis in dogs, usually within the first week.[3] It is advised to distend the abdomen with warmed dialysate solution infused via needle puncture prior to placement of the catheter in order to decrease the likelihood of trauma to abdominal organs. A small scalpel incision is made through skin/subcutaneous tissues and the catheter with stylet is inserted into the abdomen. Following puncture through the abdominal wall the stylet is retracted slightly before advancing the catheter caudally, adjacent to the urinary bladder.

The Cohen acute pediatric peritoneal dialysis catheter system (Cook, Bloomington, IN) consists of a semiflexible fenestrated tube and wire stylet. Local anesthesia with 2% lidocaine is infused at the site of catheter placement (2 cm caudal to the umbilicus and just off the midline) and the urinary bladder is emptied prior to catheter placement. The introducer needle is placed first (after shifting the skin to allow a tunnel), then the stylet is threaded through the needle. The needle is removed, leaving the stylet in place. The catheter is threaded down the stylet, twisting slightly to facilitate its passage through the peritoneum. All catheter holes are ascertained to be within the abdomen and the stylet is removed. A purse-string suture is placed at the entry site. The catheter is secured, and a sterile bandage is applied. Although designed for acute access, this catheter has been successfully employed in dogs for as long as 30 days.[49]

Chronic access—surgically placed catheters

Two catheters designed for long-term peritoneal dialysis in dogs are commercially available. The Parker peritoneal dialysis cannula (CPA Vet, Marysville, CA) consists of a trocar, guide tube, a stainless steel needle, and a silicone rubber dialysis cannula. This catheter can be placed with local anesthesia if the animal is severely depressed and is transfixed across the flank in a bowed manner ventral to the bladder. Leakage of dialysate is minimal because of the dorsal flank exit site for the catheter. A Dacron cuff is present at the level of the body wall to decrease ascending infection.

This system for chronic catheter placement in dogs has been shown to be highly successful in the reduction of uremic solutes and in its ability to freely drain dialysate.[1] Unfortunately, this catheter has not achieved widespread use due to limited commercial availability initially.

The column disk peritoneal dialysis catheter represents the device used most commonly for long-term placement and rapid drainage of dialysate in dogs[3] (Vet Cath, Physio-Control Dialysis, Products Division, Redmond, WA). The catheter is made of silicone and consists of a single tube opening between two parallel disks separated by numerous pillars (Fig. 39-1). Advantages for this catheter include excellent effluent drainage and minimal leakage of dialysate. The pillars help prevent catheter-outflow occlusion by omentum, fibrin, and abdominal organs. The disks are secured into a nonmovable position along the body wall. Two Dacron cuffs are placed on the catheter to allow fibrous tissue growth and prevent ascending bacterial migration.

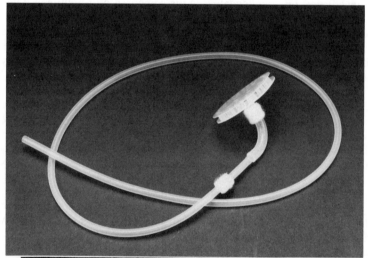

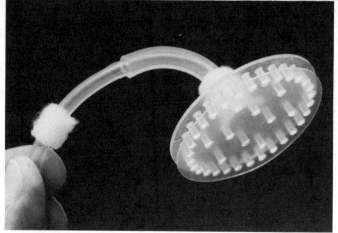

A

B

Fig. 39-1 Column-disk peritoneal dialysis catheter. **A,** Entire catheter with disk, Dacron cuffs, and tubing for subcutaneous tunneling. **B,** Closeup of the disk showing two parallel silastic plates separated by pillars to ensure that the central drainage hole does not become occluded. The disk remains entirely within the peritoneal cavity, pulled flush against the abdominal wall. (Vet Cath, Physio-Control Dialysis, Products Division, Redmond, WA.)

Placement of column disk peritoneal dialysis catheter

The column disk catheter can be placed with the animal under local anesthesia, through a small incision, particularly if the animal is severely depressed or moribund. However, general anesthesia is recommended for most patients in order to allow for ideal column disk catheter placement.[50] This surgical procedure combines catheter placement (from inside the abdominal cavity outward), partial omentectomy, and renal biopsy. Partial omentectomy has been instrumental to the success of dialysis treatments[4,50] because of improved outflow of dialysate (less omental occlusion). A renal biopsy should be performed in all animals undergoing chronic peritoneal dialysis to facilitate prognosis and treatment.

A left paramedian incision enables a wedge biopsy of the left kidney to be done at the time of catheter placement. The caudal two thirds of the omentum is removed unless peritonitis is present or the animal has recently had bowel surgery. In these cases an omentopexy is performed instead. The disk of the catheter is placed just cranially to the pelvic brim and the tubing is pulled through a midline stab incision made 2 to 3 cm cranially to the pelvic brim. The disk is pulled flush with the parietal peritoneum and the dacron cuff closest to the disk is placed in the abdominal musculature. A purse-string suture is placed in the rectus fascia around the catheter tubing and the tubing is tunneled subcutaneously 6 to 8 cm cranially before exiting the skin via a ventral midline stab incision. The second Dacron cuff is placed in the subcutaneous tissue. The subcutaneous tissue is meticulously closed to eliminate dead space, using absorbable suture material in a simple continuous pattern. The skin is closed routinely with monofilament nylon.

The dialysis catheter should be flushed with heparinized saline at the time of placement. The abdomen should be lavaged to remove fibrin clots that might occlude the dialysis catheter. It is suggested that heparinized lactated Ringer's solution or heparinized commercial peritoneal dialysis solution be instilled into the abdominal cavity and proper drainage capability verified at the time of closure. A residual volume of 10 to 20 ml/kg of heparinized peritoneal fluid should remain to minimize clotting within the dialysis catheter. Dialysis is delayed for 12 to 24 hours following catheter placement to enable a tighter seal to develop at the catheter exit site. Dialysis may be started immediately if it is imperative because of life-threatening metabolic disturbances and uremia.

SELECTION AND PREPARATION OF DIALYSATE

Dialysate is generally chosen to approximate normal plasma composition (with the exception of proteins).[7] Dialysate should be tailored, however, to the individual patient for sodium, chloride, potassium, and alkali needs. The concentration gradient between blood and dialysate largely determines what substances are removed from or added to the animal's blood. A large concentration gradient from blood to dialysate favors solute removal from the body, whereas a large concentration gradient from dialysate to blood favors uptake of solute to the body. The concentration gradient between blood and dialysate should be nonexistent for substances not desired to be removed from or added to the body.

Commercial dialysate solution

Commercially available peritoneal dialysis solutions designed for use in humans work well in dogs and cats (Table 39-1). These polyelectrolyte peritoneal dialysis solutions approximate normal plasma electrolyte concentrations and contain dextrose at 1.5%, 2.5%, and 4.5% concentrations. Dialysate containing 1.5% dextrose is usually effective, but 2.5% or 4.5% dextrose solutions may be needed to correct overhydration or when effluent dialysate volume declines because of marked hyperosmolality of patient serum. Hypernatremia occurs commonly during peritoneal dialysis and is attributed to ultrafiltration of solute-free water. For this reason it may be advantageous or necessary to choose dialysate solutions that are lower in sodium concentrations than plasma during the course of dialysis.

Table 39-1 Composition of peritoneal dialysis solutions

	Dianeal	Lactated Ringer's	0.9% Saline
Sodium	132	130	154
Chloride	96	109	154
Potassium	0	4	0
Calcium	3.5	3	0
Magnesium	0.5	0	0
Lactate	40	28	0
Osmolality:			
0% Dextrose	272	308	
1.5% Dextrose	360	396	
2.5% Dextrose	411	447	
4.5% Dextrose	522	558	

All values reported in milliequivalents per liter, except for osmolality, which is reported in milliosmoles per kilogram.

Home-made dialysate solutions

Home-made dialysate using lactated Ringer's, 0.45% sodium chloride, or 0.9% sodium chloride as base solutions can be individually tailored to the patient as an alternative to commercial fluids. Commercial dialysate fluids are generally preferred, since alterations of the dialysate (additives) increase the risk for bacterial contamination during preparation. All home-prepared solutions require the addition of glucose. Thirty milliliters of 50% dextrose is added to each liter to achieve a 1.5% dextrose solution, or 50 ml of 50% dextrose to achieve a 2.5% dextrose solution.

Magnesium

Magnesium should also be added to home-made dialysate after the first several days of dialysis if anorexia persists, at 72 mg per liter of fluids to achieve a standard concentration of 1.5 mEq/L. Magnesium chloride may not be readily available as a sterile commercial solution; consequently, magnesium chloride powder may be dissolved in dextrose and then millipore-filtered prior to injection into dialysate.

Sodium bicarbonate

Sodium bicarbonate at 30 to 45 mEq/L should be added to home-made 0.45% or 0.9% sodium chloride base dialysate to provide a source of alkali. Lactated Ringer's solution contains lactate equivalent to 28 mEq/L alkali; bicarbonate should not be added to this solution because of potential for calcium salt precipitation.

Heparin

Heparin is added to commercial and home-made dialysate solutions just prior to infusion (dose, 1000 units/L) to decrease clot formation and outflow obstruction.

Antibiotics

There is no advantage to the use of prophylactic antibiotics in the dialysate to prevent bacterial peritonitis, but antibiotics should be added to dialysate if peritonitis is diagnosed (see "Peritonitis").

Potassium

Commercial dialysate for use in CAPD is usually potassium-free. Potassium-free dialysate is ideal for the treatment of hyperkalemia during initial dialysis and can be continued as maintenance dialysate in animals that are able to take in food. Hypokalemia can result during aggressive dialysis, particularly when hourly exchanges are used or when more than 4 daily exchanges are given during anorexia. In these instances it is necessary to add potassium supplementation to parenteral fluids or to dialysate. Potassium chloride (4 mEq/L) can be added to potassium-free solutions to help prevent hypokalemia in animals that are not eating after the first 24 to 48 hours of aggressive dialysis. As much as 10 to 20 mEq/L of potassium chloride can be added to dialysate to correct hypokalemia, the amount required will depend on the severity of the hypokalemia and the number of daily exchanges. It is advisable to supplement potassium in dialysate cautiously to avoid the development of hyperkalemia. Serum potassium concentrations should be measured frequently during the initial phases of supplementation.

Calcium

Calcium-free commercial dialysate solutions are not available. In cases with hypercalcemia or those with severe hyperphosphatemia it may be advisable initially to choose a home-made preparation that is lacking in calcium (0.9% sodium chloride with glucose added).

Prewarming fluids

Prewarming of fluids is recommended when exchanges will be conducted frequently during aggressive dialysis (every 1 to 3 hours). Fluids 1 to 2°C higher than body temperature have been recommended in an effort to vasodilate the vasculature to enhance solute exchange.[1] Warming of fluids becomes less important with longer dwell times, as heat dissipation occurs.[6] Cold fluids are avoided so that vasoconstriction of peritoneal vessels does not occur. Prewarmed dialysate fluids are recommended for all hypothermic animals. Dialysate contained in plastic bags can be warmed in a microwave oven for a few minutes until warm to the touch. Hot water baths can also be used, but bacterial contamination is common.[6]

INFUSION OF DIALYSATE

Rapid infusion of dialysate at 200 to 300 ml per minute by gravity flow is well tolerated by animals.[1,3] Infusion volumes of 250, 500, 1000, and 2000 ml are often chosen based on body weight to approximate a dose of 40 ml/kg.[3] The abdomen should be palpably distended following dialysate infusion to ensure maximal contact of fluid with peritoneal surfaces.[51] The abdomen should not be overdistended so as to reduce ventilatory excursions or cause patient discomfort. Excessive fluid volume is undesirable since it enhances peritoneal capillary/lymphatic uptake of fluid and solute from the increased hydrostatic pressure within the peritoneal cavity and may reduce peritoneal membrane permeability by reducing the pore size.[3] Immediate drainage of dialysate should take place if dyspnea occurs during infusion. Dialysate volume should be reduced when leakage from infused peritoneal fluid into subcutaneous tissues is substantial.

Commercial dialysate is available in 1- or 2-L bags. Following infusion and dwell the empty dialysate bag can be used to collect effluent through the same administration line, the bag discarded, and a fresh bag of dialysate attached to the infusion line. Alternatively, when only a portion of the bag will be infused during an exchange, it is advised to infuse through one opening of a three-way stopcock and drain through another into a sterile empty bag. After drainage of effluent in this instance, further fresh dialysate can be infused from the original bag, which minimizes waste of dialysate and lessens chances for contamination by lessening the number of times that bags must be changed.

It is difficult to deliver accurately a small volume of dialysate to a patient by estimating the fluid line in a plastic bag. Accurate delivery can be accomplished by serially weighing the bag on a gram scale during delivery of dialysate (1 g of fluid equals approximately 1 ml). For example, 100 ml of dialysate from a 1-L bag will be administered when the bag has lost 100 g during infusion.

DWELL TIME FOR DIALYSATE

Dwell time for dialysate is based on the urgency of need to correct uremic abnormalities. Animals with life-threatening conditions such as hyperkalemia and metabolic acidosis may require hourly exchanges until stabilization has occurred. Animals with AIRF may require 12 to 48 consecutive hourly exchanges before a marked decline in uremic solute (blood urea nitrogen, serum creatinine, serum phosphorus) can be demonstrated. Frequent exchanges allow for greater efficiency in the removal of uremic solutes, since a more favorable concentration gradient is maintained for diffusion into fresh dialysate. Vigorous gentle palpation of peritoneal fluid during the dwell period may help to mix stagnant dialysate with fresh solution, which will facilitate diffusion in situations in which maximal exchange of solute is considered essential. Dwell time can be increased to 4 to 8 hours (three to six daily exchanges) during maintenance chronic dialysis following initial stabilization of the uremic animal.

DRAINAGE OF EFFLUENT

Dialysate is drained by gravity usually within 15 minutes following an appropriate dwell time.[3] It is best to drain effluent into the same bag used to infuse dialysate so that chances for bacterial contamination are minimized during manipulations of the mechanical apparatus. Too rapid drainage of dialysate can be painful for dogs, as the abdomen is rapidly decompressed,[1] but this phenomenon does not occur often. Effluent volume during the first one or two exchanges may be less than that which was infused due to sequestration within the abdomen or absorption of some fluid. Effluent volume should closely match or exceed the volume infused during subsequent hourly exchanges with 1.5% dextrose solutions.

Failure to retrieve 90% or more of infused dialysate following hourly exchanges usually indicates a mechanical problem with drainage. In these instances it may be necessary to change the animal's posture to enhance drainage or to vigorously flush the dialysis catheter with heparinized saline to remove occluding clots, fibrin strands, omentum, or gut. In some instances, obstruction of the catheter will persist, which necessitates replacing the catheter. Occasionally, reduced effluent volume is the result of increased peritoneal absorption of fluid and solute. This can follow marked dehydration (low capillary hydrostatic pressure), increased plasma osmolality, or increased plasma protein concentration (increased oncotic pressure) such that fluid absorption into the blood vessels is favored. Intravenous fluid therapy will help restore adequate capillary hydrostatic pressure and reduce oncotic pressure within peritoneal vessels, while increasing dialysate osmolality (2.5% or 4.5% dextrose solutions) will establish the necessary osmotic gradient to favor ultrafiltration in these instances. Peritonitis also results in reduced recovery of effluent due to enhanced absorption of glucose and water.

PERITONITIS

Bacteria can colonize the peritoneal cavity if they ascend through or around the dialysis catheter.[46,47] Impaired phagocytic function of polymorphonuclear leukocytes associated with the low pH and high osmolality of dialysate may be a predisposing factor.[6]

Effluent is often blood-tinged for 1 to 2 days following catheter placement. Effluent should be monitored daily for visual clarity, as cloudiness can be an early indication of peritonitis. Cytologic evaluation, including Gram stain and bacterial culture (anaerobic and aerobic), should be obtained whenever the effluent appears cloudy. Frequent cytologic examination and Gram stain (two to three times weekly) of effluent in the absence of turbidity may allow early detection of peritonitis. Normal effluent contains less than 50 white cells per microliter, most of which are mononuclear cells. Effluent turbidity due to bacterial peritonitis is associated with white cell counts in excess of 100 to 200 cells/μl with neutrophils predominant.[52,53] Weekly bacteriologic culture of effluent is recommended for monitoring in the absence of signs and effluent turbidity.

Cultures of dialysate following millipore filtration have been advocated to increase the likelihood for isolation of small numbers of bacteria causing peritonitis. In this technique, 60 ml of dialysate is suctioned through a 0.2-μm filter and the filter is placed onto a blood agar plate for bacterial isolation. This technique is considered the most sensitive for isolation of bacteria following antibacterial treatments, superior to either direct agar plate or broth isolation.[52]

The use of a once daily dilute iodine solution flush is recommended to prevent bacterial peritonitis during the first 5 days following catheter placement. This technique has also proven useful when breaks in sterile technique occur during preparation, infusion, or drainage of dialysate. Iodine in combination with water forms hypoiodous acid, which is microbiocidal.[3] The routine addition of antibiotics to dialysate as a prophylactic measure is not recommended during this period.

The following protocol is recommended if breaks in sterile technique occur: The dialysate solution is drained, isotonic saline solution (40 ml/kg up to 1 L) is then instilled and immediately drained to remove dextrose (dextrose converts iodine to inactive iodide), 0.2 ml of 2% iodine solution USP is added to 1 L of 0.9% sodium chloride (do not substitute povidone iodine for USP iodine since the povidone portion is associated with toxicity[54]) and the iodine flush is infused, allowed a 4-minute dwell time, drained, and dialysis resumed. If bacterial peritonitis is present, double the amount of iodine added to the saline flush or increase the flushes to twice daily for 24 hours. If peritonitis is not resolved after this period, discontinue iodine flushes.

Depression, anorexia, fever, abdominal pain, diarrhea, and vomiting are clinical signs of bacterial peritonitis that may be observed in animals. Gram-positive organisms predominated in reports from one author,[52,53] but gram-negative organisms predominated in another.[24] Treatment with broad-spectrum antibiotics should be instituted following diagnosis of peritonitis and adjustments made based on results of organism antibacterial susceptibility testing. Systemic antimicrobial administration may not achieve therapeutic antibacterial concentrations in peritoneal fluid. Consequently, it is recommended to add at least a portion of the daily antimicrobial dose to the dialysate.

Cephalothin is recommended as an initial choice for empirical treatment of peritonitis while awaiting return of culture and susceptibility results. Aminoglycosides have been recommended for treatment of gram-negative or multiple-organism peritonitis,[52,53] but because of the potential for further renal injury from these drugs they should not be used unless absolutely necessary

(life-threatening sepsis, or culture and susceptibility results indicate no alternative).

Rapid therapeutic systemic concentrations of cephalothin can be achieved solely with peritoneal administration. A dosage of 250 mg per 2-L bag has been recommended during maintenance dialysis.[52,53] One loading dose of gentamicin or tobramycin is recommended at 4 mg/kg intramuscularly followed by a dosage of 10 mg per 2-L bag of dialysate to maintain systemic therapeutic concentrations.[52,53] Drugs that can be added to the dialysate at the following dosages extrapolated from humans include penicillin G (50,000 units/L), ampicillin (50 mg/L), cloxacillin (100 mg/L), ticarcillin (100 mg/L), vancomycin (30 mg/L), amikacin (50 mg/L), clindamycin (50 mg/L), and sulfadiazine/trimethoprim (25/5 mg/L). Heparin should not be mixed with penicillin, vancomycin, or aminoglycosides.[52,53]

Peritonitis may not respond to the above management recommendations in some instances. Removal of the current peritoneal dialysis catheter and replacement with a new one may be necessary if peritonitis is nonresponsive to medical therapy. Nonresponsive peritonitis can be severe enough to cause death or warrant euthanasia.

EVALUATING EFFECTIVENESS OF DIALYSIS
Record keeping

It is important to keep accurate records during peritoneal dialysis, documenting exchange volumes and patient weight. This procedure ensures that progressive overhydration or dehydration does not develop. Patient weights should be obtained at least twice daily (utilizing the same scale) after the animal's bladder is emptied. The times of infusion, dwell, and drainage, as well as the precise volumes infused and drained should be accurately recorded for each exchange (see Fig. 39-2 for flow chart). Net fluid balance to the patient includes fluid flux of dialysate and any intravenous fluid administration. Fluid balance to the patient is calculated both for each individual exchange and cumulatively. The ideal is to have zero fluid balance to the patient when the intravenous fluid volume administered is considered. If the patient has positive fluid balance (less dialysate drained than infused and weight gain) and mechanical obstruction has been ruled out, it is necessary to alter the composition of dialysate by increasing osmolality (add more dextrose). If the patient has negative fluid balance (more dialysate is drained than infused and weight loss) then it becomes necessary either to increase intravenous fluid infusion or to decrease dialysate osmolality. Increasing the dwell time will also lessen effluent volume. Serial packed cell volume and total se-

Clinician _____

Date _____ ICU day # _____

Weight _____ lbs/kg _____ AM

Weight _____ lbs/kg _____ PM

Comments:

Exch.	Inflow			Outflow			Balance
#	Time start	Time Finish	Vol (ml)	Time Start	Time Finish	Vol (ml)	Per exch./cum.

Fig. 39-2 Flow chart to facilitate recording of input/output volumes during exchanges of dialysate. Accurate body weights at the start and finish of dialysis are also very helpful to ensure that overhydration or dehydration is not developing.

rum protein measurements may provide additional useful information about the animal's intravascular hydration.

Laboratory evaluation

Serial laboratory evaluations should include measurement of blood urea nitrogen, serum creatinine, serum phosphorus, and electrolyte (sodium, potassium, chloride, calcium) concentrations, and blood gas analysis to monitor effectiveness of dialysis (Table 39-2). Resolution of severe hyperkalemia, azotemia, and metabolic acidosis represents an initial success of dialysis that is mandatory for patient survival. Activity level, strength, appetite, interest in life, vomiting, and anemia are other facets of uremia that can sometimes be successfully improved or managed with peritoneal dialysis in dogs and cats. Improved renal function

Table 39-2 Monitoring interval for peritoneal dialysis*

	Acute	Maintenance
Body weight	8-12 hours	Daily
Packed cell volume and total serum protein	12-24 hours	Weekly
Sodium and potassium	12 hours, if hyperkalemic	Weekly
	24 hours, if hypokalemic	
	48 hours, if normokalemic	
Blood gases	8 to 12 hours, first day;	Optional
	48 to 72 hours thereafter	
Blood urea nitrogen and serum creatinine	12 hours, first day;	Weekly
	24-48 hours thereafter	
Serum phosphorus	48 hours	Weekly
Effluent culture	Weekly	2 weeks
Complete blood count	3-5 days	2 weeks

*Measurement intervals should be adjusted so that more frequent monitoring is taken in the initial phases of dialysis and when an animal's condition is unstable or deteriorating. Less frequent monitoring may be warranted when an animal's condition is stable.

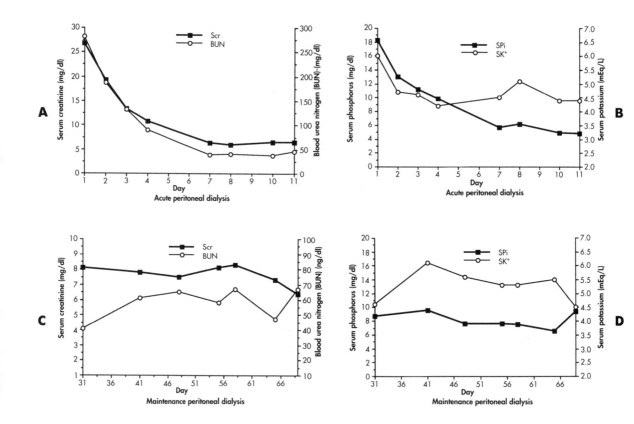

Fig. 39-3 Time course of selected biochemical parameters during peritoneal dialysis in a uremic dog treated using the column disk catheter. Primary renal failure in this dog was from ethylene glycol poisoning. Values for blood urea nitrogen, serum creatinine, and serum phosphorus declined dramatically, but did not enter the normal range. Exchanges were performed every 1 to 2 hours during the first several days of dialysis (acute) (**A** and **B**) and were performed every 4 to 6 hours during maintenance dialysis (**C** and **D**).

(increased glomerular filtration rate, decreased serum creatinine or blood urea nitrogen levels) as dialysis is withdrawn represents the desirable overall measure of successful dialysis.

The serum concentration of uremic solutes (blood urea nitrogen, creatinine, and phosphorus) reflects clearance from the extracellular water into dialysate, the rate of new solute generation, and solute redistribution from intracellular to extracellular water (Fig. 39-3, *A* and *B*). It is common to see what appears to be a rebound increase in blood urea nitrogen and serum creatinine concentrations shortly following interruption of acute dialysis (Fig. 39-3, *C*). This effect is attributed to redistribution of these solutes from intracellular to extracellular water. Peritoneal dialysis is a cumulative process, and removal of only a portion of total body uremic solute occurs during each exchange. Animals with severe catabolism are expected to generate blood urea nitrogen at increased rates. This factor has not been well studied in clinical cases involving dogs or cats.

The level of azotemia achieved that is considered successful or appropriate during dialysis is debatable. Survival is the first priority, followed by allowing the animal to feel better and to begin oral nutritional intake. Is there a certain level of azotemia and retention of associated waste products that either hinders or facilitates renal repair? The answer has yet to be established. Most dogs dramatically improve clinically when peritoneal dialysis lowers the blood urea nitrogen levels to less than 90 mg/dl and serum creatinine concentrations to less than 9 mg/dl.

Individual animals tolerate the same level of azotemia differently. For example, one dog with a serum creatinine concentration of 7.0 mg/dl may exhibit minimal clinical signs and be eating while another dog with the same creatinine level may still be exhibiting severe signs of uremia. Dialysis must be individually tailored to alleviate the signs of uremia.

Acute intrinsic renal failure (AIRF) patients in the maintenance phase with severe azotemia have a relatively poor prognosis for the return of normal renal structure and function, with or without dialysis. This fact may be a consequence of inadequate control of the uremic environment despite improving the animal's condition and decreasing the uremic solute concentrations during dialysis. Too few patients with AIRF and peritoneal dialysis have been critically evaluated to determine if more aggressive dialysis treatments to control uremic solute concentrations will result in increased renal healing, diminished development of further renal lesions, or improved renal function and survival.

Maintenance regimens of CAPD do not result in normal serum phosphorus, blood urea nitrogen, or creatinine concentration (Fig. 39-3, *C* and *D*). Intestinal phosphate binders are usually necessary as an additional treatment measure along with low-phosporus, low-protein foods in order to maintain normal serum phosphorus concentrations.

Peritoneal dialysis is usually performed on critically ill uremic animals. Although dialysis can result in dramatic alterations in uremic solute concentration and in fluid, electrolyte, or acid-base balance, parenteral fluid therapy must be continued for several days until adequate control of the uremic environment has been accomplished by dialysis. Parenteral fluid therapy is not usually necessary during maintenance dialysis treatments.

COMPLICATIONS

Hypoalbuminemia and dialysate retention or catheter obstruction are the most common complications in dogs and cats undergoing peritoneal dialysis.[24] A complete listing of complications is given in Table 39-3. Most of these complications are manageable. Dialysate retention, catheter obstruction, and subcutaneous leakage have been reduced since the use of the modified technique of catheter placement. Loss of proteins into effluent can account for development of hypoalbuminemia, and this effect is magnified during peritonitis. Other reports of complications include a case of *Candida albicans* peritonitis in a dog[14] and pleural effusion in a dog.[4] Pleural effusion following peritoneal dialysis has been observed in people.[55,56]

ENDING DIALYSIS

Ideally, dialysis is continued until renal function

Table 39-3 Frequency of complications during peritoneal dialysis

Hypoalbuminemia	41%
Dialysate retention/catheter obstruction	30%
Peritonitis	22%
Hypochloremia	22%
Subcutaneous leakage of dialysate	22%
Limb edema	19%
Hypokalemia	19%
Hyponatremia	19%
Hypomagnesemia*	15%
Hyperkalemia	11%

*Serum magnesium concentration measured in 4 of 27 animals.

Reprinted with permission from Crisp MS, Chew DJ, DiBartola SP, Birchard SJ. Peritoneal dialysis in dogs and cats: 27 Cases (1976-1987). J Am Vet Med Assoc 1989; 1266.

returns to normal or until enough renal excretory function is reclaimed so that the patient can survive without dialysis. In veterinary medicine, dialysis is rarely continued until the patient is metabolically stable enough to undergo renal transplantation.

If it is apparent that renal function cannot return to a level to support life without dialysis, euthanasia is recommended. This decision is made after evaluation of serial serum biochemistries and renal biopsy.

Dialysis is terminated if the quality of life is not improved to an acceptable level over several days despite successful mechanics of dialysis. This circumstance would include patients that fail to improve biochemically, those whose uremic signs do not improve despite decreased levels of azotemia, and those with nonmanageable peritonitis.

REFERENCES

1. Parker HR, Gourley IM, Bell RL. Current developments in peritoneal and hemo dialysis. Presented at the Gaines 22nd Veterinary Symposium, Stillwater, Oklahoma, March 15, 1972.
2. Parker HR. Current status of peritoneal dialysis. In Kirk RW, ed. Current veterinary therapy VII. Philadelphia: WB Saunders, 1980:1106-1111.
3. Thornhill JA. Peritoneal dialysis in the dog and cat: an update. Compend Contin Educ Pract Vet 1981;3:20-34.
4. Carter LJ, Wingfield WE, Allen TA. Clinical experience with peritoneal dialysis in small animals. Compend Contin Educ Pract Vet 1989;11:1335-1343.
5. Maher JF. Peritoneal transport rates: mechanisms, limitations, and methods for augmentation. Kidney Int 1980;18(Suppl 10):S117-S120.
6. Nolph KD. Peritoneal dialysis. In Brenner BM, Rector FC, eds. The Kidney, ed. 3. Philadelphia: WB Saunders, 1986:1847-1906.
7. Rudnick MR, Cohen RM, Gordon A, Maxwell MH. fluid-electrolyte complications of dialysis. In Maxwell MH, Kleeman CR, Narins RG, eds. Clinical disorders of fluid and electrolyte metabolism, ed. 4. New York: McGraw-Hill, 1987:1053-1103.
8. Rose BD. Physiology of body Fluids. fluids. In rose Rose BD, ed. Clinical physiology of acid-base and electrolyte disorders, ed. 3. New York: McGraw-Hill, 1989:1-27.
9. Henderson LW. Peritoneal ultrafiltration dialysis: enhanced urea transfer using hypertonic peritoneal dialysis fluid. J Clin Invest 1966;45:950-955.
10. Henderson LW, Nolph KD. Altered permeability of the peritoneal membrane after using hypertonic peritoneal dialysis fluid. J Clin Invest 1969;48:992-1001.
11. DiBartola SP, Chew DJ, Tarr MJ, Sams RA. Hemodialysis of a dog with acute renal failure. J Am Vet Med Assoc 1985;186:1323-1326.
12. Twardowski ZJ. Peritoneal dialysis current technology and techniques. Postgrad Med 1989;85:161-182.
13. Grollman A, Turner LB, McLean JA. Intermittent peritoneal lavage in nephrectomized dogs and its application to the human being. Arch Intern Med 1951;87:379-390.
14. Seligman AM, Frank HA, Fine J. Treatment of experimental uremia by means of peritoneal irrigation. J Clin Invest 1946;25:211-219.
15. Rubin J, Jones Q, Quillen E, Bower JD. A model of long-term peritoneal dialysis in the dog. Nephron 1983;35:259-263.
16. Wells IC, Durr MP, Grabner BJ, Holladay FP, Campbell AS, Zielinski CM, Hammeke MD, Egan JD. Experimental study of chronic ambulatory peritoneal dialysis. Clin Physiol Biochem 1985;3:8-15.
17. Simmons EE, Lockard BS, Moncrief JW, Hiatt MP, McCollough WS, Popovich RP. Experience with continuous ambulatory peritoneal dialysis and maintenance of a surgically anephric dog. Southwest Vet 1980;33:129-135.
18. Thornhill JA, Hartman J, Boon GD, Riviere JE, Jacobs D, Ash SR. Support of an anephric dog for 54 days with ambulatory peritoneal dialysis and a newly designed peritoneal catheter. Am J Vet Res 1984;45(6):1156-1161.
19. Johnson RC, Bock F, Knab W, Martis L. A model for study of the kinetics of continuous ambulatory peritoneal dialysis (CAPD). Trans Am Soc Artif Organs 1983;29:67-70.
20. Kirk RW. Peritoneal lavage in uremia in dogs. J Am Vet Med Assoc 1957;131:101-103.
21. Jackson RF. The use of peritoneal dialysis in the treatment of uremia in dogs. Vet Rec 1964;76:1481-1486.
22. Fox LE, Grauer GF, Dubielzig RR, Bjorling DE. Reversal of ethylene glycol-induced nephrotoxicosis in a dog. J Am Vet Med Assoc 1987;191:1433-1435.
23. Thornhill JA, Ash SR, Dhein CR, Polzin DJ, Osborne CA. Peritoneal dialysis with the Purdue column disc catheter. Minn Vet 1980;20:27-33.
24. Crisp MS, Chew DJ, DiBartola SP, Birchard SJ. Peritoneal dialysis in dogs and cats: 27 cases (1976-1987). J Am Vet Med Assoc 1989;195(9):1262-1266.
25. Shahar R, Holmberg DL. Pleural dialysis in the management of acute renal failure in two dogs. J Am Vet Med Assoc 1985;187:952-954.
26. Rubin J, Jones Q, Planch A, Rushton F, Bower J. The importance of the abdominal viscera to peritoneal dialysis in the dog. Am J Med Sci 1986;292:203-208.
27. Kliger AS. Current concepts in peritoneal dialysis. Nephron 1981;27:209-214.
28. Mactier RA, Khanna R, Twardowski ZJ, Nolph KD. Role of peritoneal cavity lymphatic absorption in peritoneal dialysis. Kidney Int 1987;32:165-172.
29. Mactier RA, Khanna R. Absorption of fluid and solutes from the peritoneal cavity, theoretic and therapeutic implications and applications. Trans Am Soc Artif Intern Organs 1989;35:122-131.
30. Rubin J, McFarland S, Hellems EW, Bower JD. Peritoneal dialysis during peritonitis. Kidney Int 1981;19:460-464.
31. Meengs W, Greene JA, Weller JM. Peritoneal clearance of urea and potassium and protein removal during acute peritonitis in dogs. J Lab Clin Med 1970;76:903-906.
32. Elzouki AY, Gruskin AB, Baluarte HJ, Polinsky MS, Prebis JW. Developmental aspects of peritoneal dialysis kinetics in dogs. Pediatr Res 1981;15:853-858.
33. Zelman A, Gisser D, Whittman PJ, Parsons RH, Schuyler R. Augmentation of peritoneal dialysis efficiency with programmed hyper/hyposmotic dialysates. Trans Am Soc Artif Organs 1977;23:203-209.
34. Brown EA, Kliger AS, Finkelstein FO. Peritoneal dialysis clearances, a practical approach to the measurement of small and middle-molecule clearances. Nephron 1978;21:310-316.
35. Brown EA, Kliger AS, Goffinet J, Finkelstein FO. Effect of hypertonic dialysate and vasodilators on peritoneal dialysis clearances in the rat. Kidney Int 1978;13:271-277.
36. Hain H, Kessel M. Aspects of new solutions for peritoneal dialysis. Nephrol Dial Transplant 1987;2:67-72.
37. Miller FN, Nolph KD, Joshua IG, Wiegman DL, Harris PD, Anderson DB. Hyperosmolality, acetate, and lactate:

dilatory factors during peritoneal dialysis. Kidney Int 1981;20:397-402.

38. Nolph KD, Rubin J, Wiegman DL, Harris PD, Miller FN. Peritoneal clearances with three types of commercially available peritoneal dialysis solutions. Nephron 1979;24:35-40.

39. Felt J, Richard C, McCaffrey C, Levy M. Peritoneal clearance of creatinine and inulin during dialysis in dogs: effect of splanchnic vasodilators. Kidney Int 1979;16:459-469.

40. Chew DJ. Urogenital emergencies. In Sherding RG, ed. Medical emergencies. New York: Churchill Livingstone, 1985:187-212.

41. Zager RA. Hyperphosphatemia: a factor that provokes severe experimental acute renal failure. J Lab Clin Med 1982;100:230-239.

42. Reuler JB. Peritoneal dialysis in the management of hypothermia. JAMA 1978;240:2289-2290.

43. Welton DE, Mattox KL, Miller RR, Petmecky FF. Treatment of profound hypothermia. JAMA 1978;240:2291-2292.

44. Hamilton JW, Lasrich M, Hirszel P. Peritoneal dialysis in the treatment of severe hypercalcemia. J Dial 1980;4:129-138.

45. Vale JA, Widdop B, Bluett NH. Ethylene glycol poisoning. Postgrad Med 1976;52:598-602.

46. Copley JB. Prevention of peritoneal dialysis catheter-related infections. Am J Kidney Dis 1987;10:401-407.

47. Werner HP. Disinfectants in dialysis: dangers, drawbacks and disinformation. Nephron 1988;49:1-8.

48. Parks J. Peritoneal lavage. J Am Vet Med Assoc 1974;165:148-149.

49. Kaufman G. Personal communication, 1990.

50. Birchard S, Chew DJ, Crisp MS, Fossum T. Modified technique for placement of a column disc peritoneal dialysis catheter. J Am Anim Hosp Assoc 1988;24:663-666.

51. Robson M, Oreopoulos DG, Izatt S, Ogilvie R, Rapoport A, deVeber GA. Influence of exchange volume and dialysate flow rate on solute clearance in peritoneal dialysis. Kidney Int 1978;14:486-490.

52. Thornhill JA. Peritonitis associated with peritoneal dialysis: diagnosis and treatment. J Am Vet Med Assoc 1983;182:721-724.

53. Thornhill JA. Therapeutic strategies involving antimicrobial treatment of small animals with peritonitis. J Am Vet Med Assoc 1984;185:1181-1184.

54. Lagarde MC, Balton JS: Intraperitoneal povidone-iodine in experimental peritonitis. Ann Surg 1978;186:613.

55. Lorentz WB. Acute hydrothorax during peritoneal dialysis. Pediatrics 1979;94:417-419.

56. Rudnick MR, Coyle JF, Beck LH, McCurdy DK: Acute massive hydrothorax complicating peritoneal dialysis, report of 2 cases and a review of the literature. Clin Nephrol 1979;12:38-44.

40 Hypertension

Linda A. Ross

Hypertensive emergencies are situations in which greatly elevated systemic arterial blood pressure must be rapidly lowered to prevent extensive end-organ damage or death. In humans, severe hypertension is divided into two categories: hypertensive emergencies, which require blood pressure reduction within 1 hour, and hypertensive urgencies, which are less acute. In the latter situation, the blood pressure is extremely elevated but end-organ damage is not evident. Blood pressure reduction in hypertensive urgencies can therefore be accomplished over a somewhat longer time interval (up to 24 hours).[1-8] Severe systemic arterial hypertension has infrequently been diagnosed in veterinary medicine. This may be attributed in part to the failure of clinicians to consider hypertension as a possible cause of certain organ-system dysfunction, and to the historic lack of systemic arterial blood pressure measurements in small animals. The determination of blood pressure in clinical small animal practice has become more common during the past few years. This is attributable to the advent of equipment that enhances the ease, accuracy, and reproducibility of such measurements and to increased recognition of hypertension as a clinical entity. It may be projected that situations constituting hypertensive emergencies and urgencies will be recognized with increasing frequency in the future.

Conditions constituting hypertensive emergencies have been well described in humans. Some of these, such as hypertension associated with pregnancy toxemia, dissecting aortic aneurysms, and refractory hypertension following renal transplantation, are relatively common in humans but have not been described in small animals. Nevertheless, there are a number of situations in which blood pressure reduction must be accomplished rapidly. These include severe accelerated (malignant) hypertension; hypertension complicated by acute left ventricular failure, intracranial hemorrhage, intraocular hemorrhage, retinal detachment, or postoperative bleeding; hypertensive encephalopathy; uncontrolled hypertension in an animal that requires emergency surgery; hypertensive crisis produced by a functional pheochromocytoma; and hypertension associated with acute renal failure (see box below).[1,2,4,6-11]

CLINICAL CONSEQUENCES OF HYPERTENSION

Restoration of normal blood pressure in animals with hypertension is necessary to minimize the clinical consequences of persistently or severely elevated pressures. The organs most affected by hypertension are the brain, eyes, heart, and kidneys, i.e., organs that regulate blood flow or contain extensive capillary networks. Initially, increases in blood pressure trigger autoregulatory mechanisms that result in arteriolar vasoconstriction. Sustained elevations in blood pressure result in arterial and arteriolar hypertrophy and hyperplasia of the tunica media, loss of the internal elastic lamina, and fibrinoid necrosis.[12]

HYPERTENSIVE EMERGENCIES

Hypertension associated with any of the following:
    Malignant hypertension
    Acute left ventricular failure
    Intracranial hemorrhage
    Hypertensive encephalopathy
    Intraocular hemorrhage
    Retinal detachment
    Preoperatively (urgent surgery indicated within 12 to 24 hours)
    Postoperative hemorrhage
    Acute renal failure
    Pheochromocytoma

Clinical neurologic abnormalities associated with hypertension are most commonly the result of intracerebral hemorrhages that result from ruptures of weakened arterial or arteriolar walls. Clinical signs will depend on the size and location of the hemorrhage, but most commonly include vomiting, neurologic deficits, alterations in level of consciousness, coma, and death.[1,6,13] A syndrome of hypertensive encephalopathy has been described in humans. It is most commonly seen in patients that have an acute, severe increase in blood pressure, such as that which occurs in acute renal failure. Clinical signs include acute onset of headache, nausea, vomiting, mental confusion, and apprehension; focal neurologic signs (including seizures) may occur in a waxing and waning pattern.[13,14] The mechanism is not known, and

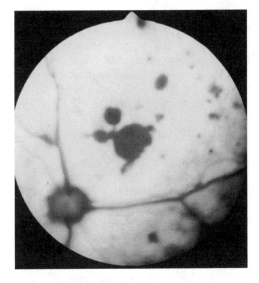

Fig. 40-1 Multiple retinal hemorrhages in a cat with hypertension and chronic renal failure.

two schools of thought exist as to the pathogenesis. The first attributes the neurologic signs to cerebral ischemia resulting from autoregulatory vasoconstriction. The second argues for a "breakthrough" of autoregulation at high pressures, leading to vasodilation and cerebral edema.[13-16] The diagnosis is made in a patient with hypertension and neurologic signs if no other organic cause can be demonstrated and if the signs remit promptly with lowering of blood pressure. The prevalence and character of neurologic abnormalities in dogs and cats with hypertension is not known.

Ocular lesions associated with hypertension have been described in dogs and cats, and appear to parallel those in humans. A grading system is used to assess the severity of the lesions in people.[17] While such a system has not yet been applied to animals, the lesions can be characterized as mild (early), moderate, and severe (late). Arteriolar vasoconstriction occurs early in the course of hypertension and is visualized as straightening and narrowing of the retinal vessels. Sustained elevations in blood pressure produce characteristic changes in retinal arterioles, which eventually lead to vascular smooth muscle necrosis and vascular dilation. Funduscopic examination at this time shows dilated, tortuous retinal vessels. Progression of hypertensive retinopathy to the moderate stage reveals lesions characterized by retinal hemorrhages (Fig. 40-1), "cotton wool" spots representing areas of infarction, and retinal edema. Severe changes may include any of the above as well as retinal exudates, detachments (Fig. 40-2), and papilledema.[17-19] Changes in vision or ocular lesions may be the presenting complaint in dogs or cats with severe hypertension.[18,20]

The cardiac response to hypertension is left ventricular hypertrophy, which enables the heart to overcome the increased afterload resulting from increased peripheral vascular resistance. Cardiac

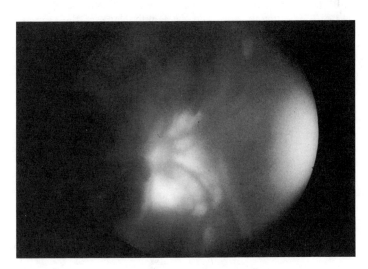

Fig. 40-2 Retinal detachment in a dog with hypertension and chronic renal failure.

dysfunction or left-sided congestive heart failure may occur with severe hypertrophy.[21]

Renal pathology that occurs as the result of hypertension includes focal and segmental glomerular proliferation, and glomerulosclerosis. Severe, untreated hypertension in humans can lead to renal failure.[12] While it is presumed that a similar situation exists in animals, clinical cases have not been documented.[22] Systemic hypertension may contribute to glomerular hyperfiltration in animals with renal insufficiency, hastening the rate of progression of renal failure.[23] While lowering blood pressure is important in the prevention of renal lesions, it is rarely an emergency situation. In fact, rapid reductions of blood pressure in animals with renal failure may worsen renal function, at least temporarily, due to decreased renal blood flow.[7] This is apparently due to upward shifting of the autoregulatory curve during chronic hypertension.[2]

Malignant hypertension in humans is a syndrome characterized by severe hypertension, retinopathy with papilledema, impairment of renal function, fibrinoid necrosis in the kidneys, and a rapidly progressive and fatal course. Virtually all of the clinical manifestations can be attributed to lesions in small arteries and arterioles of various organs.[12] Malignant hypertension has not been described in small animal patients; however, there are published reports of cats and dogs with clinical signs and a clinical course that fit this syndrome.[18,24]

Normal blood pressure in dogs and cats

Hypertension is defined as the elevation of arterial blood pressure above the level generally considered normal for the population of the species. Two components of blood pressure are usually recorded. The systolic pressure is the highest pressure that occurs during ventricular ejection of blood, and the diastolic pressure is the lowest pressure that occurs during ventricular filling. Mean arterial pressure is recorded by some instruments. This value is not an average of the systolic and diastolic pressures, since the heart remains in diastole longer than it remains in systole; the mean pressure is closer to the diastolic reading.

Surveys of clinically normal conscious dogs have reported mean systolic arterial pressures from 112 to 192 mm Hg and mean diastolic pressures of 56 to 110 mm Hg.[22] Blood pressures greater than 160/95 in dogs are taken to indicate hypertension by most investigators. Relatively few studies have been performed in cats, and the results are not consistent. One investigator reported a mean systolic pressure (±range) of 171±22 mm Hg and a mean diastolic pressure of 123±17 mm Hg in 10 normal cats. Another study

reported the mean systolic and diastolic pressures to be 113/85; a third found systolic pressure to range from 139±8 to 146±9 mm Hg, and diastolic from 91±9 to 118±16 mm Hg. Studies by Labato and Ross in 6 normal cats determined the mean systolic pressure to be 127.5±7 mm Hg and the mean diastolic pressure 71±3.7 mm Hg.[25] These disparate findings make it more difficult to recommend maximum values for normal blood pressure in the cat; however, values above 190/140 should exclude most normal cats from being hypertensive.

MEASUREMENT OF BLOOD PRESSURE

Arterial blood pressure can be measured by either indirect or direct techniques. A number of studies have shown good correlation between the two methods as long as careful attention is paid to technique.[22] Indirect methods have the advantage of being noninvasive, while direct measurement allows access to the arterial circulation for additional sampling (blood gas analysis). Animals with hypertensive emergencies will require frequent blood pressure determinations over several days, which makes repeated arterial punctures for direct measurements impractical if not impossible. Direct measurement through an indwelling arterial catheter is probably the method of choice in these animals, although indirect measurement is acceptable.

Indirect blood pressure measurements involve the occlusion of a peripheral artery by inflation of a cuff. The closing and opening of the artery is detected as the cuff is inflated and deflated. This is accomplished by palpatory, auscultatory, ultrasonic, or oscillometric means (Fig. 40-3). The cranial tibial artery is usually the best choice for indirect blood pressure measurements (Fig. 40-4), although the brachial artery may prove more satisfactory in chondrodystrophic breeds of dogs and in some cats. The cuff width should be approximately 40% and the length 150% of the circumference of the limb. Oversized cuffs produce artifactually low readings, while undersized cuffs produce artifactually high readings. The cuff should be inflated to a pressure 30 to 40 mm Hg higher than that necessary to obliterate the pulse. As the cuff is gradually deflated, blood begins to flow through the artery and a series of sounds can be detected (Korotkoff sounds, see box on p. 651). The first appearance of the sound (Phase I) indicates initiation of blood flow through the artery and represents the systolic pressure. Diastolic pressure is usually measured at Phase IV, although Phases IV and V are usually close. It is recommended that several indirect readings be taken at 1-minute intervals and the results averaged, since

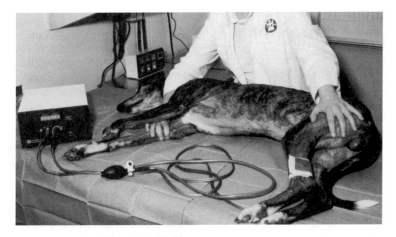

Fig. 40-3 A dog correctly positioned for indirect blood pressure measurement using an ultrasonic Doppler flow detector. (From Ettinger SJ: Textbook of veterinary internal medicine, ed. 3. Philadelphia: WB Saunders, 1989.)

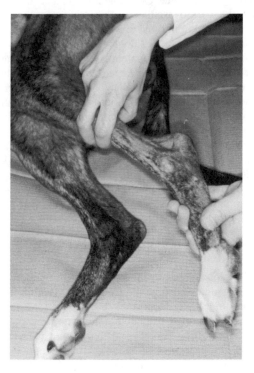

Fig. 40-4 Placement of the flow detector for indirect blood pressure measurement is determined by palpation of the pulse through the cranial tibial artery.

HYPERTENSIVE EMERGENCIES

Hypertension associated with any of the following:
   Malignant hypertension
   Acute left ventricular failure
   Intracranial hemorrhage
   Hypertensive encephalopathy
   Intraocular hemorrhage
   Retinal detachment
   Preoperatively (urgent surgery indicated within
      12 to 24 hours)
   Postoperative hemorrhage
   Acute renal failure
   Pheochromocytoma

---

there is some minute-to-minute variation in pressure due to respiration, movement, and heart rate.

DIAGNOSIS OF HYPERTENSIVE EMERGENCIES

A hypertensive emergency should be suspected and the blood pressure measured in animals exhibiting signs of hypertension-induced end-organ damage. These include encephalopathy and other neurologic signs, loss of vision, retinal hemorrhages or detachment, and pulmonary edema from congestive heart failure. In addition, animals with diseases known to be associated with hypertension (see the box on p. 652) should be considered

DISEASES ASSOCIATED WITH HYPERTENSION

Endocrine diseases
    Hyperadrenocorticism
    Pheochromocytoma
    Hyperthyroidism
    Hypothyroidism*
    Hyperparathyroidism*
    Acromegaly*
Renal failure
    Acute oliguric failure, any cause
    Chronic failure
    Chronic interstitial nephritis
    Glomerulonephritis
    Congenital renal dysplasia
Neurologic disorders*
    Trauma
    Neoplasia
Severe body burns*

*Not yet documented as causes of hypertension in dogs or cats.

at risk for hypertensive crises. These animals should have base-line blood pressure measurements taken as soon as the disease is recognized.

Diseases associated with hypertension

A brief review of the disorders known to be associated with hypertension will alert the clinician to situations in which blood pressure should be measured. While primary, or essential hypertension, has been documented in dogs, the prevalence is extremely low.[22] Most of the dogs and cats with elevations in arterial blood pressure have secondary hypertension.[22,25]

Acute renal failure may be associated with severe hypertension, particularly in oliguric animals that have been treated with fluid therapy. Sixty percent of dogs and cats with chronic renal failure are hypertensive,[22] although the mechanism is not known. Ocular lesions constituting hypertensive emergencies have been reported in both dogs[20,24] and cats[18] with chronic renal failure.

Various endocrine diseases have been associated with hypertension in small animals. Hyperadrenocorticism in dogs has been associated with hypertension in 59%[26] to 82%[27] of the cases studied. The thromboembolic phenomenon sometimes seen in affected animals could be partially attributed to vascular pathology caused by increased blood pressure. Hyperthyroidism, a common endocrine disorder of aged cats, has been reported to be associated with hypertension in 87% of affected animals.[28] Hypothyroidism has also been associated with in-

creased blood pressure in humans.[29] The prevalence of hypertension in animals with hypothyroidism is not known. There is one report of a dog with hypertension and hypothyroidism.[24] Acromegaly is the result of persistently elevated growth hormone levels, and has been associated with hypertension in humans.[29] Acromegaly is seen in dogs that have been chronically treated with progestagens for contraception and in cats as a spontaneous disease.[30] The prevalence of hypertension in these animals is not known, although the high prevalence of cardiomyopathy and congestive heart failure in cats with acromegaly could be related to underlying hypertension.[30] Hyperparathyroidism is another disorder associated with elevated blood pressure in humans,[29] but the occurrence of hypertension in animals with hyperparathyroidism is unknown. Pheochromocytomas (rare tumors of the adrenal medulla) are considered a classic cause of hypertension. They produce catecholamines that act directly on the cardiovascular system to increase blood pressure, although the elevations may be paroxysmal.[31] Two reports of dogs with pheochromocytomas found similar prevalences of hypertension (approximately 50% of affected animals).[32,33] Other published series of canine cases did not report blood pressures, but did describe clinical and pathologic findings consistent with those caused by hypertension.[34,35]

Several miscellaneous conditions have been associated with severe hypertension in humans, including intracranial hemorrhage, head injuries, and severe body burns.[7] Although a similar association has not been reported in animals, it is possible that it could occur.

THERAPY OF HYPERTENSIVE EMERGENCIES

The blood pressure in animals with hypertensive emergencies must be reduced rapidly (within minutes to 1 hour) to normal levels[2,7,8,11] and takes precedence over extensive diagnostic procedures. An indwelling venous catheter should be placed for administration of parenteral antihypertensive agents, and an arterial line established if blood pressure is to be measured directly (see Chapter 4). The choice of antihypertensive agent depends more on the degree of hypertension and the severity of clinical signs than on the underlying cause, with the exception of animals with pheochromocytomas (see box above).

Most vasodilator and adrenergic antagonistic drugs used to lower blood pressure in hypertensive emergencies cause sodium and water retention by the kidney.[6,7,9] A diuretic should be administered concomitantly with the antihypertensive agents unless the animal is dehydrated. Fu-

Table 40-1 Drugs used in the treatment of hypertensive emergencies

Drug	Dosage	Maximum Response (Minutes)	Mechanism of Action
Acepromazine	0.05-0.1 mg/kg intravenous bolus	60	Alpha-adrenergic blocker
Sodium nitroprusside	0.5-3.0 μg/kg/minute IV initially; maximum 10 μg/kg/minute	1-2	Balanced vasodilator
Diazoxide	5 mg/kg intravenous bolus (humans)	3-5	Arteriolar vasodilator
Nifedipine	10 mg PO (humans)	30	Vasodilation through calcium channel blockade
Labetalol	1-2 mg/kg IV infused over 10 minutes (humans)	5-10	Alpha- and beta-adrenergic blocker
Phentolamine	0.02-0.1 mg/kg IV	1-3	Alpha-adrenergic blocker
Phenoxybenzamine	0.2-1.5 mg/kg PO every 12 hours	60-120?	Alpha-adrenergic blocker
Prazosin	0.25-2.0 mg PO every 8-12 hours	60-180	Balanced vasodilator
Hydralazine	0.5-2.0 mg/kg PO every 12 hours	30-120	Arteriolar vasodilator
Captopril	0.5-2.0 mg/kg PO every 8-12 hours	60-90	Inhibition of angiotensin II-mediated vasoconstriction, natriuresis

IV = intravenously; PO = orally.

rosemide is the diuretic of choice at a dosage of 0.5 to 2.2 mg/kg every 8 to 12 hours.

Acepromazine, administered as an intravenous bolus of 0.05 to 0.1 mg/kg body weight, is probably the most readily available drug for initial therapy.[36] Acepromazine lowers blood pressure by alpha-adrenergic blockade causing peripheral arterial vasodilation. If this therapy is unsuccessful in reducing blood pressure, there are several antihypertensive agents that may be tried (Table 40-1). Although these drugs have been evaluated in hypertensive emergencies in humans, their efficacy in animals with similar conditions is unproven. It would seem logical to use these drugs since their pharmacologic action in both animals and humans is similar.

Sodium nitroprusside is considered the most potent and most predictably effective agent for treatment of hypertensive crises in humans.[2,5-9,37] It is a rapid-acting, balanced vasodilator whose potency is such that arterial pressure can be maintained at almost any level by appropriate adjustment of the infusion rate.[9] Nitroprusside has the advantage of reducing blood pressure rapidly in almost any situation, but the disadvantage of requiring very close monitoring of blood pressure. Sedation does not occur because nitroprusside does not cross the blood-brain barrier. It is administered as a constant intravenous infusion at a rate of 0.5 to 3 μg/kg per minute; this rate may be increased to a maximum of 10 μg/kg per minute in an attempt to reduce blood pressure.[38] Use of a variable-rate fluid infusion pump is recommended for accurate dose delivery. The blood pressure will begin to fall within 1 or 2 minutes after the initiation of the infusion. The duration of action of sodium nitroprusside is extremely short, so that blood pressure will return to pretreatment levels within 5 minutes after cessation of infusion.[37] The drug is light sensitive after dilution, and bottles or bags of fluid as well as the intravenous administration tubing must be covered. Solutions several hours old should be discarded.[9,38] Sodium nitroprusside is metabolized to cyanide, which is then converted to thiocyanate by the liver and excreted by the kidneys.[37] Administration of sodium nitroprusside to an animal with liver or kidney disease could conceivably result in cyanide or thiocyanate toxicity, especially with prolonged infusions or high doses.

Diazoxide is a benzothiadiazine derivative that directly relaxes arteriolar smooth muscle and reduces blood pressure. It does not impair baroreceptor reflexes, and reflex tachycardia as well as increases in stroke volume and cardiac output occur as blood pressure decreases.[2,6,9,39] Diazoxide is more convenient to administer than sodium nitroprusside because it is given by intravenous bolus. The dosage used in humans is 5 mg/kg; dosages in veterinary patients have not been established. A rapid and profound drop in blood pressure occurs within 3 to 5 minutes of diazoxide administration and lasts 12 to 18 hours.[7,39] Close monitoring of the animal would be required only during the first 15 to 20 minutes after injection.[9] This drug has limited usage in human medicine because of the inability to modulate the rapid and sustained drop in blood pressure that may compromise renal, cardiac, or cerebral blood flow. Hyperglycemia routinely occurs with diazoxide use, as insulin secretion by pancreatic beta cells is suppressed, although this effect is not usually of clinical significance.[39]

Nifedipine is a calcium-channel blocker and vasodilator. It acts directly on vascular smooth muscle cells to decrease intracellular calcium ions.[40] The use of oral or sublingual nifedipine for hypertensive emergencies in humans has been advocated as an equally efficacious but more cost-effective alternative to sodium nitroprusside.[2,40-43] In dogs, intravenous administration produces a reduction in blood pressure but also causes an increase in heart rate and cardiac output via sympathetic activation.[44] Oral administration produced variable and only mild reductions in blood pressure.[44] In addition, the half-life of nifedipine in dogs by either intravenous or oral administration is very short (1 hour).[44] These species differences suggest that nifedipine may not have a role in the therapy of hypertensive crises in small animals.

Labetalol is an alpha- and beta-blocking agent whose administration causes a decrease in peripheral vascular resistance and a fall in blood pressure without reflex tachycardia. It has been shown to reduce blood pressure within 5 to 10 minutes when administered as an intravenous bolus of 20 mg, followed by 40- or 80-mg boluses every 10 minutes until normal blood pressure is attained.[7,45] Doses of 1 to 2 mg/kg infused over 10 minutes have also been reported to be effective.[46] Its use in dogs and cats has not been investigated.

Phentolamine, an alpha-receptor antagonist, is the drug of choice for animals with pheochromocytomas and hypertensive crises associated with elevated levels of circulating catecholamines. It is administered as an initial intravenous bolus of 1 to 5 mg followed by intravenous infusion.[7,31] Administration of labetalol could also be considered. Oral phenoxybenzamine (an alpha-blocker) or prazosin (a balanced vasodilator) may be administered to maintain blood pressure, prior to surgical intervention, once normal levels are achieved.[31] In the presence of tachyarrhythmias associated with pheochromocytomas an alpha-antagonist must be given prior to beta-blocker administration

to prevent a hypertensive crisis (Chapter 18).

If severe end-organ damage does not seem imminent within a few hours, reduction of blood pressure by administration of potent oral antihypertensive agents may be the therapy of choice. Prazosin is an alpha-adrenergic antagonist that produces balanced vasodilation. It consistently reduces blood pressure in dogs within several hours of administration; in fact, the first dose has been associated with hypotension and syncope when administered to dogs with congestive heart failure. The effect in cats is somewhat less predictable. The suggested dose is 0.25 to 2.0 mg orally every 8 to 12 hours.[47,48]

Hydralazine is a potent direct-acting arteriolar vasodilator. Reductions in blood pressure are accompanied by reflex tachycardia and activation of the renin-angiotensin aldosterone system, necessitating concurrent therapy with diuretics. The suggested dosage in dogs is 0.5 to 2.0 mg/kg orally every 12 hours.[48]

Angiotensin-converting-enzyme inhibitors (captopril, enalapril) represent another class of antihypertensive agents that reduce blood pressure through several mechanisms.[22,47,49] These drugs inhibit the conversion of angiotensin I to angiotensin II. Reductions in blood pressure are primarily the result of loss of angiotensin II-mediated vasoconstriction and suppression of aldosterone secretion with subsequent natriuresis. Other effects, such as increased concentrations of bradykinin and prostaglandin E_2 resulting in vasodilation, play a minor role. The suggested dosage for captopril in dogs and cats is 0.5 to 2.0 mg/kg orally every 8 to 12 hours. This dosage must be reduced in animals with renal failure because the drug is excreted by the kidneys.[22,47]

CHRONIC THERAPY FOR SYSTEMIC HYPERTENSION

Once blood pressure has been reduced, the cause of the hypertension should be determined by appropriate diagnostic procedures. Since most hypertension in dogs and cats is secondary in origin, elimination of the primary disease should result in normalization of blood pressure. If the disease cannot be corrected, or if diagnostics will be prolonged, oral antihypertensive drugs should be administered. Drugs are administered in sequence as necessary to maintain blood pressure.[22,47,49] Diuretics are generally the first line of therapy, and should already have been administered to animals that have been treated for a hypertensive crisis. Beta-adrenergic blocking agents such as propranolol constitute the second class of drugs. The third class consists of the vasodilators, including hydralazine, prazosin, and calcium-channel blockers such as verapamil. Angiotensin-converting-enzyme inhibitors represent a fourth class of antihypertensive drugs. In order to prevent a second hypertensive crisis, animals that initially presented as hypertensive emergencies should be hospitalized until it is determined that normal blood pressure can be maintained with oral antihypertensive drugs.

REFERENCES

1. Alpert MA, Bauer JH. Hypertensive emergencies: recognition and pathogenesis. Cardiovasc Rev Reports 1985;6:407-427.
2. Ferguson RK, Vlasses PH. Hypertensive emergencies and urgencies. JAMA 1986;255:1607-1623.
3. Anderson RJ, Reed WG. Current concepts in treatment of hypertensive urgencies. Am Heart J 1986;111:211-219.
4. Houston M. Hypertensive emergencies and urgencies: pathophysiology and clinical aspects. Am Heart J 1986;111:205-210.
5. Vidt DG. Current concepts in treatment of hypertensive emergencies. Am Heart J 1986;111:220-225.
6. Garcia JY, Vidt DG. Current management of hypertensive emergencies. Drugs 1987;34:263-278.
7. Gifford RW Jr. Management and treatment of essential hypertension, including malignant hypertension and emergencies. In Genest J, Kuchel O, Hamet P, Cantin M, eds. Hypertension, ed. 2. New York: McGraw-Hill, 1983;1127-1170.
8. Grim CE. Emergency treatment of severe or malignant hypertension. Geriatrics 1980;35:57-60.
9. Koch-Weser J. Hypertensive emergencies. N Engl J Med 1974;290:211-214.
10. Keith TA III. Hypertension crisis. JAMA 1977;237:1570-1577.
11. Vaamonde CA, David NJ, Palmer RF. Hypertensive emergencies. Med Clin North Am 1971;55:325-334.
12. Kincaid-Smith P. Malignant hypertension: mechanisms and management. Pharmacol Ther 1980;9:245-269.
13. Sandok BA, Whisnant JP. Hypertension and the brain: clinical aspects. In Genest J, Kuchel O, Hamet P, Cantin M, eds. Hypertension, ed. 2. New York: McGraw-Hill, 1983;777-791.
14. Gifford RW, Westbrook E. Hypertensive encephalopathy: mechanisms, clinical features, and treatment. Prog Cardiovasc Dis 1974;17:115-124.
15. Johansson B, Strandgaard S, Lassen NA. On the pathogenesis of hypertensive encephalopathy. Circ Res 1974;34(suppl 1):167-174.
16. Skinhoj E, Strandgaard S. Pathogenesis of hypertensive encephalopathy. Lancet 1973;1:461-462.
17. Dollery CT. Hypertensive retinopathy. In Genest J, Kuchel O, Hamet P, Cantin M, eds. Hypertension, ed. 2. New York: McGraw-Hill, 1983;723-732.
18. Morgan RV. Systemic hypertension in four cats: ocular and medical findings. J Am Anim Hosp Assoc 1985;22:615-621.
19. Garner A, Ashton N, Tripathi R, Kohner EM, Bulpitt CJ, Dollery CT. Pathogenesis of hypertensive retinopathy: an experimental study in the monkey. Br J Ophthalmol 1975;59:3.
20. Blanchard, GL, Eyster GE, Carrig CB, Rovner DR, Barlie MD, Padgett GA. Primary essential hypertension in a Siberian Husky dog [abstract]. Fed Proc 1979;38:1450.
21. Frohlich ED. The heart in hypertension. In Genest J, Kuchel O, Hamet P, Cantin M, eds. Hypertension, ed. 2. New York: McGraw-Hill, 1983;791-810.

22. Ross LA. Hypertensive disease. In Ettinger SJ, ed. Textbook of veterinary internal medicine, ed. 3. Philadelphia: WB Saunders, 1989;2047-2056.
23. Baldwin DS, Neugarten J. Blood pressure control and progression of renal insufficiency. Contemp Issues Nephrol 1986;14:81-110.
24. Gwin RM, Gelatt KN, Terrell TG, Hood CI. Hypertensive retinopathy associated with hypothyroidism, hypercholesterolemia, and renal failure in a dog. J Am Anim Hosp Assoc 1978;14:200-209.
25. Labato MA, Ross LA. Diagnosis and management of hypertension. In August J, ed. Consultations in feline internal medicine. Philadelphia: WB Saunders. In press.
26. Kallet A, Cowgill LD. Hypertensive states in the dog. In Proceedings of the American College of Veterinary Internal Medicine. Salt Lake City: American College of Veterinary Internal Medicine, 1982;79.
27. Peterson ME. Hyperadrenocorticism. Vet Clin North Am Small Anim Pract 1984;14:731-749.
28. Kobayashi DL, Graves TK, Nichols CE, Peterson ME. Blood pressure is elevated in hyperthyroid cats and cats with renal disease [abstract]. In Proceedings of the Sixth Annual Veterinary Medical Forum. Washington DC: American College of Veterinary Internal Medicine, 1988;723.
29. Hamet P. Endocrine hypertension: Cushing's syndrome, acromegaly, hyperparathyroidism. In Genest J, Kuchel O, Hamet P, Cantin M, eds. Hypertension, ed. 2. New York: McGraw-Hill, 1983;964-976.
30. Petersen ME, Taylor RS, Greco DS, Lothrop CD. Spontaneous acromegaly in the cat [abstract]. In Proceedings of the Fourth Annual Veterinary Medical Forum. Washington DC: American College of Veterinary Internal Medicine, 1986;14-43.
31. Kuchel O. Adrenal medulla: pheochromocytoma. In Genest J, Kuchel O, Hamet P, Cantin M, eds. Hypertension, ed. 2. New York: McGraw-Hill, 1983;947-963.
32. Feldman EC, Nelson RW. Canine and feline endocrinology and reproduction. Philadelphia: WB Saunders, 1987.
33. Twedt DC, Wheeler SL. Pheochromocytoma in the dog. Vet Clin North Am Small Anim Pract 1984;14:767-782.
34. Bouayad H, Feeney DA, Caywood DD, Hayden DW. Pheochromocytoma in dogs: 13 cases (1980-1985). J Am Vet Med Assoc 1987;1610-1615.
35. Howard EB, Nielsen SW. Pheochromocytomas associated with hypertensive lesions in dogs. J Am Vet Med Assoc 1965;147:245-252.
36. Cowgill LD, Kallet AJ. Systemic hypertension. In Kirk RW, ed. Current veterinary therapy IX. Philadelphia: WB Saunders, 1986;360-364.
37. Palmer RF, Lasseter KC. Sodium nitroprusside. N Engl J Med 1975;292:294-297.
38. Nipride. In: Physicians' desk reference. Oradell, NJ: Medical Economics, 1989;1741-1742.
39. Koch-Weser J. Diazoxide. N Engl J Med 1976;294:1271-1274.
40. Bertel O, Conen LD. Treatment of hypertensive emergencies with the calcium channel blocker nifedipine. Am J Med 1985;79(suppl 4A):31-35.
41. Houston MC. Treatment of hypertensive urgencies and emergencies with nifedipine. Am Heart J 1986;111:963-969.
42. Ellrodt AG, Ault MJ, Riedinger MS, Murata GH. Efficacy and safety of sublingual nifedipine in hypertensive emergencies. Am J Med 1985;79(suppl 4A):19-25.
43. Franklin C, Nightingale S, Mamdani B. A randomized comparison of nifedipine and sodium nitroprusside in severe hypertension. Chest 1986;90:500-503.
44. Keene BW, Hamlin RL. Calcium antagonists. In Kirk, RW, ed. Current veterinary therapy IX. Philadelphia: WB Saunders, 1986;340-342.

45. Cressman M, Moore S, Wilson D, Vidt DG. Intravenous labetalol for the rapid control of severe hypertension [abstract]. Clin Pharmacol Ther 1982;31:213-214.

46. Brogden RN, Heel RC, Speight TM, Avery GS. Labetalol: a review of its pharmacology and therapeutic use in hypertension. Drugs 1978;15:251-270.

47. Ross LA, Labato MA. Use of drugs to control hypertension in renal failure. In Kirk RW, ed. Current veterinary therapy X. Philadelphia: WB Saunders, 1989;1201-1204.

48. Bonagura JD, Muir W. Vasodilator therapy. In Kirk, RW, ed. Current veterinary therapy IX. Philadelphia: WB Saunders, 1986;329-333.

49. Allen, TA. The treatment of hypertension. In Proceedings of the American College of Veterinary Internal Medicine Forum. Washington, DC: American College of Veterinary Internal Medicine, 1986;3-105-3-107.

41 Cardiac Pacing

John E. Rush and James N. Ross, Jr.

Artificial cardiac pacing is the repetitive delivery of low electrical energy to the heart to initiate and maintain the cardiac rhythm. Animals occasionally have cardiac arrhythmias that are best corrected by cardiac pacing. Cardiac pacing can be a life-saving technique and it is useful in animals with either bradycardias or tachycardias. Although some specialized equipment is required to perform cardiac pacing, the procedure to insert a temporary cardiac pacing catheter into the right ventricle is not difficult. We strongly believe that animals with clinical signs of cardiac insufficiency due to bradycardia should have a temporary pacemaker quickly inserted. With appropriate equipment and technical training, cardiac pacing is a technique that can be performed at many emergency facilities.

Bradycardia is the most common indication for cardiac pacing in veterinary patients. Bradyarrhythmias that commonly require pacing include third-degree atrioventricular (AV) block, high-grade second-degree AV block, type II second-degree AV block in association with bifascicular bundle-branch block, sinus arrest (especially in association with sick sinus syndrome), persistent sinus bradycardia, and permanent atrial standstill due to atrial muscular dystrophy.[1-11] Arrhythmias requiring pacemaker therapy can usually be identified from the resting electrocardiogram. In some cases, further studies such as exercise electrocardiogram or Holter monitor recordings are required to diagnose transient arrhythmias.

When considering which animals with bradyarrhythmias require pacemaker therapy, one must determine whether there is clinical evidence of low cardiac output. Diminished cardiac output resulting from bradycardia can lead to lethargy, exercise intolerance, weakness, oliguria, syncope (Stokes-Adams attacks) and congestive heart failure. The indications for cardiac pacing in critically ill animals are broader than those for otherwise healthy patients with a normal cardiovascular reserve. Critically ill patients with drug-resistant sinus bradycardia and less advanced forms of AV block may benefit from pacemaker therapy, especially if antiarrhythmic drugs that might depress automaticity or conduction are to be used.

Marked reductions in cardiac output attend most bradyarrhythmias. Cardiac output is the product of stroke volume and heart rate. The ability of the heart to increase stroke volume acutely is limited, yet over a wide range, increases in heart rate are directly related to increases in cardiac output. This increase in cardiac output is independent of contractility and cardiac loading conditions (preload and afterload). Therefore, simply increasing the heart rate of a animal with bradycardia by inserting a temporary pacemaker will result in a marked increase in cardiac output. The resulting increase in blood flow is beneficial to all organs and tissues. Although medical therapy with anticholinergic or sympathomimetic drugs may improve bradyarrhythmias in some patients (see Chapter 17), most are unresponsive or become refractory to drugs. If drug therapy is ineffective or only partially effective, a temporary pacing catheter should be placed without hesitation. Unnecessary delays in pacemaker placement often result in deterioration of the patient's condition.

PACING MODES

Several pacemaker types are available. Temporary pacing is accomplished by using a temporary intracardiac pacing catheter and a nonimplantable pulse generator or pacing unit located outside the body (Fig. 41-1). This pacing catheter remains in the heart until a permanent pacemaker is implanted or until the arrhythmia has resolved. With permanent pacemakers, both the pacing lead and

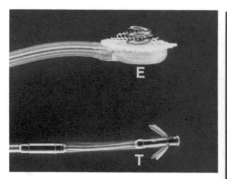

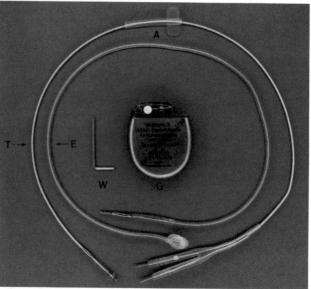

Fig. 41-1 Equipment for cardiac pacemaker implantation. G = pulse generator; T = bipolar transvenous lead; E = unipolar epicardial lead; A = lead anchor sleeve; W = Allen wrench. Upper left-hand corner close-up of transvenous endocardial pacing lead = T and epicardial screw-in pacing lead = E.

pulse generator are surgically implanted beneath the skin. The pulse generator is the source of the delivered electrical impulse and acts as the brain of the pacing unit. A permanent pulse generator is composed of a battery source and complex electrical pacing circuitry housed within a sealed titanium case. The pacing leads are attached to the pulse generator using recessed screws inside of a sealed epoxy connector to minimize contact with body fluids and prevent interruption of the electrical circuit.

Depending on the type of arrhythmia, atrial pacing, ventricular pacing, or dual pacing (both atrial and ventricular) may be appropriate. Atrial pacing alone relies on intact conduction through the AV node. Ventricular pacing is used most frequently in veterinary patients as the atrial or AV node are commonly diseased, precluding effective transmission of an atrial impulse to the ventricles. One significant disadvantage to ventricular pacing is the loss of an atrial "kick" to prime the heart with blood in late diastole. The loss of this atrial contribution to cardiac output (15% to 20%) can be overcome with dual chamber pacing, in which the atria and ventricle are activated in sequence, permitting coordination of atrial and ventricular contractions. Dual pacing is used infrequently in dogs because of the necessity of a double-lead system, the potential for "cross talk," and the added expense.[6,11] Cross talk occurs when the

atrial pacemaker output is incorrectly identified by the ventricular sensor as a spontaneous ventricular depolarization. This results in inhibition of all ventricular pacing, a disastrous consequence if the patient has complete heart block. Cardiac pacing can be accomplished using endocardial or epicardial pacing. Endocardial pacing, currently the most common technique in dogs, is accomplished by passing the pacing lead into the heart through systemic veins.[2,6,9-11] Epicardial pacing can only be accomplished by surgically invading the thorax and placing a pacing lead electrode in contact with the epicardial surface of the heart.[1,3-5,7-10] Transcutaneous pacemakers are also available for use in humans; however, they are associated with significant patient discomfort[12] in dogs and are not well tolerated by them.

The earliest cardiac pacemakers had limited functions and were programmed to discharge at a fixed rate, independent of the underlying cardiac rhythm. This mode of pacing, described as asynchronous pacing, is available on temporary pacing units but is no longer used in permanent pacemakers. Asynchronous pacing could result in stimulating the heart during the vulnerable period of the T wave, thus inducing fatal ventricular arrhythmias. With demand or inhibited pacing, the pacemaker senses the animal's natural cardiac rhythm and delivers a pacing stimulus only when the inherent cardiac rhythm falls below a desired

Table 41-1 ICHD generic pacemaker code

1st Letter Chamber(s) Paced	2nd Letter Chamber(s) Sensed	3rd Letter Mode of Response	4th Letter Programmable Functions	5th Letter Tachycardia Functions
V = Ventricle	V = Ventricle	I = Inhibited	P = simple programmable	S = Scanning
A = Atrium	A = Atrium	T = Triggered	M = Multi-programmable	E = External
D = Dual	D = Dual	D = Dual (both triggered/inhibited)	O = None	B = Burst pacing
O = None	O = None	O = None		O = None

heart rate. Pacemaker technology has progressed such that multiprogrammable pacemakers now allow for transcutaneous adjustment of heart rate, degree of cardiac sensing, and stimulus output. Some pacemakers even have the ability to sense tachycardias and deliver a pacing burst to terminate the tachycardia and/or deliver an internal defibrillatory shock.[13-18]

CODING OF PACEMAKERS

To simplify identification of pacemakers and communication about pacing modes, a five-letter code was designed to describe the type and mode of action (Table 41-1). The first letter indicates which cardiac chambers are stimulated, with *V* referring to the ventricle, *A* atrium, and *D* dual (both atrium and ventricle). The second letter identifies the chamber(s) that are sensed, again *V, A,* and *D* (ventricle, atrium, or both). The letter *O* indicates that this capability is lacking. The third letter defines the pacemaker's mode of response to sensed events. Sensing an intrinsic cardiac event may either inhibit *(I)* or trigger *(T)* pacing output and/or resetting of the timing circuit. The letter *D* in the third position indicates that the pacemaker is both inhibited by sensed ventricular activity and triggered by spontaneous atrial activity (after a preset delay to coordinate atrial and ventricular contraction). The fourth and fifth letters describe whether the unit has programmable functions or tachycardia functions. Most pacemakers implanted into veterinary patients are *VVIPO* (ventricular inhibited, demand, rate and output programmable) or *VVIMO* (ventricular inhibited, demand, multiprogrammable). These pacemakers with the *VVI* designation act by sensing the electrical activity of the ventricle and deliver an impulse only when the inherent rate of the chamber falls below the programmed rate, usually between 80 and 110 beats per minute in the dog.

LEAD SYSTEMS

The electrical circuit of the pacemaker and lead wire combination may be unipolar or bipolar.[10,19]

Both systems can be used reliably with permanent pacing; however, temporary pacing requires a bipolar lead. A bipolar lead has two wires extending from the pulse generator to the heart. Both wires exit a short distance from each other at the tip of the lead with the cathode usually located at the tip of the catheter and the anode located just proximally (Fig. 41-2). Unipolar lead systems contain a single wire with the cathode exiting at the distal tip of the lead. Current flows from the pulse generator down the lead wire to the cathode, causing depolarization of the heart. The electrical current then flows through the animal's body fluids back to the casing of the pulse generator, which acts as the anode.

In animals with unipolar lead systems, skeletal muscle in proximity to the pulse generator may be stimulated by the impulse returning from the heart. This possibility is reduced by placing the pulse generator in a pouch,[11] though the twitching usually diminishes without this intervention in the first few weeks as the pulse generator becomes encapsulated. An additional disadvantage of unipolar systems is their tendency (incorrectly) to sense skeletal muscle myopotentials as cardiac action potentials, causing inhibition of pacemaker discharge.

A disadvantage of bipolar-lead systems is their failure to sense low-amplitude ventricular premature depolarizations, potentially resulting in cardiac pacing during the vulnerable period of the T wave.[19,20]

TEMPORARY PACING

Temporary pacing is indicated in a number of clinical situations in which symptomatic bradycardia is present or expected to occur. Temporary pacing is used to stabilize patients prior to permanent pacemaker implantation. In animals with bradycardia and profound weakness, frequent syncope, or congestive heart failure, temporary pacing is commonly performed for 1 to 3 days to treat heart failure and to ensure adequate renal and cerebral perfusion prior to anesthesia and surgery for their permanent pacemaker implantation.

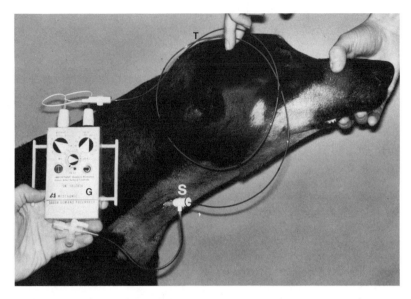

Fig. 41-2 Temporary transvenous pacing. An external pulse generator *(G)* is attached to a 5 French bipolar pacing lead *(T)*. The pacing lead is passed through the sheath introducer *(S)* into the jugular vein.

Because ventricular asystole and ventricular fibrillation are reported during induction of anesthesia in dogs with heart block and atrial standstill,[5,10,11] temporary pacing is routinely performed prior to anesthetic induction for permanent pacemaker implantation. Additional indications for temporary cardiac pacing include drug intoxications causing bradycardia, right heart catheterization in patients with preexisting left bundle-branch block, bradycardia following cardiac surgery, neurologic causes of bradycardia, and heart failure associated with a slow heart rate.

As with most emergency procedures, preparedness and careful planning are the keys to successful placement of a temporary pacemaker. All of the necessary equipment, including a spare battery, must be ready and at arm's reach. This is especially true in the treatment of patients who develop bradyarrhythmias during cardiopulmonary arrest (CPA). Several investigations in humans document the need to place the pacing catheter within the first 5 minutes of bradycardic CPA if a favorable outcome is to be achieved during cardiopulmonary resuscitation.[12,21,22] These studies emphasize the point that a pacing catheter should be placed without delay in cases in which pacemaker therapy is anticipated.

Placement

In some weak or moribund patients, a temporary pacing catheter can be placed with local anesthesia and manual restraint alone. Mild sedation is required in others and administration of a reversible narcotic agent (oxymorphone, 0.1 to 0.2 mg/kg intramuscularly) is recommended. Electrocardiography should be performed continuously during the procedure.

Temporary pacing is achieved via a transvenous route from the jugular vein (usually the left) or a femoral vein. Because of patient movement and a higher potential for lead dislodgment, the femoral vein is less desirable except when the patient is going directly to anesthesia for a permanent pacemaker. Following sterile skin preparation, vascular access is achieved by either surgical exposure of the vein or by percutaneous introduction of an indwelling vascular sheath introducer (8.5 French Percutaneous Sheath introducer set, (Arrow International, Reading, PA) with a hemostasis port using a modified Seldinger technique. The pacing lead (5 French electrode catheter [USCI, C.R. Bard, Billerica, MA] for right ventricular pacing) is inserted in the vein directly or through the sheath introducer. Measurement of the approximate distance from the jugular vein to the right ventricle may aid placement. The bipolar pacing lead is passed toward the heart with the assistance of fluoroscopic guidance or by electrocardiographic monitoring alone. Alternative catheter pacing systems are available, including balloon-tipped pacing catheters and multipurpose Swan-Ganz catheters.

Fluoroscopy monitored placement. Fluoroscopic guidance is ideal for quick and accurate lead placement and is the procedure of choice when available. The lead is passed to the right

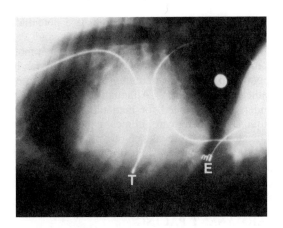

Fig. 41-3 Thoracic radiograph from a dog with a temporary transvenous pacemaker lead in place. The pacing lead *(T)* traverses the cranial vena cava and right atrium, and the electrode rests in the right ventricle. A previously placed permanent epicardial pacing lead *(E)* had pulled out of the myocardium and at surgery was found to be in contact with only the pericardium.

atrium and is directed ventrally through the tricuspid valve. The catheter is gently manipulated until it rests securely in the apex of the right ventricle, lodged under the trabeculae carnae when possible (Fig. 41-3). A small amount of "slack" should be permitted in the catheter as it courses through the right atrium. The pacing lead outside the body is connected to the temporary pulse generator. The electrocardiogram should document successful pacing when the temporary pacing device is activated (Fig. 41-4). The manual controls on the temporary pacemaker are adjusted to suit the patient's needs. The heart rate is typically set at 100 beats per minute in the dog and 140 beats per minute in the cat. The pacing stimulus is adjusted to at least twice the minimum current needed to maintain ventricular capture consistently, commonly from 2 to 5 mA. The mode is set on demand so that spontaneous ventricular activity is sensed to avoid stimulus delivery during the vulnerable period of the T wave.

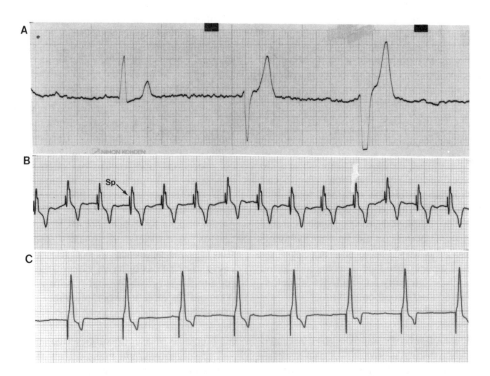

Fig. 41-4 Electrocardiogram before **(A)** and after **(B)** temporary and permanent **(C)** cardiac pacing in a Springer spaniel with atrial standstill. In **A** (Lead II, 50 mm/per second, 1 cm = 1 mV), the rhythm was atrial standstill with a ventricular escape rhythm originating from several foci, with a ventricular rate of approximately 55 beats per minute. In **B** (Lead II, 25 mm per second, 1 cm = 1 mV), the right ventricle is being paced by a temporary pacemaker and transvenous lead at approximately 135 beats per minute. The positive spike *(Sp)* just preceding the QRS is the pacing spike, and in each instance it generates ventricular depolarization. **C** (Lead II, 25 mm per second, 1 cm = 1 mV), electrocardiogram after permanent endocardial pacemaker placement in same dog (70 beats per minute).

ECG monitored placement. Placement of the pacing lead with electrocardiographic monitoring alone is somewhat more difficult. The temporary pacing unit is attached to the pacing catheter lead wire and pacing is initiated as the lead wire is passed toward the heart. A 45-degree bend in the tip of the catheter may aid passage through the tricuspid valve into the right ventricle. The operator should be aware that the wire may pass into several locations before successfully lodging in the right ventricle. Atrial pacing may be noted when the catheter reaches the atrium and diaphragmatic pacing may provide a clue to the operator that the catheter has passed into the caudal vena cava. Alternatively to external electrocardiographic monitoring, the pacing electrodes on the catheter tip can be used to monitor the electrogram as the catheter is advanced.

Once ventricular pacing is achieved, the lead is secured to the neck with either suture material, glue, or tape. We prefer application of waterproof adhesive tape to the catheter and suturing of the tape to the skin. The excess lead wire is gently coiled and bandaged to the neck. Areas of sharp angulation, especially as the catheter leaves the neck and as it attaches to the pulse generator, are to be avoided, as these bends cause increased mechanical stress and predispose to wire fracture. The external pulse generator is incorporated in the neck bandage or bandaged to the body, depending on the size of the patient. A thoracic radiograph is obtained to confirm correct placement of the pacing catheter. On the lateral view, the catheter should curve gently from the top of the heart ventrally and the tip of the pacing wire should lie over the apex of the right ventricle. A 12-lead electrocardiogram should be obtained for future reference and continuous electrocardiographic monitoring is employed to monitor cardiac rhythm. Spare batteries should be readily available in case of battery failure in the temporary pacing unit. The neck bandage is changed and the skin site is inspected daily for evidence of catheter-related infection (thrombophlebitis).

Complications

The prevalence of severe complications associated with temporary pacing is low.[13,15] Lead dislodgment causing intermittent failure to sense and/or pace has been reported in up to 25% of cases in humans.[15] Lead fracture, loose lead connections, and change in myocardial threshold can also cause failure to pace. Arrhythmias resulting from local myocardial irritation by the catheter are often observed, but they can usually be managed by changing the position of the catheter in the ventricle. Myocardial perforation of the right ventricular wall or interventricular septum is a potential, but uncommon complication. Phlebitis and venous thrombosis are also potential but uncommon complications. A high prevalence of bacteremia is reported in human patients by the third day after catheter placement.[15] Although this occurrence underscores the need for meticulous sterile technique and catheter care, clinical experience would indicate that the prevalence of catheter-related infection in animals is quite low. Implantation of the permanent pacemaker by the third day of temporary pacing is recommended in order to reduce the risk of catheter-related infections.

PERMANENT PACING

Systems for permanent cardiac pacing have been employed in veterinary patients since 1968.[1] Epicardial pacing was commonly used during the early years, but as the technology of pacemakers and lead wire tips improved, transvenous pacing has gained popularity.[10,11] Lead wires for permanent pacemakers are usually made of polyurethane or silicone coated multifilament helical coiled wires. The type of lead tip depends on whether endocardial or epicardial pacing is selected. Both systems are still used, and selection of the type of system may be based on individual preferences or pacemaker availability.

Permanent transvenous (endocardial) pacing

A major advantage of transvenous pacemakers is the obviation of an invasive thoracotomy or celiotomy for lead placement. Implantation of a transvenous pacemaker is usually a shorter surgical procedure, and for this reason it may be less expensive than epicardial techniques. A potential disadvantage is the need for fluoroscopic guidance to place the lead. While some authors have reported successful placement of permanent transvenous pacemakers using only local anesthesia,[10,11] this approach is not recommended because of the possibility of patient movement disrupting the surgical site and resulting in increased potential for infectious complications. In most animals, general anesthesia can be performed safely during temporary pacing, thus facilitating the maintenance of aseptic surgical technique.

The surgeon should make certain that the pacemaker and lead wire are compatible and that an appropriate wrench is available to connect them. Availability of a backup pulse generator, lead wire, and wrench is a desirable safeguard. Following placement of a temporary pacing catheter and anesthetic induction, the skin is surgically prepared. Access to the jugular vein can be achieved by surgical isolation or by percutaneous puncture with a large-bore, peel-away sheath introducer. We find that the surgical approach to the jugular vein results in easier manipulation of the lead wire, better hemostasis and reduced hematoma formation, which can be a potential nidus of bacterial infection.

Transvenous pacemakers may be unipolar or bipolar, and there is no definitive advantage to either design. However, the characteristics of the tip of the lead wire are important.[10,11,20] Catheter tips can have an active method of fixation in which a metal screw is embedded into the ventricular myocardium or may provide passive fixation with flanged or winged tips, or flexible tines. We prefer the flexible-tined leads, which provide passive fixation by lodging within the ventricular trabeculae (Fig. 41-1).

After entering the vein, the lead is passed into the right ventricle under fluoroscopic guidance. A bend of about 45 degrees in the inner guide wire 1 to 3 cm from the tip will facilitate passage through the tricuspid valve. When the tined lead is used, the lead is manipulated or rotated until the tines are securely entrapped in trabeculae muscles. The guide wire is removed, the rate on the temporary pacemaker is reduced to a rate less than the permanent pacemaker to avoid competition, and the permanent pacemaker is attached to the pacing lead using the sterile Allen wrench (Fig. 41-1). The permanent pacemaker will immediately control the rhythm in bipolar systems; however, the pacemaker must be in contact with the patient's body to complete the circuit in unipolar designs. The electrocardiogram and peripheral arterial pulse should verify pacing by the permanent device. When vascular access is via a surgical approach, a lead anchoring sleeve is useful to anchor the lead to the vein and prevent lead migration. Two grooves or holes in the lead anchoring sleeve permit double ligation with nonabsorbable sutures at the site of vessel entry (see Fig. 41-1).

The pulse generator is usually implanted in the neck (Fig. 41-5). In smaller dogs and cats, the lead wire can be tunneled beneath the skin to the lateral thorax behind the front limb. A pocket large enough to accommodate the pacemaker is made in the subcutaneous tissues by blunt dissection. Some authors have advocated the use of a polypropylene mesh pouch to help prevent seroma formation and fix the pacemaker in place.[11] Placement of the pacemaker below the latissimus dorsi muscle may help prevent seroma formation and improve cosmetic appearance in small dogs.

A potential early complication of endocardial pacing is lead dislodgment, which usually occurs within the first 2 weeks. Lead-wire displacement should be suspected if there is a failure to pace,

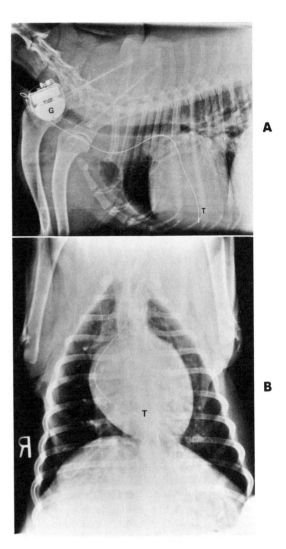

Fig. 41-5 Thoracic radiographs (lateral, **A**; ventrodorsal, **B**) of a dog after cardiac pacemaker implantation. The pulse generator *(G)* rests in the subcutaneous tissues of the neck. The pacing lead *(T)* enters the right jugular vein in the neck and traverses the cranial vena cava, right atrium and the tined leads are fixed within the trabecular muscle of the right ventricle.

or if an unexpected electrocardiographic pattern or alteration in the morphology of the paced QRS complex occurs. These possibilities make the importance of obtaining a 10-lead electrocardiogram immediately after pacemaker implantation imperative. Replacement of the lead into the ventricular trabecula is required. Animals with marked right ventricular dilation are more likely to have this problem develop; therefore epicardial pacing should be considered in these patients. The development of tined leads to secure the lead to trabecular muscle has greatly diminished the occurrence of lead dislodgment in dogs.

Permanent epicardial pacing

One of the potential advantages of permanent epicardial pacing is more secure placement of the epicardial lead wire. These leads usually have a corkscrew design, enabling the electrode to be screwed into the myocardium and/or sutured to the epicardium (see Fig. 41-1). Although this design would seem to confer an advantage in lead stability, it is still possible for these leads to become dislodged. Additionally, in some dogs fibrous tissue develops around the electrode in the ventricular myocardium, resulting in failure to pace (exit block) and/or sense (entrance block) ventricular activity. A major disadvantage of epicardial pacing is the need for an invasive thoracotomy.

Surgical exposure to implant epicardial pacemakers can be via a lateral intercostal thoracotomy approach[3,4]; via a technique combining a caudal median sternotomy and cranial midline celiotomy[5,23]; or via an abdominal transdiaphragmatic approach.[7,8] Postoperative infection is reportedly less frequent using the more recently developed abdominal transdiaphragmatic approach. Once the heart is surgically exposed, the pericardium is incised and retracted. The site for epicardial-lead attachment is selected to avoid epicardial coronary vessels. The lead is usually placed in the left ventricle, as its larger ventricular mass better accommodates the "screw-in" type electrodes. The lead should also avoid contact with either the phrenic nerve or the diaphragm as contact may result in unsightly and uncomfortable diaphragmatic pacing. Once the site is selected, the lead is screwed clockwise into the myocardium using the disposable insertion tool.

A pocket for the pulse generator is formed, usually in the lateral flank between the external and internal abdominal oblique muscles. The lead is tunneled through the subcutaneous tissues from the thorax to the subcutaneous pocket, allowing for some redundant lead wire at the electrode and pulse-generator sites to avoid undue tension. The rate of the temporary pacemaker is reduced, and the lead wire and pulse generator are attached as previously described. As unipolar leads are employed with epicardial pacemakers, pacing will not actually begin until the pulse generator is in contact with body fluids to complete the electrical circuit.

Some authors suggest leaving the pacemaker free in the abdomen[7,8]; however this has several disadvantages. If the pulse generator fails or needs to be replaced, a laparotomy is required instead of subcutaneous dissection. Further, when the pacemaker is located superficially, reprogramming can be consistently accomplished transcutaneously without surgery or sedation. When reprogramming is necessary in dogs with intraabdominal pulse-generator placement, an additional laparotomy may be required. Finally, migration of the pulse generator within the abdomen of larger dogs may result in excessive traction, twisting, or bending on the lead wire, causing it to pull out of the myocardium or to fracture (see Fig. 41-3).

Potential complications

Permanent pacemaker implantation is not without risk, and the possibility for both early and late complications is widely recognized. Pacemaker complications reported frequently include postoperative infection and/or seroma formation, muscle twitching, postoperative cardiac arrhythmias, failure of the pulse generator (battery failure), lead-wire fracture, and lead displacement.[3-11] Additionally, the disease that led to the original failure of impulse formation and/or conduction (myocarditis, neoplasia, cardiomyopathy, endocarditis) may progress to intractable heart failure. Pacemaker complications and/or progression of heart disease are reported in approximately 60% of dogs with pacemakers.[3-5,7,8,11]

Postoperative infection surrounding the pulse generator or lead wire is an infrequent but serious complication. As with implantation of any foreign material, the infection is rarely cured unless the foreign material is removed. Long-term antibiotic therapy may control the infection in selected patients; however, antibiotic therapy in combination with pacemaker and lead-wire replacement is the treatment of choice.

Ventricular arrhythmias in the postoperative period have also been reported and may lead to sudden death.[3,5,7,8] Postoperative electrocardiographic monitoring for arrhythmias is always indicated. Antiarrhythmic therapy is sometimes required, although the ventricular dysrhythmias often abate within 7 to 10 days without therapy.

Failure of the pulse generator, or battery failure, is a common complication, especially when using the older (or even previously used) pacemakers that are available and economically feasible for most veterinary applications. Impending battery failure may be indicated by a change in the heart rate (usually a decrease), a change in the pulse amplitude (usually a reduction), or an increase in the pulse duration detected by a change in morphology of the stimulus artifact on the electrocardiogram. Battery failure ultimately results in a failure to pace, usually with recurrence of clinical signs from bradycardia.

Lead-wire complications occur with both endocardial and epicardial pacing systems. Fracture of the lead wire or a break in the insulation leading

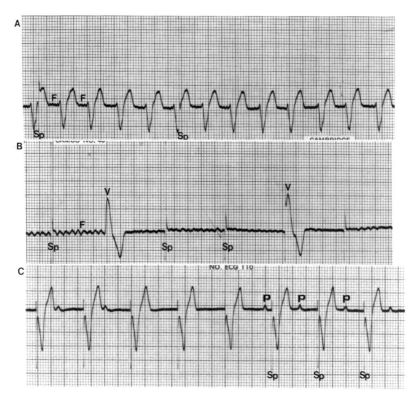

Fig. 41-6 Serial electrocardiograms of pacemaker failure in a German shepherd with recurrence of syncope. **A,** Ventricular tachycardia with fibrillation waves *(F)* in the base line indicative of atrial fibrillation; several pacing spikes *(Sp)* are present, which fail to produce a QRS complex (exit block). The fact that the pacing spikes occur without regard to the ventricular arrhythmia indicates failure to sense as well (entrance block). **B,** Later, atrial fibrillation and third-degree AV block with a ventricular escape rhythm *(V)* are present. Pacemaker spikes are present but fail to stimulate the heart (exit block). Large pacing spikes are indicative of an epicardial pacing system. Failure to pace was a result of scar tissue in the myocardium at the site of the pacing lead. **C,** Electrocardiogram obtained after replacement of pacing lead at a new site in the ventricle. Atrial fibrillation has converted, P waves are noted *(P)*, third-degree AV block is still present; pacemaker system is functioning properly at 96 beats per minute. (Courtesy of Dr. Johanna M. Reimer, University of Pennsylvania, New Bolton Center, Kewett Square, PA.)

to electrical leakage is possible with both systems. Lead-wire fracture is most common in an area of mechanical stress, often either near the pacemaker or where the catheter enters the blood vessel or chest cavity. Replacement of the lead wire is necessary and curative. Lead-wire fracture can often be documented by radiography or fluoroscopy. Epicardial electrodes sometimes cause fibrosis at the site of implantation, which causes exit and/or entrance block and a failure in pacing, sensing, or both functions (Fig. 41-6). Replacement of the lead in another location on the ventricle is curative; however, fibrosis may recur. The use of corticosteroids to minimize scar-tissue formation has been proposed, but their use may predispose to infection.

Progression of cardiac disease is also a common cause for patient demise. Dogs requiring pacemaker implantation are often elderly and many have concurrent endocardiosis and mitral regurgitation. Some animals develop atrioventricular block as a result of myocarditis, which can cause progressive cardiac failure. Regardless of the cause, many dogs with pacemakers eventually develop heart failure that requires concomitant drug therapy with furosemide, vasodilators, or digitalis (see Chapter 17).

Postoperative care and monitoring

Continuous electrocardiographic monitoring should be performed for at least the initial 24 hours after surgery both to ensure proper pacemaker system function and to watch for ventricular arrhythmias. A radiogram and a 10-lead electrocardiogram are obtained in the immediate postoperative period as a reference for future evaluations. The pacemaker specifications (model and manufacturer, pacing rate, and pulse current) are placed in the patient's permanent record. Others recommend administration of a broad-spectrum antibiotic for 10 days after surgery; however, we routinely administer antibiotics, usually cephalothin only in the perioperative period (one dose before surgery and two doses afterward). Animals are confined to a cage for 24 hours, and owners are instructed to limit activity to leash walking for 2 weeks to allow the electrode to heal in place.

The routine reevaluations indicated in animals with pacemakers include electrocardiographic, radiographic, and echocardiographic monitoring. An electrocardiogram is obtained 2 and 4 weeks after surgery, then every 3 months. Thoracic radiographs should be obtained every 6 months and an echocardiogram at least once a year to monitor for pacemaker malfunction, progression of cardiac disease or the development of congestive heart failure. Owners are instructed about pacemakers and they are trained to monitor heart and pulse rates.

Survival of dogs after pacemaker implantation has been reported in several studies, but most of the data reported does not reflect current techniques and devices. Additionally, in all of these studies several dogs were still alive at the time of publication, preventing accurate calculation of survival data. In one early study, 9 of 31 dogs died within the first 2 weeks of pacemaker implantation.[3] Although survival times longer than 3 years are now quite common, the mean and median survival times in published studies are at least 14 months and 11 months, respectively.[3-5,7,11] If those that died within the first 2 weeks are excluded, the mean and median survival times increase to at least 17 months and 14 months, respectively.

PACEMAKER SELECTION

There have been a number of advances in pacemaker and electrode design over the past two decades that have greatly expanded the potential use of pacemaker therapy in human medicine. Although these developments are not yet commonly employed in clinical veterinary patients, primarily because of the expense involved, some are mentioned here to spark interest, as these innovations may be used more by veterinarians in the future.

Dual-chambered pacemakers were developed to more closely approximate the normal physiologic function of the heart. These pacemakers are attached to both right atrial and right ventricle electrodes, and they can sense and/or stimulate either chamber or both of them. Sequential activation of the atria and ventricles means that the "atrial kick" is preserved. Physiologic increases in the rate of sinus-node discharge are sensed and result in increased ventricular pacing rate to meet demands for increased cardiac output. Thus, while VVI pacing has provided symptomatic relief for many animals with sick-sinus syndrome or impaired AV conduction, considerable evidence suggests that appropriately timed atrial systole is important to ventricular performance.[24-31] With ventricular pacing only, atrial contractions may be absent, dissociated, or improperly coupled to ventricle events such that cardiac output is not only reduced but valve function is impaired.[13,26,27] These adverse hemodynamic effects are obviously more important in critically ill patients than in the animal with a normal cardiovascular reserve. AV sequential (DVI), atrial sequential (VAT, VDD) and optimal sequential (DDD) pacemakers have been shown to improve cardiac output up to 67% in human patients as compared with ventricular pacemakers alone.[27-30] Ventricular pacing (VVI) is consistently associated with lower mean systemic arterial blood pressures, lower cardiac output, and higher ventricular filling pressures as compared with dual-chamber pacing.[13,31,32] Dual chamber pacemakers should be considered in young animals, in animals that need to be active, or in animals with VVI pacemakers if they have inadequate exercise tolerance.

Proper and precise pacemaker mode selection, however, requires complex electrophysiologic testing of the animal to gain knowledge and assess performance of the sinus node, conduction pathways, and hemodynamic parameters. Programmed electrical stimulation studies often precede pacemaker implantation in humans.[33] Such studies not only are helpful in selecting an appropriate pacemaker, but these studies also help localize the origin of the arrhythmias and have been useful in extending the use of pacemakers for the therapy of tachyarrhythmias.

Temporary pacing has been useful in terminating a variety of supraventricular and ventricular tachycardias.[15,17,34-40] The use of moderately elevated pacing rates may suppress premature beats and prevent some tachycardias from recurring (overdrive suppression). Tachycardias that occur only in the setting of bradycardias (i.e., sick sinus bradyarrhythmic-tachyarrhythmic dogs) can be prevented by pacing at normal rates. Pacemakers designed to produce an appropriate sequence of electrical stimuli when sensing a tachycardia have been used successfully in human patients.[17,34,35] Some of these devices produce pairs or bursts of stimuli to terminate the tachycardia. The paced impulse terminates a tachycardia by depolarizing part of the reentrant pathway responsible for the arrhythmia, thus making it refractory to the reentrant impulse. Some "dual demand" pacemakers automatically deliver stimuli at a fixed, relatively slow rate when either a bradycardia or tachycardia is sensed; and the tachycardia is terminated when the properly timed stimulus occurs at appropriate sequela in the tachycardia cycle (under drive termination).[36,37] Two additional advances in electrical treatment for sustained ventricular and supraventricular arrhythmias are devices that can deliver synchronized cardioversion shocks via a transvenous catheter electrode, and implantable defibrillators that sense and terminate ventricular fibrillation.[16,18,38-40]

It seems clear that rate adaptive pacemaker systems increase the patient's physical capability and quality of life. Rather than the complexity of dual-chamber pacemakers, an approach that shows much promise and may be preferable for animals is single-chambered pacing with the pacing rate varying with a physiologically sensed parameter such as activity,[41] respiratory rate,[42] oxygen saturation,[43] pH value,[44] or blood temperature.[45,46] The latter seems particularly relevant and is commercially available in a unit (Nova MR, Intermedics, Freeport, TX) that is single-chambered and varies its pacing rate according to central venous blood temperature. Temperature is sensed by a small thermistor near the distal end of the transvenous pacing electrode in the right ventricle. Blood temperature increases with activity, and rate changes per degree temperature change can be fixed telemetrically. The algorithm in the pacemaker also distinguishes between the steeper brief temperature change during exercise and the slower fluctuation of circadian rhythm temperature changes, and the pacemaker responds to each appropriately.[46]

In the future, pacing may be used for treating cardiovascular diseases seemingly unrelated to arrhythmia control. A novel approach, demonstrated experimentally in animals, is that chronic atrial bradycardial pacing increased capillary density and maximal cardiac minute work and performance in normal and in pathologically hypertrophied hearts.[47] Chronic bradycardial pacing, therefore, may be useful in a number of cardiac diseases by inducing angiogenesis in hypertrophied or diseased myocardium, thus improving oxygen delivery to myocytes. Extensive investigation of the chronic bradycardial pacing technique is necessary, however, before clinical use of this method is indicated.

REFERENCES

1. Buchanan JW, Dear MG, Pyle RL. Medical and pacemaker therapy of complete heart block and congestive heart failure in a dog. J Am Vet Med Assoc 1968;1528:1099-1109.
2. Musselman EE, Rouse GP, Parker AJ. Permanent pacemaker implantation with a transvenous electrode placement in a dog with complete heart block, congestive heart failure, and Stokes-Adams syndrome. J Small Anim Pract 1976;17:149-162.
3. Lombard CW, Tilley LP, Yoshioka M. Pacemaker implantation in the dog: survey and literature review. J Am Anim Hosp Assoc 1981;17:751-758.
4. Yoshioka MM, Tilley LP, Harvey HJ, Wayne ES, Lombard CW, Schollmeyer M. Permanent pacemaker implantation in the dog. J Am Anim Hosp Assoc 1981;17:746-750.
5. Bonagura JD, Helphrey ML, Muir WM. Complications associated with permanent pacemaker implantation in the dog. J Am Vet Med Assoc 1983;182:149-155.
6. Darke PGG, Been M, Marks A. Use of a programmable, 'physiological' cardiac pacemaker in a dog with total atrioventricular block (with some comments on complications associated with cardiac pacemakers). J Small Anim Pract 1985;26:295-303.
7. Fox PR, Mathiesen DT, Purse D, Brown NO. Ventral abdominal, transdiaphragmatic approach for implantation of cardiac pacemakers in the dog. J Am Vet Med Assoc 1986;189:1303-1308.
8. Fingeroth JM, Birchard SJ SSJ. Transdiaphragmatic approach for permanent pacemaker implantation in dogs. Vet Surg 1986;15:329-333.
9. Schollmeyer M. Pacemaker therapy. In Fox PR, ed. Canine and feline cardiology. New York: Churchill Livingstone, 1988.
10. Sisson DD. Bradyarrhythmias and cardiac pacing. In Kirk RW, ed. Current veterinary therapy X. Philadelphia: WB Saunders, 1989;286-294.
11. Darke PGG, Been M. Transvenous cardiac pacing in 19 dogs and one cat. J Small Anim Pract 1989;30:491-499.
12. Noe R, Cockrell W, Moses HW, Dove JT, Batchelder JE. Transcutaneous pacemaker use in a large hospital. Pace 1986;9:101-104.
13. Donovan KD. Cardiac pacing in intensive care. Anaesth Intensive Care 1984;13:41-62.
14. Sharma AD, Klein GJ. Pathophysiology and management of atrial and ventricular arrhythmias in the critically ill. Crit Care Clin 1985;1:677-697.
15. Silver MD, Goldschlager N. Temporary transvenous cardiac pacing in the critical care setting. Chest 1988;93:607-613.
16. Rosenthal ME, Josephson ME. Current status of antitachycardia devices. Circulation 1990;82:1889-1899.
17. Griffin J, Mason J, Calfee R. Clinical use of an implantable automatic tachycardia-terminating pacemaker. Am Heart J 1980;100:1093.
18. Zipes D, Jackman W, Heger J, et al. Clinical transvenous cardioversion of recurrent life-threatening ventricular tachyarrhythmias: low energy synchronized cardioversion of ventricular tachycardia and termination of ventricular fibrillation in patients using a catheter electrode. Am Heart J 1982;103:789.
19. Harthorne JW, Eisenhauer AC, Steinhaus DM. Cardiac pacing. In Eagle KA, Haber E, DeSanctis RW, Austen WG, eds. The practice of cardiology. Boston: Little, Brown, 1980;287-336.

20. Miller MS. Pacemaker therapy. In 1990 Academy of Veterinary Cardiology Proceedings, Ralston Purina Co. St. Louis: Academy of Veterinary Cardiology, 1990;30-35.

21. Syverud SA, Dalsey WC, Hedges JR, Hanslits ML. Radiologic assessment of transvenous pacemaker placement during CPR. Ann Emerg Med 1986;15:131-137.

22. Syverud SA, Dalsey WC, Hedges JR. Transcutaneous and transvenous cardiac pacing for early bradyasystolic cardiac arrest. Ann Emerg Med 1986;15:121-124.

23. Helphrey ML, Schollmeyer M. Pacemaker therapy. In Kirk RW, ed. Current veterinary therapy VIII. Philadelphia: WB Saunders, 1983;373-376.

24. Ogawa S, Breifus L, Shenoy P, Brockman S, Berkovits B. Hemodynamic consequences of atrioventricular and ventriculoatrial pacing. Pace 1:8, 1978.

25. Rosenqvist M, Brandt J, Schuller H. Atrial versus ventricular pacing in sinus node disease: A treatment comparison. Am Heart J 1986;111:292.

26. Samet P, Bernstein W, Levine S. Significance of the atrial contribution to ventricular filling. Am J Cardiol 1965-B;15:195.

27. Samet P, Castillo C, Bernstein W. Hemodynamic sequelae of atrial, ventricular, and sequential atrioventricular pacing in cardiac patients. Am Heart J 1966;72:725.

28. Karlof I. Hemodynamic effect of atrial triggered versus fixed rate pacing at rest and during exercise in complete heart block. Acta Med Scand 1975;197:195.

29. Samet P, Castillo C, Bernstein W. Hemodynamic consequences of sequential atrioventricular pacing. Am J Cardiol 1968;21:207.

30. Hartzler G, Maloney J, Curtis J, Barnhorst D. Hemodynamic benefits of atrioventricular sequential pacing after cardiac surgery. Am J Cardiol 1977;40:232.

31. Kruse I, Arnman K, Conradson TB, Ryden L. A comparison of the acute and long-term haemodynamic effects of ventricular inhibited and atrial synchronous ventricular inhibited pacing. Circulation 1982;65:846-855.

32. Kruse I, Ryden L. A comparison of physical work capacity and systolic time intervals with ventricular inhibited and atrial synchronous ventricular inhibited pacing. Br Heart J 1981;46:129.

33. Zipes DP, Duffin EG: Cardiac pacemakers. In Braunwald E, ed. Heart disease, ed. 2. Philadelphia: WB Saunders, 1984;744-772.

34. Newmann G, Funke HD, Bakels N, Kirchoff PG, Schaede A. A new atrial demand pacemaker for the management of supraventricular tachycardias. In Proceedings of the Sixth World Symposium on Cardiac Pacing. 1979;27-37.

35. Camm A, Nathan A, Hellestrand K, Ward D, Spurrell R. The clinical evaluation of tachycardia termination by utilizing autodecremental atrial pacing. Pace 1981;4:A-84.

36. Curry P, Rowland E, Krikler D. Dual-demand pacing for refractory atrioventricular reentry tachycardia. Pace 1979;2:137.

37. Maloney J, Medina-Ravell V, Pieretti O et al. Follow-up assessment of dual-demand, dualchamber DVI-DVO pacing for automatic conversion, control, and prevention of refractory paroxysmal supraventricular tachycardia. Pace 1981;4:A-57.

38. Jackman WM, Zipes DP. Low energy synchronous cardioversion of ventricular tachycardia using a catheter electrode in a canine model of subacute myocardial infarction. Circulation 1982;66:187.

39. Zipes D, Prystowsky E, Browne K, Chilson D, Heger J. Additional observations on transvenous cardioversion of recurrent ventricular tachycardia. Am Heart J 1982;104:163.

40. Mirowski M, Reid PR, Watkins L, Weisfeldt ML, Mower MM. Clinical treatment of life-threatening ventricular tachyarrhythmias with the automatic implantable defibrillator. Am Heart J 1981;102:265.

41. Humen DP, Anderson K, Brumwell D, et al. A pacemaker which automatically increases its rate with physical activity. In Proceedings of the World Symposium on Cardiac Pacing. Darmstadt, Germany: Steinkopff Verlag, 1983;259-264.

42. Rossi P, Plicchi G, Canducci GC, Rognoni G, Aina F. Respiratory rate as a determinant of optimal pacing rate. Pace 1983;6:502-510.

43. Wirtzfeld A, Goedel-Meinen L, Bock T, Heinze R, Liss HD, Munteanu J. Central venous oxygen saturation for the control of automatic rate-responsive pacing. Pace 1982;5:829-835.

44. Cammilli L, Alcidi L, Papeschi G, et al. Preliminary experience with the pH-triggered pacemaker. Pace 1978;1:448-457.

45. Alt E, Hirgstetter C, Heinz M. Blomer H. Rate control of physiologic pacemakers by central venous blood temperature. Circulation 1986;73:1206-1212.

46. Alt E, Volker R, Hogl B, MacCarter D. First clinical results with a new temperature-controlled rate-responsive pacemaker. Circulation 1988;78(Suppl III):III116-III124.

47. Wright AJA, Hudlicka O, Brown MD. Beneficial effect of chronic bradycardial pacing on capillary growth and heart performance in volume overload heart hypertrophy. Circ Res 1989;64:1205-1212.

Index